T0294573

COLOR ATLAS OF VETERINARY AN

Volume 2

THE HORSE

Commissioning Editor: Robert Edwards
Development Editor: Lynn Watt/Ailsa Laing
Project Manager: Nancy Arnott
Designer/Design Direction: Stewart Larking
Illustration Manager: Merlyn Harvey
Illustrator: Samantha Elmhurst

Color Atlas of Veterinary Anatomy

Volume 2

The Horse

Second Edition

Raymond R. Ashdown
BVSc PhD MRCVS
Emeritus Reader in Veterinary Anatomy
University of London
London

Stanley H. Done
BA BVetMed PhD DECPHM DECVP FRCVS FRCPath
Visiting Professor of Veterinary Pathology
University of Glasgow Veterinary School, Glasgow
Former Lecturer in Veterinary Anatomy
Royal Veterinary College
London

Photography by
Susan A. Evans
MIScT AIMI MIAS
Former Chief Technician in Anatomy
Department of Veterinary Basic Sciences
Royal Veterinary College
London

With radiographs provided by
Elizabeth A. Baines
MA VetMB DVR DipECVDI MRCVS
Lecturer in Veterinary Radiology
Department of Veterinary Clinical Sciences
Royal Veterinary College
London

MOSBY

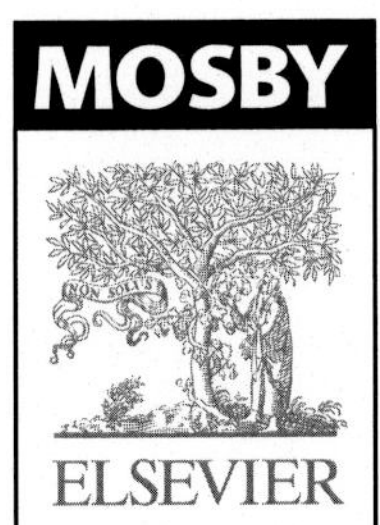
ELSEVIER

Edinburgh London New York Oxford Philadelphia St Louis Sydney Toronto 2011

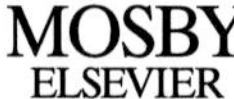

First edition 1987
Second edition 2011

ISBN 978-0-7234-3414-6

British Library Cataloguing in Publication Data
A catalogue record for this book is available from the British Library

Library of Congress Cataloging in Publication Data
A catalog record for this book is available from the Library of Congress

Notices

Knowledge and best practice in this field are constantly changing. As new research and experience broaden our understanding, changes in research methods, professional practices, or medical treatment may become necessary.

Practitioners and researchers must always rely on their own experience and knowledge in evaluating and using any information, methods, compounds, or experiments described herein. In using such information or methods they should be mindful of their own safety and the safety of others, including parties for whom they have a professional responsibility.

With respect to any drug or pharmaceutical products identified, readers are advised to check the most current information provided (i) on procedures featured or (ii) by the manufacturer of each product to be administered, to verify the recommended dose or formula, the method and duration of administration, and contraindications. It is the responsibility of practitioners, relying on their own experience and knowledge of their patients, to make diagnoses, to determine dosages and the best treatment for each individual patient, and to take all appropriate safety precautions.

To the fullest extent of the law, neither the Publisher nor the authors, contributors, or editors, assume any liability for any injury and/or damage to persons or property as a matter of products liability, negligence or otherwise, or from any use or operation of any methods, products, instructions, or ideas contained in the material herein.

Printed in Great Britain
Last digit is the print number: 15

PREFACE

This book is intended for veterinary students and practising veterinary surgeons. Important features of topographical anatomy are presented in a series of full-colour photographs of detailed dissections. The structures are identified in accompanying coloured line drawings, and the nomenclature is based on that of the *Nomina Anatomica Veterinaria* (1992). Latin terms are used for muscles, arteries, veins, lymphatics and nerves, but anglicized terms are used for most other structures. When necessary, information needed for interpretation of the photographs is given in the captions. Each section begins with photographs of regional surface features taken before dissection, and complementary photographs of an articulated equine skeleton illustrate the important palpable bony features of these regions. The dissections and photographs have been specially prepared for this book.

The horses used for this work were ponies of various ages and types (two stallions, one gelding, three mares and several colt foals). The specimens were embalmed, for the most part, in the standing position using methods routinely employed in the Department of Anatomy at the Royal Veterinary College. Every effort was made to ensure that the final position corresponded to that of normal level standing. In four cases red neoprene latex was injected into the arteries and blue neoprene latex was also injected into the veins of the pregnant mare. The dissections follow the pattern of prosections that were used for teaching at the Royal Veterinary College for many years.

The aim of these dissections and photographs is to reveal the topography of the animal as it would be presented to the veterinary surgeon during a routine clinical examination. Therefore, lateral views predominate and we have, as far as possible, avoided photographs of parts removed from the body or the use of views from unusual angles, or of unusual body positions. It is our earnest hope that this book will enable students and veterinary surgeons to see, beneath the outer surface of the animals entrusted to their care, the muscles, bones, vessels, nerves and viscera that go to make up each region of the body and each organ system.

A significant difference between this and previous editions of the volume is the addition of radiographs and scans which are placed in a new chapter at the end of the book. A second major difference is the inclusion of clinical notes at the beginning of each main chapter. These notes highlight the areas of anatomy which are of particular clinical significance. Finally, over 100 self-assessment questions are available online with this new edition.

We feel that these additions to the book add considerably to its usefulness, especially to the aspiring veterinary surgeon.

ACKNOWLEDGEMENTS

The dissections and photography for this book were carried out at the Royal Veterinary College, University of London. We are grateful to the Department of Anatomy for the provision of specialized facilities, without which this work could not have been possible. In particular we would like to thank Stephen W. Barnett, BA, MIST, formerly Chief Technician in Anatomy, for advice and assistance. The task of preparing and caring for the specimens before and during dissection was undertaken by Douglas Hopkins and Andrew Crook. The photographs for Figs 8.31–8.35 were taken by Alan Coombs (Department of Veterinary Anatomy, University of Bristol) and those for Figs 8.48–8.53 were taken by Malcolm Parsons (Department of Veterinary Surgery, University of Bristol).

The idea of producing an atlas of equine anatomy was based on our yearly teaching program of equine prosection. And we are very grateful to the project editor, designer and illustrator for their hard work and for sustaining us with their optimism and enthusiasm.

Lizza Baines provided the radiographs for this new edition with Elsevier and we are very grateful to her for help with all aspects of the new chapter on radiographical imaging.

London 2011

RRA
SD

BIBLIOGRAPHY

Numerous original papers have been consulted during this work, but our studies have mainly been supported by a range of anatomical textbooks. We would especially acknowledge our debt to the following, which were our constant companions throughout the preparation of the specimens and the text.

Berg R (1973) *Angewandete und topographische Anatomie der Haustiere.* Jena: Fisher.

Bradley O C, Grahame T (1946) *The Topographical Anatomy of the Limbs of the Horse.* 2nd Edn. Edinburgh: Green & Son Ltd.

Bradley O C, Grahame T (1946) *The Topographical Anatomy of the Thorax and Abdomen of the Horse.* 2nd Edn. Edinburgh: Green & Son Ltd.

Bradley O C, Grahame T (1946) *The Topographical Anatomy of the Head and Neck of the Horse.* 2nd Edn. Edinburgh: Green & Son Ltd.

Butler J, Colles C, Dyson S, Kold S, Poules P (2008) Clinical radiology of the horse, 3rd Edn. Chichester-Oxford: Wiley-Blackwell.

Calderon W F (n.d.) *Animal Painting and Anatomy.* London: Seeley Service.

Chauveau A, Arloing S, Lesbre F-X (1903) *Traité d'Anatomie Comparée des Animaux Domestiques.* 5e édition. Paris: Baillière-Tindall.

Dittrich H, Ellenberger W, Baum H (1907) *The Horse. A Pictorial Guide to its Anatomy.* Translated by Sisson S. London: Fisher Unwin. Leipsic: Dieterich.

Ellenberger W, Baum H (1943) *Handbuch der vergleichenden Anatomie der Haustiere.* 18th Edn. Edited by Zeitzschmann O, Ackernecht E & Grau H. Berlin: Springer-Verlag.

Field E J, Harrison R J (1968) *Anatomical Terms. Their origin and derivation.* 3rd Edn. Cambridge: Heffer.

Ghoshal N G, Koch T, Popesko P (1981) *The Venous Drainage of the Domestic Animals.* Philadelphia: W.B. Saunders Company.

Goubaux A, Barrier G (1892) *The Exterior of the Horse.* Translated and edited by Harger SJJ. Philadelphia: J.B. Lippincott Co.

Habel R E (1973) *Applied Veterinary Anatomy.* Ithaca: Habel.

Hayes M H (1903) *Veterinary notes for horse owners.* 6th Edn. London: Hurst, Blackett (54 good photographs of the teeth of horses of known ages [birth to 42 years] in Ch. 33, which is not included in earlier Edns).

Hayes M H (1952) *Points of the Horse.* 6th Edn. Edited by Brooke G & Sanders M. London: Hurst, Blackett.

International Committee on Veterinary Anatomical Nomenclature, World Association of Veterinary Anatomists (1992). *Nomina Anatomica Veterinaria.* 4th Edn. Gent: International Committee on Veterinary Gross Anatomical Nomenclature.

Kovács G (1963) *The Equine Tarsus, Topographic and Radiographic Anatomy.* Translated by McKay P. Budapest: Akademiai Kiadó.

Lydekker R (1912) *The Horse and its Relatives.* London: Allen.

McFadyean J (1922) *The Anatomy of the Horse. A Dissection Guide.* 3rd Edn. Edinburgh: Johnstone.

McFadyean J (1964) *Osteology and Arthrology of the Domesticated Animals.* 4th Edn. Edited by Hughes H V & Dransfield J W. London: Baillière Tindall, Cox.

Martin P, Schauder W (1938) *Lehrbuch der Anatomie der Haustiere.* Bd. III. Anatomie der Hauswiederkäuer. 3rd Edn. Stuttgart: Schickhardt, Ebner.

Nickel R, Schummer A, Seiferle E (1973) *The Viscera of the Domestic Animals.* Translated and revised by Sack WO. Berlin, Hamburg: Paul Parey.

Nickel R, Schummer A, Seiferle E (1975) *Lehrbuch der Anatomie der Haustiere* Bd. IV. Nervensystem, Sinnesorgane, Endokrine Drusen. 2 Auflage. Seiferle E & Böhme G. Berlin, Hamburg: Paul Parey.

Nickel R, Schummer A, Seiferle E (1981) *The Anatomy of the Domestic Animals* Vol 3. The circulatory system, the skin and the cutaneous organs of the domestic mammals. Schummer A, Wilkens H, Vollmerhaus BK & Habermehl KH. Translated by Siller WG & Wright PAL. Berlin, Hamburg: Paul Parey.

Nickel R, Schummer A, Seiferle E (1984) *Lehrbuch der Anatomie der Haustiere* Bd. I Bewegungsapparat. 5 Auflage. Frewein J, Wille K-H & Wilkens H. Berlin, Hamburg: Paul Parey.

Popesko P (1971) *Atlas of topographical anatomy of the domestic animals.* Vols I–III. Translated by Getty R & Brown J. Philadelphia: W.B. Saunders Company.

Sack W O, Habel R E (1977) *Rooney's Guide to the Dissection of the Horse.* Ithaca: Veterinary Textbooks.

Schebitz H, Wilkens H (1978) *Atlas der Röntgenanatomie des Pferdes.* Berlin, Hamburg: Paul Parey.

Schmaltz R (1909) *Atlas der Anatomie des Pferdes.* 2 Teil. Topographische Myologie. Berlin: Schoetz.

Schmaltz R (1924) *Atlas der Anatomie des Pferdes.* 1 Teil. Das Skelett des Rumpfes und der Gleidmassen. 4,5 Auflage. Berlin: Schoetz

Share-Jones J T (1907) *The Surgical Anatomy of the Horse.* London: Williams, Norgate.

Sisson S, Grossman J D (1953) *The Anatomy of the Domestic Animals.* 4th Edn, revised Philadelphia: W.B. Saunders Company.

Sisson S, Grossman J D (1975) *The Anatomy of the Domestic Animals.* Vol. 1. Edited by Getty R. 5th Edn. Philadelphia: W.B. Saunders Company.

Tagand R, Barone R (1950–1957) *Anatomie des Equides Domestiques.* Lyon: École Nationale Vètèrinaire.

Taylor J A (1955–1970) *Regional and Applied Anatomy of the Domestic Animals.* Parts I-III. Edinburgh: Oliver & Boyd.

Vollmerhaus B, Habermehl K H (n.d.) *Topographical Anatomical Diagrams of Injection Technique in Horses, Cattle, Dogs and Cats.* Marburg, Lahn: Hoechst, Behringwerke A.G.

CONTENTS

Introduction xi

1 The Head (including the skin) 1

2 The Neck 55

3 The Forelimb 73

4 The Thorax 109

5 The Abdomen 143

6 The Hindlimb 185

7 The Foot 225

8 The Pelvis (including the spine) 269

9 Diagnostic Imaging of the Head, Withers, Manus and Pes 325

Index 345

INTRODUCTION

The range of the Veterinary Curriculum is continually expanding, and in many subjects its depth is continually increasing, yet the overall length of the course remains constant. As a result, there is pressure to allocate less and less time to some subjects, of which anatomy is a notable example. Furthermore, within departments of anatomy the desire to give greater emphasis to functional and applied aspects of the discipline, to radiological anatomy and to teratology, makes it increasingly difficult to allocate adequate time to personal dissection of each species by each student. An obvious solution to this problem is to rely more and more upon prepared dissections for the teaching of topographical anatomy. This saves much student time, but has several major disadvantages. Firstly, the student loses the chance to gain manipulative skills and is unable to see and feel the structures as they are progressively revealed by scalpel and scissors. Secondly, it means that the student must rapidly and in quick succession master complexities that were more surely understood by the leisurely methods of 40 years ago. Nothing can fully compensate for the lack of personal dissection by the skilled dissector supplemented by the intelligent use of graphic methods to record the work as it progresses. However, our experience at the Royal Veterinary College over many years has convinced us that the work of the skilful prosector, carefully studied, recorded and annotated, can be more useful than personal dissections of large animals carried out hurriedly by a group of inexpert students.

One problem in the teaching of topographical anatomy from prepared specimens has been the difficulty of providing students with enough good preparations of a full range of dissection stages of specific regions. It is our sincere hope that this photographic atlas of dissections will help to compensate for this deficiency in prepared specimens. For those students who are able to carry out their own detailed dissections, this atlas will provide a permanent reminder of what they saw, or should have seen, during each stage (often transitory) of the dissection.

The sequence of dissections presented in this volume is an expanded version of that used by us for a series of twenty 3-hour sessions on the topographical anatomy of the horse. Each stage of the work has been photographed in order to show many more stages of each major dissection than could be shown in our practical demonstration classes. We hope that this will compensate for the loss of the third dimension that is inevitable in photographs of dissections. We have tried to present the progression of required dissections as they occurred. Where the specimen was unusual or where we were not completely successful in demonstrating all of the structures as planned, we have not substituted a different specimen in the sequence; this would have broken the thread of the narrative. Occasionally, for the sake of clarity, we have reversed photographs of dissections made on one side, so that they fit more readily into the major sequence, but when this has been done it is clearly indicated in the legends. In every dissection room it is, from time to time, advantageous to mount extra demonstrations. For some regions we also have done this to show a different dissection procedure or a different specimen. Students should beware of treating these extras as optional or unnecessary complications – often they are of considerable importance.

A comment is needed on the technique of dissection shown in these photographs. In many instances we have not cleaned away all of the connective tissue from the structures being displayed. In 'complete' dissections it is often impossible to preserve accurately the original topographical relationships of vessels and nerves. Also, such dissections encourage the student to think that textbook drawings are real and that adipose, fascial and areolar tissues should not exist. We have tried to make the photographs represent the structures as they really appear during the course of an actual dissection.

It is no part of our plan, as teachers of veterinary anatomy, to entice the students out of the dissection room, away from the specimens, and into the comfort of armchairs for their study of practical topographical anatomy. Rather, we have attempted to provide an atlas with which they can extend their own personal study of dissections of the horse at times when the dissections are no longer readily available.

This is not an atlas of applied veterinary anatomy, but it is intended for veterinary students; considerable emphasis is given to those regions and structures that seem important for the veterinarian in practice. As far as possible, the photographs have been taken to provide information about the animal as it is seen during a routine clinical examination – other views have been used only occasionally, even though they are sometimes more informative from a strictly anatomical standpoint. It is hoped that the clinical student and the practising veterinarian may find this approach of value in examination, diagnosis and treatment of the standing animal. The experimentalist may also find that some of his problems of topographical anatomy are illuminated by these photographs of dissections. We realize that his requirements are diverse and unpredictable and have made our labelling of the various series of dissections as complete as possible with this in mind.

Radiographs and scans have been added to this new edition in the hope that they will give a useful introduction to an increasingly important aspect of veterinary anatomy.

RRA
SD

1. THE HEAD (INCLUDING THE SKIN)

Clinical importance of the skin

The surface of the horse is clinically important. Any part is liable to trauma because of the activities in which a horse participates. For example, ponies collide with obstacles, thoroughbreds with fences, and hunters with any hazard in the field. Therefore, the skin of the horse can be easily damaged. Horses react with violence to stress, especially to the presence of other horses, so there is a real possibility of being kicked. Head trauma is always a risk; brain damage as well as skull fractures may result, and the neurological effects can be detected by a full neurological examination.

The skin is one of the largest and most important systems of the body in the horse. Physical examination of the surface of the horse will help to assess general bodily condition. Also, the skin itself may be examined and the distribution and sizes of lesions may be noted. Clinical manifestations may include alopecia (hair loss) and pruritis (itching). Physical examination may also detect signs of trauma in the form of wounds, bites, burns, thermal injuries, acute swellings (oedema), insect stings and bites particularly midge bites from *Culicoides*, and the consequences of any initial injury. There are many consequences of surface trauma and these include inflammation, infection, oedema, haematomas, chronic wound infections, lymphangitis (swollen lymphatics, particularly in the lower limbs) and purpura (immunological disorders).

The skin will also show evidence of generalized systemic disturbances. It may show dehydration, congestion, oedema, possibly jaundice etc. and will be visibly affected when the horse is suffering from any form of malnutrition. Many of these conditions will require treatment, and a thorough knowledge of anatomy will be important, particularly if diagnostic techniques (e.g. radiography, ultrasonography, diagnostic nerve blocks), treatments (bandaging, corrective farriery) and surgery are required. There are also diagnostic techniques that can be applied to the skin – these include skin scrapings, stains, microbiological culture and biopsy techniques.

One of the important truisms is that the horse has four feet on the ground; these are easily damaged. Always remember the old adage that the first place to look for the seat of lameness is in the foot. Puncture wounds are common, and these may progress to solar abscesses and other abnormalities discussed in the section on the foot. Piercing of the feet by nails from incorrect shoeing, or from losing a shoe traumatically, is also a relatively common accident.

Treatment of wounds is a whole subject in itself. There are four phases: inflammation and debridement, repair, maturation and wound healing. The approach to wounds is important. Wounds to the trunk often heal by contraction and are treated by daily cleaning (wound lavage and debridement), because they cannot be dressed easily. Wounds in distal parts of the limbs are often complicated by oedema, and often heal with 'proud flesh'. 'First intention' wound healing follows suturing, but wounds that are either infected, or too extensive to suture, heal by 'second intention' and these repair, ultimately, by granulation tissue. Wounds require treatment and lots of time – in the horse, poor wound healing is a feature of a number of cases. There are many factors which delay wound healing, and these are beyond the scope of this introduction. Nowadays, a whole new field of equine surgery is possible, using skin grafting to repair these abnormalities of wound healing.

There is a multitude of skin conditions in the horse. Many of these are parasitic and include lice, mange of various types, and miscellaneous parasitic skin conditions including onchocerciasis, harvest mite infestation, equine ventral midline dermatitis and parafilariasis. Bacterial skin diseases are widespread and include specific exotic infections such as glanders (a zoonosis). Much more likely is one of a whole range of opportunistic bacterial infections including those involving *Dermatophilus* (rainscald); in many cases where there are pyogenic organisms involved, wounds progress to form an abscess. Mycoses include *Sporothrix*, histoplasmosis and, much more routinely, ringworm infections. A variety of hypersensitivity or similar reactions are also seen, including *Culicoides* hypersensitivity, urticaria pemphigus, and lupus erythematosus. Nodular skin disease and neoplastic papillomatosis may be seen, but are not common. The exception is probably sarcoids which are very common in all horses; they are a type of fibroblastic skin tumour. In addition, melanomas occur in grey horses. Other miscellaneous skin conditions include sunburn and photosensitization which may be of hepatogenous origin and associated with poisonous plants, especially ragwort (*Senecio*).

Clinical importance of the head

We will now consider the various regions and structures in the equine head, but disorders of the larynx and guttural pouch are discussed in Chapter 2.

The mucous membranes of the eye, mouth and nose give a good assessment of the cardiovascular system and general bodily state. They may reveal cyanosis (blue colour), which is a failure of oxygenation, pallor (anaemia), or even yellow as in jaundice, of which there are various causes in the horse. The ear is often involved in surface injuries but may also suffer from infections. There may be pain on handling, discharges, swellings and abnormal head/ear carriage. Specific diseases include parasitic infections such as *Otodectes* and also lesions from small biting flies. Sarcoids (fibroblastic tumours) are found throughout the body. They occur in many forms on the skin and are often found in the ear. They may be occult, verrucose, nodular, fibroblastic, malevolent or of a mixed type. *Otitis media* (inflammation of the middle ear within the tympanic cavity) may result in rupture of the ear drum and may be associated with extension of guttural pouch disease or haematogenous spread of pus-forming bacteria.

The eye is often examined to give a general assessment of health. The 'sunken eye' (loss of the periorbital fat from the eye socket) may be caused by dehydration or by wasting and emaciation. It is often one of the first abnormalities detected at a full clinical examination. The eye may also be discoloured. Pale ocular mucous membranes may suggest one of several types of anaemia. There may be excessive red cell destruction, resulting from renal or hepatic failure. Neonatal isoerythrolysis, in which foals have acquired immunity to red blood cells, is also a possibility. The mare produces antibodies to the RBCs of the foal, which are then concentrated in the colostrum and the foal receives these antibodies when suckled.

Examination of the eye is performed quite frequently as part of a pre-purchase examination. The eye is often involved in fractures of the orbit and periorbital region, associated with trauma in racing or hunting. Young horses falling over backwards may fracture the basisphenoid or basioccipital bone and, occasionally, the petrous temporal bones. There is a good prognosis for these fractures if the eyeball itself is not involved in the process. There are several developmental abnormalities of the eye that may be found, including microphthalmos, anopthalmos and endophthalmos up to the sclera. The sclera is involved in pion. Orbital neoplasia can also occur, but is very rare. The eyelids are often affected by trauma (eyelid lacerations are quite common) which causes inflammation. Entropion and ectropion (inturning and out-turning of the eyelashes on the abnormal lids) are also seen in the horse.

There are a whole variety of eye conditions, most of which require specialist ophthalmological investigations and are beyond the scope of this chapter. More straightforward diagnoses include inflammation of the conjunctiva (conjunctivitis). Foreign bodies may be found in the conjuctival sac. The lacrimal duct may be narrowed or blocked. Corneal problems may include inflammation (keratitis), ulceration and foreign bodies. Bacterial, viral and mycotic keratitis may occur. The uveal tract (iris, ciliary body and choroid) may be involved in disease processes such as acute or recurrent equine uveitis. Neoplasia, such as squamous cell carcinoma of the third eyelid, is rare. Congenital and acquired cataracts are not common, neither is glaucoma. The fundus of the eye of the horse is subject to a considerable range of variations. Pathological changes may include retinal detachment, retinal haemorrhage, retinal atrophy and inflammation. Optic nerve neuropathy, optic neuritis and optic nerve atrophy are rarely diagnosed.

The mucous membrane of the nose should be inspected in a general assessment of health. Discharges at the nostril can be very variable and include serous fluid, mucus, mucopurulent or purulent discharges and frank haemorrhage. They can originate from the nose itself or from any part of the respiratory tract, including the sinuses and the guttural pouches or even from the lung.

The nostrils should be examined, as they may show a variety of changes including hypertrophy of the alar folds, atheroma of the nasal diverticulum (false nostril) or trauma and necrosis of the alar cartilage. Foreign bodies and nasal polyps are commonly found, but amyloidosis, 'wry nose', fungal diseases and atheroma are rare. At the nostrils a specific haemorrhage, called epistaxis (idiopathic), may be seen in racehorses. It is associated with racing. Exercise-induced pulmonary haemorrhage (EIPM) is also seen at the nostrils. The nostrils are a common site for nasal lacerations.

The upper respiratory tract is really important in equine practice. Horses that have run into objects, or have been kicked, may suffer from serious trauma to the nasal cavity. Many types of injury can occur and new diagnoses are being added all the time, particularly as a result of imaging techniques. These injuries include fractures to the walls of the paranasal sinuses or nasal passages; in these cases epistaxis will most obviously be a feature.

The nasal cavity provides a pathway through which the stomach tube or endoscope can be passed. The endoscope can be used to examine the sinuses, pharynx, larynx, Eustachian tube, guttural pouch, trachea and major bronchi of the lower respiratory tract, and also the oesophagus and stomach. It can be used to take pictures of anatomical abnormalities or lesions. It can be used to wash out structures and collect lavage fluids and tissues or discharges for culture, or cytology. It can also be used for biopsy. Nasotracheal intubation is a very useful technique for the investigation of respiratory disorders. Dynamic airway collapse can be revealed by tracheal endoscopy. The alar fold is reflected and the tube is passed along the ventral nasal meatus into the pharynx and then into the trachea, with the head elevated to prevent the tube being swallowed. For orotracheal intubation the tongue must be pulled out, a speculum is placed in the mouth, and the tube is advanced gently to allow swallowing. Radiography, ultrasonics and exercise tests including exercise endoscopy, are also used to examine these structures.

The head is obviously the most rostral part of the body and therefore particularly prone to trauma. In these cases there may be facial deformity or swelling. Jaw fractures occur reasonably commonly, especially to the body and the incisive region of the mandible. In the upper jaw, the incisive bone is most commonly affected. These fractures are often repaired surgically, possibly under nerve block and sedation, and may require braces, splints or pins and long screw fixation. These fractures may be accompanied by dental problems and other problems may follow extraction. Infections of the gingival margins may lead to dental alveolitis.

One of the key anatomical relationships in the head of the horse is between the nasal cavity, paranasal sinuses and teeth. The paranasal sinuses develop as progressive invasions of the diploë of the bones of the skull by the epithelium of the nasal cavity. The sinuses lighten the skull, insulate the brain from outside temperature variation and facilitate mucociliary clearance of the inhaled debris (look at the dust in a stable after the bedding or hay has been shaken out!). These sinus cavities are normally air-filled, resonant, and lined by mucoperiosteum. The presence of nasal discharge may be the first indication of a sinusitis that can subsequently be confirmed by radiography and endoscopy. Sinusitis may be associated with mycoses or neoplasia. The discharge may be mucopurulent, mucoid or serous.

Left and right sides of the head have paranasal sinuses that are separated by midline septa. On each side, two maxillary sinuses (rostral and caudal) extend progressively into the diploë of the maxilla from the middle nasal meatus through the nasomaxillary opening. The large *caudal maxillary sinus* extends caudally into the sphenoid and palatine bones to form the sphenopalatine sinus. It also extends through the frontomaxillary opening to form the frontal sinus. The frontal sinus extends into the caudal part of the first ethmoidal endoturbinate bone (the dorsal nasal concha) to form the dorsal conchal sinus. The frontal sinus also extends into the second ethmoidal endoturbinate bone to form the middle conchal sinus. The smaller *rostral maxillary sinus* also extends caudally into the caudal part of the ventral nasal concha through the conchomaxillary opening to form the ventral conchal sinus. (The anatomy is complicated by the presence of the conchal bulla which lies ventral to the conchomaxillary opening).

The frontal sinus has a conchal part and a frontal part; drainage goes into the caudal maxillary sinus through the frontomaxillary foramen. The ethmoidal and sphenopalatine sinuses also drain into the caudal maxillary sinuses and thus into the middle meatus. The rostral maxillary sinus has a drainage pathway into the middle nasal meatus through the nasomaxillary opening. This sinus is divided into a lateral bony compartment and a medial conchal compartment (within the ventral concha). These compartments are separated by the infra-orbital canal and a sheet of bone joining it ventrally to the roots of the teeth. In the young horse, the lateral component is almost entirely occupied by the roots of the cheek teeth. With age, the roots recede towards the floor of the sinus and the sinus increases in size. The ventral conchal sinus is accessible for surgery through the floor of the concho-frontal sinus.

Inflammation of the sinuses can occur by extension from the other mucosal surfaces. If they become filled with mucopurulent exudates these must be drained by trephination because the natural drainage ostia are not at the lowest points of the sinus system. Treatment of sinusitis involves trephining a hole in the bone over the sinus. The frontal sinus, dorsal and medial to the orbit, can be trephined along a line from the medial ocular angle (canthus) to the mid-line, about 1 cm caudal to the mid-point of this line. The caudal maxillary sinus is trephined 3 cm lateral to the medial canthus and 3 cm dorsal to the facial crest. The rostral maxillary sinus can be trephined at a point half way along the line from the medial canthus to the rostral extremity of the facial crest. Through these trephination sites, samples can be collected from the sinuses and can be cultured for bacterial examination and antibiotic sensitivity testing. The sinus can then be flushed out and treated. Sinus cysts, sinus polyps and neoplasia occur infrequently.

Four other conditions involving the head require some knowledge of anatomy. Occasional horses may show acute salivation (idiopathic sialo-adenitis). Even more rarely do we find occlusion of the salivary ducts and possible mucocoele. Head shaking is also an equine phenomenon. 'Crib biting' is a habitual neurotic vice which can produce extreme wear in the incisor teeth. It can suggest an abnormality of diet. It fulfils a functional digestive need in that it helps to meet the demand for unsatisfied foraging behaviour. Lastly, there may be masseter myopathy. In this, there is atrophy of the muscles, probably caused by damage to the masseteric nerve, which is superficial and easily damaged in accidents.

The lymph nodes are important. The streptococcal infection known as strangles (caused by *Streptococcus equi*) is a particularly severe purulent infection of the submandibular nodes, but may extend to other nodes of the head and neck and even into the thorax. The former epizootic disease (glanders) caused by *Pfeifferella mallei* also severely affects the lymph nodes of the head. Any local infection may cause swelling of the parotid, retropharyngeal and submandibular lymph nodes.

Alimentary tract disorders affecting the oral cavity are less common than disorders of the teeth or nasal cavity. Traumatic injuries to the tongue may or may not include glossal nerve damage. Paralysis of the tongue may indicate botulism. Viral stomatitis and oral ulceration are also sporadically diagnosed.

The teeth of the horse are hypsodont (high-crowned), composed of enamel (hard and brittle, 98% inorganic), dentine (slightly softer, 70–80% inorganic), cementum (with structural affinities to bone) and the pulp (soft). Deciduous incisor teeth erupt soon after birth. The central incisor teeth (i1) erupt at less than 2 weeks, the second incisors (i2) at about 6 weeks, and third incisors (i3) at around 6–9 months (you can remember 8 days, 8 weeks and 8 months more easily). Two-year-olds then shed the central deciduous incisors, 3-year-olds the second (lateral) incisors and 4-year-olds the third (corner) incisors. If all permanent incisor teeth (I1, I2, I3) are in wear, the horse is over 5 years old. Foals have three deciduous premolar cheek teeth. The permanent premolar teeth (P2, P3, P4) are usually called 'cheek teeth 1,2 and 3' in clinical work. They erupt at approx. 2.5, 3 and 3.5–4 years. The molar teeth (M1, M2 and M3) are usually called 'cheek teeth 4,5 and 6' in clinical work. They erupt at 1, 2 and 3.5–4 years of age.

In the young horse, developmental disorders of the teeth may include retained deciduous teeth, displacement of cheek teeth, and dentigerous cysts which are usually manifest as a discharging tract at the base of the ear. Teeth may also acquire disorders such as sharp edges (which require rasping – an energetic sport for the young and fit!), undulating occlusal surfaces ('wave mouth'), or loss of enamel ridges ('shear mouth' or '18-month mouth'). In cases of tramautic injury, teeth may be split.

Dental diseases may show as 'quidding' (drooling of the food from the corners of the mouth), facial distortion, facial swelling and a nasal discharge. Overgrown teeth occur if the opposing tooth is missing. Periodontal disease is also possible. Occasionally, cheek teeth may be displaced and there may be supplementary teeth. Dental caries may occur, accompanied by alveolar periosteitis, as a result of bacterial fermentation leading to erosion of the enamel.

The rostral cheek teeth can be removed by oral extraction, principally by lateral buccotomy. This involves removal of alveolar bone, taking care not to damage the facial nerve. Retropulsion, with a punch, is also used for removing the mandibular and maxillary teeth. The upper cheek teeth 4 and 5 (M^1, M^2) are taken out through the maxillary sinus and 6 (M^3) through the frontal sinus. In this you have to trephine (make a hole in the bone) over the tooth to be extracted and then punch it out. Care must be taken to avoid damage to the adjacent teeth. Complications do occur, including collateral damage, dental sequestration, alveolar bone sequestra and oronasal fistulae. In the mandible, retropulsion needs to be performed carefully because the parotid duct runs along the ventromedial edge of the body of the mandible, with the facial vessels. They turn laterally and dorsally close to the roots of the molar teeth.

Peripheral nerve or cranial nerve damage is not common. There are probably two exceptions: damage to the facial nerve and damage to the nerves associated with the guttural pouch (i.e. those traversing the *foramen lacerum*). The facial nerve can be damaged by trauma and this leads to paresis and paralysis. All three branches can be affected together at the nucleus level (in the pons) but the auricular, palpebral and buccal branches may be damaged separately on the face. The site of the damage on the face determines which nerve, and therefore which muscles, are affected. The buccal branches are probably the most exposed, over the body of the mandible and the masseter muscle. Damage to the facial nerve at any point will lead to abnormalities of facial expression. All of the branches will be affected if the lesions (such as fractures of the hyoid bone, or the cranial floor, or damage to the guttural pouch) occur near the base of the brain.

Local nerve blocks may be performed on the head, principally for facilitating wound repair (e.g. auriculopalpebral, lacrimal, zygomatic or infratrochlear nerves). In the past, mental and mandibular nerve blocks for dental surgery were also performed but general anaesthesia is now a much safer option. Occasionally, both are used together. A detailed analysis of the disorders of the central nervous system, especially the infectious diseases, is beyond the scope of this clinical introduction but a brief list would have to include Japanese B encephalitis, equine protozoal encephalitis, rabies, Western, Eastern and Venezuelan encephalitis and equine herpes virus infections and now, of course, West Nile virus infections.

Recently, a specific protozoal myeloencephalomyelitis (associated with *Sarcocystis neurona*) has become a problem in the USA. Generalized non-specific disorders such as vasculitis, epilepsy, ataxia and equine degenerative myeloencephalopathy should be listed. Equine motor neuron disease, botulism, tetanus and organophosphorus poisoning should be included in the list.

Pharyngeal lymphoid hyperplasia is an inflammatory condition of the pharyngeal mucosa. Pharyngeal trauma, lacerations and foreign bodies may be seen. Dorsal displacement of the soft palate occurs normally during swallowing, but can occur abnormally during racing or fast exercise; it is diagnosed by endoscopy. In this condition, the free border of the palatal arch becomes dislodged from its normal, subepiglottic, position. Unsupported soft tissue is then inhaled into the *rima glottidis* causing acute respiratory obstruction. It may be caused by fatigue or by disorders of the soft palate itself, or by disorders of the epiglottis and conditions that cause mouth breathing and pharyngeal discomfort. Remember the horse is an ***obligate*** nose breather.

The temporomandibular joint is of considerable veterinary importance. It may be fractured, leading to displacement, but disease in this joint can follow bacteraemia or septicaemia. If infected, it can be palpated; quite often there is swelling in the joint capsule and the fluid can be aspirated. Clinically, there is considerable difficulty in swallowing (dysphagia) leading to 'quidding' (dropping of food) and possibly asymmetry of the masseter muscles.

The larynx and the auditory tube, including the guttural pouch, are discussed in the section dealing with the neck and the clinical problems of airway obstruction.

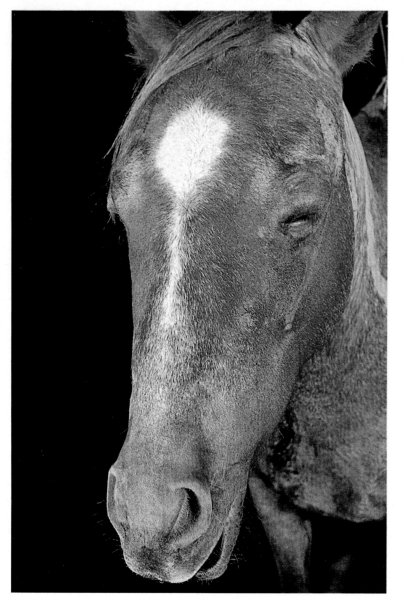

Fig. 1.1 Surface features of the head: rostral view. The palpable bony features have been shaved. This young gelding was a red roan, with conjoined star and stripe on frontal and dorsal nasal regions. The position of the hair vortex is variable and there may be two vortices.

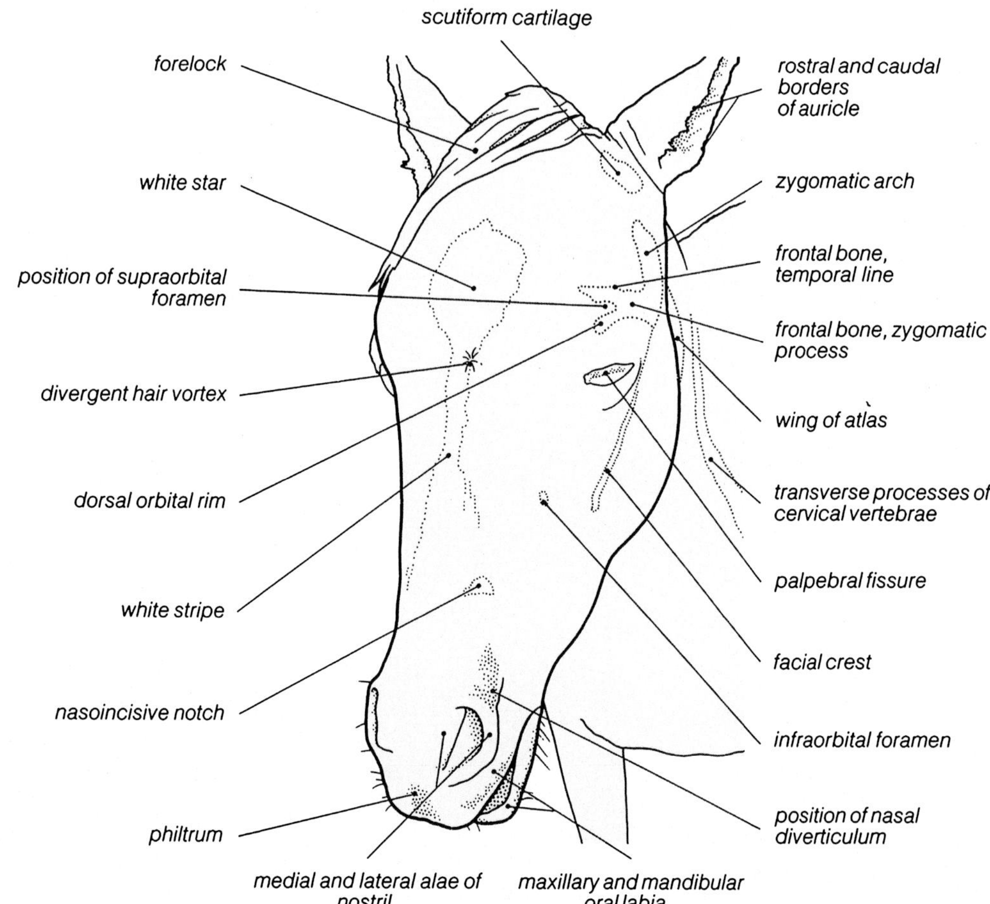
scutiform cartilage
forelock
rostral and caudal borders of auricle
white star
zygomatic arch
position of supraorbital foramen
frontal bone, temporal line
frontal bone, zygomatic process
divergent hair vortex
wing of atlas
dorsal orbital rim
transverse processes of cervical vertebrae
palpebral fissure
white stripe
facial crest
nasoincisive notch
infraorbital foramen
position of nasal diverticulum
philtrum
medial and lateral alae of nostril
maxillary and mandibular oral labia

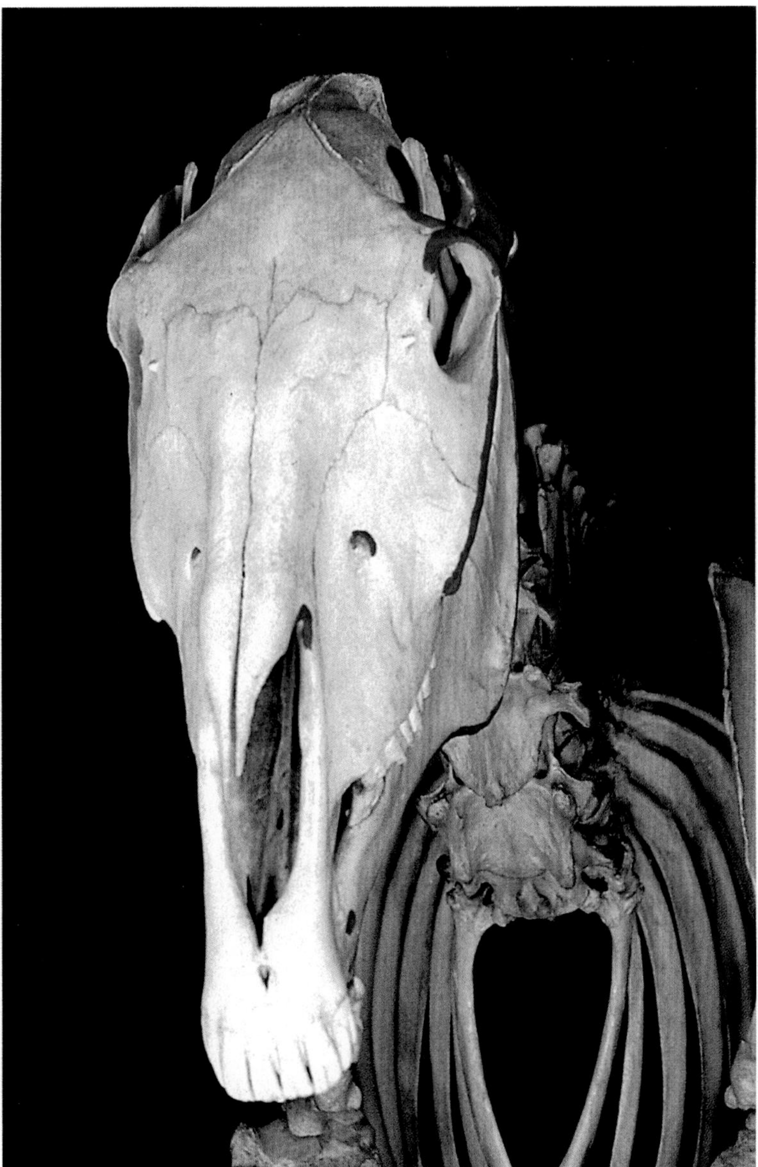

Fig. 1.2 Bones of the head: rostral view. The palpable bony features shown in Fig. 1.1 are coloured red. The mental foramen is also shown (see Figs. 1.4 and 1.5).

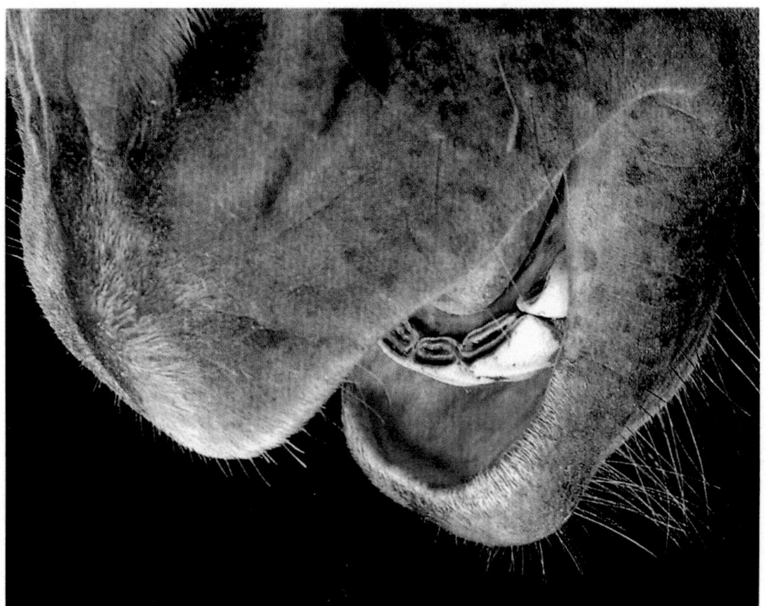

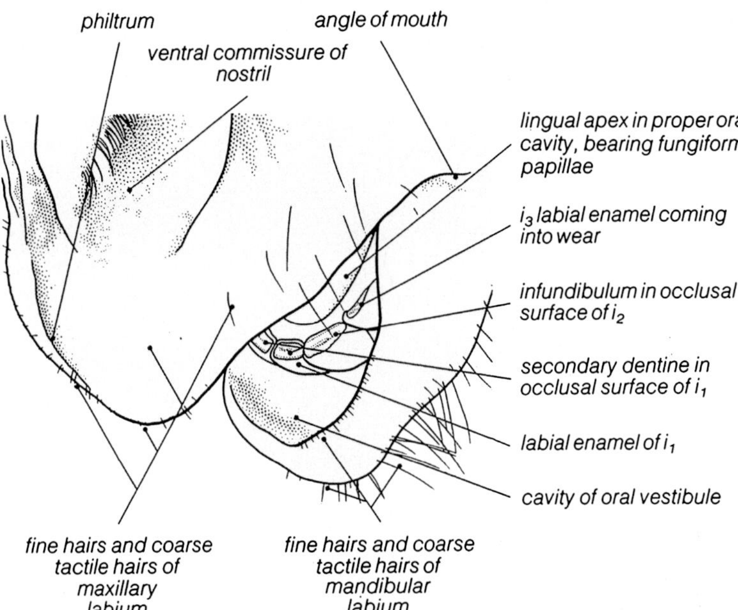
philtrum
angle of mouth
ventral commissure of nostril
lingual apex in proper oral cavity, bearing fungiform papillae
i_3 labial enamel coming into wear
infundibulum in occlusal surface of i_2
secondary dentine in occlusal surface of i_1
labial enamel of i_1
cavity of oral vestibule
fine hairs and coarse tactile hairs of maxillary labium
fine hairs and coarse tactile hairs of mandibular labium

Fig. 1.3 The lips and incisor teeth: left rostrolateral view. The third temporary mandibular incisor tooth erupts at about 6–9 months of age, and by 18 months this tooth is usually well in wear. The hairs of both labia form divergent hair vortices and those on the maxillary labium may be long forming a 'moustache'.

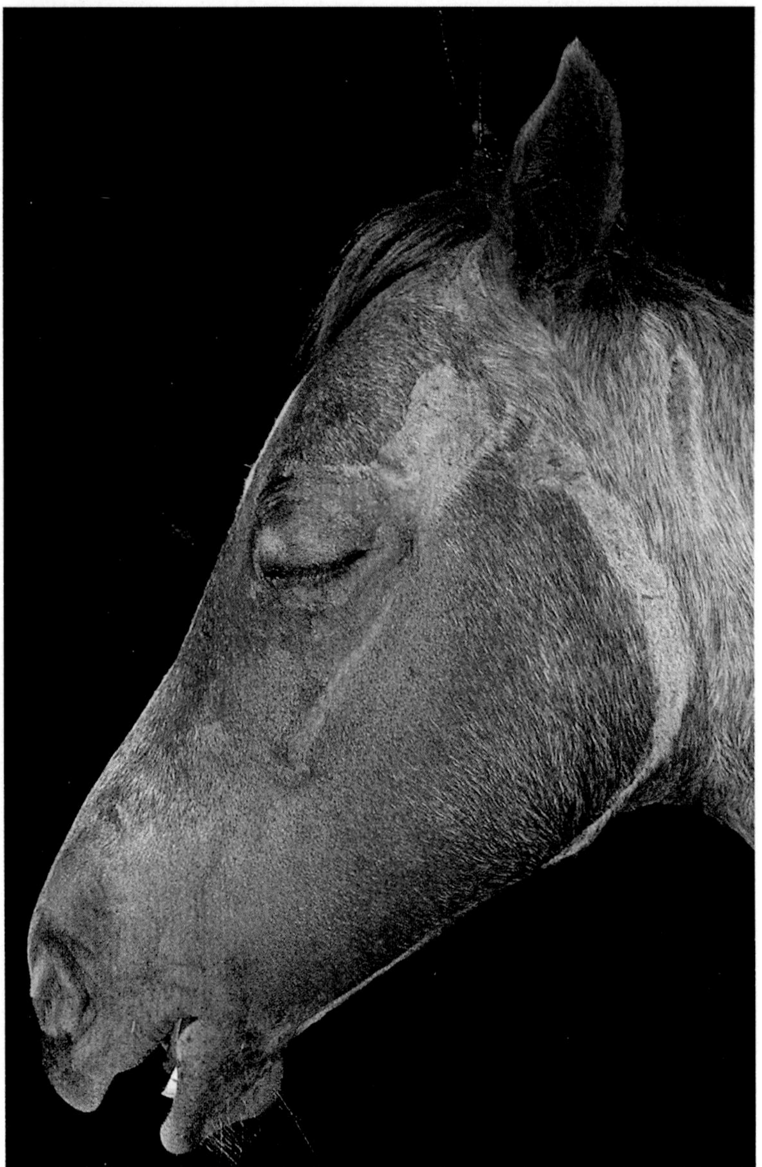

Fig. 1.4 Surface features of the head: left lateral view. The palpable bony features have been shaved. The nasal region is markedly concave and the frontal region is rather convex. This dished shape is characteristic of Arab horses.

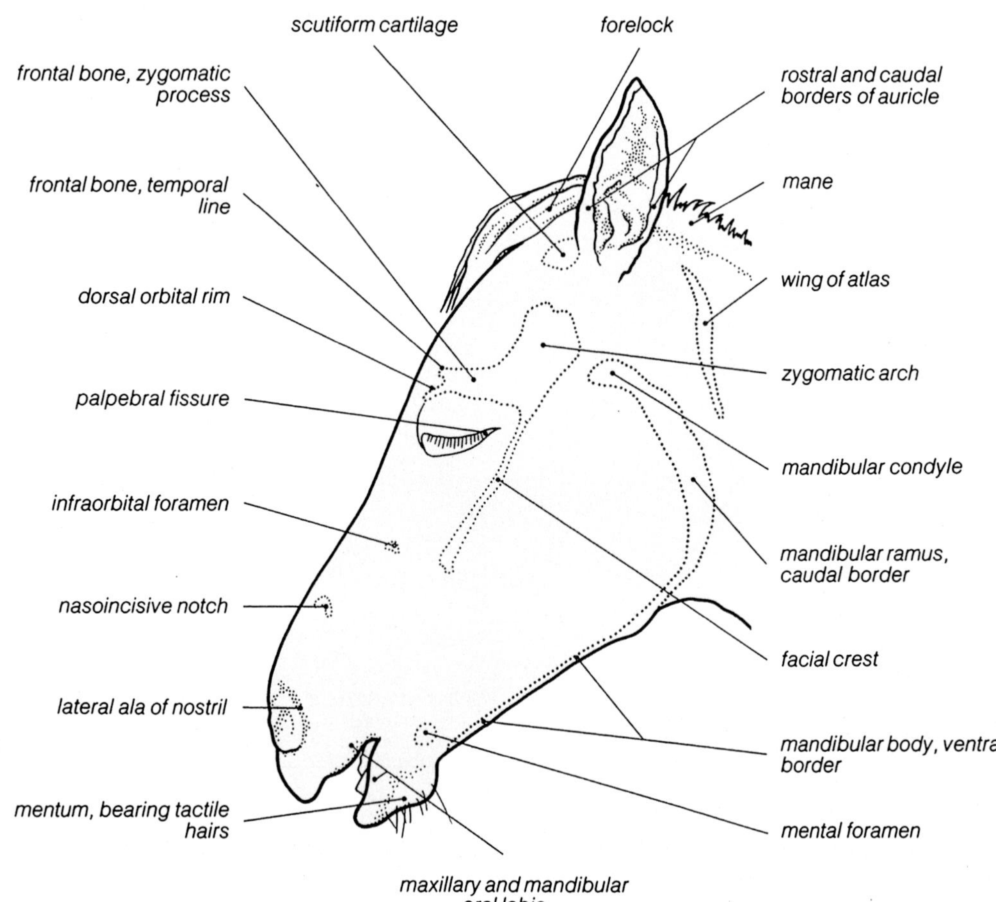
scutiform cartilage
forelock
frontal bone, zygomatic process
rostral and caudal borders of auricle
frontal bone, temporal line
mane
wing of atlas
dorsal orbital rim
zygomatic arch
palpebral fissure
mandibular condyle
infraorbital foramen
mandibular ramus, caudal border
nasoincisive notch
facial crest
lateral ala of nostril
mandibular body, ventral border
mentum, bearing tactile hairs
mental foramen
maxillary and mandibular oral labia

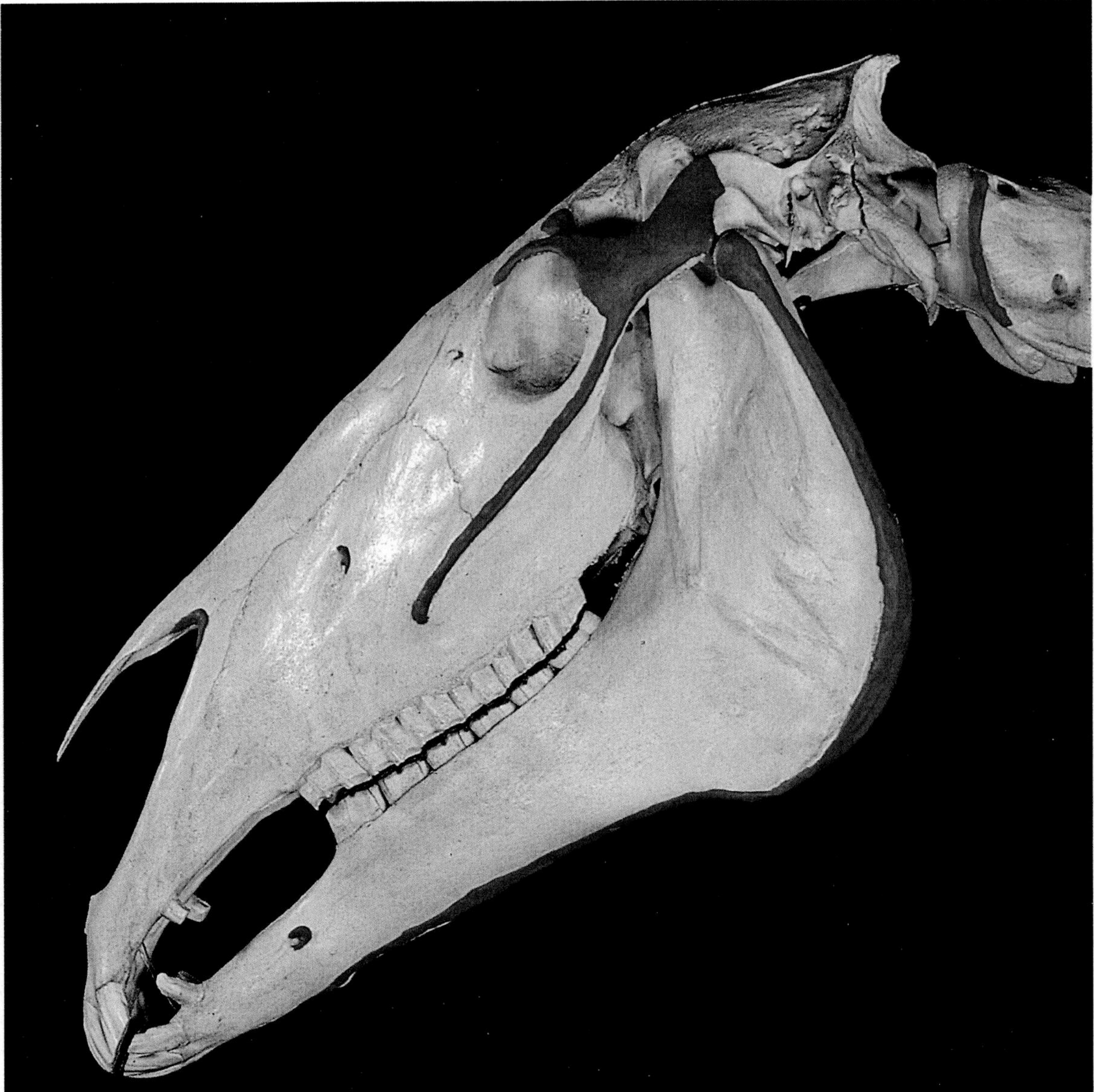

Fig. 1.5 Bones of the head: left lateral view. The palpable bony features shown in Fig. 1.4 are coloured red. The skull is not, however, of the same dished shape.

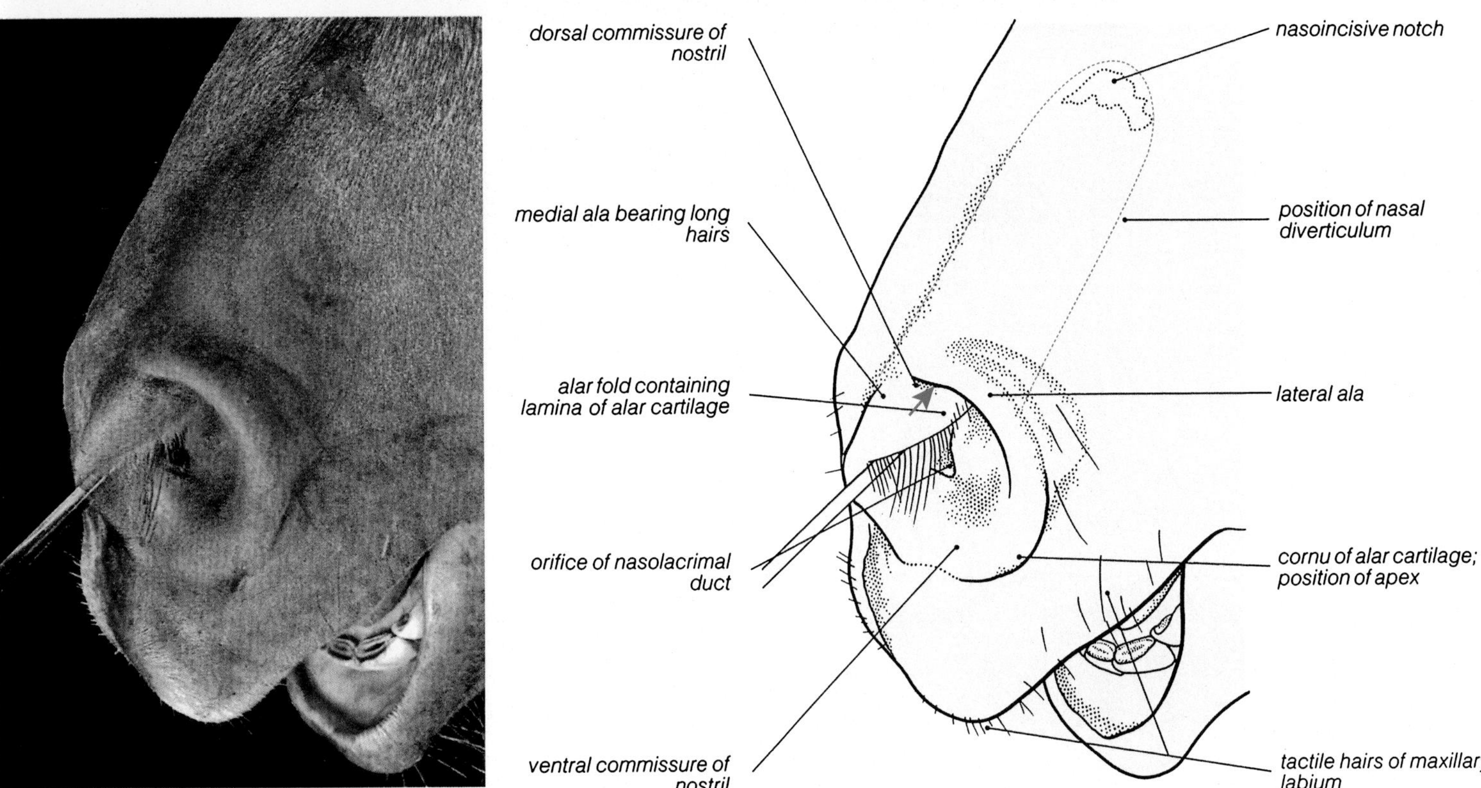
dorsal commissure of nostril
nasoincisive notch
medial ala bearing long hairs
position of nasal diverticulum
alar fold containing lamina of alar cartilage
lateral ala
orifice of nasolacrimal duct
cornu of alar cartilage; position of apex
ventral commissure of nostril
tactile hairs of maxillary labium

Fig. 1.6 The nostril: left rostro-lateral view. The medial ala has been lifted to display the nasolacrimal orifice, using a glass rod placed in the dorsal nasal meatus. A blue arrow indicates the dorsal entrance into the nasal diverticulum. The cavity of the diverticulum is shown in Fig. 1.7. Further details of the nostrils in the fresh state are shown in Figs. 1.39–1.41, including the relationships of the alar cartilage.

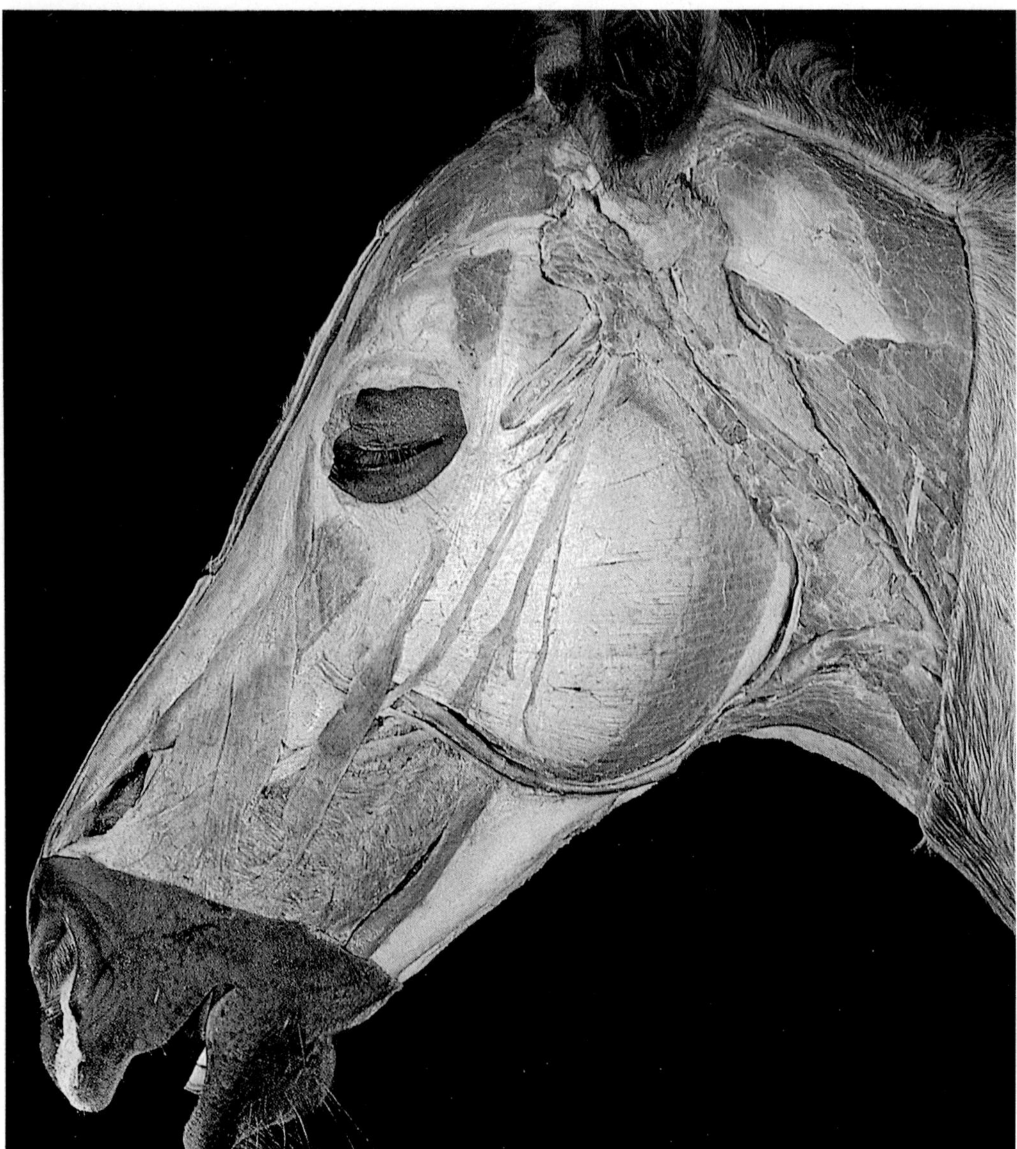

Fig. 1.7 Superficial structures of the head: left lateral view. Further details of this dissection are shown in Figs. 1.8–1.11. The lateral wall of the nasal diverticulum has been cut away. A yellow paste was injected into the left guttural pouch, and this appears at the left nostril.

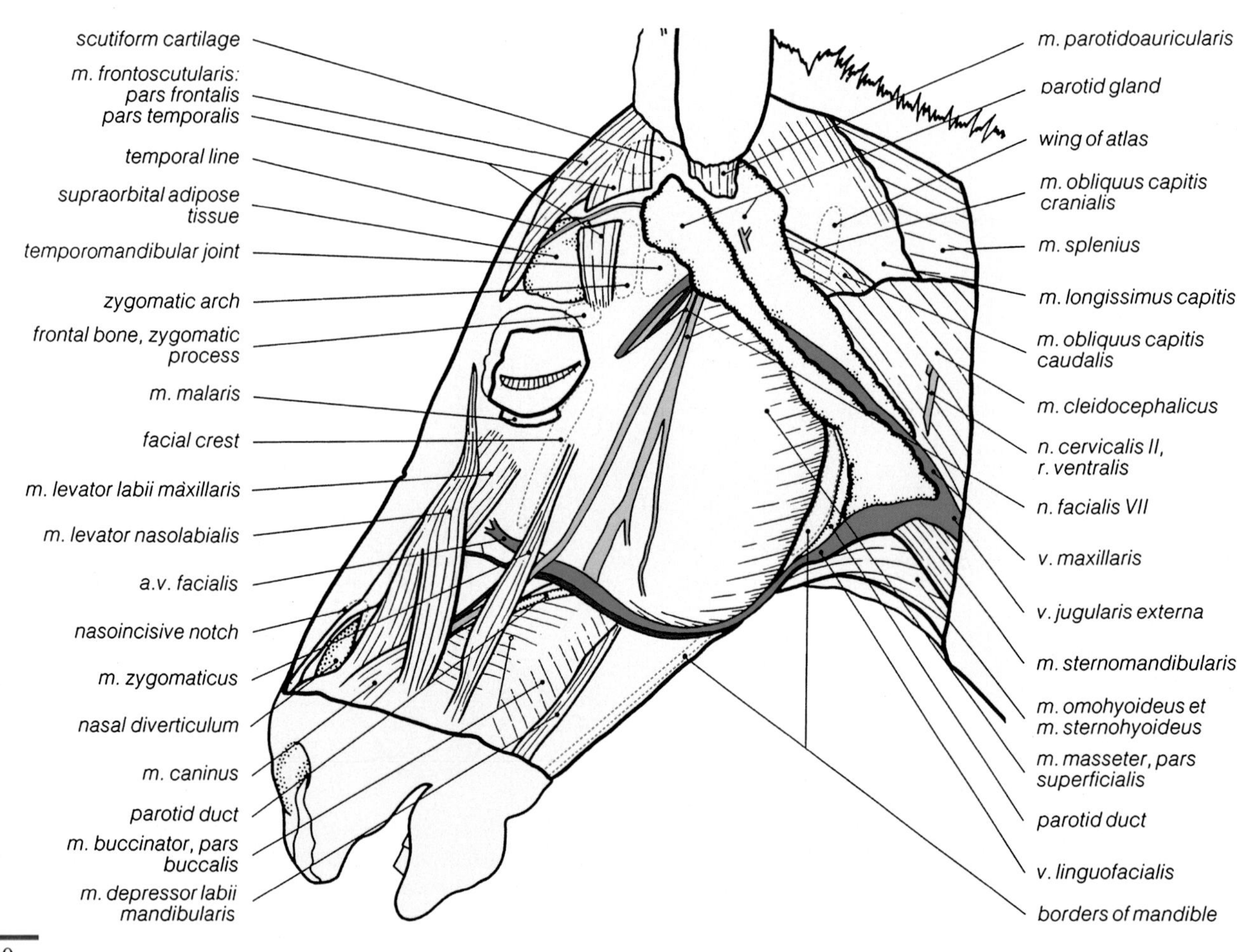

scutiform cartilage
m. frontoscutularis:
pars frontalis
pars temporalis
temporal line
supraorbital adipose tissue
temporomandibular joint
zygomatic arch
frontal bone, zygomatic process
m. malaris
facial crest
m. levator labii maxillaris
m. levator nasolabialis
a.v. facialis
nasoincisive notch
m. zygomaticus
nasal diverticulum
m. caninus
parotid duct
m. buccinator, pars buccalis
m. depressor labii mandibularis
m. parotidoauricularis
parotid gland
wing of atlas
m. obliquus capitis cranialis
m. splenius
m. longissimus capitis
m. obliquus capitis caudalis
m. cleidocephalicus
n. cervicalis II, r. ventralis
n. facialis VII
v. maxillaris
v. jugularis externa
m. sternomandibularis
m. omohyoideus et m. sternohyoideus
m. masseter, pars superficialis
parotid duct
v. linguofacialis
borders of mandible

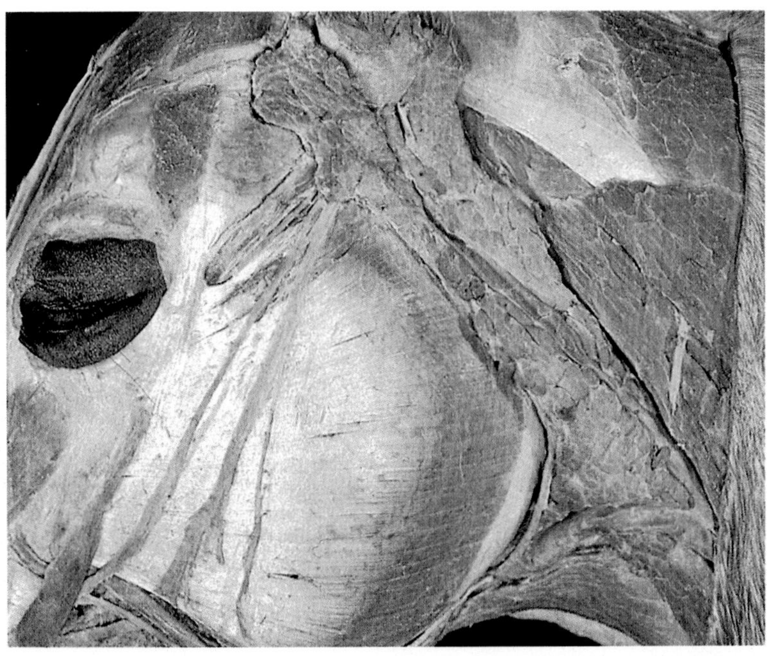

Fig. 1.8 Superficial structures of the parotid and masseteric regions: left lateral view. This is a closer view of a part of the dissection shown in Fig. 1.7.

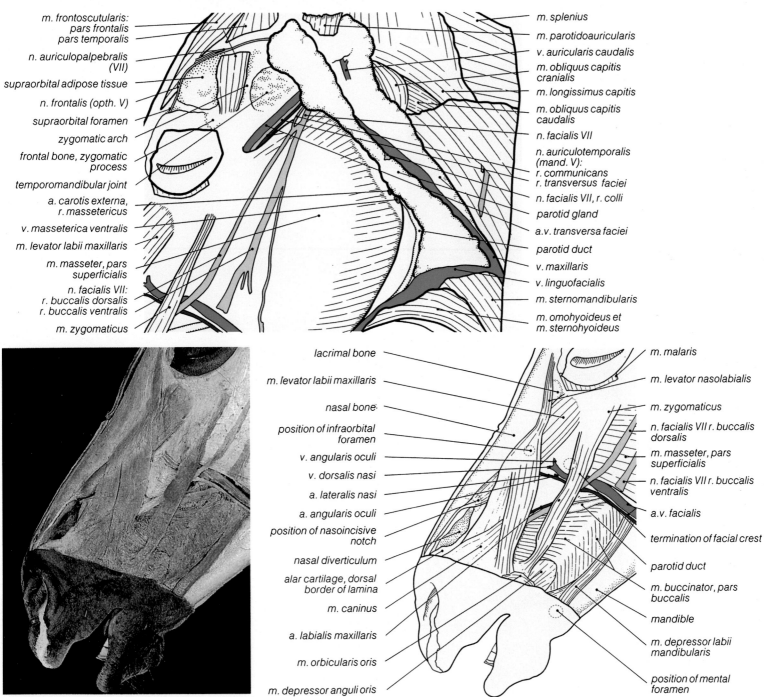

m. frontoscutularis:
pars frontalis
pars temporalis
n. auriculopalpebralis (VII)
supraorbital adipose tissue
n. frontalis (opth. V)
supraorbital foramen
zygomatic arch
frontal bone, zygomatic process
temporomandibular joint
a. carotis externa, r. massetericus
v. masseterica ventralis
m. levator labii maxillaris
m. masseter, pars superficialis
n. facialis VII:
r. buccalis dorsalis
r. buccalis ventralis
m. zygomaticus

m. splenius
m. parotidoauricularis
v. auricularis caudalis
m. obliquus capitis cranialis
m. longissimus capitis
m. obliquus capitis caudalis
n. facialis VII
n. auriculotemporalis (mand. V):
r. communicans
r. transversus faciei
n. facialis VII, r. colli
parotid gland
a.v. transversa faciei
parotid duct
v. maxillaris
v. linguofacialis
m. sternomandibularis
m. omohyoideus et m. sternohyoideus

lacrimal bone
m. levator labii maxillaris
nasal bone
position of infraorbital foramen
v. angularis oculi
v. dorsalis nasi
a. lateralis nasi
a. angularis oculi
position of nasoincisive notch
nasal diverticulum
alar cartilage, dorsal border of lamina
m. caninus
a. labialis maxillaris
m. orbicularis oris
m. depressor anguli oris

m. malaris
m. levator nasolabialis
m. zygomaticus
n. facialis VII r. buccalis dorsalis
m. masseter, pars superficialis
n. facialis VII r. buccalis ventralis
a.v. facialis
termination of facial crest
parotid duct
m. buccinator, pars buccalis
mandible
m. depressor labii mandibularis
position of mental foramen

Fig. 1.9 Superficial structures of the facial regions: left lateral view. This is a closer view of the dissection shown in Fig. 1.7. The nerve foramina are revealed in Fig. 1.12. Further details of the nostrils are shown in Figs. 1.39–1.41.

Fig. 1.10 Superficial structures of the cranial and facial regions: left craniolateral view. This figure does not show the fine branches of the lacrimal nerve which, together with those of the auriculopalpebral and frontal nerves, form a superficial nerve plexus. On the right hand side, the skin incisions which expose the paranasal sinuses (Fig. 1.35–1.38) are shown.

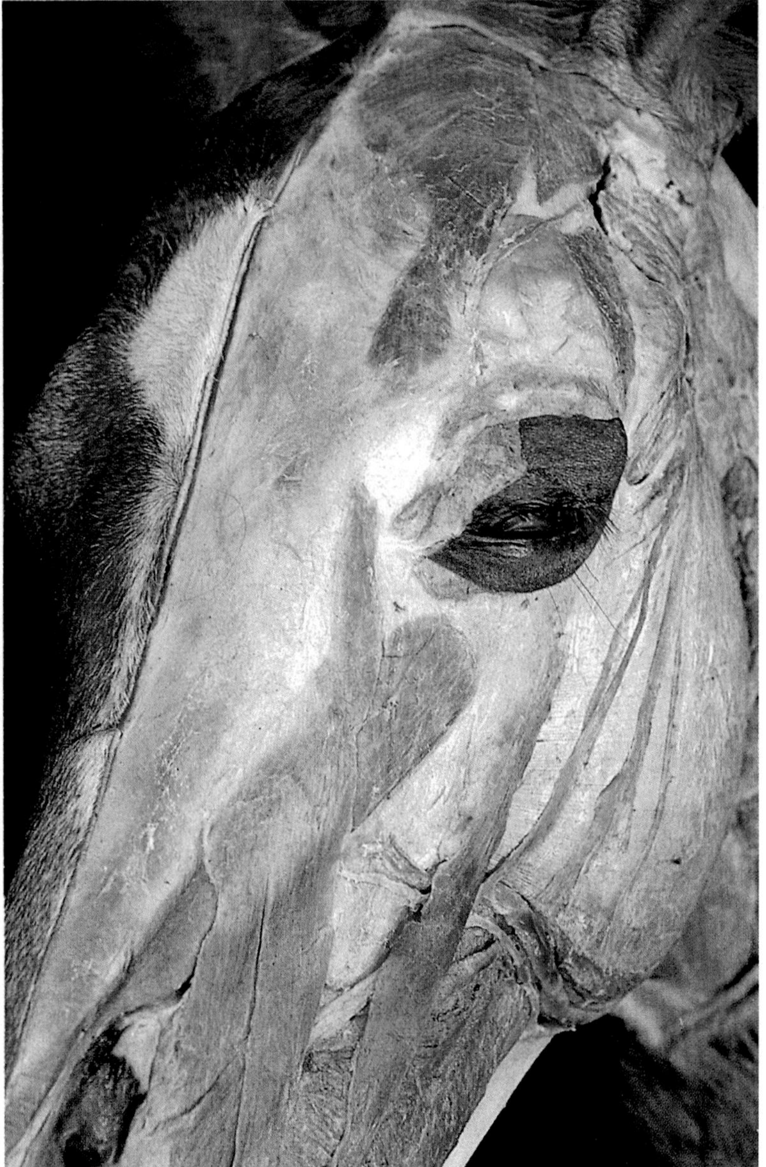

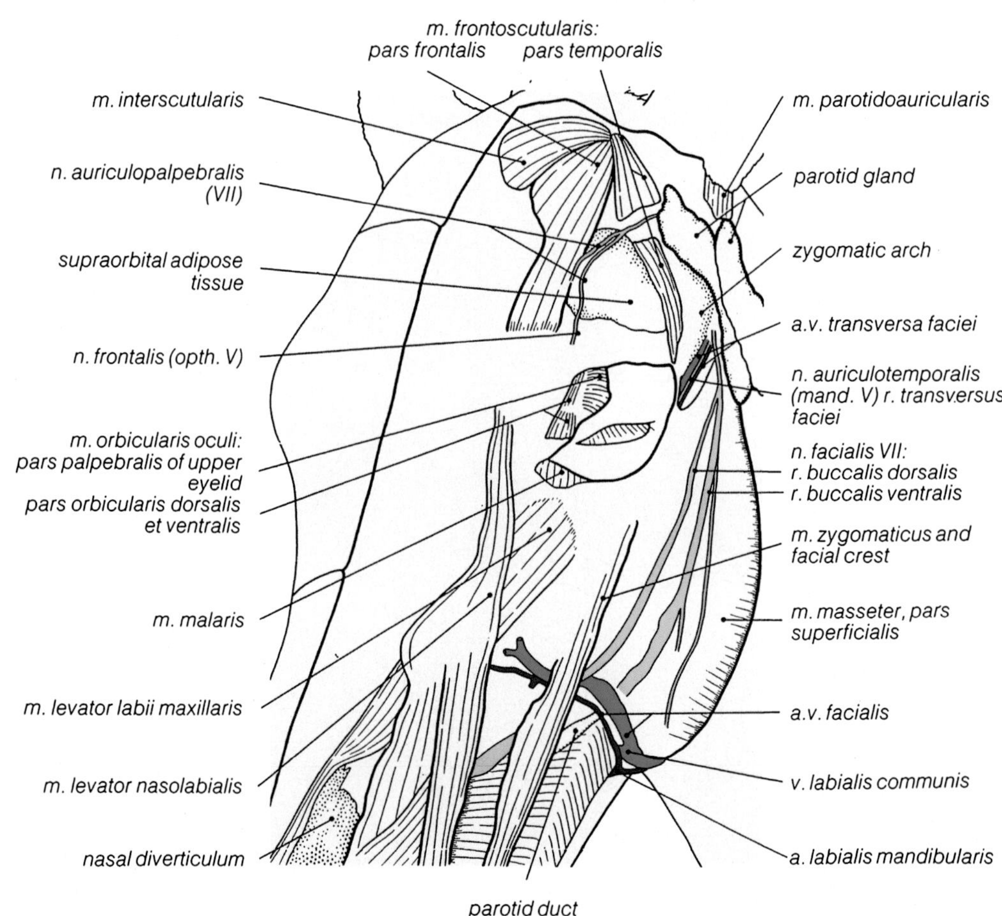
m. frontoscutularis:
pars frontalis
pars temporalis
m. interscutularis
n. auriculopalpebralis (VII)
supraorbital adipose tissue
n. frontalis (opth. V)
m. orbicularis oculi:
pars palpebralis of upper eyelid
pars orbicularis dorsalis et ventralis
m. malaris
m. levator labii maxillaris
m. levator nasolabialis
nasal diverticulum
parotid duct
m. parotidoauricularis
parotid gland
zygomatic arch
a.v. transversa faciei
n. auriculotemporalis (mand. V) r. transversus faciei
n. facialis VII:
r. buccalis dorsalis
r. buccalis ventralis
m. zygomaticus and facial crest
m. masseter, pars superficialis
a.v. facialis
v. labialis communis
a. labialis mandibularis

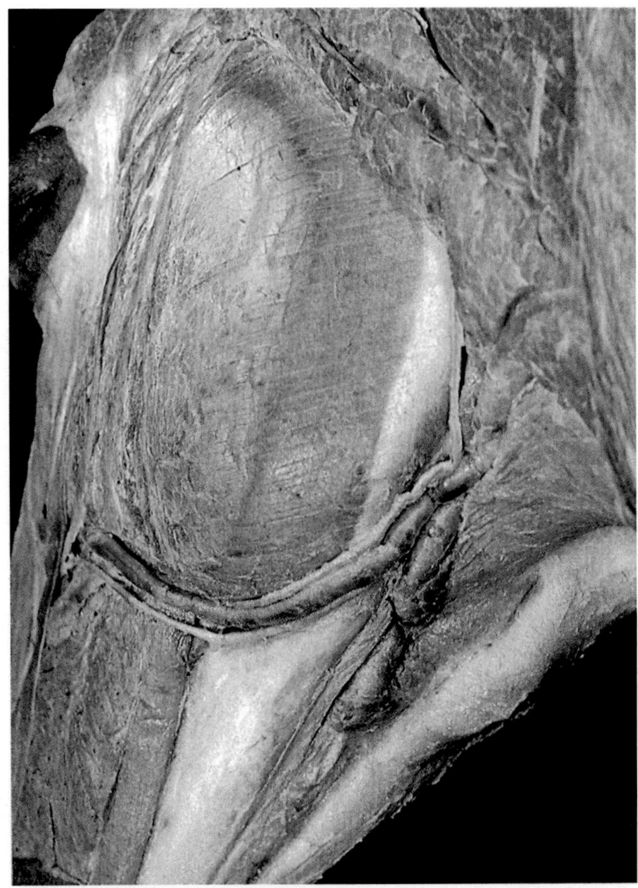

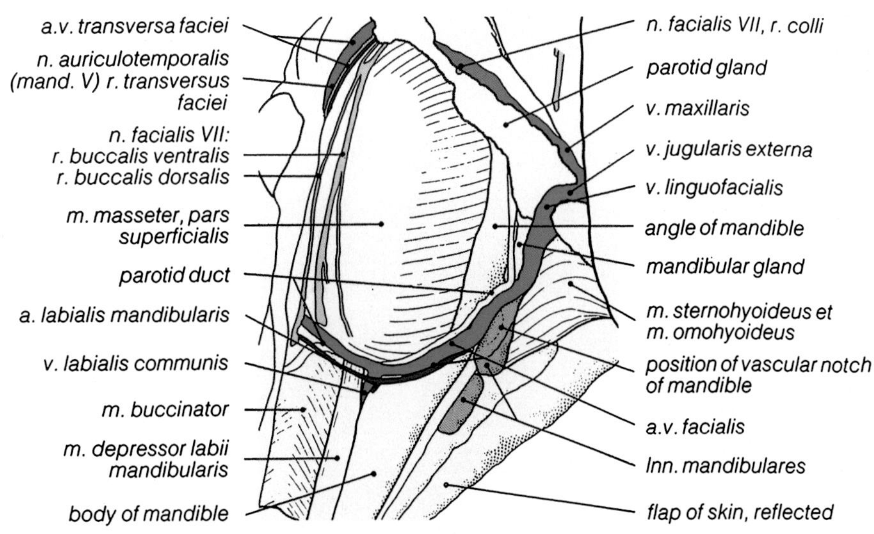
a.v. transversa faciei
n. auriculotemporalis (mand. V) r. transversus faciei
n. facialis VII:
r. buccalis ventralis
r. buccalis dorsalis
m. masseter, pars superficialis
parotid duct
a. labialis mandibularis
v. labialis communis
m. buccinator
m. depressor labii mandibularis
body of mandible
n. facialis VII, r. colli
parotid gland
v. maxillaris
v. jugularis externa
v. linguofacialis
angle of mandible
mandibular gland
m. sternohyoideus et m. omohyoideus
position of vascular notch of mandible
a.v. facialis
lnn. mandibulares
flap of skin, reflected

Fig. 1.11 Structures traversing the mandibular vascular notch: left ventrolateral view. This view, which is a part of the dissection shown in Fig. 1.7, shows the palpable structures at the ventral and caudal borders of the mandible. The vascular notch is a distinct groove in the ventral border of the mandible; shown in Fig. 1.23.

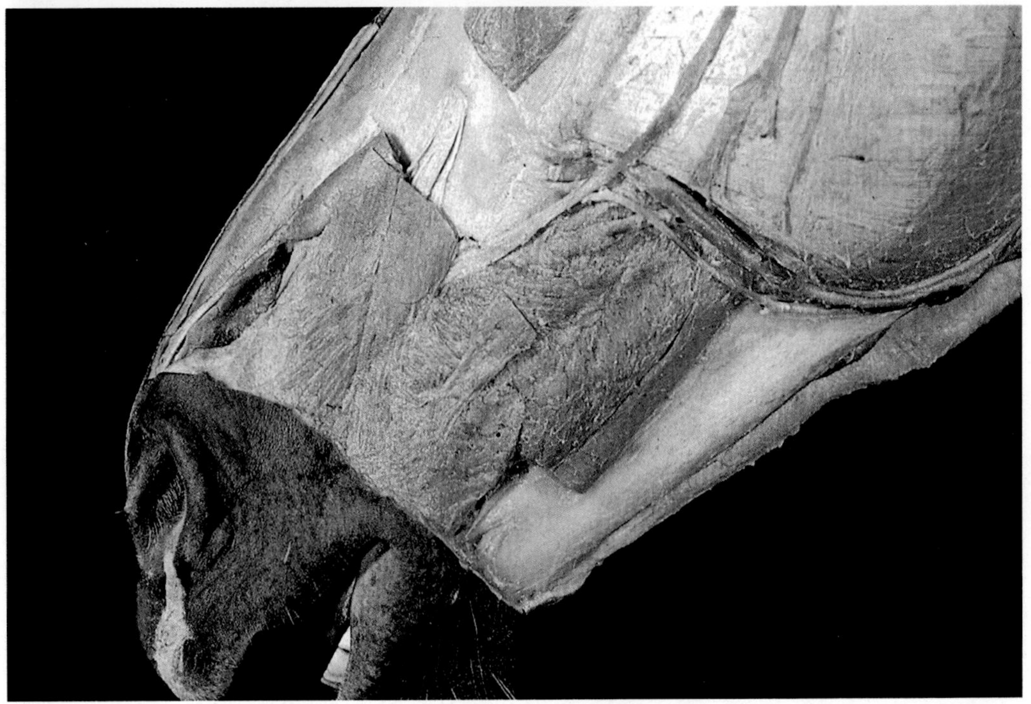

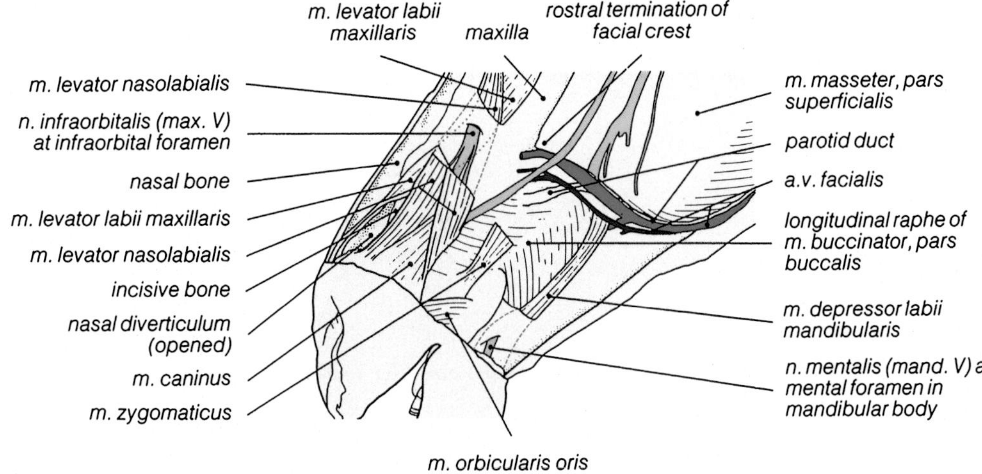
m. levator labii maxillaris
maxilla
rostral termination of facial crest
m. levator nasolabialis
n. infraorbitalis (max. V) at infraorbital foramen
nasal bone
m. levator labii maxillaris
m. levator nasolabialis
incisive bone
nasal diverticulum (opened)
m. caninus
m. zygomaticus
m. orbicularis oris
m. masseter, pars superficialis
parotid duct
a.v. facialis
longitudinal raphe of m. buccinator, pars buccalis
m. depressor labii mandibularis
n. mentalis (mand. V) at mental foramen in mandibular body

Fig. 1.12 The infraorbital and mental foramina and nerves: left lateral view. The overlying parts of the labial muscles (shown by dotted blue lines) have been resected to expose the foramina and reveal the relationships between muscles and foramina.

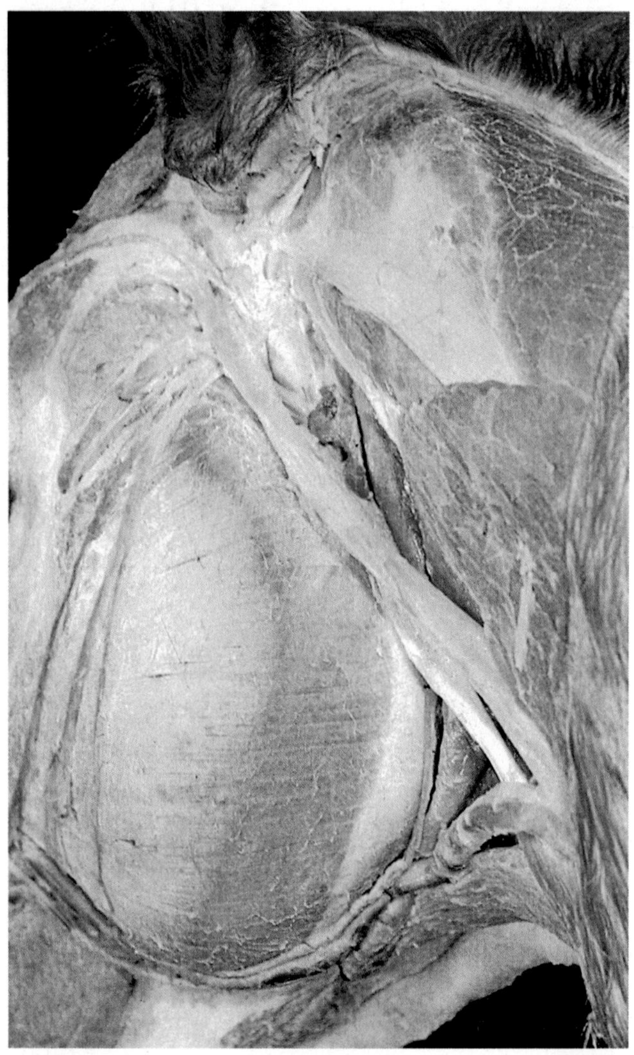

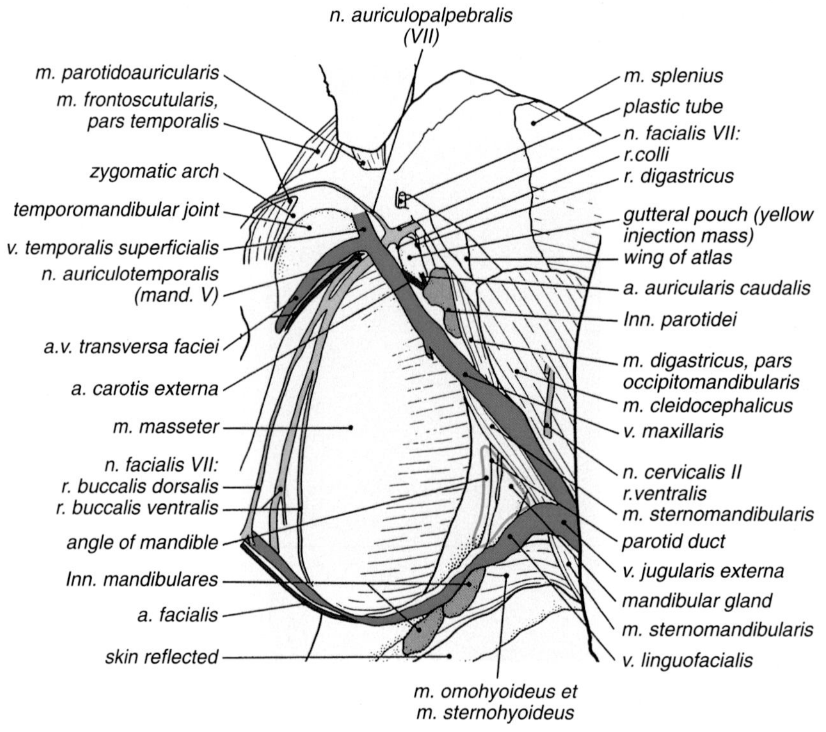
n. auriculopalpebralis (VII)
m. parotidoauricularis
m. frontoscutularis, pars temporalis
zygomatic arch
temporomandibular joint
v. temporalis superficialis
n. auriculotemporalis (mand. V)
a.v. transversa faciei
a. carotis externa
m. masseter
n. facialis VII:
r. buccalis dorsalis
r. buccalis ventralis
angle of mandible
lnn. mandibulares
a. facialis
skin reflected
m. omohyoideus et m. sternohyoideus
m. splenius
plastic tube
n. facialis VII:
r.colli
r. digastricus
gutteral pouch (yellow injection mass)
wing of atlas
a. auricularis caudalis
lnn. parotidei
m. digastricus, pars occipitomandibularis
m. cleidocephalicus
v. maxillaris
n. cervicalis II r.ventralis
m. sternomandibularis
parotid duct
v. jugularis externa
mandibular gland
m. sternomandibularis
v. linguofacialis

Fig. 1.13 The parotid region after removal of the parotid gland: left caudolateral view. The parotid duct has been pinned in place after removal of the gland. A plastic tube was inserted into the most dorsal part of the guttural pouch and a paste of yellow plaster was injected to fill the pouch and the auditory tube (see Fig. 1.7). The boundaries of the triangle of Viborg are shown in green.

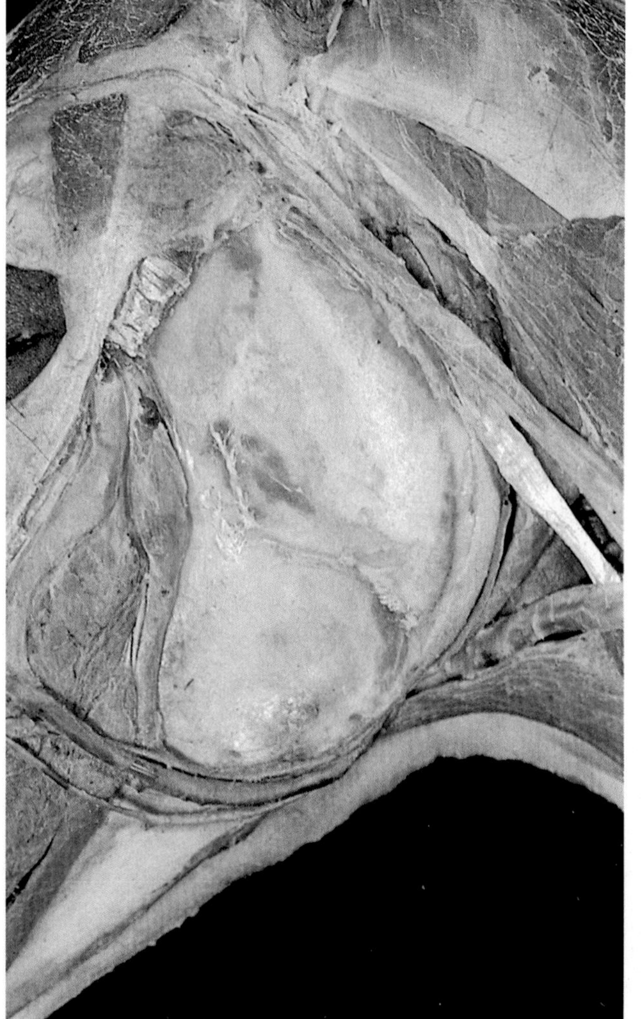

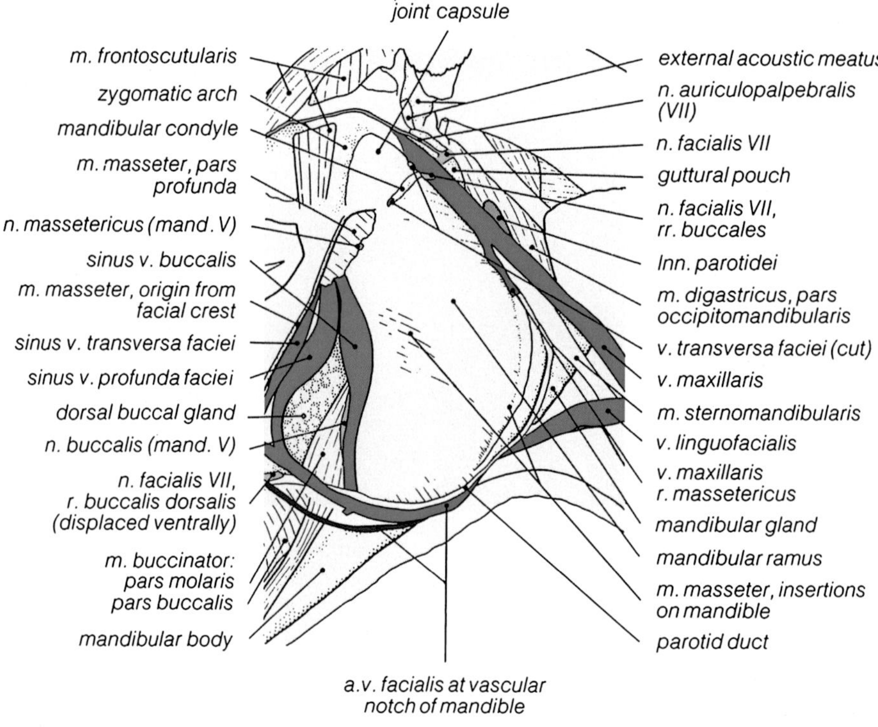
temporomandibular joint capsule
m. frontoscutularis
zygomatic arch
mandibular condyle
m. masseter, pars profunda
n. massetericus (mand. V)
sinus v. buccalis
m. masseter, origin from facial crest
sinus v. transversa faciei
sinus v. profunda faciei
dorsal buccal gland
n. buccalis (mand. V)
n. facialis VII, r. buccalis dorsalis (displaced ventrally)
m. buccinator: pars molaris pars buccalis
mandibular body
a.v. facialis at vascular notch of mandible
external acoustic meatus
n. auriculopalpebralis (VII)
n. facialis VII
guttural pouch
n. facialis VII, rr. buccales
lnn. parotidei
m. digastricus, pars occipitomandibularis
v. transversa faciei (cut)
v. maxillaris
m. sternomandibularis
v. linguofacialis
v. maxillaris r. massetericus
mandibular gland
mandibular ramus
m. masseter, insertions on mandible
parotid duct

Fig. 1.14 The mandible after removal of the masseter muscle: left lateral view. Most of the masseter muscle has been removed and the transverse facial vein has been transected to expose the condyle, ramus and body of the mandible. The veins of this region are shown injected with blue latex in Fig. 1.43.

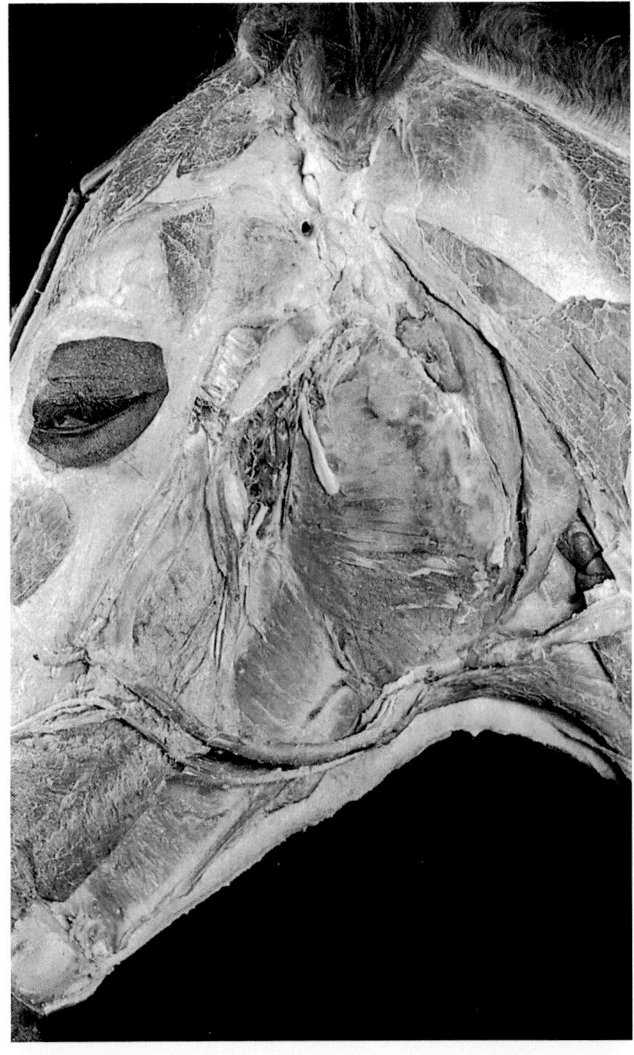

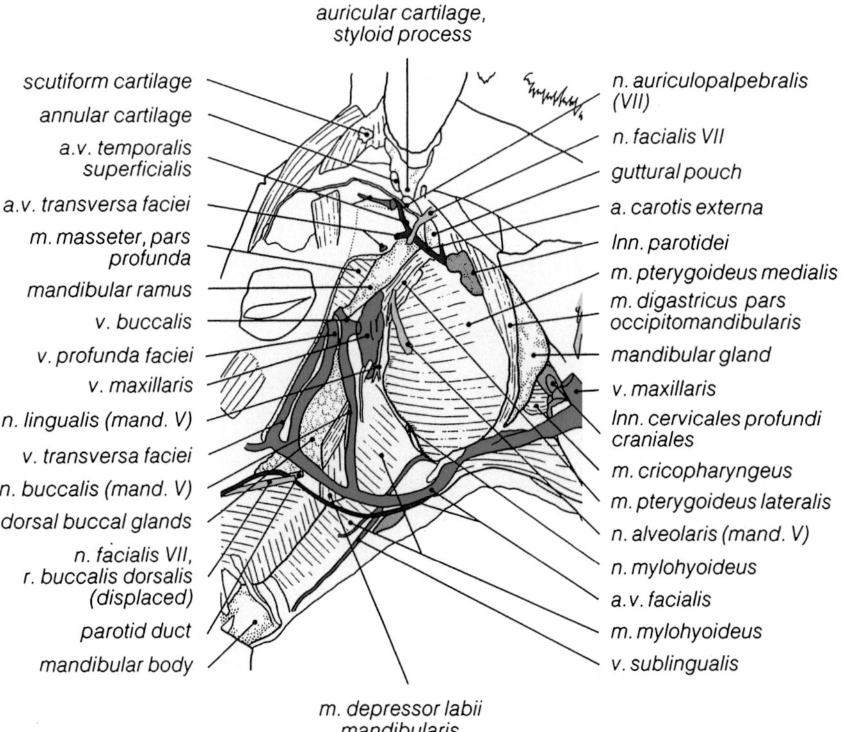
auricular cartilage,
styloid process
scutiform cartilage
annular cartilage
a.v. temporalis superficialis
a.v. transversa faciei
m. masseter, pars profunda
mandibular ramus
v. buccalis
v. profunda faciei
v. maxillaris
n. lingualis (mand. V)
v. transversa faciei
n. buccalis (mand. V)
dorsal buccal glands
n. facialis VII, r. buccalis dorsalis (displaced)
parotid duct
mandibular body
m. depressor labii mandibularis
n. auriculopalpebralis (VII)
n. facialis VII
guttural pouch
a. carotis externa
lnn. parotidei
m. pterygoideus medialis
m. digastricus pars occipitomandibularis
mandibular gland
v. maxillaris
lnn. cervicales profundi craniales
m. cricopharyngeus
m. pterygoideus lateralis
n. alveolaris (mand. V)
n. mylohyoideus
a.v. facialis
m. mylohyoideus
v. sublingualis

Fig. 1.15 Structures lying medial to the mandible: left lateral view. Removal of most of the left side of the mandible reveals the pterygoid muscles and associated structures. The mandibular alveolar nerve was cut at the mandibular foramen; the cut end, therefore, demonstrates the level of the foramen on the medial aspect of the mandible.

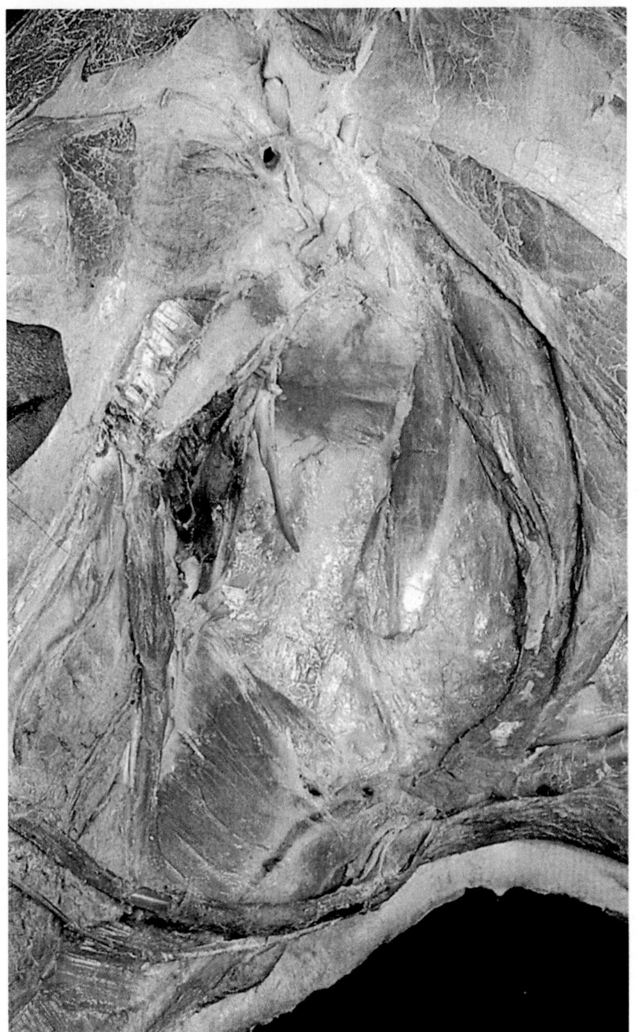

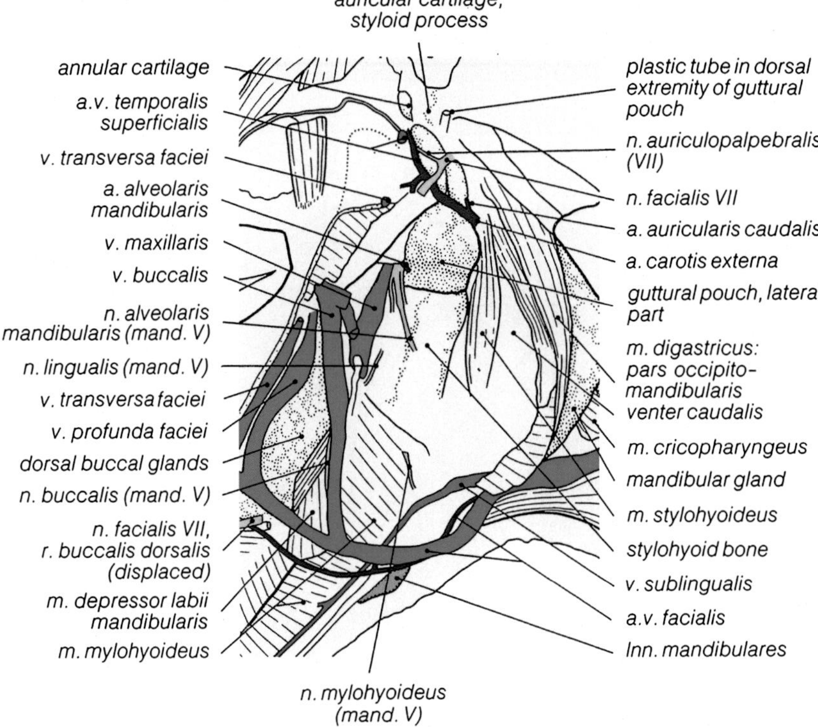
auricular cartilage,
styloid process
annular cartilage
a.v. temporalis superficialis
v. transversa faciei
a. alveolaris mandibularis
v. maxillaris
v. buccalis
n. alveolaris mandibularis (mand. V)
n. lingualis (mand. V)
v. transversa faciei
v. profunda faciei
dorsal buccal glands
n. buccalis (mand. V)
n. facialis VII, r. buccalis dorsalis (displaced)
m. depressor labii mandibularis
m. mylohyoideus
n. mylohyoideus (mand. V)
plastic tube in dorsal extremity of guttural pouch
n. auriculopalpebralis (VII)
n. facialis VII
a. auricularis caudalis
a. carotis externa
guttural pouch, lateral part
m. digastricus: pars occipito-mandibularis venter caudalis
m. cricopharyngeus
mandibular gland
m. stylohyoideus
stylohyoid bone
v. sublingualis
a.v. facialis
lnn. mandibulares

Fig. 1.16 Structures lying medial to the pterygoid muscles: left lateral view (1). The medial pterygoid muscle has been removed, but the pharyngeal fascia, which covers the stylohyoid bone and associated structures, has been preserved. The dissection of the structures lying in the pharyngeal fascia is shown in Figs. 1.17–1.21.

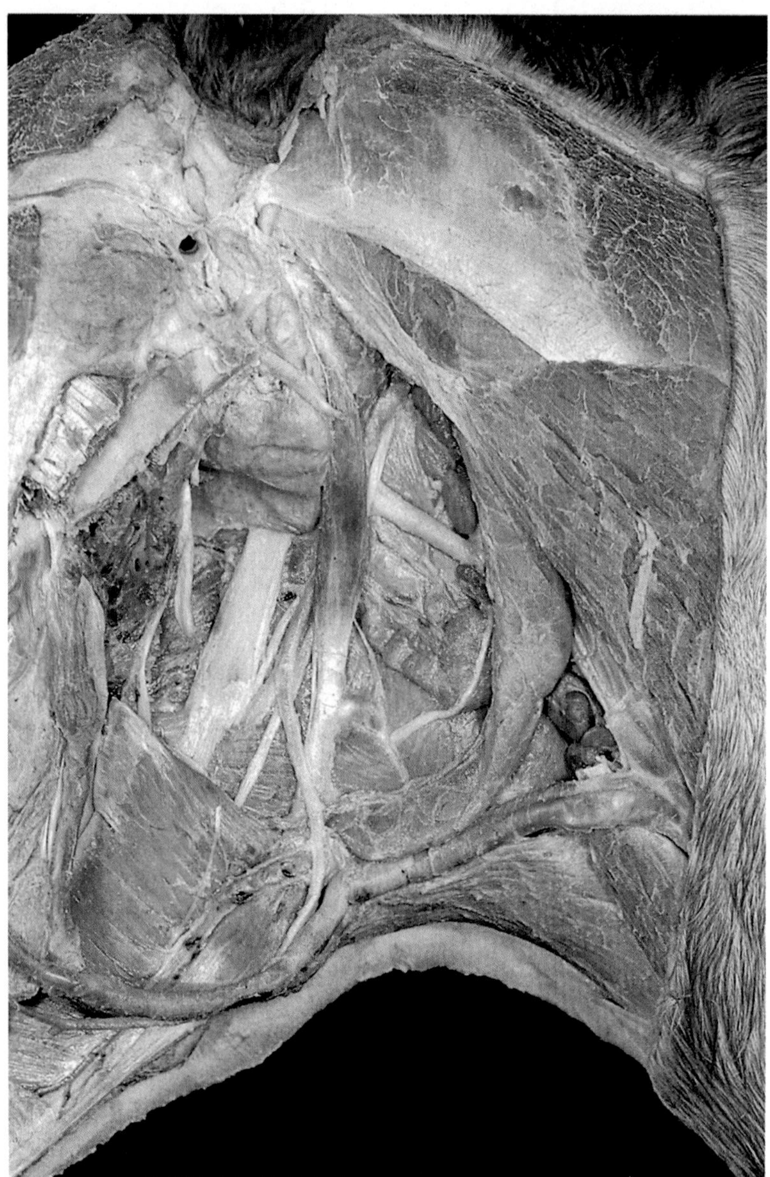

Fig. 1.17 Structures lying medial to the pterygoid muscles: left lateral view (2). Removal of the pharyngeal fascia and two parts of the digastricus muscle exposes the structures lying around the wall of the pharynx. This figure illustrates the general anatomy of bones, muscles, blood vessels and lymph nodes. Fig. 1.18 shows the nerves of the region.

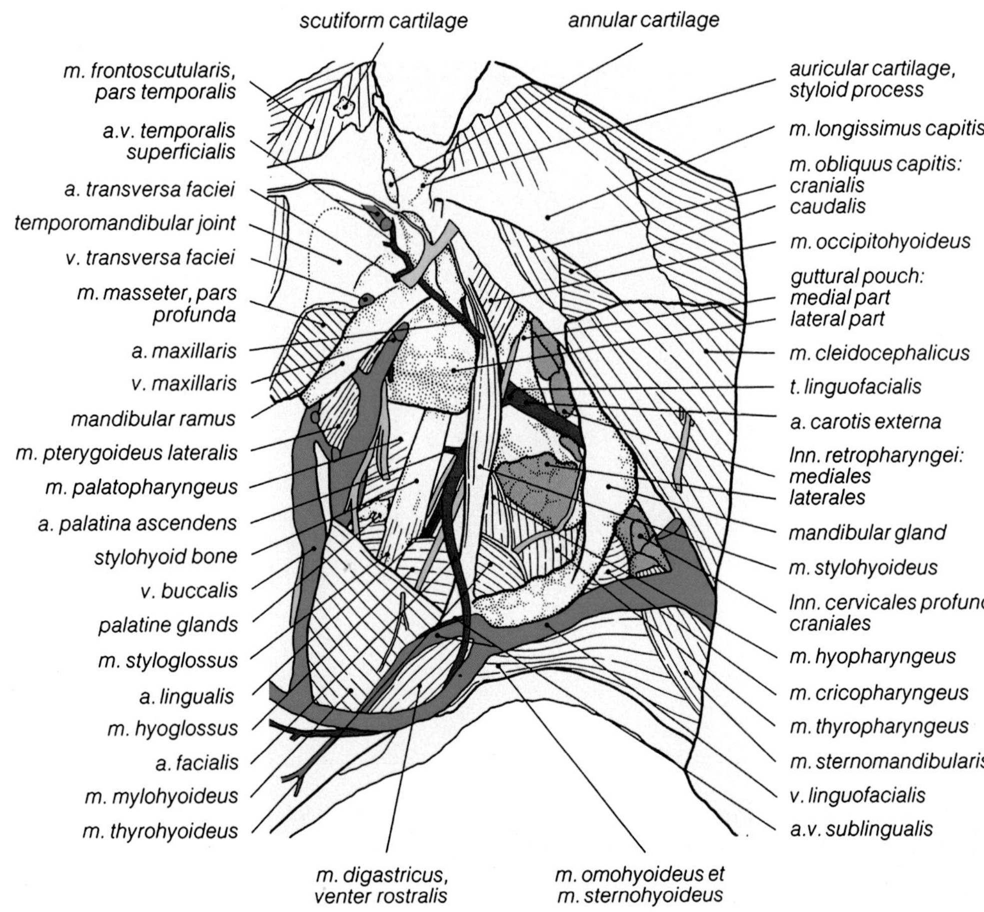
scutiform cartilage
annular cartilage
m. frontoscutularis, pars temporalis
a.v. temporalis superficialis
a. transversa faciei
temporomandibular joint
v. transversa faciei
m. masseter, pars profunda
a. maxillaris
v. maxillaris
mandibular ramus
m. pterygoideus lateralis
m. palatopharyngeus
a. palatina ascendens
stylohyoid bone
v. buccalis
palatine glands
m. styloglossus
a. lingualis
m. hyoglossus
a. facialis
m. mylohyoideus
m. thyrohyoideus
m. digastricus, venter rostralis
m. omohyoideus et m. sternohyoideus
auricular cartilage, styloid process
m. longissimus capitis
m. obliquus capitis: cranialis caudalis
m. occipitohyoideus
guttural pouch: medial part lateral part
m. cleidocephalicus
t. linguofacialis
a. carotis externa
lnn. retropharyngei: mediales laterales
mandibular gland
m. stylohyoideus
lnn. cervicales profundi craniales
m. hyopharyngeus
m. cricopharyngeus
m. thyropharyngeus
m. sternomandibularis
v. linguofacialis
a.v. sublingualis

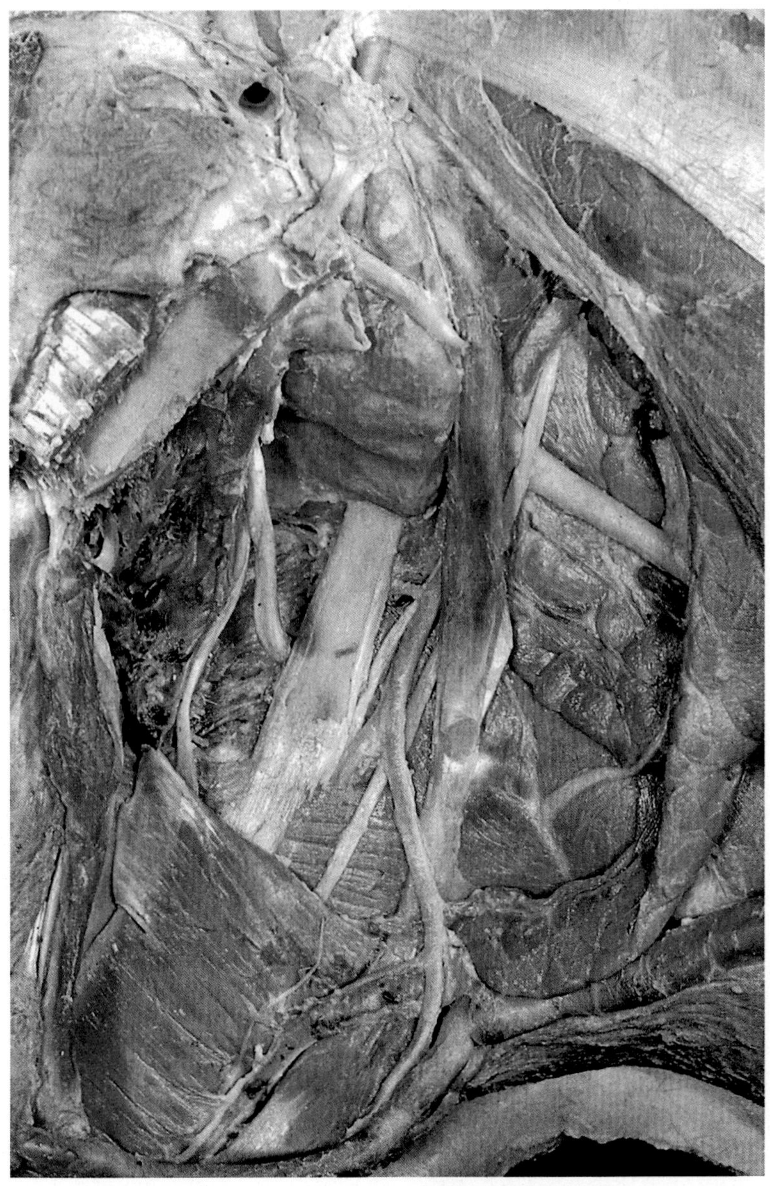

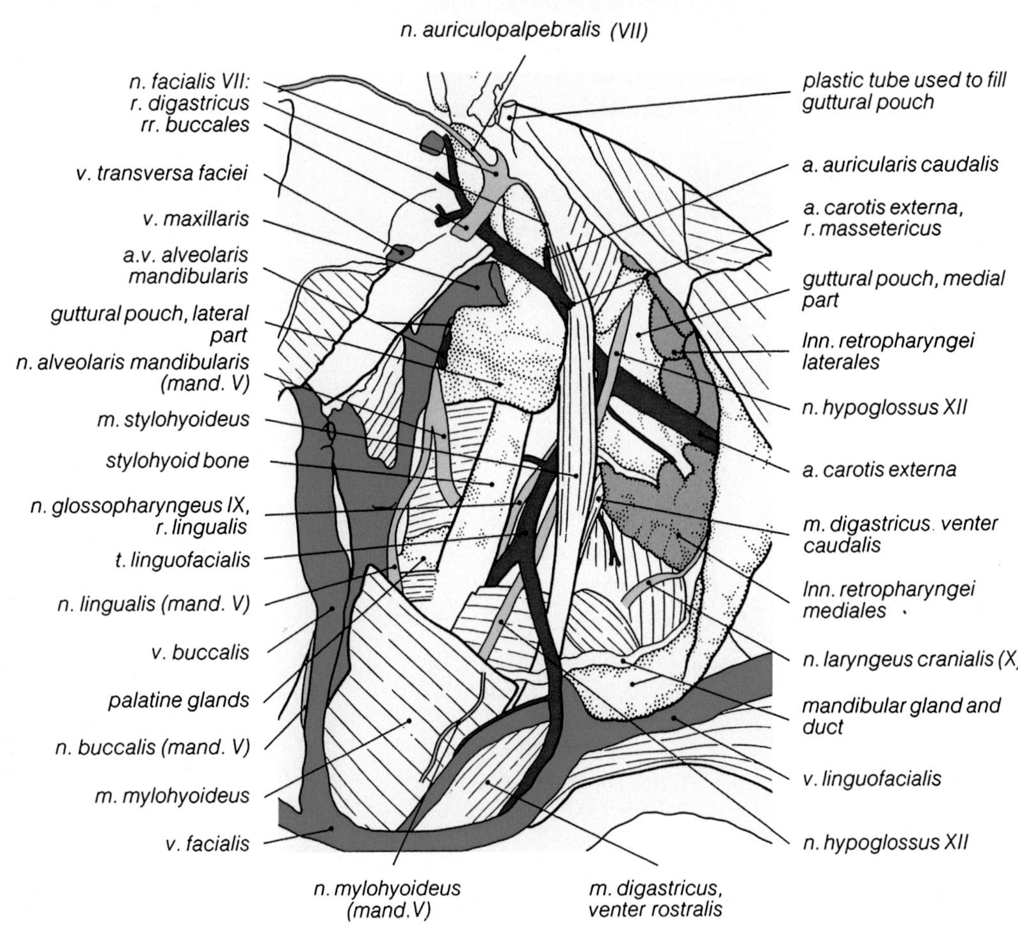

n. auriculopalpebralis (VII)
n. facialis VII:
r. digastricus
rr. buccales
v. transversa faciei
v. maxillaris
a.v. alveolaris mandibularis
guttural pouch, lateral part
n. alveolaris mandibularis (mand. V)
m. stylohyoideus
stylohyoid bone
n. glossopharyngeus IX, r. lingualis
t. linguofacialis
n. lingualis (mand. V)
v. buccalis
palatine glands
n. buccalis (mand. V)
m. mylohyoideus
v. facialis
n. mylohyoideus (mand.V)
m. digastricus, venter rostralis
plastic tube used to fill guttural pouch
a. auricularis caudalis
a. carotis externa, r. massetericus
guttural pouch, medial part
lnn. retropharyngei laterales
n. hypoglossus XII
a. carotis externa
m. digastricus. venter caudalis
lnn. retropharyngei mediales
n. laryngeus cranialis (X)
mandibular gland and duct
v. linguofacialis
n. hypoglossus XII

Fig. 1.18 Structures lying medial to the pterygoid muscles: left lateral view (3). This is a closer view of the dissection in Fig. 1.17 to show the nerves of the region. Further details are shown in Figs. 1.20, 1.21 and 1.25–1.27.

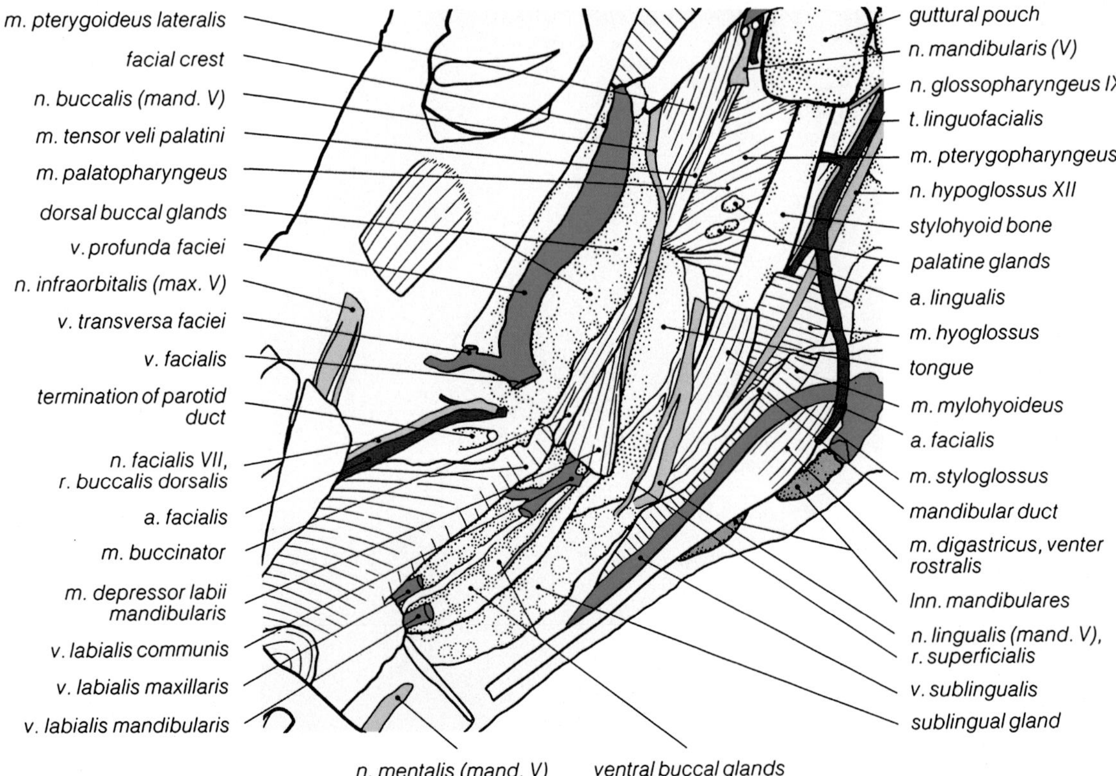
m. pterygoideus lateralis
facial crest
n. buccalis (mand. V)
m. tensor veli palatini
m. palatopharyngeus
dorsal buccal glands
v. profunda faciei
n. infraorbitalis (max. V)
v. transversa faciei
v. facialis
termination of parotid duct
n. facialis VII, r. buccalis dorsalis
a. facialis
m. buccinator
m. depressor labii mandibularis
v. labialis communis
v. labialis maxillaris
v. labialis mandibularis
n. mentalis (mand. V)
ventral buccal glands
guttural pouch
n. mandibularis (V)
n. glossopharyngeus IX
t. linguofacialis
m. pterygopharyngeus
n. hypoglossus XII
stylohyoid bone
palatine glands
a. lingualis
m. hyoglossus
tongue
m. mylohyoideus
a. facialis
m. styloglossus
mandibular duct
m. digastricus, venter rostralis
lnn. mandibulares
n. lingualis (mand. V), r. superficialis
v. sublingualis
sublingual gland

Fig. 1.19 The buccal wall: left lateral view. The mylohyoid and buccinator muscles have been partially resected.

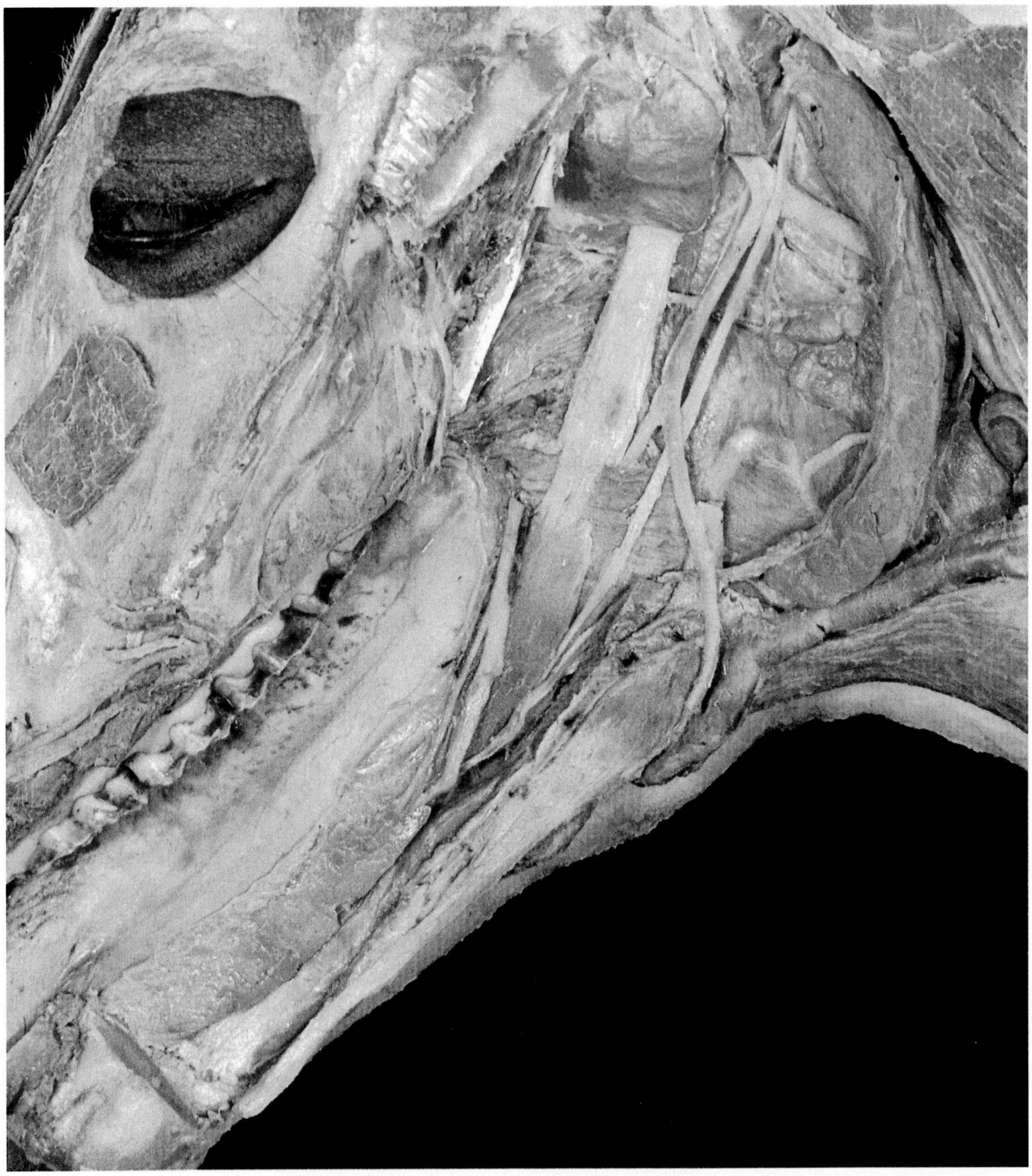

Fig. 1.20 The mandibular and sublingual glands: left lateral view. The buccal wall has been removed, exposing the labial surface of the tongue and the maxillary cheek teeth. The mandibular gland has been displaced slightly rostrally, to display the vessels and nerves lying caudal to it.

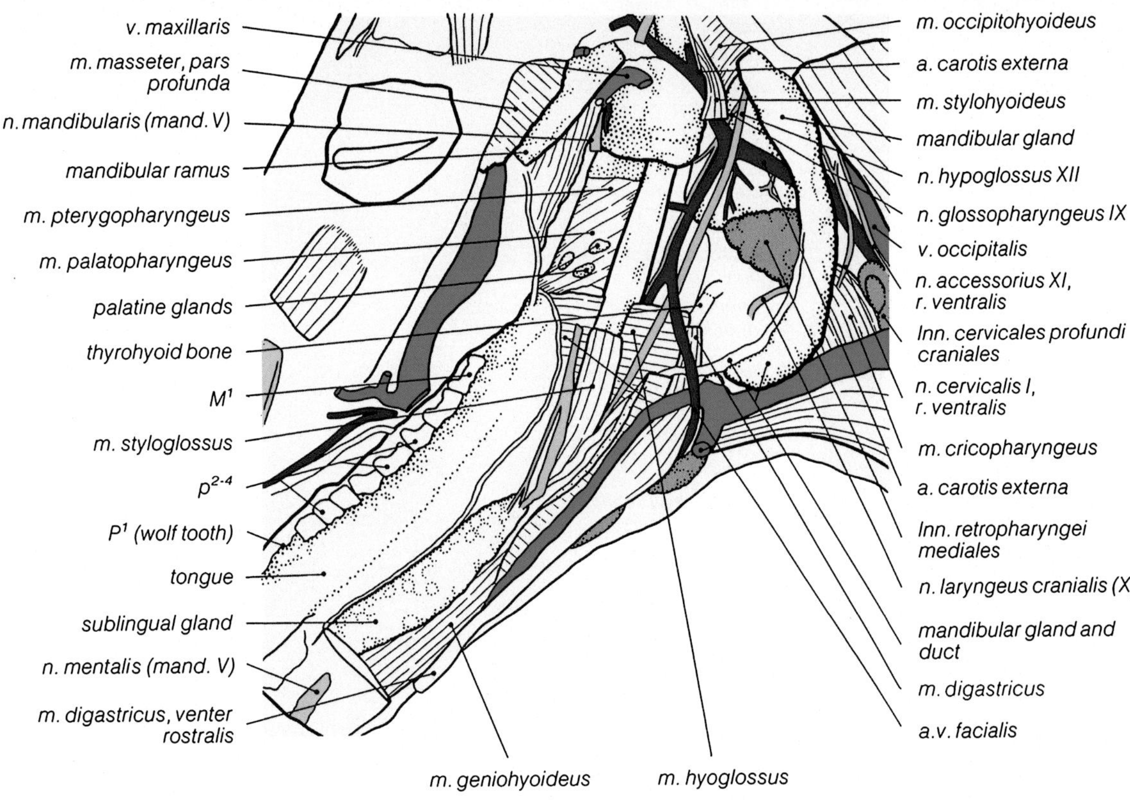
v. maxillaris
m. masseter, pars profunda
n. mandibularis (mand. V)
mandibular ramus
m. pterygopharyngeus
m. palatopharyngeus
palatine glands
thyrohyoid bone
M¹
m. styloglossus
P²⁻⁴
P¹ (wolf tooth)
tongue
sublingual gland
n. mentalis (mand. V)
m. digastricus, venter rostralis
m. geniohyoideus
m. hyoglossus
m. occipitohyoideus
a. carotis externa
m. stylohyoideus
mandibular gland
n. hypoglossus XII
n. glossopharyngeus IX
v. occipitalis
n. accessorius XI, r. ventralis
lnn. cervicales profundi craniales
n. cervicalis I, r. ventralis
m. cricopharyngeus
a. carotis externa
lnn. retropharyngei mediales
n. laryngeus cranialis (X)
mandibular gland and duct
m. digastricus
a.v. facialis

Fig. 1.21 Structures lying medial to the mandibular gland: left lateral view. The mandibular gland has been displaced ventrally to reveal the vessels, lymph nodes and nerves. Further details of the structures lying caudal to the guttural pouch are shown in Fig. 1.26.

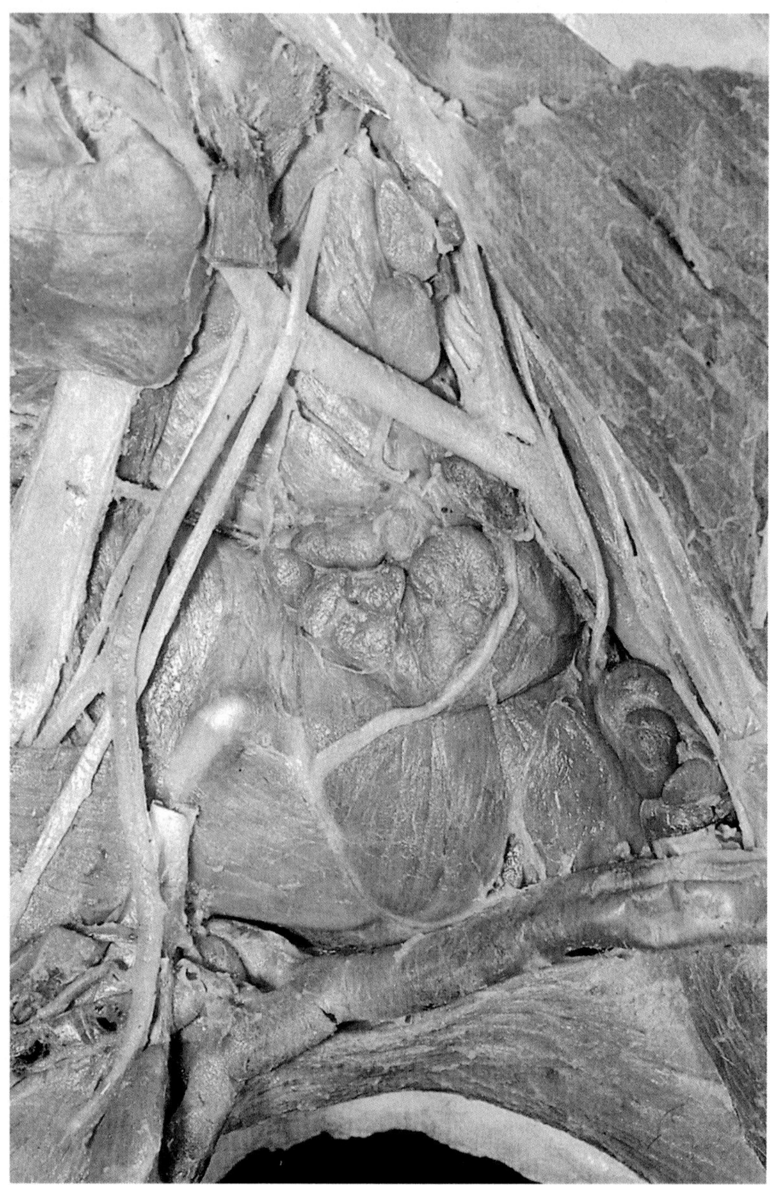

m. occipitohyoideus
m. longissimus capitis

a. auricularis caudalis
v. maxillaris
a. carotis externa
r. massetericus
m. stylohyoideus
n. hypoglossus XII
guttural pouch:
lateral part
medial part
n. glossopharyngeus IX:
r. pharyngeus
r. lingualis
stylohyoid bone
m. stylopharyngeus
a. palatina ascendens
t. linguofacialis
a. lingualis
thyroid cartilage,
cranial cornu
thyrohyoid bone
a. facialis
m. stylohyoideus
m. mylohyoideus
a.v. sublingualis
mandibular duct
lnn. mandibulares

m. obliquus capitis:
cranialis
caudalis
lnn. retropharyngei
laterales
a. carotis interna
n. laryngeus cranialis (X)
n. cervicalis I,
r. ventralis
n. accessorius XI,
r. ventralis
a.v. occipitalis
n. glossopharyngeus IX
r. sinus carotici
a. carotis externa
r. glandularis
n. vagus X, r. pharyngeus
a. carotis communis
n. laryngeus cranialis (X)
v. maxillaris
lnn. cervicales profundi
craniales
m. sternomandibularis
lnn. retropharyngei
mediales
m. cricopharyngeus
m. hyopharyngeus
m. thyropharyngeus

mandibular
gland (reflected)
v. linguofacialis
m. omohyoideus et
m. sternohyoideus

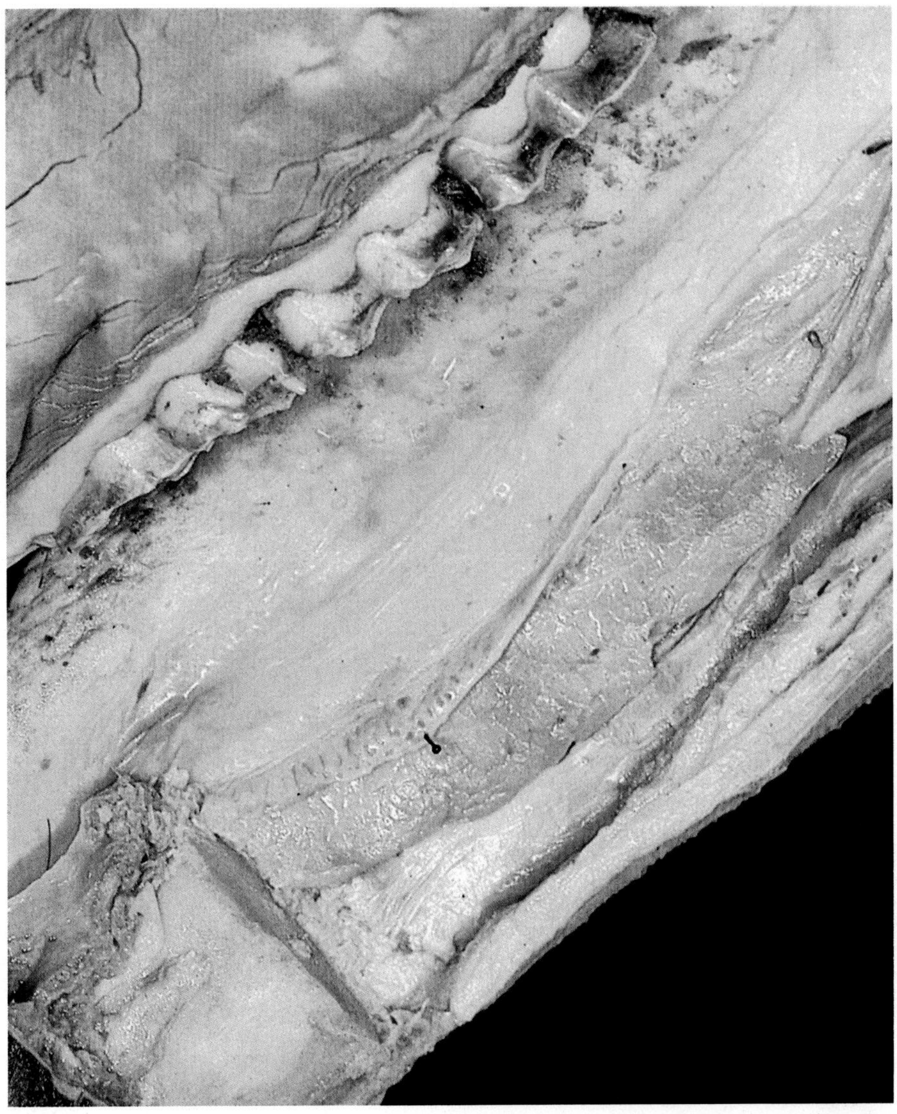

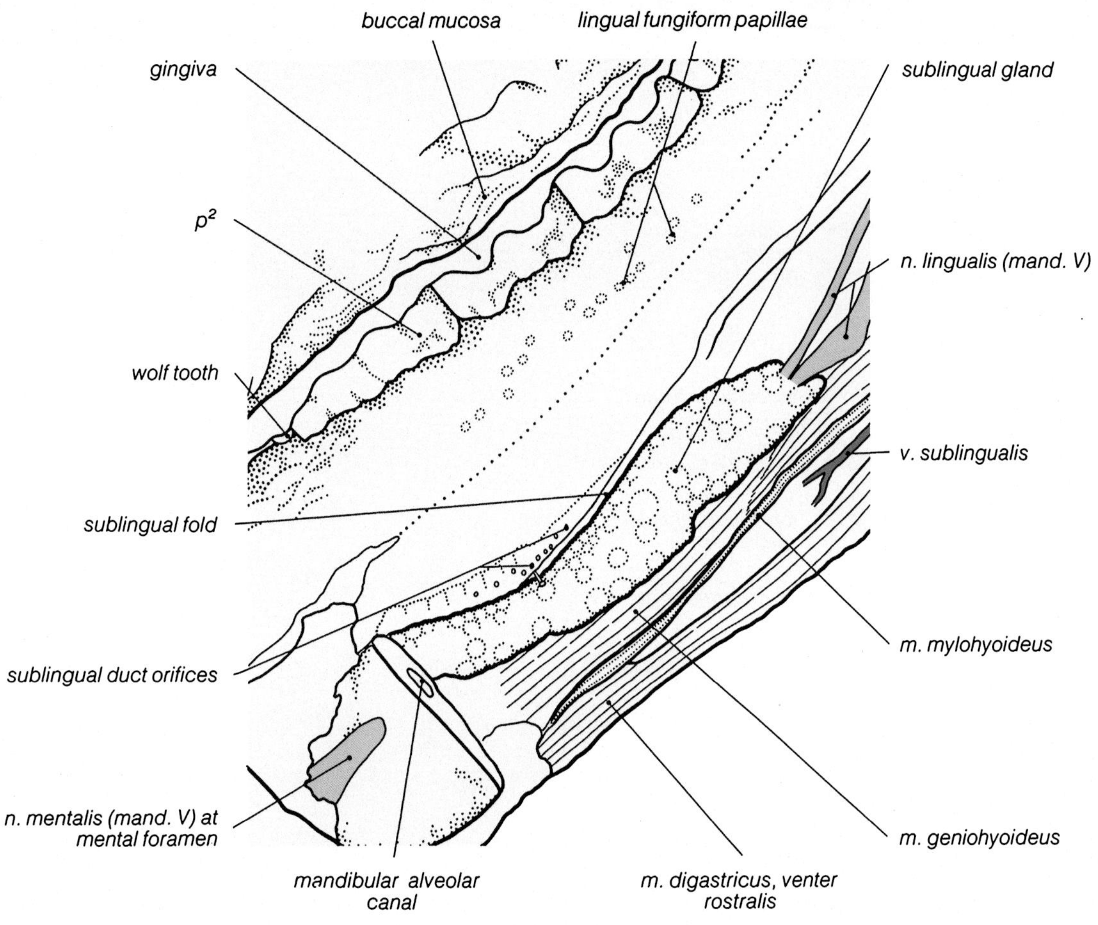
buccal mucosa
lingual fungiform papillae
gingiva
sublingual gland
p^2
n. lingualis (mand. V)
wolf tooth
v. sublingualis
sublingual fold
m. mylohyoideus
sublingual duct orifices
n. mentalis (mand. V) at mental foramen
m. geniohyoideus
mandibular alveolar canal
m. digastricus, venter rostralis

Fig. 1.22 The sublingual gland and maxillary cheek teeth: left lateral view. The sublingual fold and the buccal wall have been pinned back. For details of the dentition of this young horse, see Fig. 1.24.

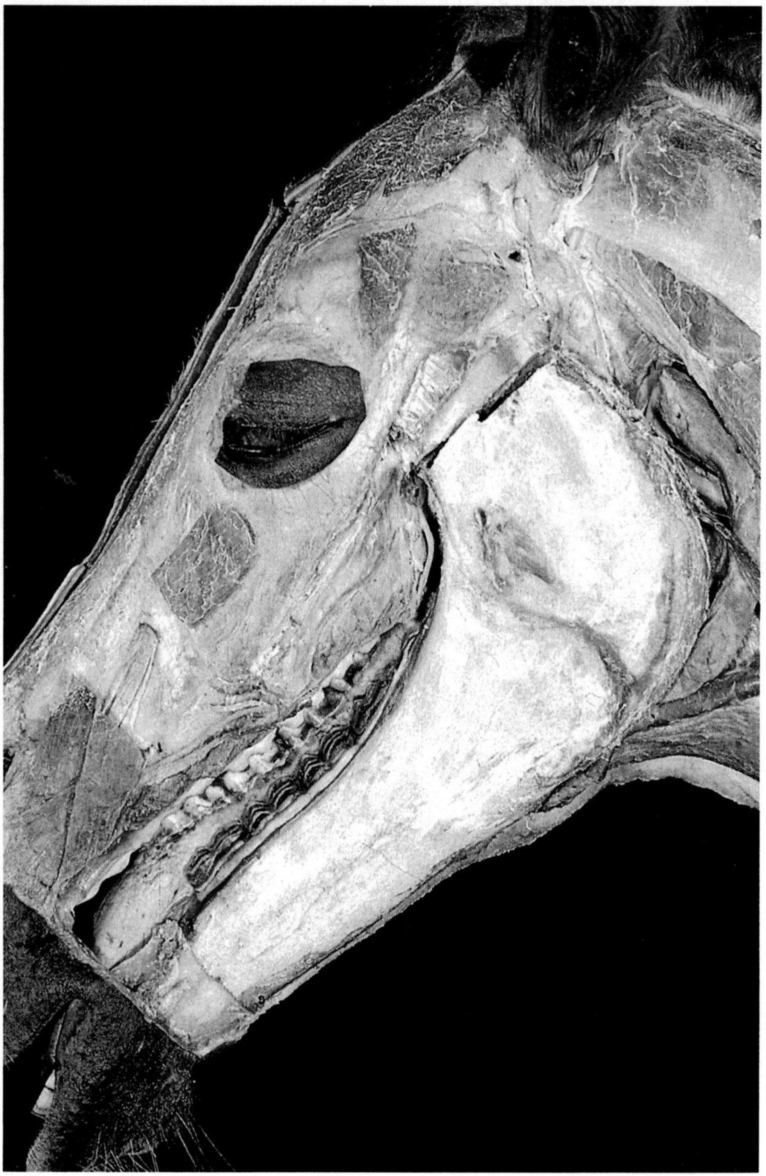

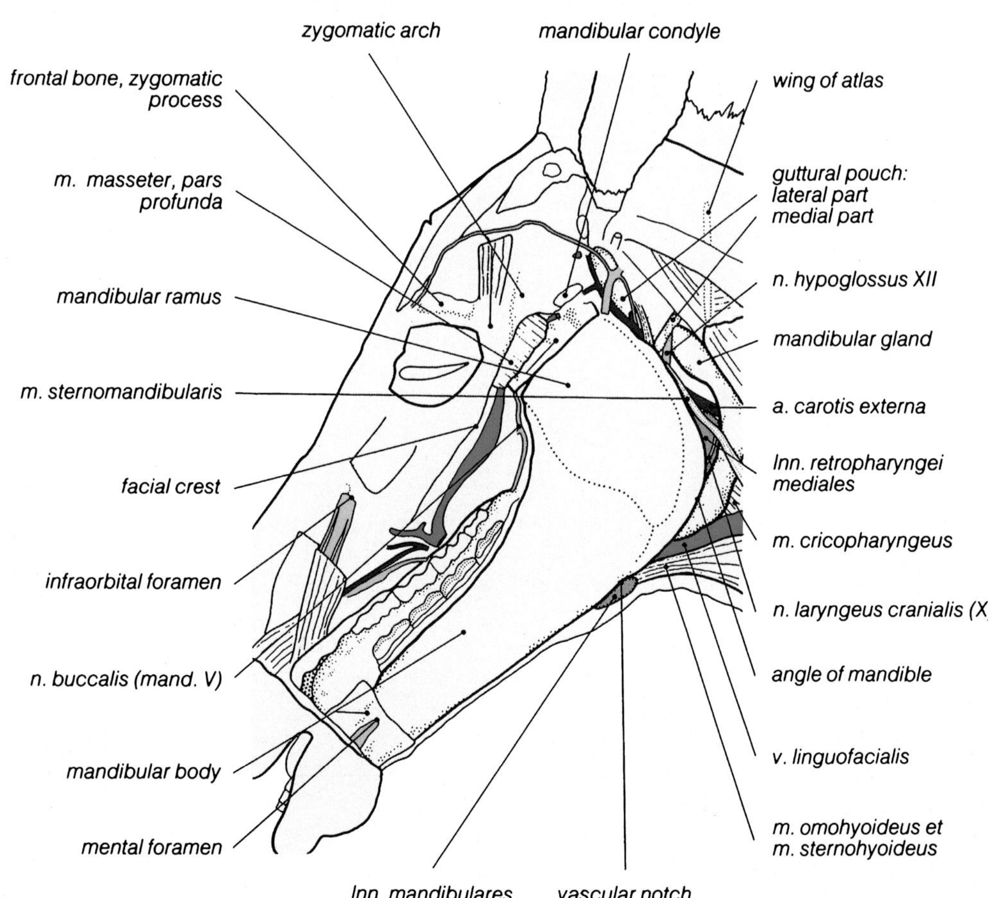
zygomatic arch
mandibular condyle
frontal bone, zygomatic process
wing of atlas
m. masseter, pars profunda
guttural pouch:
lateral part
medial part
n. hypoglossus XII
mandibular ramus
mandibular gland
m. sternomandibularis
a. carotis externa
facial crest
lnn. retropharyngei mediales
m. cricopharyngeus
infraorbital foramen
n. laryngeus cranialis (X)
n. buccalis (mand. V)
angle of mandible
mandibular body
v. linguofacialis
mental foramen
m. omohyoideus et m. sternohyoideus
lnn. mandibulares
vascular notch

Fig. 1.23 The mandible and its relationships: left lateral view. After dissecting the deeper structures (Fig. 1.20) the mandible has been replaced to show its relationships to those structures and to the adjacent landmarks. The relationships to surface and superficial features are shown in Figs. 1.4 and 1.7.

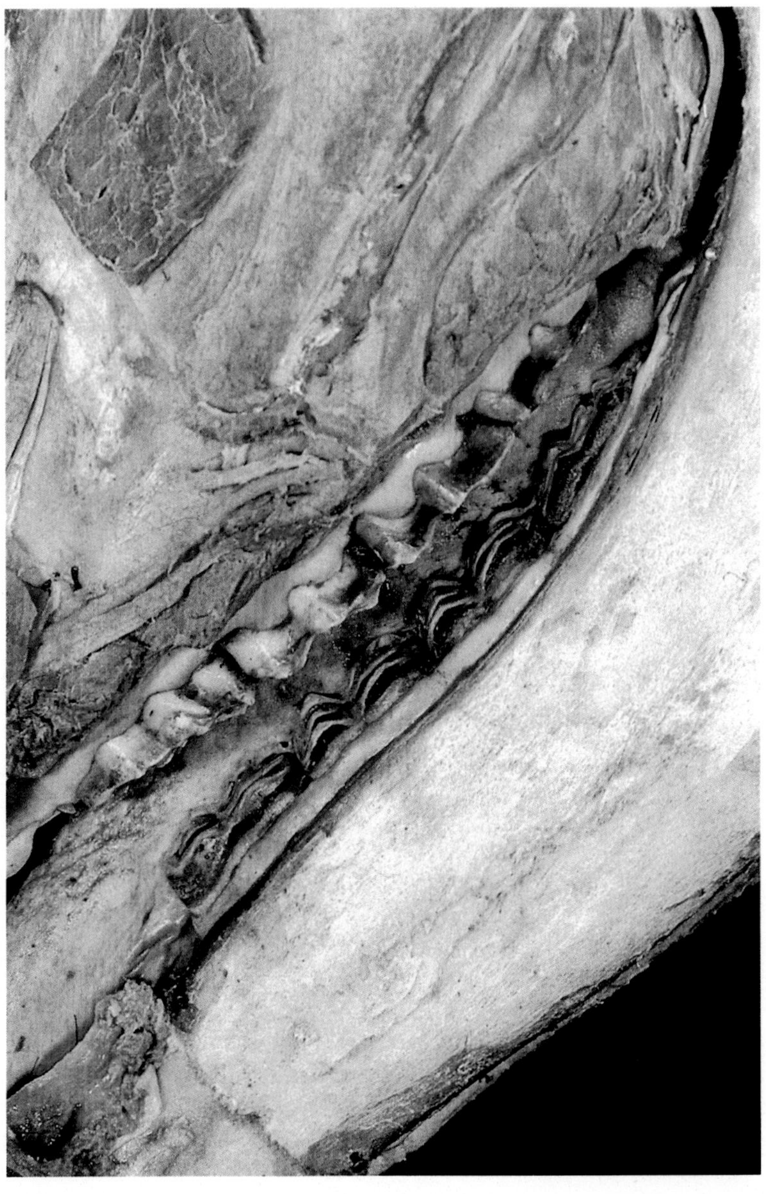

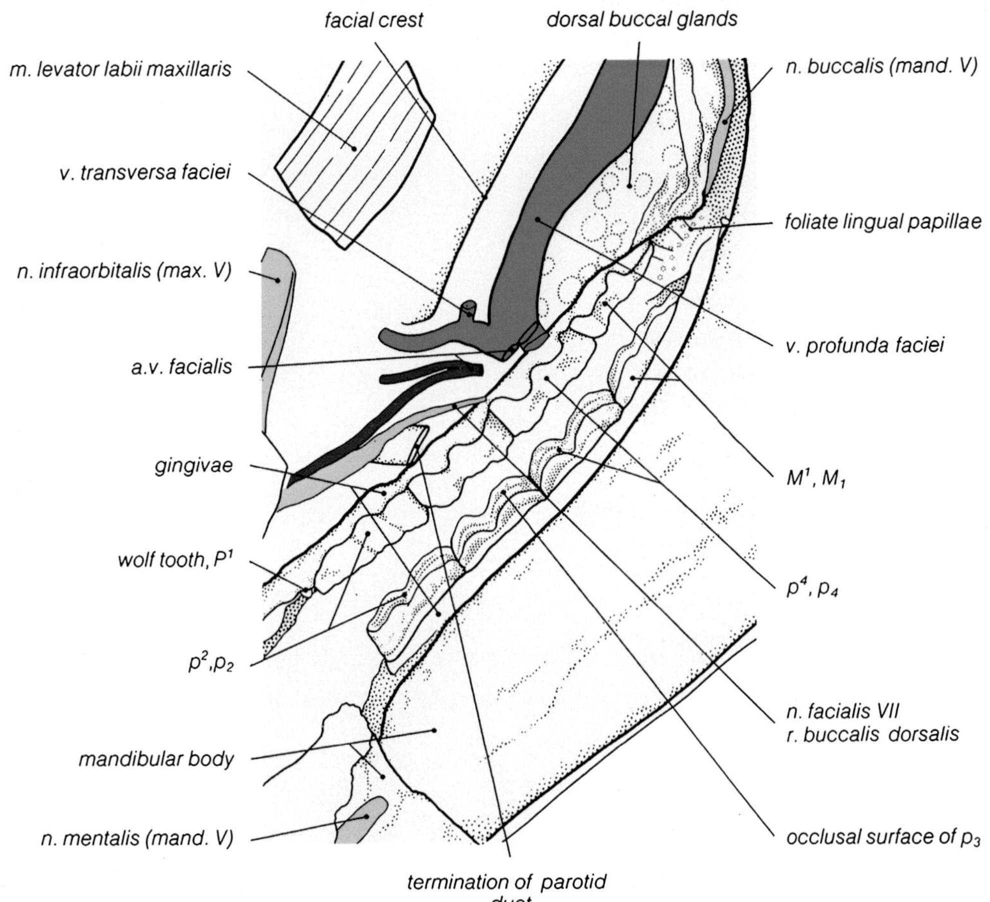
facial crest
dorsal buccal glands
m. levator labii maxillaris
n. buccalis (mand. V)
v. transversa faciei
foliate lingual papillae
n. infraorbitalis (max. V)
v. profunda faciei
a.v. facialis
gingivae
M^1, M_1
wolf tooth, P^1
p^4, p_4
p^2,p_2
n. facialis VII
r. buccalis dorsalis
mandibular body
n. mentalis (mand. V)
occlusal surface of p_3
termination of parotid
duct

Fig. 1.24 The maxillary and mandibular cheek teeth: left lateral view. This is a closer view of part of Fig. 1.23. The first premolar tooth erupts at about 6 months and the first molar tooth at about 12 months. The second premolars will be replaced at about 2½ years of age. Note that the parotid duct opens opposite the rostral (mesial) border of the third premolar in this individual.

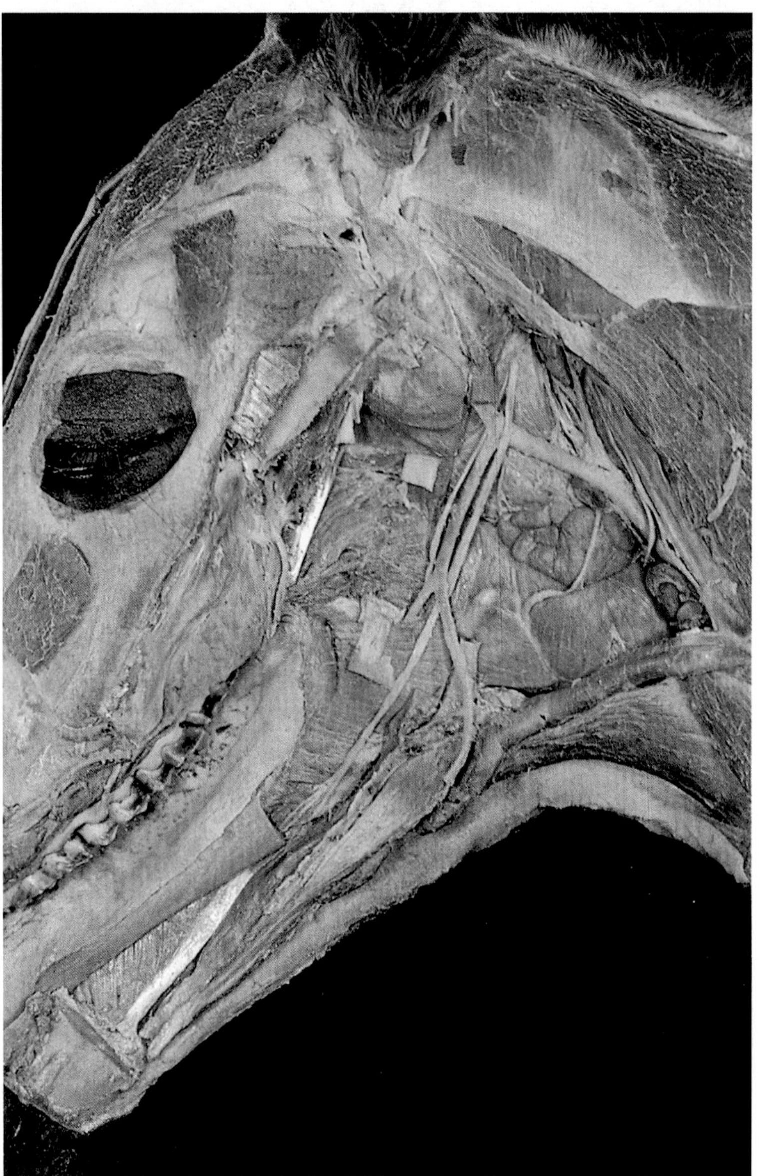

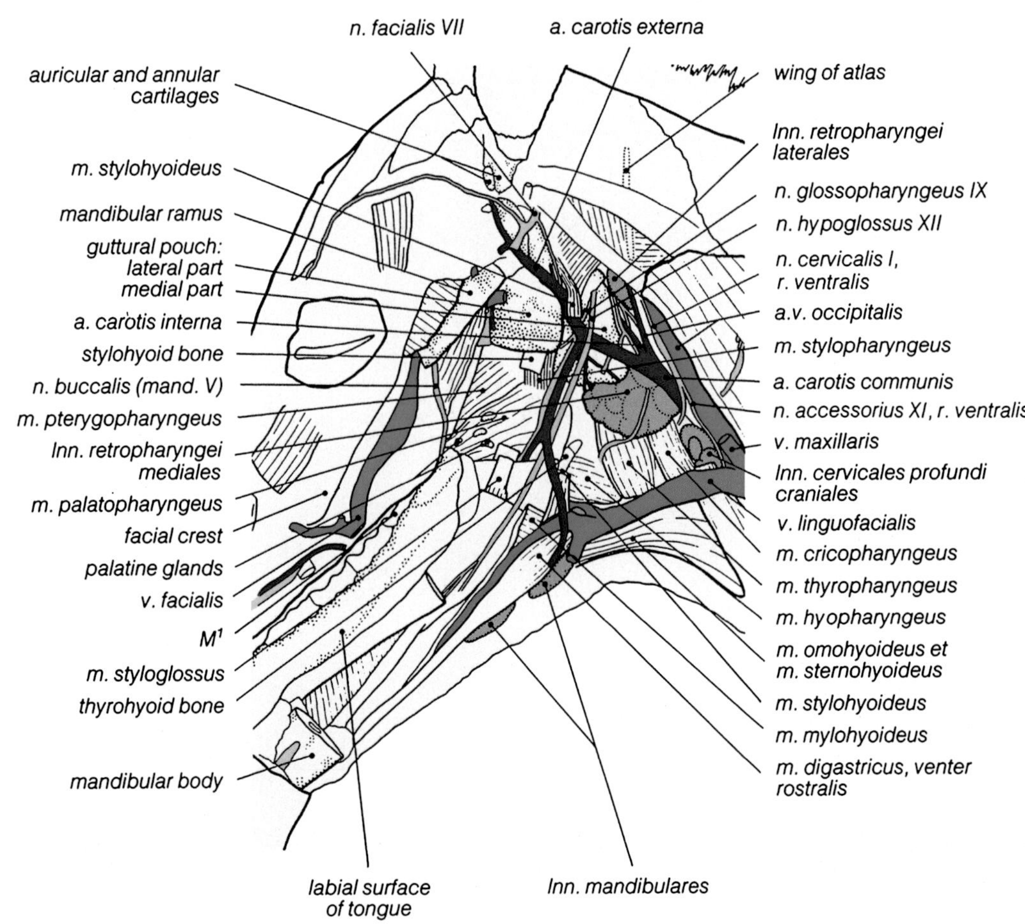
n. facialis VII
a. carotis externa
auricular and annular cartilages
m. stylohyoideus
mandibular ramus
guttural pouch:
lateral part
medial part
a. carotis interna
stylohyoid bone
n. buccalis (mand. V)
m. pterygopharyngeus
lnn. retropharyngei mediales
m. palatopharyngeus
facial crest
palatine glands
v. facialis
M¹
m. styloglossus
thyrohyoid bone
mandibular body
labial surface of tongue
lnn. mandibulares
wing of atlas
lnn. retropharyngei laterales
n. glossopharyngeus IX
n. hypoglossus XII
n. cervicalis I, r. ventralis
a.v. occipitalis
m. stylopharyngeus
a. carotis communis
n. accessorius XI, r. ventralis
v. maxillaris
lnn. cervicales profundi craniales
v. linguofacialis
m. cricopharyngeus
m. thyropharyngeus
m. hyopharyngeus
m. omohyoideus et m. sternohyoideus
m. stylohyoideus
m. mylohyoideus
m. digastricus, venter rostralis

Fig. 1.25 Relationships of the pharynx: left lateral view. The middle part of the stylohyoid bone, the mandibular and sublingual glands and parts of the lateral retropharyngeal lymph nodes have been removed. Further details of this dissection are shown in Figs. 1.26–1.28.

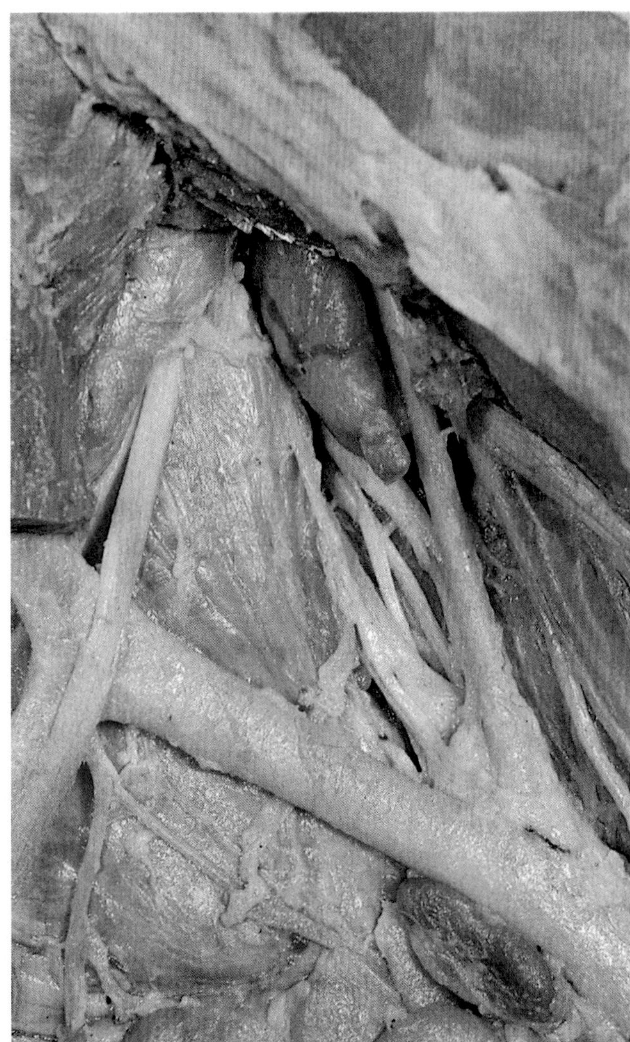

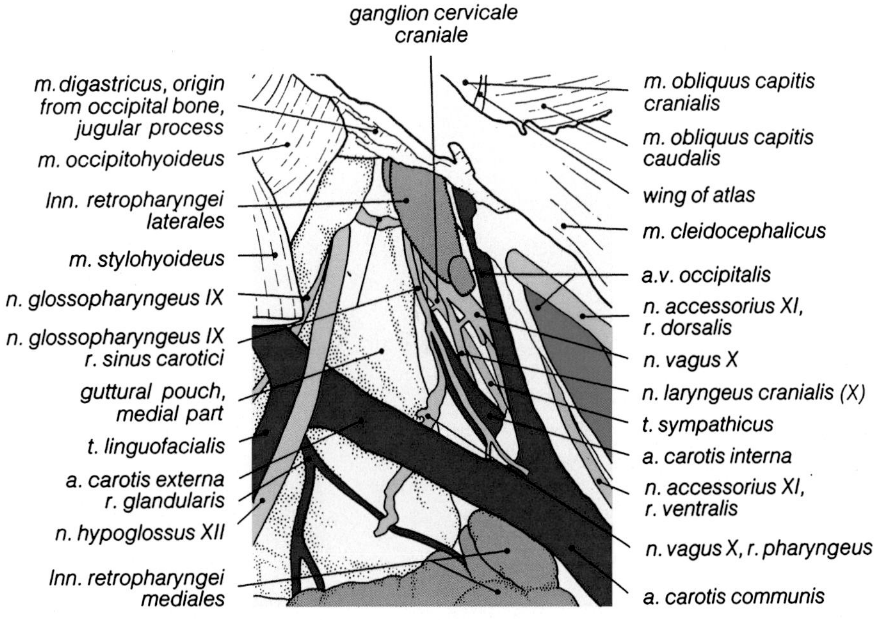
ganglion cervicale craniale
m. digastricus, origin from occipital bone, jugular process
m. occipitohyoideus
lnn. retropharyngei laterales
m. stylohyoideus
n. glossopharyngeus IX
n. glossopharyngeus IX r. sinus carotici
guttural pouch, medial part
t. linguofacialis
a. carotis externa r. glandularis
n. hypoglossus XII
lnn. retropharyngei mediales
m. obliquus capitis cranialis
m. obliquus capitis caudalis
wing of atlas
m. cleidocephalicus
a.v. occipitalis
n. accessorius XI, r. dorsalis
n. vagus X
n. laryngeus cranialis (X)
t. sympathicus
a. carotis interna
n. accessorius XI, r. ventralis
n. vagus X, r. pharyngeus
a. carotis communis

Fig. 1.26 Structures lying caudal to the guttural pouch: left lateral view. This is a closer view of a part of the specimen shown in Fig. 1.25. The vessels and nerves have been slightly separated from each other; this has disturbed the normal relationships of the structures (compare with Fig. 1.21).

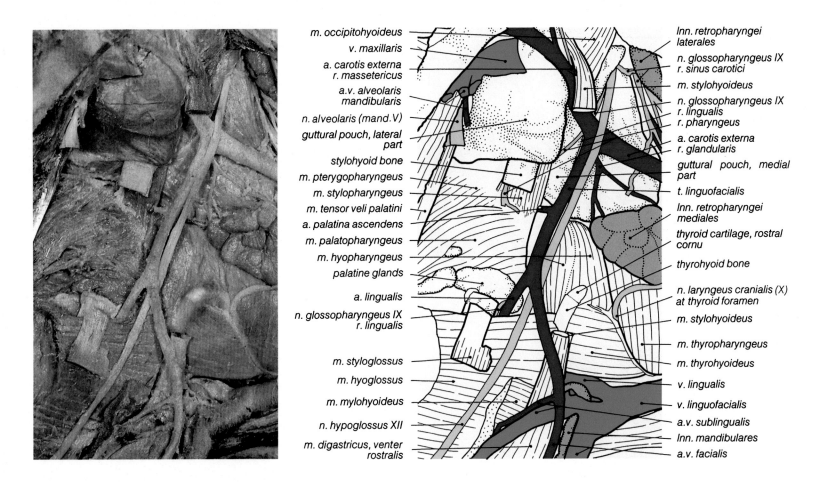

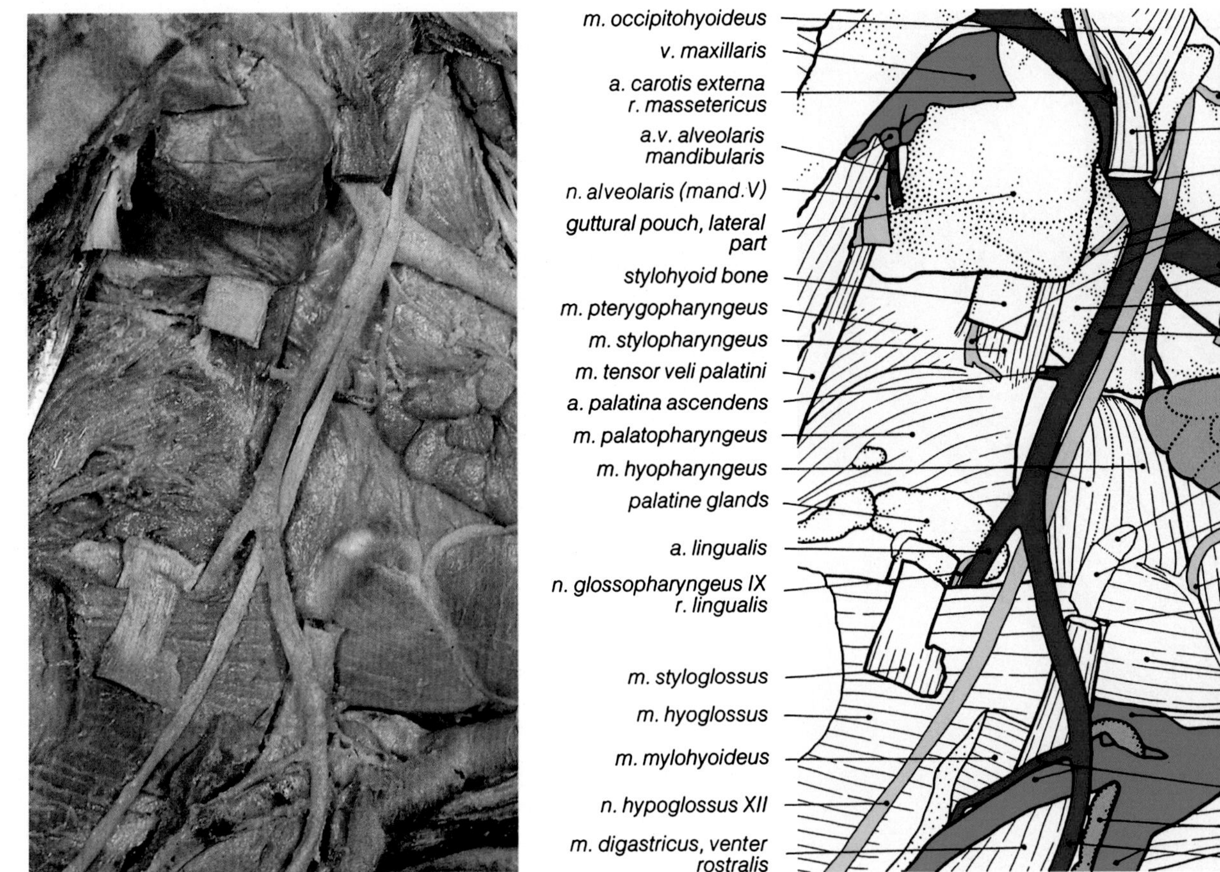
m. occipitohyoideus
v. maxillaris
a. carotis externa r. massetericus
a.v. alveolaris mandibularis
n. alveolaris (mand. V)
guttural pouch, lateral part
stylohyoid bone
m. pterygopharyngeus
m. stylopharyngeus
m. tensor veli palatini
a. palatina ascendens
m. palatopharyngeus
m. hyopharyngeus
palatine glands
a. lingualis
n. glossopharyngeus IX r. lingualis
m. styloglossus
m. hyoglossus
m. mylohyoideus
n. hypoglossus XII
m. digastricus, venter rostralis
lnn. retropharyngei laterales
n. glossopharyngeus IX r. sinus carotici
m. stylohyoideus
n. glossopharyngeus IX r. lingualis r. pharyngeus
a. carotis externa r. glandularis
guttural pouch, medial part
t. linguofacialis
lnn. retropharyngei mediales
thyroid cartilage, rostral cornu
thyrohyoid bone
n. laryngeus cranialis (X) at thyroid foramen
m. stylohyoideus
m. thyropharyngeus
m. thyrohyoideus
v. lingualis
v. linguofacialis
a.v. sublingualis
lnn. mandibulares
a.v. facialis

Fig. 1.27 The pharyngeal wall and guttural pouch: left lateral view. This is a closer view of a part of the specimen shown in Fig. 1.25. Fig. 1.26 shows further details of the caudodorsal region of this dissection.

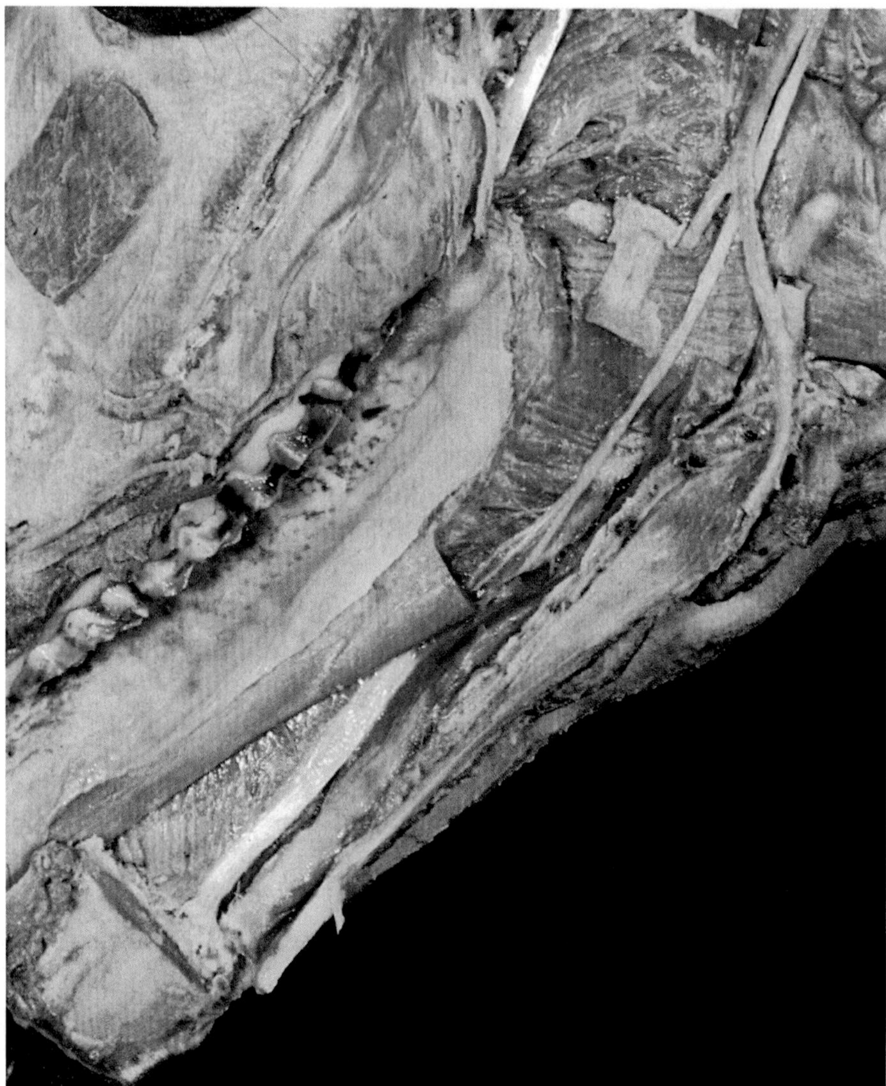

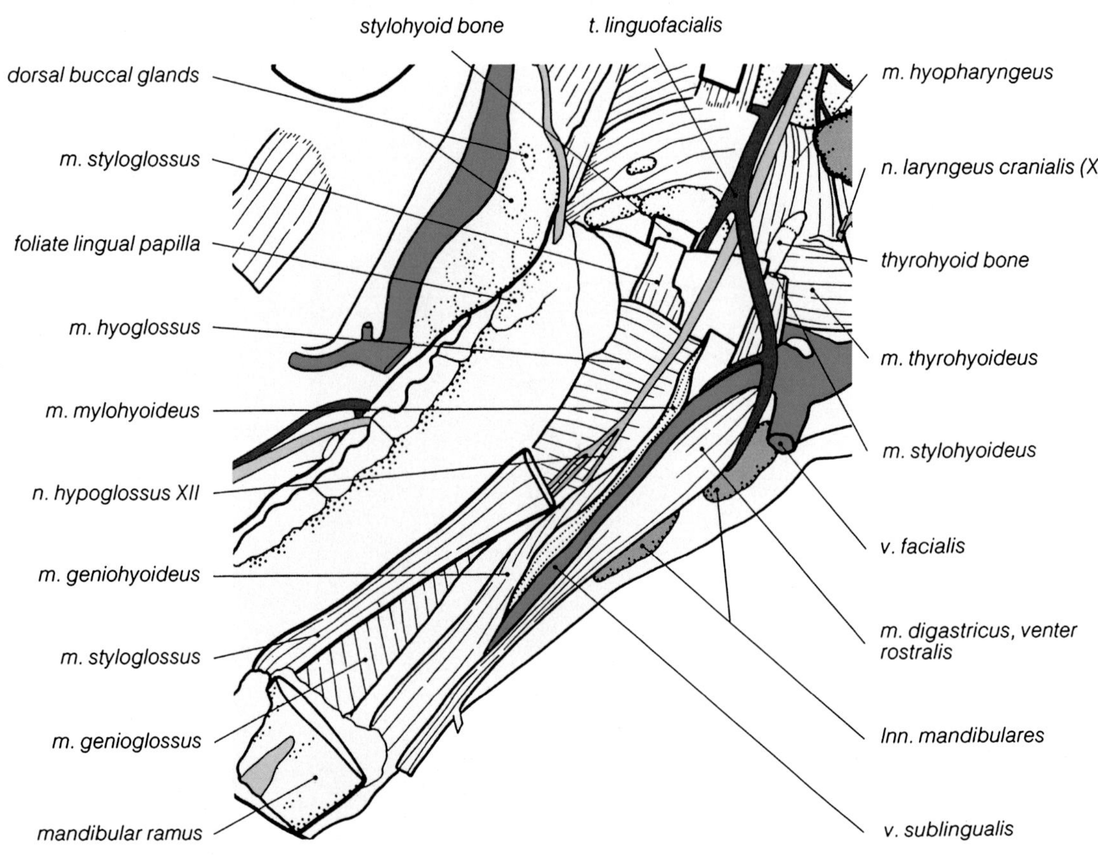
stylohyoid bone
t. linguofacialis
dorsal buccal glands
m. styloglossus
foliate lingual papilla
m. hyoglossus
m. mylohyoideus
n. hypoglossus XII
m. geniohyoideus
m. styloglossus
m. genioglossus
mandibular ramus
m. hyopharyngeus
n. laryngeus cranialis (X)
thyrohyoid bone
m. thyrohyoideus
m. stylohyoideus
v. facialis
m. digastricus, venter rostralis
lnn. mandibulares
v. sublingualis

Fig. 1.28 The lingual muscles: left lateral view. The sublingual gland (Fig. 1.20) has been removed to expose the muscles of the tongue.

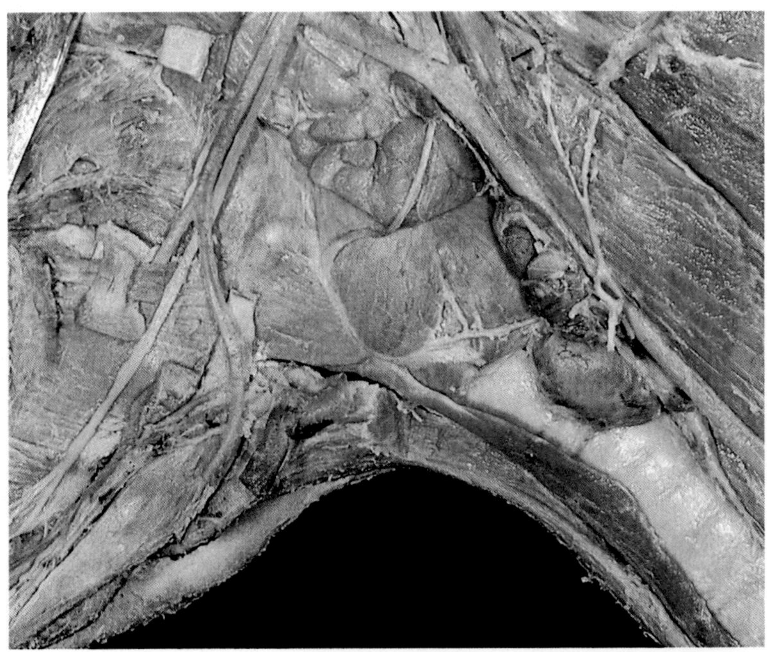

Fig. 1.29 The pharyngeal muscles and thyroid gland: left lateral view. The sternomandibularis muscle and the main tributaries of the external jugular veins have now been removed. The structures hidden by the large lymph nodes are shown in Fig. 1.30.

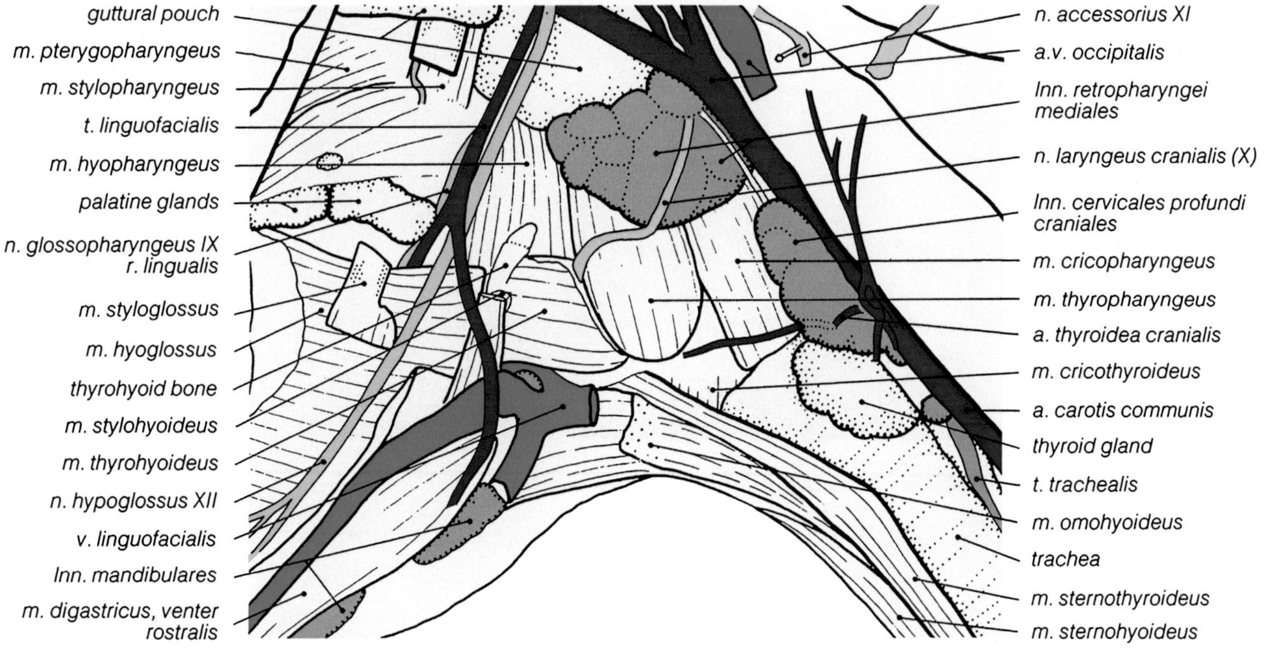

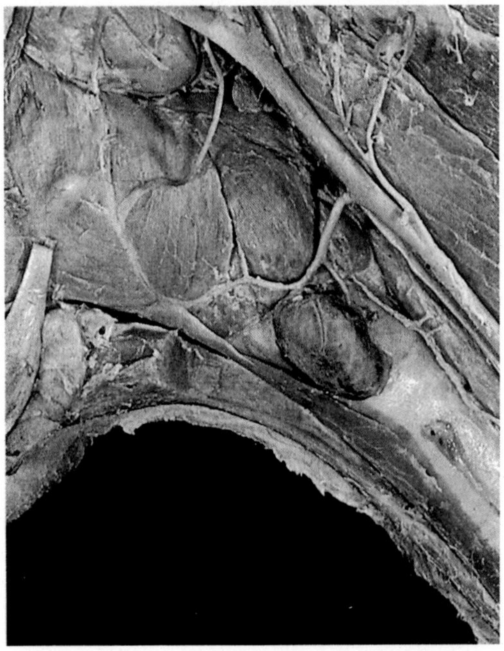

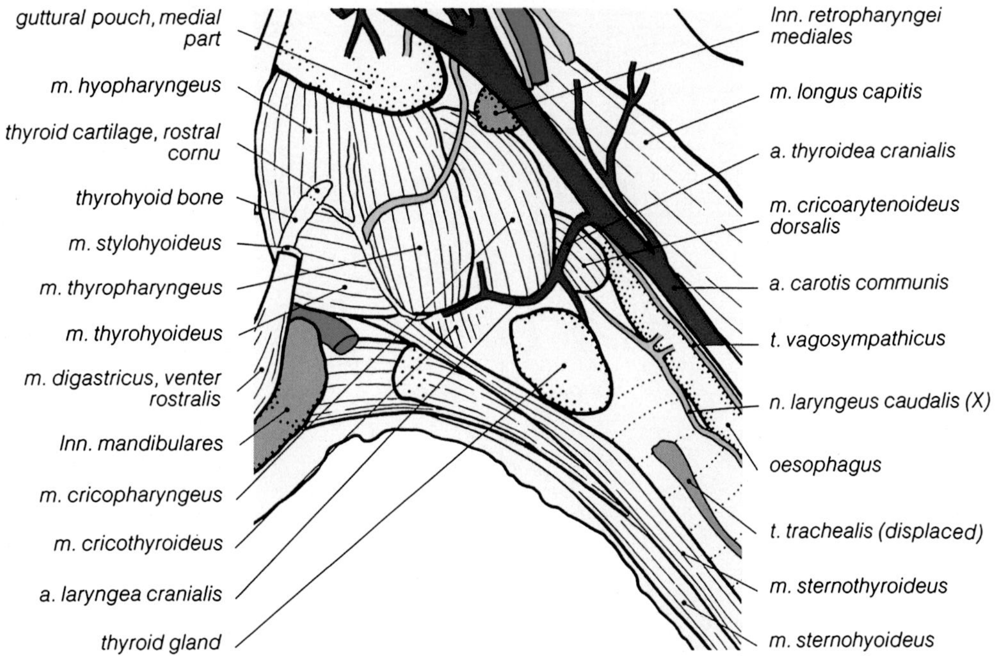

guttural pouch
m. pterygopharyngeus
m. stylopharyngeus
t. linguofacialis
m. hyopharyngeus
palatine glands
n. glossopharyngeus IX
r. lingualis
m. styloglossus
m. hyoglossus
thyrohyoid bone
m. stylohyoideus
m. thyrohyoideus
n. hypoglossus XII
v. linguofacialis
lnn. mandibulares
m. digastricus, venter
rostralis
n. accessorius XI
a.v. occipitalis
lnn. retropharyngei
mediales
n. laryngeus cranialis (X)
lnn. cervicales profundi
craniales
m. cricopharyngeus
m. thyropharyngeus
a. thyroidea cranialis
m. cricothyroideus
a. carotis communis
thyroid gland
t. trachealis
m. omohyoideus
trachea
m. sternothyroideus
m. sternohyoideus

guttural pouch, medial
part
m. hyopharyngeus
thyroid cartilage, rostral
cornu
thyrohyoid bone
m. stylohyoideus
m. thyropharyngeus
m. thyrohyoideus
m. digastricus, venter
rostralis
lnn. mandibulares
m. cricopharyngeus
m. cricothyroideus
a. laryngea cranialis
thyroid gland
lnn. retropharyngei
mediales
m. longus capitis
a. thyroidea cranialis
m. cricoarytenoideus
dorsalis
a. carotis communis
t. vagosympathicus
n. laryngeus caudalis (X)
oesophagus
t. trachealis (displaced)
m. sternothyroideus
m. sternohyoideus

Fig. 1.30 The pharyngeal and laryngeal muscles: left lateral view. Removal of almost all of the large lymph nodes lying dorsal to the pharynx and larynx reveals the dorsal cricoarytenoid muscle and the caudal laryngeal nerve.

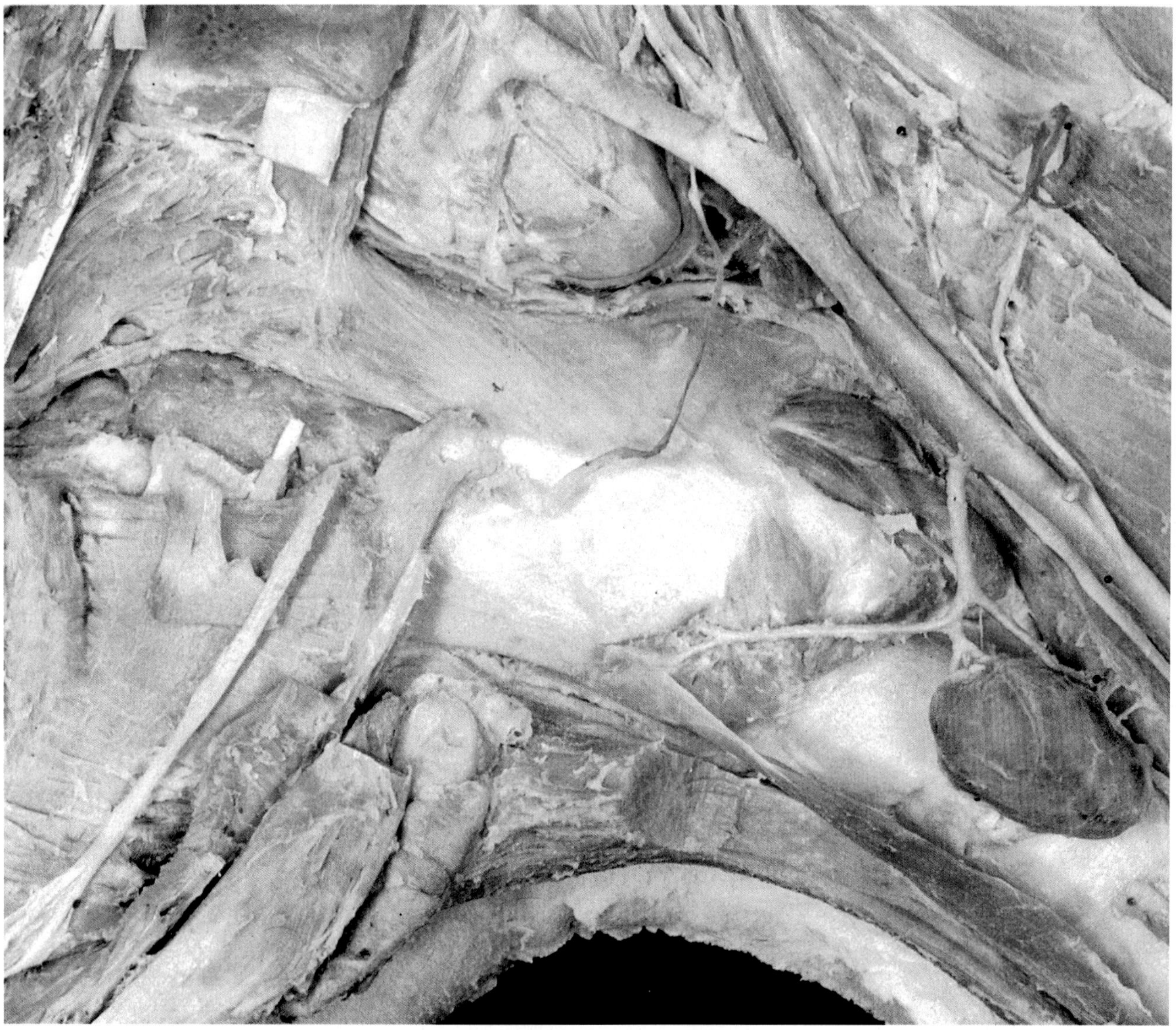

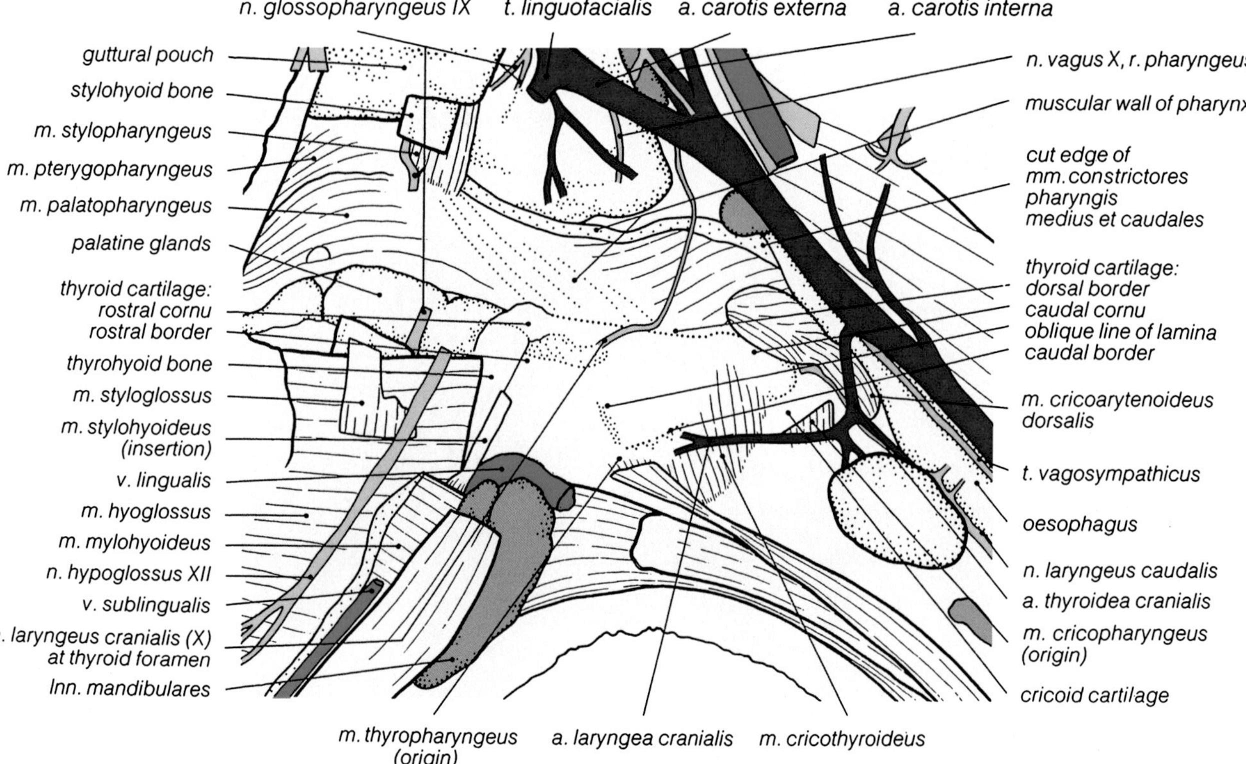
n. glossopharyngeus IX
t. linguofacialis
a. carotis externa
a. carotis interna
guttural pouch
stylohyoid bone
m. stylopharyngeus
m. pterygopharyngeus
m. palatopharyngeus
palatine glands
thyroid cartilage:
rostral cornu
rostral border
thyrohyoid bone
m. styloglossus
m. stylohyoideus
(insertion)
v. lingualis
m. hyoglossus
m. mylohyoideus
n. hypoglossus XII
v. sublingualis
n. laryngeus cranialis (X)
at thyroid foramen
lnn. mandibulares
n. vagus X, r. pharyngeus
muscular wall of pharynx
cut edge of
mm. constrictores
pharyngis
medius et caudales
thyroid cartilage:
dorsal border
caudal cornu
oblique line of lamina
caudal border
m. cricoarytenoideus
dorsalis
t. vagosympathicus
oesophagus
n. laryngeus caudalis
a. thyroidea cranialis
m. cricopharyngeus
(origin)
cricoid cartilage
m. thyropharyngeus
(origin)
a. laryngea cranialis
m. cricothyroideus

Fig. 1.31 The pharynx and larynx: left lateral view. The caudal (cricopharyngeal, thyropharyngeal) and middle (hyopharyngeal) constrictors of the pharynx have been removed to expose the thyroid cartilage and other laryngeal structures, and the deep muscles of the pharynx ('rostral constrictors').

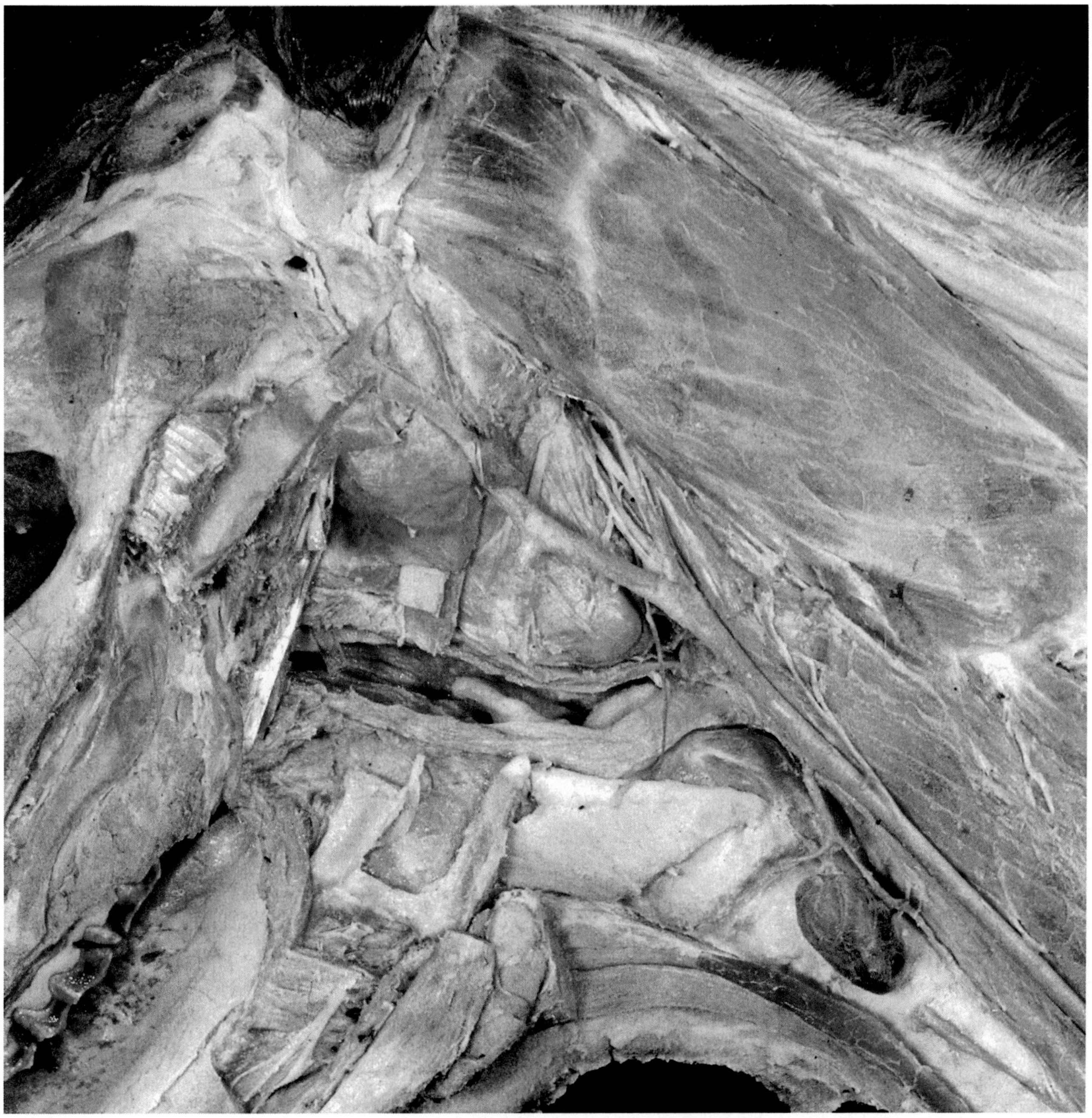

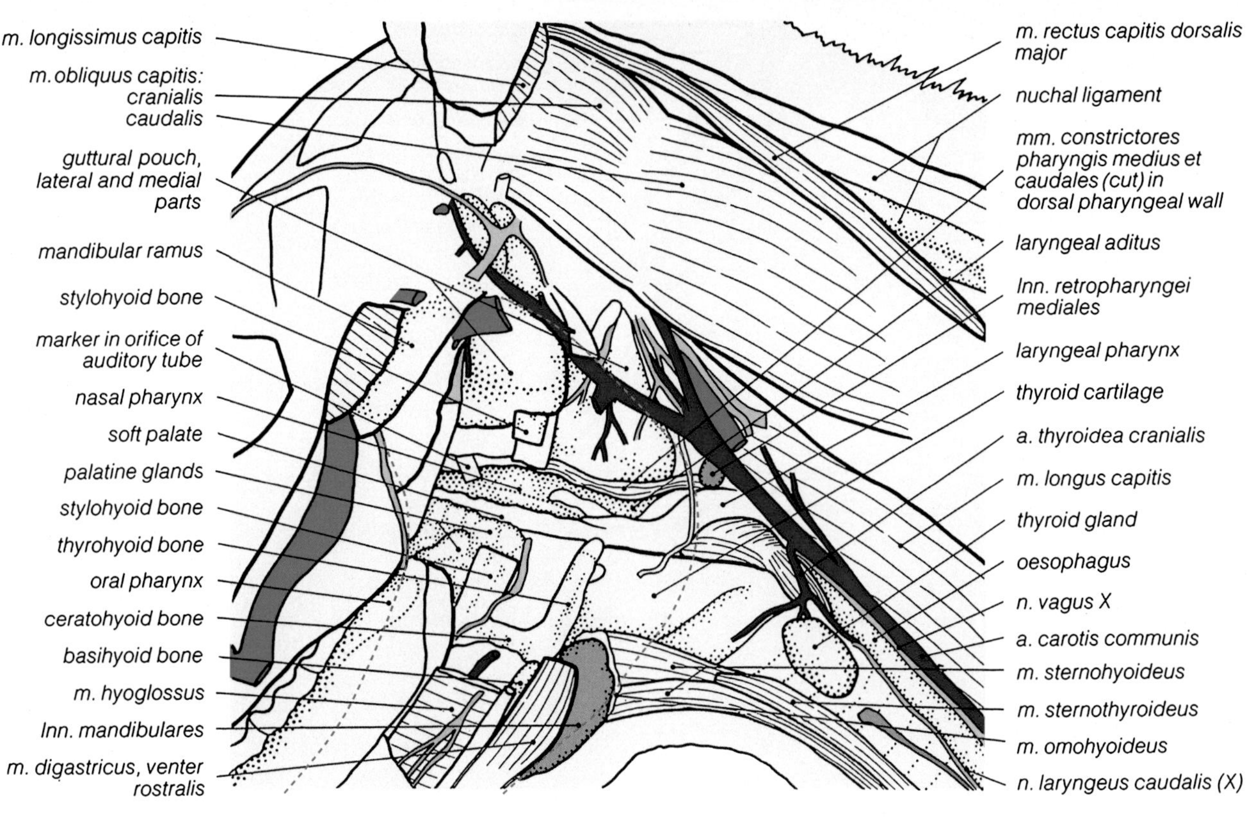
m. longissimus capitis
m. obliquus capitis:
cranialis
caudalis
guttural pouch, lateral and medial parts
mandibular ramus
stylohyoid bone
marker in orifice of auditory tube
nasal pharynx
soft palate
palatine glands
stylohyoid bone
thyrohyoid bone
oral pharynx
ceratohyoid bone
basihyoid bone
m. hyoglossus
lnn. mandibulares
m. digastricus, venter rostralis
m. rectus capitis dorsalis major
nuchal ligament
mm. constrictores pharyngis medius et caudales (cut) in dorsal pharyngeal wall
laryngeal aditus
lnn. retropharyngei mediales
laryngeal pharynx
thyroid cartilage
a. thyroidea cranialis
m. longus capitis
thyroid gland
oesophagus
n. vagus X
a. carotis communis
m. sternohyoideus
m. sternothyroideus
m. omohyoideus
n. laryngeus caudalis (X)

Fig. 1.32 The topography of the larynx: left lateral view. The lateral wall of the nasal and laryngeal parts of the pharynx has been excised. The cricothyroid muscle has been removed, and the rostral cornu of the thyroid cartilage has been cut (see Fig. 1.34). The outline of the mandible (broken blue line) has been traced from Fig. 1.23; its relationship to the larynx varies with flexion and extension of the atlanto-occipital joint.

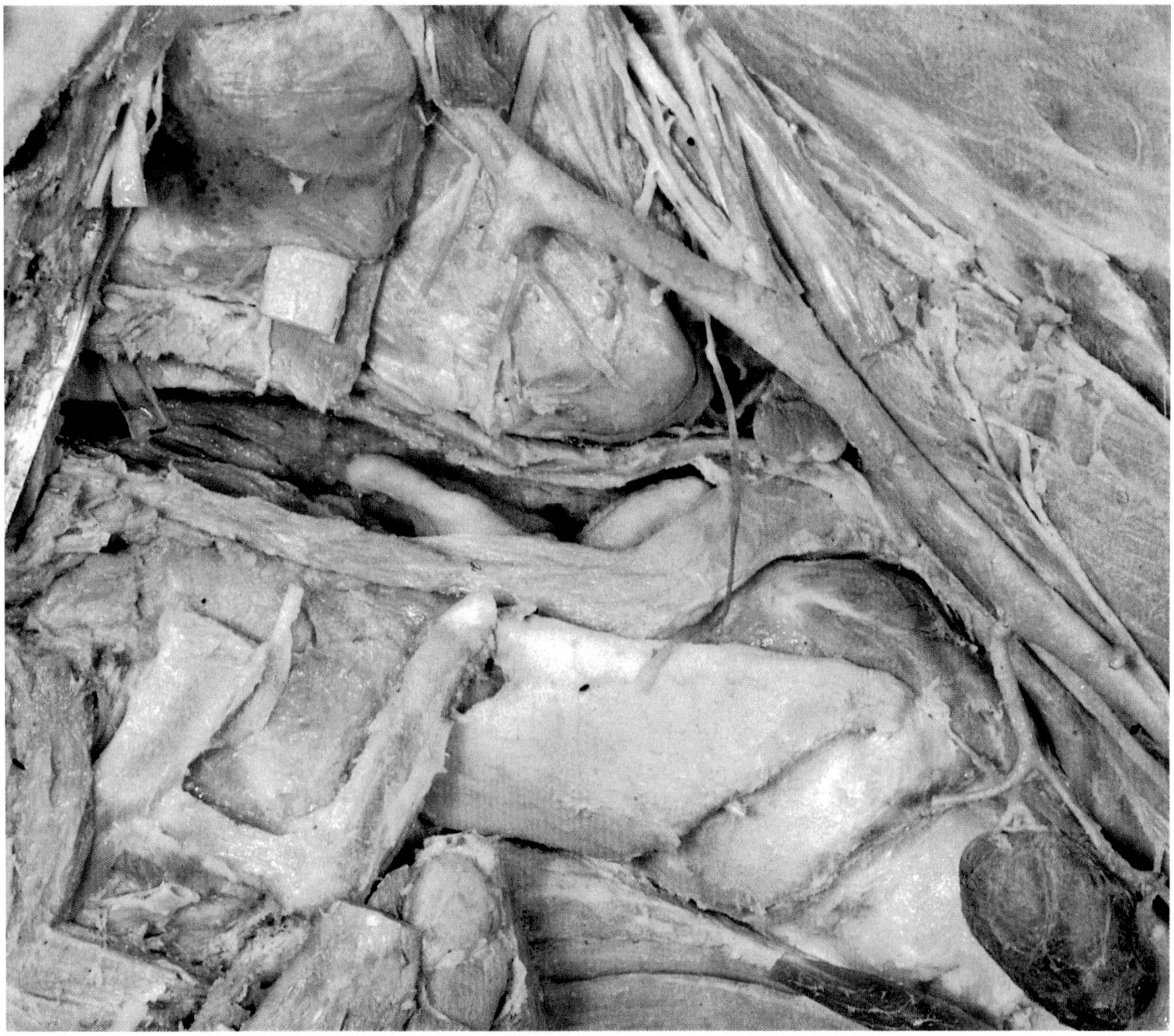

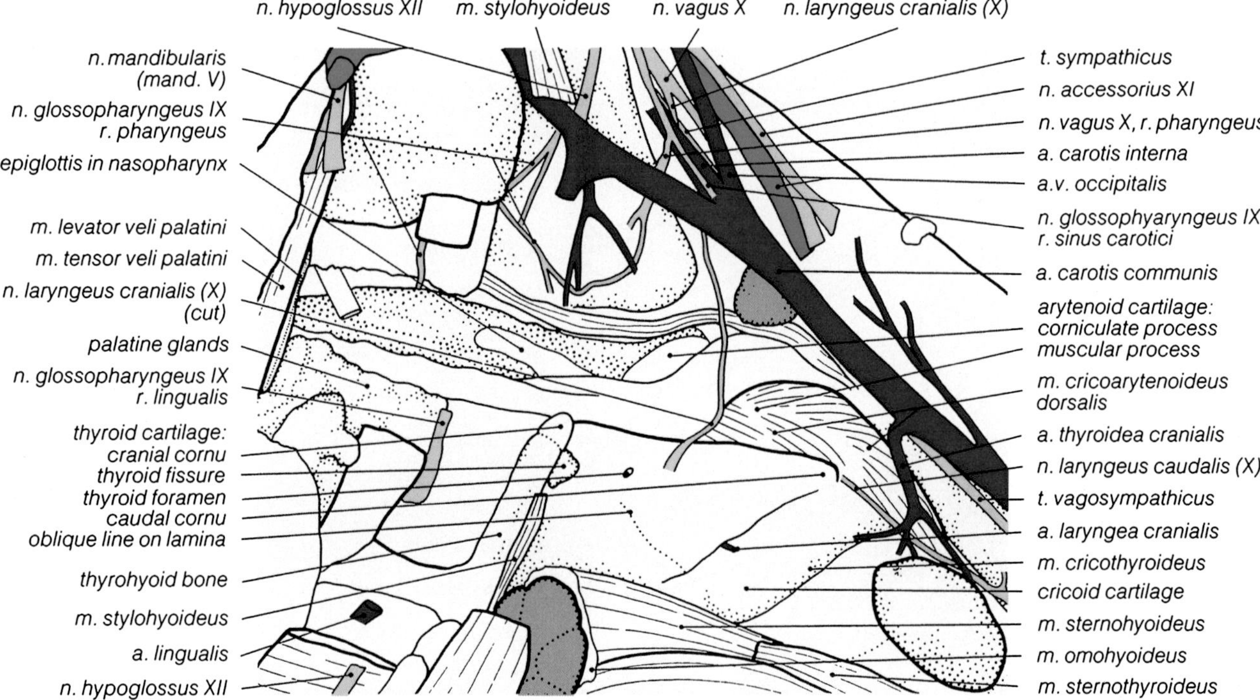
n. hypoglossus XII
m. stylohyoideus
n. vagus X
n. laryngeus cranialis (X)
n. mandibularis (mand. V)
n. glossopharyngeus IX r. pharyngeus
epiglottis in nasopharynx
m. levator veli palatini
m. tensor veli palatini
n. laryngeus cranialis (X) (cut)
palatine glands
n. glossopharyngeus IX r. lingualis
thyroid cartilage:
cranial cornu
thyroid fissure
thyroid foramen
caudal cornu
oblique line on lamina
thyrohyoid bone
m. stylohyoideus
a. lingualis
n. hypoglossus XII
t. sympathicus
n. accessorius XI
n. vagus X, r. pharyngeus
a. carotis interna
a.v. occipitalis
n. glossophyaryngeus IX r. sinus carotici
a. carotis communis
arytenoid cartilage:
corniculate process
muscular process
m. cricoarytenoideus dorsalis
a. thyroidea cranialis
n. laryngeus caudalis (X)
t. vagosympathicus
a. laryngea cranialis
m. cricothyroideus
cricoid cartilage
m. sternohyoideus
m. omohyoideus
m. sternothyroideus

Fig. 1.33 Superficial structures of the larynx: left lateral view. This is a closer view of the specimen shown in Fig. 1.32. The cranial laryngeal nerve has been cut and displaced to reveal the thyroid foramen.

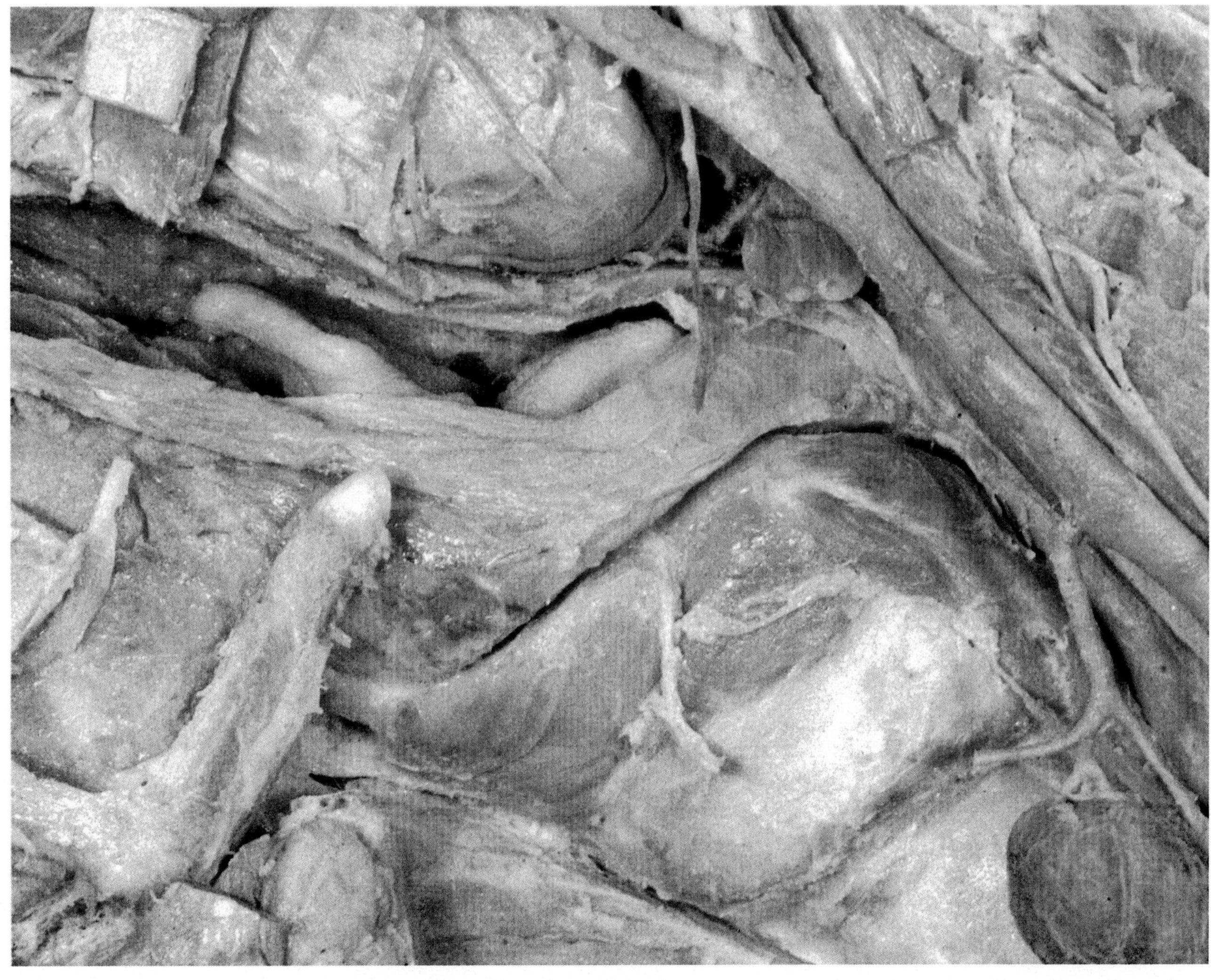

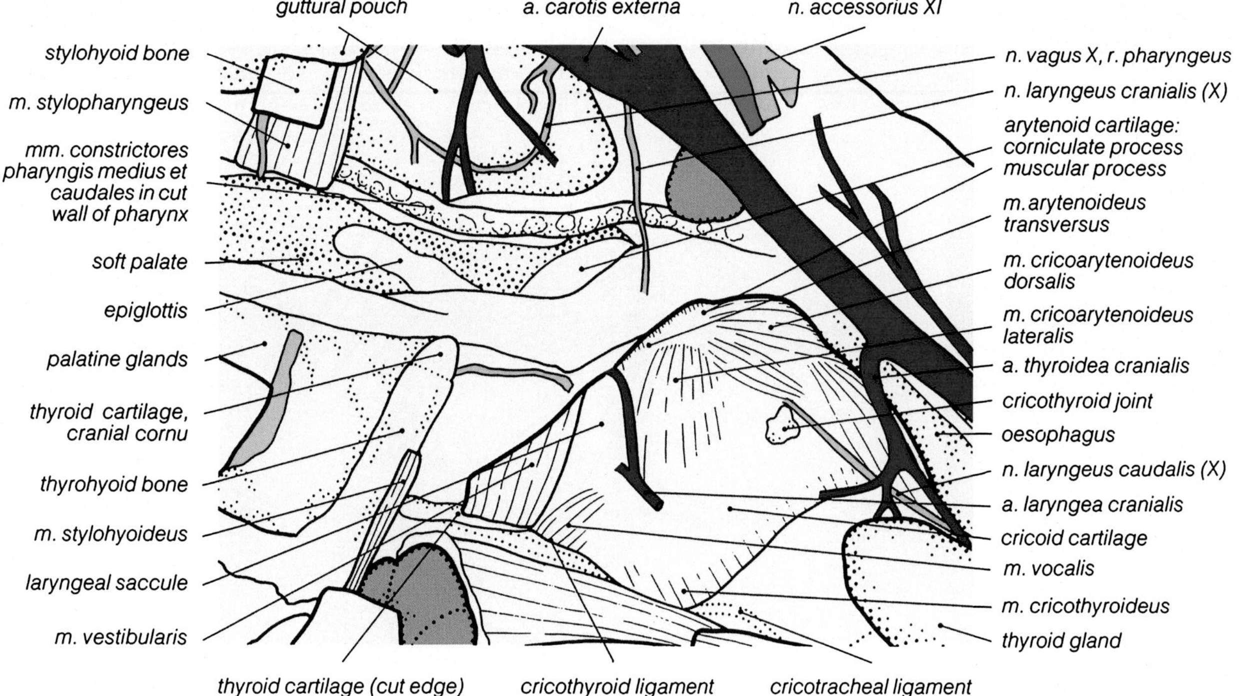
guttural pouch
a. carotis externa
n. accessorius XI
stylohyoid bone
m. stylopharyngeus
mm. constrictores pharyngis medius et caudales in cut wall of pharynx
soft palate
epiglottis
palatine glands
thyroid cartilage, cranial cornu
thyrohyoid bone
m. stylohyoideus
laryngeal saccule
m. vestibularis
n. vagus X, r. pharyngeus
n. laryngeus cranialis (X)
arytenoid cartilage: corniculate process muscular process
m. arytenoideus transversus
m. cricoarytenoideus dorsalis
m. cricoarytenoideus lateralis
a. thyroidea cranialis
cricothyroid joint
oesophagus
n. laryngeus caudalis (X)
a. laryngea cranialis
cricoid cartilage
m. vocalis
m. cricothyroideus
thyroid gland
thyroid cartilage (cut edge)
cricothyroid ligament
cricotracheal ligament

Fig. 1.34 The larynx after removal of the thyroid lamina: left lateral view. The rostral thyroid cornu was cut (see Fig. 1.33). The caudal cornu was disarticulated from the cricoid cartilage, exposing the synovial joint. Finally, the cartilage was cut close to the median plane and removed.

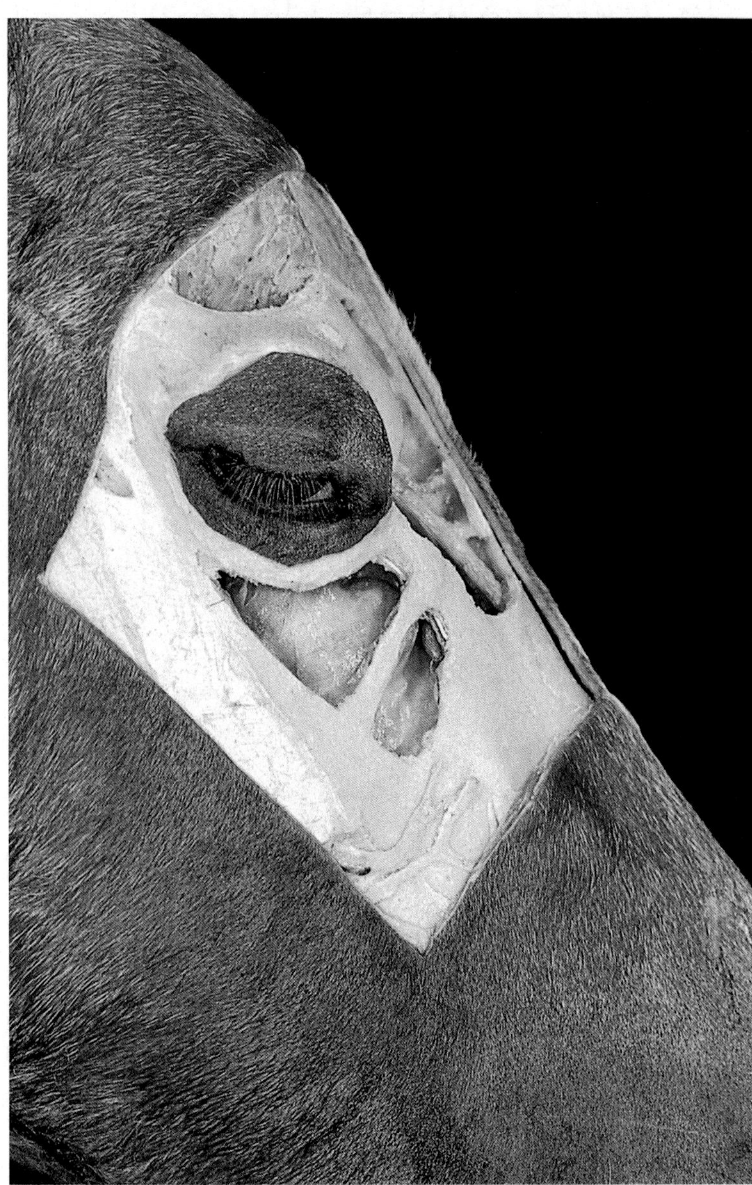

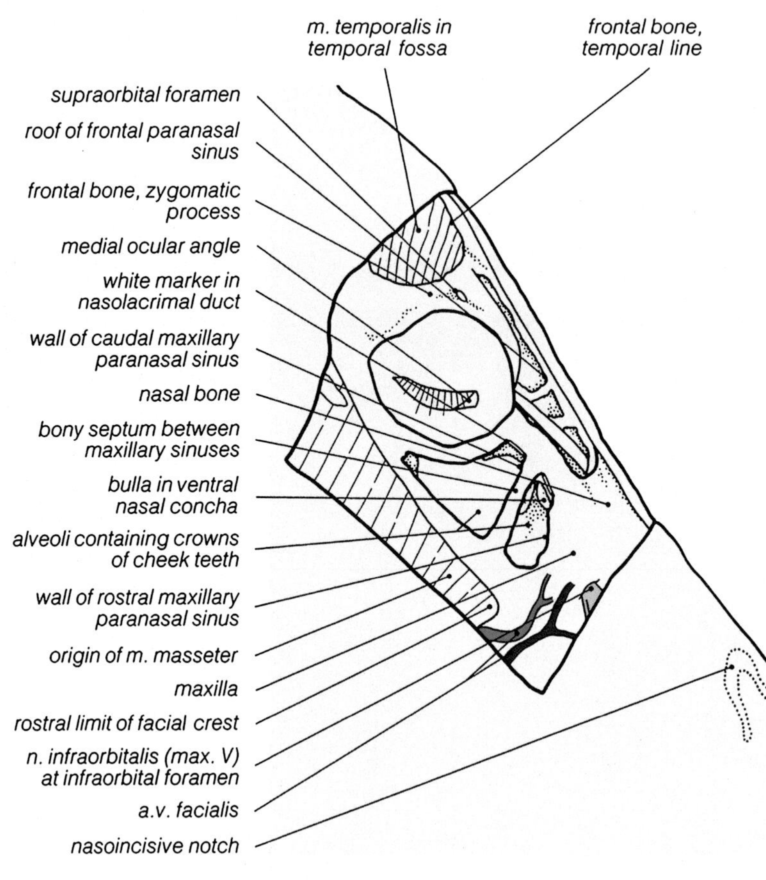
m. temporalis in temporal fossa
frontal bone, temporal line
supraorbital foramen
roof of frontal paranasal sinus
frontal bone, zygomatic process
medial ocular angle
white marker in nasolacrimal duct
wall of caudal maxillary paranasal sinus
nasal bone
bony septum between maxillary sinuses
bulla in ventral nasal concha
alveoli containing crowns of cheek teeth
wall of rostral maxillary paranasal sinus
origin of m. masseter
maxilla
rostral limit of facial crest
n. infraorbitalis (max. V) at infraorbital foramen
a.v. facialis
nasoincisive notch

Fig. 1.35 Frontal and maxillary paranasal sinuses: right lateral view (1). The outer layers of compact bone of the frontal, nasal, maxillary and lacrimal bones have been removed from the parts occupied by the sinuses, and the outer walls of the sinuses have been cut away. Associated external landmarks are shown in this figure. This horse was about 1¼ years old; a series of dissections of the paranasal sinuses of a horse aged under 9 months is shown in Figs. 1.54–1.59. The sinuses of older animals are shown in Figs. 1.44–1.47.

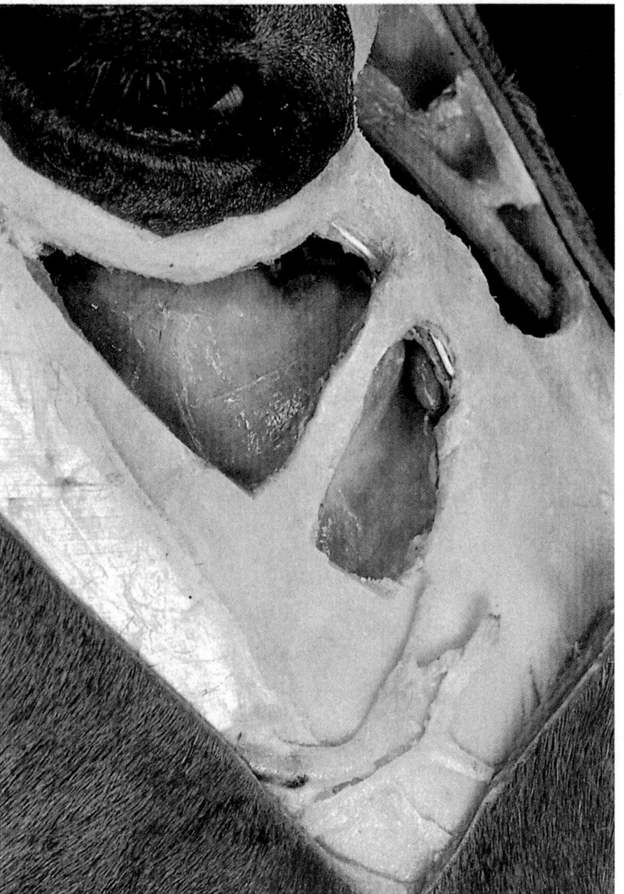

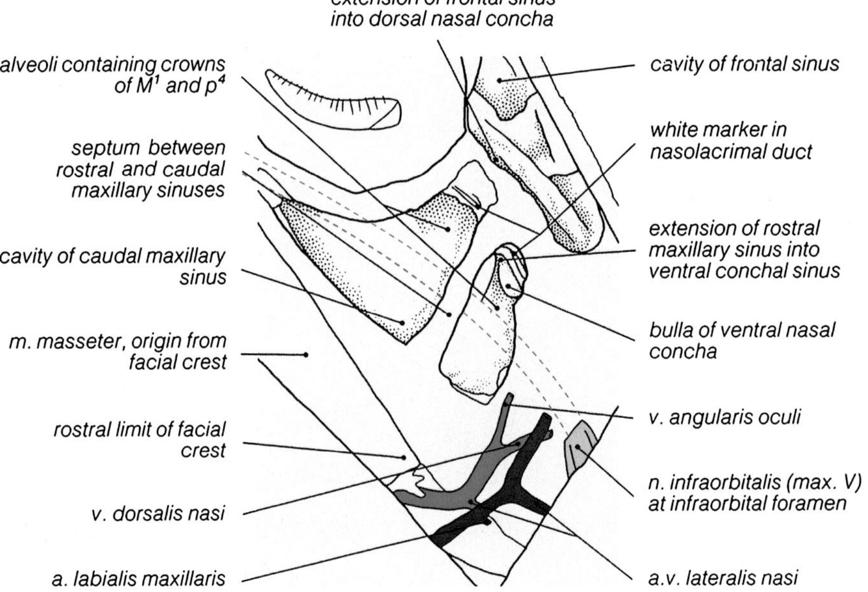
extension of frontal sinus into dorsal nasal concha
alveoli containing crowns of M^1 and p^4
septum between rostral and caudal maxillary sinuses
cavity of caudal maxillary sinus
m. masseter, origin from facial crest
rostral limit of facial crest
v. dorsalis nasi
a. labialis maxillaris
cavity of frontal sinus
white marker in nasolacrimal duct
extension of rostral maxillary sinus into ventral conchal sinus
bulla of ventral nasal concha
v. angularis oculi
n. infraorbitalis (max. V) at infraorbital foramen
a.v. lateralis nasi

Fig. 1.36 Frontal and maxillary paranasal sinuses: right lateral view (2). This is a closer view of a part of Fig. 1.35. In this young horse, the crowns of the cheek teeth, enclosed by bony alveoli, reduce the sizes of the maxillary sinuses and hide the infraorbital canal which traverses these sinuses. The position of the infraorbital canal is indicated by the broken blue lines.

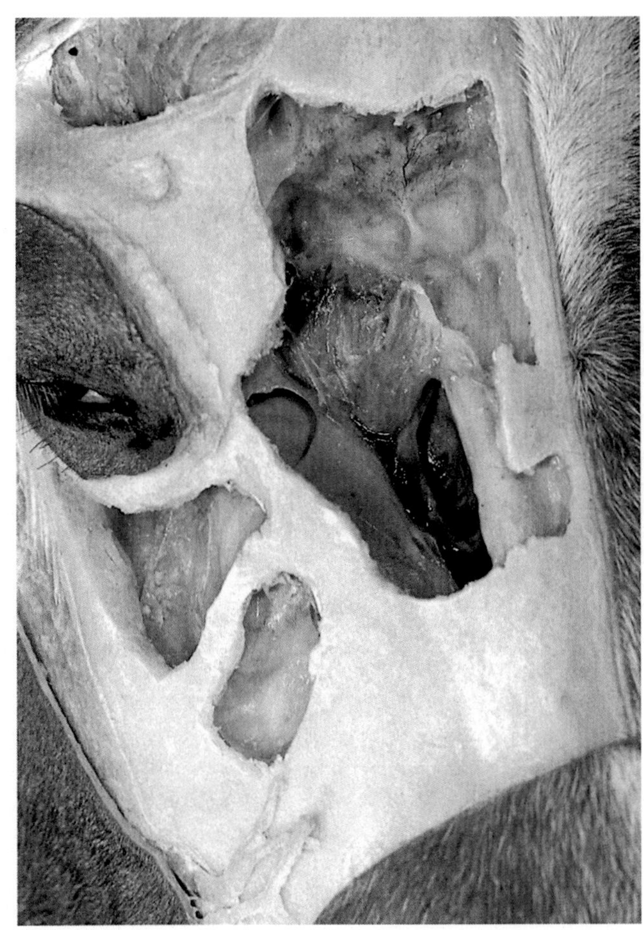

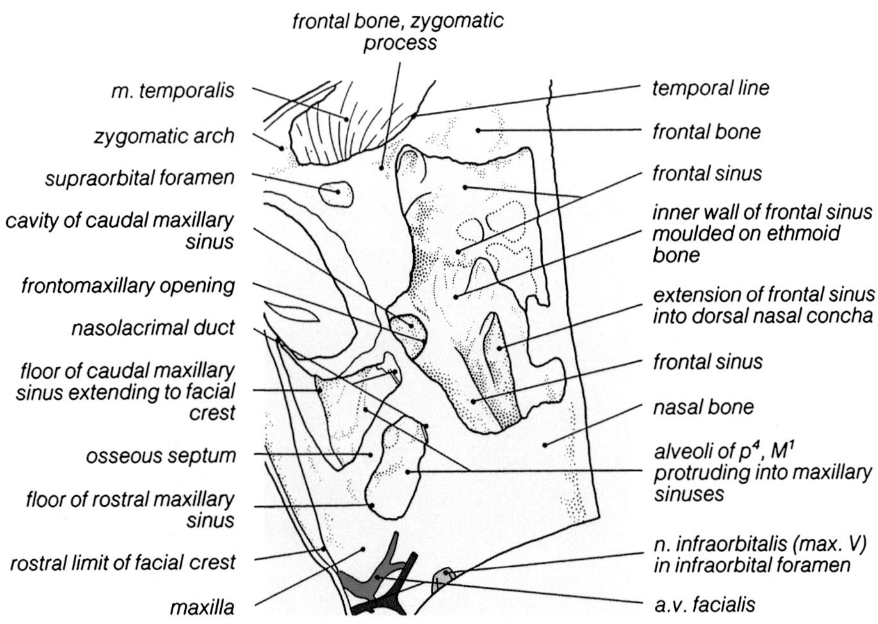
frontal bone, zygomatic process
m. temporalis
zygomatic arch
supraorbital foramen
cavity of caudal maxillary sinus
frontomaxillary opening
nasolacrimal duct
floor of caudal maxillary sinus extending to facial crest
osseous septum
floor of rostral maxillary sinus
rostral limit of facial crest
maxilla
temporal line
frontal bone
frontal sinus
inner wall of frontal sinus moulded on ethmoid bone
extension of frontal sinus into dorsal nasal concha
frontal sinus
nasal bone
alveoli of p4, M1 protruding into maxillary sinuses
n. infraorbitalis (max. V) in infraorbital foramen
a.v. facialis

Fig. 1.37 Frontal and maxillary paranasal sinuses: right dorsolateral view. In some individuals, the frontal sinus extends considerably further caudally at its medial aspect. This view of the maxillary sinuses shows that at this age (about 1¼ years) the ventral limit of the sinus is restricted by the cheek teeth but in older animals it extends well below the facial crest. The infraorbital canal is not visible but a small part of the caudal maxillary sinus can be seen through the frontomaxillary opening.

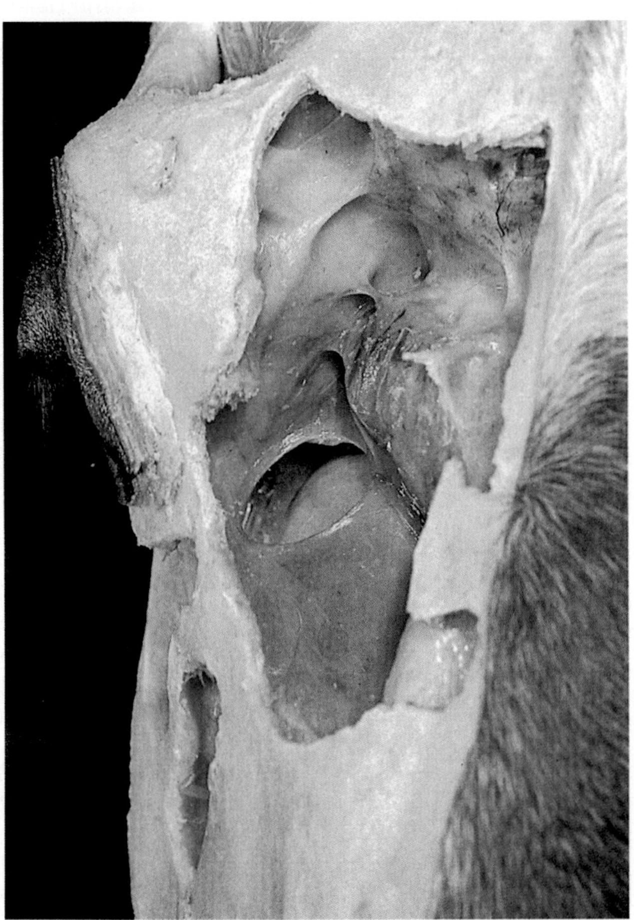

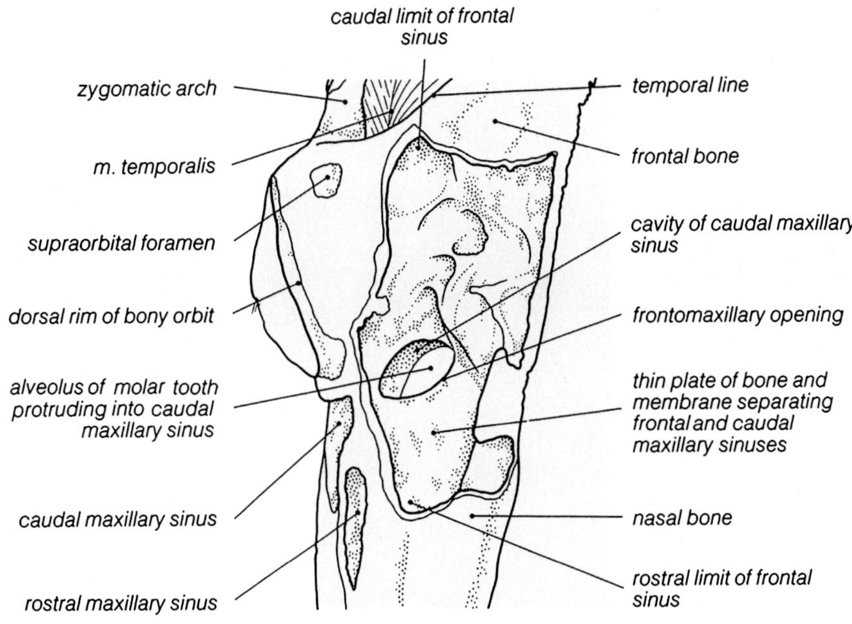
caudal limit of frontal sinus
zygomatic arch
m. temporalis
supraorbital foramen
dorsal rim of bony orbit
alveolus of molar tooth protruding into caudal maxillary sinus
caudal maxillary sinus
rostral maxillary sinus
temporal line
frontal bone
cavity of caudal maxillary sinus
frontomaxillary opening
thin plate of bone and membrane separating frontal and caudal maxillary sinuses
nasal bone
rostral limit of frontal sinus

Fig. 1.38 The frontal paranasal sinus and frontomaxillary opening: dorsal view. In this yearling horse, the infraorbital canal cannot be seen from the frontomaxillary opening. In older horses it is clearly visible, lying just medial to the alveolus of the last molar tooth. Compare with Figs. 1.47 and 1.59.

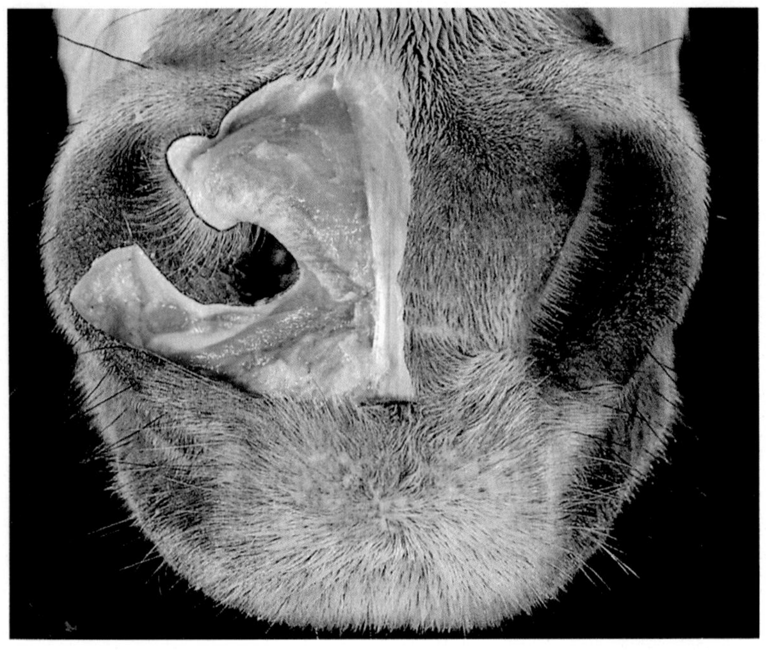

Fig. 1.39 The nostrils: rostral view. This figure, and Figs. 1.40, 1.41 are of an unembalmed pony, to supplement those of embalmed specimens (Figs. 1.1, 1.6).

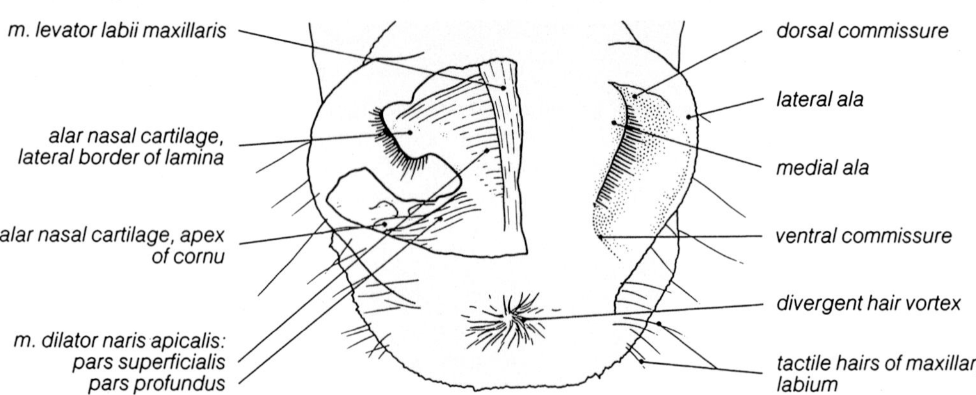
m. levator labii maxillaris
alar nasal cartilage, lateral border of lamina
alar nasal cartilage, apex of cornu
m. dilator naris apicalis: pars superficialis pars profundus
dorsal commissure
lateral ala
medial ala
ventral commissure
divergent hair vortex
tactile hairs of maxillary labium

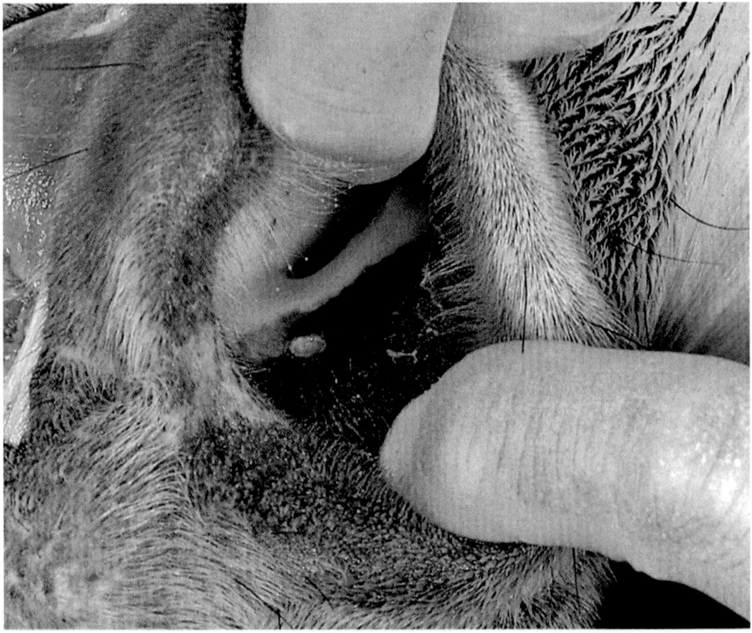

Fig. 1.40 The nasal vestibule and nasolacrimal duct: left rostrolateral view. The left nostril is being held open to reveal the nasolacrimal orifice. In some horses, two or even three nasolacrimal orifices may be present.

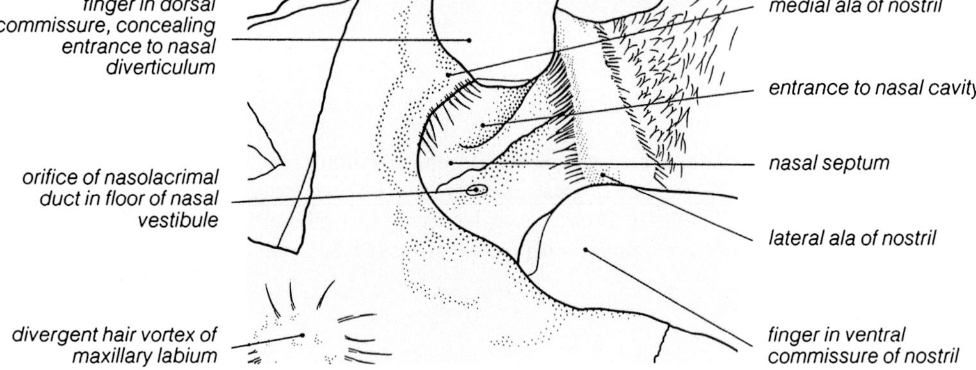
finger in dorsal commissure, concealing entrance to nasal diverticulum
orifice of nasolacrimal duct in floor of nasal vestibule
divergent hair vortex of maxillary labium
medial ala of nostril
entrance to nasal cavity
nasal septum
lateral ala of nostril
finger in ventral commissure of nostril

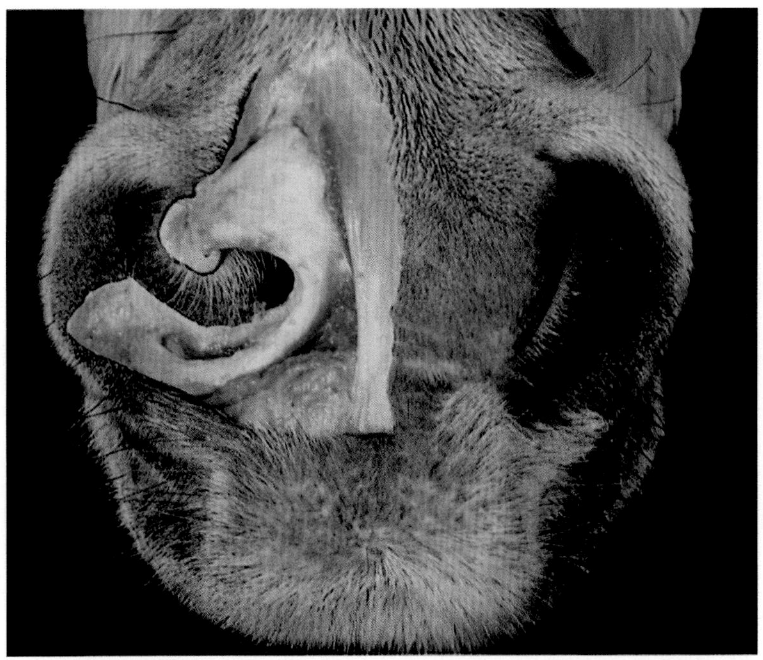

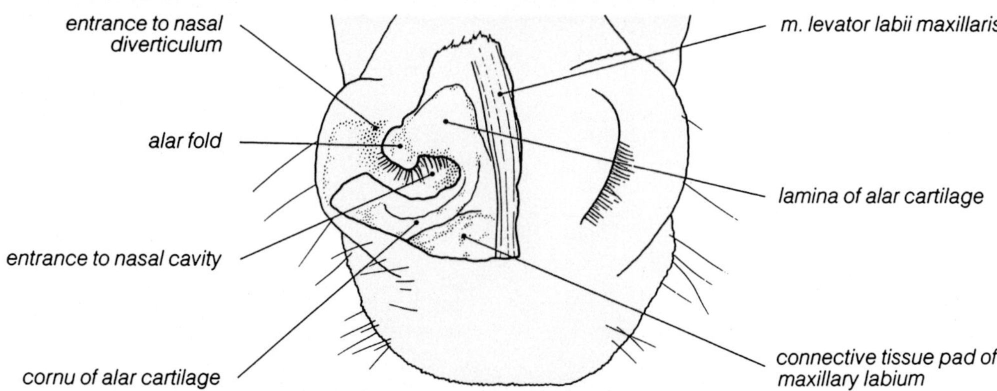
entrance to nasal diverticulum
alar fold
entrance to nasal cavity
cornu of alar cartilage
m. levator labii maxillaris
lamina of alar cartilage
connective tissue pad of maxillary labium

Fig. 1.41 The alar cartilage of the nostril: rostral view. The cartilage is readily palpable in the medial ala and at the ventral commissure of the nostril.

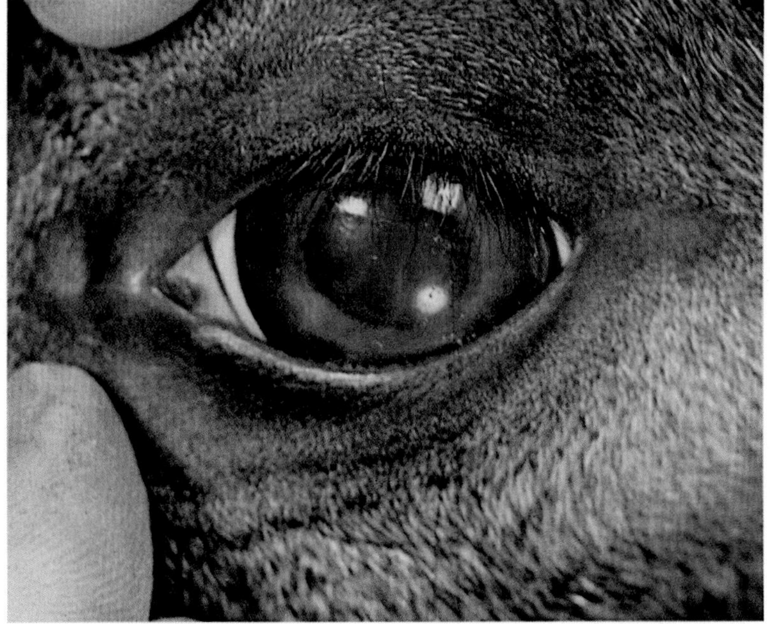

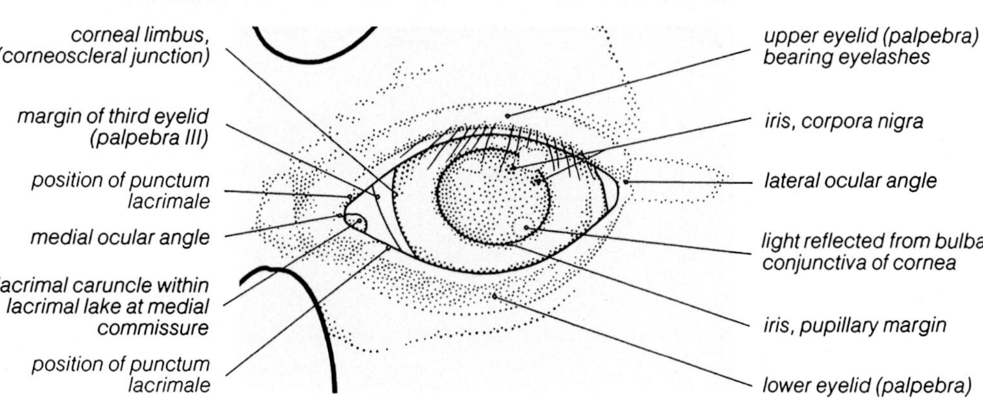
corneal limbus, (corneoscleral junction)
margin of third eyelid (palpebra III)
position of punctum lacrimale
medial ocular angle
lacrimal caruncle within lacrimal lake at medial commissure
position of punctum lacrimale
upper eyelid (palpebra) bearing eyelashes
iris, corpora nigra
lateral ocular angle
light reflected from bulbar conjunctiva of cornea
iris, pupillary margin
lower eyelid (palpebra)

Fig. 1.42 Surface features of the eye: left lateral view. This specimen was photographed shortly after exsanguination and death to supplement the surface features shown in Fig. 1.64. The eyelids are held apart to open up the angles and commissures between them. The upper corpora nigra (granula iridica) are just visible; the lower corpora nigra cannot be seen.

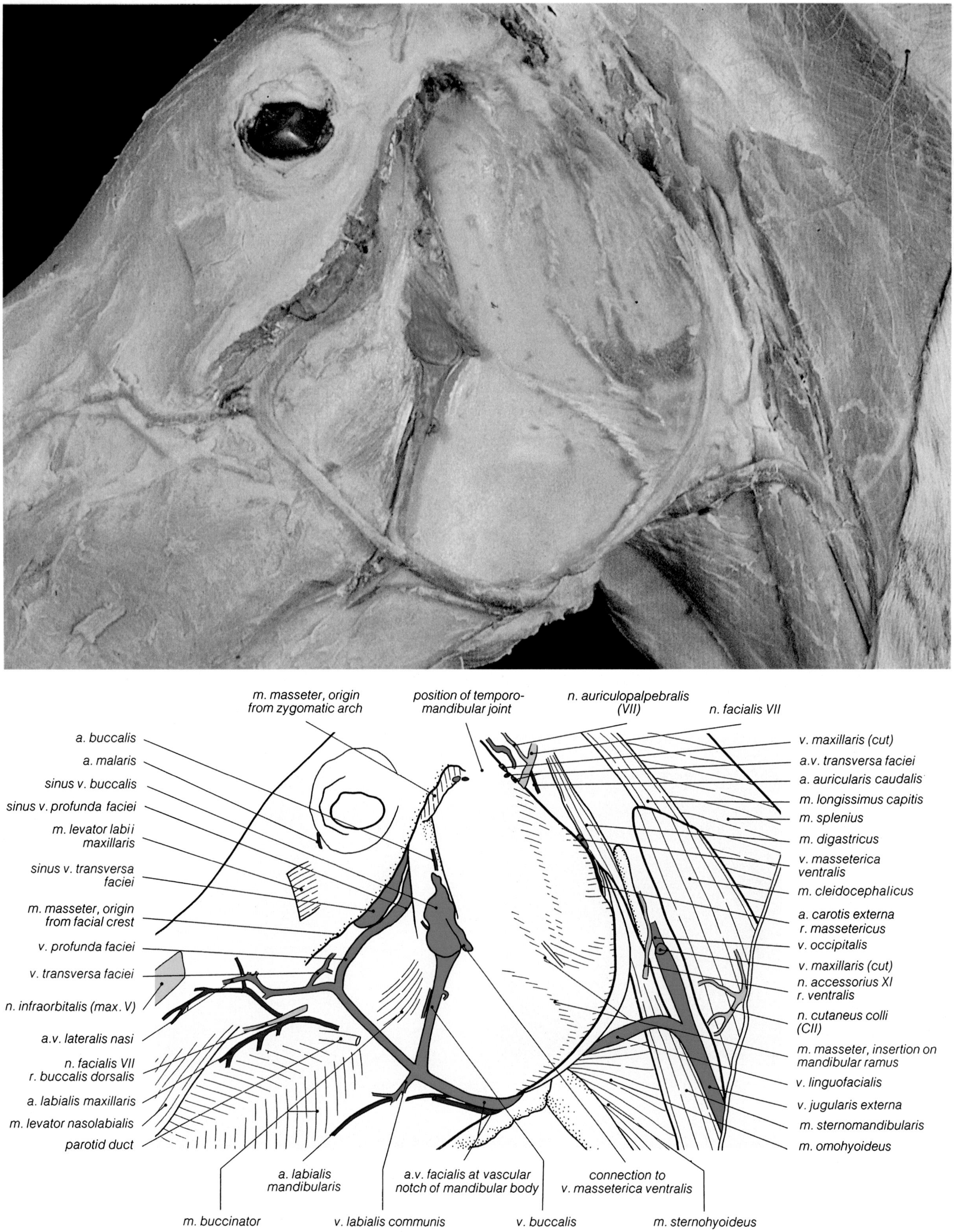

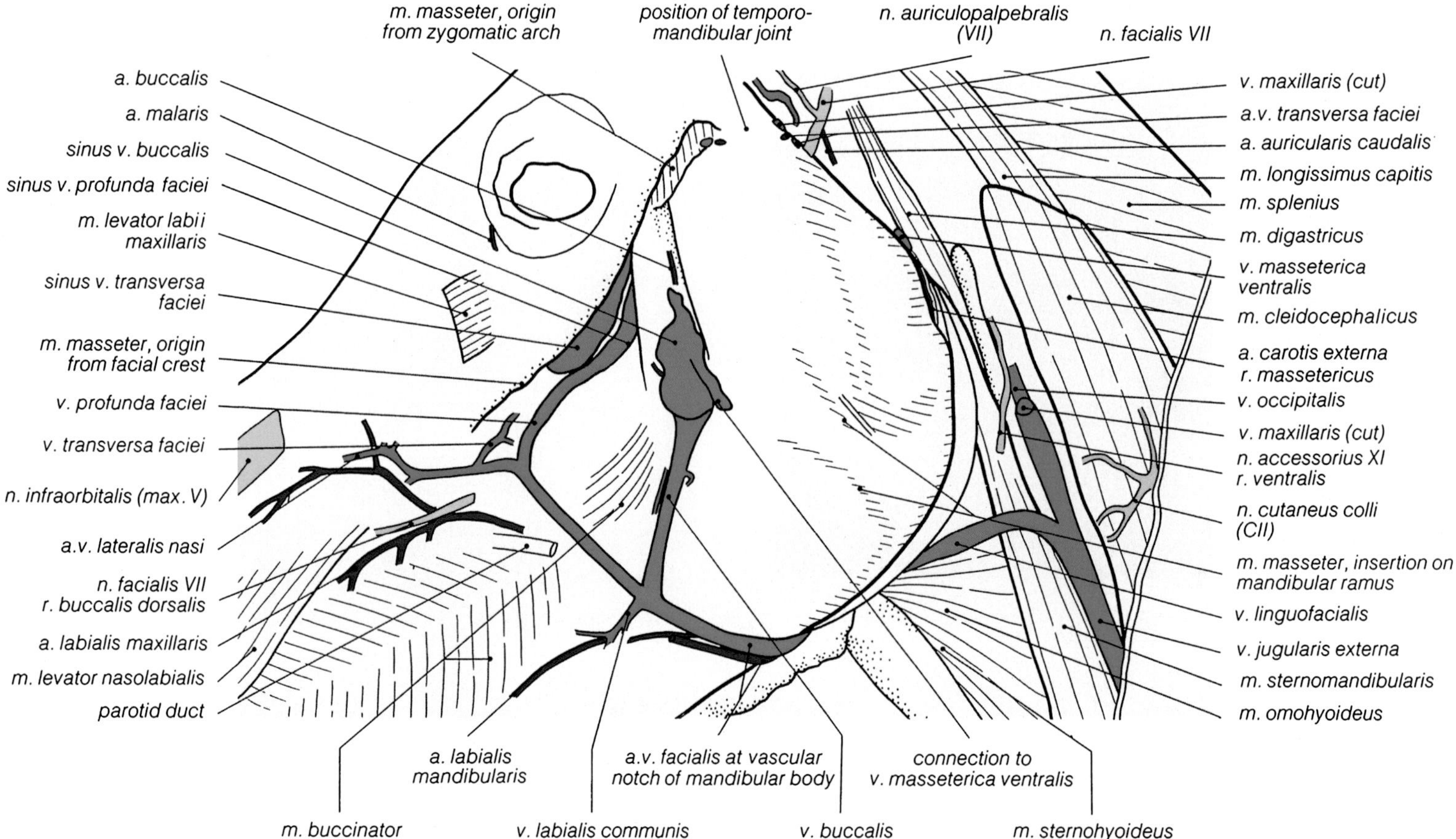
m. masseter, origin from zygomatic arch
position of temporo-mandibular joint
n. auriculopalpebralis (VII)
n. facialis VII
a. buccalis
a. malaris
sinus v. buccalis
sinus v. profunda faciei
m. levator labii maxillaris
sinus v. transversa faciei
m. masseter, origin from facial crest
v. profunda faciei
v. transversa faciei
n. infraorbitalis (max. V)
a.v. lateralis nasi
n. facialis VII r. buccalis dorsalis
a. labialis maxillaris
m. levator nasolabialis
parotid duct
v. maxillaris (cut)
a.v. transversa faciei
a. auricularis caudalis
m. longissimus capitis
m. splenius
m. digastricus
v. masseterica ventralis
m. cleidocephalicus
a. carotis externa r. massetericus
v. occipitalis
v. maxillaris (cut)
n. accessorius XI r. ventralis
n. cutaneus colli (CII)
m. masseter, insertion on mandibular ramus
v. linguofacialis
v. jugularis externa
m. sternomandibularis
m. omohyoideus
a. labialis mandibularis
a.v. facialis at vascular notch of mandibular body
connection to v. masseterica ventralis
m. buccinator
v. labialis communis
v. buccalis
m. sternohyoideus

Fig. 1.43 The veins of the masseteric region: left lateral view. The veins have been injected with blue latex via the cephalic vein, and the masseter muscle has been removed.

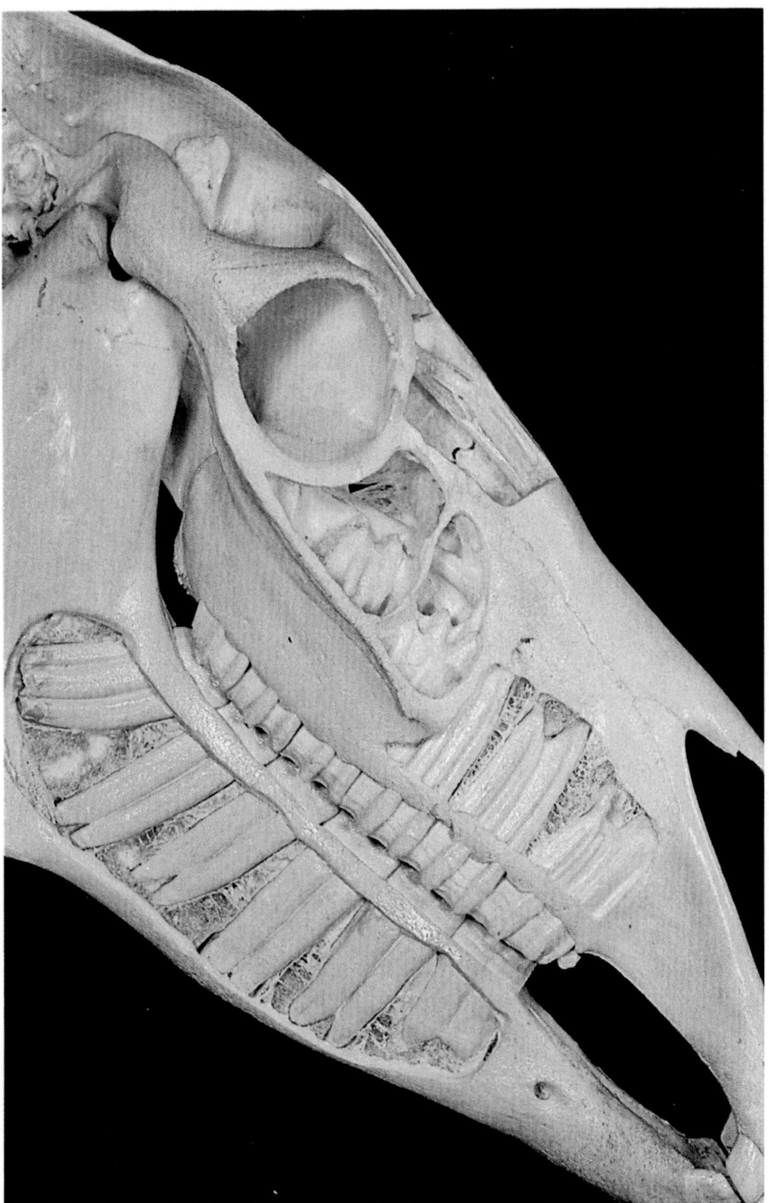

Fig. 1.44 The cheek teeth of a 6-year-old horse: right lateral view. The outer tables of the maxilla, zygomatic and lacrimal bones and mandible have been partially removed from this macerated skull to demonstrate the dental alveoli and the unerupted parts of the high-crowned cheek teeth. Calcified roots have formed in all of the teeth except the third molars. The paranasal sinuses are shown in Fig. 1.45.

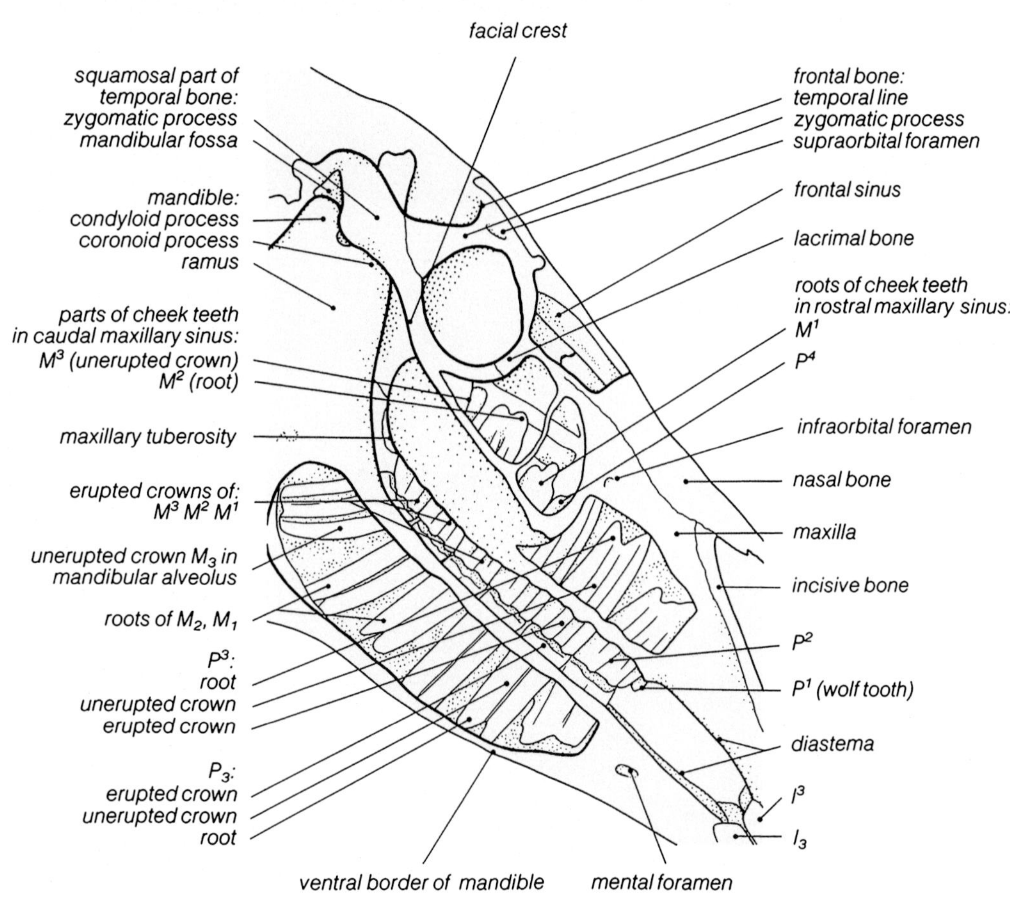
facial crest
squamosal part of temporal bone:
zygomatic process
mandibular fossa
mandible:
condyloid process
coronoid process
ramus
parts of cheek teeth in caudal maxillary sinus:
M^3 (unerupted crown)
M^2 (root)
maxillary tuberosity
erupted crowns of: M^3 M^2 M^1
unerupted crown M_3 in mandibular alveolus
roots of M_2, M_1
P^3:
root
unerupted crown
erupted crown
P_3:
erupted crown
unerupted crown
root
ventral border of mandible
mental foramen
frontal bone:
temporal line
zygomatic process
supraorbital foramen
frontal sinus
lacrimal bone
roots of cheek teeth in rostral maxillary sinus:
M^1
P^4
infraorbital foramen
nasal bone
maxilla
incisive bone
P^2
P^1 (wolf tooth)
diastema
I^3
I_3

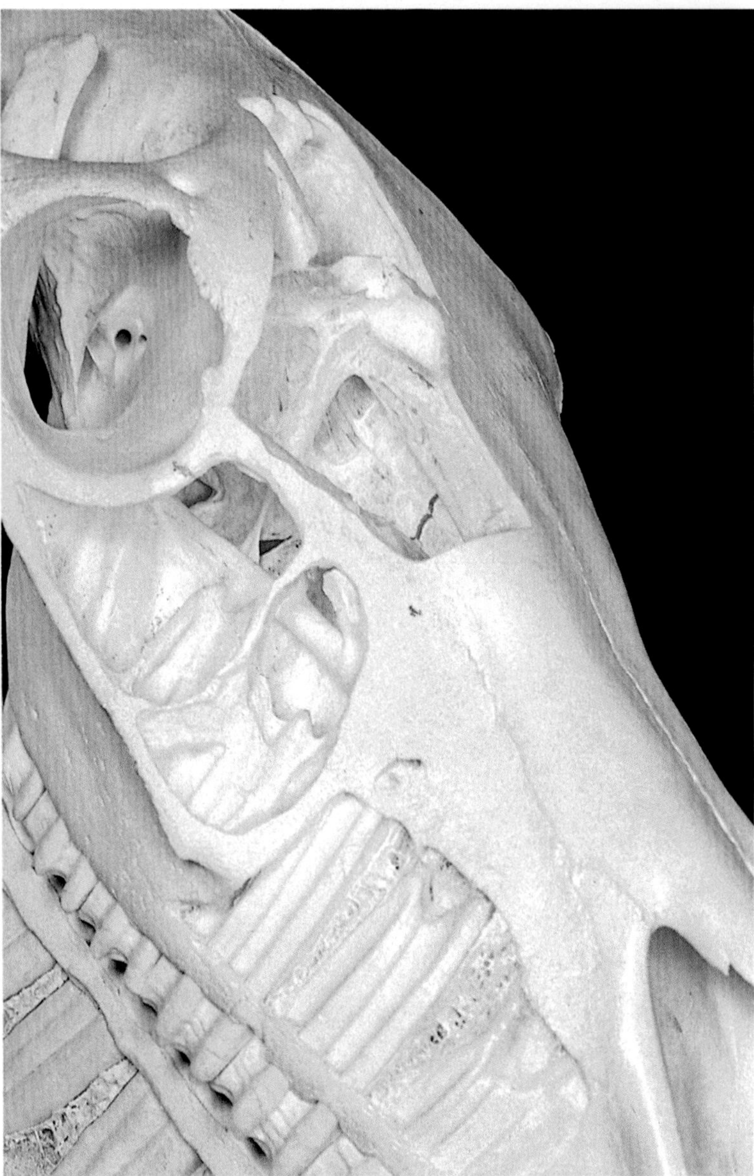

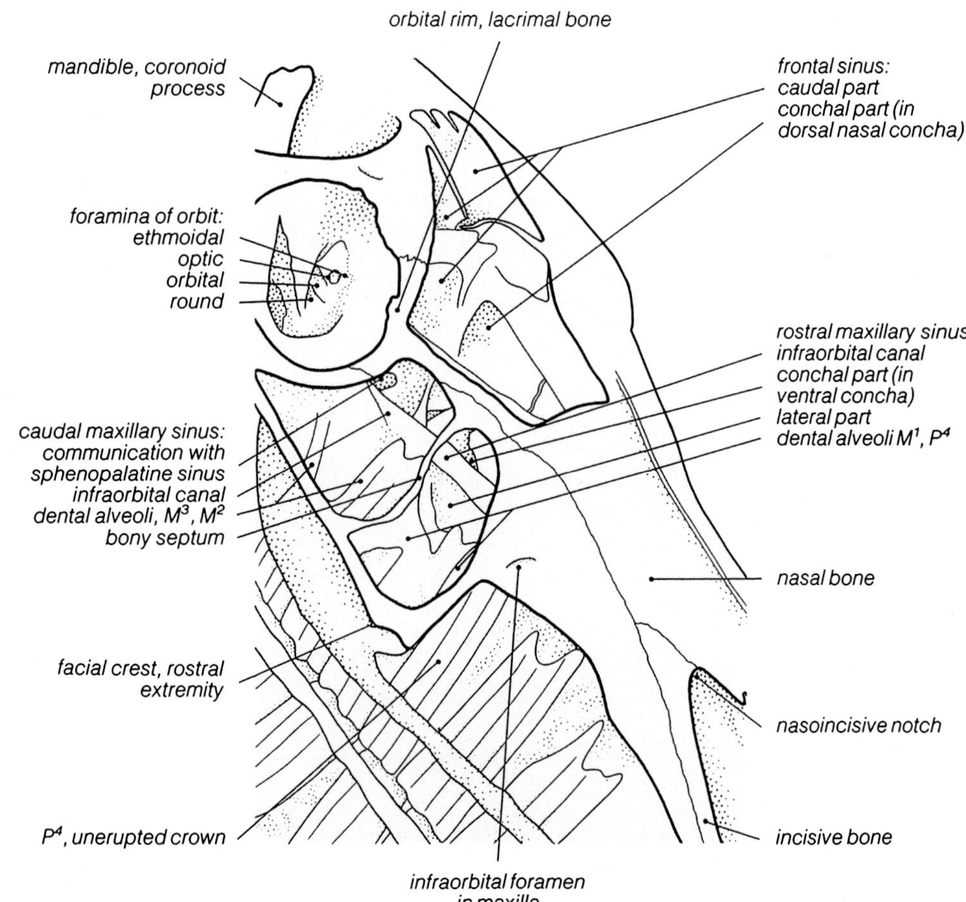
orbital rim, lacrimal bone
mandible, coronoid process
frontal sinus:
caudal part
conchal part (in dorsal nasal concha)
foramina of orbit:
ethmoidal
optic
orbital
round
rostral maxillary sinus:
infraorbital canal
conchal part (in ventral concha)
lateral part
dental alveoli M¹, P⁴
caudal maxillary sinus:
communication with sphenopalatine sinus
infraorbital canal
dental alveoli, M³, M²
bony septum
nasal bone
facial crest, rostral extremity
nasoincisive notch
P⁴, unerupted crown
incisive bone
infraorbital foramen in maxilla

Fig. 1.45 The paranasal sinuses of the 6-year-old horse: right dorsolateral view. This is a part of the skull shown in Fig. 1.44. The relationships of the dental alveoli to the maxillary sinuses are clearly seen, but it should be remembered that the membranous walls of the sinuses have been lost during maceration (compare with Fig. 1.46). The conchal extensions of the frontal and rostral maxillary sinuses are often named as separate sinuses (dorsal and ventral conchal sinuses of the NAV).

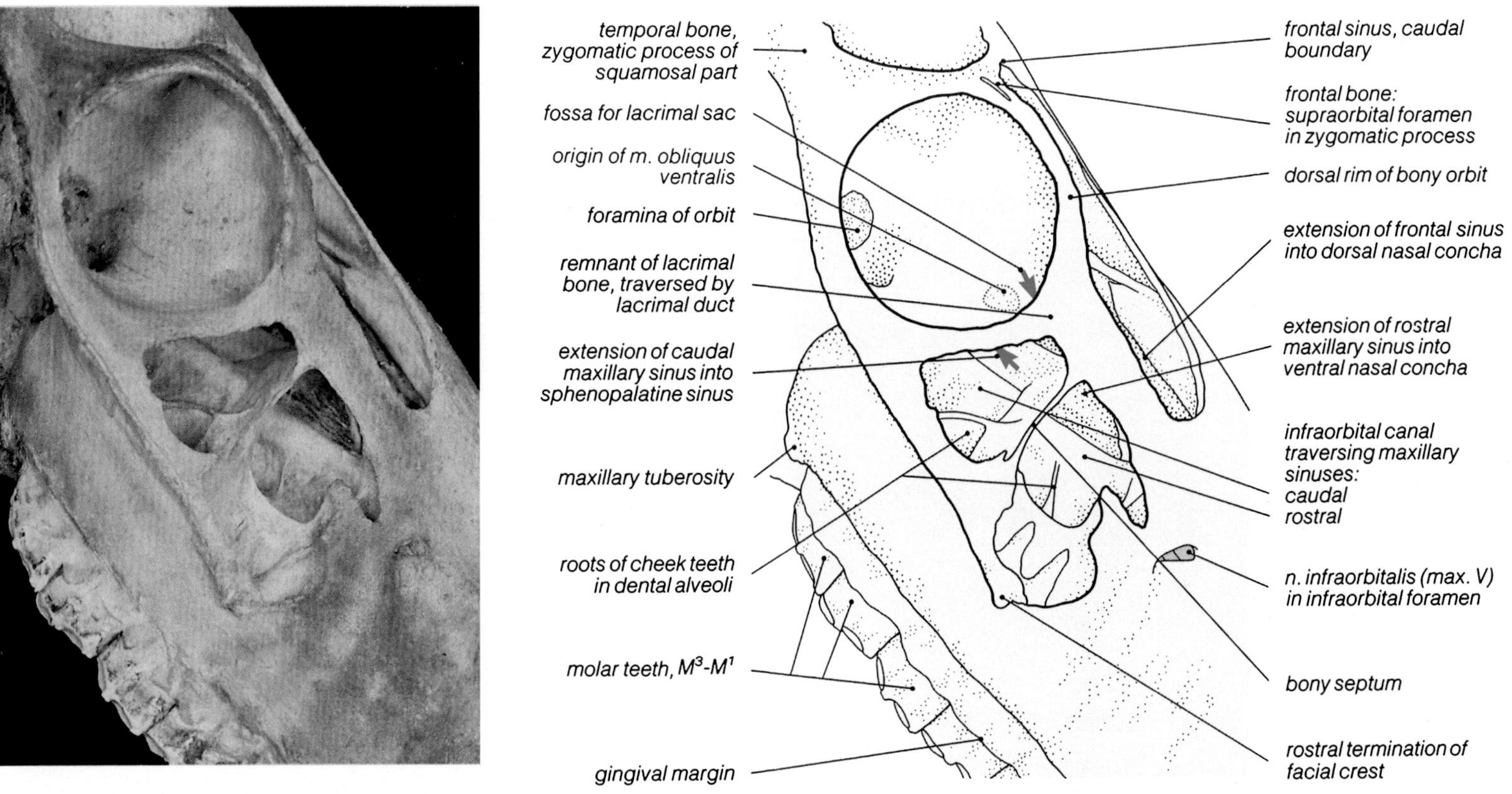
temporal bone, zygomatic process of squamosal part
fossa for lacrimal sac
origin of m. obliquus ventralis
foramina of orbit
remnant of lacrimal bone, traversed by lacrimal duct
extension of caudal maxillary sinus into sphenopalatine sinus
maxillary tuberosity
roots of cheek teeth in dental alveoli
molar teeth, M3-M1
gingival margin
frontal sinus, caudal boundary
frontal bone: supraorbital foramen in zygomatic process
dorsal rim of bony orbit
extension of frontal sinus into dorsal nasal concha
extension of rostral maxillary sinus into ventral nasal concha
infraorbital canal traversing maxillary sinuses:
caudal
rostral
n. infraorbitalis (max. V) in infraorbital foramen
bony septum
rostral termination of facial crest

Fig. 1.46 The infraorbital canal and paranasal sinuses of a 9-year-old horse: right lateral view. In older animals, the crowns of the cheek teeth have become shorter and the dental alveoli do not obscure the infraorbital canals when seen in lateral view. (Compare with dissections of younger animals shown in Figs. 1.35 and 1.59). In this dried specimen, the mucous membrane of the paranasal sinuses has been preserved. The frontal sinus is shown in Fig. 1.47.

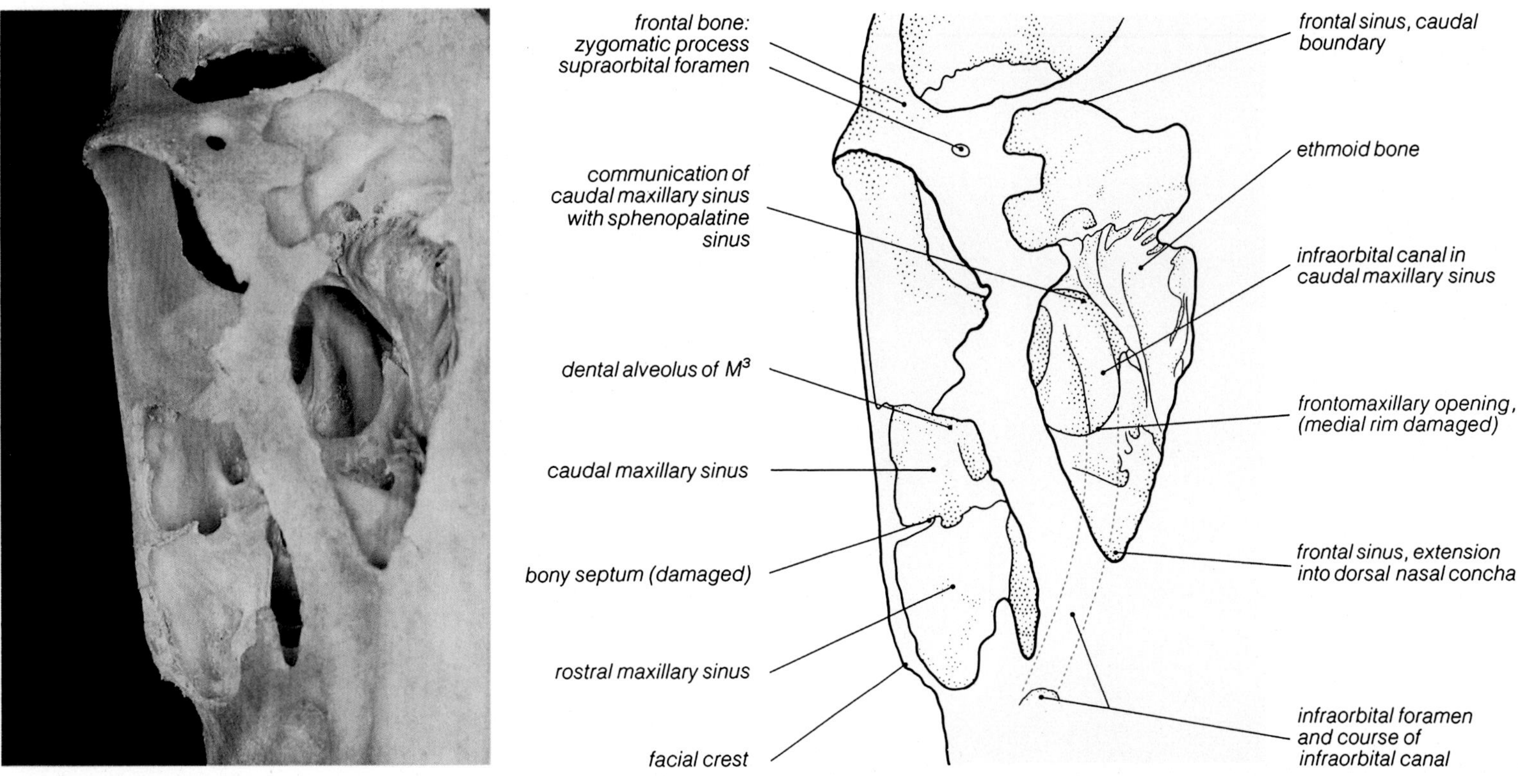
frontal bone: zygomatic process supraorbital foramen
communication of caudal maxillary sinus with sphenopalatine sinus
dental alveolus of M3
caudal maxillary sinus
bony septum (damaged)
rostral maxillary sinus
facial crest
frontal sinus, caudal boundary
ethmoid bone
infraorbital canal in caudal maxillary sinus
frontomaxillary opening, (medial rim damaged)
frontal sinus, extension into dorsal nasal concha
infraorbital foramen and course of infraorbital canal

Fig. 1.47 The infraorbital canal and paranasal sinuses of a 9-year-old horse: dorsal view. The canal traversing the caudal maxillary sinus is clearly visible through the nasomaxillary opening in this older animal (compare with Figs. 1.38 and 1.59). This dried specimen is shown in lateral view in Fig. 1.46.

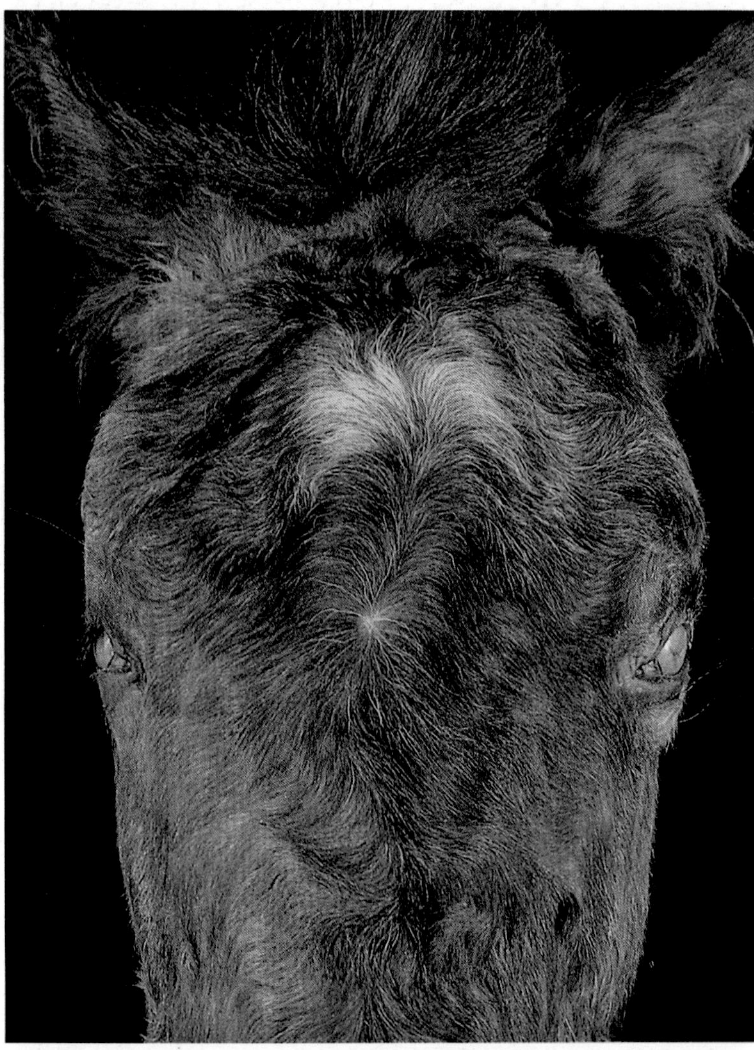

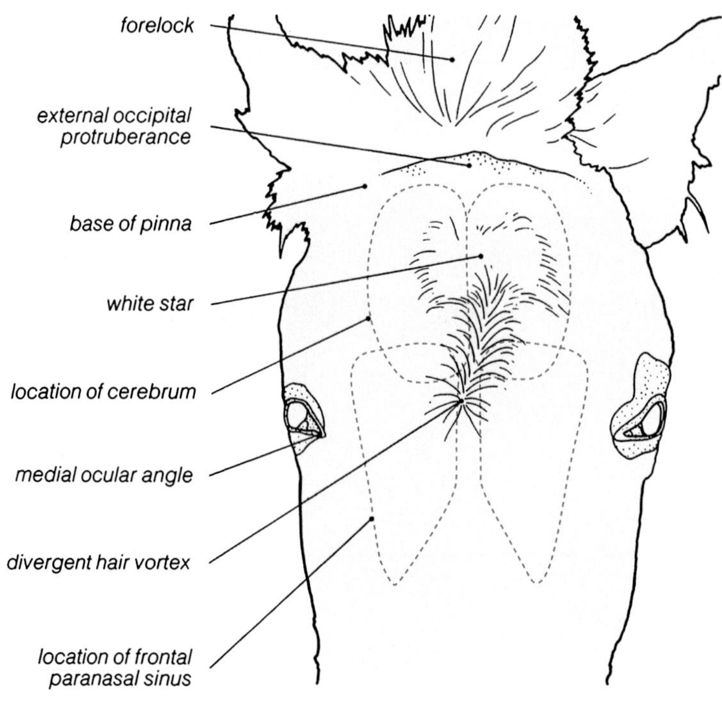
forelock
external occipital protruberance
base of pinna
white star
location of cerebrum
medial ocular angle
divergent hair vortex
location of frontal paranasal sinus

Fig. 1.48 Surface features of the cranial regions in a yearling horse: dorsal view. The position of the divergent hair vortex in relation to the medial ocular angle varies between individuals. The estimated positions of frontal sinuses and cerebrum indicated here are based on the dissection shown in Fig. 1.52. Lines drawn from the base of each pinna to the medial ocular angle of the opposite side will cross in the middle of the cerebrum.

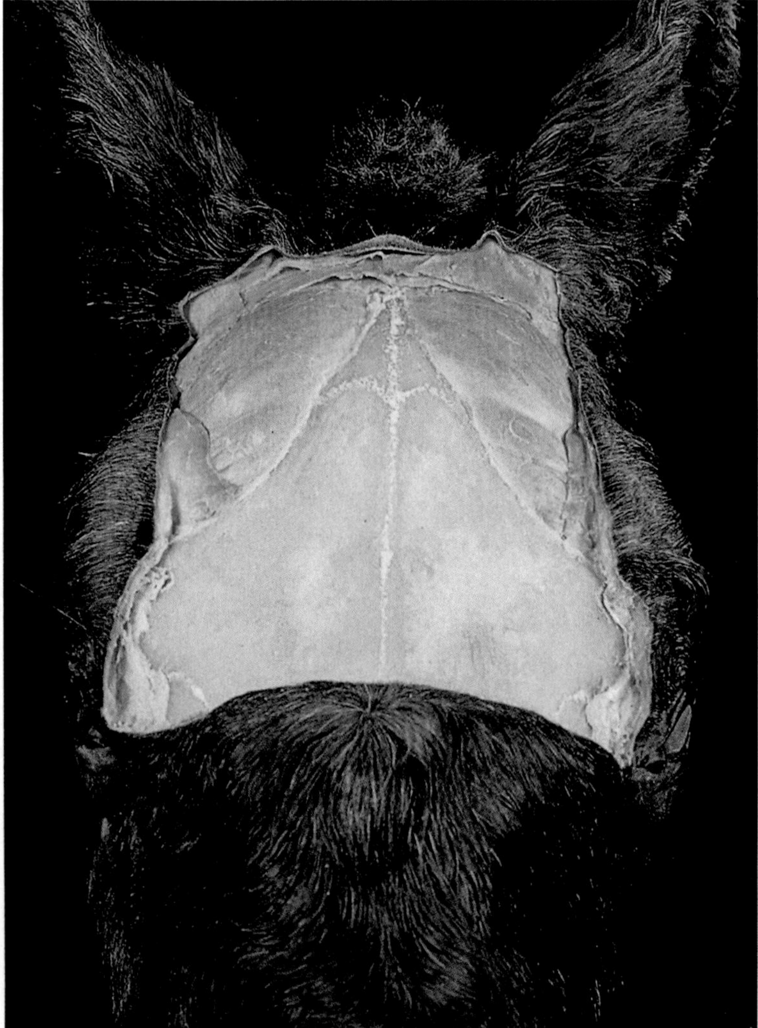

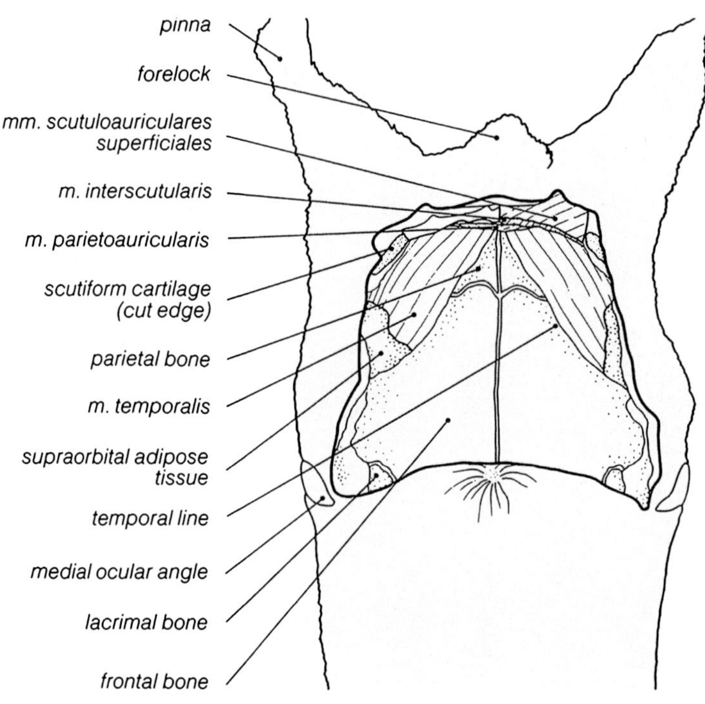
pinna
forelock
mm. scutuloauriculares superficiales
m. interscutularis
m. parietoauricularis
scutiform cartilage (cut edge)
parietal bone
m. temporalis
supraorbital adipose tissue
temporal line
medial ocular angle
lacrimal bone
frontal bone

Fig. 1.49 Superficial structures of the cranial regions in the yearling horse: dorsal view. The muscles of the external ear have been cut away to reveal the frontal bones and the temporalis muscles.

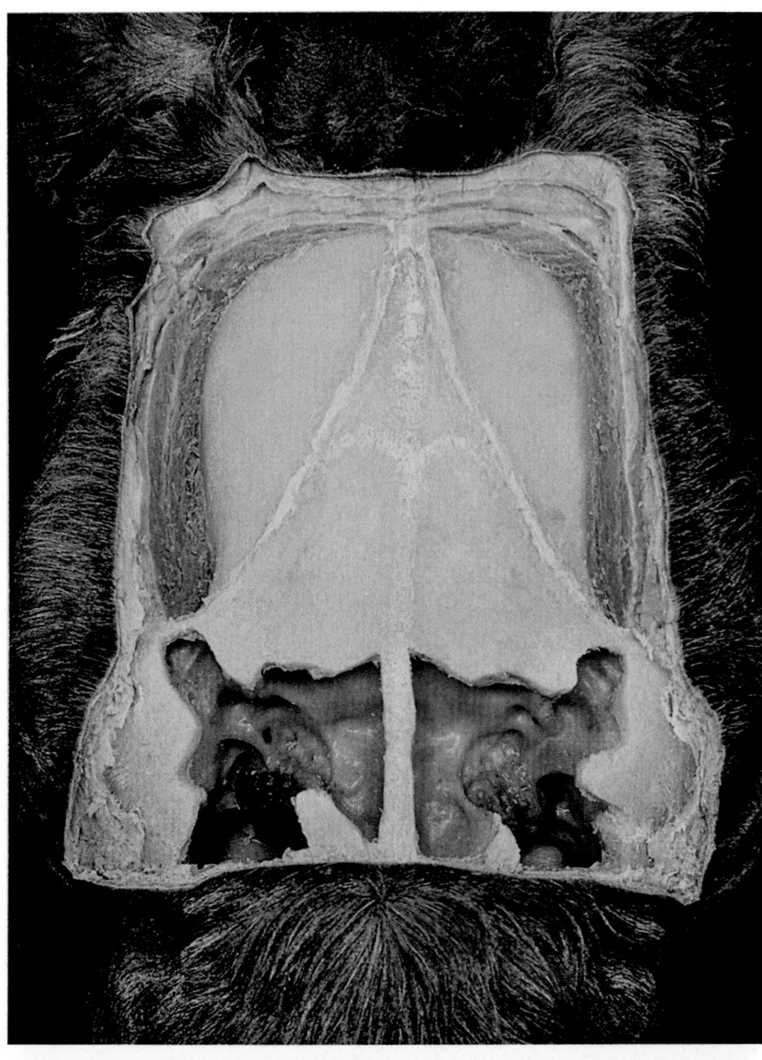

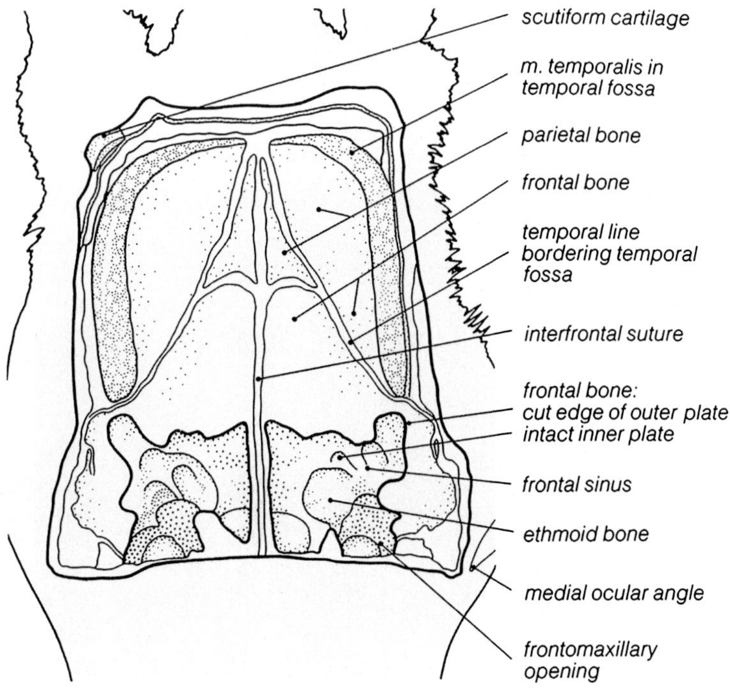
scutiform cartilage
m. temporalis in temporal fossa
parietal bone
frontal bone
temporal line bordering temporal fossa
interfrontal suture
frontal bone: cut edge of outer plate intact inner plate
frontal sinus
ethmoid bone
medial ocular angle
frontomaxillary opening

Fig. 1.50 The temporal fossae and frontal paranasal sinuses of the yearling horse: dorsal view. The dorsal parts of the temporalis muscles have been resected, and the caudal parts of the frontal sinuses have been exposed by removal of the outer plates of the frontal bones. The coronoid processes of the mandible are not visible in the temporal fossae.

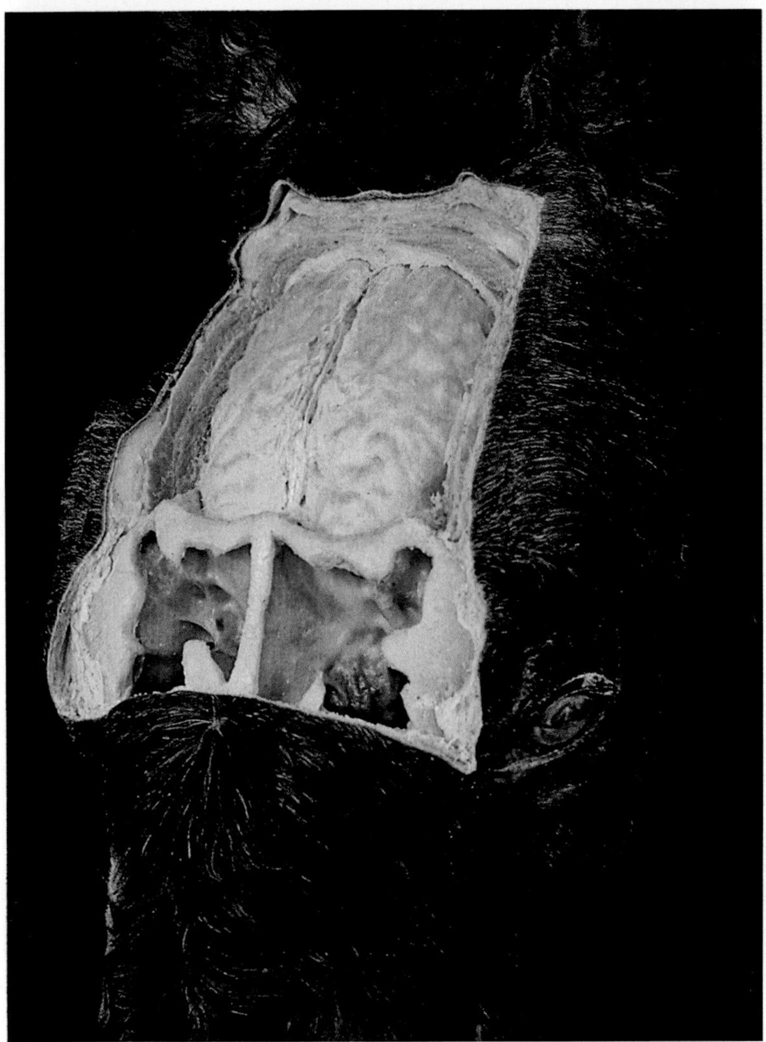

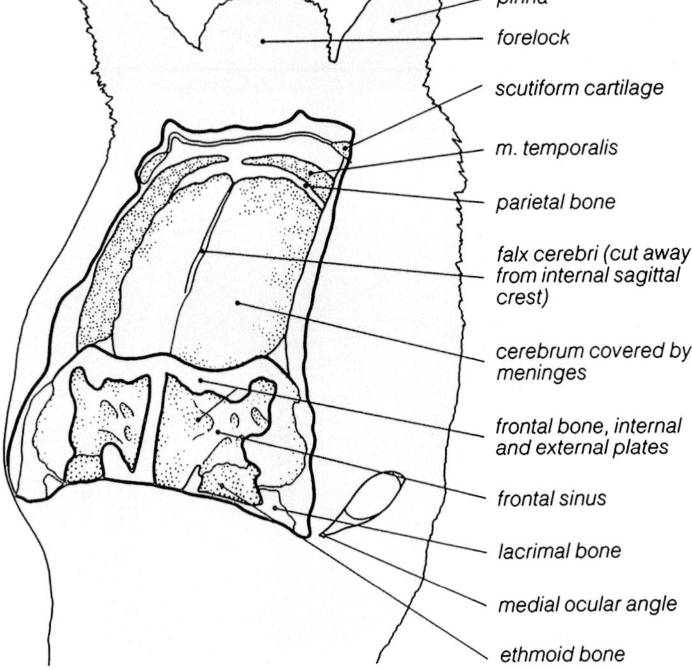
pinna
forelock
scutiform cartilage
m. temporalis
parietal bone
falx cerebri (cut away from internal sagittal crest)
cerebrum covered by meninges
frontal bone, internal and external plates
frontal sinus
lacrimal bone
medial ocular angle
ethmoid bone

Fig. 1.51 The topography of the cerebrum in the yearling horse: left dorsolateral view. The roof of the cranium has been removed. The fused layer of dura mater and cranial endosteum was readily separated from the bone except in the midsagittal plane where the falx cerebri is adherent to the internal sagittal crest of the cranium.

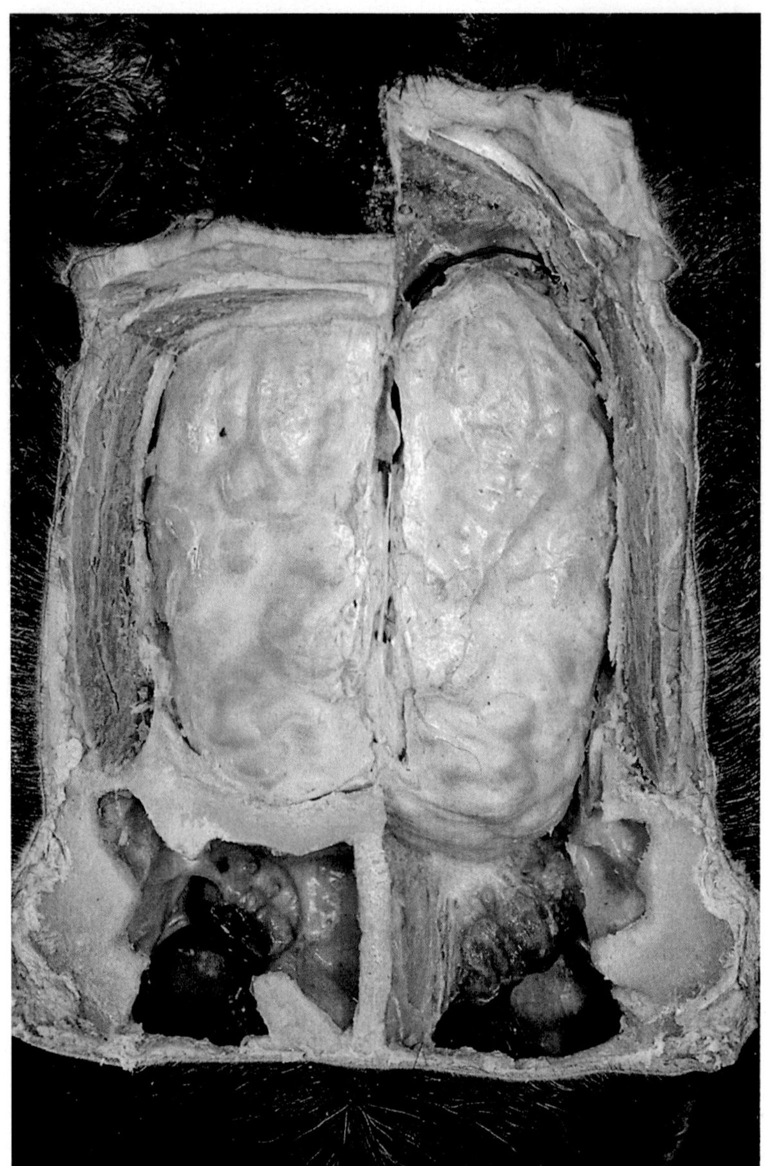

Fig. 1.52 The topography of the cerebrum in the yearling horse: dorsal view. The parietal, frontal and ethmoid bones have been cut away further to display the full extent of the left cerebral hemisphere and the degree to which the frontal paranasal sinus overlaps the cranial cavity.

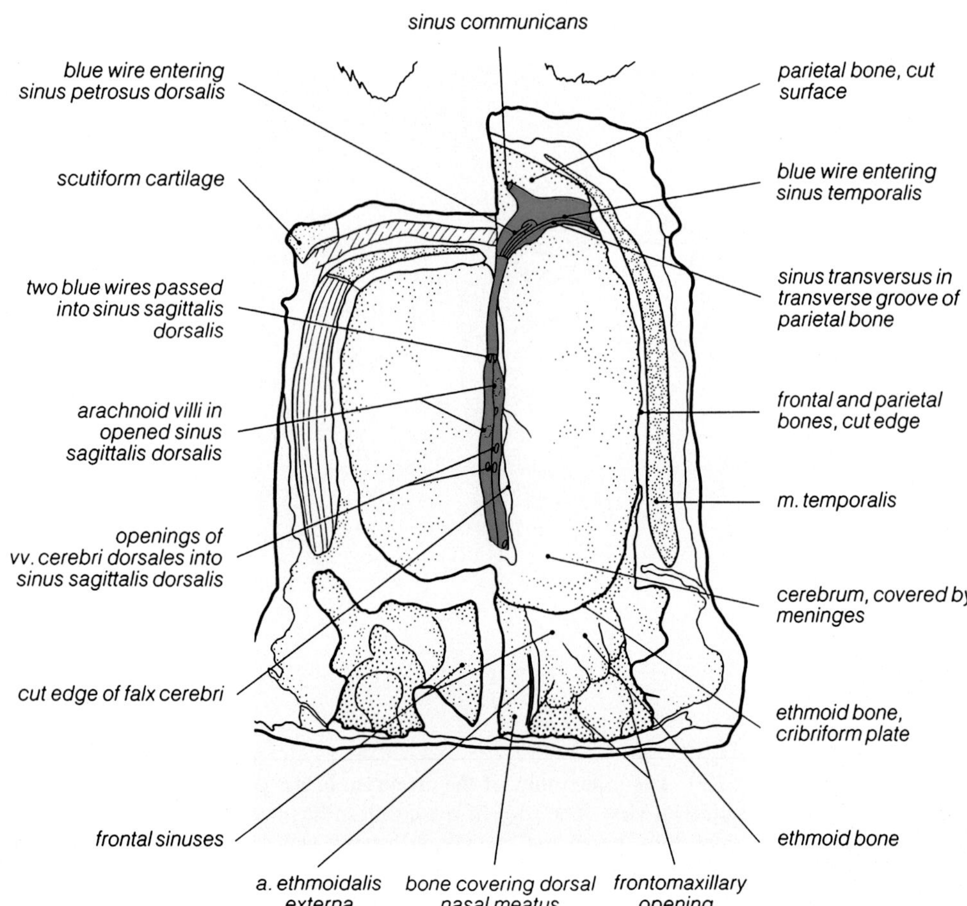
sinus communicans
blue wire entering sinus petrosus dorsalis
scutiform cartilage
two blue wires passed into sinus sagittalis dorsalis
arachnoid villi in opened sinus sagittalis dorsalis
openings of vv. cerebri dorsales into sinus sagittalis dorsalis
cut edge of falx cerebri
frontal sinuses
a. ethmoidalis externa
bone covering dorsal nasal meatus
frontomaxillary opening
parietal bone, cut surface
blue wire entering sinus temporalis
sinus transversus in transverse groove of parietal bone
frontal and parietal bones, cut edge
m. temporalis
cerebrum, covered by meninges
ethmoid bone, cribriform plate
ethmoid bone

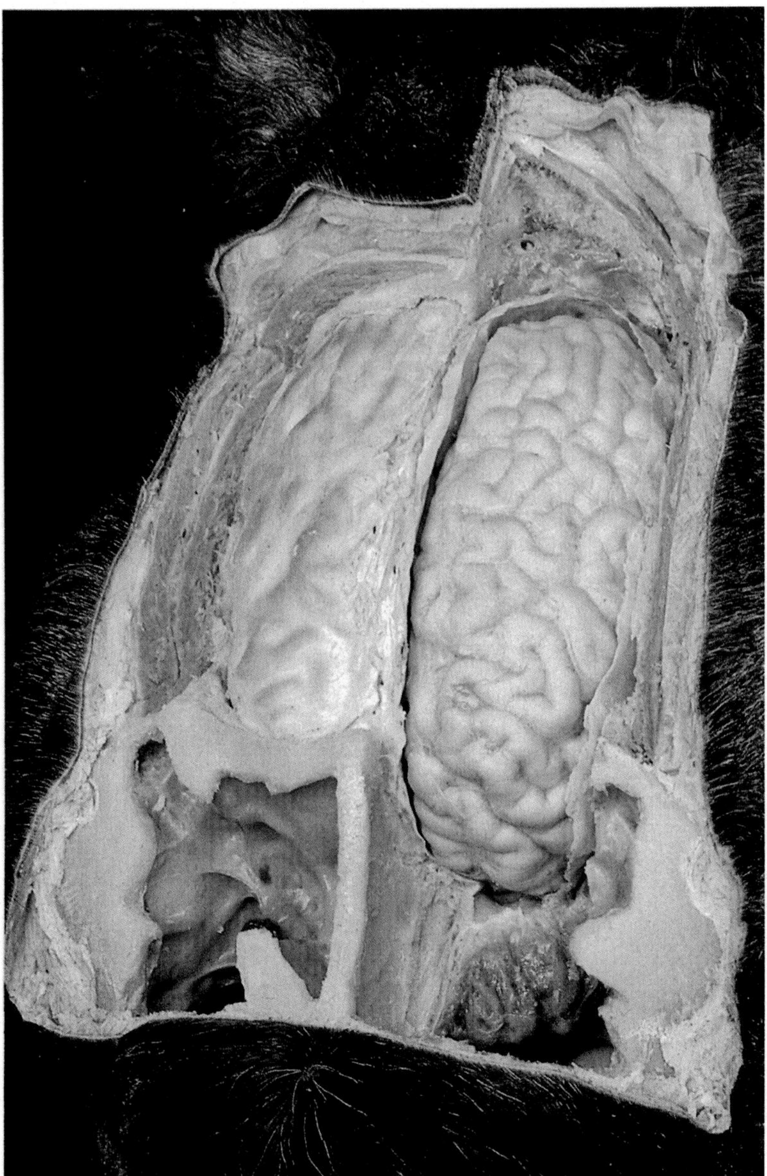

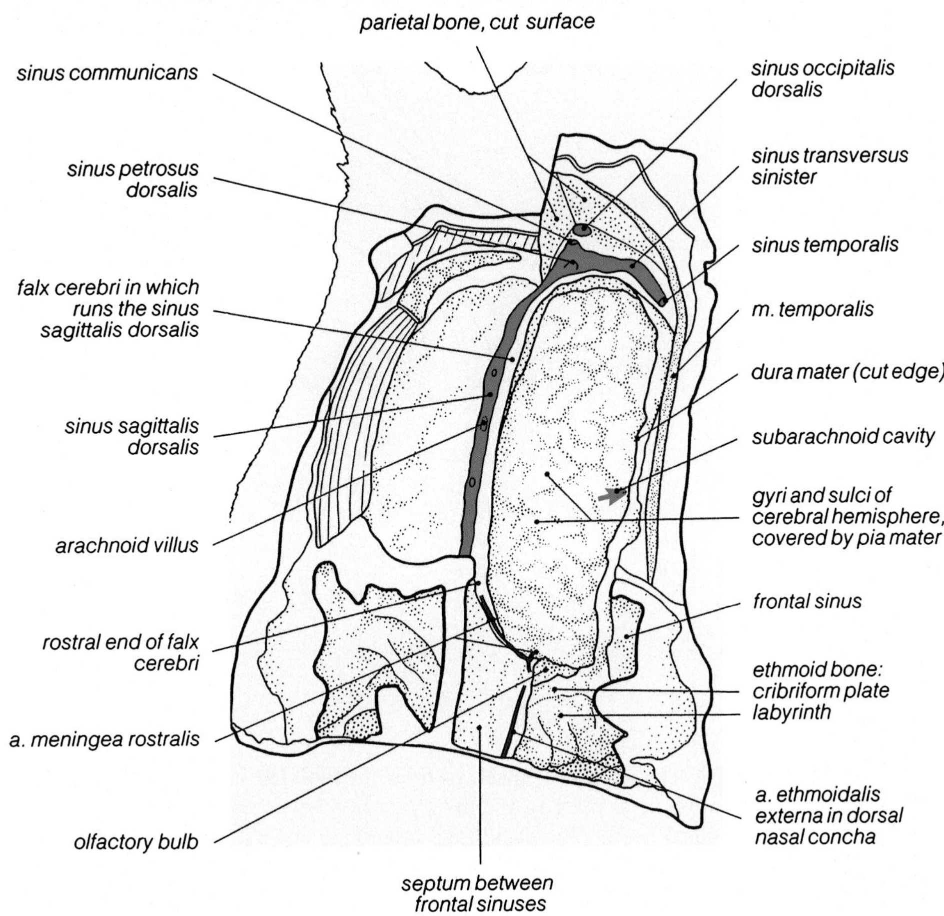
parietal bone, cut surface
sinus communicans
sinus petrosus dorsalis
falx cerebri in which runs the sinus sagittalis dorsalis
sinus sagittalis dorsalis
arachnoid villus
rostral end of falx cerebri
a. meningea rostralis
olfactory bulb
septum between frontal sinuses
sinus occipitalis dorsalis
sinus transversus sinister
sinus temporalis
m. temporalis
dura mater (cut edge)
subarachnoid cavity
gyri and sulci of cerebral hemisphere, covered by pia mater
frontal sinus
ethmoid bone: cribriform plate labyrinth
a. ethmoidalis externa in dorsal nasal concha

Fig. 1.53 The left cerebral hemisphere in a yearling horse: left dorsolateral view. The outer layer of meninges (dura mater and fused cranial endosteum together with the arachnoid membrane) has been removed on the left side to expose the subarachnoid cavity in which lies the brain, surrounded by the delicate pia mater.

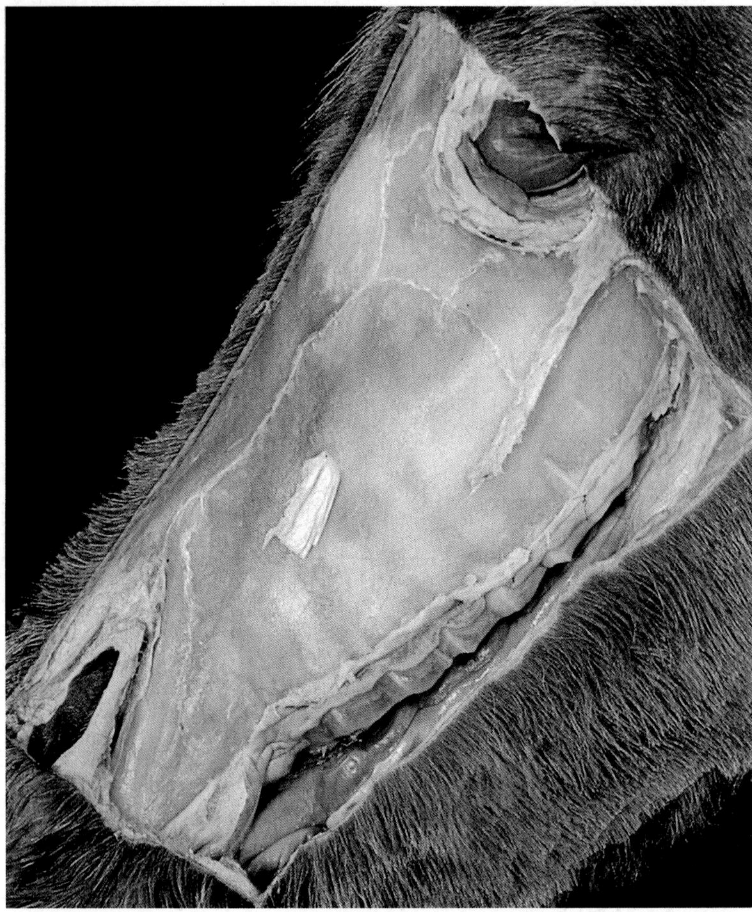

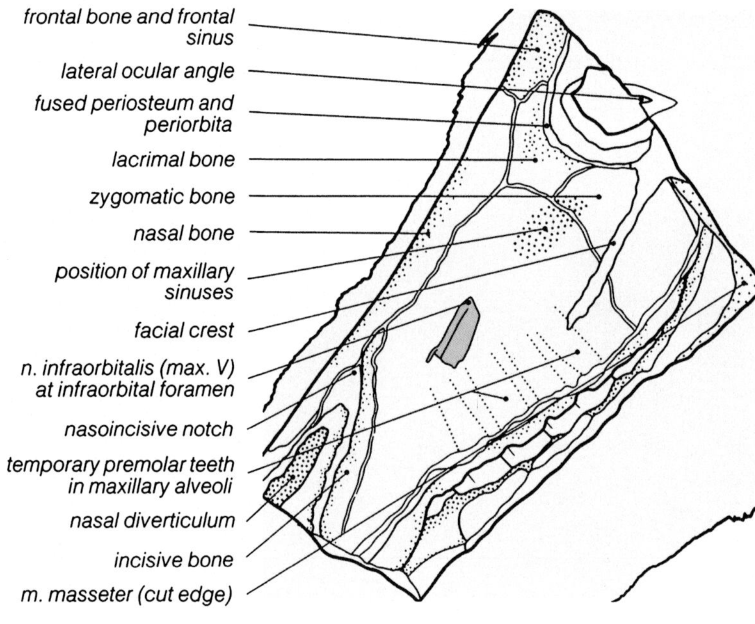
frontal bone and frontal sinus
lateral ocular angle
fused periosteum and periorbita
lacrimal bone
zygomatic bone
nasal bone
position of maxillary sinuses
facial crest
n. infraorbitalis (max. V) at infraorbital foramen
nasoincisive notch
temporary premolar teeth in maxillary alveoli
nasal diverticulum
incisive bone
m. masseter (cut edge)

Fig. 1.54 The bones of the facial region of the foal: left lateral view. Removal of the periosteum from the facial bones of this foal shows the positions of paranasal sinuses and dental alveoli lying between superficial and deep plates of the flat bones. The bony sutures were painted white.

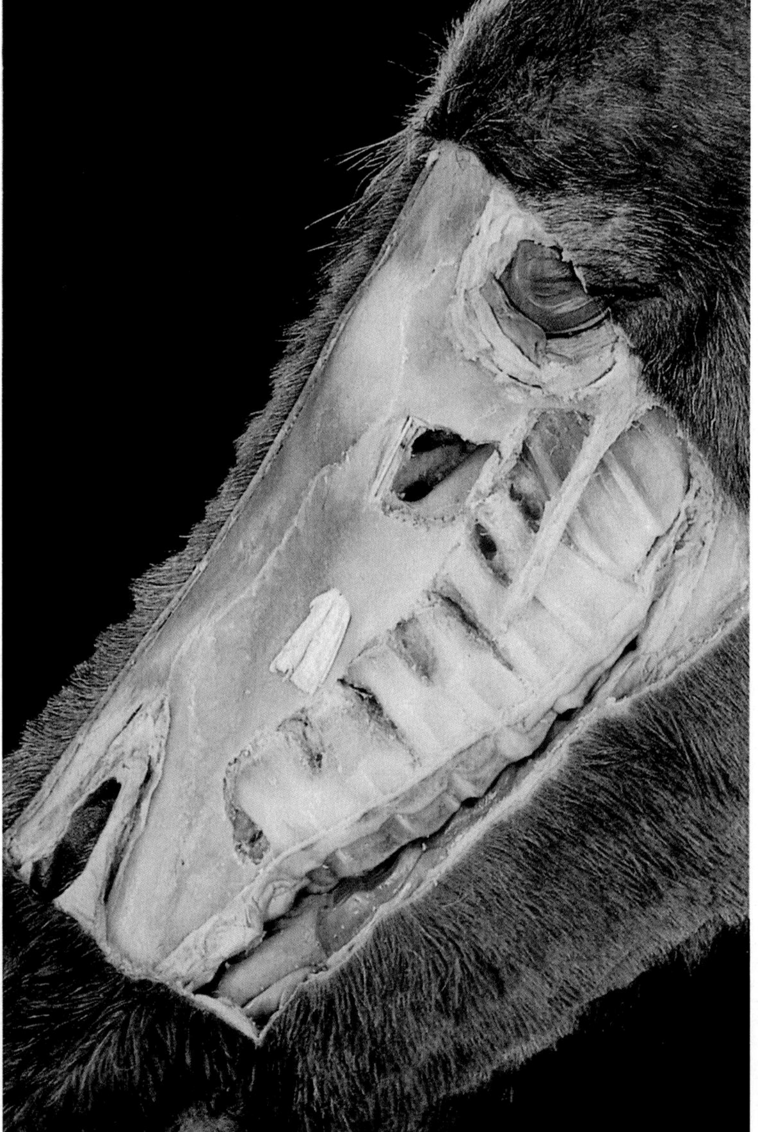

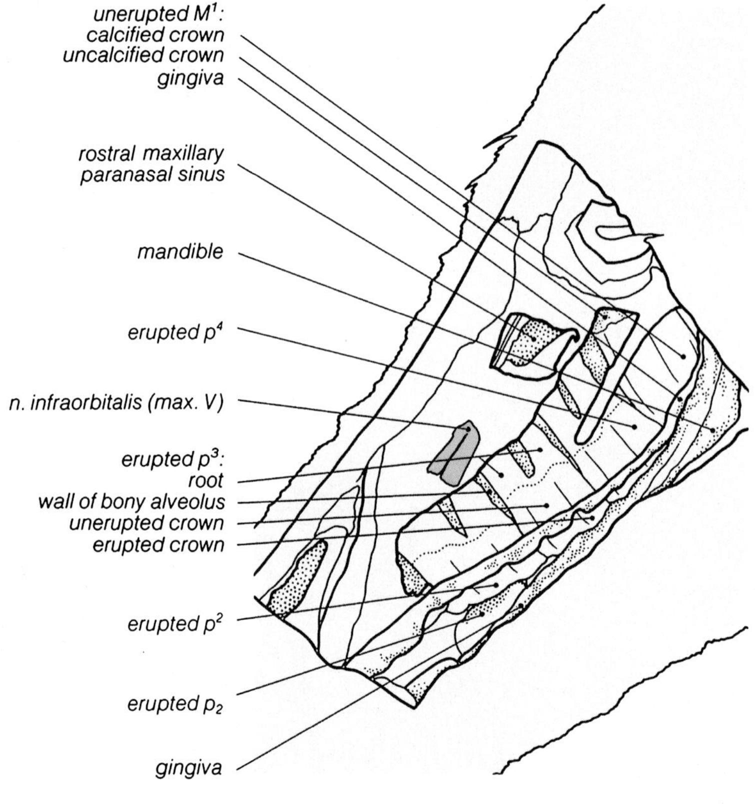
unerupted M^1:
calcified crown
uncalcified crown
gingiva
rostral maxillary paranasal sinus
mandible
erupted p^4
n. infraorbitalis (max. V)
erupted p^3:
root
wall of bony alveolus
unerupted crown
erupted crown
erupted p^2
erupted p_2
gingiva

Fig. 1.55 The maxillary cheek teeth of the foal: left lateral view. Removal of the superficial plate of the maxillary bone exposes the crowns and roots of the cheek teeth. The deciduous premolars erupt at about the time of birth. The first molar tooth erupts at 6–9 months of age. The mandibular cheek teeth and the incisors of this foal are shown in Figs. 1.57 and 1.63.

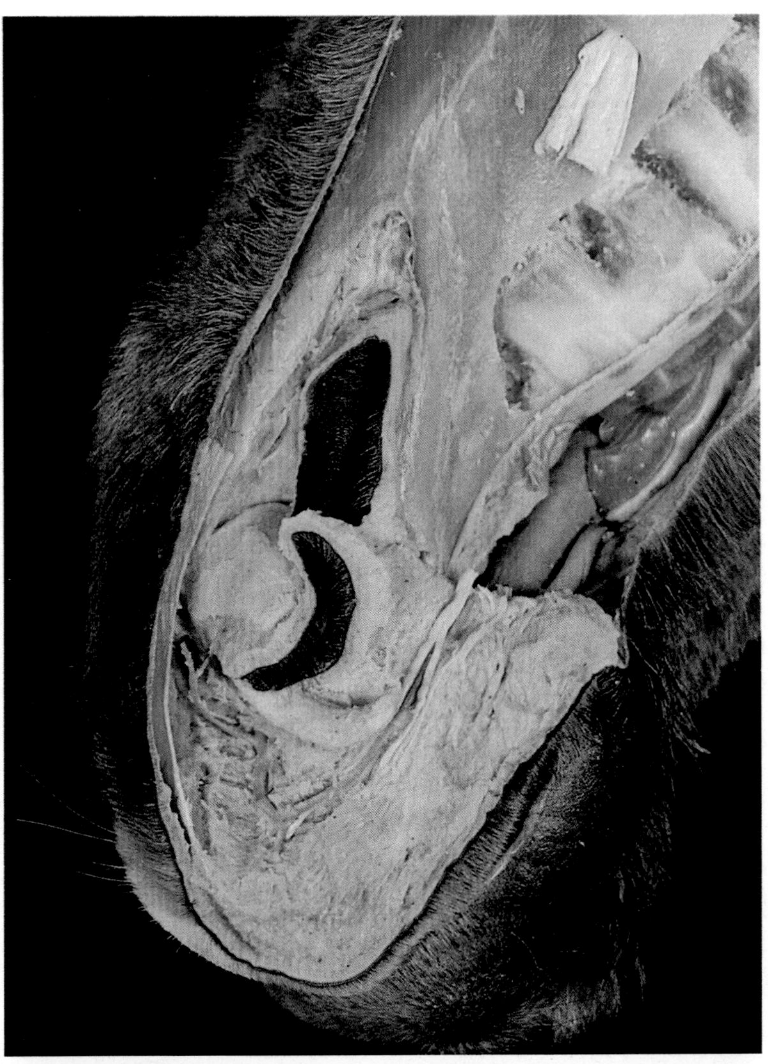

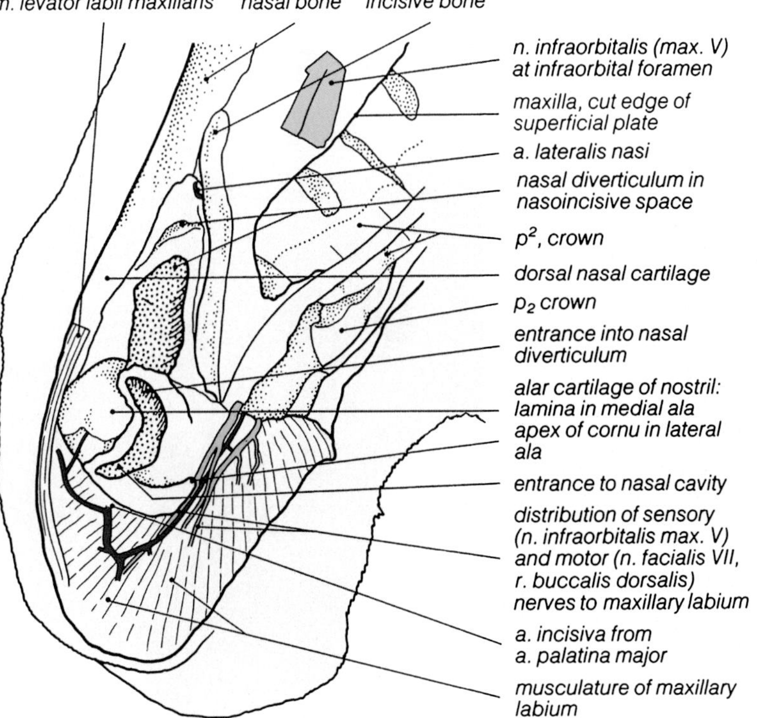
m. levator labii maxillaris
nasal bone
incisive bone
n. infraorbitalis (max. V) at infraorbital foramen
maxilla, cut edge of superficial plate
a. lateralis nasi
nasal diverticulum in nasoincisive space
p², crown
dorsal nasal cartilage
p₂ crown
entrance into nasal diverticulum
alar cartilage of nostril: lamina in medial ala
apex of cornu in lateral ala
entrance to nasal cavity
distribution of sensory (n. infraorbitalis max. V) and motor (n. facialis VII, r. buccalis dorsalis) nerves to maxillary labium
a. incisiva from a. palatina major
musculature of maxillary labium

Fig. 1.56 The maxillary labium and nostril of the foal: left rostrolateral view. Further details of this region are shown in Fig. 1.57. See also Fig. 1.6 for surface features and Figs. 1.39–1.41; Fig. 1.12 for dissections of muscles.

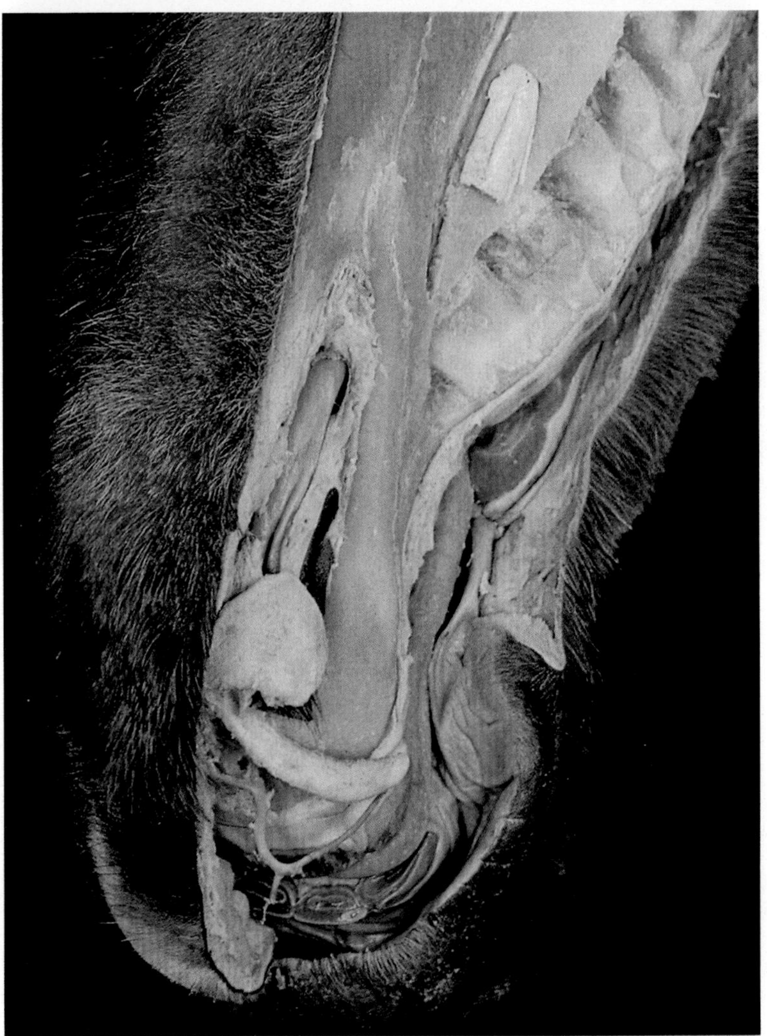

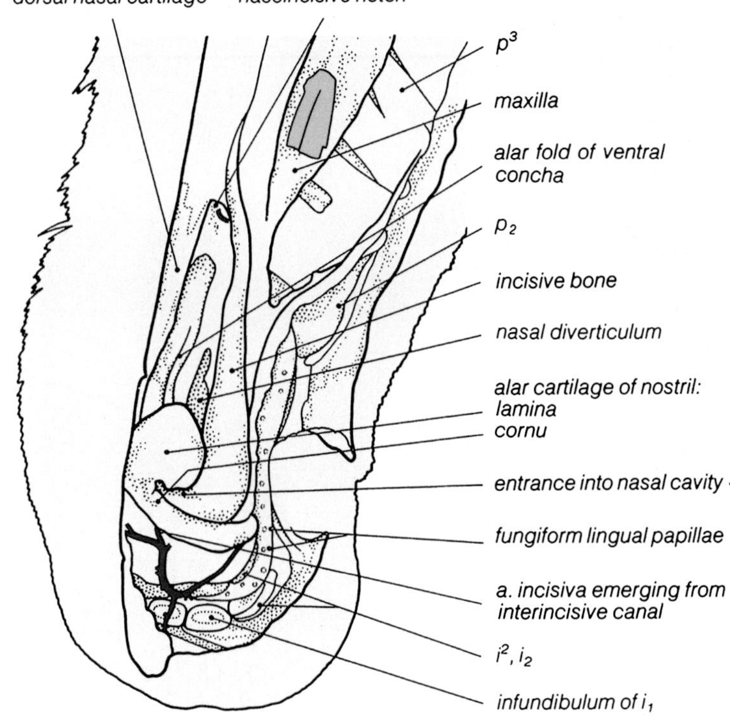
dorsal nasal cartilage
nasoincisive notch
p³
maxilla
alar fold of ventral concha
p₂
incisive bone
nasal diverticulum
alar cartilage of nostril: lamina
cornu
entrance into nasal cavity
fungiform lingual papillae
a. incisiva emerging from interincisive canal
i², i₂
infundibulum of i₁

Fig. 1.57 Structures of the nostril and nasoincisive space of the foal: left rostrolateral view. The nostril has been dissected to expose the alar cartilage and the incisive bone. The wall of the nasal cavity lying in the nasoincisive space has been resected to show the alar fold and the ventral part of the nasal diverticulum. The third deciduous incisors erupt at 6–9 months of age.

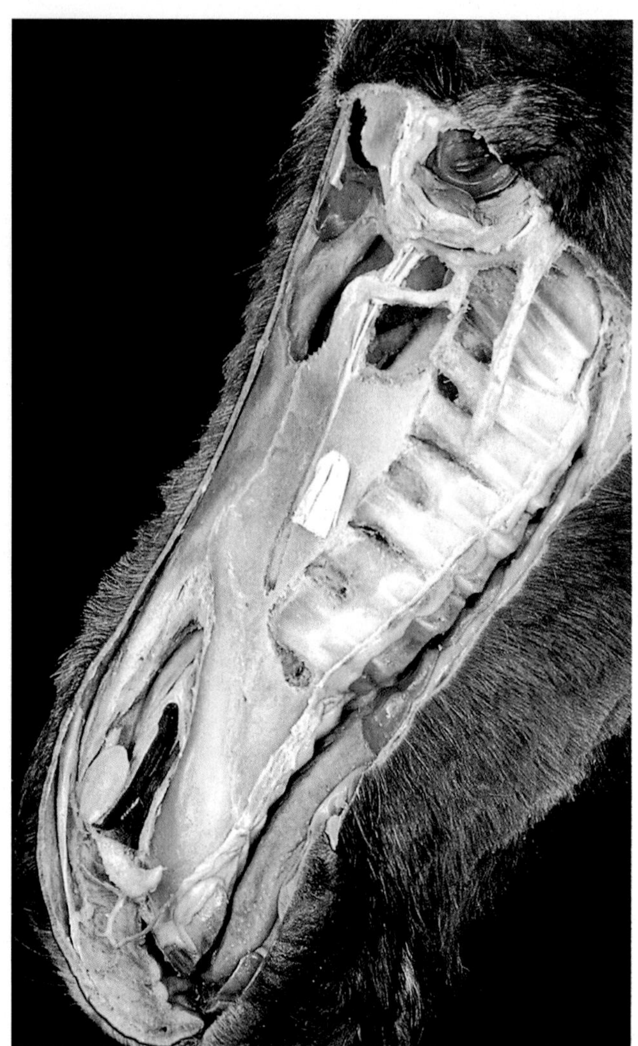

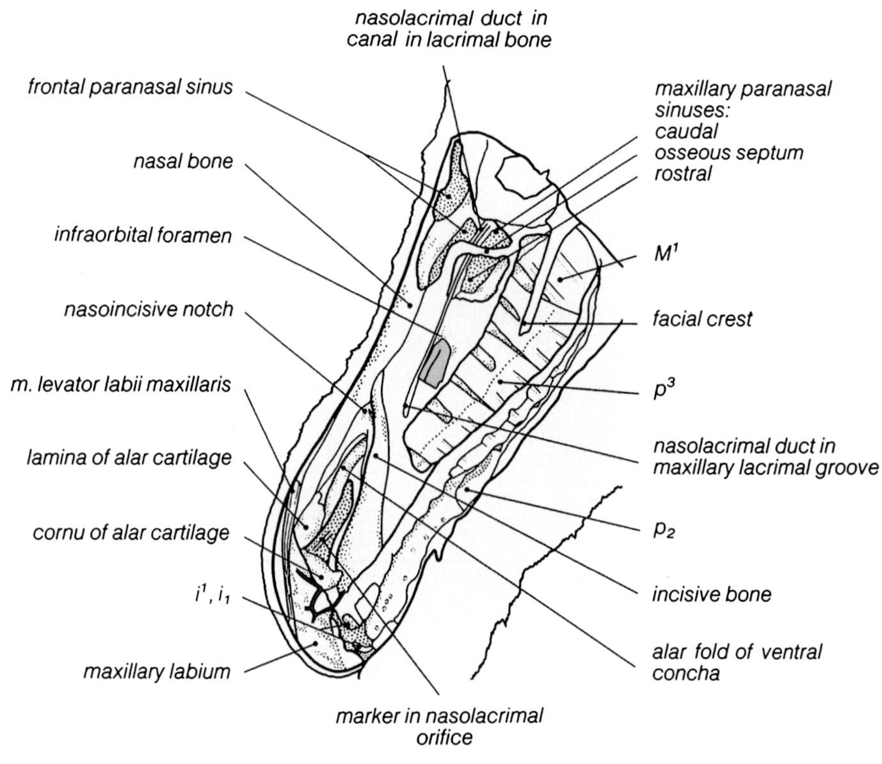

nasolacrimal duct in canal in lacrimal bone
frontal paranasal sinus
nasal bone
infraorbital foramen
nasoincisive notch
m. levator labii maxillaris
lamina of alar cartilage
cornu of alar cartilage
i^1, i_1
maxillary labium
marker in nasolacrimal orifice
maxillary paranasal sinuses:
caudal
osseous septum
rostral
M^1
facial crest
p^3
nasolacrimal duct in maxillary lacrimal groove
p_2
incisive bone
alar fold of ventral concha

Fig. 1.58 The paranasal sinuses and nasolacrimal duct of the foal: left lateral view. A white marker has been placed in the nasolacrimal duct. Further details of this dissection are shown in Fig. 1.59.

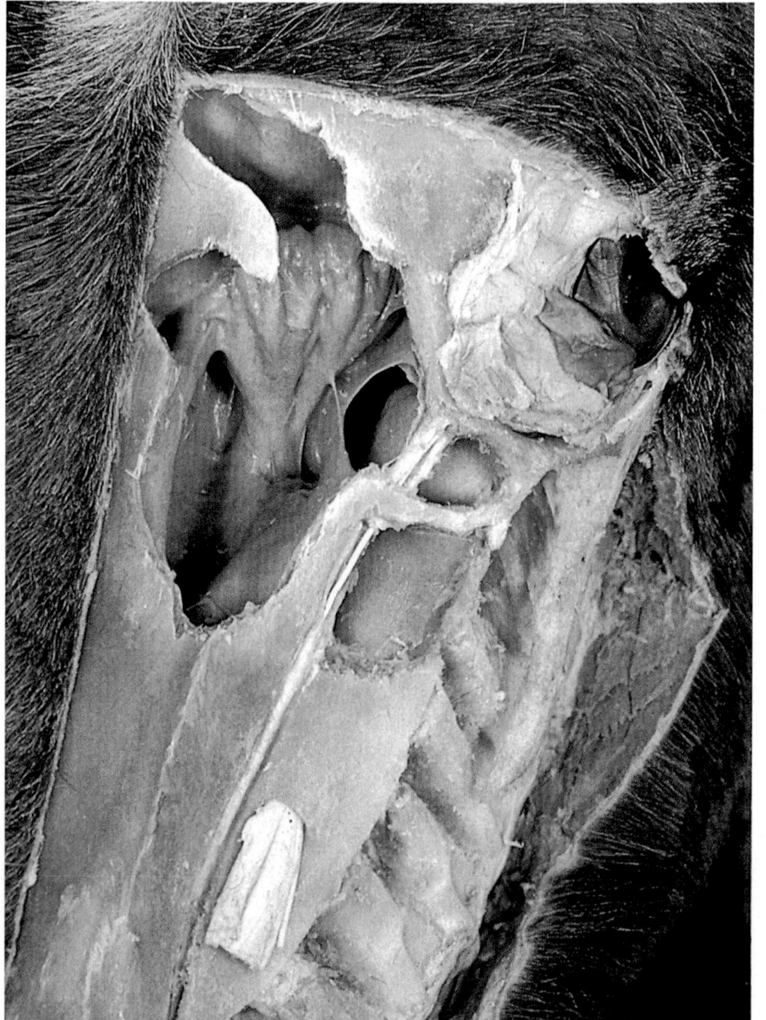

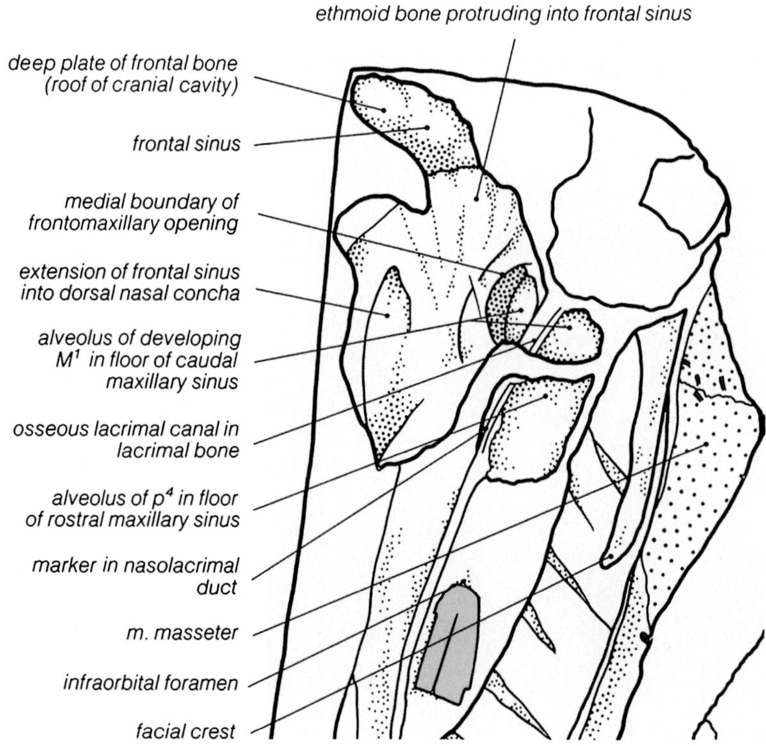

ethmoid bone protruding into frontal sinus
deep plate of frontal bone (roof of cranial cavity)
frontal sinus
medial boundary of frontomaxillary opening
extension of frontal sinus into dorsal nasal concha
alveolus of developing M^1 in floor of caudal maxillary sinus
osseous lacrimal canal in lacrimal bone
alveolus of p^4 in floor of rostral maxillary sinus
marker in nasolacrimal duct
m. masseter
infraorbital foramen
facial crest

Fig. 1.59 The frontal and maxillary paranasal sinuses of the foal: left dorsolateral view. In this foal, aged about 6 months, the maxillary sinuses are small and the developing teeth bulge into their ventral floors. The infraorbital canal is hidden by these teeth; in later life it becomes a conspicuous feature of the maxillary sinuses, as shown in Figs.1.45 and 1.46.

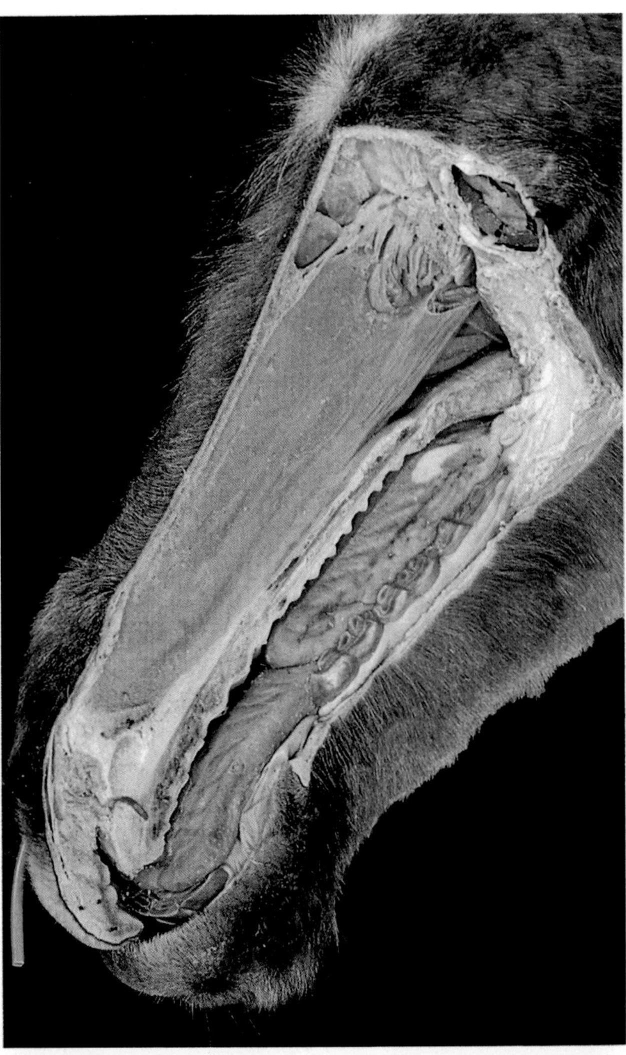

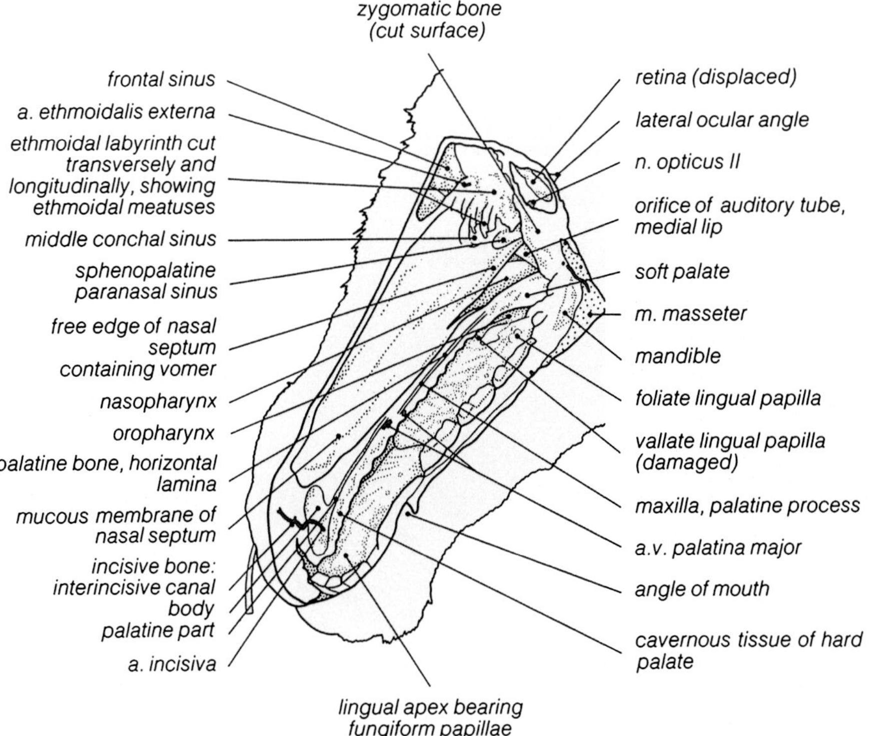

zygomatic bone (cut surface)
frontal sinus
a. ethmoidalis externa
ethmoidal labyrinth cut transversely and longitudinally, showing ethmoidal meatuses
middle conchal sinus
sphenopalatine paranasal sinus
free edge of nasal septum containing vomer
nasopharynx
oropharynx
palatine bone, horizontal lamina
mucous membrane of nasal septum
incisive bone: interincisive canal
body
palatine part
a. incisiva
lingual apex bearing fungiform papillae
retina (displaced)
lateral ocular angle
n. opticus II
orifice of auditory tube, medial lip
soft palate
m. masseter
mandible
foliate lingual papilla
vallate lingual papilla (damaged)
maxilla, palatine process
a.v. palatina major
angle of mouth
cavernous tissue of hard palate

Fig. 1.60 The nasal septum of the foal: left dorsolateral view. The left nasal cavity and maxillary dental arcade have been removed by a transverse and a median incision. The pattern of blood vessels in the submucosa of the septum is just visible. A green tube has been passed through the right nasal cavity and the nasopharynx to enter the orifice of the auditory tube. The apparent dorsal lingual torus is an artefact in this specimen; see Fig. 1.74.

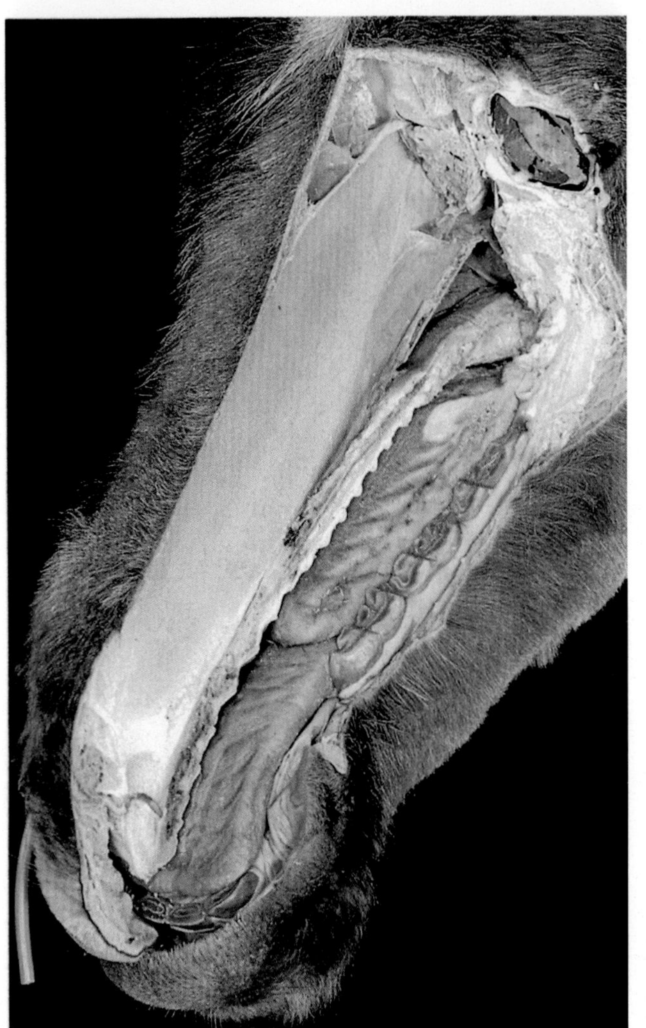

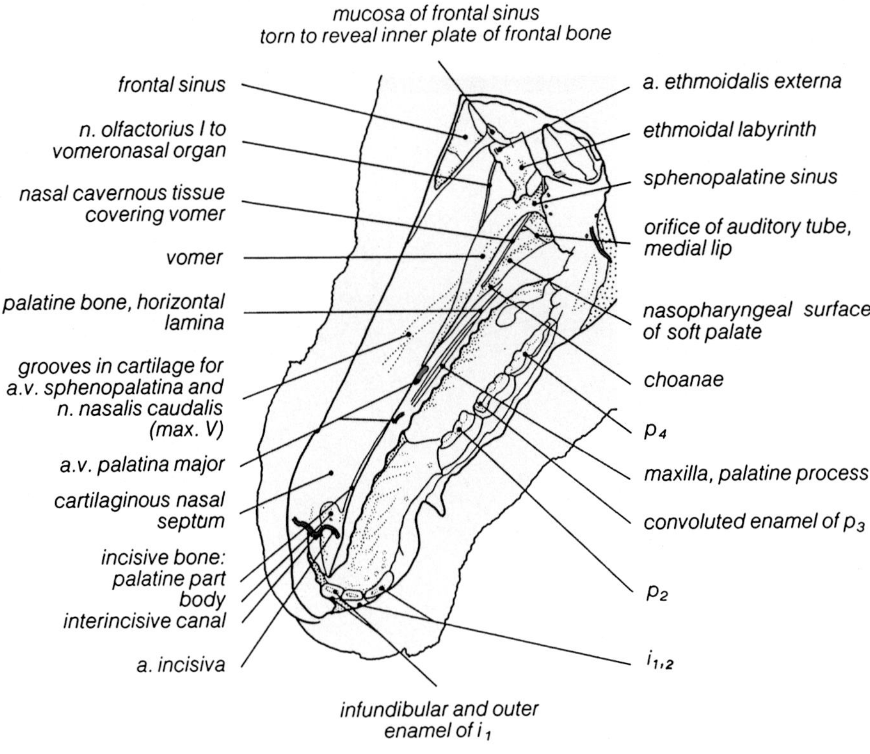

mucosa of frontal sinus torn to reveal inner plate of frontal bone
frontal sinus
n. olfactorius I to vomeronasal organ
nasal cavernous tissue covering vomer
vomer
palatine bone, horizontal lamina
grooves in cartilage for a.v. sphenopalatina and n. nasalis caudalis (max. V)
a.v. palatina major
cartilaginous nasal septum
incisive bone: palatine part
body
interincisive canal
a. incisiva
infundibular and outer enamel of i_1
a. ethmoidalis externa
ethmoidal labyrinth
sphenopalatine sinus
orifice of auditory tube, medial lip
nasopharyngeal surface of soft palate
choanae
p_4
maxilla, palatine process
convoluted enamel of p_3
p_2
$i_{1,2}$

Fig. 1.61 The cartilaginous nasal septum and mandibular teeth of the foal: left dorsolateral view. The nasal mucous membrane has been removed to show that in this foal little ossification of the nasal septum has occurred; at a later stage the caudal part of the nasal septum will ossify to form the perpendicular ethmoidal plate. The first mandibular molar erupts at 9–12 months and the third deciduous incisor at 6–9 months. No mandibular 'wolf tooth' is visible.

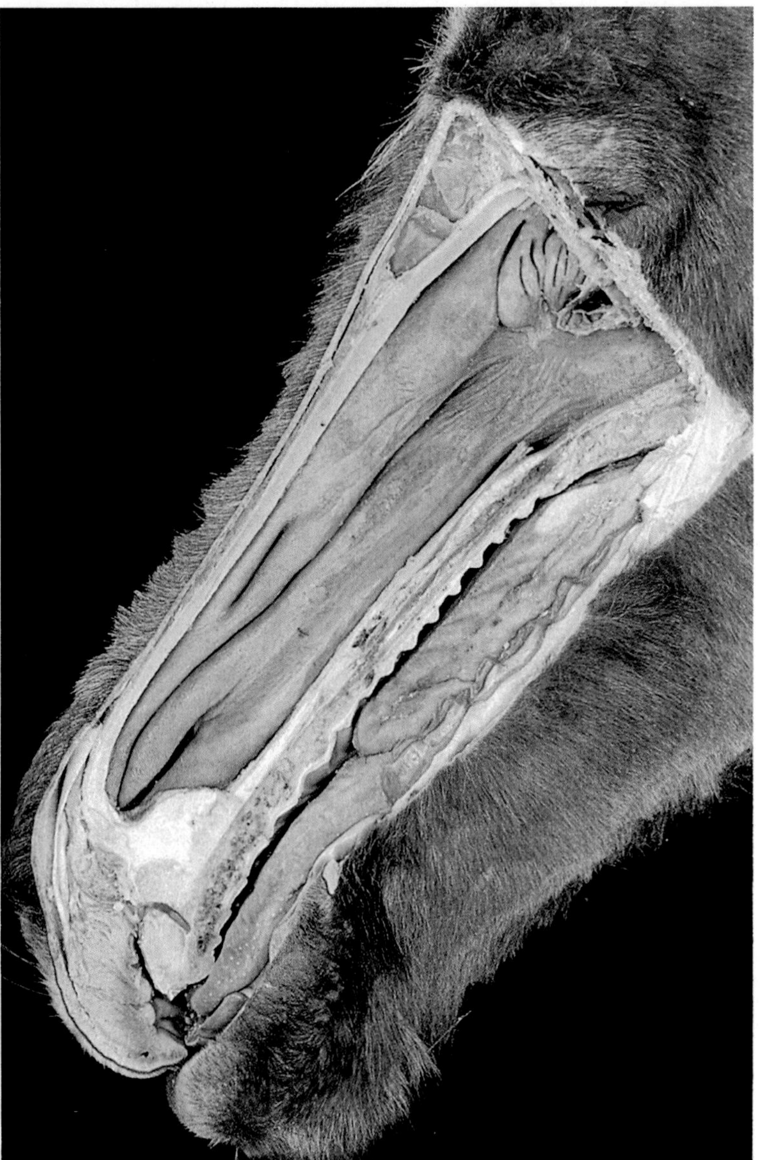

Fig. 1.62 The right nasal cavity of the foal: left lateral view. Most of the nasal septum has now been removed to reveal the structures of the right lateral wall of the nasal cavity. The common nasal meatus cannot be satisfactorily labelled; it lies between the nasal conchae and the nasal septum.

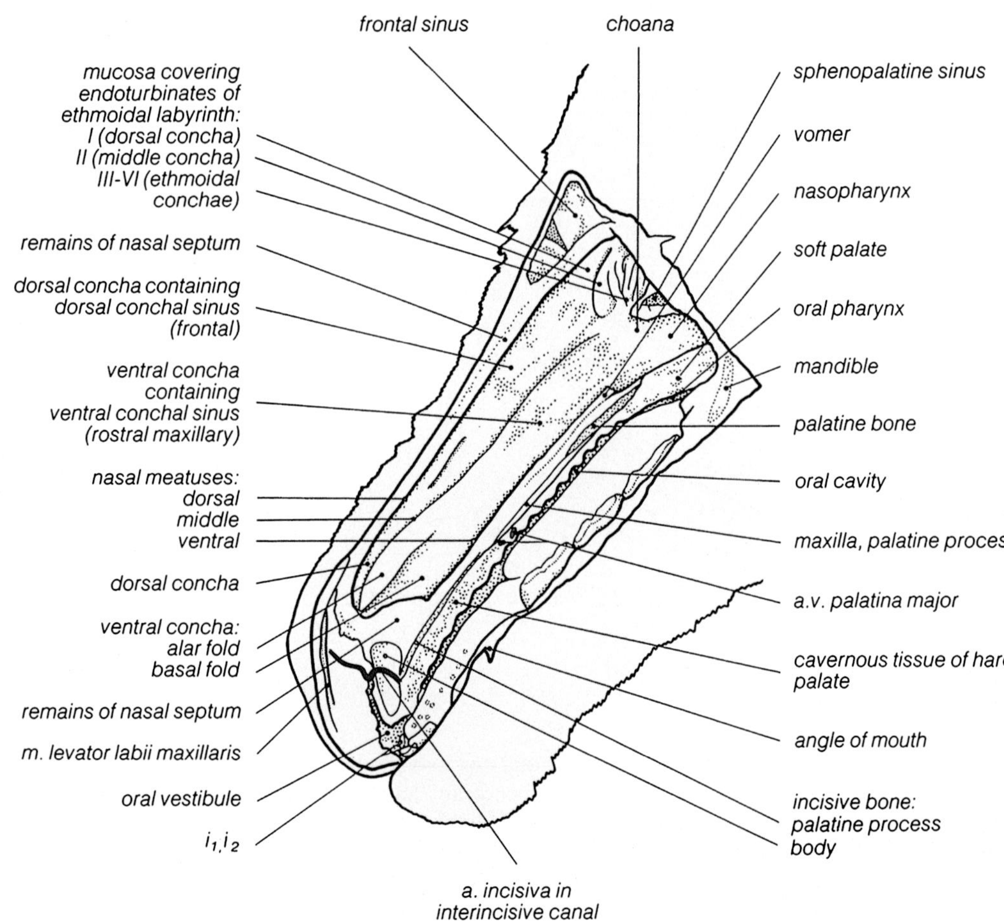
frontal sinus
choana
mucosa covering endoturbinates of ethmoidal labyrinth:
I (dorsal concha)
II (middle concha)
III-VI (ethmoidal conchae)
remains of nasal septum
dorsal concha containing dorsal conchal sinus (frontal)
ventral concha containing ventral conchal sinus (rostral maxillary)
nasal meatuses:
dorsal
middle
ventral
dorsal concha
ventral concha:
alar fold
basal fold
remains of nasal septum
m. levator labii maxillaris
oral vestibule
i_1, i_2
a. incisiva in interincisive canal
sphenopalatine sinus
vomer
nasopharynx
soft palate
oral pharynx
mandible
palatine bone
oral cavity
maxilla, palatine process
a.v. palatina major
cavernous tissue of hard palate
angle of mouth
incisive bone:
palatine process
body

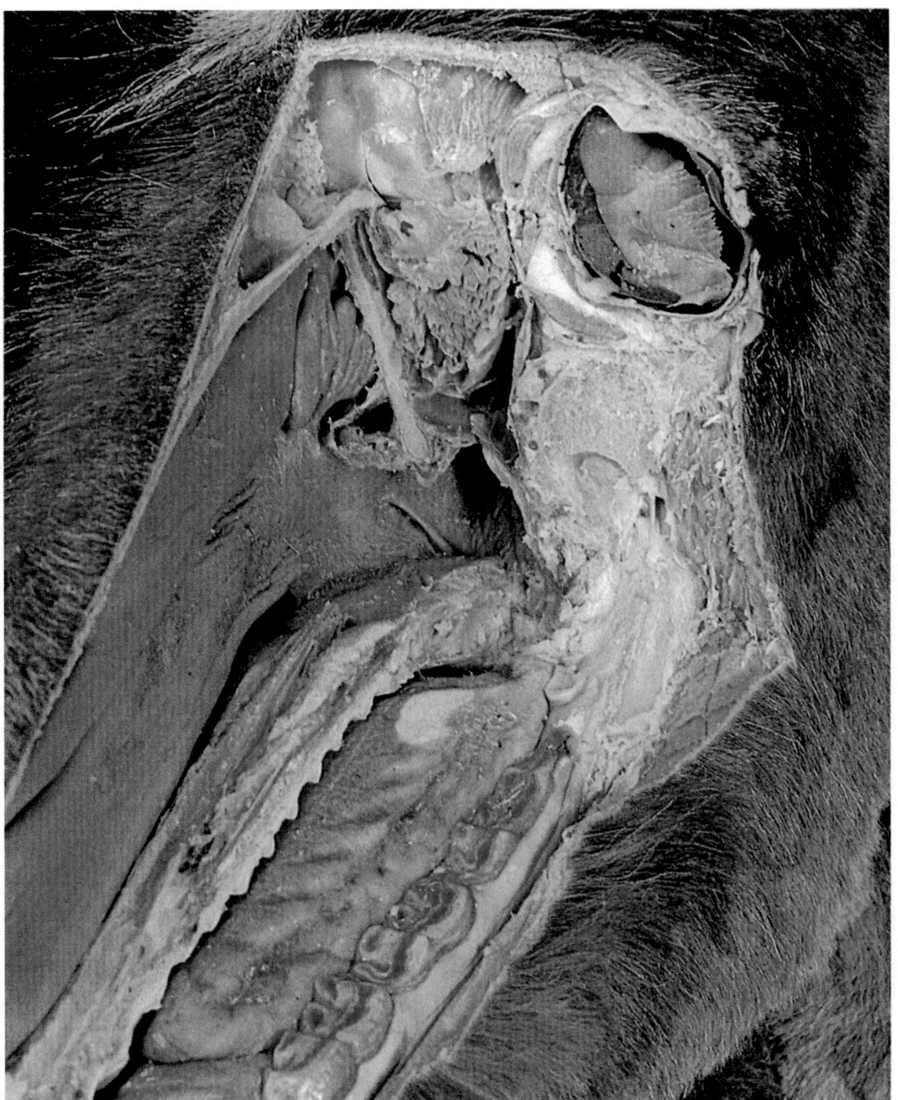

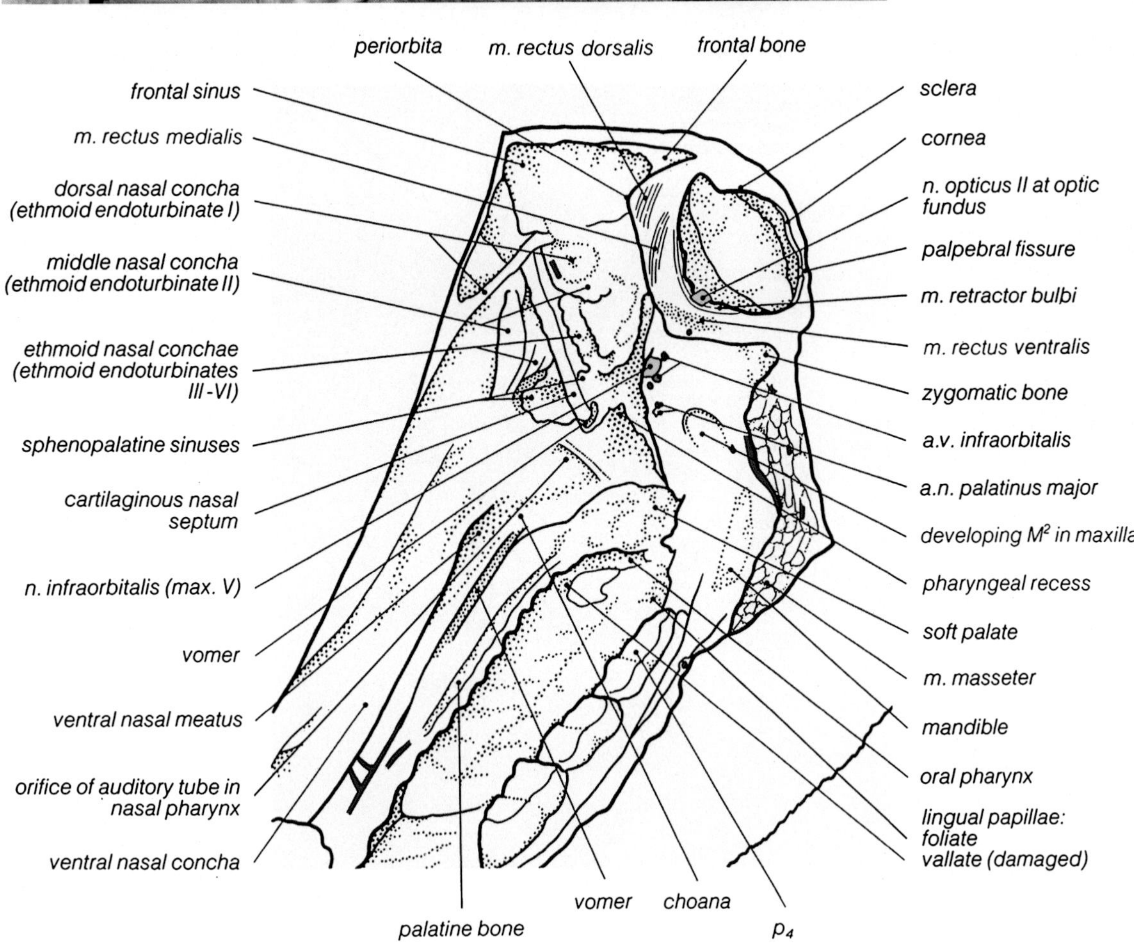

periorbita
m. rectus dorsalis
frontal bone
frontal sinus
m. rectus medialis
dorsal nasal concha (ethmoid endoturbinate I)
middle nasal concha (ethmoid endoturbinate II)
ethmoid nasal conchae (ethmoid endoturbinates III-VI)
sphenopalatine sinuses
cartilaginous nasal septum
n. infraorbitalis (max. V)
vomer
ventral nasal meatus
orifice of auditory tube in nasal pharynx
ventral nasal concha
palatine bone
vomer
choana
p_4
sclera
cornea
n. opticus II at optic fundus
palpebral fissure
m. retractor bulbi
m. rectus ventralis
zygomatic bone
a.v. infraorbitalis
a.n. palatinus major
developing M^2 in maxilla
pharyngeal recess
soft palate
m. masseter
mandible
oral pharynx
lingual papillae: foliate vallate (damaged)

Fig. 1.63 Orbital and nasal structures of the foal: left dorsolateral view. This view of the dissection shown in Fig. 1.62 shows structures on the transversely cut surface, and those of the right nasal cavity are seen in medial view. The tip of the epiglottis is just out of view in the depths of the nasopharynx (see Figs. 1.32–1.34).

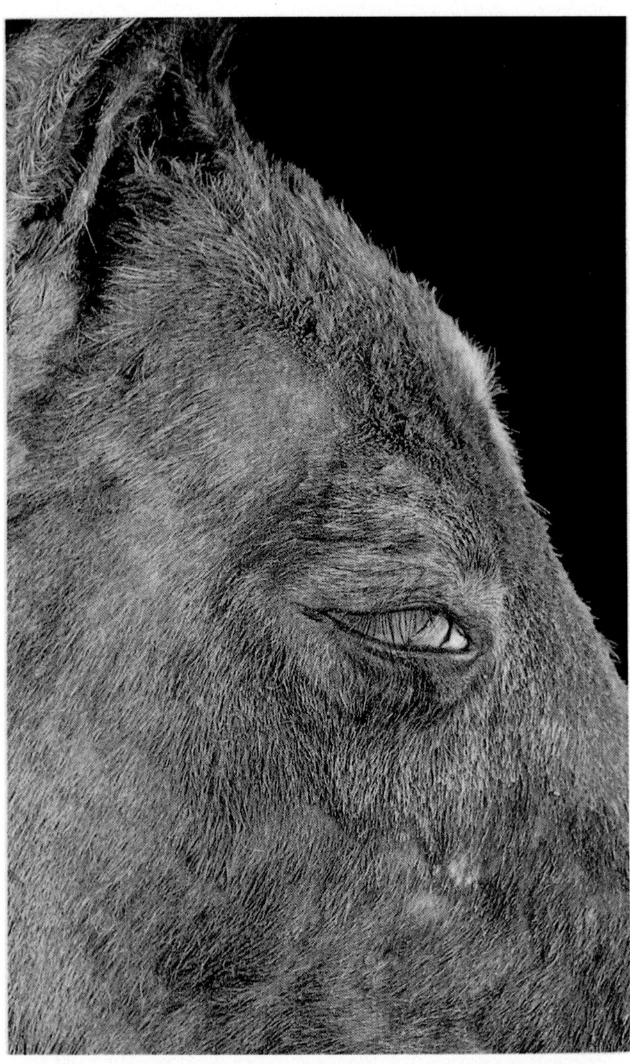

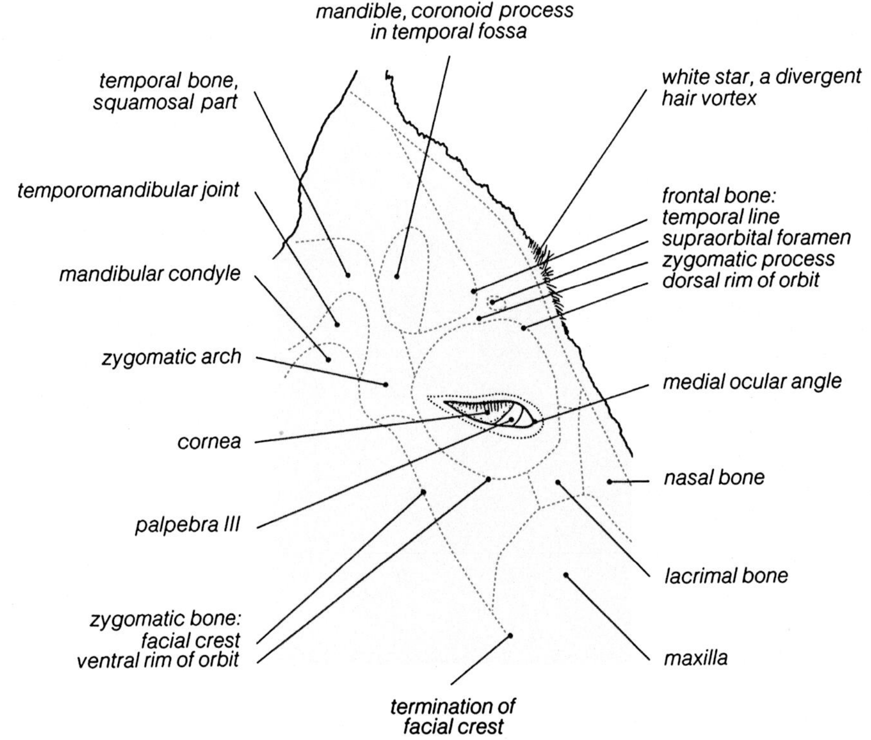
mandible, coronoid process in temporal fossa
temporal bone, squamosal part
white star, a divergent hair vortex
temporomandibular joint
frontal bone:
temporal line
supraorbital foramen
zygomatic process
dorsal rim of orbit
mandibular condyle
zygomatic arch
medial ocular angle
cornea
nasal bone
palpebra III
lacrimal bone
zygomatic bone:
facial crest
ventral rim of orbit
maxilla
termination of facial crest

Fig. 1.64 Surface features and bony landmarks of the eye of the foal: right lateral view. On the head of this young foal, the right eye (Figs. 1.64–1.71) and the left nasal cavity (Figs. 1.54–1.63) were dissected. The direction of the hairs on the eyelids has been emphasised by peroxide bleaching. The blue lines show the bones surrounding the eye, traced in part from Fig. 1.66.

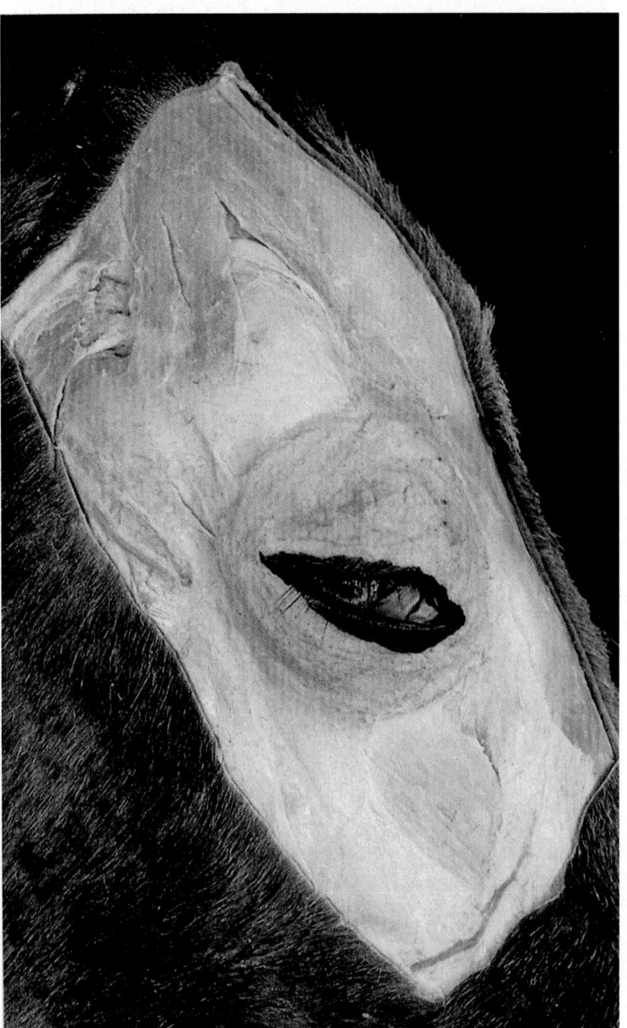

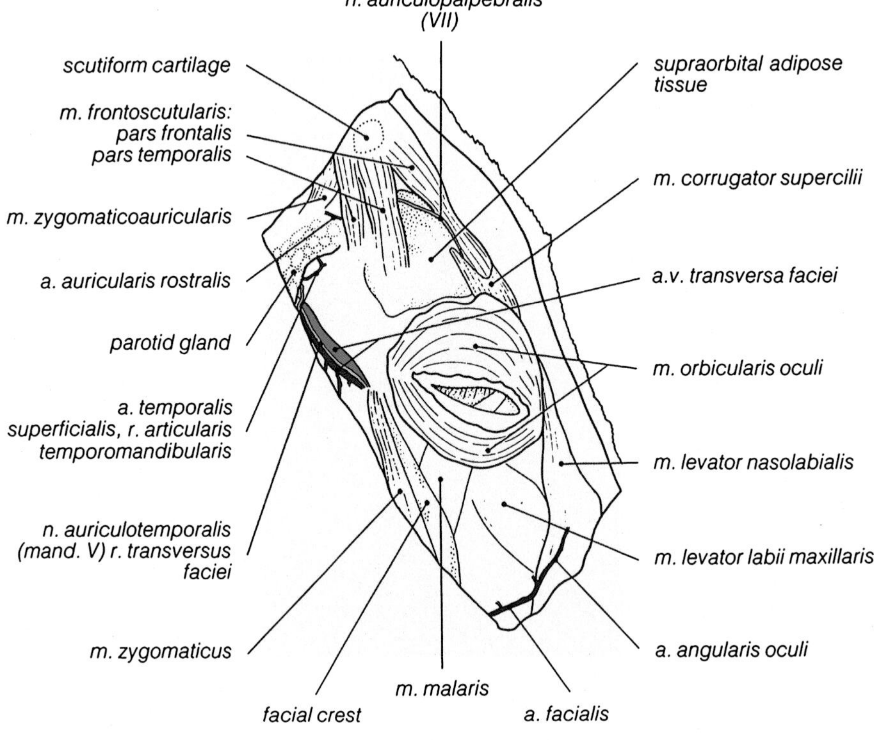
n. auriculopalpebralis (VII)
scutiform cartilage
supraorbital adipose tissue
m. frontoscutularis:
pars frontalis
pars temporalis
m. corrugator supercilii
m. zygomaticoauricularis
a. auricularis rostralis
a.v. transversa faciei
parotid gland
m. orbicularis oculi
a. temporalis superficialis, r. articularis temporomandibularis
m. levator nasolabialis
n. auriculotemporalis (mand. V) r. transversus faciei
m. levator labii maxillaris
m. zygomaticus
a. angularis oculi
m. malaris
facial crest
a. facialis

Fig. 1.65 Superficial structures of cranial and facial regions of the foal: right lateral view. Further details of the surrounding structures are shown in Figs. 1.8 and 1.9.

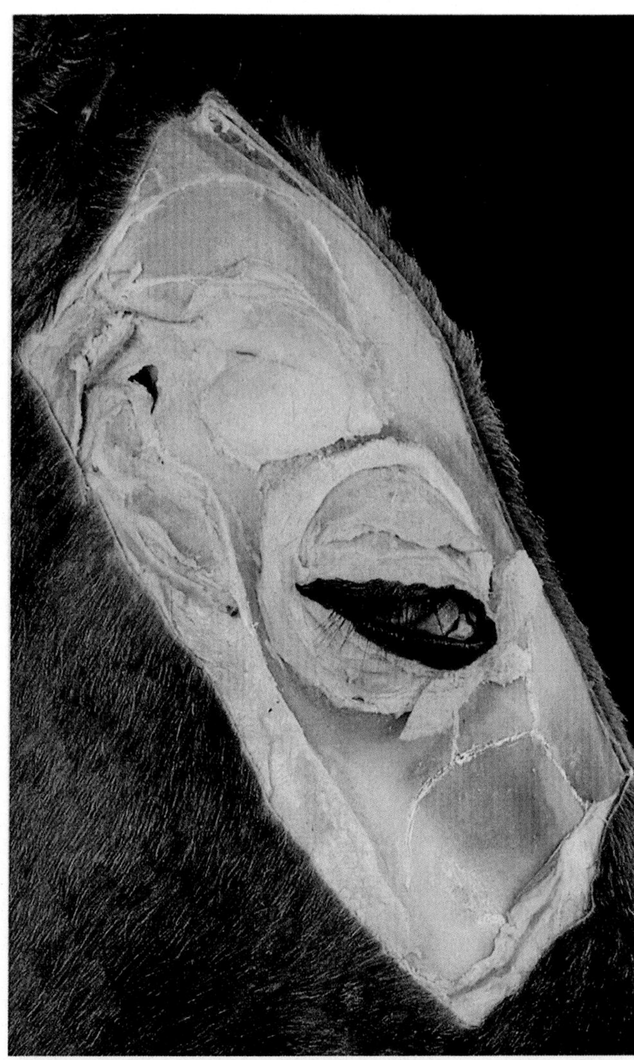

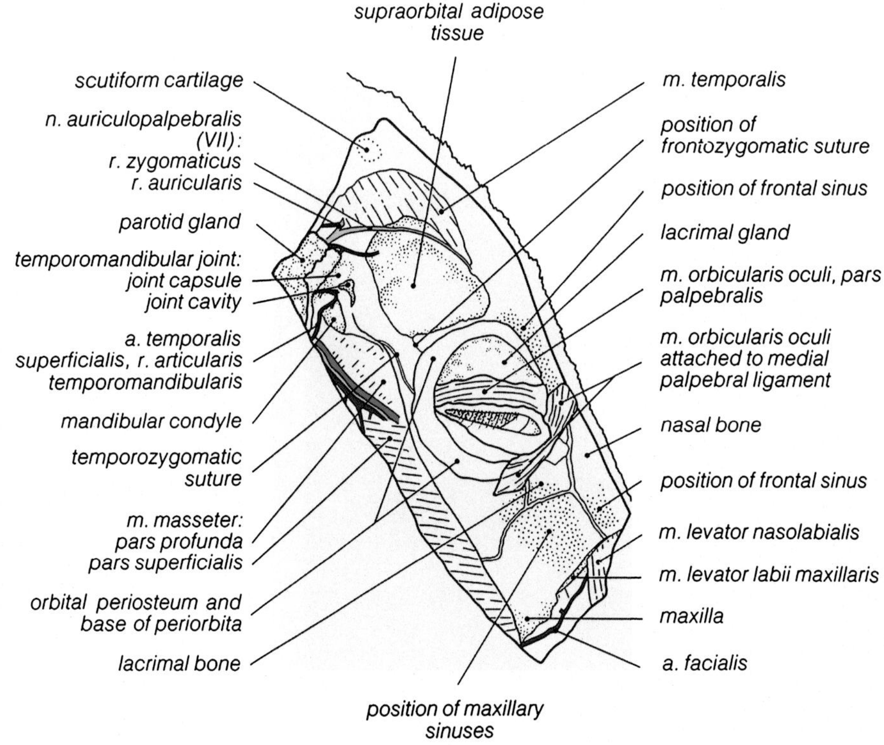
supraorbital adipose tissue
scutiform cartilage
n. auriculopalpebralis (VII):
r. zygomaticus
r. auricularis
parotid gland
temporomandibular joint:
joint capsule
joint cavity
a. temporalis superficialis, r. articularis temporomandibularis
mandibular condyle
temporozygomatic suture
m. masseter:
pars profunda
pars superficialis
orbital periosteum and base of periorbita
lacrimal bone
position of maxillary sinuses
m. temporalis
position of frontozygomatic suture
position of frontal sinus
lacrimal gland
m. orbicularis oculi, pars palpebralis
m. orbicularis oculi attached to medial palpebral ligament
nasal bone
position of frontal sinus
m. levator nasolabialis
m. levator labii maxillaris
maxilla
a. facialis

Fig. 1.66 Deeper structures of the cranial and facial regions of the foal: right lateral view. The air-filled paranasal sinuses are detectable through the thin outer tables of the facial bones in this young foal. The facial sutures were painted white.

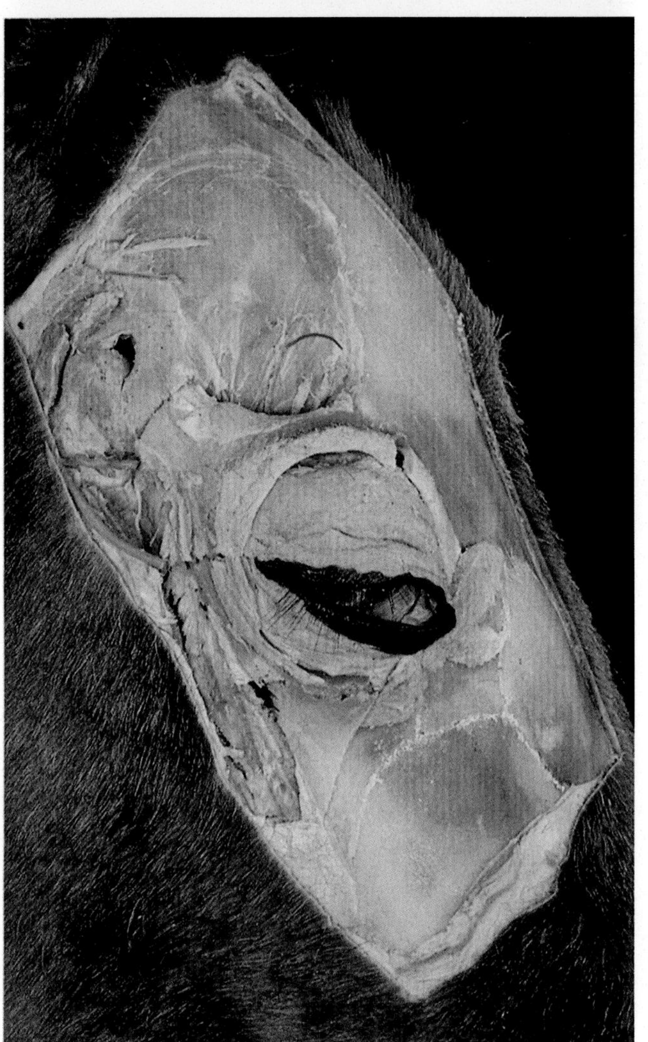

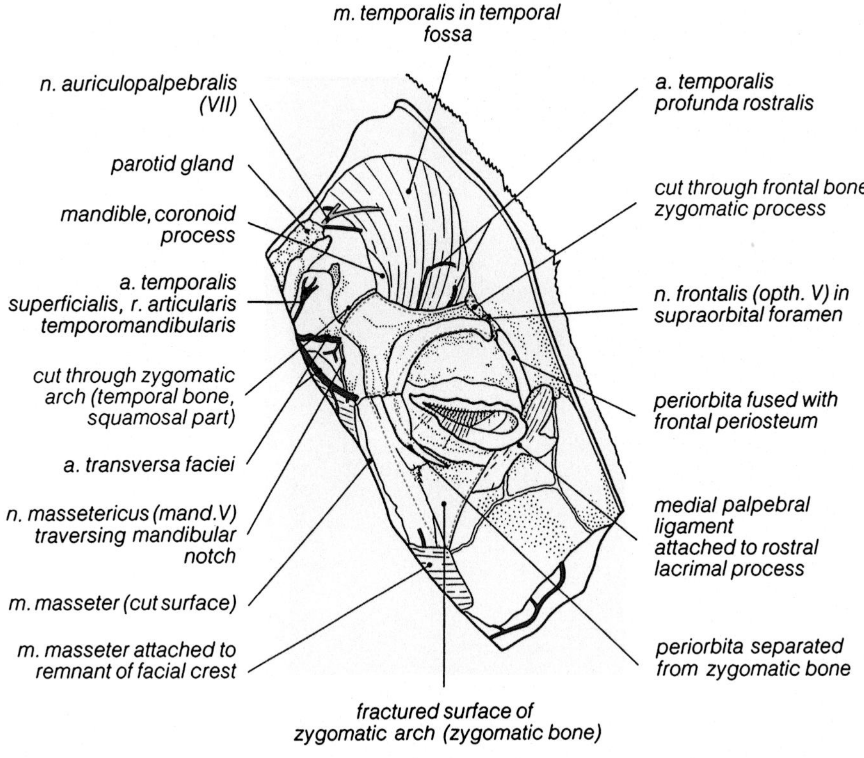
m. temporalis in temporal fossa
n. auriculopalpebralis (VII)
parotid gland
mandible, coronoid process
a. temporalis superficialis, r. articularis temporomandibularis
cut through zygomatic arch (temporal bone, squamosal part)
a. transversa faciei
n. massetericus (mand.V) traversing mandibular notch
m. masseter (cut surface)
m. masseter attached to remnant of facial crest
fractured surface of zygomatic arch (zygomatic bone)
a. temporalis profunda rostralis
cut through frontal bone, zygomatic process
n. frontalis (opth. V) in supraorbital foramen
periorbita fused with frontal periosteum
medial palpebral ligament
attached to rostral lacrimal process
periorbita separated from zygomatic bone

Fig. 1.67 Cranial and facial regions of the foal, prepared for removal of the zygomatic arch and zygomatic process: right lateral view. Parts of the frontal, zygomatic and squamosal temporal bones about to be removed are shown by the broken blue line (see also Fig. 1.66).

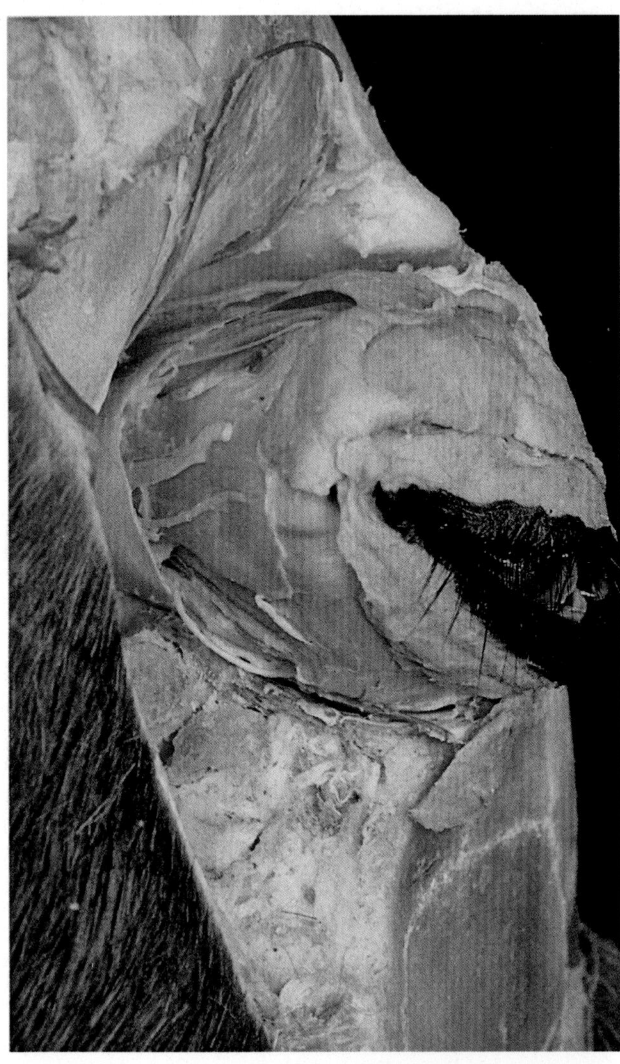

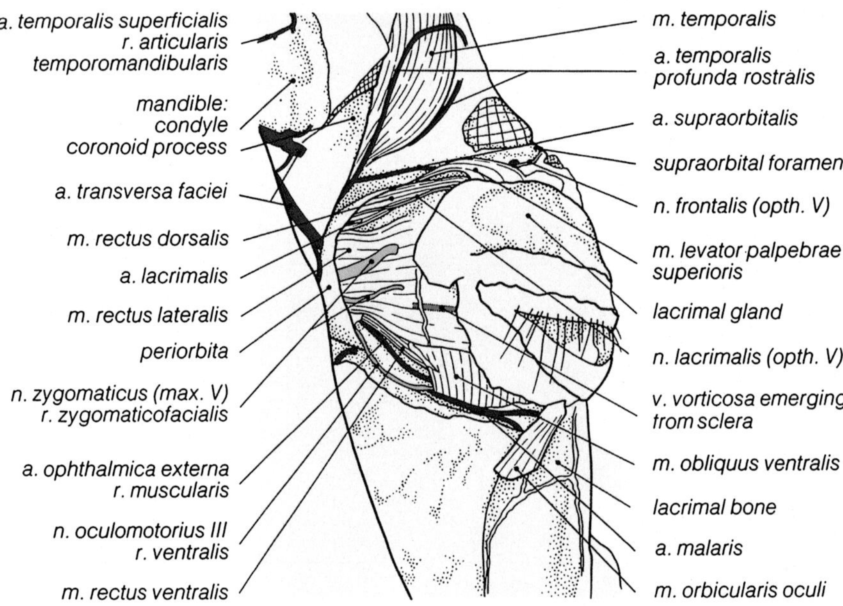
a. temporalis superficialis
r. articularis temporomandibularis
mandible: condyle
coronoid process
a. transversa faciei
m. rectus dorsalis
a. lacrimalis
m. rectus lateralis
periorbita
n. zygomaticus (max. V)
r. zygomaticofacialis
a. ophthalmica externa
r. muscularis
n. oculomotorius III
r. ventralis
m. rectus ventralis
m. temporalis
a. temporalis profunda rostralis
a. supraorbitalis
supraorbital foramen
n. frontalis (opth. V)
m. levator palpebrae superioris
lacrimal gland
n. lacrimalis (opth. V)
v. vorticosa emerging from sclera
m. obliquus ventralis
lacrimal bone
a. malaris
m. orbicularis oculi

Fig. 1.68 The orbit of the foal: right ventrolateral view (1). The cut surfaces of the zygomatic arch and the zygomatic process of the frontal bone are crosshatched on the accompanying drawing.

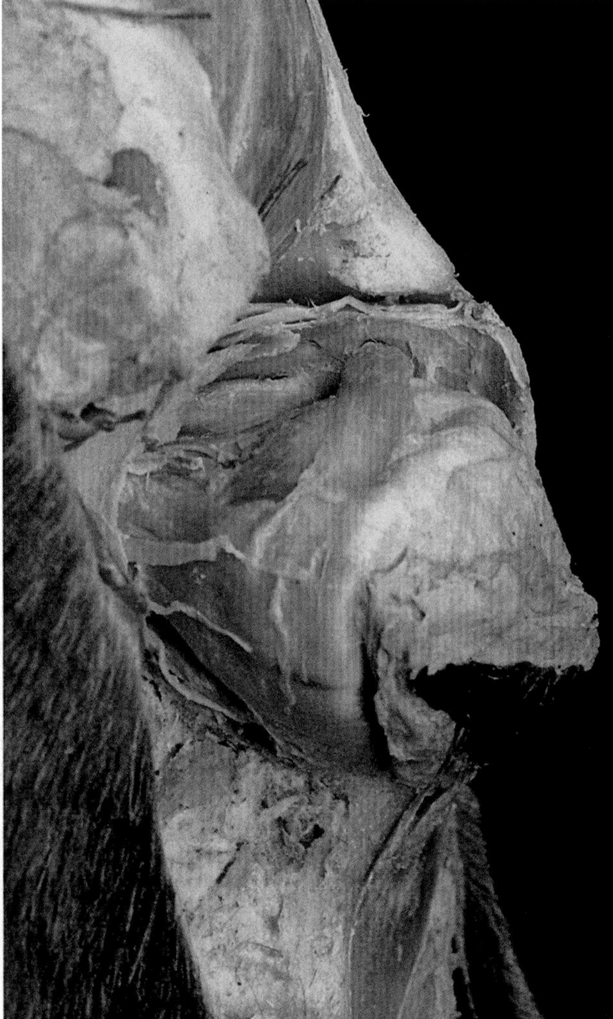

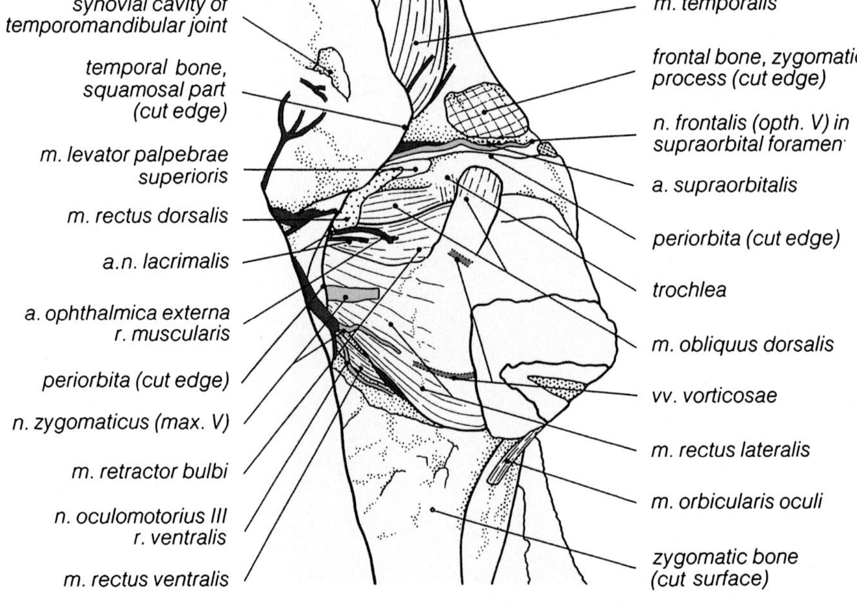
synovial cavity of temporomandibular joint
temporal bone, squamosal part (cut edge)
m. levator palpebrae superioris
m. rectus dorsalis
a.n. lacrimalis
a. ophthalmica externa
r. muscularis
periorbita (cut edge)
n. zygomaticus (max. V)
m. retractor bulbi
n. oculomotorius III
r. ventralis
m. rectus ventralis
m. temporalis
frontal bone, zygomatic process (cut edge)
n. frontalis (opth. V) in supraorbital foramen
a. supraorbitalis
periorbita (cut edge)
trochlea
m. obliquus dorsalis
vv. vorticosae
m. rectus lateralis
m. orbicularis oculi
zygomatic bone (cut surface)

Fig. 1.69 The orbit of the foal: right ventrolateral view (2). The levator muscle of the upper eyelid, the dorsal rectus muscle and the lacrimal gland have been removed. The view is slightly more dorsal than that shown in Fig. 1.68.

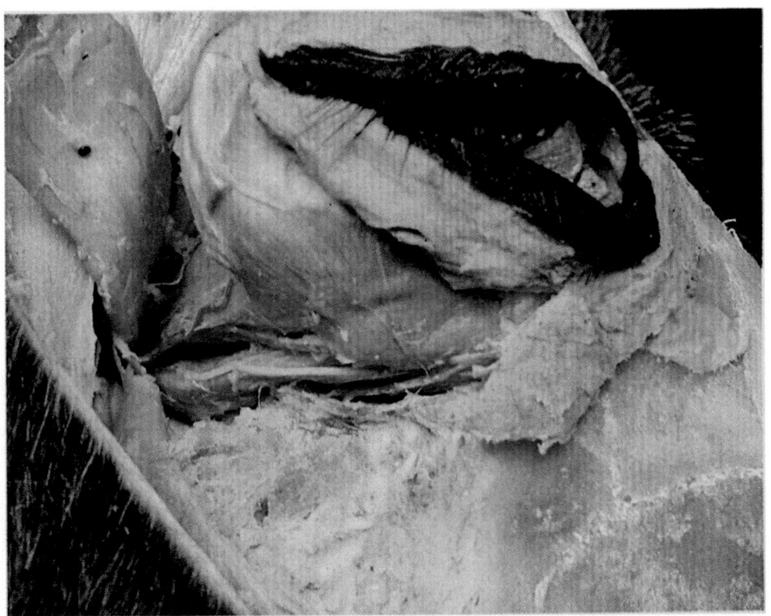

Fig. 1.70 **The abducens nerve of the foal: right lateral view.** The lateral rectus muscle has been transected and pinned back to show the nerve. Note also that where the periorbita has been resected, the deep facial vein traversing it has been slightly torn.

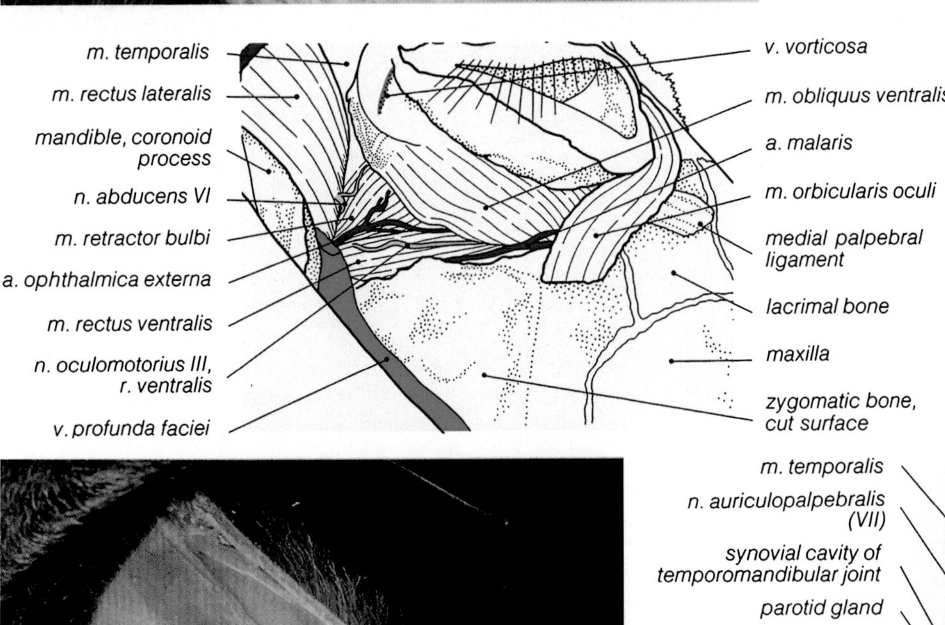

m. temporalis
m. rectus lateralis
mandible, coronoid process
n. abducens VI
m. retractor bulbi
a. ophthalmica externa
m. rectus ventralis
n. oculomotorius III, r. ventralis
v. profunda faciei
v. vorticosa
m. obliquus ventralis
a. malaris
m. orbicularis oculi
medial palpebral ligament
lacrimal bone
maxilla
zygomatic bone, cut surface

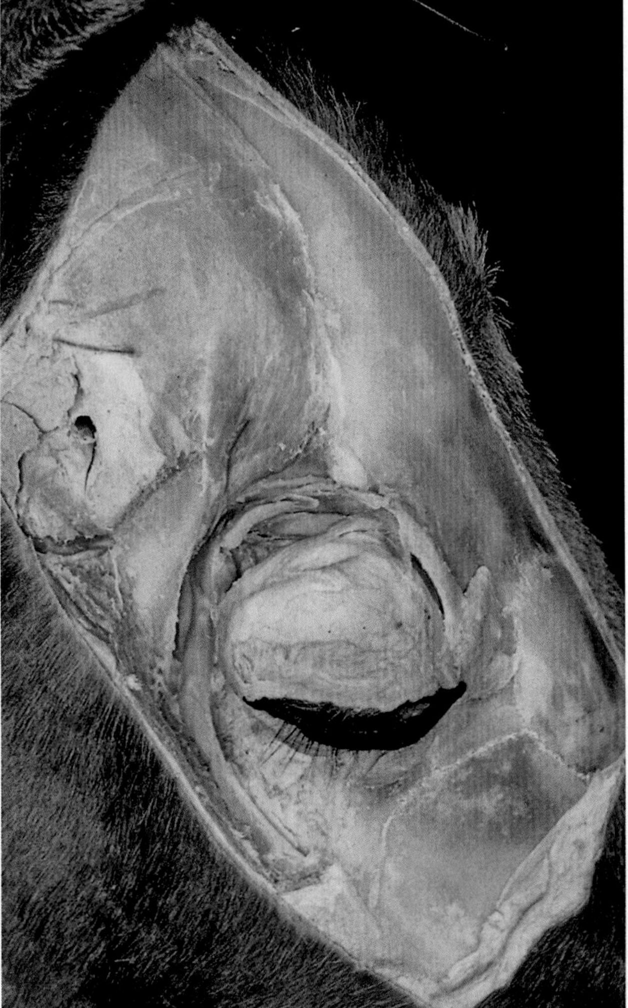

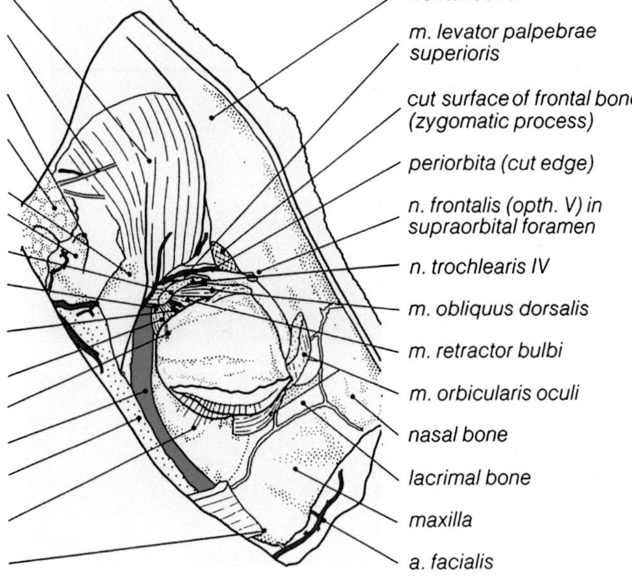

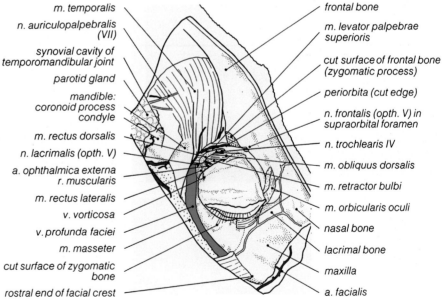

m. temporalis
n. auriculopalpebralis (VII)
synovial cavity of temporomandibular joint
parotid gland
mandible: coronoid process condyle
m. rectus dorsalis
n. lacrimalis (opth. V)
a. ophthalmica externa r. muscularis
m. rectus lateralis
v. vorticosa
v. profunda faciei
m. masseter
cut surface of zygomatic bone
rostral end of facial crest
frontal bone
m. levator palpebrae superioris
cut surface of frontal bone (zygomatic process)
periorbita (cut edge)
n. frontalis (opth. V) in supraorbital foramen
n. trochlearis IV
m. obliquus dorsalis
m. retractor bulbi
m. orbicularis oculi
nasal bone
lacrimal bone
maxilla
a. facialis

Fig. 1.71 **The dorsal oblique muscle and trochlear nerve of the foal: right lateral view.** The lateral rectus muscle has been resected from the eyeball.

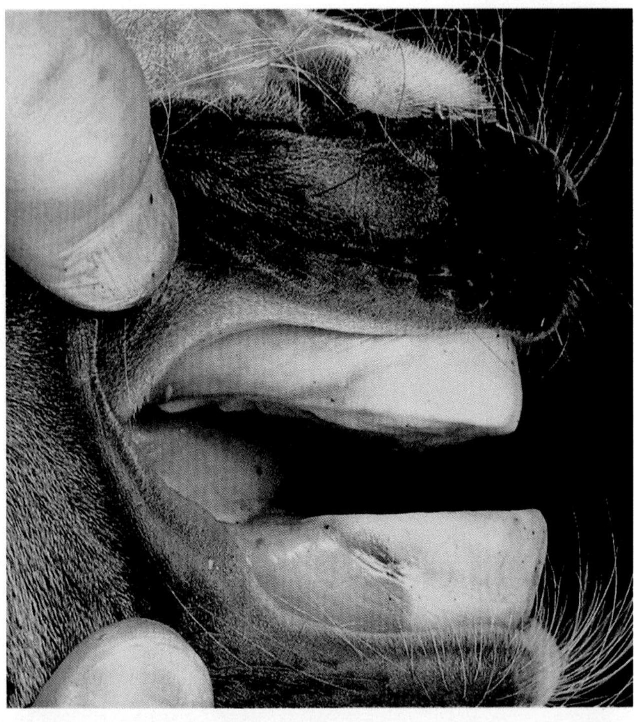
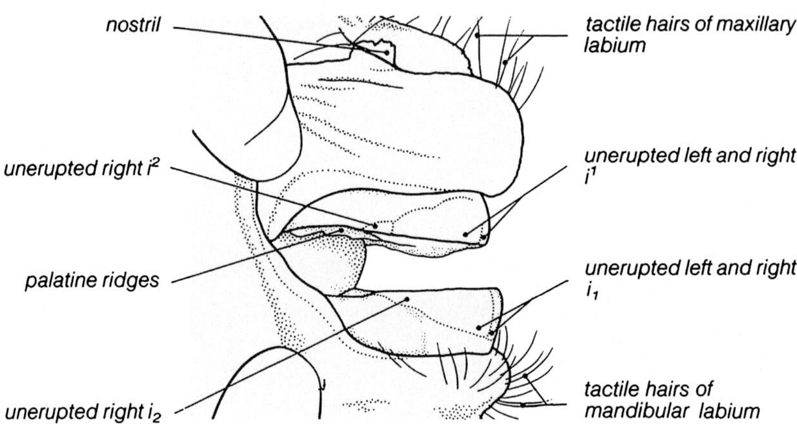
nostril
tactile hairs of maxillary labium
unerupted right i^2
unerupted left and right i^1
palatine ridges
unerupted left and right i_1
unerupted right i_2
tactile hairs of mandibular labium

Fig. 1.72 The incisor teeth of the new-born foal: right lateral view. Both first and second incisor teeth are still covered by the gingiva, and the distinction between them is not easily seen in this still-born foal. The tongue has been pulled out through the left diastema.

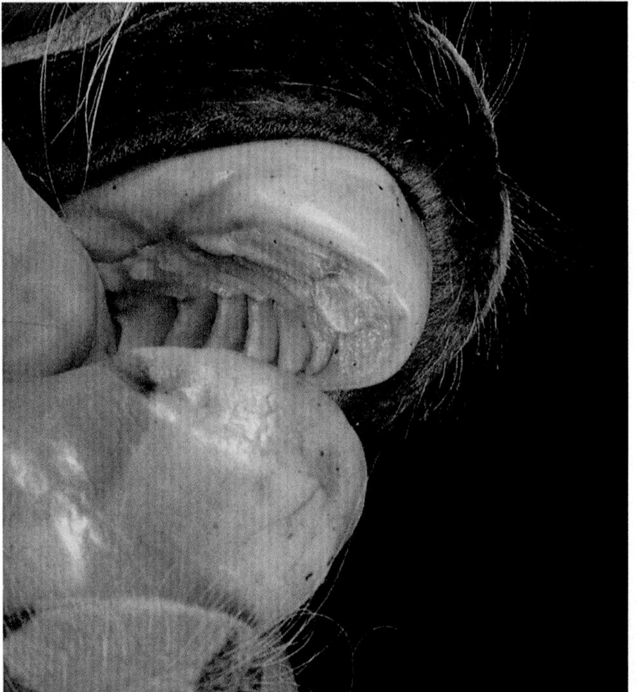
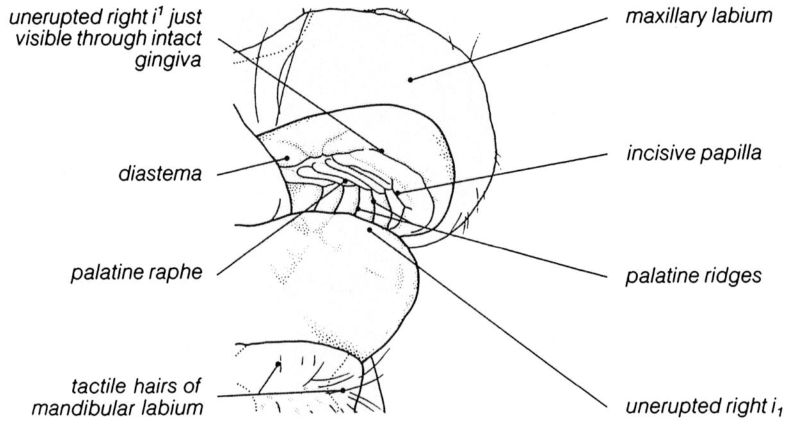
unerupted right i^1 just visible through intact gingiva
maxillary labium
diastema
incisive papilla
palatine raphe
palatine ridges
tactile hairs of mandibular labium
unerupted right i_1

Fig. 1.73 The mouth of the new-born foal: right ventrolateral view. In this still-born foal, the maxillary first temporary incisors are just beginning to cut the gingiva close to the midline. The first incisors usually erupt just before, or just after, birth. The second temporary incisors usually erupt at 3–4 weeks of age.

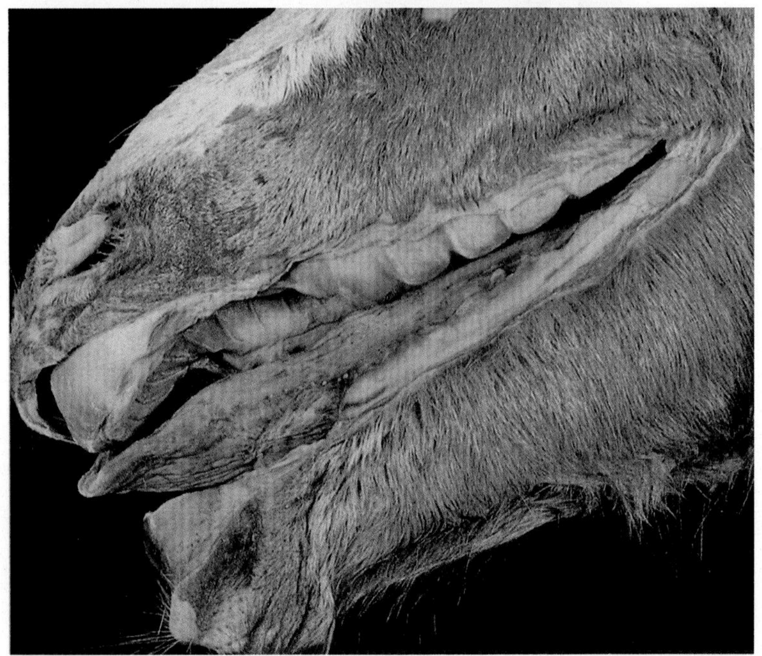
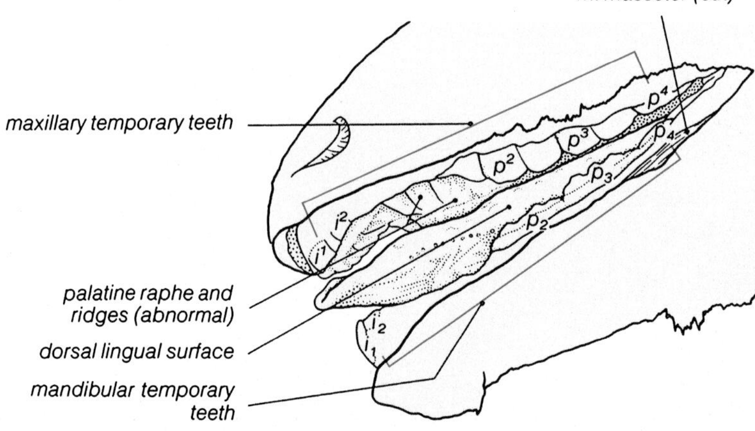
m. masseter (cut)
maxillary temporary teeth
p^4
p_4
p^3
p^2
p_3
p_2
i^2
i^1
palatine raphe and ridges (abnormal)
i_2
dorsal lingual surface
mandibular temporary teeth

Fig. 1.74 Dentition of the new-born foal: left lateral view. The discolouration of the enamel layer makes the crowns more easily visible. Considerable protrusion of the crown from the gingival surface occurs before actual penetration of the gingiva. This still born foal shows an abnormality of the hard palate but the dentition is normal. Note the flat surface of the tongue; compare with Fig. 1.60.

2. THE NECK

Clinical importance of the neck

Airway obstruction results from blockage at one or more of several sites. Choanal stenosis (at the nostrils) is the most obvious cause. Obstruction may also be caused by pharyngeal lymphoid hyperplasia, palatal cysts and defects, pharyngeal paralysis, neoplasia, pharyngeal cysts, congenital tracheal abnormalities and tracheal obstruction, and damage resulting from tracheotomy intubation. It is important to remember that lower respiratory tract disorders can become apparent as a nasal discharge or cough.

The larynx lies at the junction between head and neck. The cartilages of the larynx are locked into the caudal wall of the nasopharynx by the palato-pharyngeal arch of the soft palate in an artificial seal. This is disconnected for the act of swallowing, in which the palatopharyngeal muscles participate.

In the condition of 'roaring' or 'whistling', the horse has an excessive inspiratory noise and poor exercise tolerance. More correctly, the condition is called recurrent laryngeal neuropathy. Damage to the cranial laryngeal nerve prevents the normal, symmetrical, abduction of the arytenoid cartilages during inspiration. Air turbulence in the larynx results. It is usually left-sided. The left recurrent laryngeal nerve is significantly longer than the right. The usual aetiological suggestion is that stretching or damage to the nerve results from its course around the aorta in the thorax. There are various gradations of the disorder. It is really a progressive neurogenic atrophy. Treatment is beyond the scope of this introduction. Several surgical procedures have been developed over the years including removal of the laryngeal ventricle (ventriculectomy), prosthetic ligature, and arytenoidectomy. All of these techniques require a detailed knowledge of the anatomy of the larynx. Other defects of the larynx may include epiglottic entrapment, sub-epiglottic cysts (these are usually derived from embryonic tissue from the thyroglossal duct and are often found in an entrapment), arytenoid chondritis and defects of the 4th branchial arch leading to congenital abnormalities.

In young horses, pharyngeal lymphoid hyperplasia, probably in response to an infection, is a common problem. In epiglottic entrapment, the cartilage of the epiglottis becomes enveloped by a fold of glosso-epiglottic mucosa arising between the epiglottis and the base of the tongue and extending laterally as the aryepiglottic folds. It is not clear why it occurs. Lateral oedema is not unusual. There can be paralysis or paresis of the larynx, particularly when the lymph nodes are damaged by infection with *Streptococcus equi* (strangles).

Obstructive airway disease may involve the pharynx, but can be associated with guttural pouch problems. Other causes of obstructive airway disease include emphysema, pharyngeal paralysis, palatal defects, or displacement of the soft palate.

Occasionally the trachea is the original source of an obstructive problem, as the horse is notoriously susceptible to allergic respiratory disease. The trachea can be palpated in the neck. Its superficial position facilitates transtracheal aspiration, by which uncontaminated samples can be collected from the lower respiratory tract. An incision is made through the skin in the ventral midline; the strap muscles are separated and an incision made between the cartilaginous rings, through the annular ligament, into the trachea. Then a catheter can be used to flush with saline for a tracheal wash or for bronchoalveolar lavage. Tracheal obstruction is not common but may occur following trauma or result from a dorsal mass pressing on the trachea. The obstruction is usually cervical, occasionally thoracic. Tracheal endoscopy is used for investigating dynamic airway collapse.

Blood can be collected from the jugular vein and from other veins, including the transverse facial vein, the superficial thoracic vein caudal to the elbow, and the cephalic vein in the medial aspect of the forelimb. The saphenous vein on the medial aspect of the hind leg is also available. For arterial blood-gas analysis, the transverse facial artery, facial artery and dorsal metatarsal artery can be used. The jugular groove is important. It contains the jugular vein, an important structure for intravenous anaesthesia, administration of medications and for obtaining blood samples. The cranial third of the groove is the most accessible and likely to pose fewer hazards. It is also used for jugular catheters. The vein normally has a visible jugular pulse in the lower third of the neck. Distension of the jugular vein, or an abnormal pulse, suggests primary cardiac disease, or heart compression caused by fluid or masses in the mediastinum or pericardial sac. Thrombosis of the jugular vein (septic or non-septic) may occur after venepuncture or catheterisation and the effect on venous return from the head may ultimately produce oedema of the muzzle. The thyroid gland is important clinically. Foals rarely suffer from hypothyroidism, even though there is no build-up of iodine stores. In old horses there may be thyroid adenomas causing palpable thyroid enlargement and hyperparathyroidism also occurs.

The cervical vertebrae are clinically important. Equine accidents during racing or hunting may cause cervical vertebral trauma, particularly at the atlanto-occipital articulation. The important malformation known as cervical vertebral stenosis is more colloquially known as 'wobbler syndrome'. It occurs in 18- to 30-month-old thoroughbreds. It is probably of complex aetiology but may involve cervical vertebral displacement, developmental abnormalities of the cervical vertebrae, or cervical arthropathy. It is also possible, using ultrasonic guidance, to accomplish facet arthrocentesis for the joint spaces between the cranial and caudal processes of the vertebrae when neck pain is suspected. It is essential not to puncture the vertebral artery. The cervical musculature is readily accessible and not noticeably subject to adverse effects and so is most often the site for intramuscular injection in the horse. The cervical transverse processes can be felt, and a site 10 cm or less above the vertebrae in the middle third of the neck, a handsbreadth in front of the scapula and ventral to the nuchal ligament, is ideal. The pectoral muscles are sometimes used and also the lower half of the semimembranosus and semitendinosus muscles in the hind leg.

Dysphagia (difficulty in swallowing) may involve the mouth (oral foreign body) or pharynx, but is perhaps more likely to be associated with the oesophagus. It can also result from oral irritation, brain stem disease or cranial nerve damage, rabies, or 'grass sickness' (now known as equine dysautonomia). Oesophageal obstruction may be caused by a variety of factors, including foreign bodies, dental problems and retro-oesophageal abscesses such as guttural pouch empyaemia. Simple intraluminar oesophageal obstruction may be caused by food, woodchips or bedding and may be indicated by salivation, retching and coughing. Passing of a nasal tube will indicate the site of 'choke' and then the material can, hopefully, be flushed onward or flushed retrograde. Oesophageal perforation may result from oesophageal obstruction, foreign body perforation, external wounds, repeated intubation, extension of infection or injury, or even corrective surgery. Oesophagotomy should be carried out over the site of obstruction. It requires an 8 – 10 cm longitudinal skin incision in the ventral midline. The positions of the longus colli, sternocephalicus, and sternothyrohyoideus muscles, jugular vein, and the brachiocephalicus and omohyoideus muscles should be noted to carry out oesophagotomy successfully. The common carotid artery, recurrent laryngeal nerve and vagosympathetic trunk must be treated with the utmost care on both sides.

The lymph nodes of the neck are valuable clinical indications of pathological changes in their drainage areas. The lateral retropharyngeal lymph nodes are supposedly superficial but are not usually palpable unless enlarged with fluid or inflamed or neoplastic. The medial retropharyngeal nodes are not palpable but the deep cervical chain of lymph nodes may be palpable if enlarged. The superficial cervical (formerly pre-scapular) lymph node takes drainage from caudal neck, shoulder and most of the fore limb. It is one of the largest lymph nodes in the horse's body, and it takes drainage from a very wide area, including all of the front limbs. If often extends to a chain of accessory nodes and is palpable in thin horses, even when not enlarged.

The major clinical features of the caudal part of the head, bordering the neck, are the paired diverticula of the auditory tubes (guttural pouches). They lie ventral to the cranium and dorsal to the pharynx and oesophagus. The volume of each pouch is approximately 300 ml. Left and right pouches are in contact medially (mid-line). The architecture of each pouch is complicated by the stylohyoid bone which divides each pouch into lateral and medial compartments. The pouch is lined by pseudostratified ciliated epithelium and is therefore secretory. The drainage points of the pouches into the auditory tubes are not, unfortunately, at the lowest point of the pouch. These openings are patent during swallowing, and gravity aids drainage when the head is down. The ostia of the auditory tube are slits, under cartilage flaps, that open onto the dorsolateral wall of the pharynx. The clinical problem with the guttural pouches lies in their relationships to surrounding structures. The medial compartment is crossed by cranial nerves IX to XII and by the internal carotid artery, whereas the lateral compartment is crossed by the external maxillary artery and vein, and the facial nerve lies on the dorsal surface. Thus, any infection in the guttural pouches can potentially erode and damage these structures leading to a wide variety of clinical signs. Also, the pouch is a natural reservoir for *Streptococcus equi*, the cause of strangles. The simplest condition affecting the pouch is tympany which occurs mainly in foals, is often bilateral and can be felt and seen as swellings caudal to the mandible. In this condition, the ostium acts as a non-return valve; air enters but does not escape. It can be relieved by creating a fistula with the pharynx, or with the opposite pouch, or by dilating the ostium. There may be chronic inflammation (guttural pouch diverticulitis); mucus accumulates in the pouches and this may lead to chronic infections and the presence of solid concretions or chondroids. Far more serious is guttural pouch mycosis. This is an invasive process in the pouch, particularly in the upper part of both lateral and medial compartments (close to the vessels). The erosive process may therefore damage the internal carotid artery (medial compartment) or external maxillary artery (lateral compartment). This may result in a severe haemorrhage as the first clinical sign, which may rapidly prove fatal. In addition, the close relationship with the nerves and other structures may cause pharyngeal paralysis, laryngeal hemiplegia or facial palsy. The erosion may even extend into the temporomandibular joint. The complications can be assessed by endoscopy, ultrasonography and radiography. Treatment can be achieved through a variety of approaches such as; a) an incision cranial to the wing of the atlas; b) through Viborg's triangle which gives only restricted access; c) a parapharyngeal approach with the horse in dorsal recumbency in which a ventral midline incision is made, permitting an approach lateral to the larynx, trachea and cricopharyngeus muscle; or d) a technique known as the 'modified Whitehouse approach' which involves an incision ventral to the linguo-facial vein.

Synovial bursae deep to the funicular part of the *ligamentum nuchae* may become enlarged and infected. At the arch of the atlas vertebra (C1), the cranial nuchal (atlantal) bursa may give rise to 'poll evil'. Over the supraspinous processes of T2–T4, between the funicular and laminar parts of the ligament, lies the supraspinous bursa, which may give rise to 'fistulous withers'. These are serious conditions requiring antibacterial therapy and, possibly, surgical drainage. *Brucella abortus* has been incriminated in both conditions.

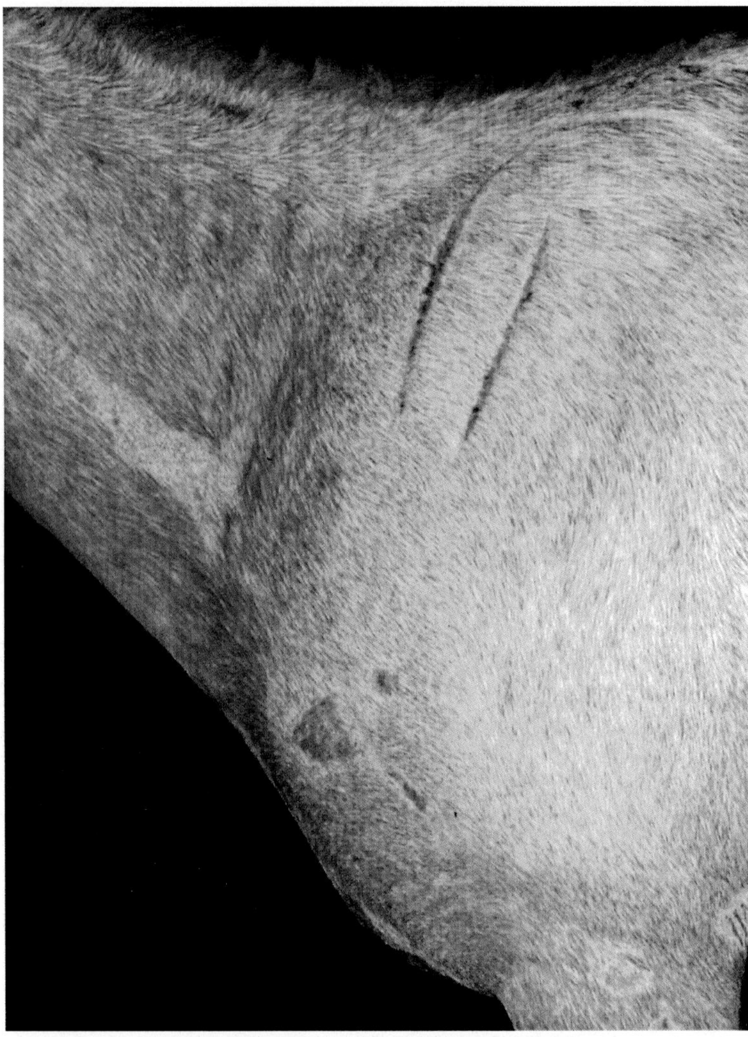

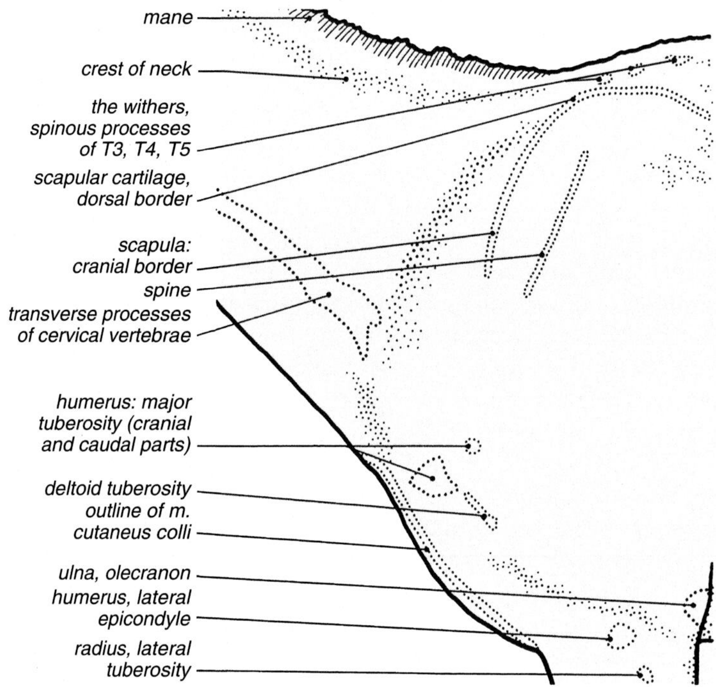
mane
crest of neck
the withers, spinous processes of T3, T4, T5
scapular cartilage, dorsal border
scapula: cranial border
spine
transverse processes of cervical vertebrae
humerus: major tuberosity (cranial and caudal parts)
deltoid tuberosity
outline of m. cutaneus colli
ulna, olecranon
humerus, lateral epicondyle
radius, lateral tuberosity

Fig. 2.1 Surface features of the neck and shoulder: left lateral view. The mane has been moved over to the right side to display the crest, which was not well developed in this young gelding. The palpable bony features have been shaved. The surface features of the cranial parts of the neck are shown in Fig. 1.4.

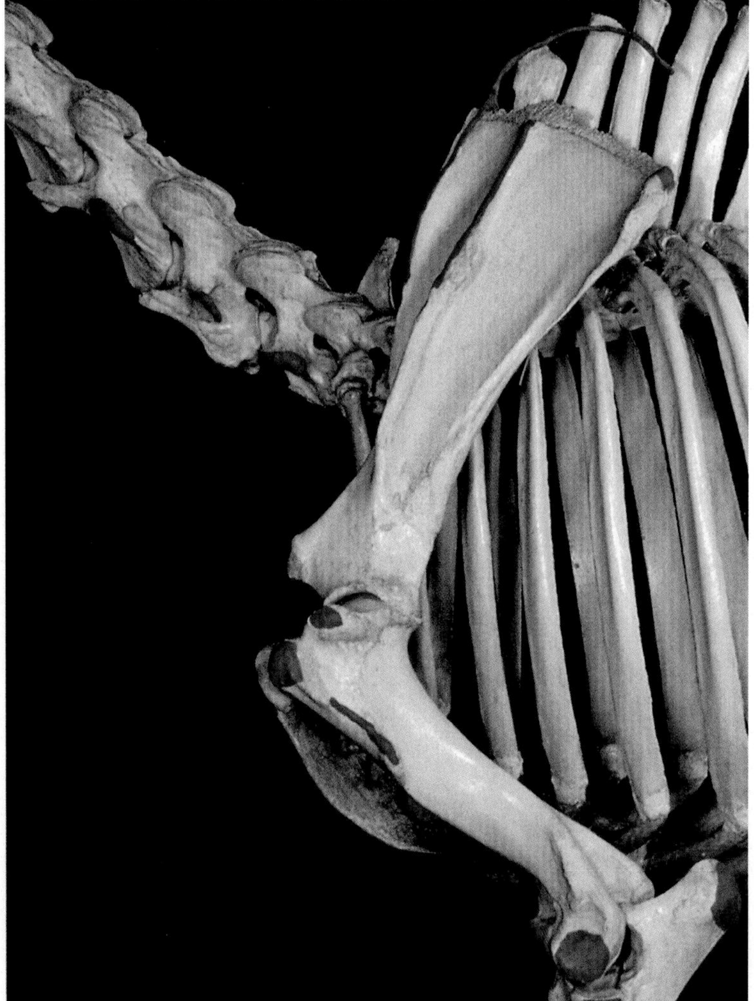

Fig. 2.2 Bones of the neck and shoulder: left lateral view. The palpable bony features shown in Fig. 2.1 have been coloured red. The dorsal border of the scapular cartilage is represented by a red wire.

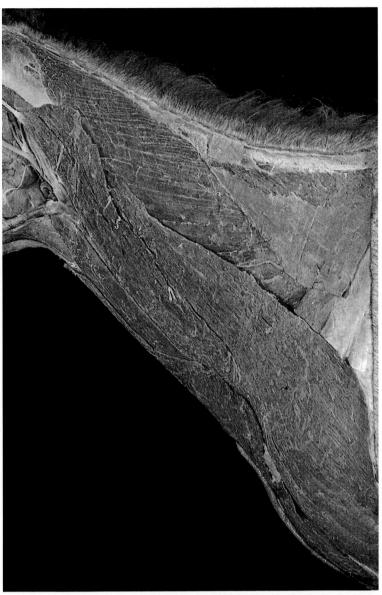

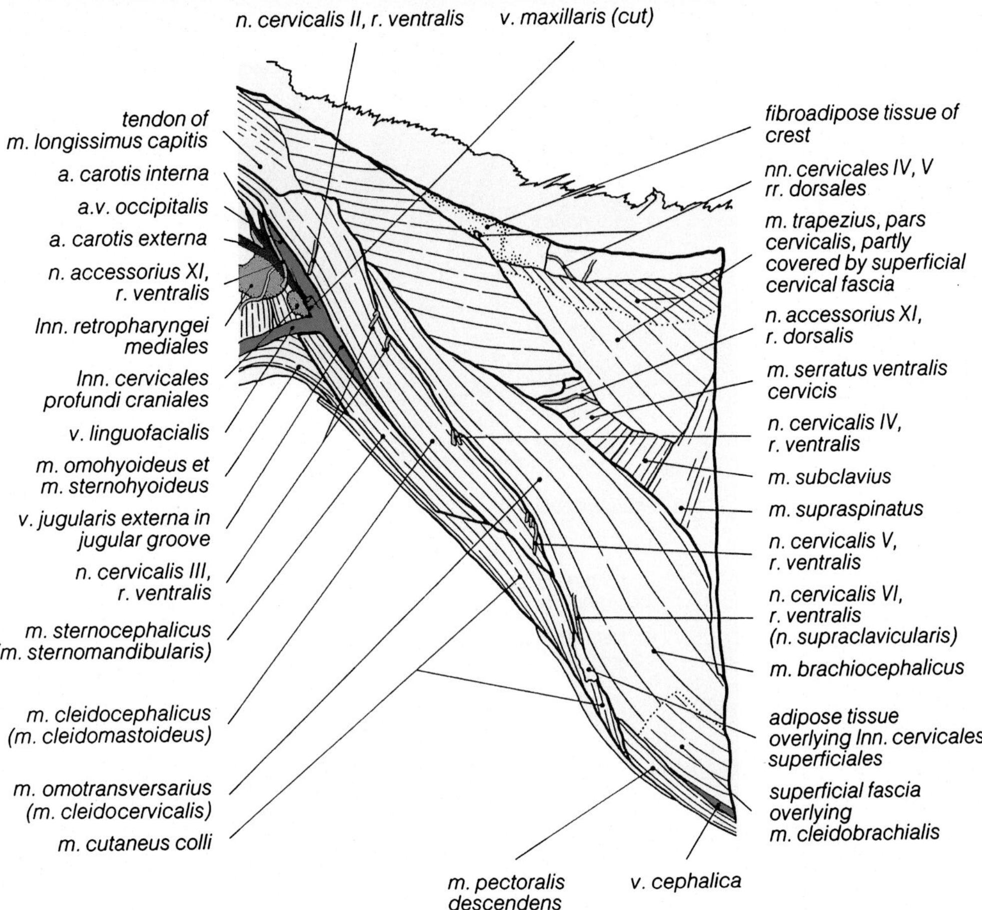
n. cervicalis II, r. ventralis
v. maxillaris (cut)
tendon of
m. longissimus capitis
a. carotis interna
a.v. occipitalis
a. carotis externa
n. accessorius XI,
r. ventralis
lnn. retropharyngei
mediales
lnn. cervicales
profundi craniales
v. linguofacialis
m. omohyoideus et
m. sternohyoideus
v. jugularis externa in
jugular groove
n. cervicalis III,
r. ventralis
m. sternocephalicus
(m. sternomandibularis)
m. cleidocephalicus
(m. cleidomastoideus)
m. omotransversarius
(m. cleidocervicalis)
m. cutaneus colli
m. pectoralis
descendens
v. cephalica
fibroadipose tissue of
crest
nn. cervicales IV, V
rr. dorsales
m. trapezius, pars
cervicalis, partly
covered by superficial
cervical fascia
n. accessorius XI,
r. dorsalis
m. serratus ventralis
cervicis
n. cervicalis IV,
r. ventralis
m. subclavius
m. supraspinatus
n. cervicalis V,
r. ventralis
n. cervicalis VI,
r. ventralis
(n. supraclavicularis)
m. brachiocephalicus
adipose tissue
overlying lnn. cervicales
superficiales
superficial fascia
overlying
m. cleidobrachialis

Fig. 2.3 Superficial musculature of the neck. The superficial fascia and the cutaneous omobrachial muscle have been removed, but the large cutaneous muscle of the neck has been preserved.

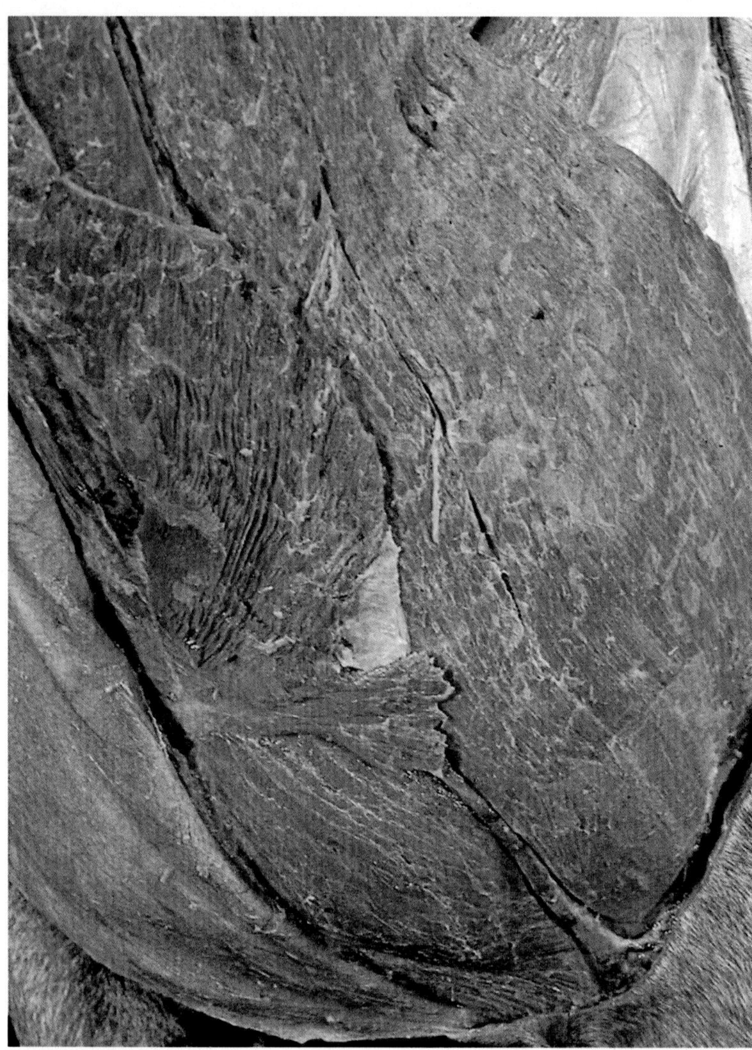

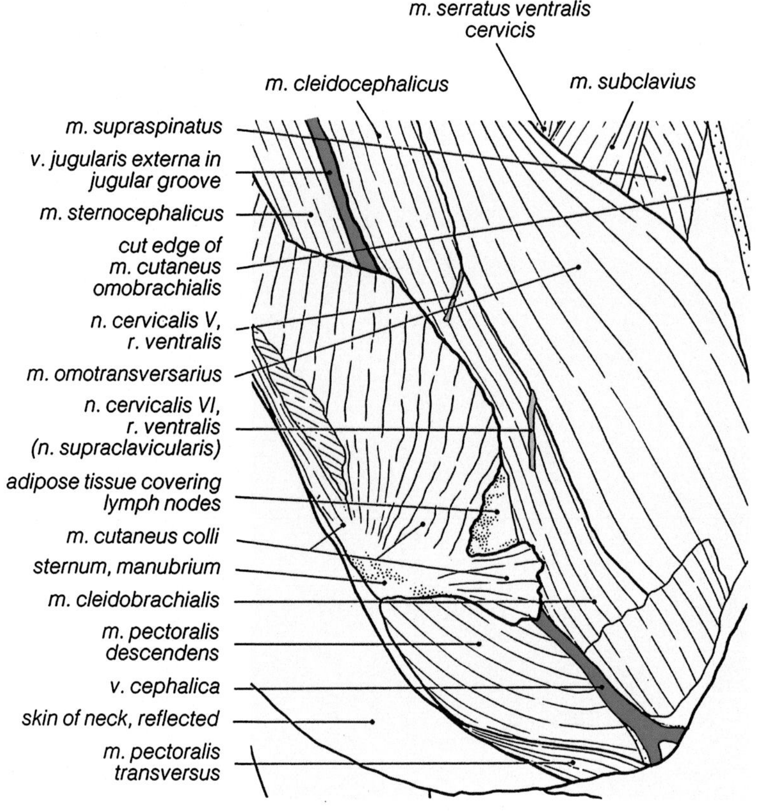
m. serratus ventralis cervicis
m. cleidocephalicus
m. subclavius
m. supraspinatus
v. jugularis externa in jugular groove
m. sternocephalicus
cut edge of m. cutaneus omobrachialis
n. cervicalis V, r. ventralis
m. omotransversarius
n. cervicalis VI, r. ventralis (n. supraclavicularis)
adipose tissue covering lymph nodes
m. cutaneus colli
sternum, manubrium
m. cleidobrachialis
m. pectoralis descendens
v. cephalica
skin of neck, reflected
m. pectoralis transversus

Fig. 2.4 The muscles covering the superficial cervical lymph nodes: left craniolateral view. The insertion of the cutaneous muscle of the neck into the cervical fascia has been removed.

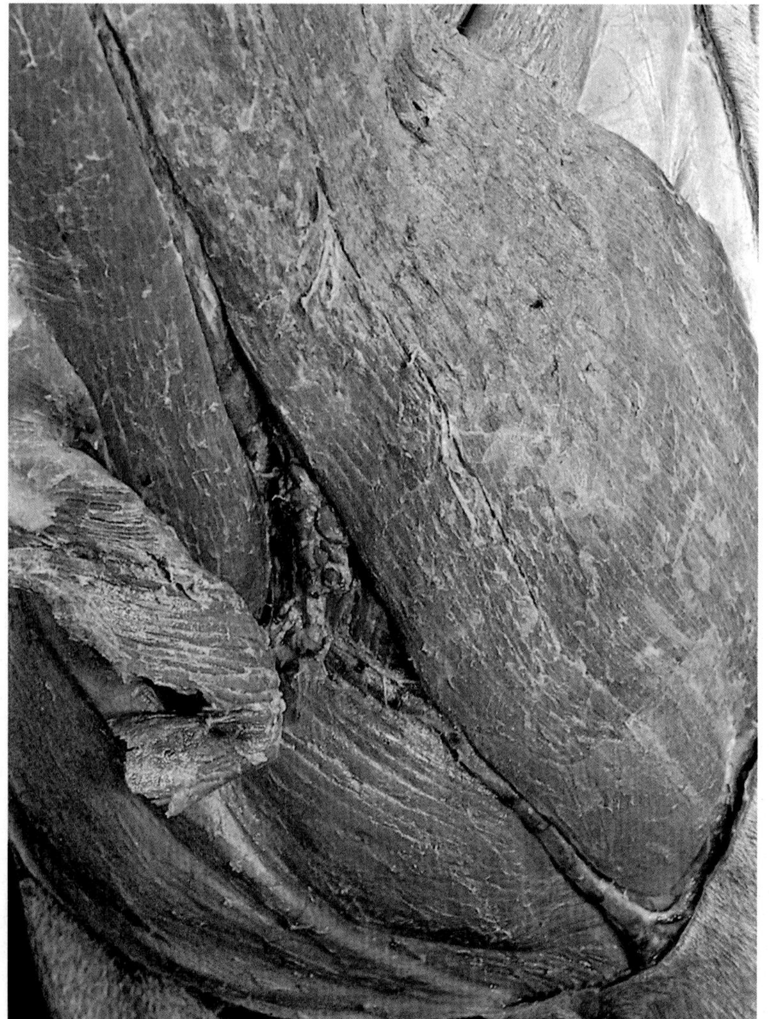

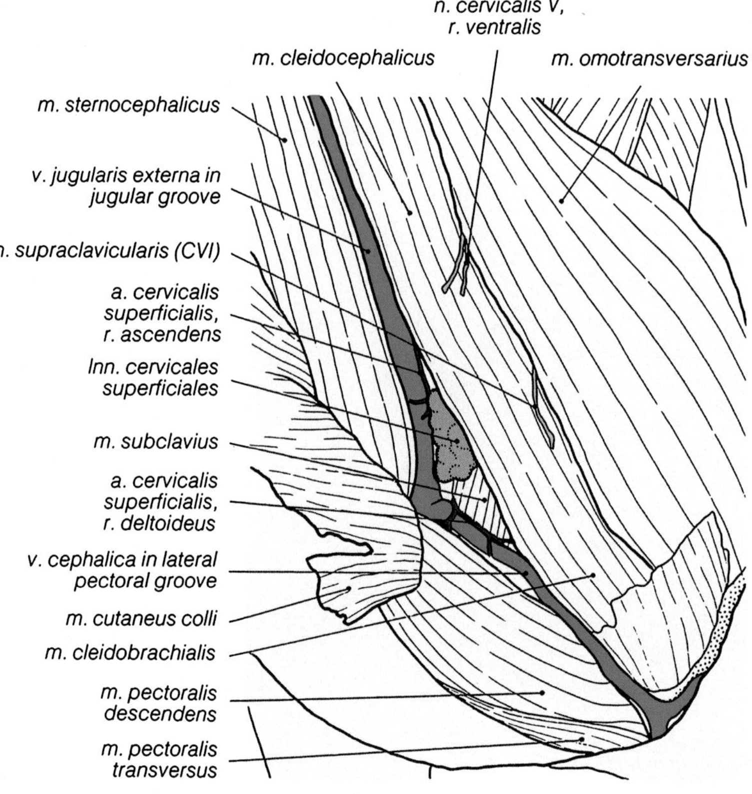
n. cervicalis V, r. ventralis
m. cleidocephalicus
m. omotransversarius
m. sternocephalicus
v. jugularis externa in jugular groove
n. supraclavicularis (CVI)
a. cervicalis superficialis, r. ascendens
lnn. cervicales superficiales
m. subclavius
a. cervicalis superficialis, r. deltoideus
v. cephalica in lateral pectoral groove
m. cutaneus colli
m. cleidobrachialis
m. pectoralis descendens
m. pectoralis transversus

Fig. 2.5 The superficial cervical lymph nodes: left craniolateral view. The cutaneous muscle of the neck has been reflected and the adipose tissue surrounding the lymph node has been removed.

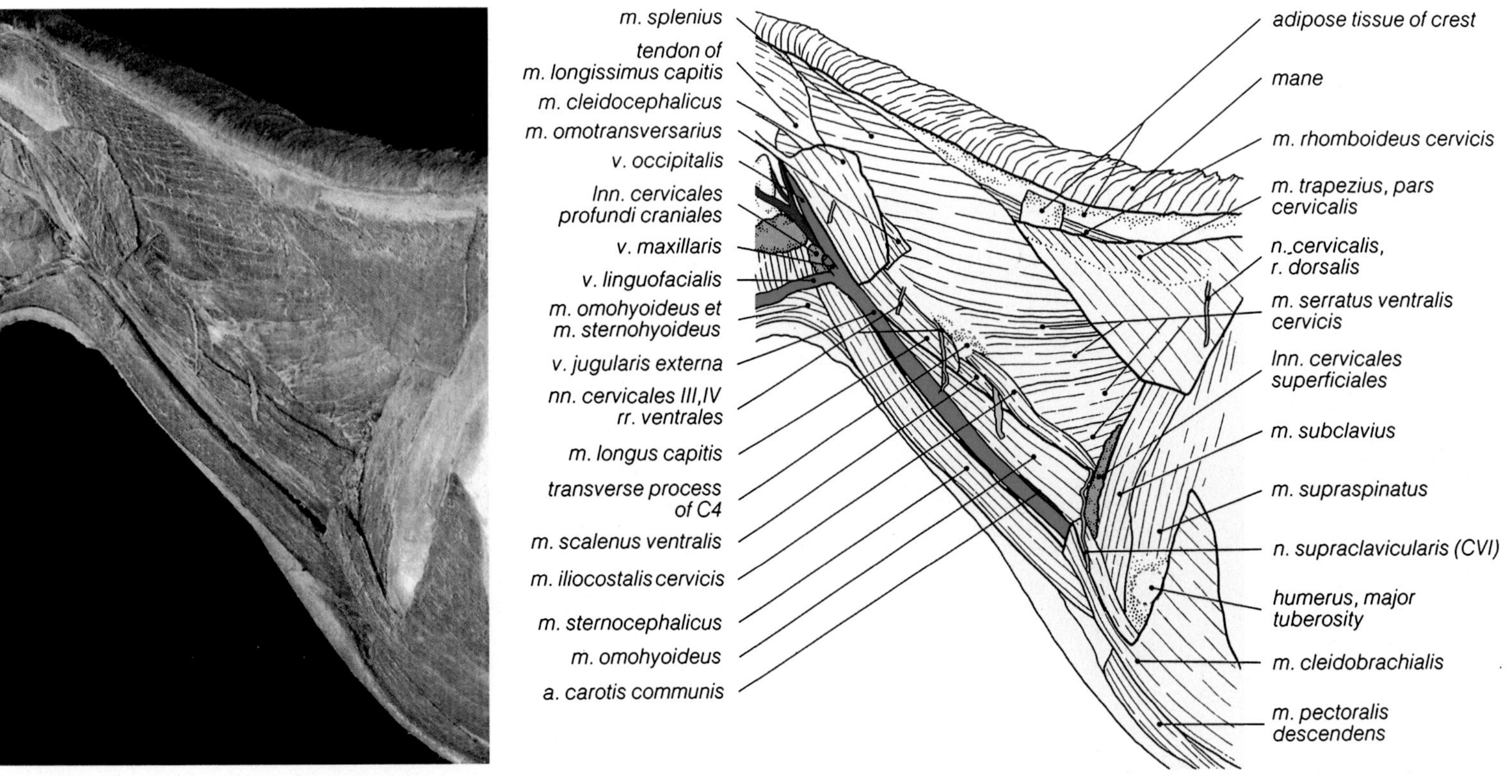
m. splenius
tendon of m. longissimus capitis
m. cleidocephalicus
m. omotransversarius
v. occipitalis
lnn. cervicales profundi craniales
v. maxillaris
v. linguofacialis
m. omohyoideus et m. sternohyoideus
v. jugularis externa
nn. cervicales III,IV rr. ventrales
m. longus capitis
transverse process of C4
m. scalenus ventralis
m. iliocostalis cervicis
m. sternocephalicus
m. omohyoideus
a. carotis communis
adipose tissue of crest
mane
m. rhomboideus cervicis
m. trapezius, pars cervicalis
n. cervicalis, r. dorsalis
m. serratus ventralis cervicis
lnn. cervicales superficiales
m. subclavius
m. supraspinatus
n. supraclavicularis (CVI)
humerus, major tuberosity
m. cleidobrachialis
m. pectoralis descendens

Fig. 2.6 Contents of the jugular groove: left lateral view. The dorsal border of the groove, formed by the brachiocephalicus muscle, has been removed, leaving the contents of the groove and its ventral border (sternocephalicus muscle) in position.

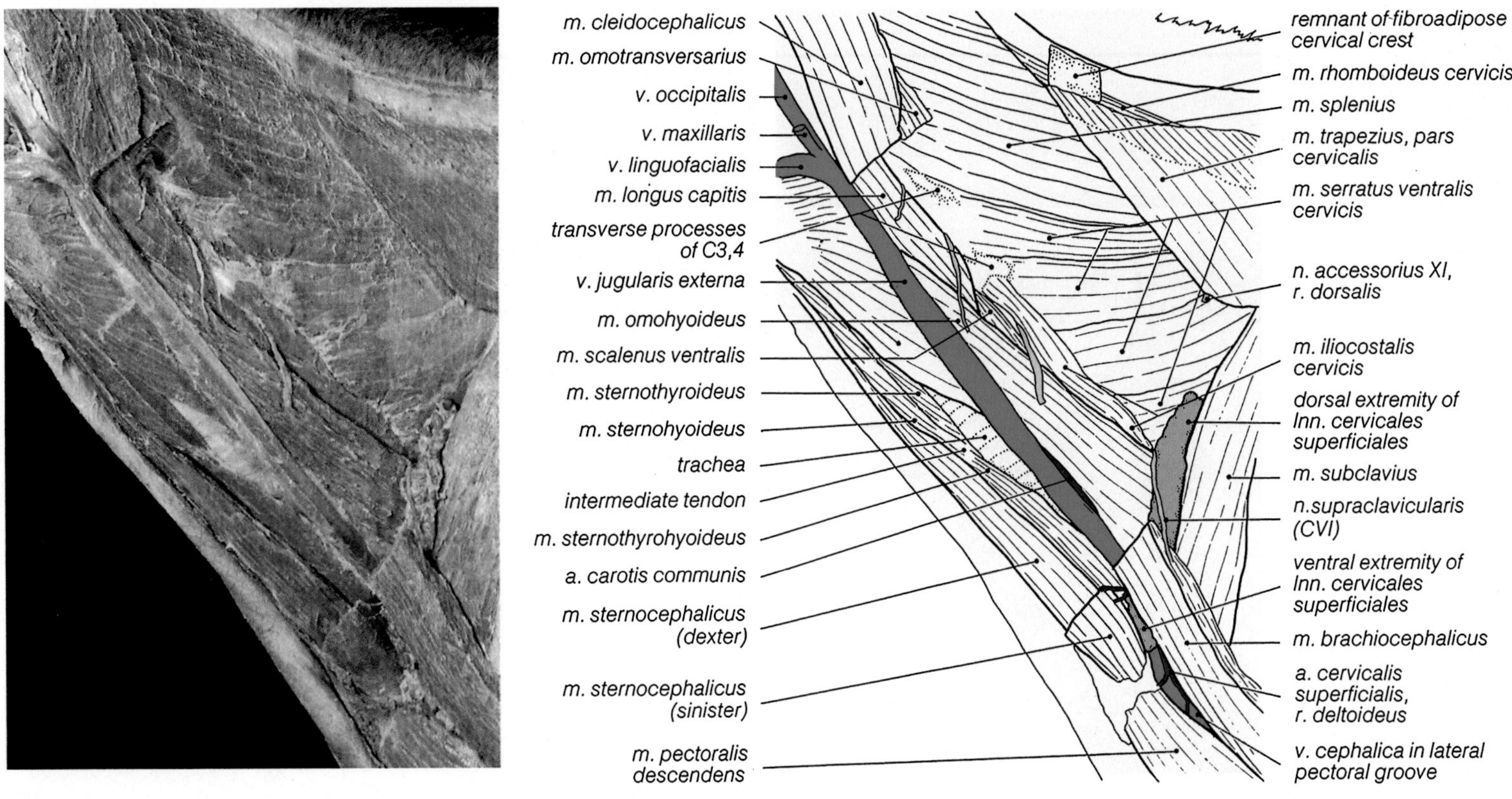
m. cleidocephalicus
m. omotransversarius
v. occipitalis
v. maxillaris
v. linguofacialis
m. longus capitis
transverse processes of C3,4
v. jugularis externa
m. omohyoideus
m. scalenus ventralis
m. sternothyroideus
m. sternohyoideus
trachea
intermediate tendon
m. sternothyrohyoideus
a. carotis communis
m. sternocephalicus (dexter)
m. sternocephalicus (sinister)
m. pectoralis descendens
remnant of fibroadipose cervical crest
m. rhomboideus cervicis
m. splenius
m. trapezius, pars cervicalis
m. serratus ventralis cervicis
n. accessorius XI, r. dorsalis
m. iliocostalis cervicis
dorsal extremity of lnn. cervicales superficiales
m. subclavius
n.supraclavicularis (CVI)
ventral extremity of lnn. cervicales superficiales
m. brachiocephalicus
a. cervicalis superficialis, r. deltoideus
v. cephalica in lateral pectoral groove

Fig. 2.7 Strap muscles of the neck: left lateral view. The brachiocephalicus and sternocephalicus muscles have been resected to display the sternohyoideus, sternothyroideus and omohyoideus muscles. The intermediate tendon is indistinct in some individuals.

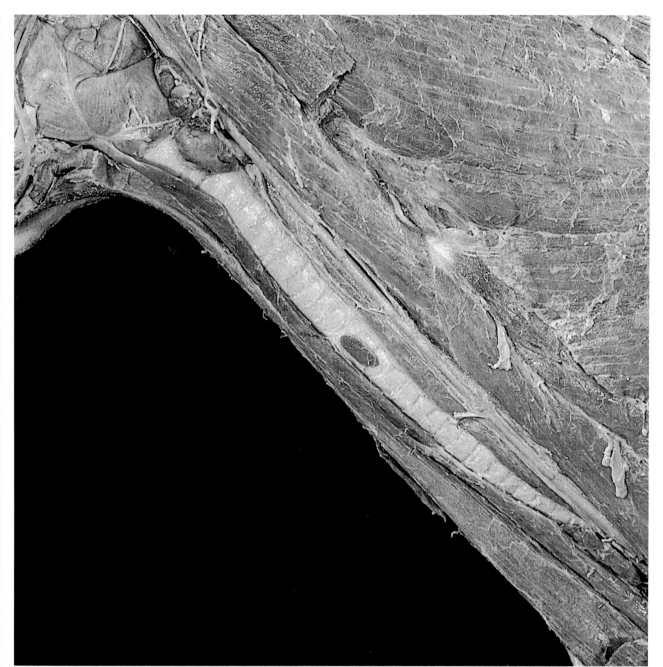

Fig. 2.8 Cervical lymph nodes and viscera: left lateral view. The deep lymph nodes and the tracheal lymph duct have been exposed by removal of the omohyoid muscle and the jugular vein.

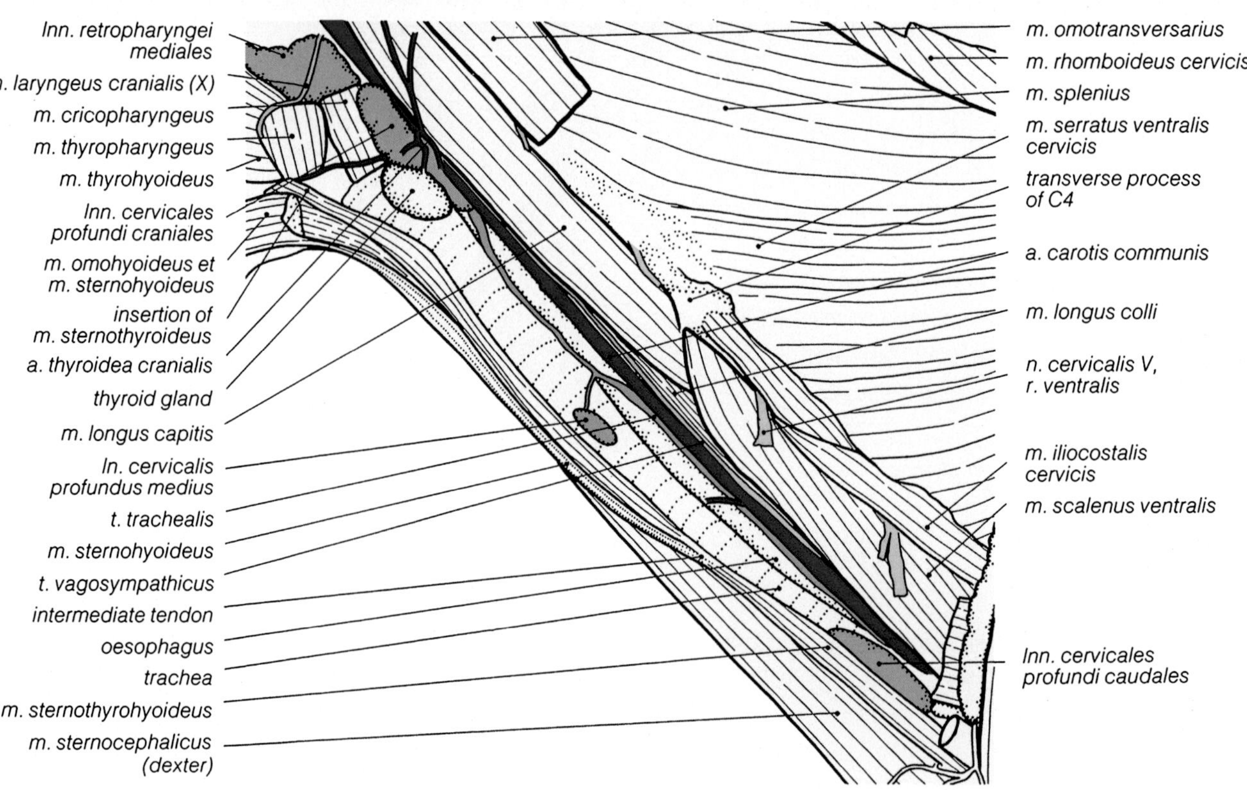
lnn. retropharyngei mediales
n. laryngeus cranialis (X)
m. cricopharyngeus
m. thyropharyngeus
m. thyrohyoideus
lnn. cervicales profundi craniales
m. omohyoideus et m. sternohyoideus
insertion of m. sternothyroideus
a. thyroidea cranialis
thyroid gland
m. longus capitis
ln. cervicalis profundus medius
t. trachealis
m. sternohyoideus
t. vagosympathicus
intermediate tendon
oesophagus
trachea
m. sternothyrohyoideus
m. sternocephalicus (dexter)
m. omotransversarius
m. rhomboideus cervicis
m. splenius
m. serratus ventralis cervicis
transverse process of C4
a. carotis communis
m. longus colli
n. cervicalis V, r. ventralis
m. iliocostalis cervicis
m. scalenus ventralis
lnn. cervicales profundi caudales

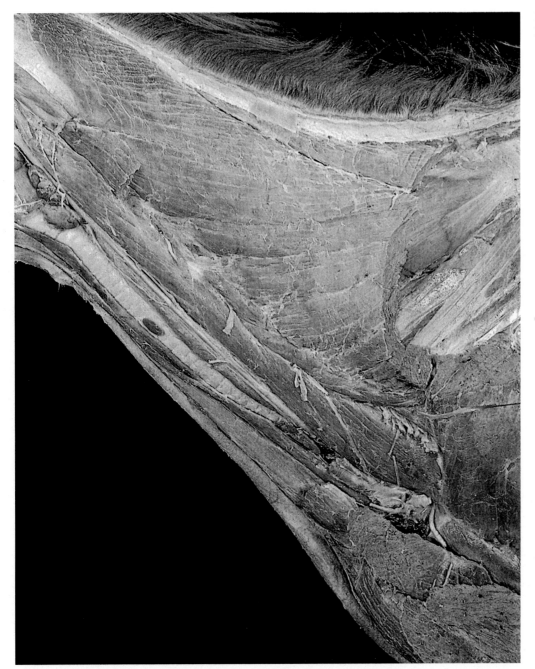

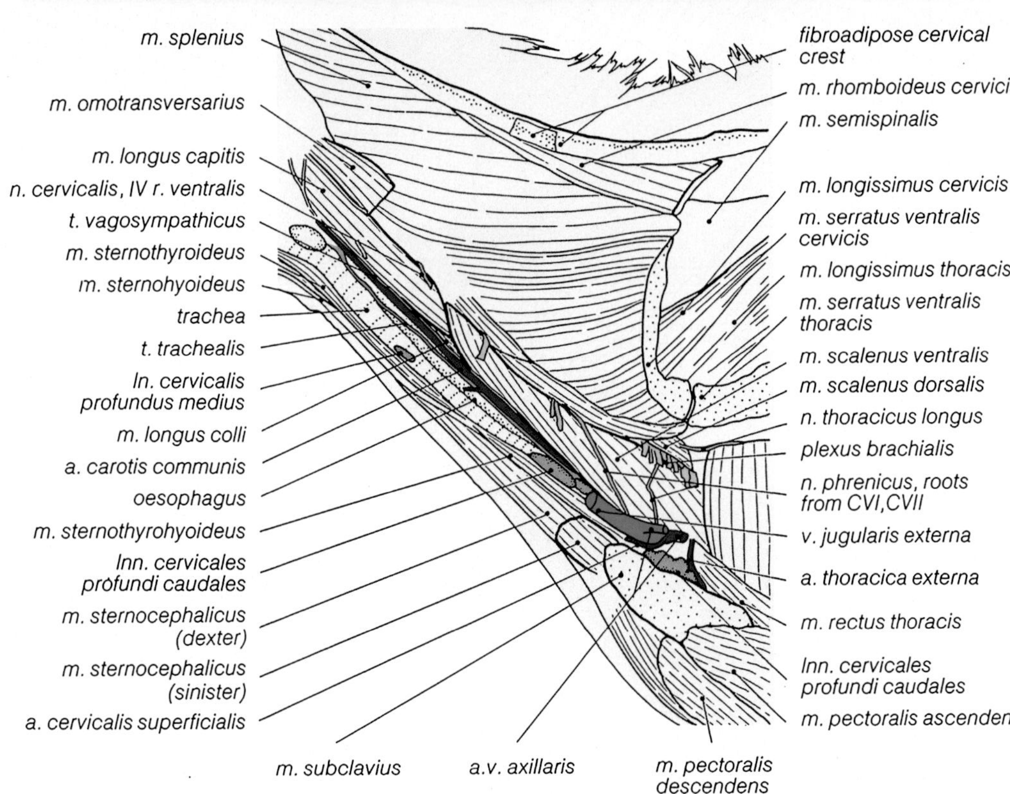

m. splenius
m. omotransversarius
m. longus capitis
n. cervicalis, IV r. ventralis
t. vagosympathicus
m. sternothyroideus
m. sternohyoideus
trachea
t. trachealis
ln. cervicalis profundus medius
m. longus colli
a. carotis communis
oesophagus
m. sternothyrohyoideus
lnn. cervicales profundi caudales
m. sternocephalicus (dexter)
m. sternocephalicus (sinister)
a. cervicalis superficialis
m. subclavius
a.v. axillaris
m. pectoralis descendens
fibroadipose cervical crest
m. rhomboideus cervicis
m. semispinalis
m. longissimus cervicis
m. serratus ventralis cervicis
m. longissimus thoracis
m. serratus ventralis thoracis
m. scalenus ventralis
m. scalenus dorsalis
n. thoracicus longus
plexus brachialis
n. phrenicus, roots from CVI,CVII
v. jugularis externa
a. thoracica externa
m. rectus thoracis
lnn. cervicales profundi caudales
m. pectoralis ascendens

Fig. 2.9 Cervical structures at the thoracic inlet: left lateral view, (1). The forelimb has been removed.

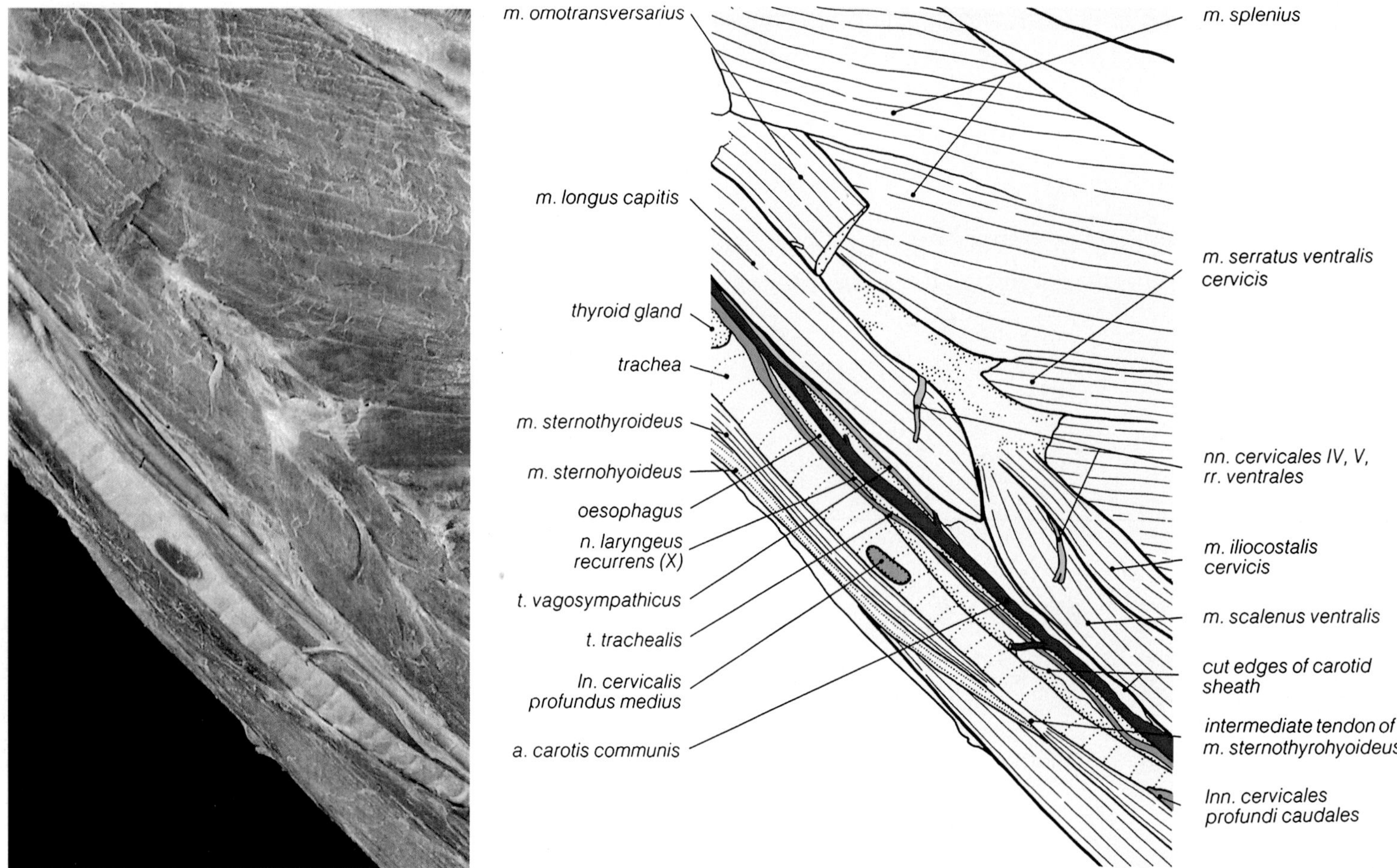
m. omotransversarius
m. longus capitis
thyroid gland
trachea
m. sternothyroideus
m. sternohyoideus
oesophagus
n. laryngeus recurrens (X)
t. vagosympathicus
t. trachealis
ln. cervicalis profundus medius
a. carotis communis
m. splenius
m. serratus ventralis cervicis
nn. cervicales IV, V, rr. ventrales
m. iliocostalis cervicis
m. scalenus ventralis
cut edges of carotid sheath
intermediate tendon of m. sternothyrohyoideus
lnn. cervicales profundi caudales

Fig. 2.10 Contents of the carotid sheath: left lateral view. The fascial sheath has been incised. The enclosed nerves, artery and the associated lymphatic trunk have been slightly separated at the position of the black pin.

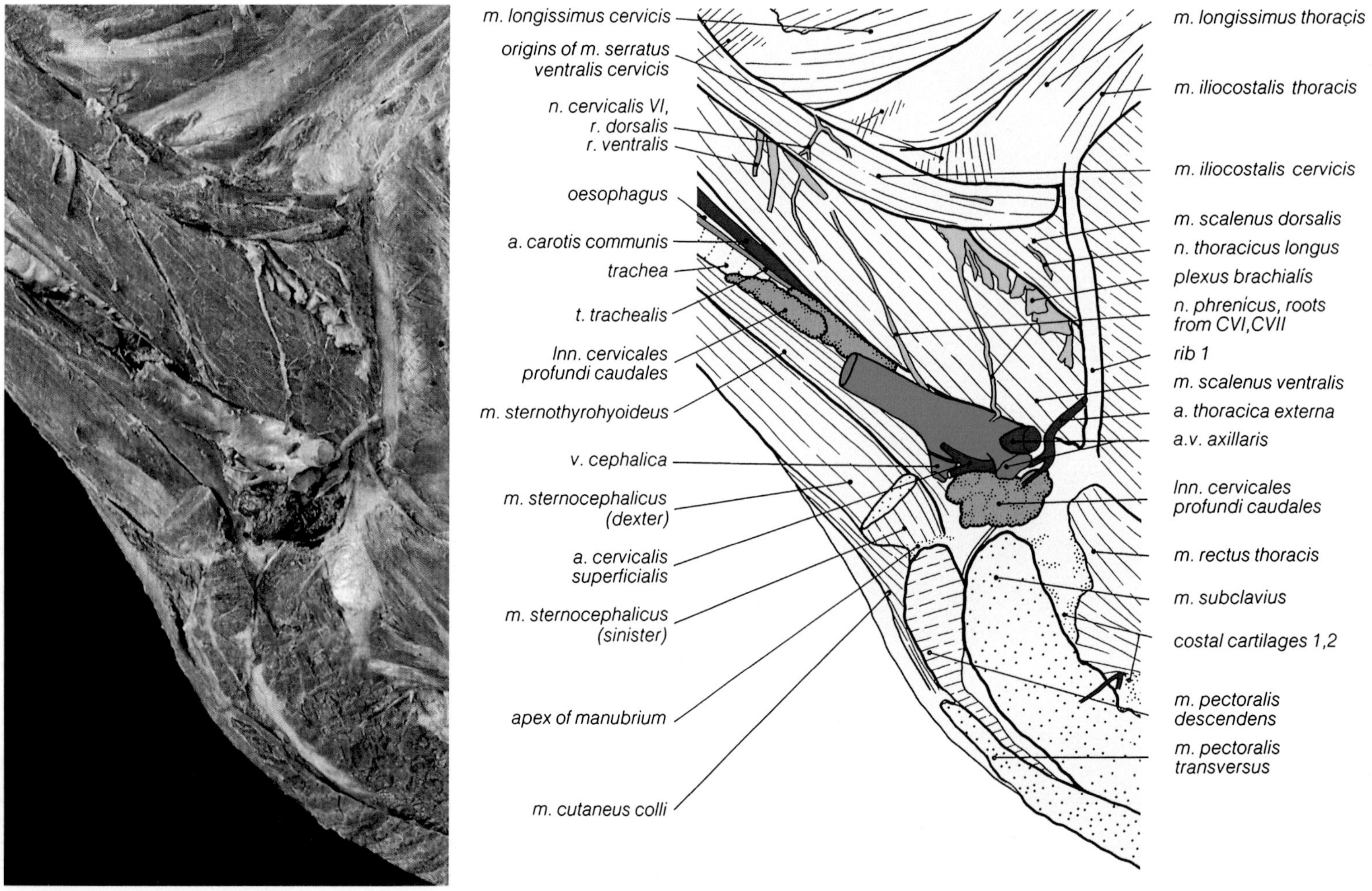

m. longissimus cervicis
origins of m. serratus ventralis cervicis
n. cervicalis VI, r. dorsalis
r. ventralis
oesophagus
a. carotis communis
trachea
t. trachealis
lnn. cervicales profundi caudales
m. sternothyrohyoideus
v. cephalica
m. sternocephalicus (dexter)
a. cervicalis superficialis
m. sternocephalicus (sinister)
apex of manubrium
m. cutaneus colli
m. longissimus thoraçis
m. iliocostalis thoracis
m. iliocostalis cervicis
m. scalenus dorsalis
n. thoracicus longus
plexus brachialis
n. phrenicus, roots from CVI,CVII
rib 1
m. scalenus ventralis
a. thoracica externa
a.v. axillaris
lnn. cervicales profundi caudales
m. rectus thoracis
m. subclavius
costal cartilages 1,2
m. pectoralis descendens
m. pectoralis transversus

Fig. 2.11 Cervical structures at the thoracic inlet: left lateral view, (2). The ventral serrate and pectoral muscles have been cut back to expose the sternum, ribs, and cervical structures at this level.

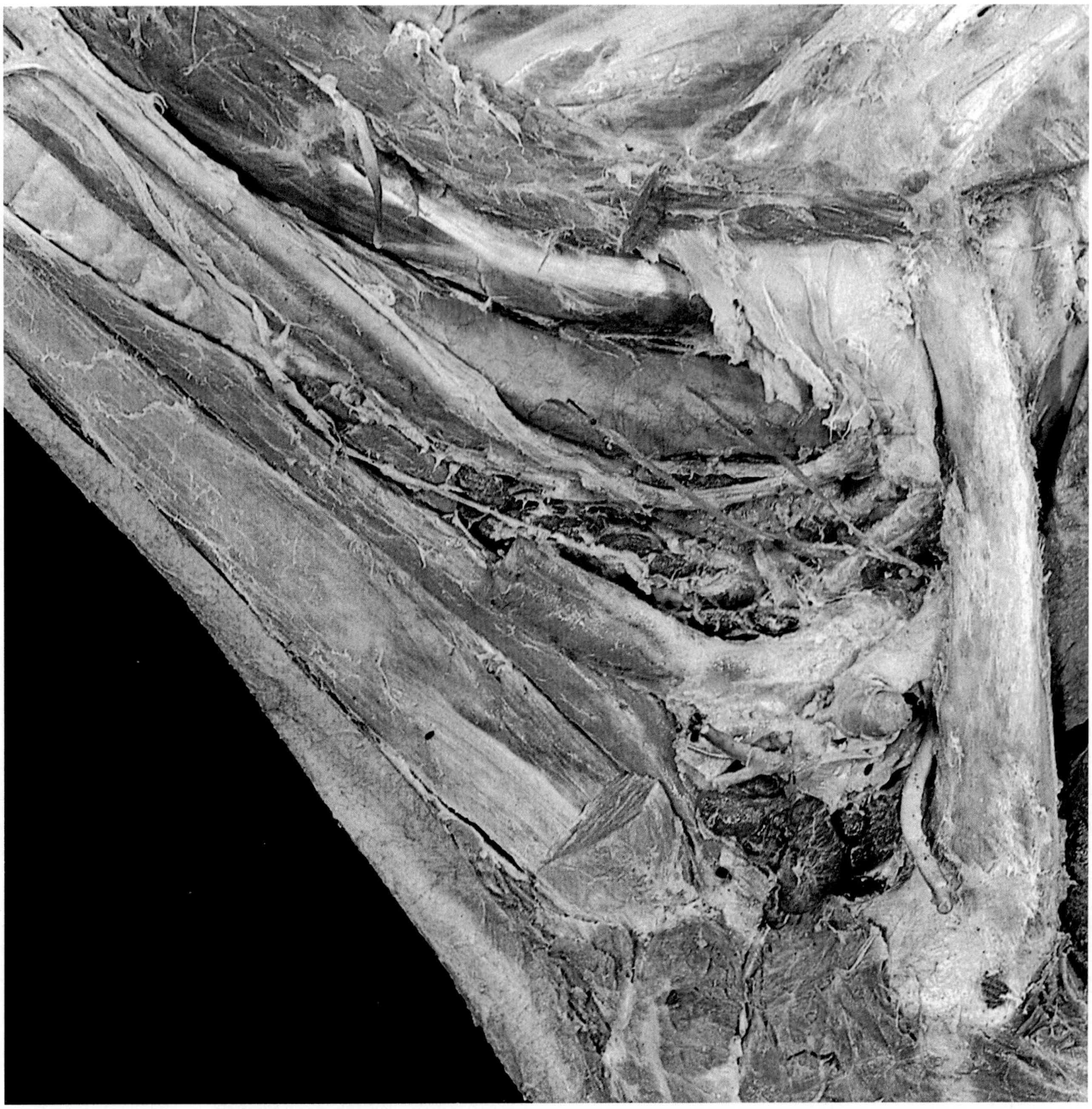

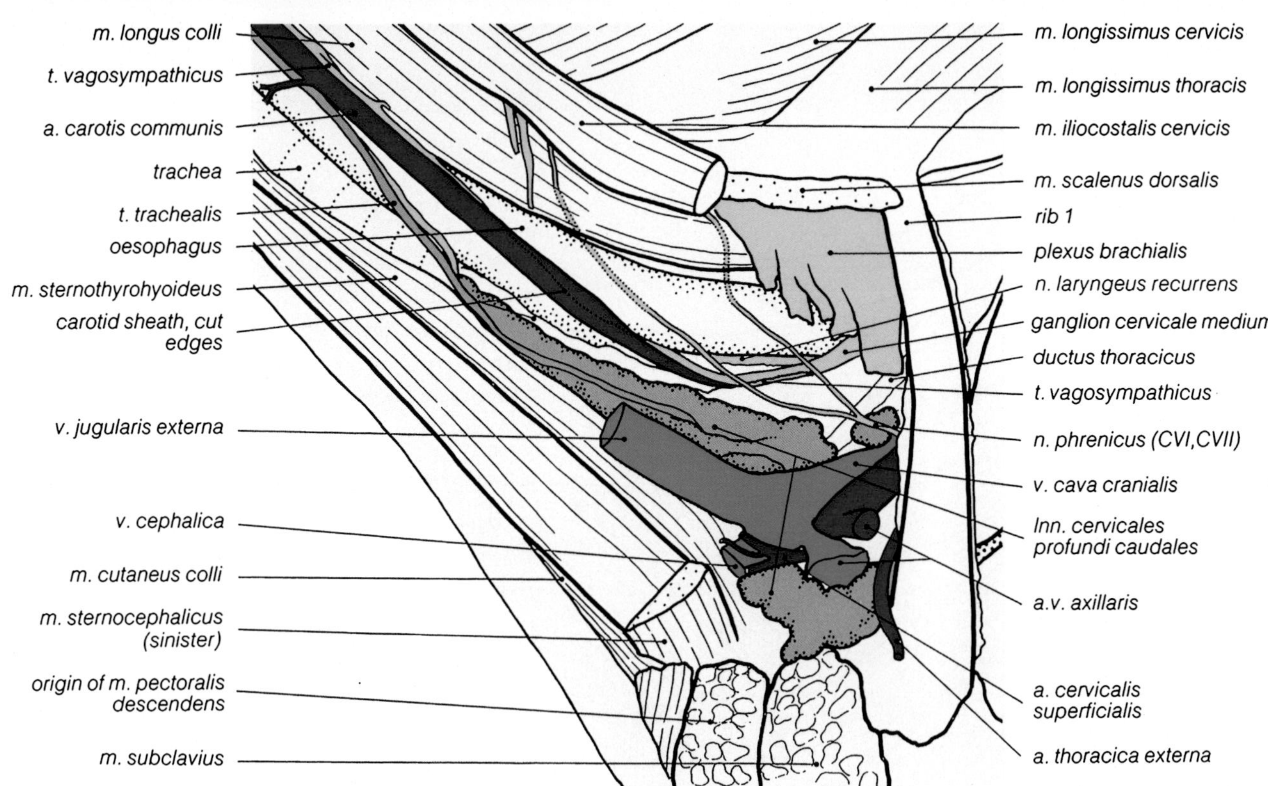
m. longus colli
t. vagosympathicus
a. carotis communis
trachea
t. trachealis
oesophagus
m. sternothyrohyoideus
carotid sheath, cut edges
v. jugularis externa
v. cephalica
m. cutaneus colli
m. sternocephalicus (sinister)
origin of m. pectoralis descendens
m. subclavius
m. longissimus cervicis
m. longissimus thoracis
m. iliocostalis cervicis
m. scalenus dorsalis
rib 1
plexus brachialis
n. laryngeus recurrens
ganglion cervicale medium
ductus thoracicus
t. vagosympathicus
n. phrenicus (CVI,CVII)
v. cava cranialis
lnn. cervicales profundi caudales
a.v. axillaris
a. cervicalis superficialis
a. thoracica externa

Fig. 2.12 Cervical structures at the thoracic inlet: left lateral view, (3). The scalenus muscles have been removed in the most caudal part of the neck.

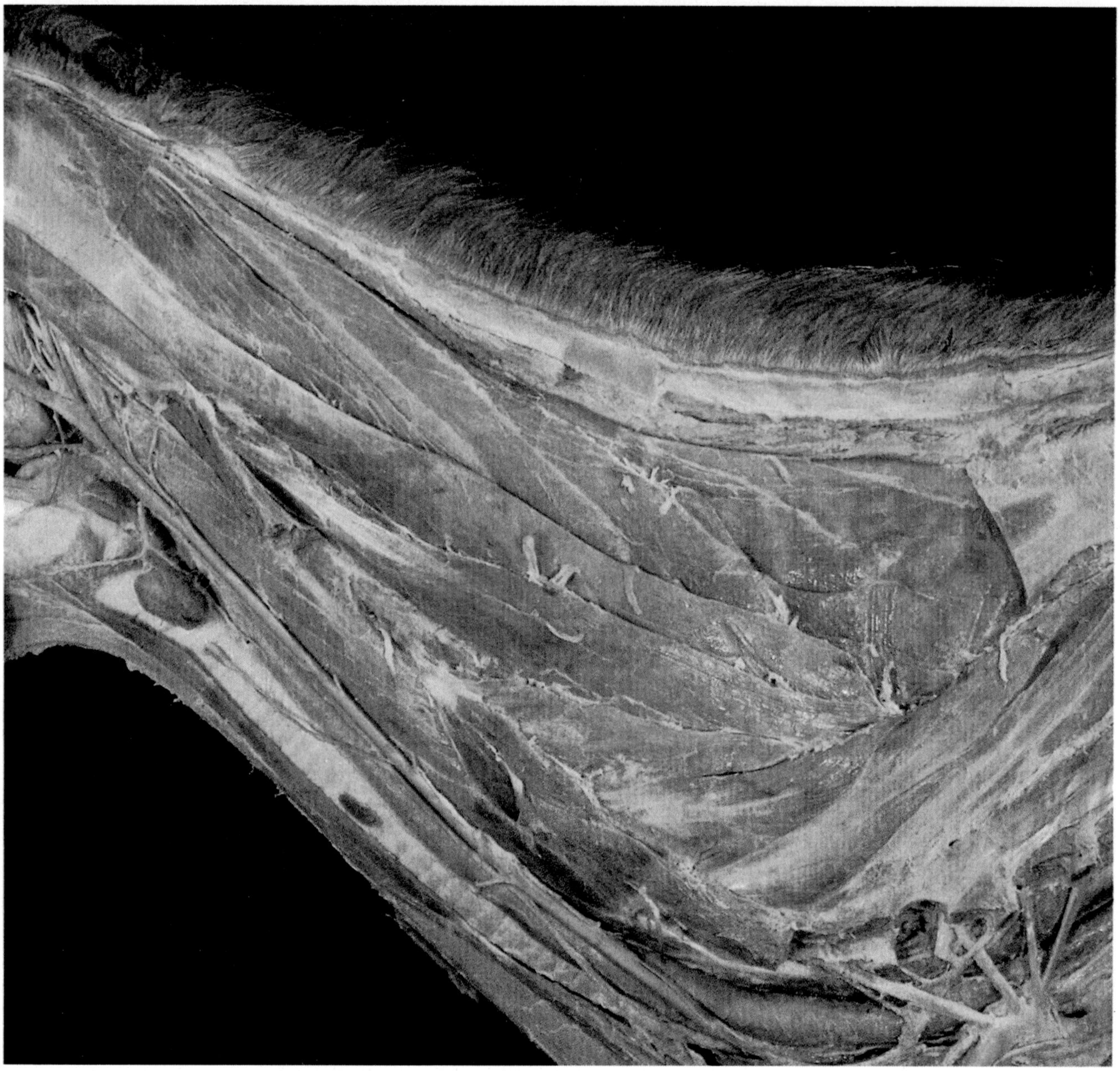

Fig. 2.13 The deeper muscles of the neck: left lateral view (1). The splenius and ventral serrate muscles have been removed. The first rib has been taken out and the second rib cut short. The cranial part of the dissection is shown in Fig. 1.31.

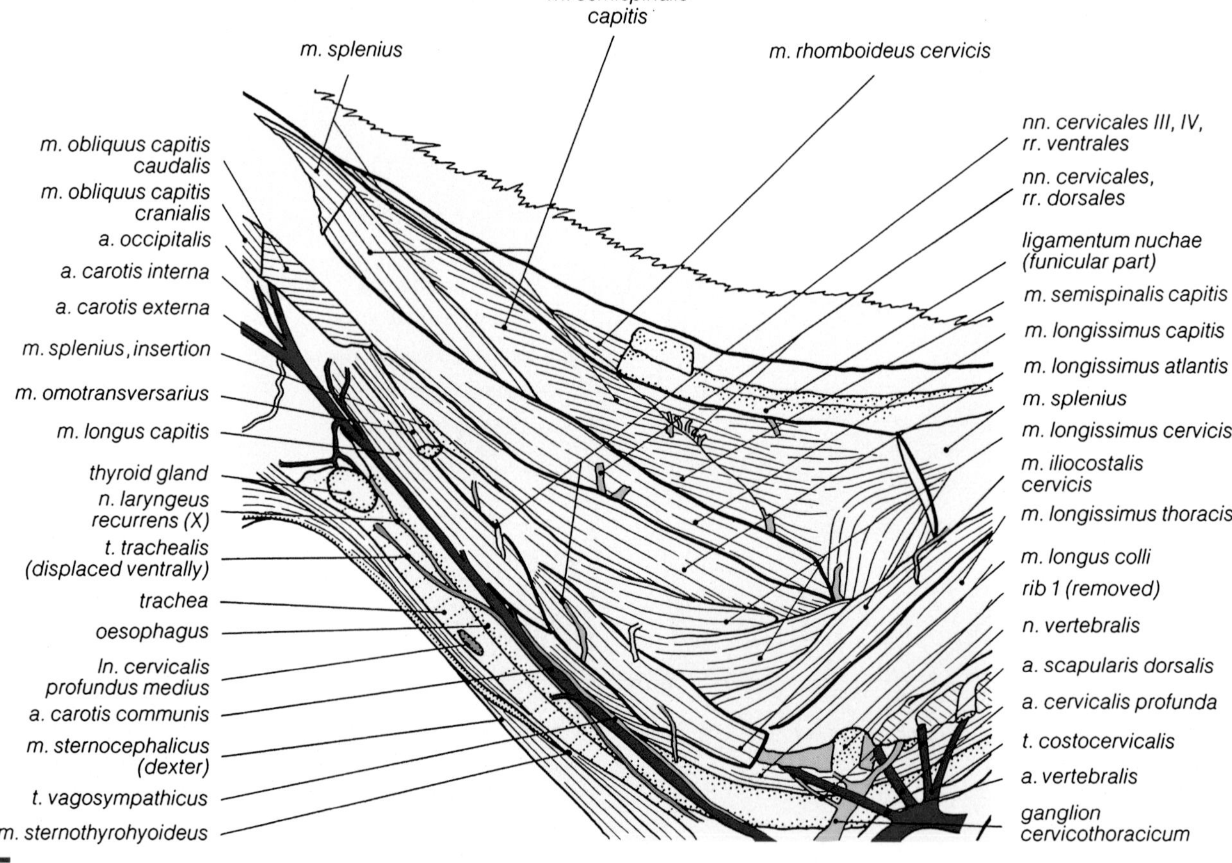
m. semispinalis capitis
m. splenius
m. rhomboideus cervicis
m. obliquus capitis caudalis
m. obliquus capitis cranialis
a. occipitalis
a. carotis interna
a. carotis externa
m. splenius, insertion
m. omotransversarius
m. longus capitis
thyroid gland
n. laryngeus recurrens (X)
t. trachealis (displaced ventrally)
trachea
oesophagus
ln. cervicalis profundus medius
a. carotis communis
m. sternocephalicus (dexter)
t. vagosympathicus
m. sternothyrohyoideus
nn. cervicales III, IV, rr. ventrales
nn. cervicales, rr. dorsales
ligamentum nuchae (funicular part)
m. semispinalis capitis
m. longissimus capitis
m. longissimus atlantis
m. splenius
m. longissimus cervicis
m. iliocostalis cervicis
m. longissimus thoracis
m. longus colli
rib 1 (removed)
n. vertebralis
a. scapularis dorsalis
a. cervicalis profunda
t. costocervicalis
a. vertebralis
ganglion cervicothoracicum

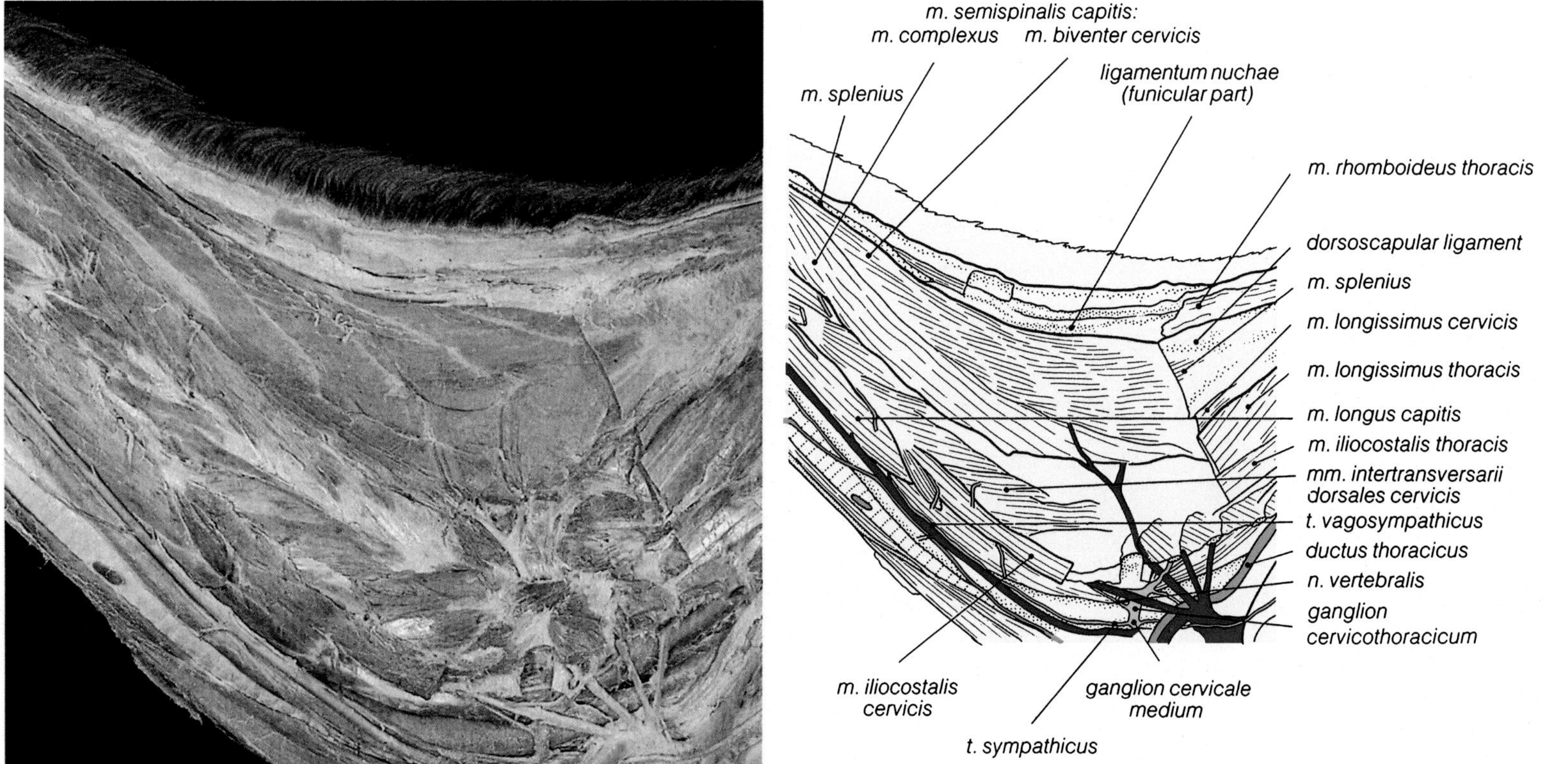
m. semispinalis capitis:
m. complexus
m. biventer cervicis
m. splenius
ligamentum nuchae (funicular part)
m. rhomboideus thoracis
dorsoscapular ligament
m. splenius
m. longissimus cervicis
m. longissimus thoracis
m. longus capitis
m. iliocostalis thoracis
mm. intertransversarii dorsales cervicis
t. vagosympathicus
ductus thoracicus
n. vertebralis
ganglion cervicothoracicum
m. iliocostalis cervicis
ganglion cervicale medium
t. sympathicus

Fig. 2.14 The deeper muscles of the neck: left lateral view (2). The cervical part of the intermediate spinal erector muscles (m. longissimus) has been removed.

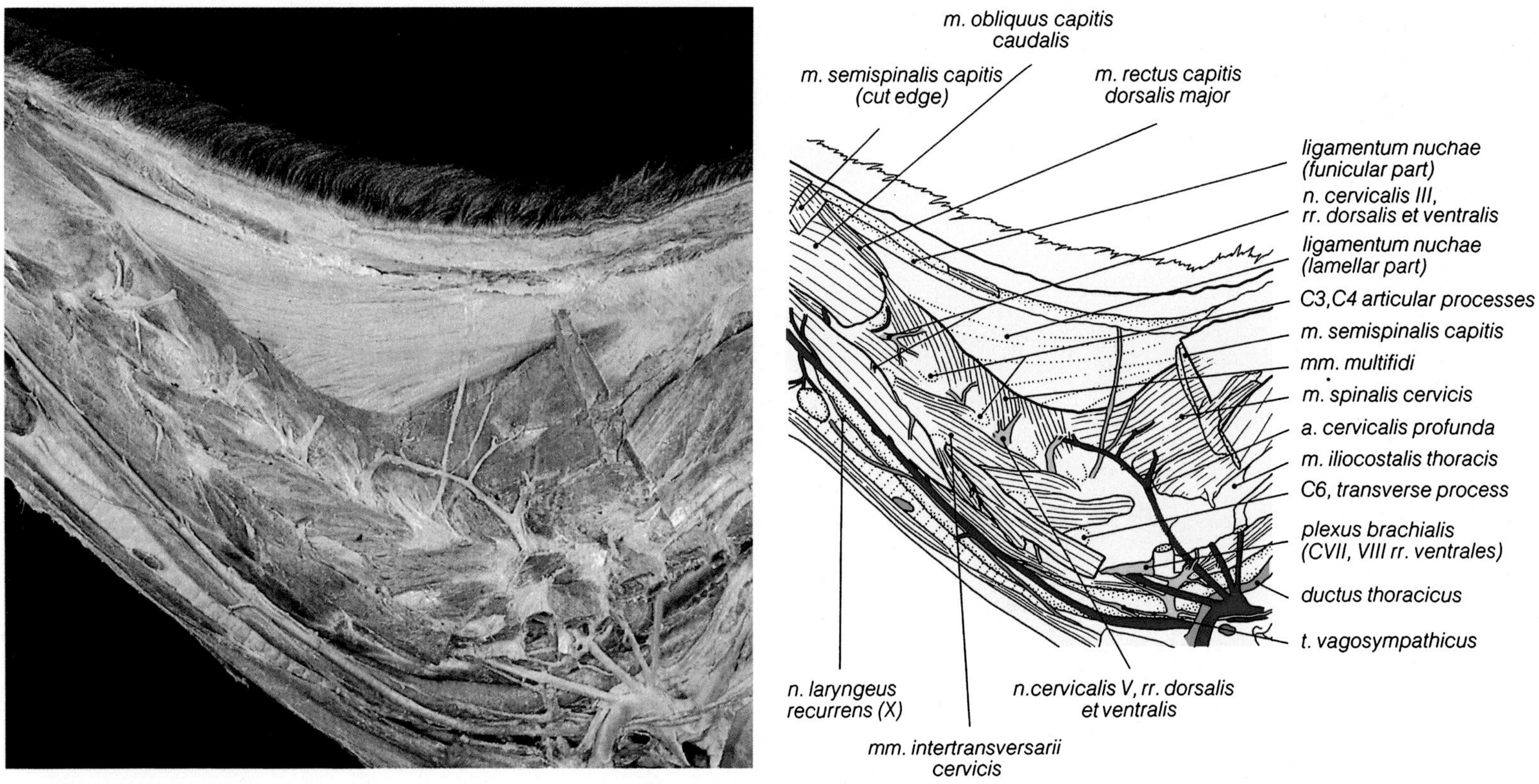
m. obliquus capitis caudalis
m. semispinalis capitis (cut edge)
m. rectus capitis dorsalis major
ligamentum nuchae (funicular part)
n. cervicalis III, rr. dorsalis et ventralis
ligamentum nuchae (lamellar part)
C3,C4 articular processes
m. semispinalis capitis
mm. multifidi
m. spinalis cervicis
a. cervicalis profunda
m. iliocostalis thoracis
C6, transverse process
plexus brachialis (CVII, VIII rr. ventrales)
ductus thoracicus
t. vagosympathicus
n. laryngeus recurrens (X)
n.cervicalis V, rr. dorsalis et ventralis
mm. intertransversarii cervicis

Fig. 2.15 The cervical nerves and nuchal ligament: left lateral view. Removal of the semispinalis capitis muscle has exposed the nuchal ligament. The dorsal branches of the cervical nerves emerge from the deepest layer of spinal muscles.

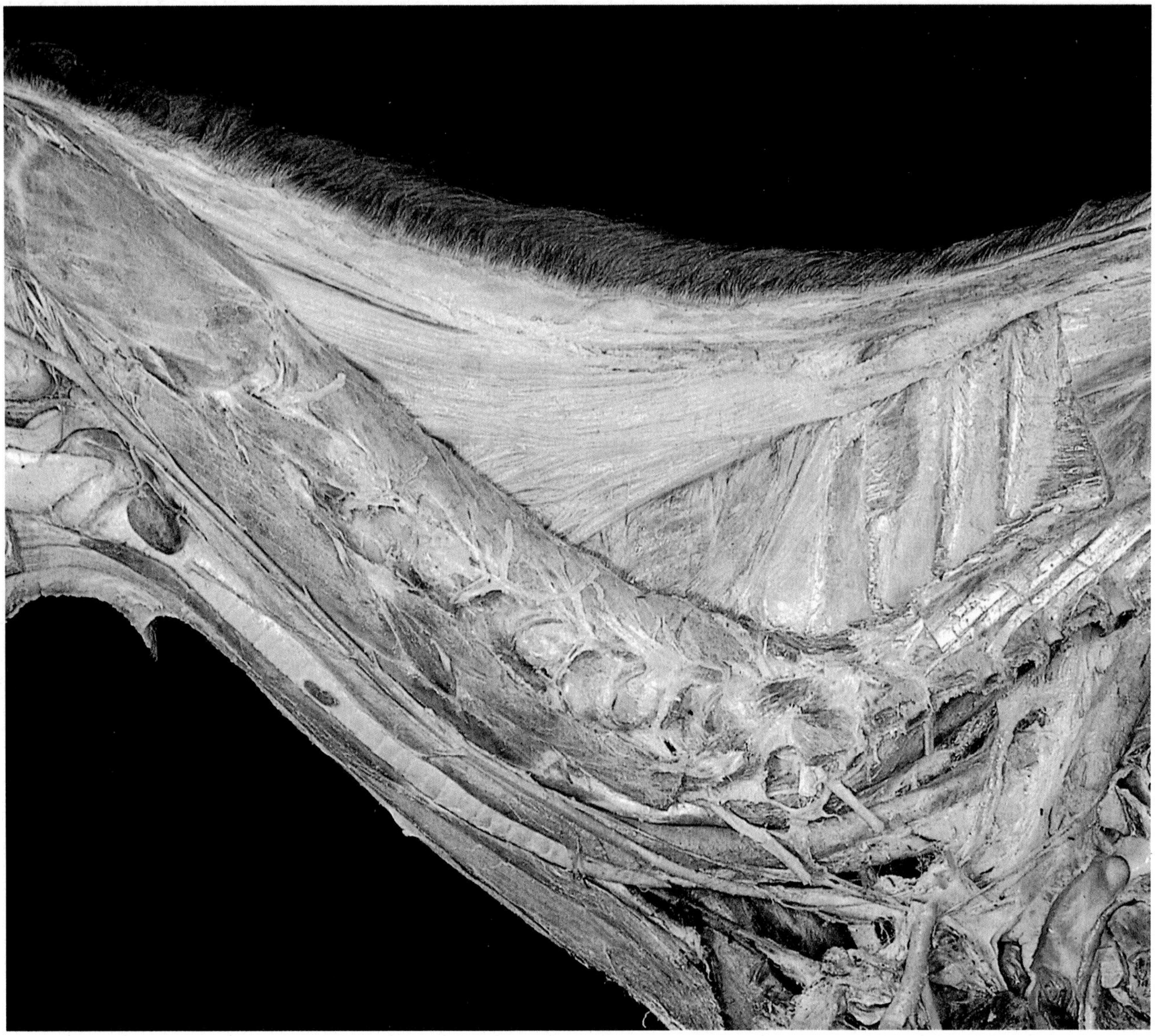

Fig. 2.16 The nuchal ligament: left lateral view. Removal of the spinalis cervicis muscle exposes the broad lamellar part of the ligament and the related thoracic interspinous ligaments. The dorsoscapular ligament (Fig. 2.14) has also been removed.

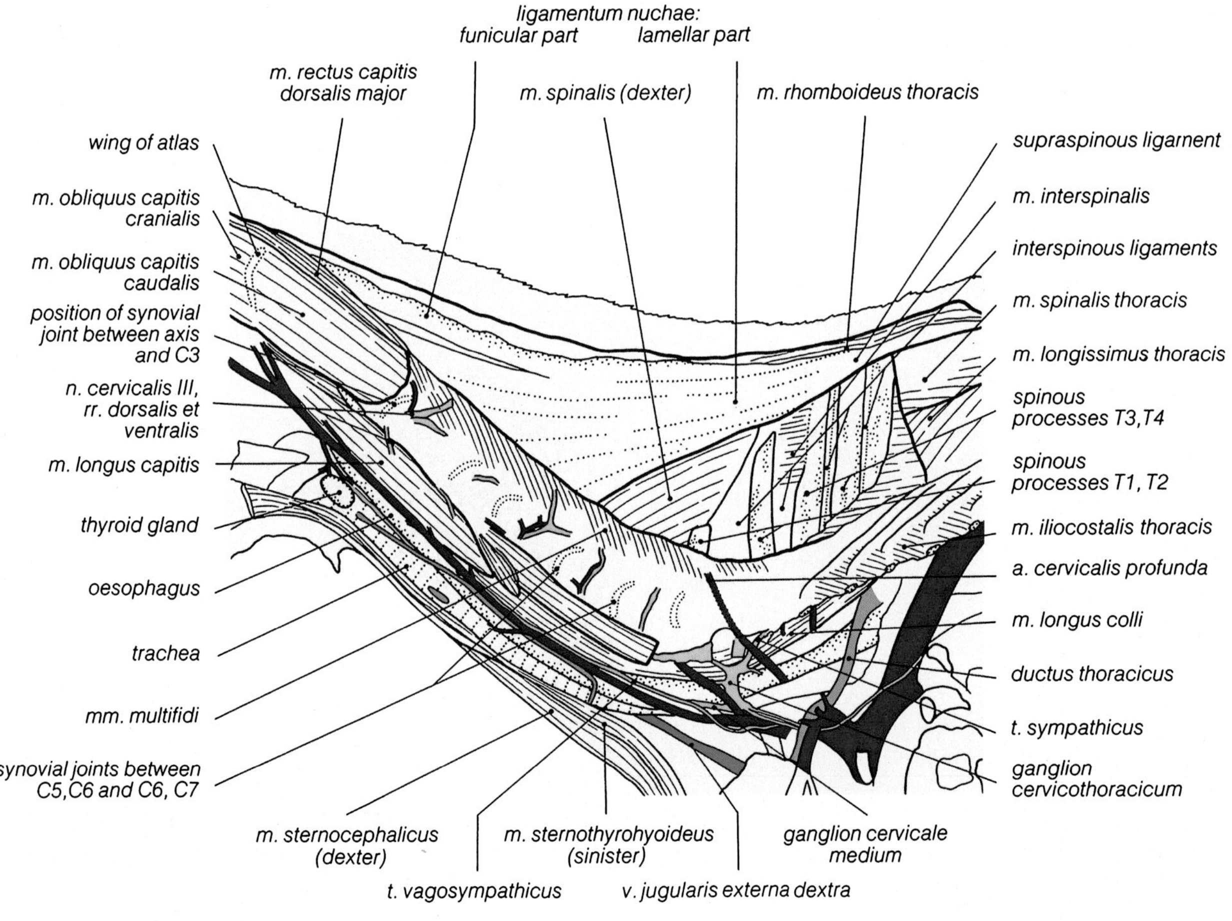
ligamentum nuchae:
funicular part
lamellar part
m. rectus capitis dorsalis major
m. spinalis (dexter)
m. rhomboideus thoracis
wing of atlas
m. obliquus capitis cranialis
m. obliquus capitis caudalis
position of synovial joint between axis and C3
n. cervicalis III, rr. dorsalis et ventralis
m. longus capitis
thyroid gland
oesophagus
trachea
mm. multifidi
synovial joints between C5,C6 and C6, C7
supraspinous ligarnent
m. interspinalis
interspinous ligaments
m. spinalis thoracis
m. longissimus thoracis
spinous processes T3,T4
spinous processes T1, T2
m. iliocostalis thoracis
a. cervicalis profunda
m. longus colli
ductus thoracicus
t. sympathicus
ganglion cervicothoracicum
m. sternocephalicus (dexter)
m. sternothyrohyoideus (sinister)
ganglion cervicale medium
t. vagosympathicus
v. jugularis externa dextra

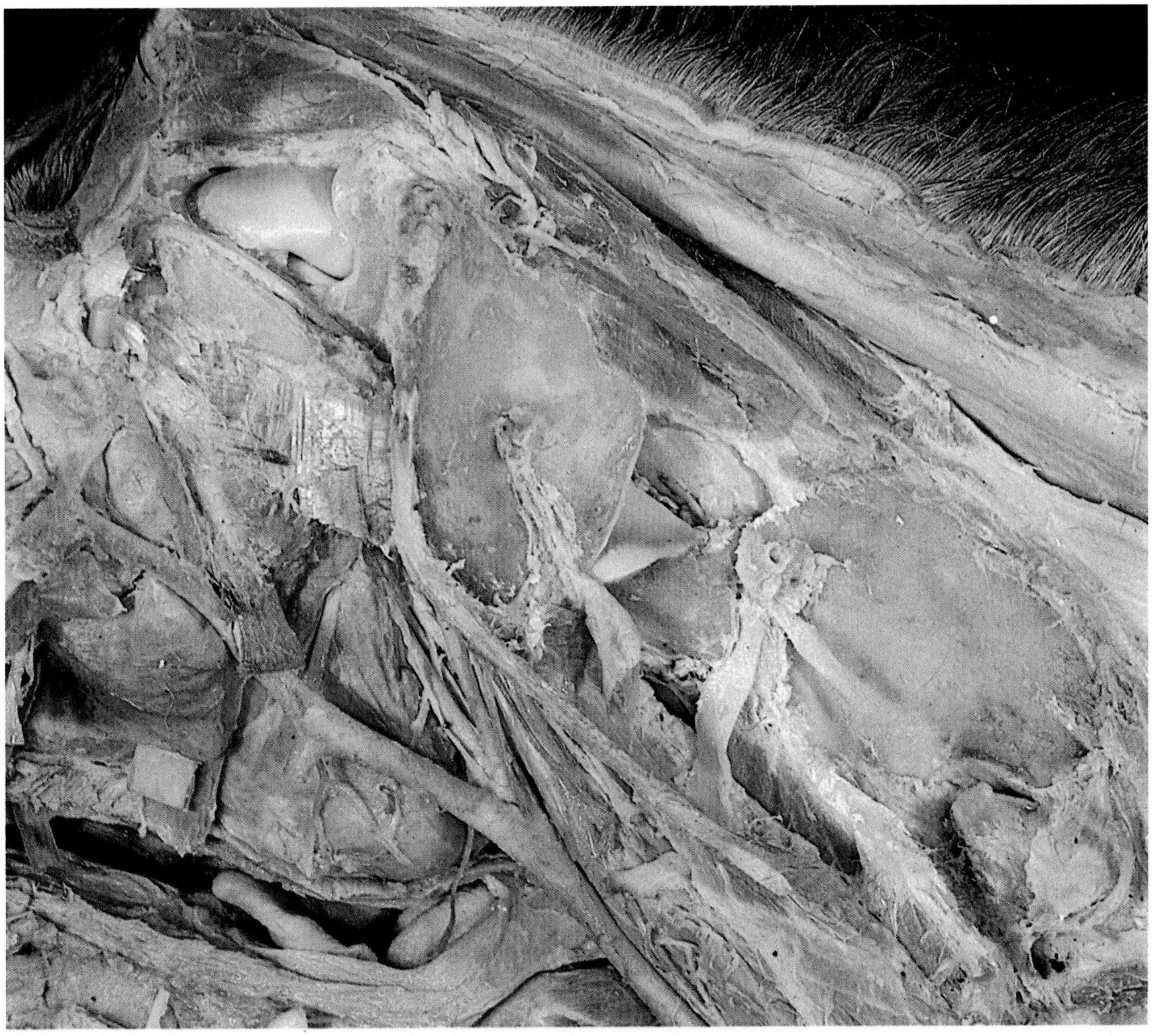

Fig. 2.17 The atlas and axis vertebrae: left lateral view. The pharyngeal structures are dealt with in detail in Fig. 1.26 and Figs. 1.32–1.34.

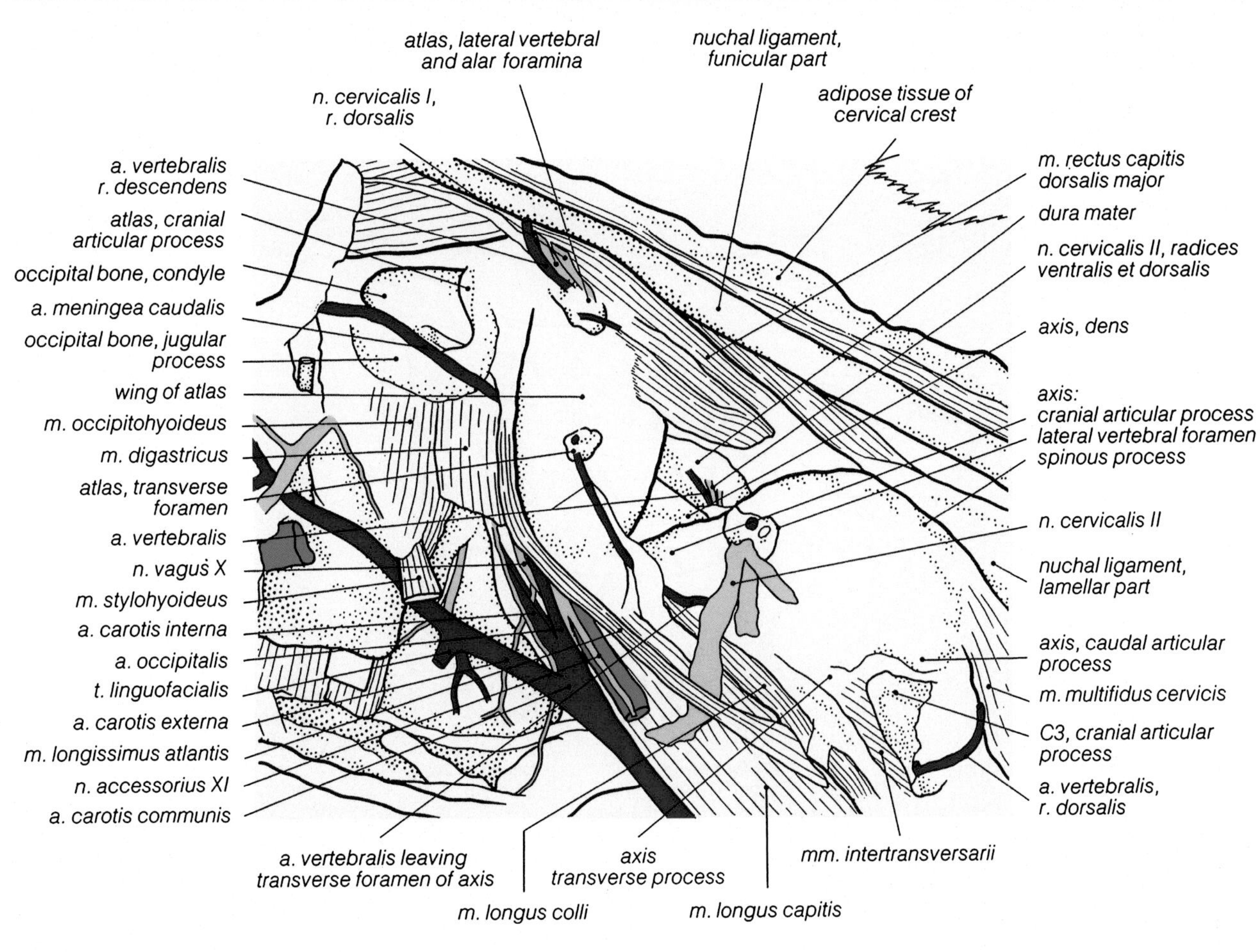
atlas, lateral vertebral and alar foramina
nuchal ligament, funicular part
n. cervicalis I, r. dorsalis
adipose tissue of cervical crest
a. vertebralis r. descendens
atlas, cranial articular process
occipital bone, condyle
a. meningea caudalis
occipital bone, jugular process
wing of atlas
m. occipitohyoideus
m. digastricus
atlas, transverse foramen
a. vertebralis
n. vagus X
m. stylohyoideus
a. carotis interna
a. occipitalis
t. linguofacialis
a. carotis externa
m. longissimus atlantis
n. accessorius XI
a. carotis communis
m. rectus capitis dorsalis major
dura mater
n. cervicalis II, radices ventralis et dorsalis
axis, dens
axis:
cranial articular process
lateral vertebral foramen
spinous process
n. cervicalis II
nuchal ligament, lamellar part
axis, caudal articular process
m. multifidus cervicis
C3, cranial articular process
a. vertebralis, r. dorsalis
a. vertebralis leaving transverse foramen of axis
axis transverse process
mm. intertransversarii
m. longus colli
m. longus capitis

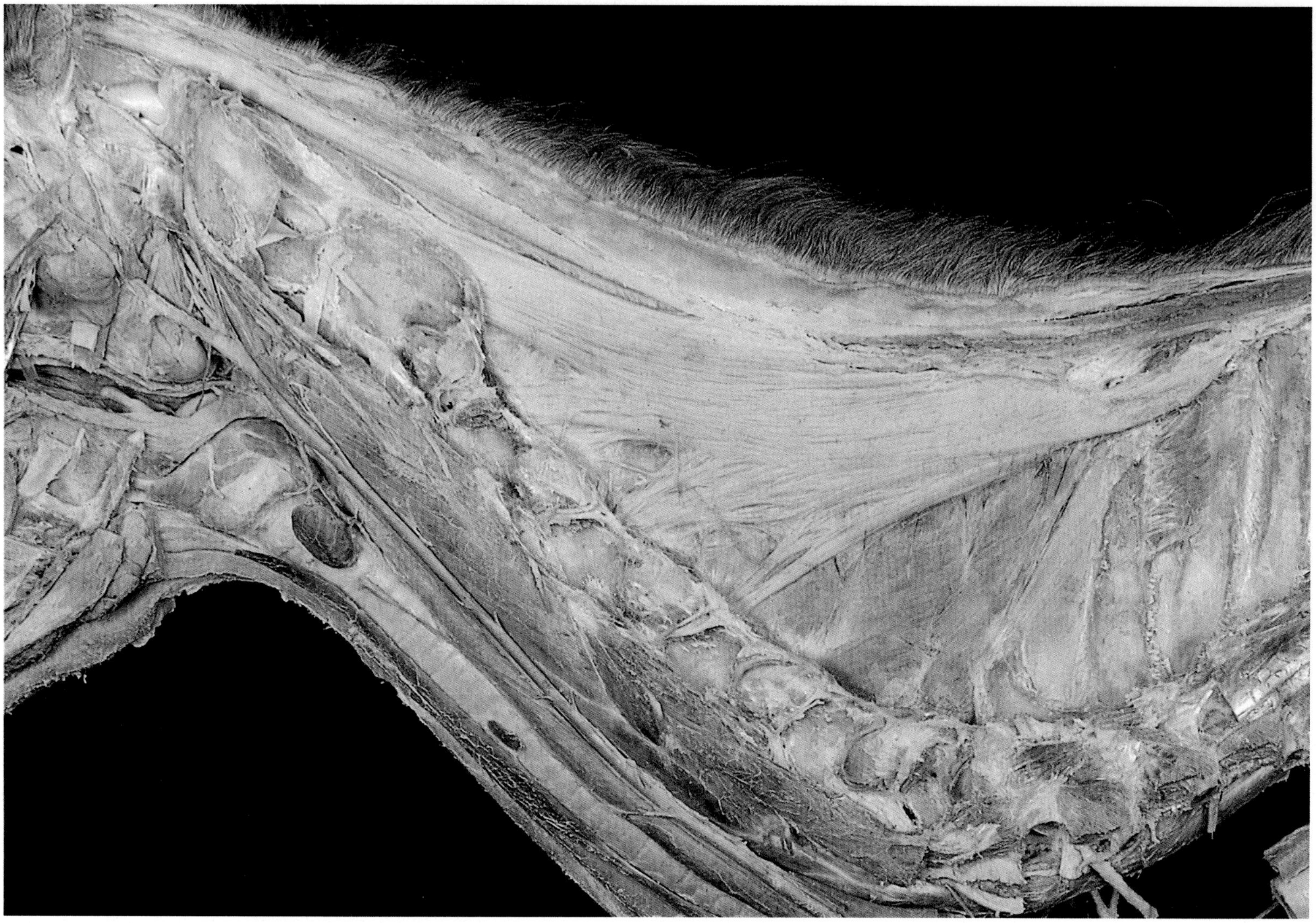

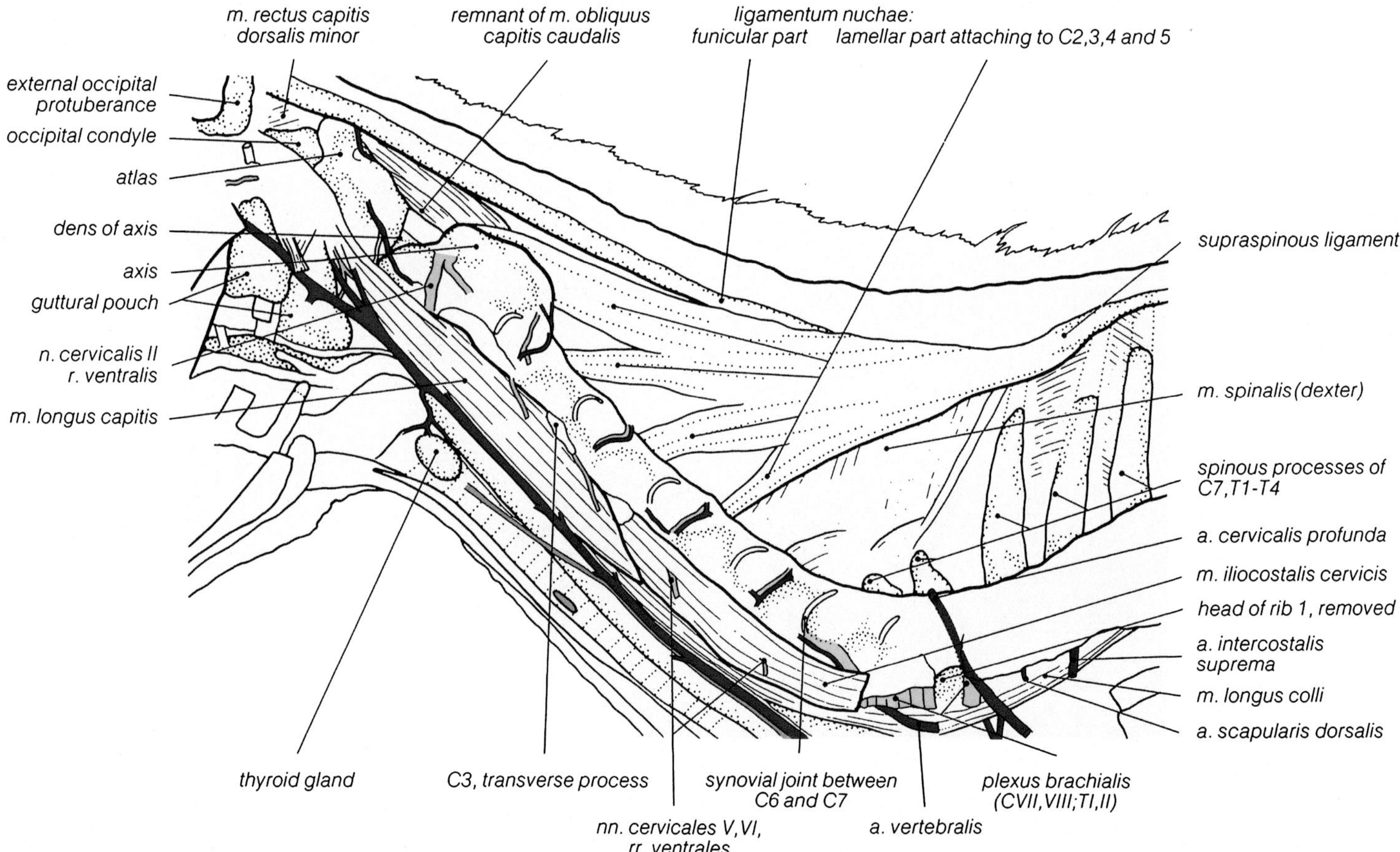
m. rectus capitis
dorsalis minor
remnant of m. obliquus
capitis caudalis
ligamentum nuchae:
funicular part
lamellar part attaching to C2,3,4 and 5
external occipital
protuberance
occipital condyle
atlas
dens of axis
axis
guttural pouch
n. cervicalis II
r. ventralis
m. longus capitis
supraspinous ligament
m. spinalis (dexter)
spinous processes of
C7,T1-T4
a. cervicalis profunda
m. iliocostalis cervicis
head of rib 1, removed
a. intercostalis
suprema
m. longus colli
a. scapularis dorsalis
thyroid gland
C3, transverse process
synovial joint between
C6 and C7
plexus brachialis
(CVII,VIII;TI,II)
nn. cervicales V,VI,
rr. ventrales
a. vertebralis

Fig. 2.18 The cervical vertebrae and nuchal ligaments: left lateral view. Removal of the deepest muscles (multifidis, intertransverse and obliquus capitis) reveals the cervical attachments of the ligament. Note that there is no attachment, in this specimen, to the dorsal spinous process of C6. Further details of this dissection are shown in Figs. 2.19 and 2.20.

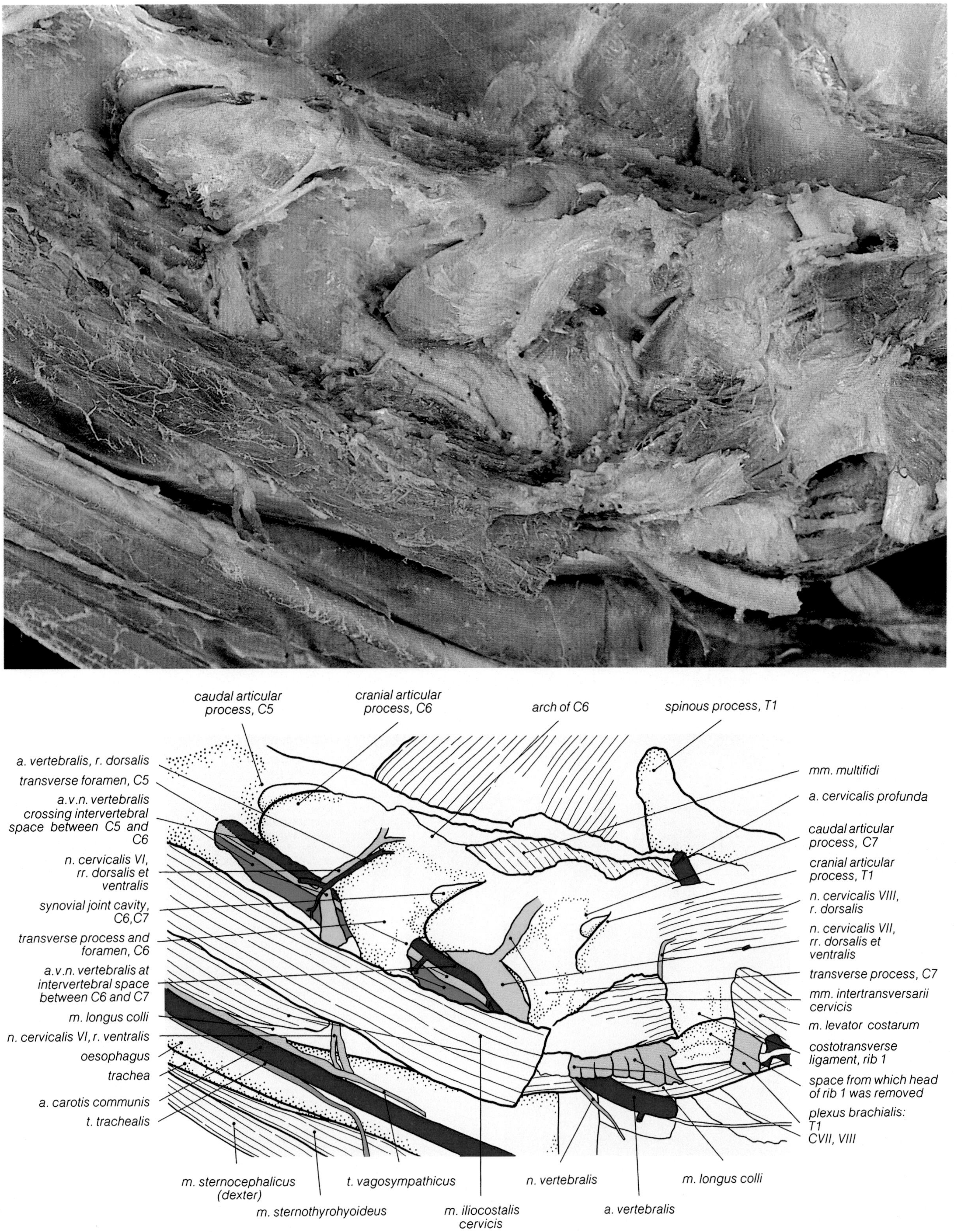

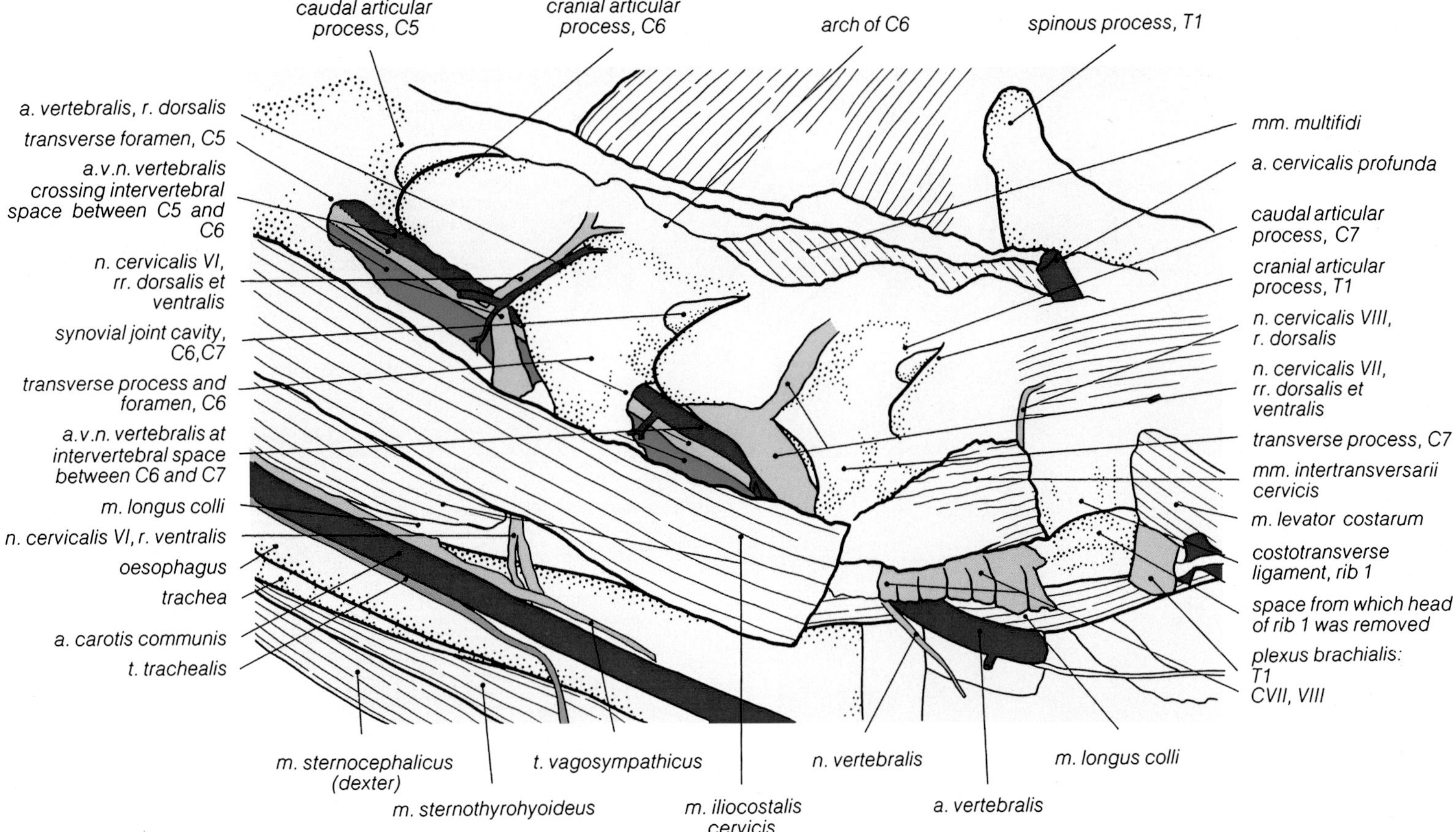
caudal articular process, C5
cranial articular process, C6
arch of C6
spinous process, T1
a. vertebralis, r. dorsalis
transverse foramen, C5
a.v.n. vertebralis crossing intervertebral space between C5 and C6
n. cervicalis VI, rr. dorsalis et ventralis
synovial joint cavity, C6,C7
transverse process and foramen, C6
a.v.n. vertebralis at intervertebral space between C6 and C7
m. longus colli
n. cervicalis VI, r. ventralis
oesophagus
trachea
a. carotis communis
t. trachealis
mm. multifidi
a. cervicalis profunda
caudal articular process, C7
cranial articular process, T1
n. cervicalis VIII, r. dorsalis
n. cervicalis VII, rr. dorsalis et ventralis
transverse process, C7
mm. intertransversarii cervicis
m. levator costarum
costotransverse ligament, rib 1
space from which head of rib 1 was removed
plexus brachialis:
T1
CVII, VIII
m. sternocephalicus (dexter)
m. sternothyrohyoideus
t. vagosympathicus
m. iliocostalis cervicis
n. vertebralis
a. vertebralis
m. longus colli

Fig. 2.19 The last two cervical and first thoracic vertebrae: left lateral view. The transverse canal houses the vertebral artery, vein and nerve. It begins at the caudal transverse foramen of C6. There is no C7 transverse foramen.

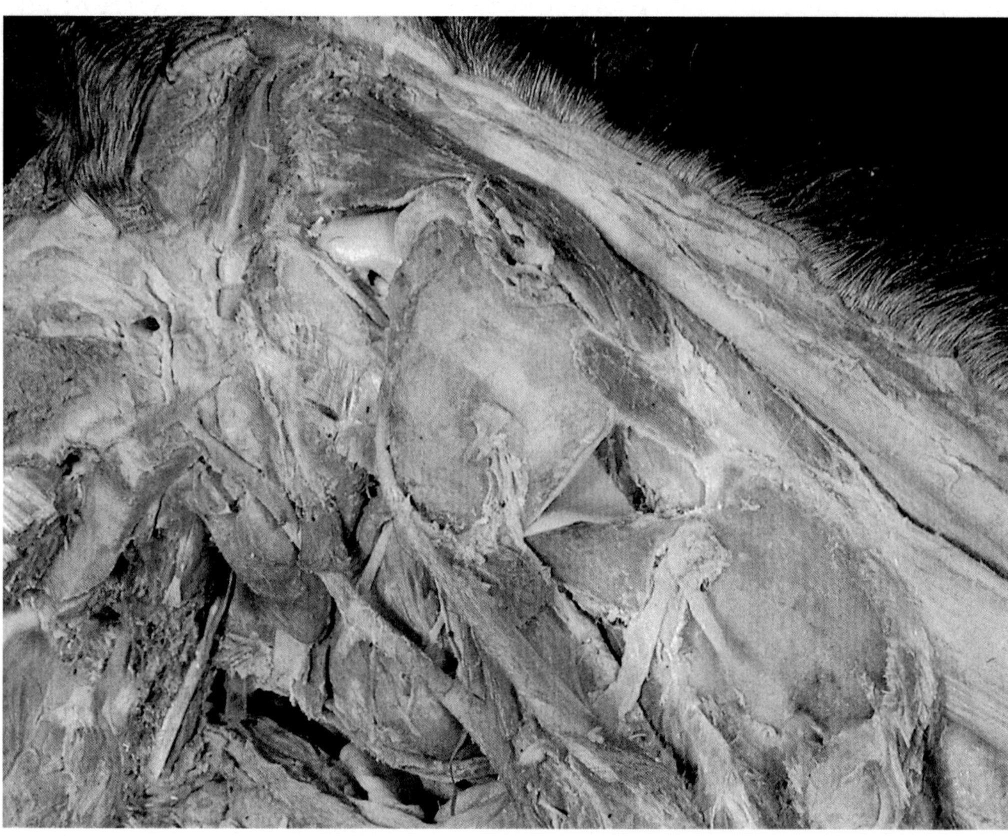

Fig. 2.20 The nuchal ligament at the atlanto-axial articulation: left lateral view. This is a closer view of part of the dissection shown in Fig. 2.18.

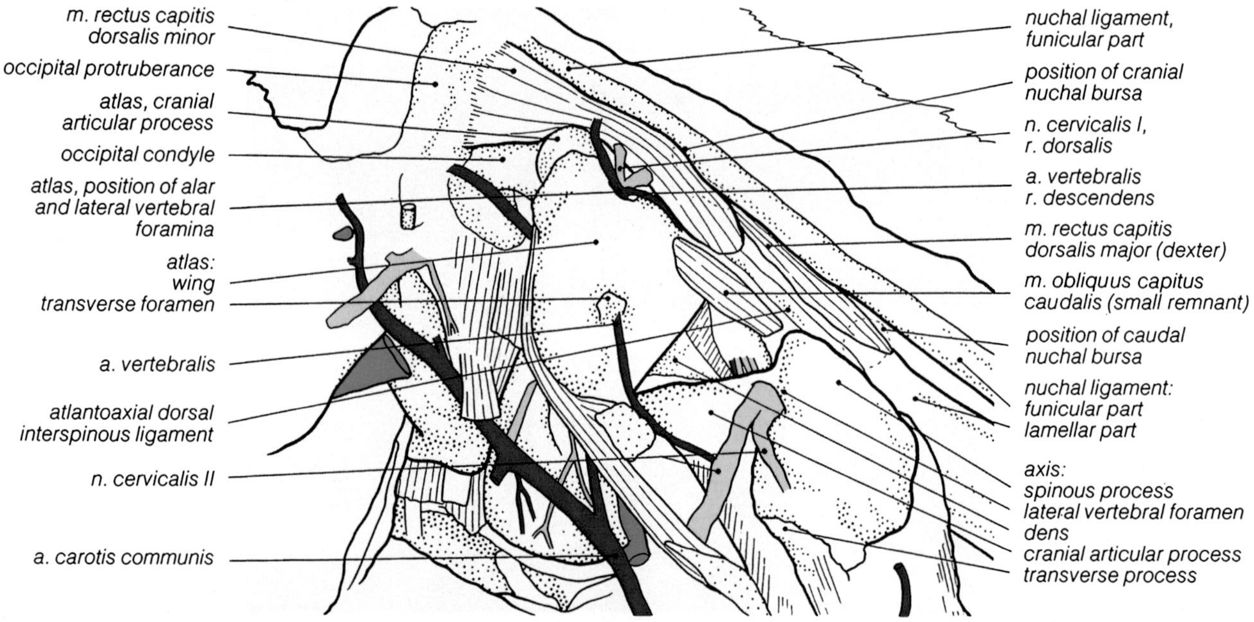

m. rectus capitis dorsalis minor
occipital protruberance
atlas, cranial articular process
occipital condyle
atlas, position of alar and lateral vertebral foramina
atlas: wing
transverse foramen
a. vertebralis
atlantoaxial dorsal interspinous ligament
n. cervicalis II
a. carotis communis
nuchal ligament, funicular part
position of cranial nuchal bursa
n. cervicalis I, r. dorsalis
a. vertebralis r. descendens
m. rectus capitis dorsalis major (dexter)
m. obliquus capitus caudalis (small remnant)
position of caudal nuchal bursa
nuchal ligament: funicular part lamellar part
axis: spinous process lateral vertebral foramen dens cranial articular process transverse process

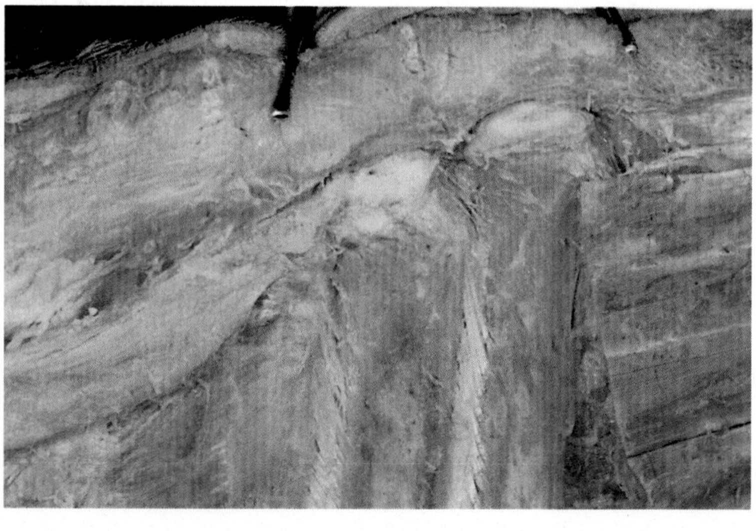

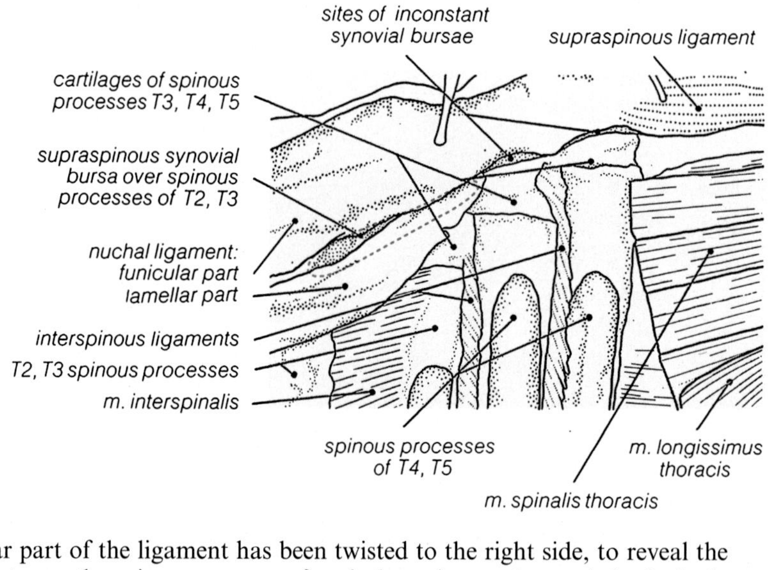

sites of inconstant synovial bursae
supraspinous ligament
cartilages of spinous processes T3, T4, T5
supraspinous synovial bursa over spinous processes of T2, T3
nuchal ligament: funicular part lamellar part
interspinous ligaments
T2, T3 spinous processes
m. interspinalis
spinous processes of T4, T5
m. longissimus thoracis
m. spinalis thoracis

Fig. 2.21 The nuchal ligament at the withers: left lateral view. The funicular part of the ligament has been twisted to the right side, to reveal the spinous processes of T4 and T5. Synovial bursae are sometimes located between the spinous process of each thoracic vertebra and the funicular part of the nuchal ligament. The supraspinous bursa lies between the two parts of the nuchal ligament.

3. THE FORELIMB

Clinical importance of the forelimb

The foal grows rapidly, especially from birth to 10 weeks-of-age. Fusion of growth plates in the limb bones gives an approximate estimation of the age of the young horse. Lighter breeds tend to fuse earlier than the heavier breeds. The proximal humeral growth plate closes at about 24–42 months of age and the distal at 12–24 months. In the radius, the proximal growth plate fuses at 12–24 months of age and the distal plate at 24 months (it has continuous growth for the first 60 weeks of life). The ulnar growth plates fuse at around 24–36 months. The proximal growth plate of metacarpal bone III is fused at birth, as are the distal growth plates of phalanges I and II. The distal growth plate of metacarpal bone III fuses at 6–9 months and the proximal growth plates of phalanges I and II fuse around 6–12 months.

In the young horse there may be abnormalities of conformation and if there are angular bone abnormalities they are best sorted out by 70 days of age. They are usually crooked legs, with flexure and contractile deformities. The young horse may also suffer from *osteochondrosis dissecans* in the shoulder and elbow and this may be unilateral or bilateral. Sub-chondral bone cysts may also affect the young horse.

Equine limbs are often subjected to trauma, especially the forelimbs.

It is not easy to separate the components that may be involved in the complex subject of lameness. It is important to localise the site(s) of the problem and to characterise the nature of the pathological changes. This requires a good history, an overall inspection, a complete physical examination which includes palpation and manipulation and, ultimately, a detailed evaluation. Clinical examination will reveal deformity, swellings or thickenings, skin wounds, and muscle wasting.

Palpation detects heat and pain as well as the precise location and consistency of swelling. Superficial pain is usually tested by poking the skin and deep pain is tested by using hoof testers, limb flexion or deep digital palpation. Analgesia is used for joints and also for diagnostic nerve blocks. In chronic disorders, the induced analgesia may not completely block out the diagnostic lesions. If more than one site, or both limbs, are involved it may be even more difficult. After using analgesia on the nerves in the upper parts of the limbs, loss of motor function and stumbling may result. Manipulation of the joints allows evaluation of movement and detects restrictions, instabilities, pain and crepitus. Abnormalities of gait may be detected. These results can then be further investigated by the available techniques such as radiology, ultrasonography, scintography, magnetic resonance imaging, computed tomography and the use of regional anaesthesia and specific nerve blocks to localise the site of lameness.

There are several types of fractures. The direction and location of the fracture line within a single bone may have a significant effect on the feasibility of repair. The relative displacement of the fractured pieces is also important. In some instances the fracture is incomplete. It may be stable or unstable, but probably the most important feature is whether it is open or closed, as an open fracture is almost invariably infected. The treatments of individual fractures are beyond our remit but fractures of proximal limb bones are difficult, often impossible, to repair and distal limb fractures are more accessible. In nearly all fracture cases there is an acute, non-weight-bearing lameness. Techniques of diagnosis and treatment continually improve, but the fact that they all require formation of a callus, followed by subsequent remodelling, will never change. Anaesthetic recovery and aftercare for these fractures following surgical repair, are the most crucial aspect of equine orthopaedics.

The scapula (four centres of ossification) is not easily fractured, but the *tuber scapulae* can be fractured and the articular surface of the glenoid cavity may be affected. The proximal humerus has three centres of ossification which fuse together at about 3–5 months of age; the distal humerus has two centres. This bone also is not commonly fractured as, like the scapula, it is supported by strong musculature, but all the other bones of the forelimb are more exposed.

A fractured radius requires a Robert Jones bandage to prevent adduction. Fracture of the ulna often involves the articular surface of the trochlear notch. This, and separation of the olecranon (also not uncommon following a fall or being kicked by another horse) are both seen as 'dropped elbow' because the triceps muscle is unable to prevent it.

Fracture of the accessory carpal bone and chip fractures of the carpus may lead to carpal sheath injuries.

The activities of the horse predispose to a wide variety of joint lesions, often associated with the extra stresses which result from galloping and jumping. There are a variety of joint diseases, including idiopathic synovitis, traumatic arthritis, and osteoarthritis. Osteoarthritis may be primary or secondary following mechanical disruptions and cytokine-mediated inflammation (antibody-associated, free radical damage, or enzyme damage). The initial sign is nearly always a result of extra fluid accumulation in the joint and appears as a soft tissue swelling around the joint. Most of the joints with great mobility have a large joint capsule from which fluid is easily aspirated, but 'low motion' joints, such as those of the carpus, are much more difficult to aspirate.

These synovial structures may also be affected by external puncture wounds. Quite often there is a small wound, followed 2–3 days later by swelling, followed by synovial fluid leaking from the joint. Joints are also affected by haematogenous spread of organisms (particularly in foals), local penetration, or local extension from peri-articular structures.

Arthrocentesis followed by intra-articular medication is commonly performed when diagnosing and treating joint disease. Synovial fluid analysis aids in the interpretation of joint disease and is particularly important in horses with septic arthritis. Synovial fluid analysis requires visual assessment, examinations of volume, total protein, inflammatory cells and a cytological analysis.

The shoulder joint may show luxation or sub-luxation, particularly if there is laxness in the ligaments of the joint and tendons of the muscles. Intra-articular analgesia of the shoulder joint requires access between the cranial and caudal prominences of the greater tubercle of the humerus, with the needle directed in a horizontal and slightly caudo-medial direction, to enter the synovial cavity.

The elbow joint is very large and is often affected by septic arthritis. Capped elbow is an acquired bursa at the point of the elbow. Intra-articular analgesia of the elbow joint is possible. The lateral humeral epicondyle and the lateral tuberosity of the radius are palpated, and the needle inserted between them, cranial or caudal to the lateral ligament, in a horizontal direction, to a depth of 4–5 cm.

Carpal joint disease is quite common. There are 7 or 8 bones in the carpus. The proximal carpal row has radial, intermediate, ulnar and accessory carpal bones. The distal row has carpal bones II, III, IV and sometimes carpal bone I. There are approximately 26–27 separate articulations between these bones. There are essentially three joints – the antebrachio-carpal, which both rotates and glides; the middle carpal joint which is a simple hinge joint and the carpo-metacarpal articulation which has very little movement.

Intra-articular analgesia of the carpal joints is possible as a diagnostic technique. With the limb fixed in a flexed position, the injection sites are easily palpable. The radio-carpal joint is found by locating the depression between the radius and the proximal row of the carpal bones. For the middle carpal joint, locate the depression between the proximal and distal rows of the carpal bones. For both joints the needle is inserted medial to the extensor carpi radialis tendon or between that tendon and the common digital extensor tendon.

Muscles and tendons, and the synovial structures associated with them, are very commonly subjected to injury in any type of working horse. Rupture of the common digital extensor, usually in the sheath over the lateral aspect of the carpus, can occur in foals with carpal contracture. The fibrous palmar carpal joint capsule is dense, and closely attached to the palmar aspect of the carpal bones. It forms the dorsal wall of the carpal canal. It continues distally to form the accessory head of the deep digital flexor tendon (the accessory or inferior check ligament). The carpal fascia on the palmar aspect of the carpal region forms the flexor retinaculum (transverse carpal ligament) between the free palmar edge of the accessory carpal bone and the medial aspect of the carpus. This completes the carpal arch, which contains the superficial digital flexor and deep digital flexor tendons. Carpal flexor tendon sheath injuries are less common than injuries to the digital flexor tendon sheath, but can be a severe cause of lameness. They often result from fractures of accessory carpal bones. The tendon sheath extends from 4–8 cm proximal to the accessory carpal bone to 5–10 cm distal to the carpal bone. The proximal sheath is caudal to the distal radius and cranial to the deep digital flexor tendon. The accessory ligament of the superficial digital flexor tendon (radial or superior check ligament) forms part of the medial wall of the sheath. The short radial head of the deep digital flexor muscle protrudes into the sheath proximally and is inserted into the dorso-medial aspect of the deep digital flexor tendon, approximately 2 cm proximal to the accessory carpal bone. Midway between the proximal recess of the sheath and the accessory carpal bone, caudal to the distal radius, the sheath extends laterally and medially to the deep digital flexor tendon.

Damage to the nerves of the forelimb is usually caused by trauma from normal activities or by aggression from other horses. Damage to the suprascapular nerve, which is motor to the supraspinatus and infraspinatus muscles, results in 'shoulder slip'. Atrophy of the shoulder muscles may take 18 months to recover.

Radial nerve damage may accompany humeral fractures. The loss of innervation to the extensor tendons of the digit causes a dropped elbow and inability to stand, resulting in long periods of lateral recumbency. Damage to the ulnar and median nerve may result in the loss of skin sensation to palmar metacarpal and to palmar and dorsodistal digital regions. Analgesia of the antebrachium can be carried out by blocking the median nerve medially, 5 cm distal to the elbow joint, where the nerve runs along the caudal aspect of the radius. The ulnar nerve is blocked 10 cm proximal to the accessory carpal bone, in a groove between the flexor carpi ulnaris and the extensor carpi radialis (ulnaris lateralis) muscles.

Damage to the musculocutaneous nerve results in an inability to flex the elbow, as there is no effective innervation of the biceps brachii, coracobrachialis and brachialis muscles. There is also a loss of sensation to the dorsomedial aspect of the limb from the carpus to the fetlock. The nerve can be blocked subcutaneously on either side of the cephalic vein, about half way between the carpus and the elbow, to anaesthetise both cranial and caudal branches of the metacarpal nerves.

The axillary nerve may be damaged. This results in reduced flexion of the shoulder and lateral instability of the shoulder joint, as there is no effective innervation of deltoid and teres major and minor muscles.

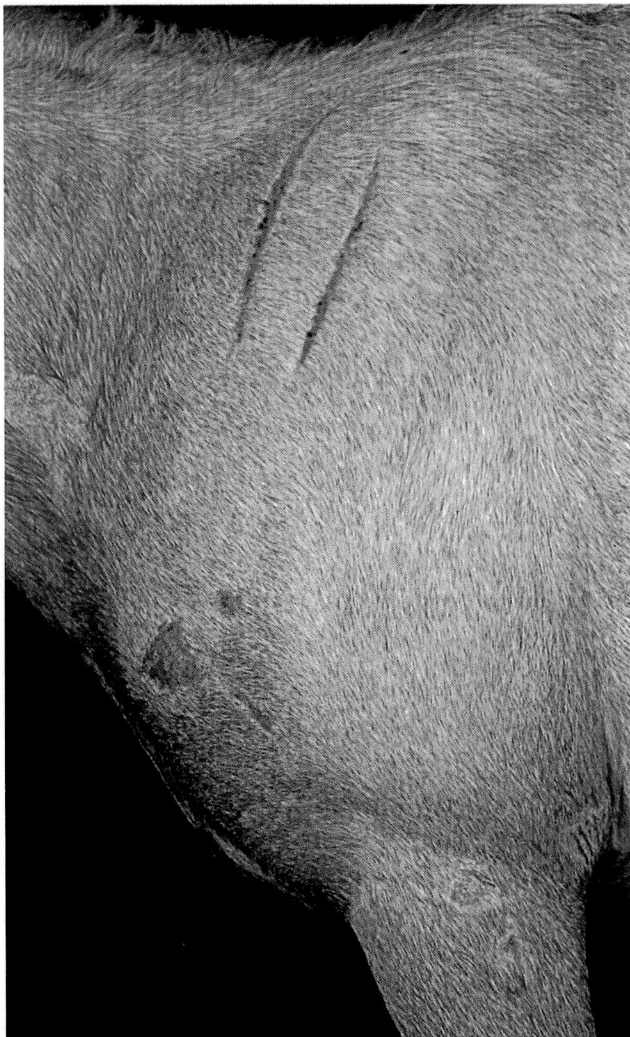

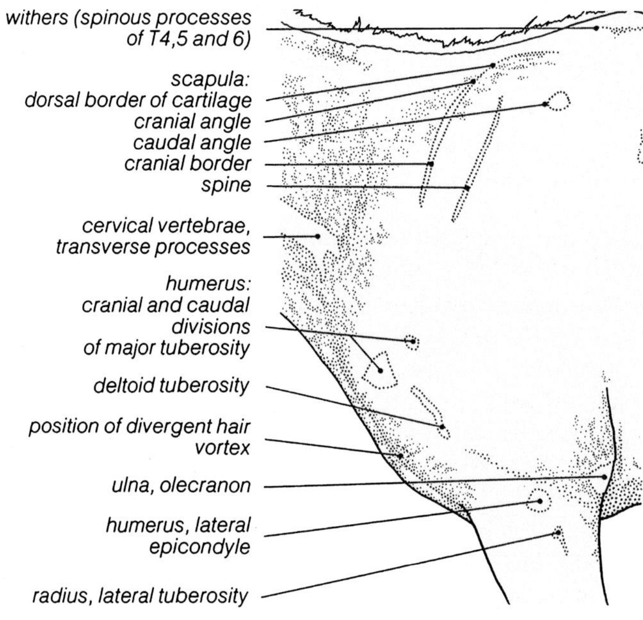
withers (spinous processes of T4,5 and 6)
scapula:
dorsal border of cartilage
cranial angle
caudal angle
cranial border
spine
cervical vertebrae, transverse processes
humerus:
cranial and caudal divisions of major tuberosity
deltoid tuberosity
position of divergent hair vortex
ulna, olecranon
humerus, lateral epicondyle
radius, lateral tuberosity

Fig. 3.1 Surface features of the scapular and brachial regions: left lateral view. The palpable bony prominences have been shaved. The cranial border of the scapula is covered by the subclavius and supraspinatus muscles and is not clearly palpable. The acromion is small or absent in the horse and is never palpable. The divergent hair vortex situated just cranial to the humerus is usually very clearly visible but it does not show well in this lateral view.

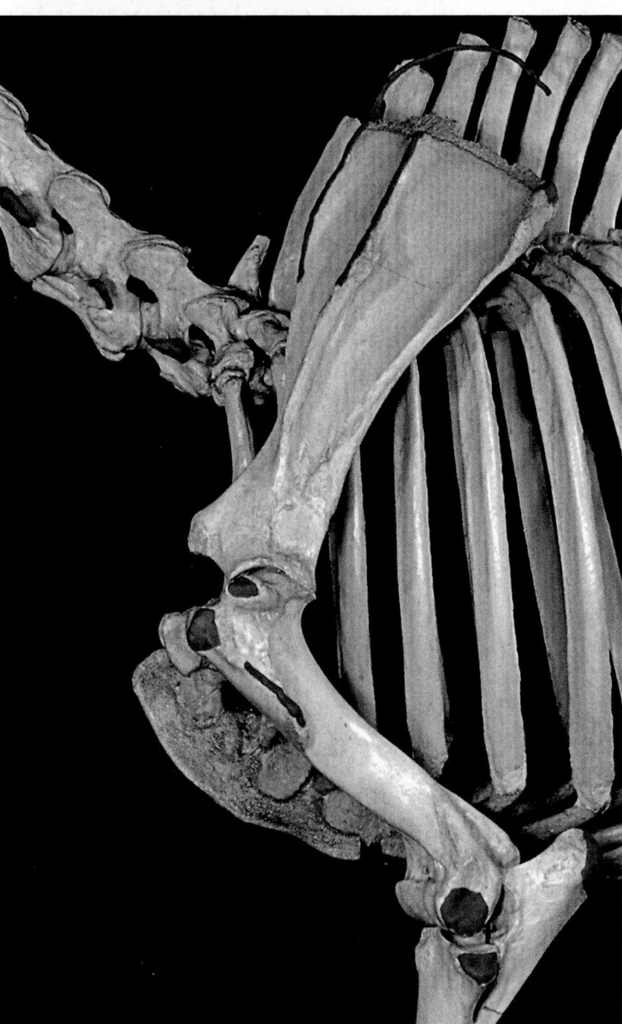

Fig. 3.2 The bones of the forelimb. Scapular and brachial regions: left lateral view. The palpable bony prominences shown in Fig. 3.1 have been coloured red. The palpable edge of the scapular cartilage is shown by a red wire. The tips of the spinous processes at the withers have not been coloured.

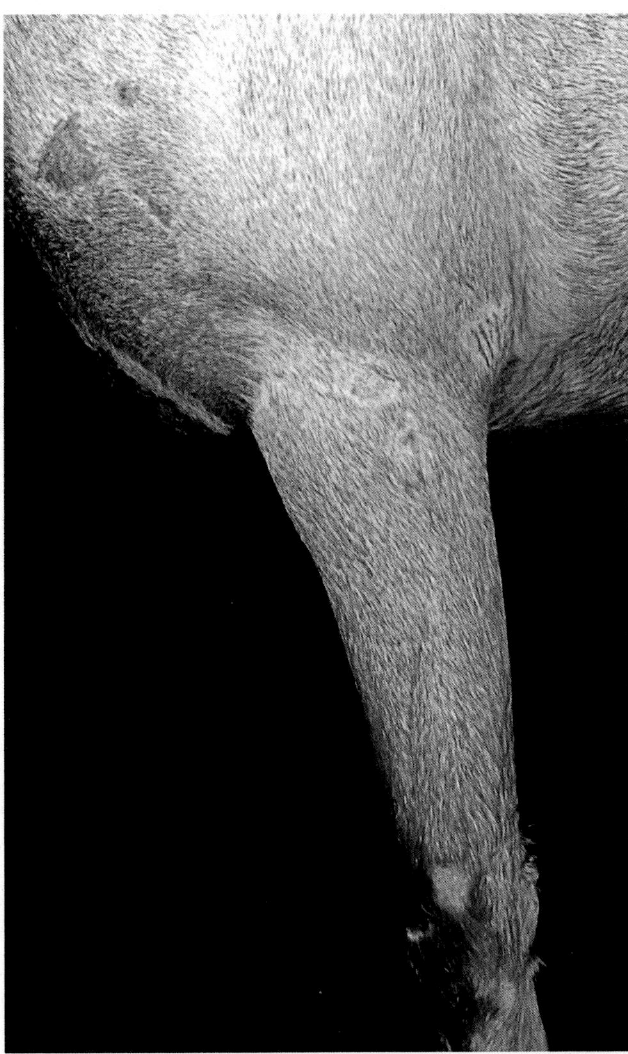

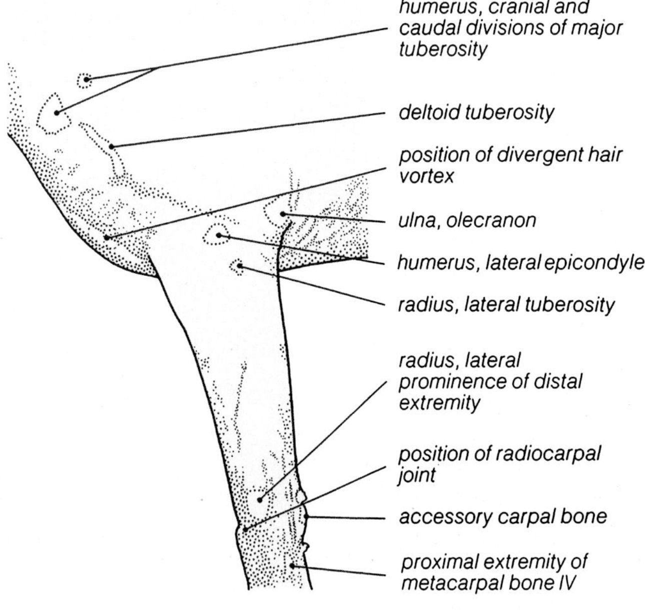
humerus, cranial and caudal divisions of major tuberosity
deltoid tuberosity
position of divergent hair vortex
ulna, olecranon
humerus, lateral epicondyle
radius, lateral tuberosity
radius, lateral prominence of distal extremity
position of radiocarpal joint
accessory carpal bone
proximal extremity of metacarpal bone IV

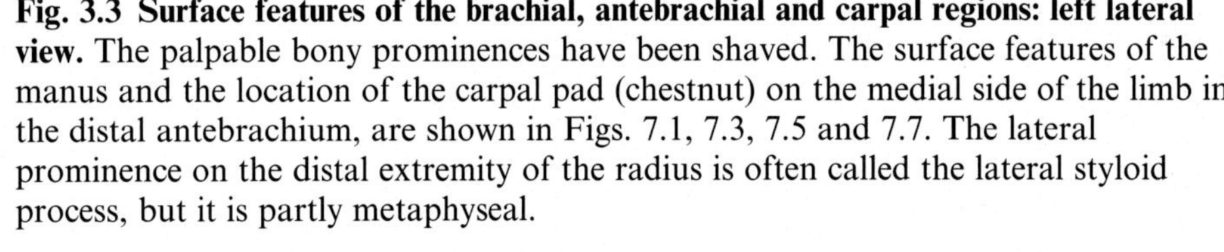
Fig. 3.3 Surface features of the brachial, antebrachial and carpal regions: left lateral view. The palpable bony prominences have been shaved. The surface features of the manus and the location of the carpal pad (chestnut) on the medial side of the limb in the distal antebrachium, are shown in Figs. 7.1, 7.3, 7.5 and 7.7. The lateral prominence on the distal extremity of the radius is often called the lateral styloid process, but it is partly metaphyseal.

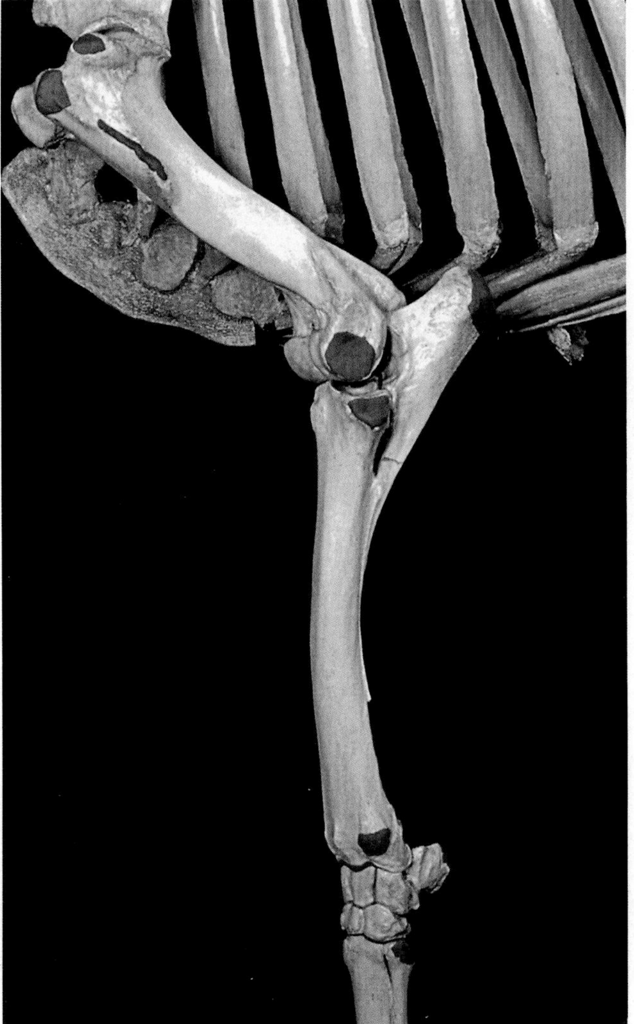

Fig. 3.4 Bones of the forelimb. Brachial, antebrachial and carpal regions: left lateral view. The palpable bony prominences shown in Fig. 3.3 have been coloured red. The articular process situated just distal to the marked metaphyseal prominence of the radius is the so-called 'lateral styloid process of the radius': it is, in fact, the distal epiphysis of the ulna and it articulates with the ulnar carpal bone.

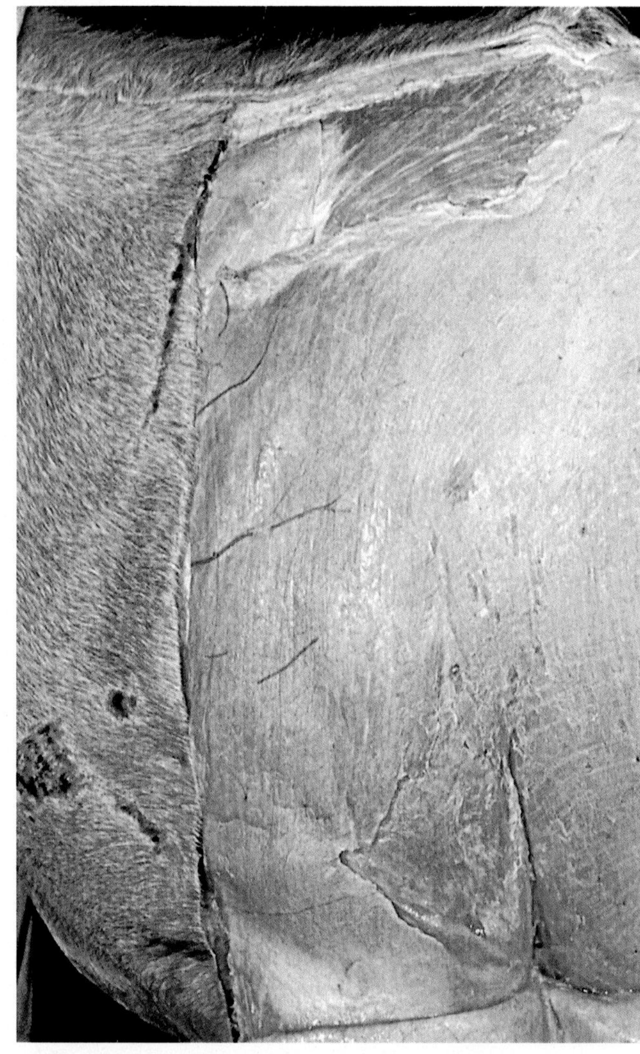

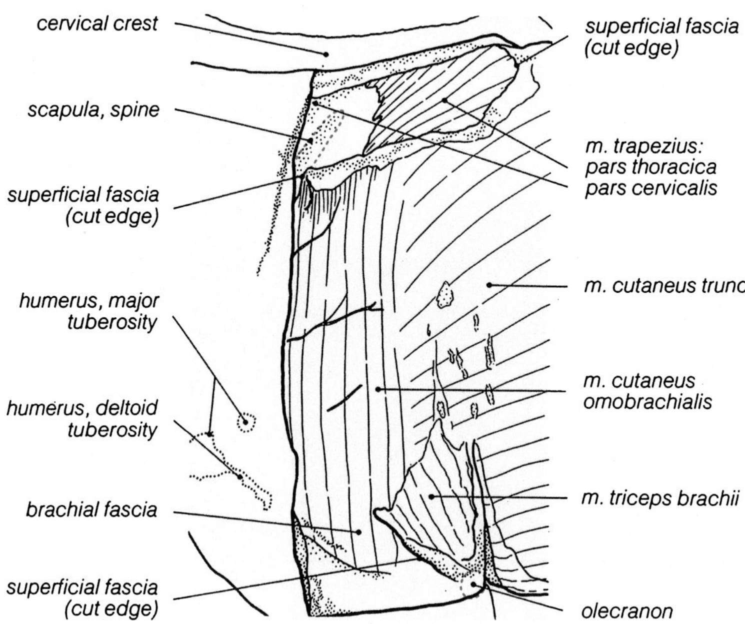
cervical crest
scapula, spine
superficial fascia (cut edge)
humerus, major tuberosity
humerus, deltoid tuberosity
brachial fascia
superficial fascia (cut edge)
superficial fascia (cut edge)
m. trapezius:
pars thoracica
pars cervicalis
m. cutaneus trunci
m. cutaneus omobrachialis
m. triceps brachii
olecranon

Fig. 3.5 Cutaneous muscles of the scapular and brachial regions: left lateral view. The superficial fascia, in which the cutaneous muscles lie, has been opened both dorsally and ventrally to show the underlying muscles. These muscles are more fully revealed in Fig. 3.6.

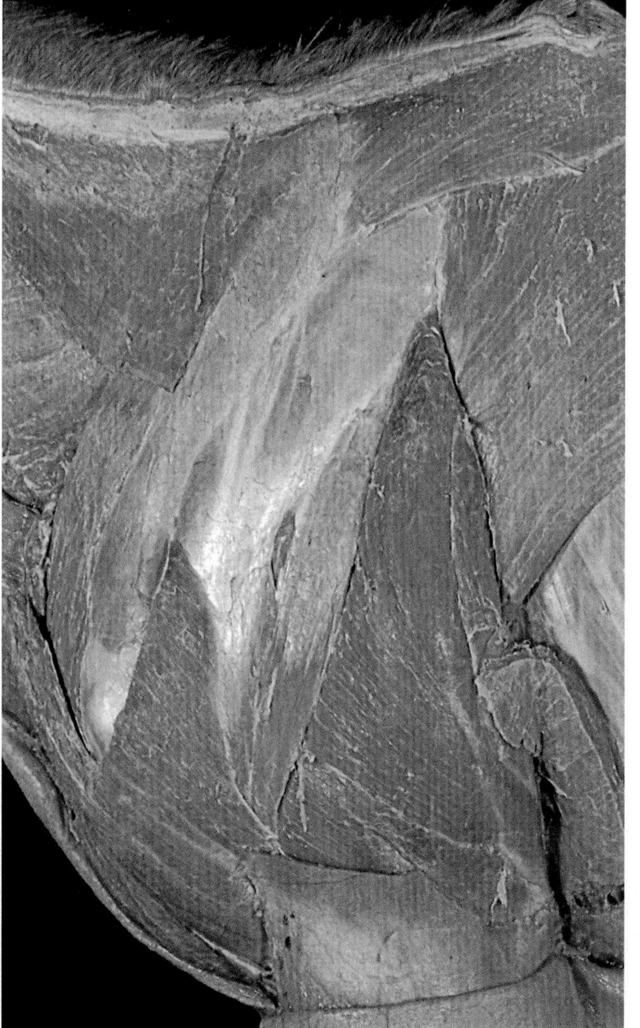

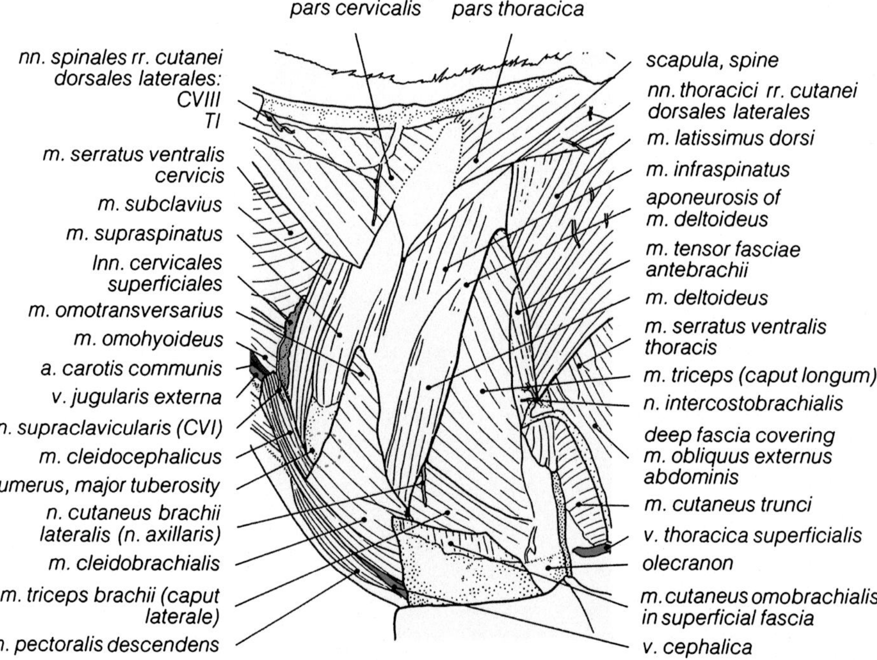
m. trapezius:
pars cervicalis
pars thoracica
nn. spinales rr. cutanei dorsales laterales:
CVIII
TI
m. serratus ventralis cervicis
m. subclavius
m. supraspinatus
lnn. cervicales superficiales
m. omotransversarius
m. omohyoideus
a. carotis communis
v. jugularis externa
n. supraclavicularis (CVI)
m. cleidocephalicus
humerus, major tuberosity
n. cutaneus brachii lateralis (n. axillaris)
m. cleidobrachialis
m. triceps brachii (caput laterale)
m. pectoralis descendens
scapula, spine
nn. thoracici rr. cutanei dorsales laterales
m. latissimus dorsi
m. infraspinatus
aponeurosis of m. deltoideus
m. tensor fasciae antebrachii
m. deltoideus
m. serratus ventralis thoracis
m. triceps (caput longum)
n. intercostobrachialis
deep fascia covering m. obliquus externus abdominis
m. cutaneus trunci
v. thoracica superficialis
olecranon
m. cutaneus omobrachialis in superficial fascia
v. cephalica

Fig. 3.6 Superficial structures of the scapular and brachial regions: left lateral view (1). The superficial fascia and the cutaneous muscles have been removed. During the previous dissection of the neck (see Chapter 2) the omotransversarius and brachiocephalicus muscles (shown intact in Figs. 2.3 and 2.4) were transected (Fig. 2.7).

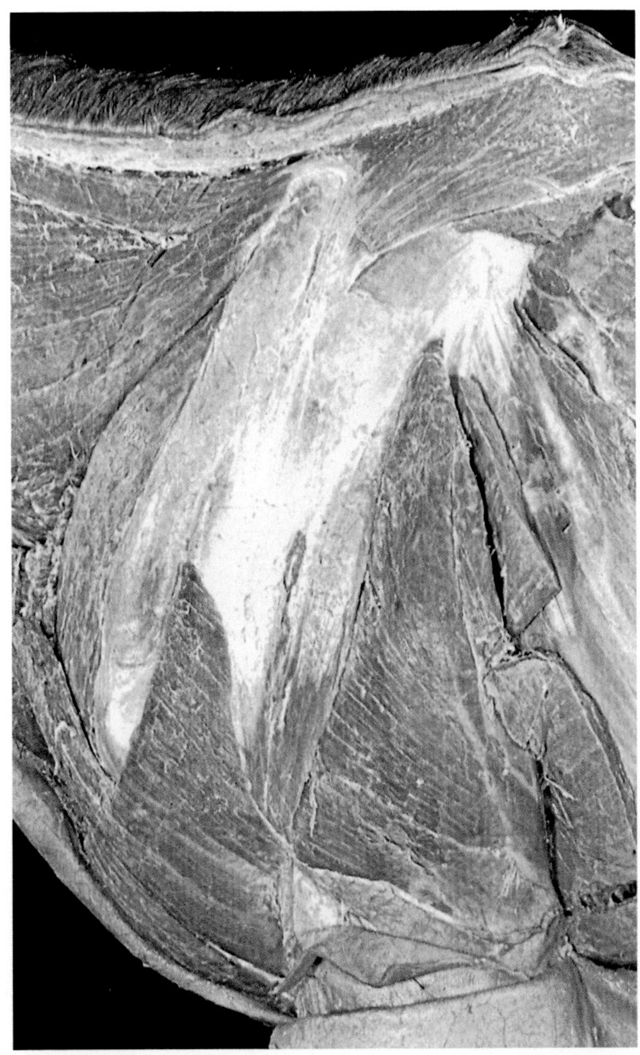

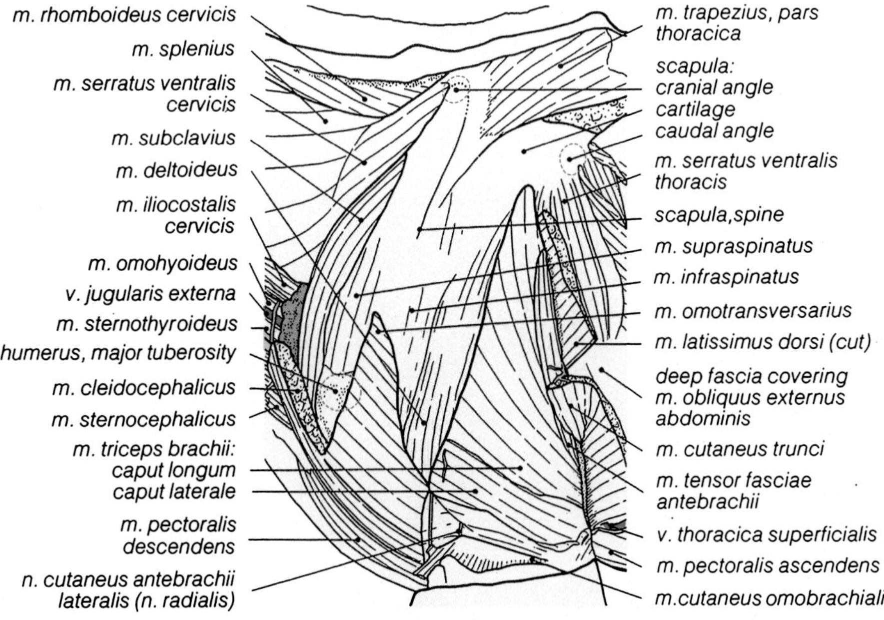
m. rhomboideus cervicis
m. splenius
m. serratus ventralis cervicis
m. subclavius
m. deltoideus
m. iliocostalis cervicis
m. omohyoideus
v. jugularis externa
m. sternothyroideus
humerus, major tuberosity
m. cleidocephalicus
m. sternocephalicus
m. triceps brachii:
caput longum
caput laterale
m. pectoralis descendens
n. cutaneus antebrachii lateralis (n. radialis)
m. trapezius, pars thoracica
scapula:
cranial angle
cartilage
caudal angle
m. serratus ventralis thoracis
scapula,spine
m. supraspinatus
m. infraspinatus
m. omotransversarius
m. latissimus dorsi (cut)
deep fascia covering m. obliquus externus abdominis
m. cutaneus trunci
m. tensor fasciae antebrachii
v. thoracica superficialis
m. pectoralis ascendens
m.cutaneus omobrachialis

Fig. 3.7 Superficial structures of the scapular and brachial regions: left lateral view (2). The cervical trapezius muscle has been removed and the latissimus dorsi transected to show the scapular attachments of the cervical and thoracic parts of the ventral serrate muscle. The full extent of this muscle is seen when the scapula is removed (Fig. 3.10).

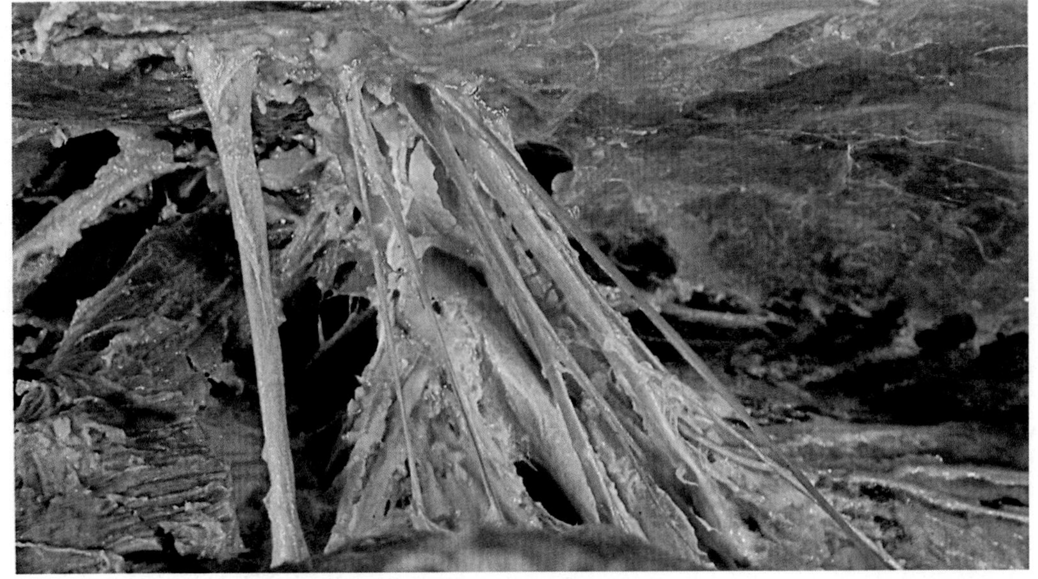

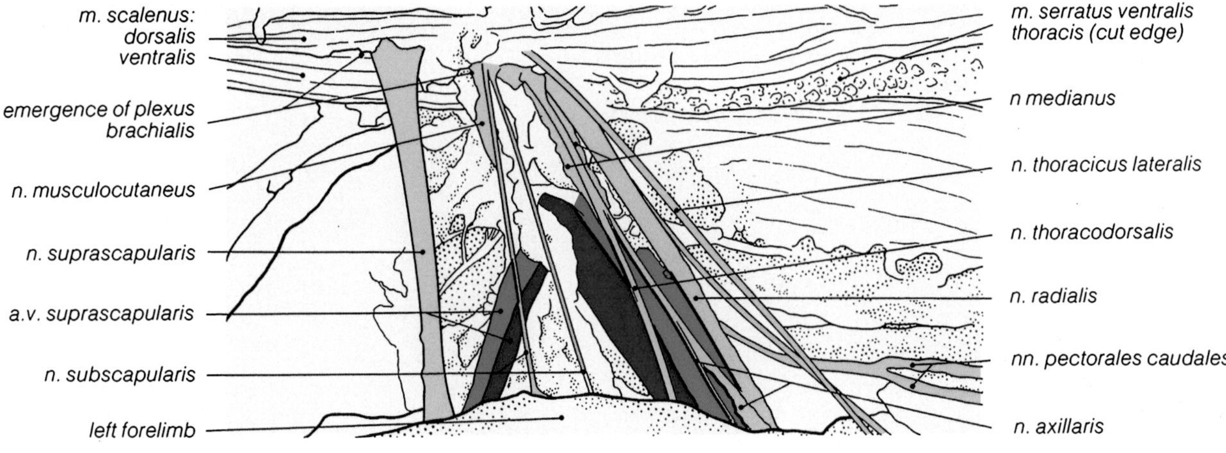
m. scalenus:
dorsalis
ventralis
emergence of plexus brachialis
n. musculocutaneus
n. suprascapularis
a.v. suprascapularis
n. subscapularis
left forelimb
m. serratus ventralis thoracis (cut edge)
n medianus
n. thoracicus lateralis
n. thoracodorsalis
n. radialis
nn. pectorales caudales
n. axillaris

Fig. 3.8 Axillary structures before removal of the left forelimb: dorsal view. The trapezius, rhomboideus and ventral serrate muscles have been cut, and the scapula has been abducted and viewed from above to display the emergence of the brachial plexus between the two parts of the scalenus muscle. Fig. 3.9 shows a further stage in this dissection of the axilla.

Fig. 3.9 Axillary structures before removal of the left forelimb: caudal view. The forelimb has now been further abducted to display the axilla more completely. The nerves and blood vessels of the axilla have been further dissected to reveal their topographical relationships. Further details of trunk and limb are shown in Figs. 3.10 and 3.15.

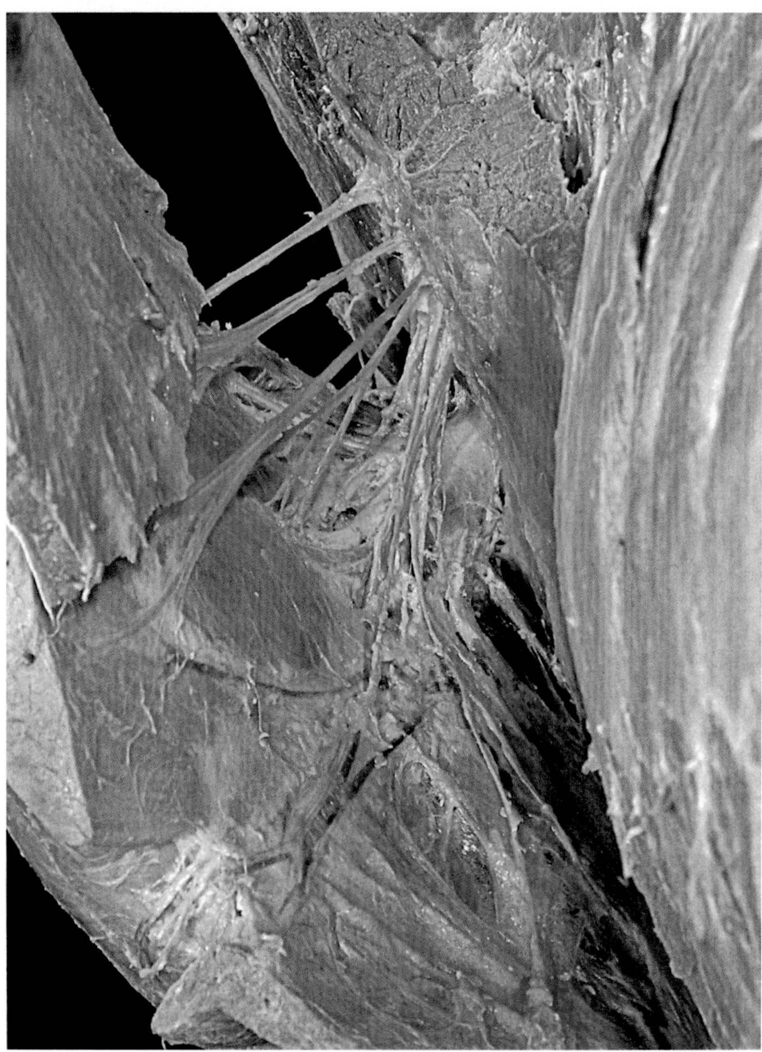

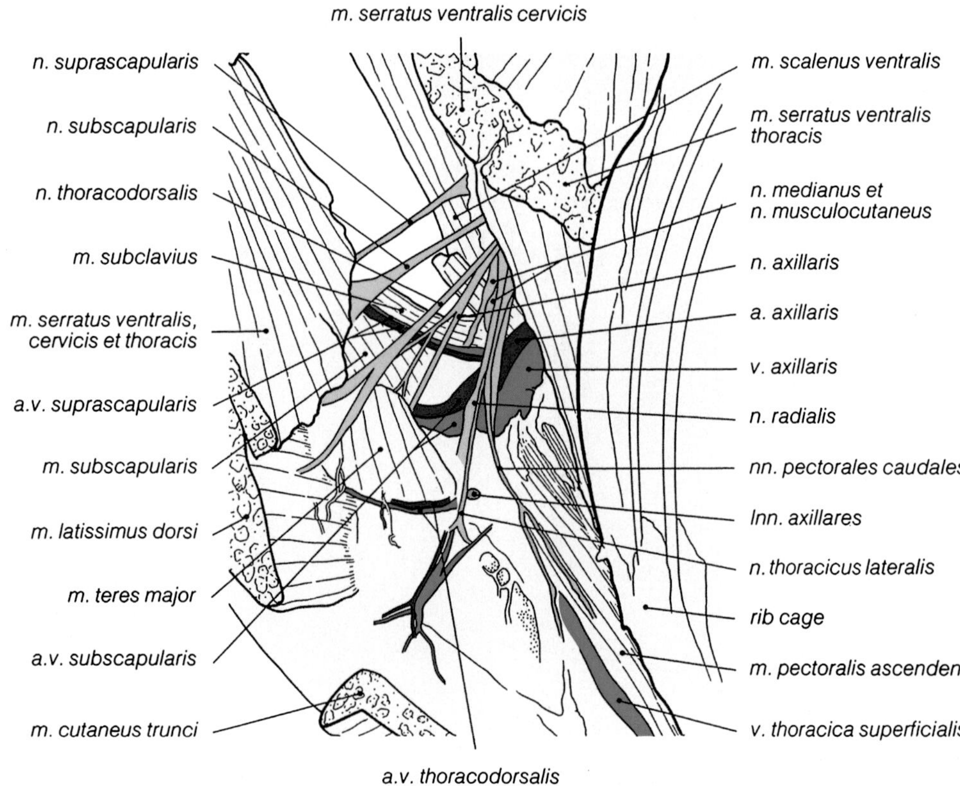
m. serratus ventralis cervicis
n. suprascapularis
n. subscapularis
n. thoracodorsalis
m. subclavius
m. serratus ventralis, cervicis et thoracis
a.v. suprascapularis
m. subscapularis
m. latissimus dorsi
m. teres major
a.v. subscapularis
m. cutaneus trunci
a.v. thoracodorsalis
m. scalenus ventralis
m. serratus ventralis thoracis
n. medianus et n. musculocutaneus
n. axillaris
a. axillaris
v. axillaris
n. radialis
nn. pectorales caudales
lnn. axillares
n. thoracicus lateralis
rib cage
m. pectoralis ascendens
v. thoracica superficialis

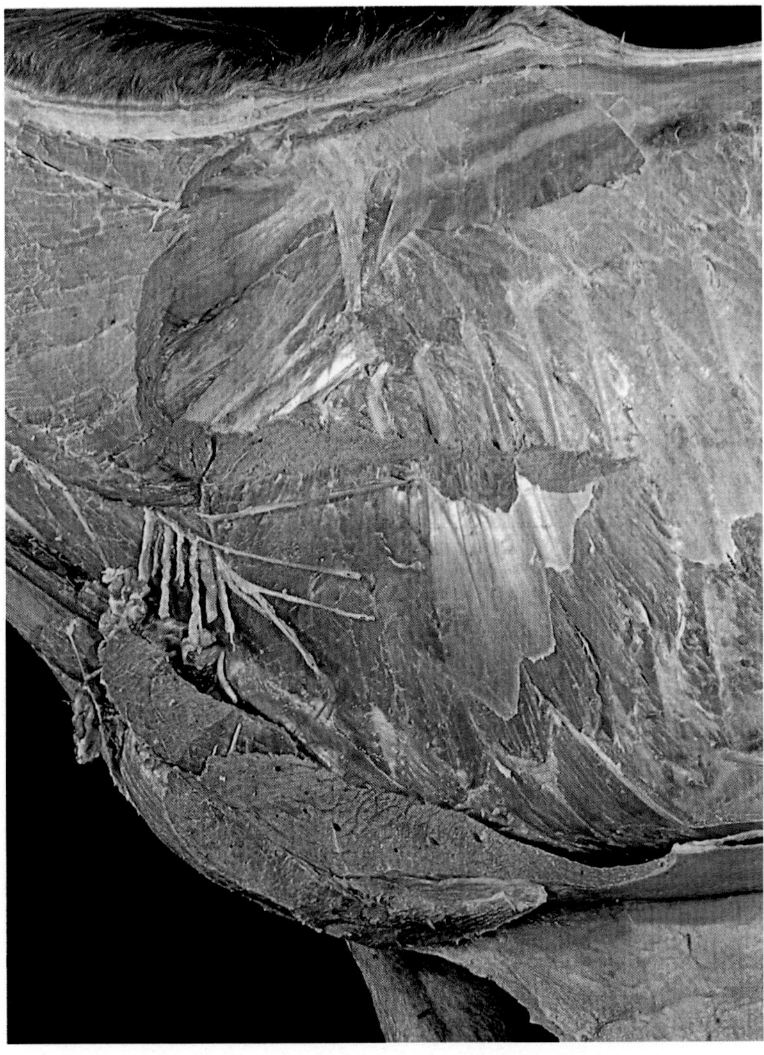

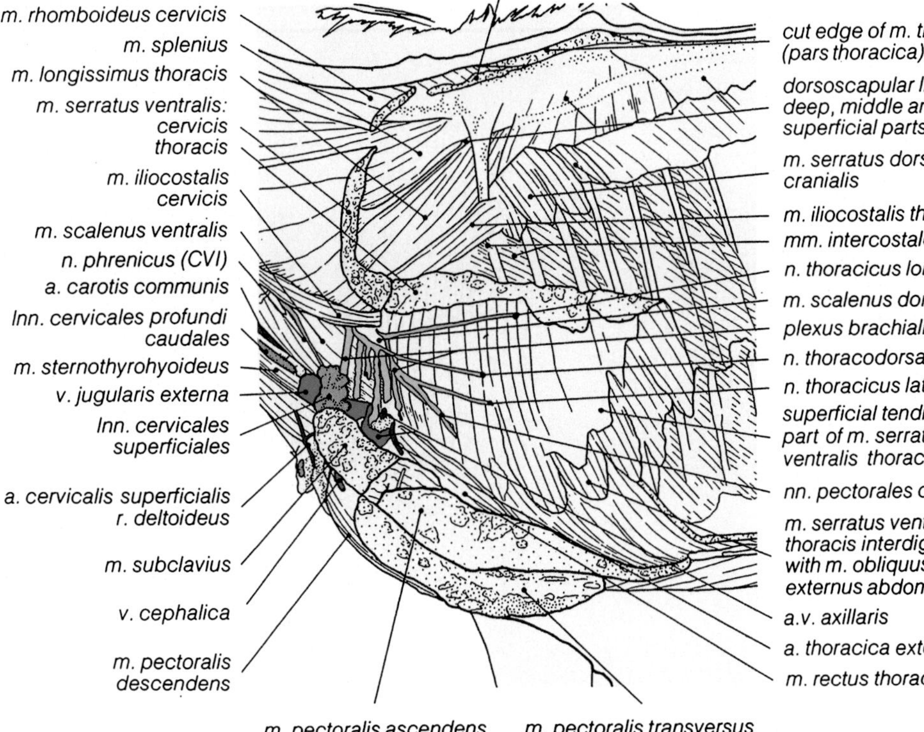
m. rhomboideus thoracis
m. rhomboideus cervicis
m. splenius
m. longissimus thoracis
m. serratus ventralis:
cervicis
thoracis
m. iliocostalis
cervicis
m. scalenus ventralis
n. phrenicus (CVI)
a. carotis communis
lnn. cervicales profundi
caudales
m. sternothyrohyoideus
v. jugularis externa
lnn. cervicales
superficiales
a. cervicalis superficialis
r. deltoideus
m. subclavius
v. cephalica
m. pectoralis
descendens
m. pectoralis ascendens
m. pectoralis transversus
cut edge of m. trapezius
(pars thoracica)
dorsoscapular ligament,
deep, middle and
superficial parts
m. serratus dorsalis
cranialis
m. iliocostalis thoracis
mm. intercostales externi
n. thoracicus longus
m. scalenus dorsalis
plexus brachialis
n. thoracodorsalis
n. thoracicus lateralis
superficial tendinous
part of m. serratus
ventralis thoracis
nn. pectorales caudales
m. serratus ventralis
thoracis interdigitating
with m. obliquus
externus abdominis (cut)
a.v. axillaris
a. thoracica externa
m. rectus thoracis

Fig. 3.10 The pectoral and ventral serrate muscles after removal of the forelimb: left lateral view. Pectoralis, rhomboideus, trapezius and ventral serrate muscles have been incised to remove the forelimb. The nerves of the brachial plexus are not arranged to show the disposition before removal of the limb. This is, however, shown in Fig. 3.48.

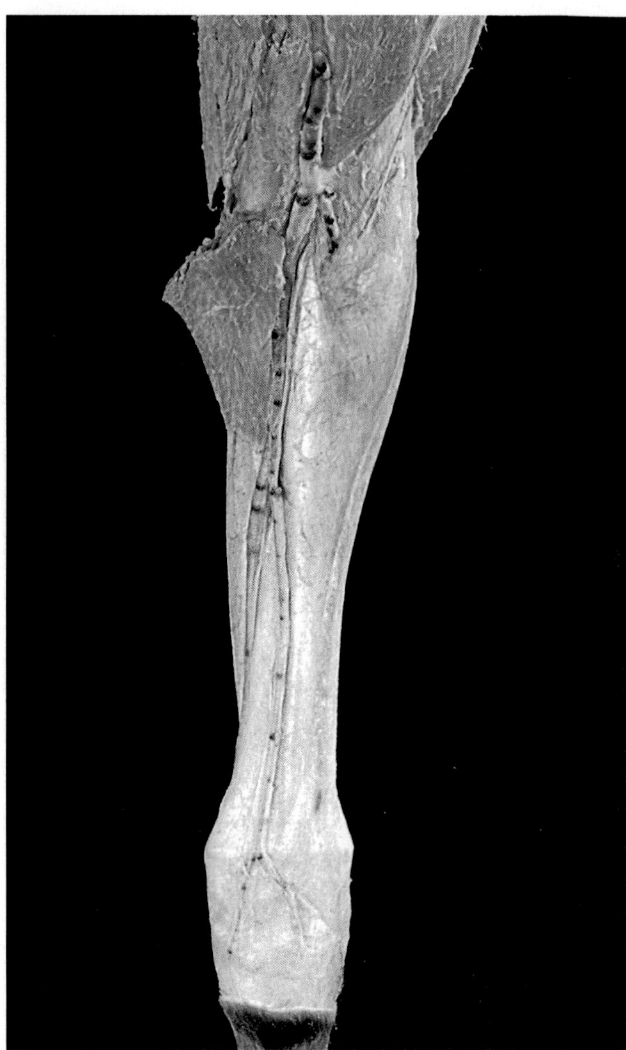

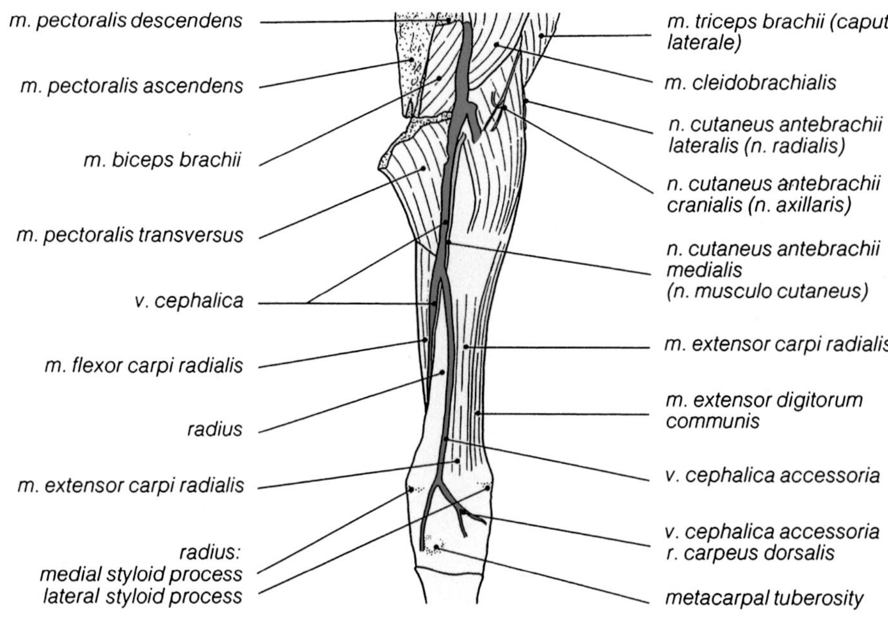
m. pectoralis descendens
m. pectoralis ascendens
m. biceps brachii
m. pectoralis transversus
v. cephalica
m. flexor carpi radialis
radius
m. extensor carpi radialis
radius:
medial styloid process
lateral styloid process
m. triceps brachii (caput laterale)
m. cleidobrachialis
n. cutaneus antebrachii lateralis (n. radialis)
n. cutaneus antebrachii cranialis (n. axillaris)
n. cutaneus antebrachii medialis
(n. musculo cutaneus)
m. extensor carpi radialis
m. extensor digitorum communis
v. cephalica accessoria
v. cephalica accessoria
r. carpeus dorsalis
metacarpal tuberosity

Fig. 3.11 Superficial structures of the left antebrachium and carpus: rostral view. The limb has been removed from the trunk. The skin and superficial fascia have been removed to show the superficial vessels and nerves, but the antebrachial muscles are still invested by the strong antebrachial fascia. The specimen at this stage of dissection is also shown in Figs. 3.12–3.14.

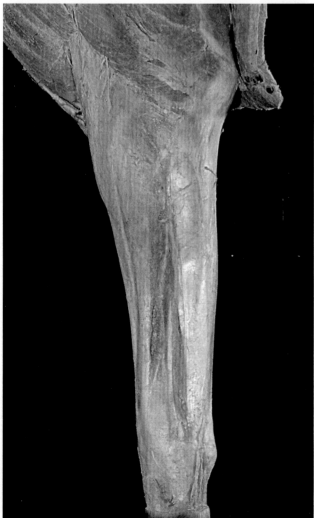

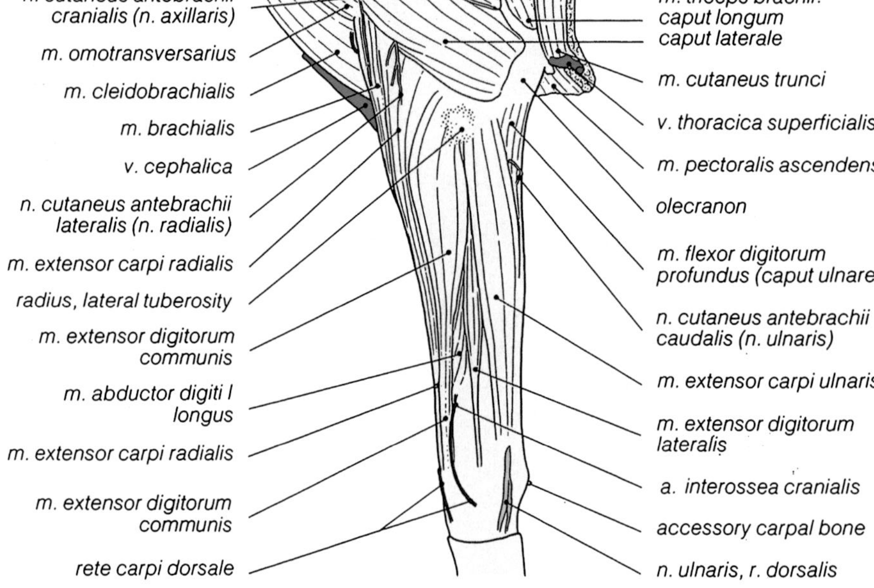
n. cutaneus antebrachii cranialis (n. axillaris)
m. omotransversarius
m. cleidobrachialis
m. brachialis
v. cephalica
n. cutaneus antebrachii lateralis (n. radialis)
m. extensor carpi radialis
radius, lateral tuberosity
m. extensor digitorum communis
m. abductor digiti I longus
m. extensor carpi radialis
m. extensor digitorum communis
rete carpi dorsale
m. triceps brachii:
caput longum
caput laterale
m. cutaneus trunci
v. thoracica superficialis
m. pectoralis ascendens
olecranon
m. flexor digitorum profundus (caput ulnare)
n. cutaneus antebrachii caudalis (n. ulnaris)
m. extensor carpi ulnaris
m. extensor digitorum lateralis
a. interossea cranialis
accessory carpal bone
n. ulnaris, r. dorsalis

Fig. 3.12 Superficial structures of the left antebrachium and carpus: lateral view. The specimen is at the same stage of dissection as that shown in Figs. 3.11, 3.13 and 3.14.

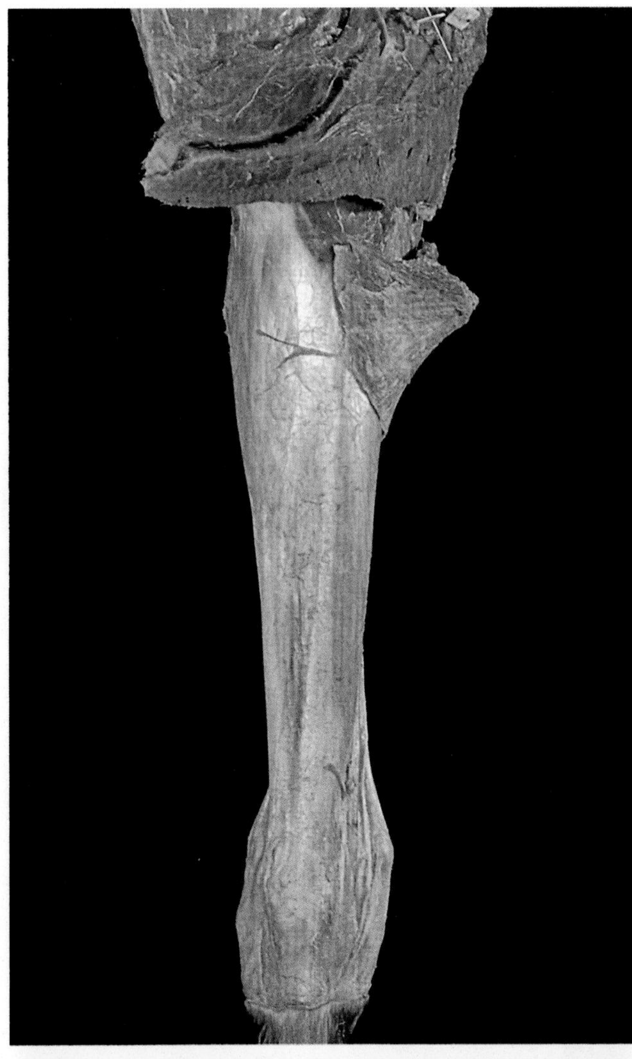

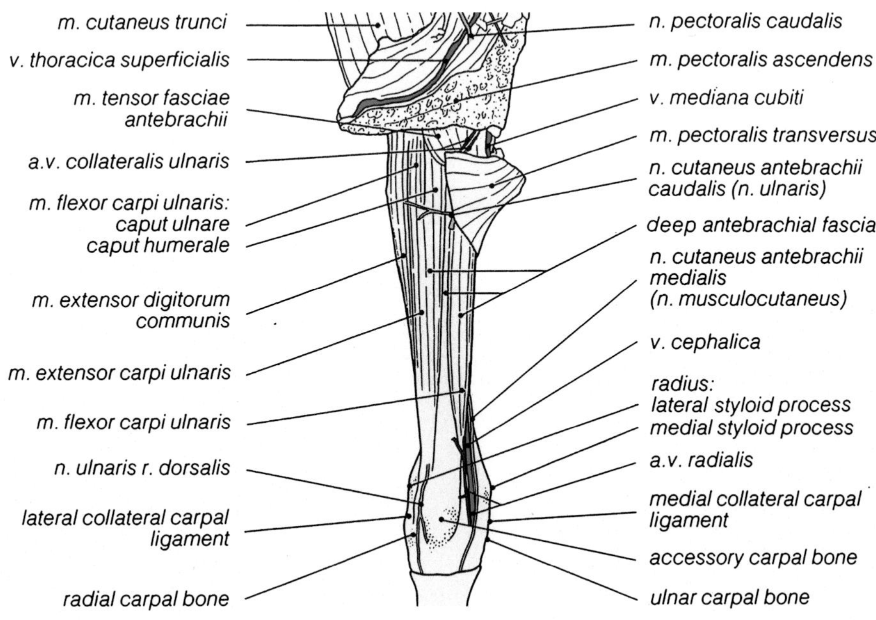
m. cutaneus trunci
v. thoracica superficialis
m. tensor fasciae antebrachii
a.v. collateralis ulnaris
m. flexor carpi ulnaris:
caput ulnare
caput humerale
m. extensor digitorum communis
m. extensor carpi ulnaris
m. flexor carpi ulnaris
n. ulnaris r. dorsalis
lateral collateral carpal ligament
radial carpal bone
n. pectoralis caudalis
m. pectoralis ascendens
v. mediana cubiti
m. pectoralis transversus
n. cutaneus antebrachii caudalis (n. ulnaris)
deep antebrachial fascia
n. cutaneus antebrachii medialis
(n. musculocutaneus)
v. cephalica
radius:
lateral styloid process
medial styloid process
a.v. radialis
medial collateral carpal ligament
accessory carpal bone
ulnar carpal bone

Fig. 3.13 Superficial structures of the left antebrachium and carpus: caudal view. The specimen is at the same stage of dissection as that shown in Figs. 3.11, 3.12, 3.14 For a comment on the use of the term 'lateral styloid process' see note on Fig. 7.4

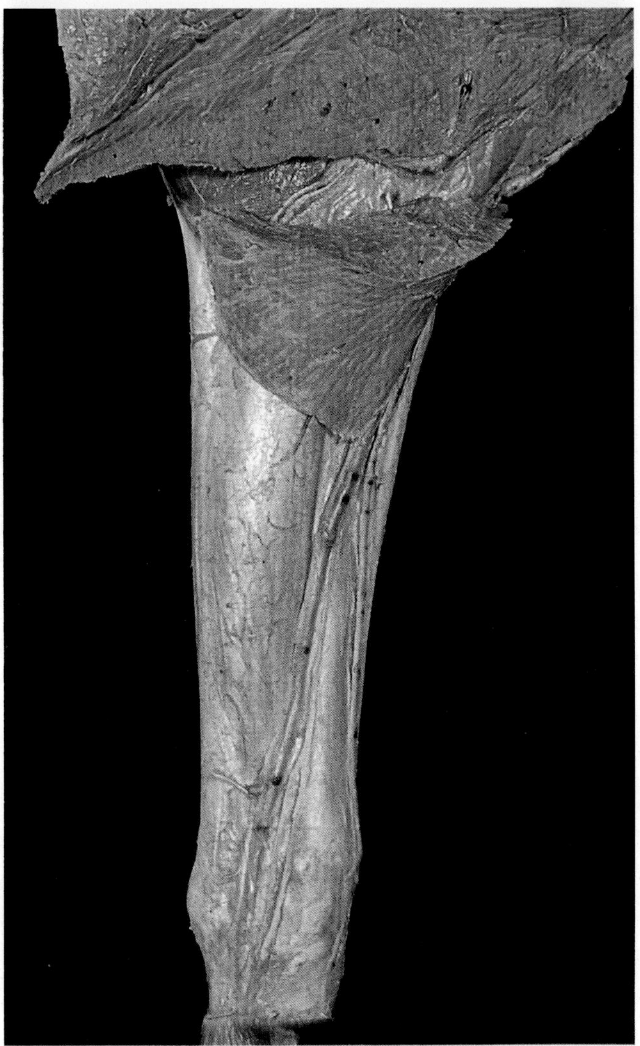

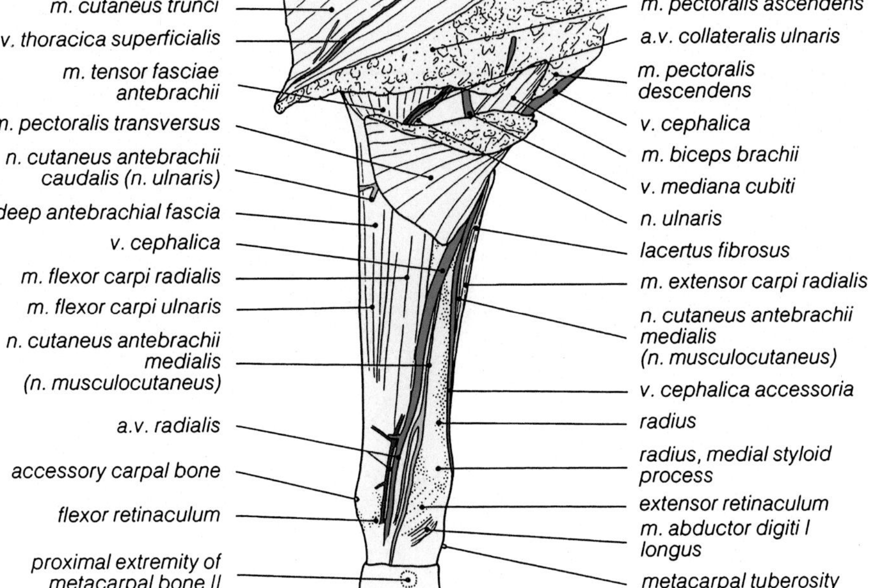
m. cutaneus trunci
v. thoracica superficialis
m. tensor fasciae antebrachii
m. pectoralis transversus
n. cutaneus antebrachii caudalis (n. ulnaris)
deep antebrachial fascia
v. cephalica
m. flexor carpi radialis
m. flexor carpi ulnaris
n. cutaneus antebrachii medialis
(n. musculocutaneus)
a.v. radialis
accessory carpal bone
flexor retinaculum
proximal extremity of metacarpal bone II
m. pectoralis ascendens
a.v. collateralis ulnaris
m. pectoralis descendens
v. cephalica
m. biceps brachii
v. mediana cubiti
n. ulnaris
lacertus fibrosus
m. extensor carpi radialis
n. cutaneus antebrachii medialis
(n. musculocutaneus)
v. cephalica accessoria
radius
radius, medial styloid process
extensor retinaculum
m. abductor digiti I longus
metacarpal tuberosity

Fig. 3.14 Superficial structures of the left antebrachium and carpus: medial view. The specimen is at the same stage of dissection as that shown in Figs. 3.11–3.13.

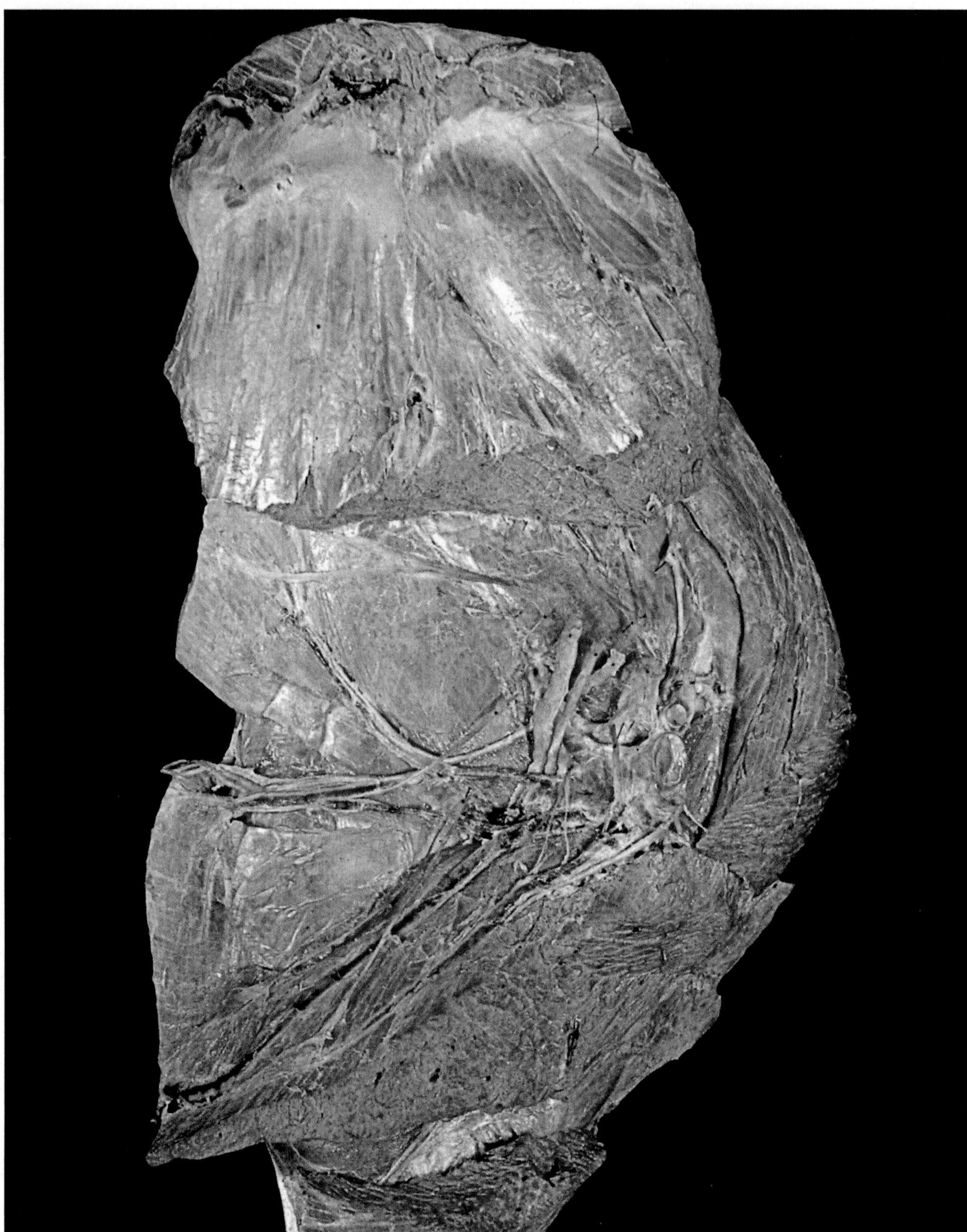

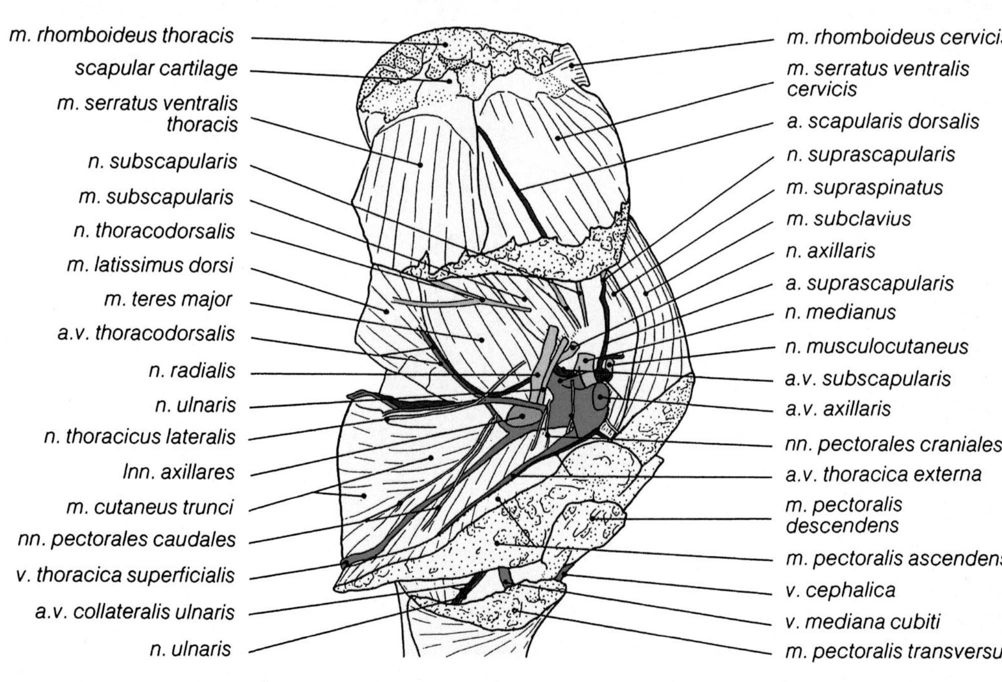
m. rhomboideus thoracis
scapular cartilage
m. serratus ventralis thoracis
n. subscapularis
m. subscapularis
n. thoracodorsalis
m. latissimus dorsi
m. teres major
a.v. thoracodorsalis
n. radialis
n. ulnaris
n. thoracicus lateralis
lnn. axillares
m. cutaneus trunci
nn. pectorales caudales
v. thoracica superficialis
a.v. collateralis ulnaris
n. ulnaris
m. rhomboideus cervicis
m. serratus ventralis cervicis
a. scapularis dorsalis
n. suprascapularis
m. supraspinatus
m. subclavius
n. axillaris
a. suprascapularis
n. medianus
n. musculocutaneus
a.v. subscapularis
a.v. axillaris
nn. pectorales craniales
a.v. thoracica externa
m. pectoralis descendens
m. pectoralis ascendens
v. cephalica
v. mediana cubiti
m. pectoralis transversus

Fig. 3.15 The left scapular and brachial regions: medial view. The muscles that join the limb to the trunk have been cut, see Fig. 3.10, but their attachments to the scapula and humerus have been preserved. No attempt has been made to display the axillary vessels and nerves in their correct topographical positions. These are shown in Figs. 3.43–3.51.

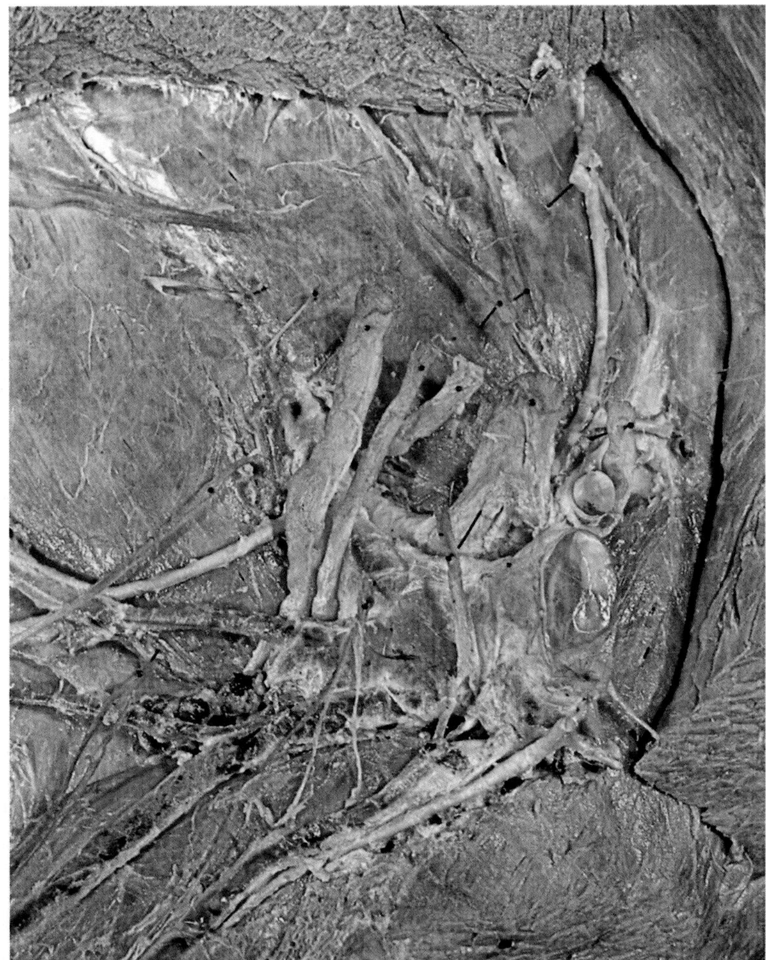

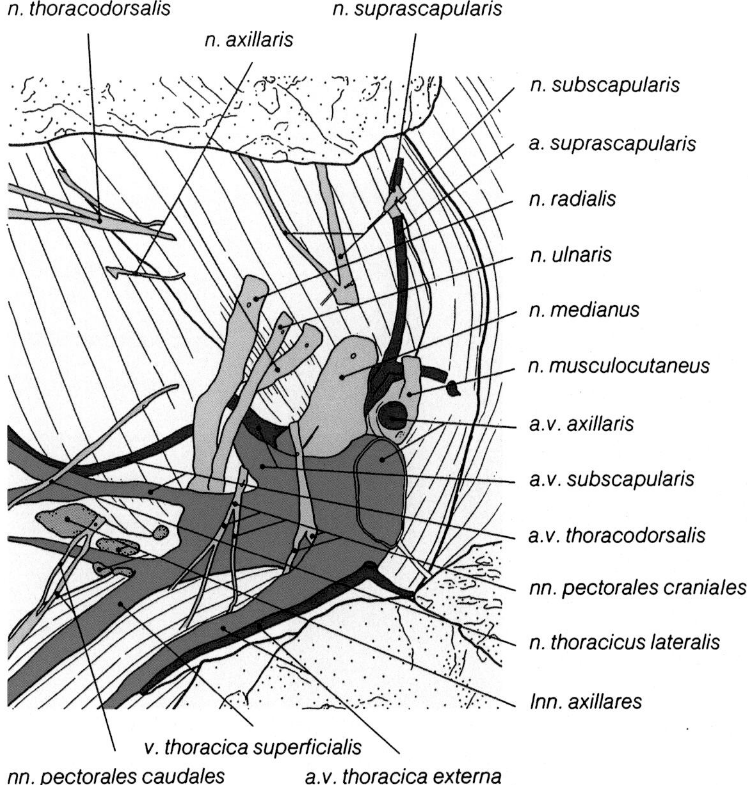
n. thoracodorsalis
n. suprascapularis
n. axillaris
n. subscapularis
a. suprascapularis
n. radialis
n. ulnaris
n. medianus
n. musculocutaneus
a.v. axillaris
a.v. subscapularis
a.v. thoracodorsalis
nn. pectorales craniales
n. thoracicus lateralis
lnn. axillares
v. thoracica superficialis
nn. pectorales caudales
a.v. thoracica externa

Fig. 3.16 The nerves of the brachial plexus of the left forelimb: medial view. This is a closer view of a part of the specimen shown in Fig. 3.15.

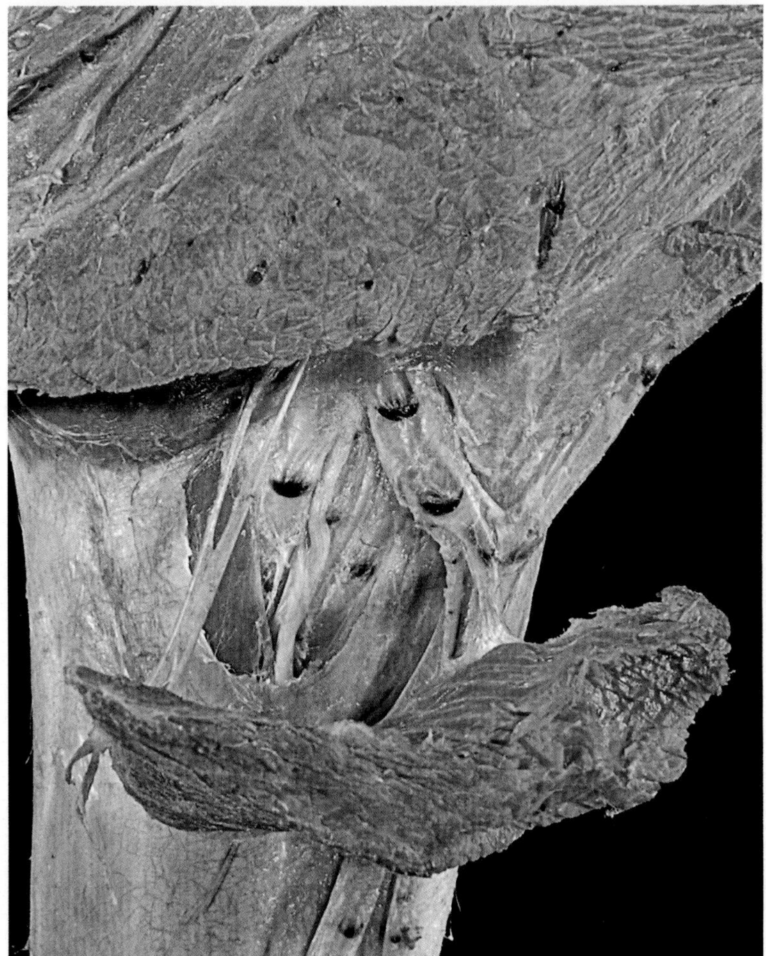

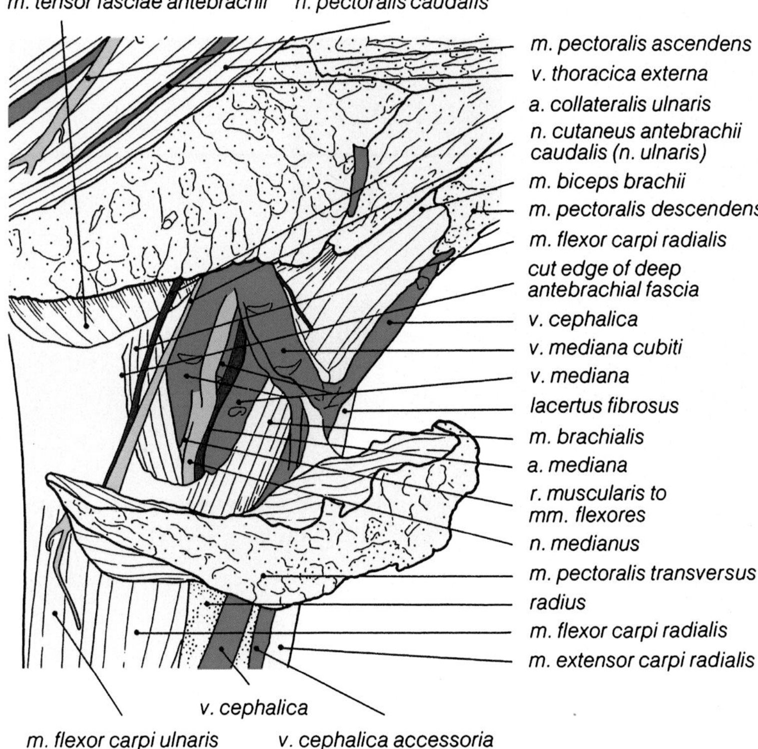
m. tensor fasciae antebrachii
n. pectoralis caudalis
m. pectoralis ascendens
v. thoracica externa
a. collateralis ulnaris
n. cutaneus antebrachii caudalis (n. ulnaris)
m. biceps brachii
m. pectoralis descendens
m. flexor carpi radialis
cut edge of deep antebrachial fascia
v. cephalica
v. mediana cubiti
v. mediana
lacertus fibrosus
m. brachialis
a. mediana
r. muscularis to mm. flexores
n. medianus
m. pectoralis transversus
radius
m. flexor carpi radialis
m. extensor carpi radialis
v. cephalica
m. flexor carpi ulnaris
v. cephalica accessoria

Fig. 3.17 The left median artery, vein and nerve at the medial cubital region: medial view. The transverse pectoral muscle has been reflected ventrally to display the position of the artery, vein and nerve. These structures, lying medial to the medial radial tuberosity and the medial humeral epicondyle, have been revealed by removal of the deep antebrachial fascia. At this site the pulse may be taken and the median nerve is surgically accessible.

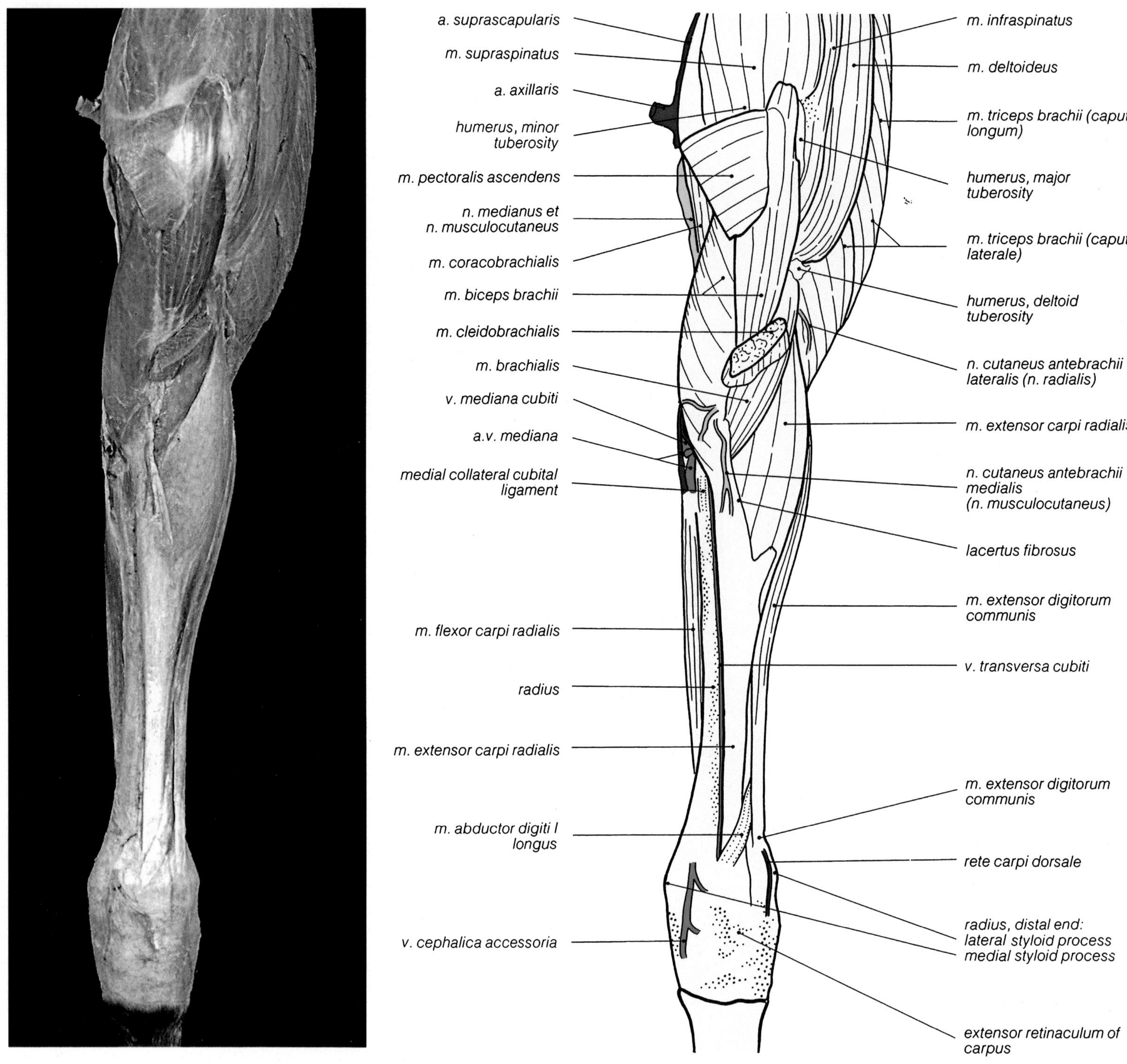
a. suprascapularis
m. supraspinatus
a. axillaris
humerus, minor tuberosity
m. pectoralis ascendens
n. medianus et n. musculocutaneus
m. coracobrachialis
m. biceps brachii
m. cleidobrachialis
m. brachialis
v. mediana cubiti
a.v. mediana
medial collateral cubital ligament
m. flexor carpi radialis
radius
m. extensor carpi radialis
m. abductor digiti I longus
v. cephalica accessoria
m. infraspinatus
m. deltoideus
m. triceps brachii (caput longum)
humerus, major tuberosity
m. triceps brachii (caput laterale)
humerus, deltoid tuberosity
n. cutaneus antebrachii lateralis (n. radialis)
m. extensor carpi radialis
n. cutaneus antebrachii medialis (n. musculocutaneus)
lacertus fibrosus
m. extensor digitorum communis
v. transversa cubiti
m. extensor digitorum communis
rete carpi dorsale
radius, distal end: lateral styloid process medial styloid process
extensor retinaculum of carpus

Fig. 3.18 Structures of the left brachial region, antebrachium and carpus: rostral view. The long tendon in the biceps muscle (lacertus fibrosus) is clearly seen inserting with the extensor carpi radialis. This specimen is also shown in Figs. 3.19–3.24.

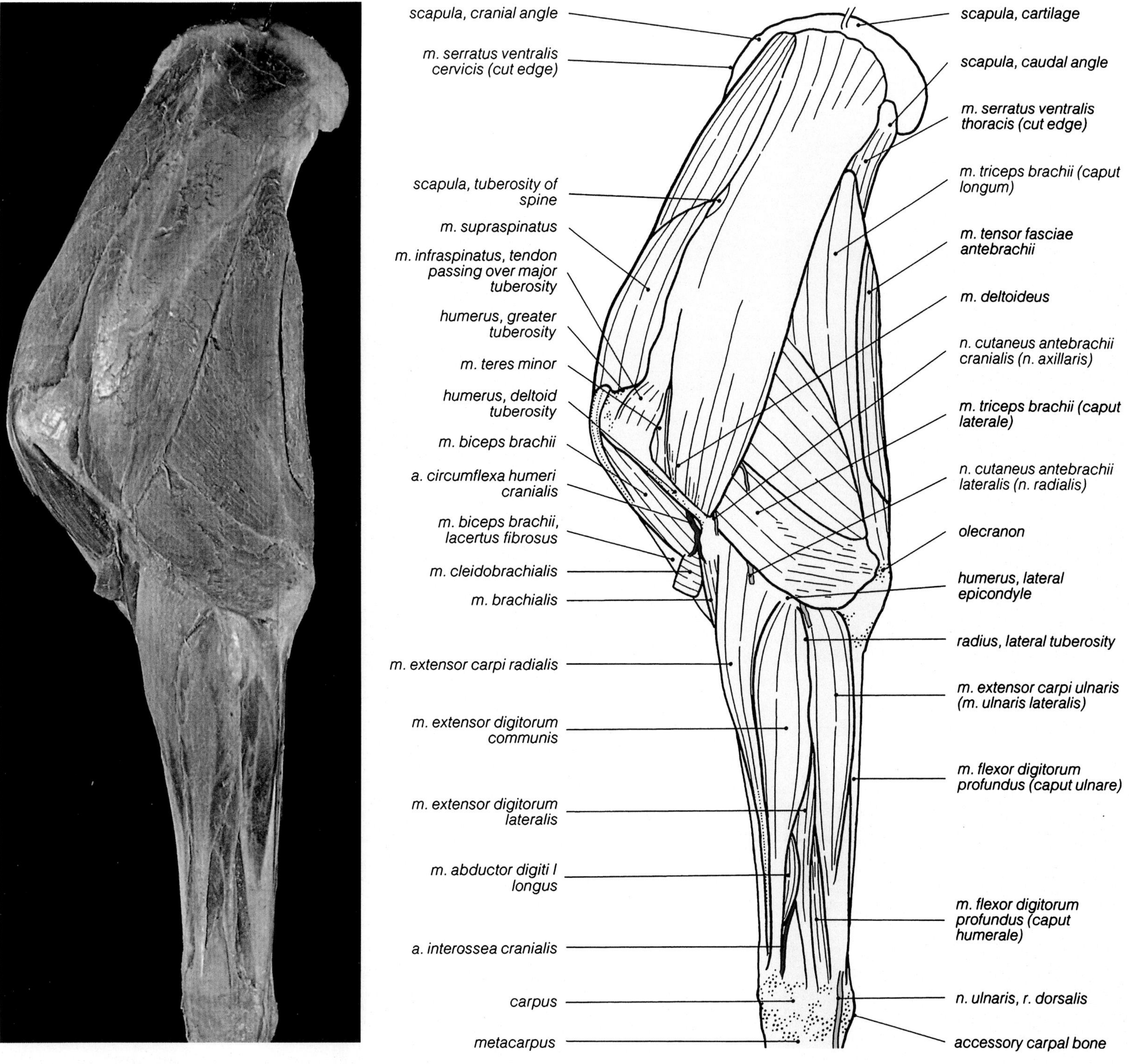
scapula, cranial angle
m. serratus ventralis cervicis (cut edge)
scapula, tuberosity of spine
m. supraspinatus
m. infraspinatus, tendon passing over major tuberosity
humerus, greater tuberosity
m. teres minor
humerus, deltoid tuberosity
m. biceps brachii
a. circumflexa humeri cranialis
m. biceps brachii, lacertus fibrosus
m. cleidobrachialis
m. brachialis
m. extensor carpi radialis
m. extensor digitorum communis
m. extensor digitorum lateralis
m. abductor digiti I longus
a. interossea cranialis
carpus
metacarpus
scapula, cartilage
scapula, caudal angle
m. serratus ventralis thoracis (cut edge)
m. triceps brachii (caput longum)
m. tensor fasciae antebrachii
m. deltoideus
n. cutaneus antebrachii cranialis (n. axillaris)
m. triceps brachii (caput laterale)
n. cutaneus antebrachii lateralis (n. radialis)
olecranon
humerus, lateral epicondyle
radius, lateral tuberosity
m. extensor carpi ulnaris (m. ulnaris lateralis)
m. flexor digitorum profundus (caput ulnare)
m. flexor digitorum profundus (caput humerale)
n. ulnaris, r. dorsalis
accessory carpal bone

Fig. 3.19 Structures of the scapular and brachial regions and the antebrachium: left lateral view. The strong omobrachial, brachial and antebrachial fasciae have been removed. This specimen is also shown in Figs. 3.18 and 3.20–3.24.

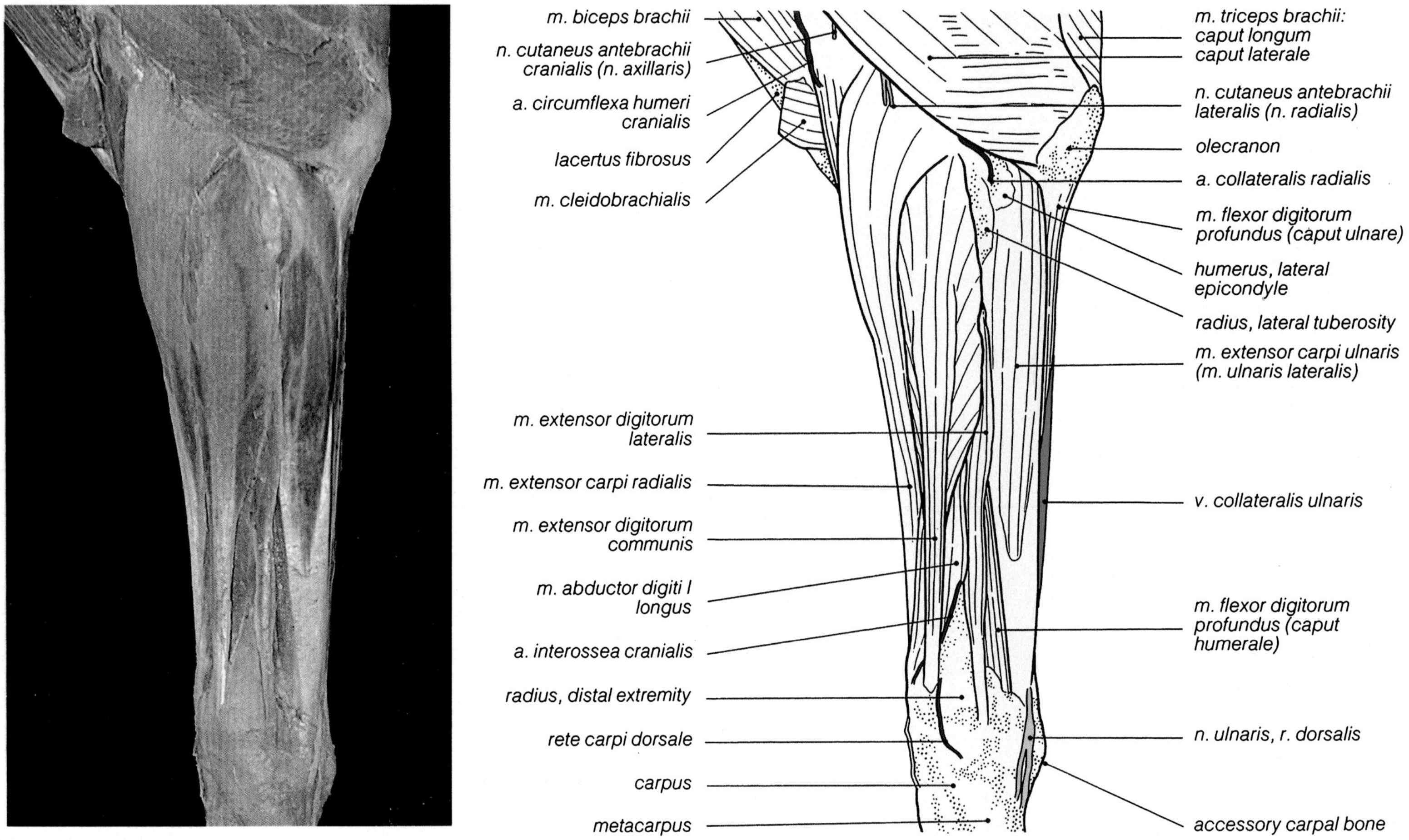

m. biceps brachii
n. cutaneus antebrachii cranialis (n. axillaris)
a. circumflexa humeri cranialis
lacertus fibrosus
m. cleidobrachialis
m. extensor digitorum lateralis
m. extensor carpi radialis
m. extensor digitorum communis
m. abductor digiti I longus
a. interossea cranialis
radius, distal extremity
rete carpi dorsale
carpus
metacarpus
m. triceps brachii:
caput longum
caput laterale
n. cutaneus antebrachii lateralis (n. radialis)
olecranon
a. collateralis radialis
m. flexor digitorum profundus (caput ulnare)
humerus, lateral epicondyle
radius, lateral tuberosity
m. extensor carpi ulnaris (m. ulnaris lateralis)
v. collateralis ulnaris
m. flexor digitorum profundus (caput humerale)
n. ulnaris, r. dorsalis
accessory carpal bone

Fig. 3.20 Structures of the antebrachium and carpus: left lateral view. This figure reveals the distal part of the specimen shown in Fig. 3.19.

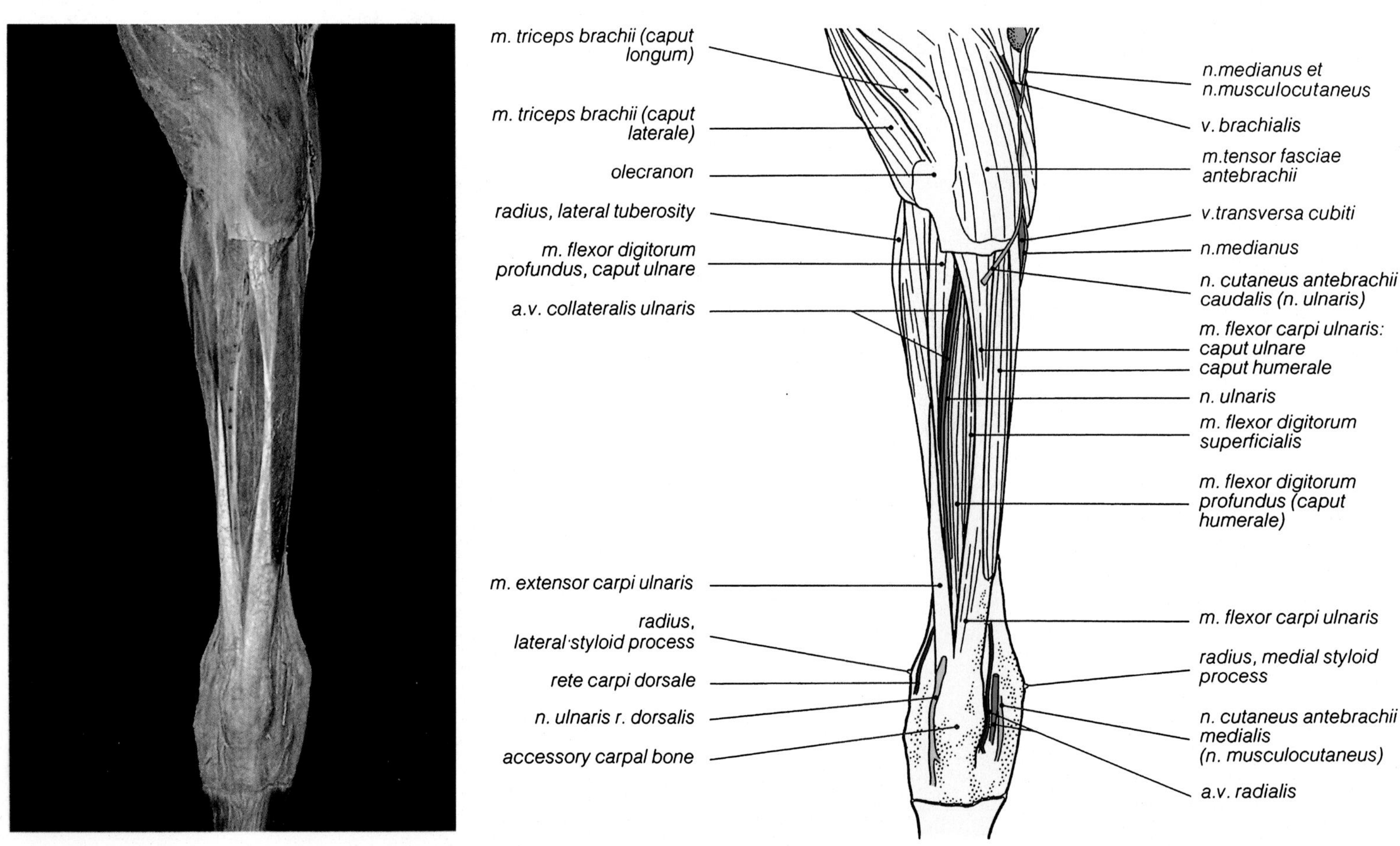
m. triceps brachii (caput longum)
m. triceps brachii (caput laterale)
olecranon
radius, lateral tuberosity
m. flexor digitorum profundus, caput ulnare
a.v. collateralis ulnaris
m. extensor carpi ulnaris
radius, lateral styloid process
rete carpi dorsale
n. ulnaris r. dorsalis
accessory carpal bone
n.medianus et n.musculocutaneus
v. brachialis
m.tensor fasciae antebrachii
v.transversa cubiti
n.medianus
n. cutaneus antebrachii caudalis (n. ulnaris)
m. flexor carpi ulnaris:
caput ulnare
caput humerale
n. ulnaris
m. flexor digitorum superficialis
m. flexor digitorum profundus (caput humerale)
m. flexor carpi ulnaris
radius, medial styloid process
n. cutaneus antebrachii medialis (n. musculocutaneus)
a.v. radialis

Fig. 3.21 Structures of the left brachial region, antebrachium and carpus: caudal view. The specimen is at the stage of dissection shown in Figs. 3.19, 3.20, 3.22, 3.23 and 3.24.

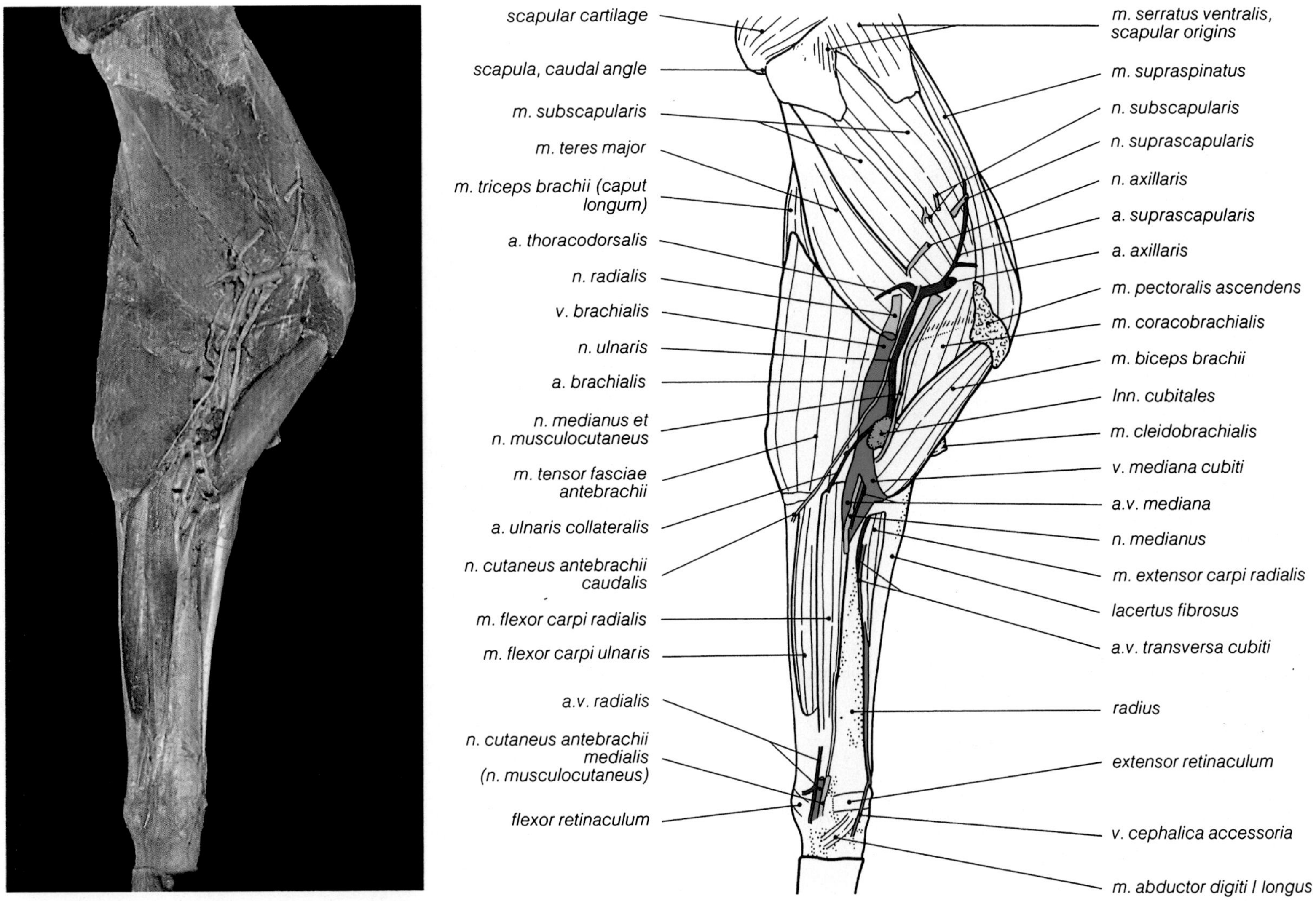

scapular cartilage
scapula, caudal angle
m. subscapularis
m. teres major
m. triceps brachii (caput longum)
a. thoracodorsalis
n. radialis
v. brachialis
n. ulnaris
a. brachialis
n. medianus et n. musculocutaneus
m. tensor fasciae antebrachii
a. ulnaris collateralis
n. cutaneus antebrachii caudalis
m. flexor carpi radialis
m. flexor carpi ulnaris
a.v. radialis
n. cutaneus antebrachii medialis (n. musculocutaneus)
flexor retinaculum
m. serratus ventralis, scapular origins
m. supraspinatus
n. subscapularis
n. suprascapularis
n. axillaris
a. suprascapularis
a. axillaris
m. pectoralis ascendens
m. coracobrachialis
m. biceps brachii
lnn. cubitales
m. cleidobrachialis
v. mediana cubiti
a.v. mediana
n. medianus
m. extensor carpi radialis
lacertus fibrosus
a.v. transversa cubiti
radius
extensor retinaculum
v. cephalica accessoria
m. abductor digiti I longus

Fig. 3.22 Structures of the left scapular and brachial regions, antebrachium and carpus: medial view. The specimen is at the stage of dissection shown in Figs. 3.18–3.21 and Figs. 3.23–3.24. Compared with the earlier stage of dissection, shown in Figs. 3.14 and 3.15, further details of the nerves, arteries and veins of the antebrachium are exposed by removal of the muscles that joined the limb to the trunk.

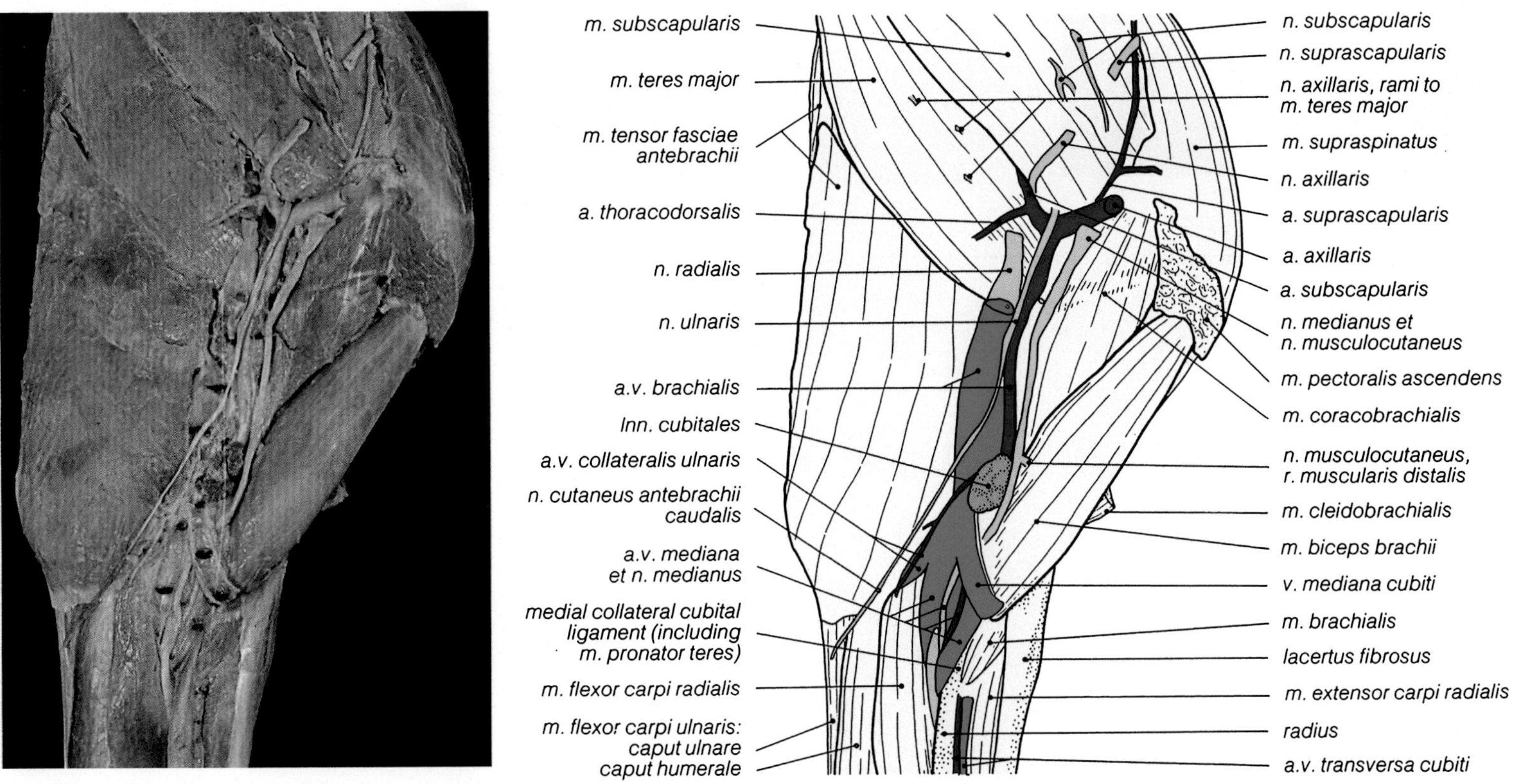
m. subscapularis
m. teres major
m. tensor fasciae antebrachii
a. thoracodorsalis
n. radialis
n. ulnaris
a.v. brachialis
lnn. cubitales
a.v. collateralis ulnaris
n. cutaneus antebrachii caudalis
a.v. mediana et n. medianus
medial collateral cubital ligament (including m. pronator teres)
m. flexor carpi radialis
m. flexor carpi ulnaris: caput ulnare caput humerale
n. subscapularis
n. suprascapularis
n. axillaris, rami to m. teres major
m. supraspinatus
n. axillaris
a. suprascapularis
a. axillaris
a. subscapularis
n. medianus et n. musculocutaneus
m. pectoralis ascendens
m. coracobrachialis
n. musculocutaneus, r. muscularis distalis
m. cleidobrachialis
m. biceps brachii
v. mediana cubiti
m. brachialis
lacertus fibrosus
m. extensor carpi radialis
radius
a.v. transversa cubiti

Fig. 3.23 The left brachial region and antebrachium: medial view. This is a closer view of a part of the specimen shown in Fig. 3.22.

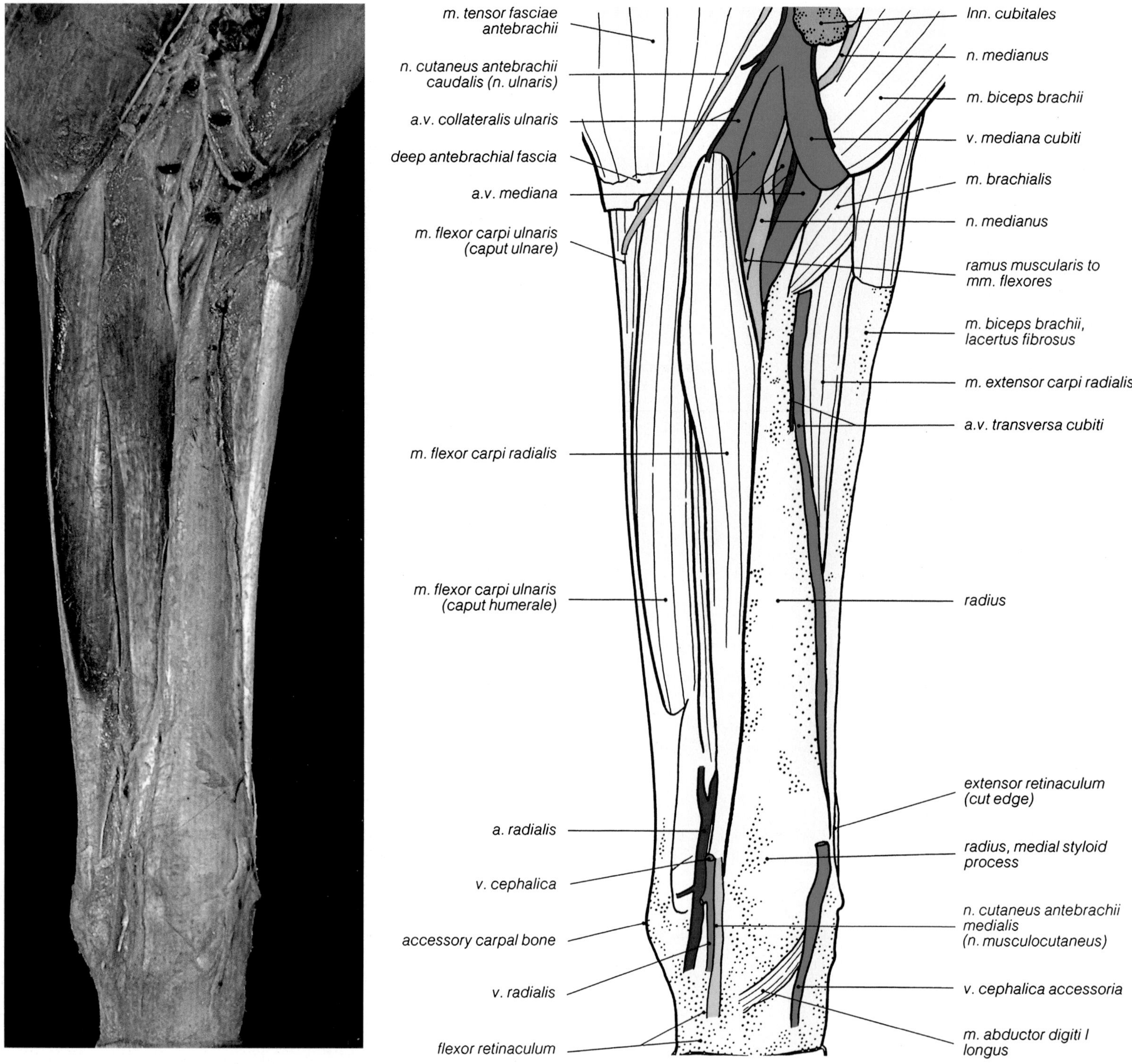
m. tensor fasciae antebrachii
n. cutaneus antebrachii caudalis (n. ulnaris)
a.v. collateralis ulnaris
deep antebrachial fascia
a.v. mediana
m. flexor carpi ulnaris (caput ulnare)
m. flexor carpi radialis
m. flexor carpi ulnaris (caput humerale)
a. radialis
v. cephalica
accessory carpal bone
v. radialis
flexor retinaculum
lnn. cubitales
n. medianus
m. biceps brachii
v. mediana cubiti
m. brachialis
n. medianus
ramus muscularis to mm. flexores
m. biceps brachii, lacertus fibrosus
m. extensor carpi radialis
a.v. transversa cubiti
radius
extensor retinaculum (cut edge)
radius, medial styloid process
n. cutaneus antebrachii medialis (n. musculocutaneus)
v. cephalica accessoria
m. abductor digiti I longus

Fig. 3.24 The left antebrachium and carpus: medial view. This is a closer view of a part of the specimen shown in Fig. 3.22.

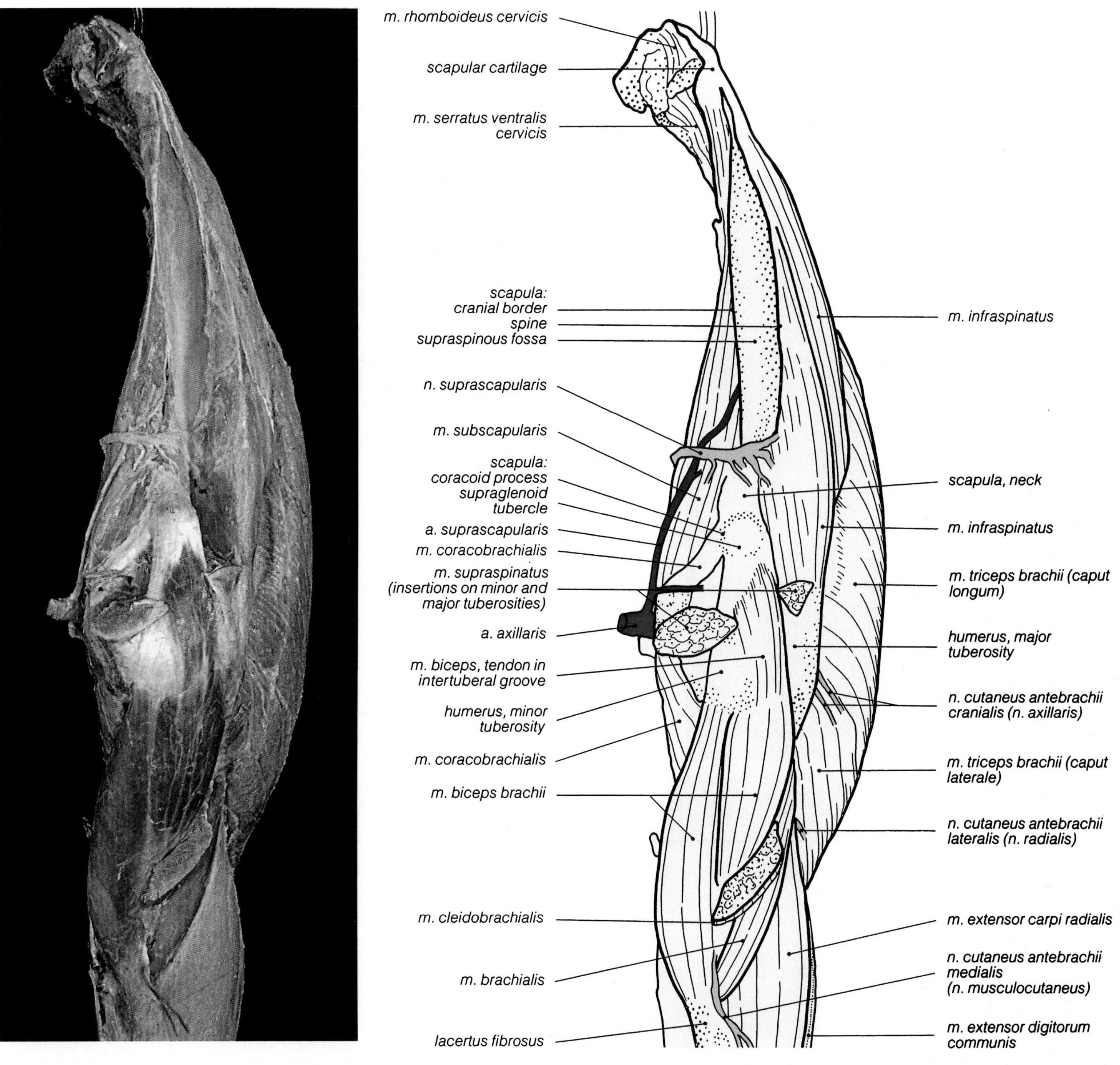
m. rhomboideus cervicis
scapular cartilage
m. serratus ventralis cervicis
scapula: cranial border
spine
supraspinous fossa
n. suprascapularis
m. subscapularis
scapula: coracoid process
supraglenoid tubercle
a. suprascapularis
m. coracobrachialis
m. supraspinatus (insertions on minor and major tuberosities)
a. axillaris
m. biceps, tendon in intertuberal groove
humerus, minor tuberosity
m. coracobrachialis
m. biceps brachii
m. cleidobrachialis
m. brachialis
lacertus fibrosus
m. infraspinatus
scapula, neck
m. infraspinatus
m. triceps brachii (caput longum)
humerus, major tuberosity
n. cutaneus antebrachii cranialis (n. axillaris)
m. triceps brachii (caput laterale)
n. cutaneus antebrachii lateralis (n. radialis)
m. extensor carpi radialis
n. cutaneus antebrachii medialis (n. musculocutaneus)
m. extensor digitorum communis

Fig. 3.25 Deeper structures of the left scapular and brachial regions: rostral view. The supraspinatus muscle has been removed from the supraspinous fossa to show the suprascapular nerve and the origin of the biceps brachii muscle. The deltoid muscle has also been removed. The intermediate tuberosity of the humerus is not visible in the intertuberal groove; it is covered by the biceps tendon which is moulded upon the double groove between major and minor tuberosities. This specimen is also shown in Figs. 3.26 and 3.28.

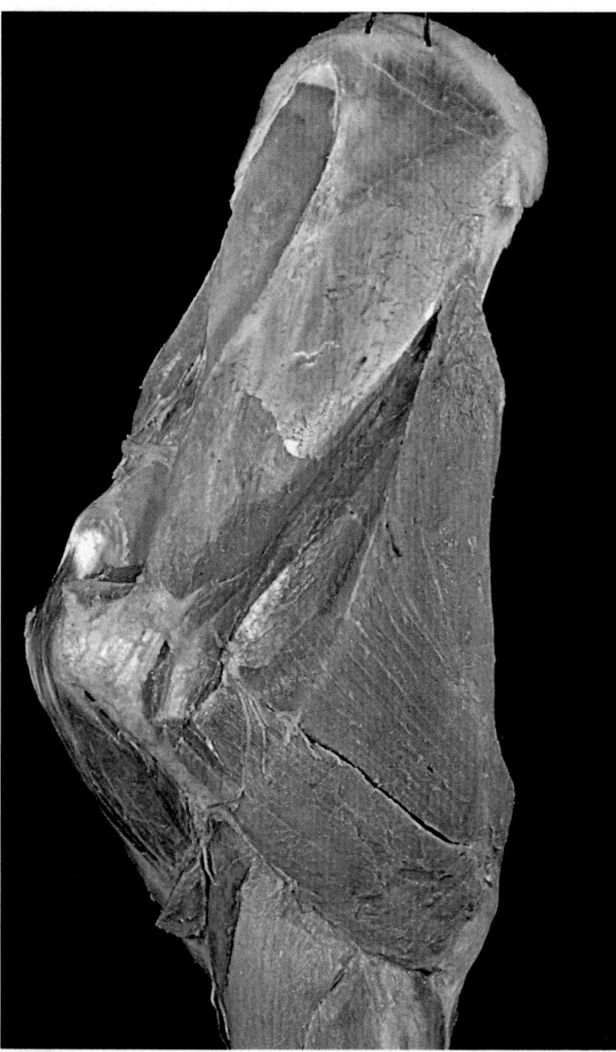

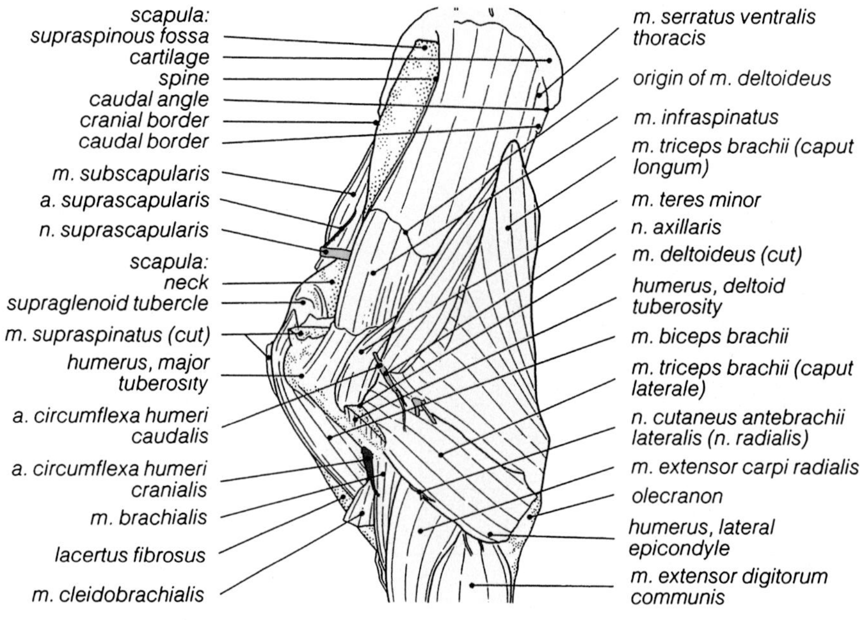
scapula:
supraspinous fossa
cartilage
spine
caudal angle
cranial border
caudal border
m. subscapularis
a. suprascapularis
n. suprascapularis
scapula:
neck
supraglenoid tubercle
m. supraspinatus (cut)
humerus, major
tuberosity
a. circumflexa humeri
caudalis
a. circumflexa humeri
cranialis
m. brachialis
lacertus fibrosus
m. cleidobrachialis
m. serratus ventralis
thoracis
origin of m. deltoideus
m. infraspinatus
m. triceps brachii (caput
longum)
m. teres minor
n. axillaris
m. deltoideus (cut)
humerus, deltoid
tuberosity
m. biceps brachii
m. triceps brachii (caput
laterale)
n. cutaneus antebrachii
lateralis (n. radialis)
m. extensor carpi radialis
olecranon
humerus, lateral
epicondyle
m. extensor digitorum
communis

Fig. 3.26 Deeper structures of the left scapular and brachial regions: lateral view. Removal of the deltoid muscle shows the full extent of the infraspinatus muscle and also the teres minor muscle.

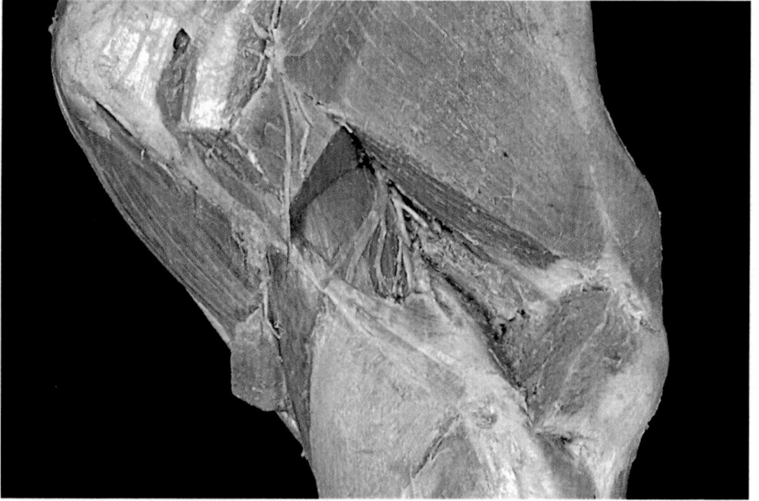

Fig. 3.27 The humeral groove, brachialis muscle and radial nerve: left lateral view. The lateral head of the triceps muscle has been resected to reveal the brachialis muscle in its humeral groove, and the associated nerve and artery. In older textbooks this feature of the shaft of the humerus is called the musculospiral groove.

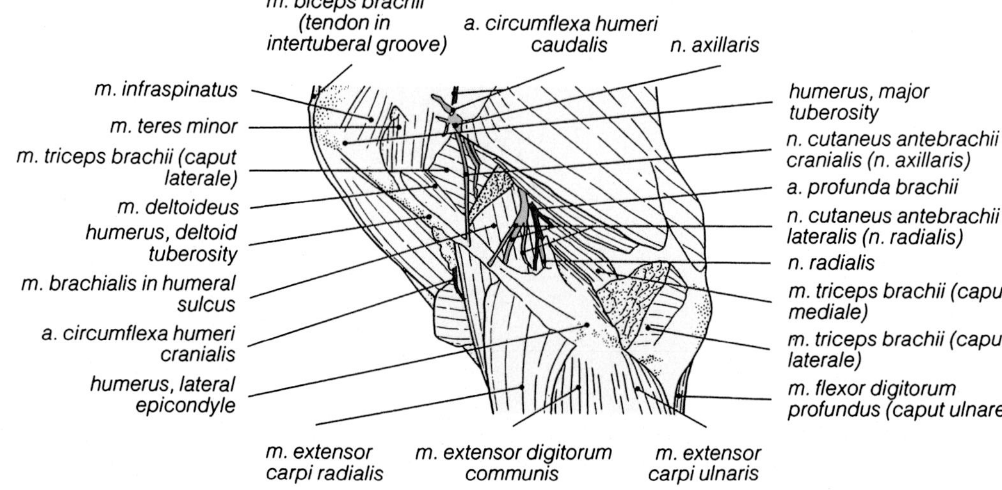
m. biceps brachii
(tendon in
intertuberal groove)
a. circumflexa humeri
caudalis
n. axillaris
m. infraspinatus
m. teres minor
m. triceps brachii (caput
laterale)
m. deltoideus
humerus, deltoid
tuberosity
m. brachialis in humeral
sulcus
a. circumflexa humeri
cranialis
humerus, lateral
epicondyle
humerus, major
tuberosity
n. cutaneus antebrachii
cranialis (n. axillaris)
a. profunda brachii
n. cutaneus antebrachii
lateralis (n. radialis)
n. radialis
m. triceps brachii (caput
mediale)
m. triceps brachii (caput
laterale)
m. flexor digitorum
profundus (caput ulnare)
m. extensor
carpi radialis
m. extensor digitorum
communis
m. extensor
carpi ulnaris

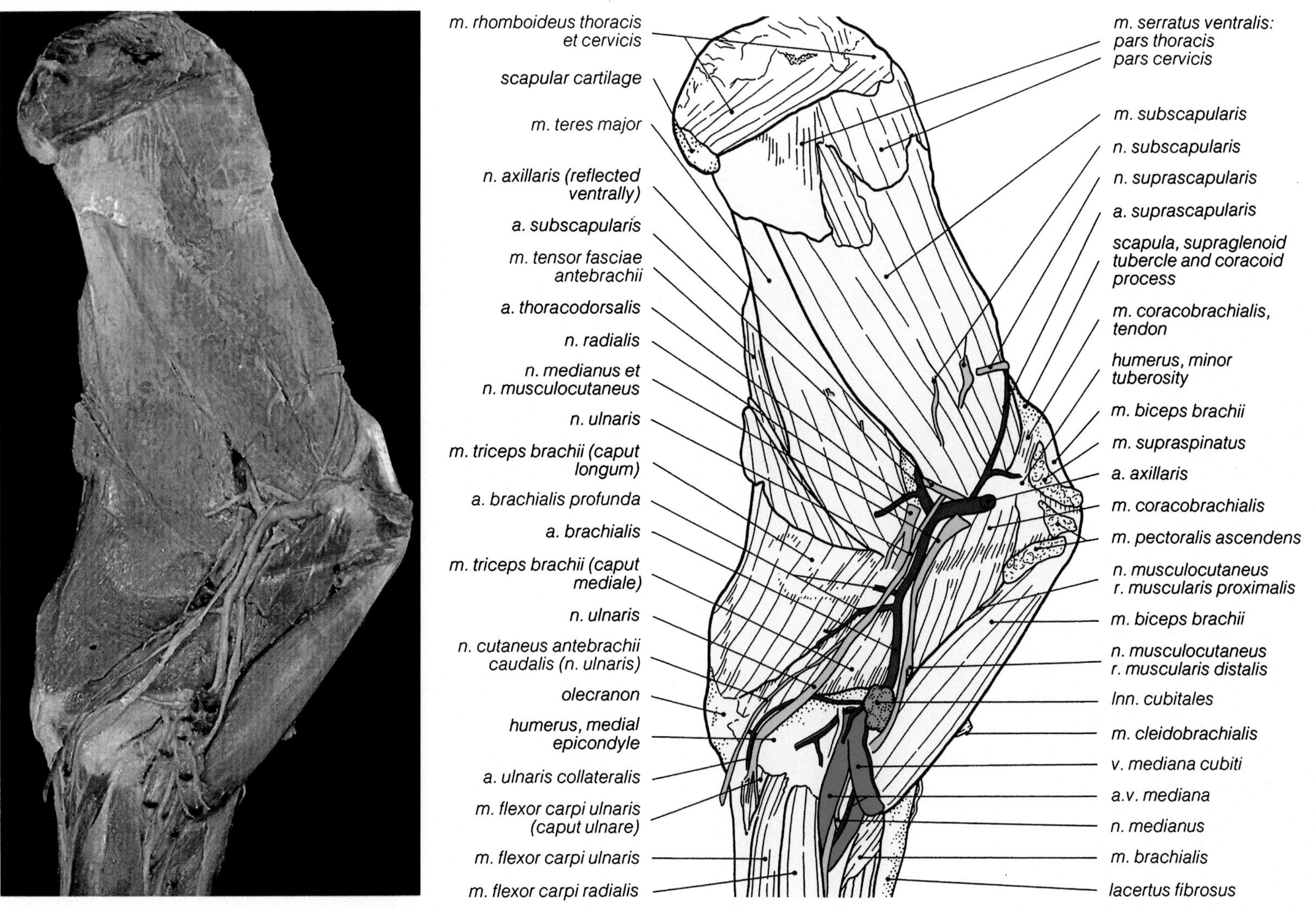

m. rhomboideus thoracis et cervicis
scapular cartilage
m. teres major
n. axillaris (reflected ventrally)
a. subscapularis
m. tensor fasciae antebrachii
a. thoracodorsalis
n. radialis
n. medianus et n. musculocutaneus
n. ulnaris
m. triceps brachii (caput longum)
a. brachialis profunda
a. brachialis
m. triceps brachii (caput mediale)
n. ulnaris
n. cutaneus antebrachii caudalis (n. ulnaris)
olecranon
humerus, medial epicondyle
a. ulnaris collateralis
m. flexor carpi ulnaris (caput ulnare)
m. flexor carpi ulnaris
m. flexor carpi radialis
m. serratus ventralis: pars thoracis pars cervicis
m. subscapularis
n. subscapularis
n. suprascapularis
a. suprascapularis
scapula, supraglenoid tubercle and coracoid process
m. coracobrachialis, tendon
humerus, minor tuberosity
m. biceps brachii
m. supraspinatus
a. axillaris
m. coracobrachialis
m. pectoralis ascendens
n. musculocutaneus r. muscularis proximalis
m. biceps brachii
n. musculocutaneus r. muscularis distalis
lnn. cubitales
m. cleidobrachialis
v. mediana cubiti
a.v. mediana
n. medianus
m. brachialis
lacertus fibrosus

Fig. 3.28 The left brachial artery and ulnar and median nerves: medial view. The specimen is at the stage of dissection shown in Figs. 3.25 and 3.26. The veins have been removed from the brachial region to show the arteries and nerves more clearly. The supraspinatus muscle has been removed to show the origins of the biceps brachii and coracobrachialis muscles from the scapula. The tensor muscle of the antebrachial fascia has been removed.

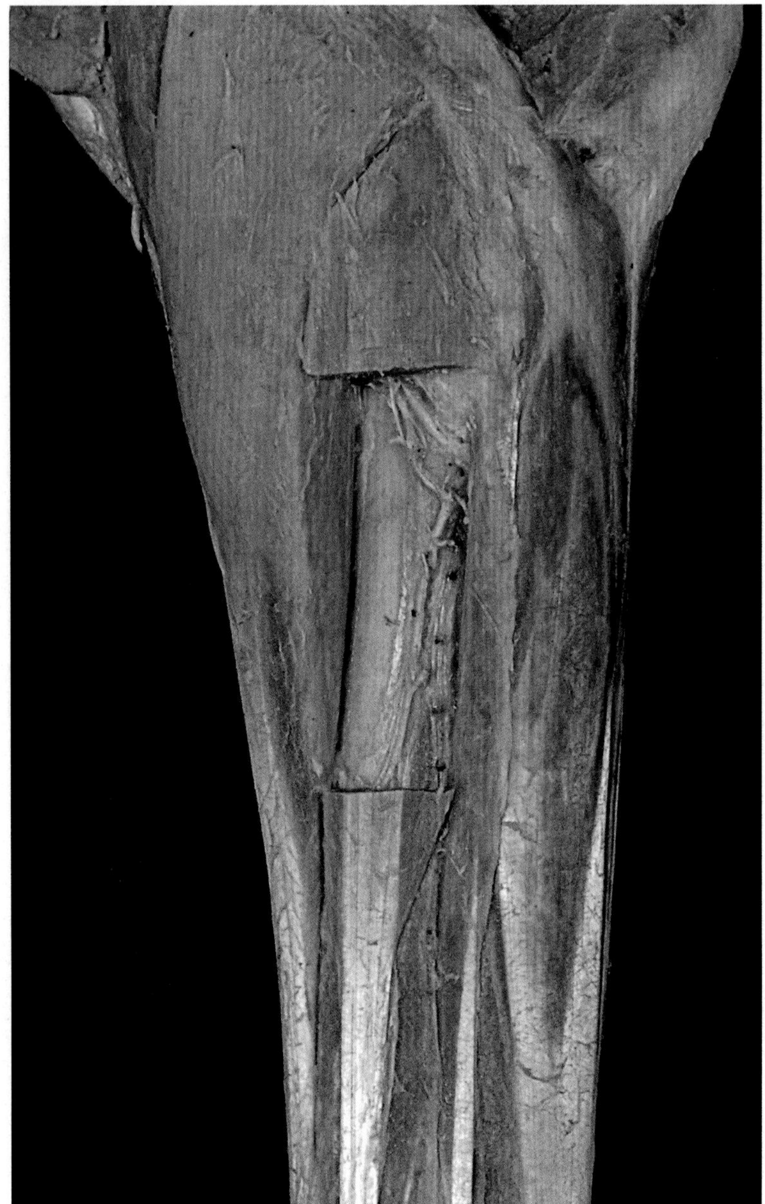

Fig. 3.29 Deep vessels and nerves of the left antebrachium: lateral view. Part of the common digital extensor muscle has been removed to show the cranial interosseous artery and branches of the radial nerve.

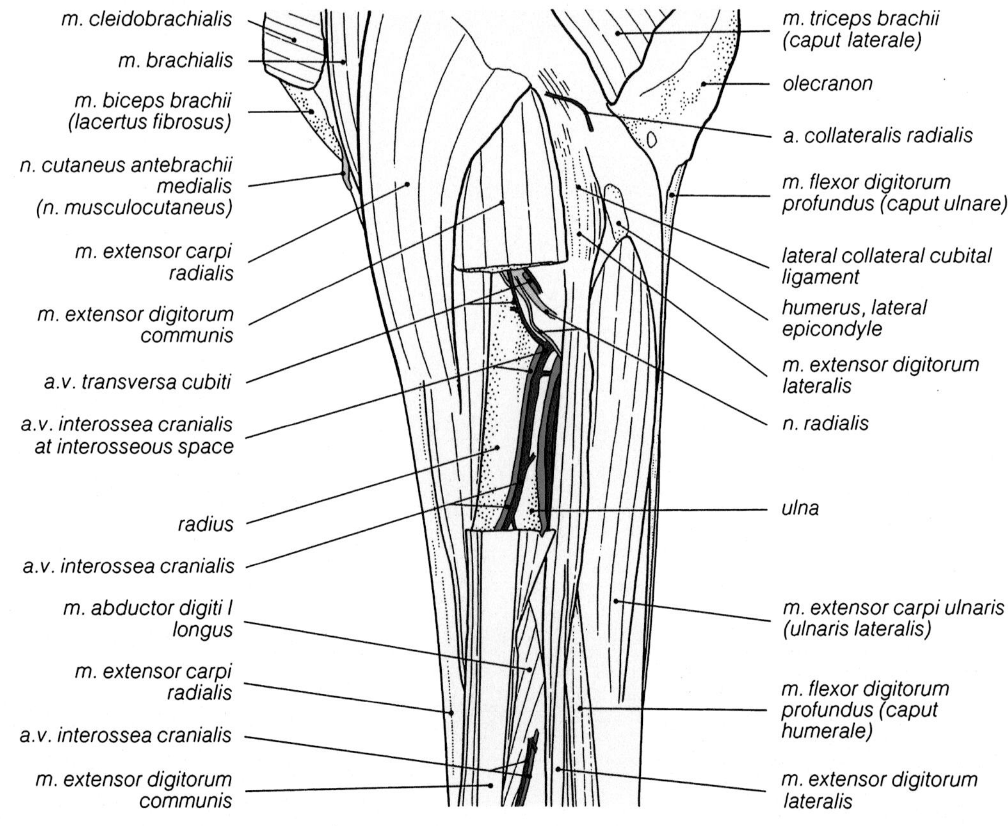
m. cleidobrachialis
m. brachialis
m. biceps brachii (lacertus fibrosus)
n. cutaneus antebrachii medialis (n. musculocutaneus)
m. extensor carpi radialis
m. extensor digitorum communis
a.v. transversa cubiti
a.v. interossea cranialis at interosseous space
radius
a.v. interossea cranialis
m. abductor digiti I longus
m. extensor carpi radialis
a.v. interossea cranialis
m. extensor digitorum communis
m. triceps brachii (caput laterale)
olecranon
a. collateralis radialis
m. flexor digitorum profundus (caput ulnare)
lateral collateral cubital ligament
humerus, lateral epicondyle
m. extensor digitorum lateralis
n. radialis
ulna
m. extensor carpi ulnaris (ulnaris lateralis)
m. flexor digitorum profundus (caput humerale)
m. extensor digitorum lateralis

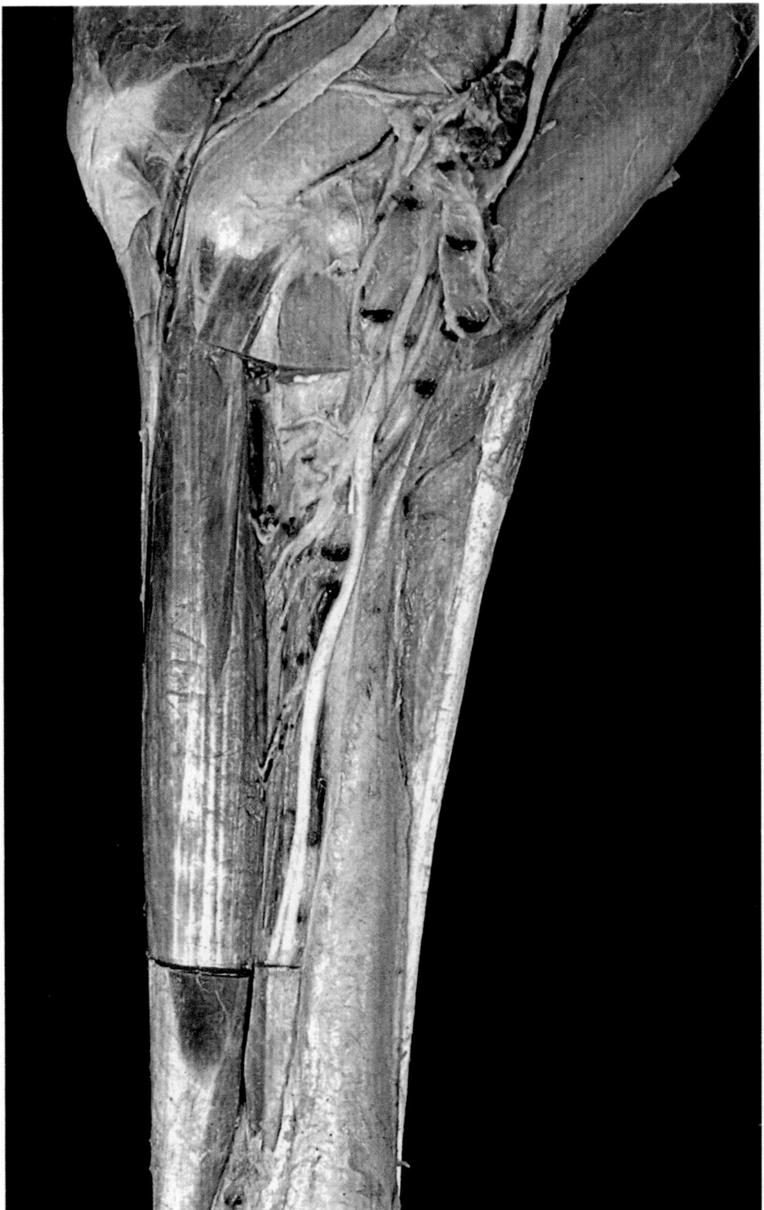

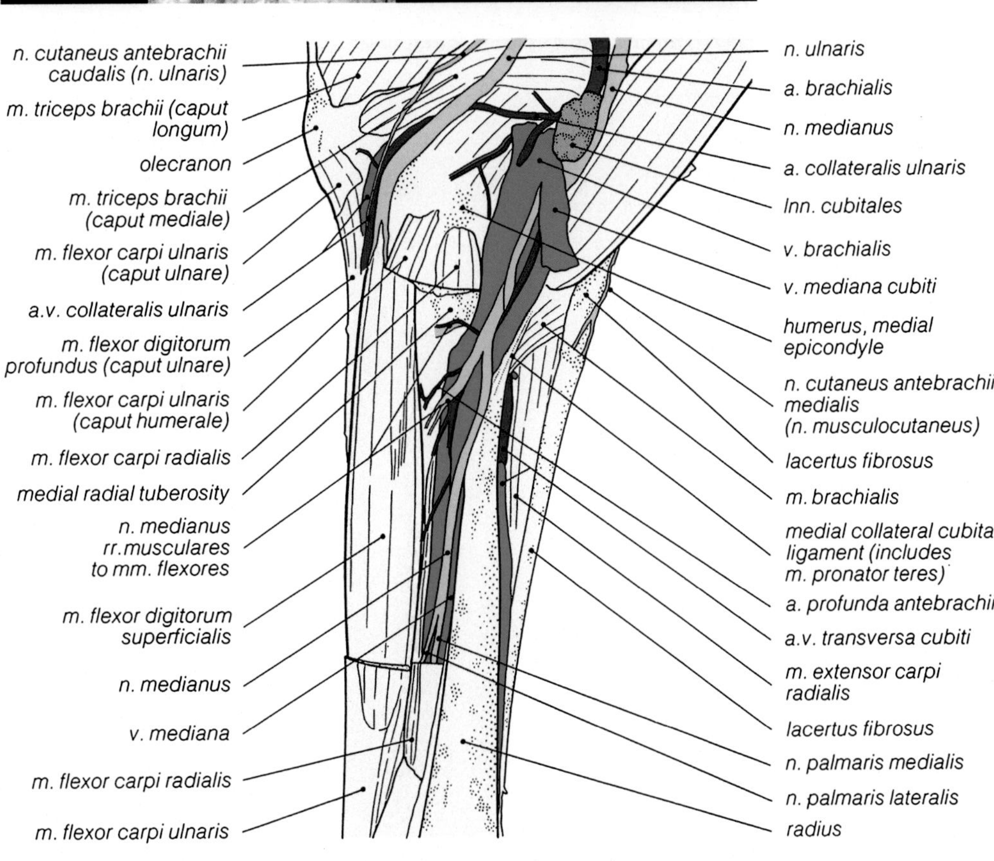

n. cutaneus antebrachii caudalis (n. ulnaris)
m. triceps brachii (caput longum)
olecranon
m. triceps brachii (caput mediale)
m. flexor carpi ulnaris (caput ulnare)
a.v. collateralis ulnaris
m. flexor digitorum profundus (caput ulnare)
m. flexor carpi ulnaris (caput humerale)
m. flexor carpi radialis
medial radial tuberosity
n. medianus rr.musculares to mm. flexores
m. flexor digitorum superficialis
n. medianus
v. mediana
m. flexor carpi radialis
m. flexor carpi ulnaris
n. ulnaris
a. brachialis
n. medianus
a. collateralis ulnaris
lnn. cubitales
v. brachialis
v. mediana cubiti
humerus, medial epicondyle
n. cutaneus antebrachii medialis (n. musculocutaneus)
lacertus fibrosus
m. brachialis
medial collateral cubital ligament (includes m. pronator teres)
a. profunda antebrachii
a.v. transversa cubiti
m. extensor carpi radialis
lacertus fibrosus
n. palmaris medialis
n. palmaris lateralis
radius

Fig. 3.30 Deep vessels and nerves of the left antebrachium: medial view (1). The flexor carpi radialis and flexor carpi ulnaris muscles have been partly removed (see also Fig. 3.22) to show the median nerve with its muscular branches and the common interosseous artery.

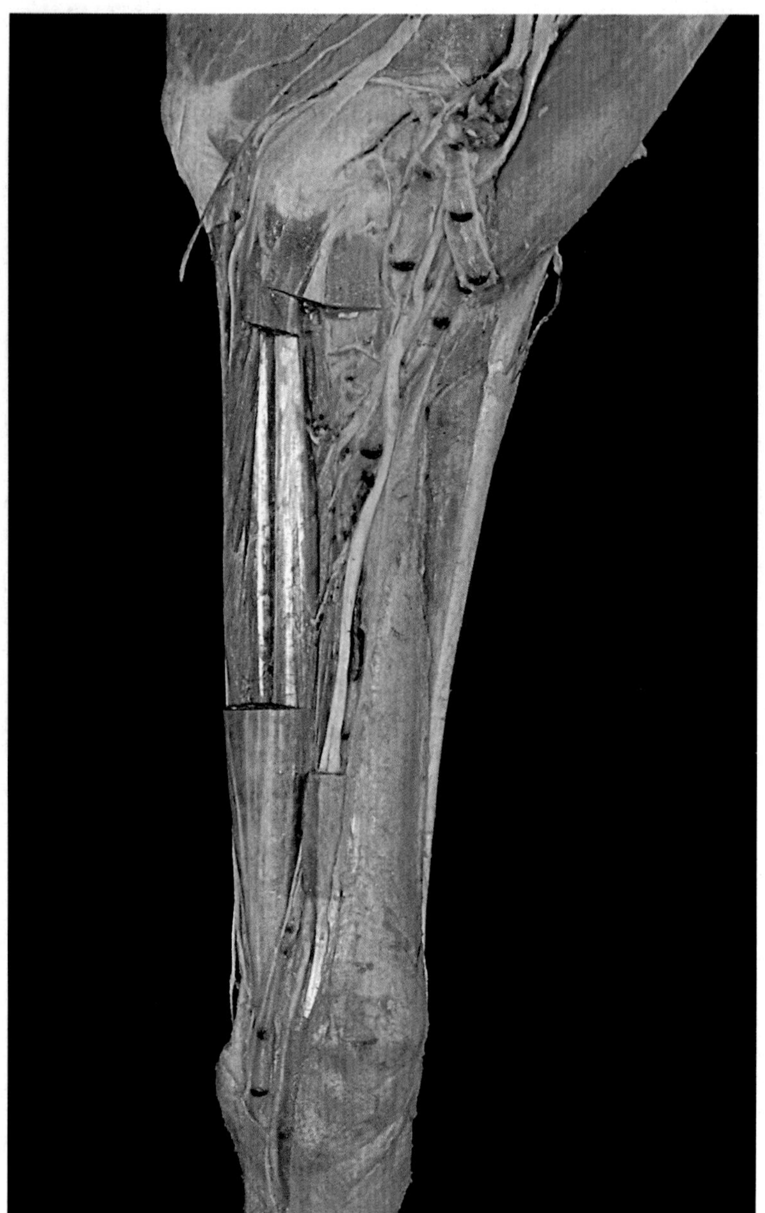

Fig. 3.31 The deep vessels and nerves of the left antebrachium: medial view (2). The flexor carpi ulnaris muscle has been removed to display the structures lying deep to its tendon of insertion (see also Fig. 3.32). A part has been removed from the superficial digital flexor muscle to show the radial and humeral heads of the deep flexor muscle.

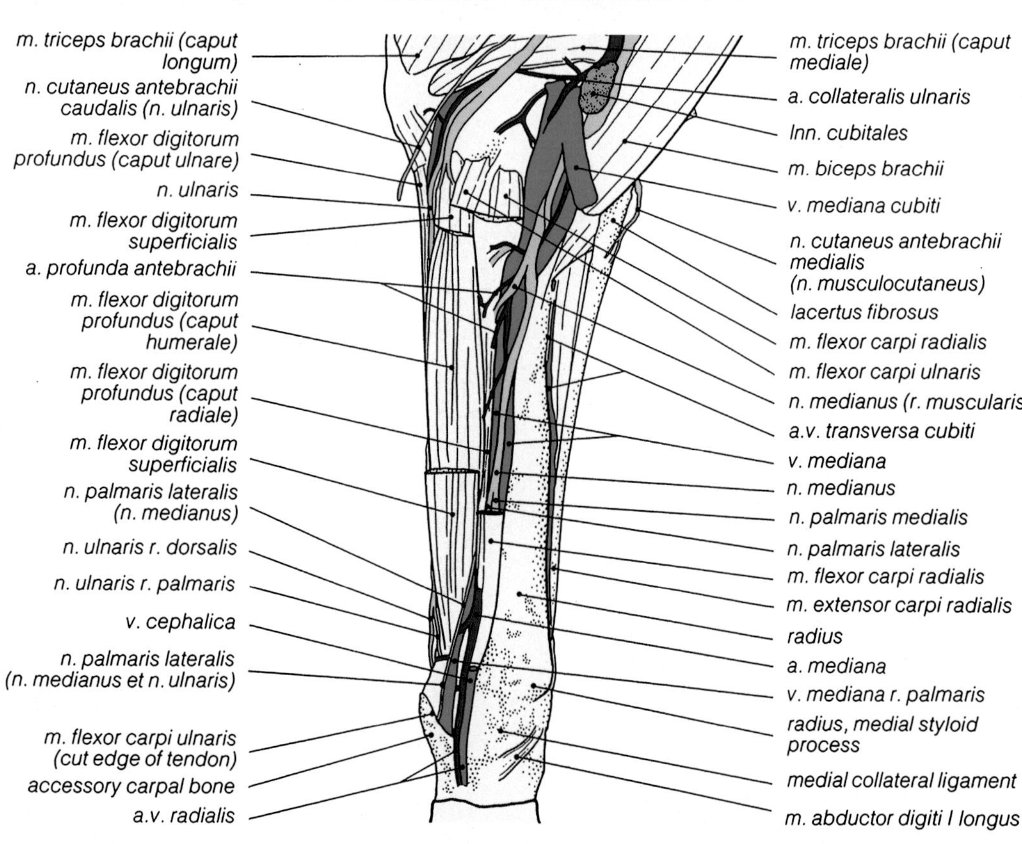
m. triceps brachii (caput longum)
n. cutaneus antebrachii caudalis (n. ulnaris)
m. flexor digitorum profundus (caput ulnare)
n. ulnaris
m. flexor digitorum superficialis
a. profunda antebrachii
m. flexor digitorum profundus (caput humerale)
m. flexor digitorum profundus (caput radiale)
m. flexor digitorum superficialis
n. palmaris lateralis (n. medianus)
n. ulnaris r. dorsalis
n. ulnaris r. palmaris
v. cephalica
n. palmaris lateralis (n. medianus et n. ulnaris)
m. flexor carpi ulnaris (cut edge of tendon)
accessory carpal bone
a.v. radialis
m. triceps brachii (caput mediale)
a. collateralis ulnaris
lnn. cubitales
m. biceps brachii
v. mediana cubiti
n. cutaneus antebrachii medialis (n. musculocutaneus)
lacertus fibrosus
m. flexor carpi radialis
m. flexor carpi ulnaris
n. medianus (r. muscularis)
a.v. transversa cubiti
v. mediana
n. medianus
n. palmaris medialis
n. palmaris lateralis
m. flexor carpi radialis
m. extensor carpi radialis
radius
a. mediana
v. mediana r. palmaris
radius, medial styloid process
medial collateral ligament
m. abductor digiti I longus

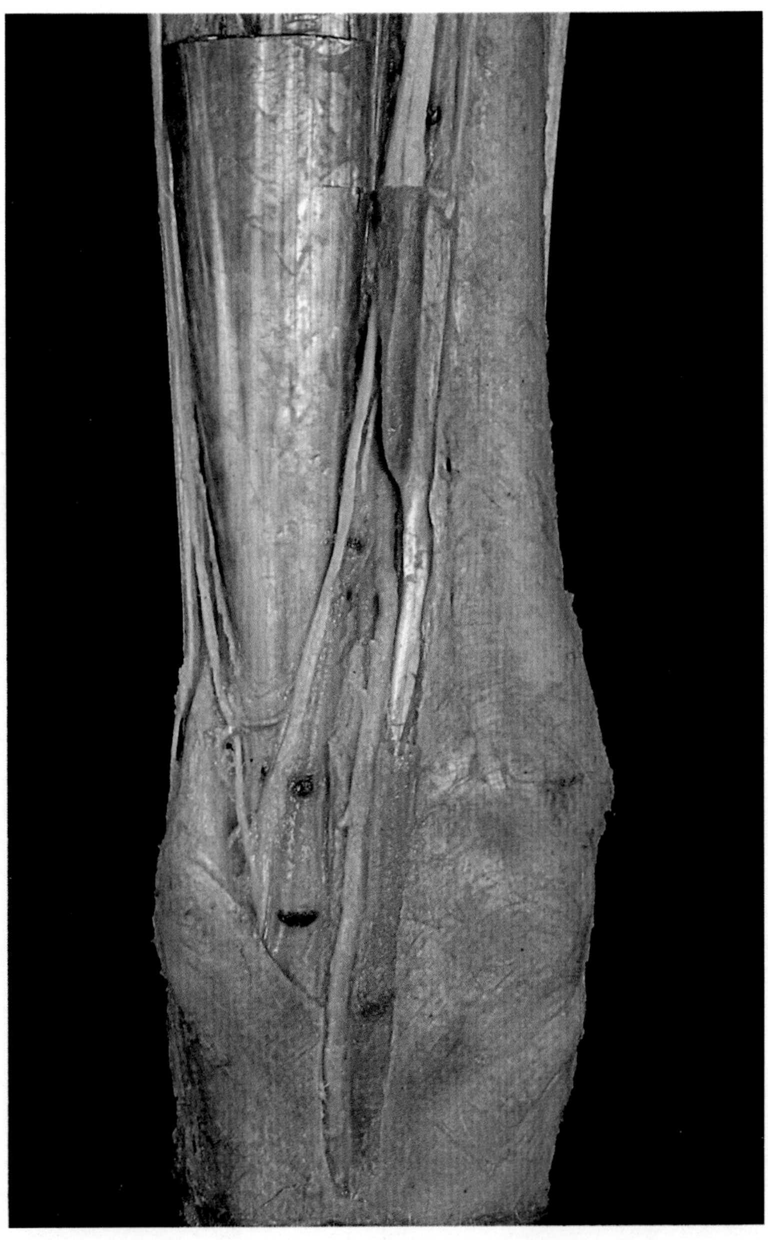

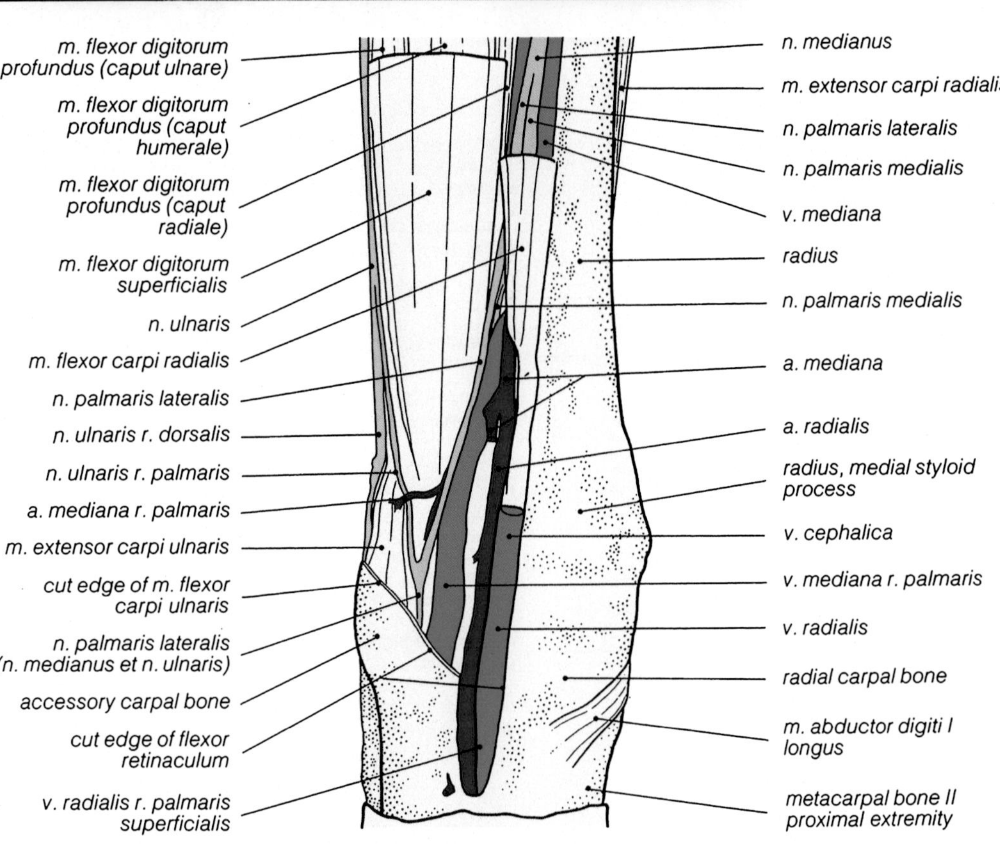
m. flexor digitorum profundus (caput ulnare)
m. flexor digitorum profundus (caput humerale)
m. flexor digitorum profundus (caput radiale)
m. flexor digitorum superficialis
n. ulnaris
m. flexor carpi radialis
n. palmaris lateralis
n. ulnaris r. dorsalis
n. ulnaris r. palmaris
a. mediana r. palmaris
m. extensor carpi ulnaris
cut edge of m. flexor carpi ulnaris
n. palmaris lateralis (n. medianus et n. ulnaris)
accessory carpal bone
cut edge of flexor retinaculum
v. radialis r. palmaris superficialis
n. medianus
m. extensor carpi radialis
n. palmaris lateralis
n. palmaris medialis
v. mediana
radius
n. palmaris medialis
a. mediana
a. radialis
radius, medial styloid process
v. cephalica
v. mediana r. palmaris
v. radialis
radial carpal bone
m. abductor digiti I longus
metacarpal bone II proximal extremity

Fig. 3.32 Vessels and nerves of the left carpus: medial view. This is a closer view of a part of the dissection shown in Fig. 3.31. The deeper structures are shown in Figs. 3.41 and 3.42. The more distal regions of the limb are shown in Figs. 3.36 and 3.40.

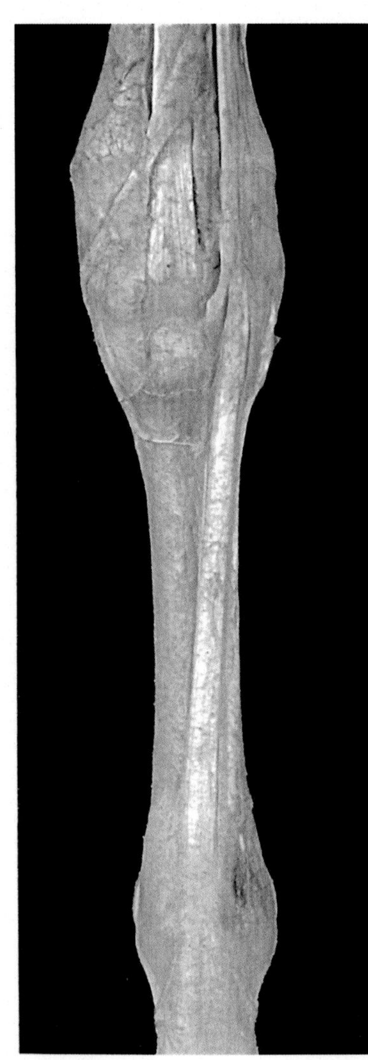

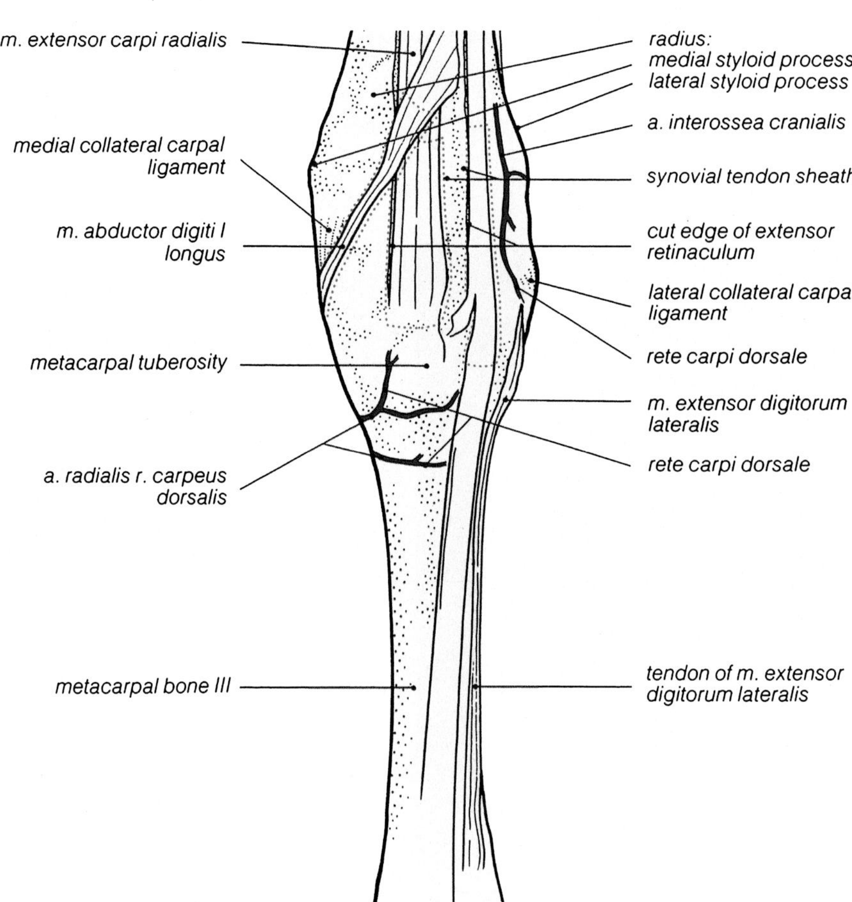
m. extensor carpi radialis
medial collateral carpal ligament
m. abductor digiti I longus
metacarpal tuberosity
a. radialis r. carpeus dorsalis
metacarpal bone III
radius:
medial styloid process
lateral styloid process
a. interossea cranialis
synovial tendon sheaths
cut edge of extensor retinaculum
lateral collateral carpal ligament
rete carpi dorsale
m. extensor digitorum lateralis
rete carpi dorsale
tendon of m. extensor digitorum lateralis

Fig. 3.33 Structures of the left carpus and proximal metacarpus: dorsal view. Figs. 3.34–3.36 show these regions at the same stage of dissection. The approximate extents of the synovial tendon sheaths are indicated by dotted blue lines.

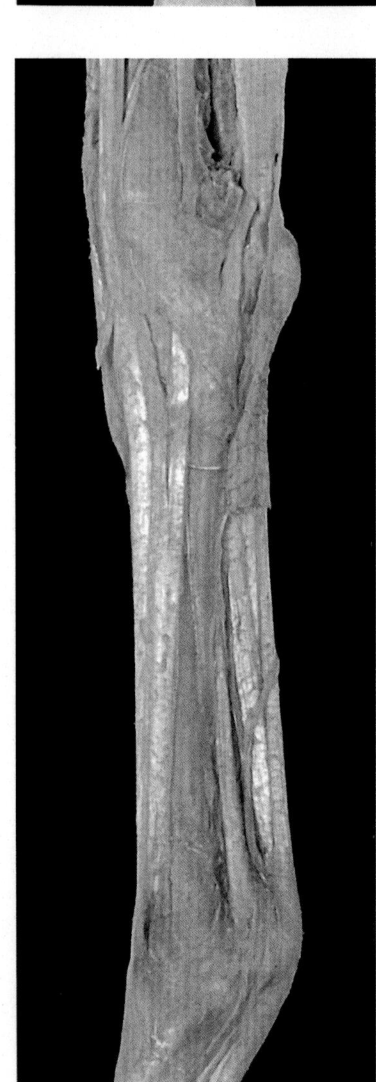

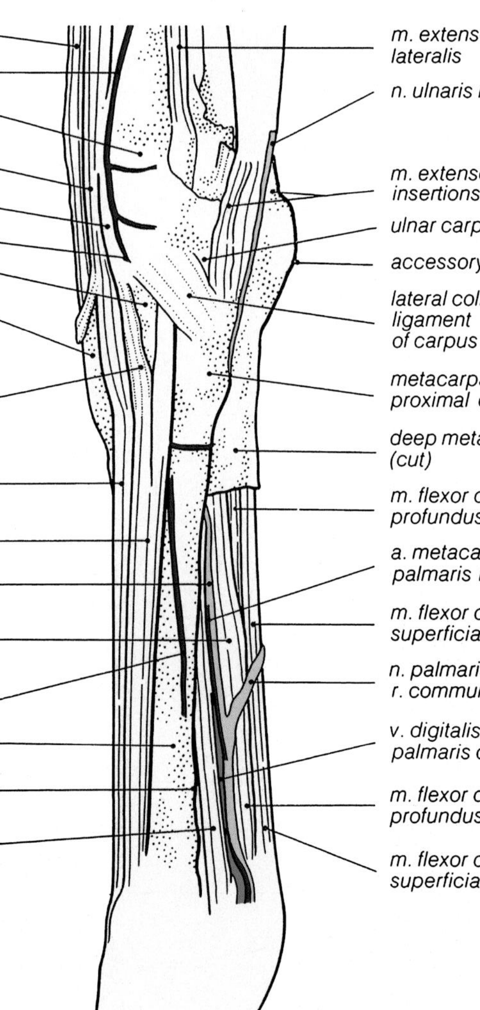
m. extensor carpi radialis
a. interossea cranialis
radius, lateral styloid process
m. extensor digitorum communis
intermediate carpal bone
rete carpi dorsale
carpal bone IV
metacarpal bone III, tuberosity
tendon from m. extensor digitorum communis (caput radiale) to m. extensor digitorum lateralis
m. extensor digitorum communis
m. extensor digitorum lateralis
n. palmaris lateralis
m. flexor digitorum profundus, ligamentum accessorium
a. metacarpea dorsalis III
metacarpal bone III
metacarpal bone IV distal extremity
m. interosseus (suspensory ligament)
m. extensor digitorum lateralis
n. ulnaris r. dorsalis
m. extensor carpi ulnaris, insertions
ulnar carpal bone
accessory carpal bone
lateral collateral ligament of carpus
metacarpal bone IV, proximal extremity
deep metacarpal fascia (cut)
m. flexor digitorum profundus
a. metacarpea palmaris III
m. flexor digitorum superficialis
n. palmaris medialis r. communicans
v. digitalis palmaris communis III
m. flexor digitorum profundus
m. flexor digitorum superficialis

Fig. 3.34 Structures of the left carpus and metacarpus: lateral view. The specimen is that shown in Figs. 3.33, 3.35 and 3.36. The accessory ligament of the deep digital flexor muscle is also known as the check ligament or carpal head of this muscle.

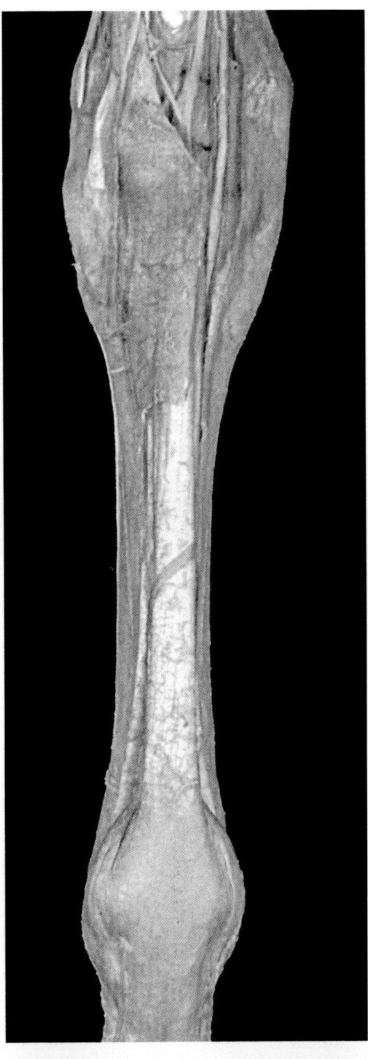

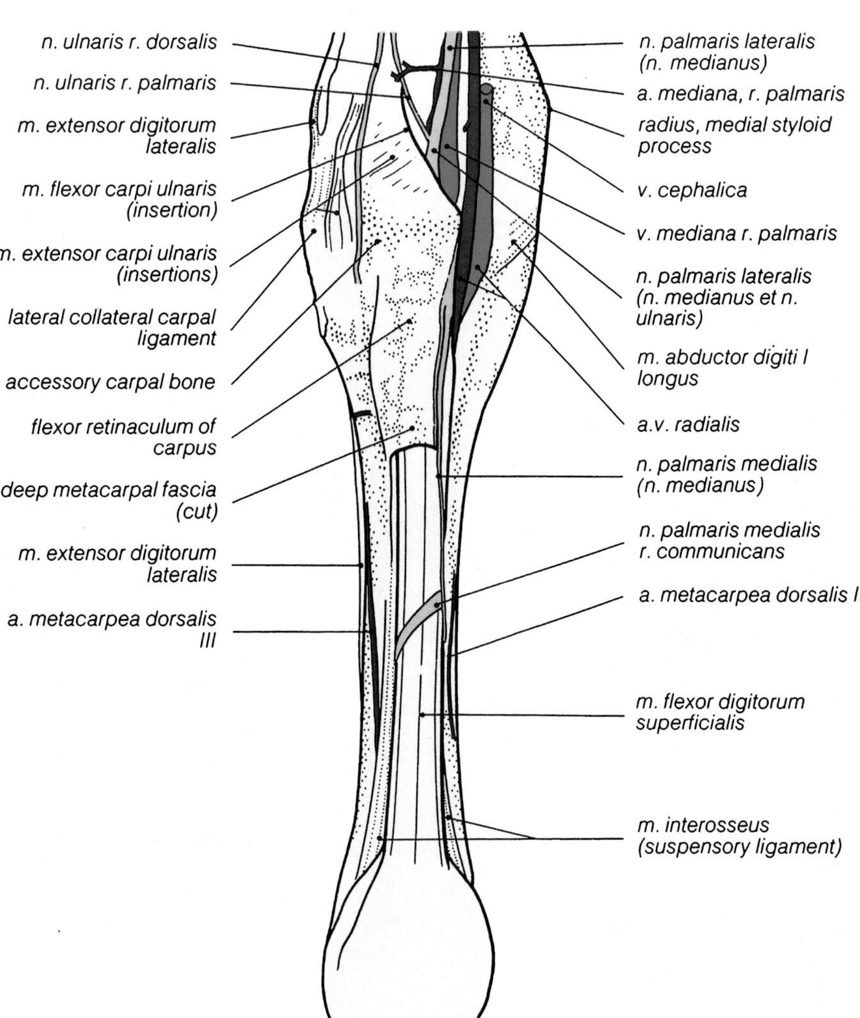

n. ulnaris r. dorsalis
n. ulnaris r. palmaris
m. extensor digitorum lateralis
m. flexor carpi ulnaris (insertion)
m. extensor carpi ulnaris (insertions)
lateral collateral carpal ligament
accessory carpal bone
flexor retinaculum of carpus
deep metacarpal fascia (cut)
m. extensor digitorum lateralis
a. metacarpea dorsalis III
n. palmaris lateralis (n. medianus)
a. mediana, r. palmaris
radius, medial styloid process
v. cephalica
v. mediana r. palmaris
n. palmaris lateralis (n. medianus et n. ulnaris)
m. abductor digiti I longus
a.v. radialis
n. palmaris medialis (n. medianus)
n. palmaris medialis r. communicans
a. metacarpea dorsalis II
m. flexor digitorum superficialis
m. interosseus (suspensory ligament)

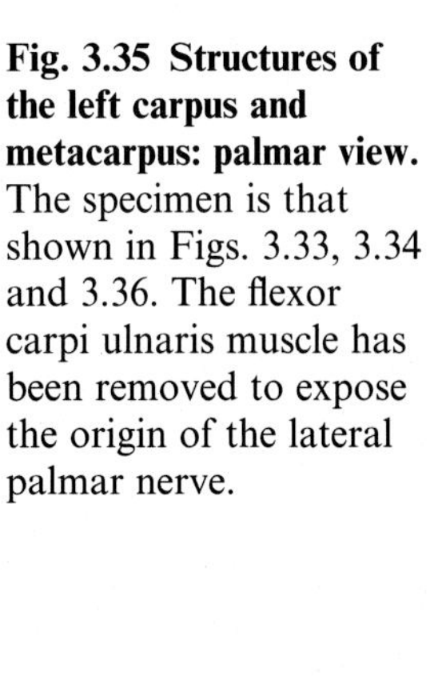

Fig. 3.35 Structures of the left carpus and metacarpus: palmar view. The specimen is that shown in Figs. 3.33, 3.34 and 3.36. The flexor carpi ulnaris muscle has been removed to expose the origin of the lateral palmar nerve.

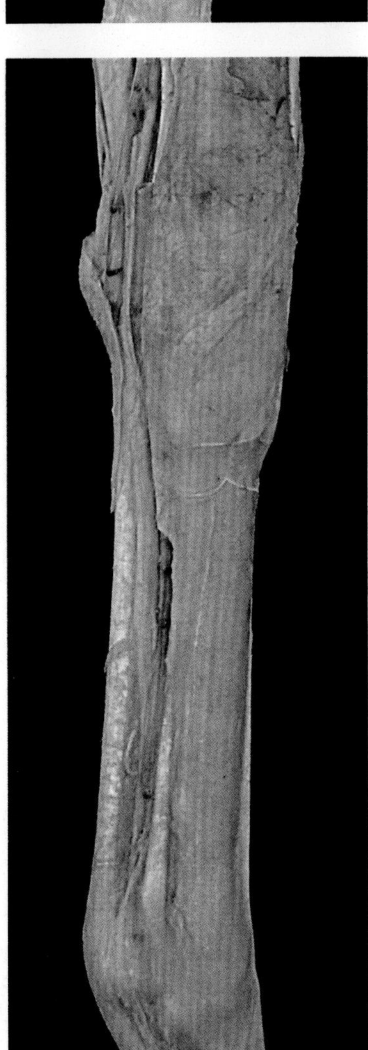

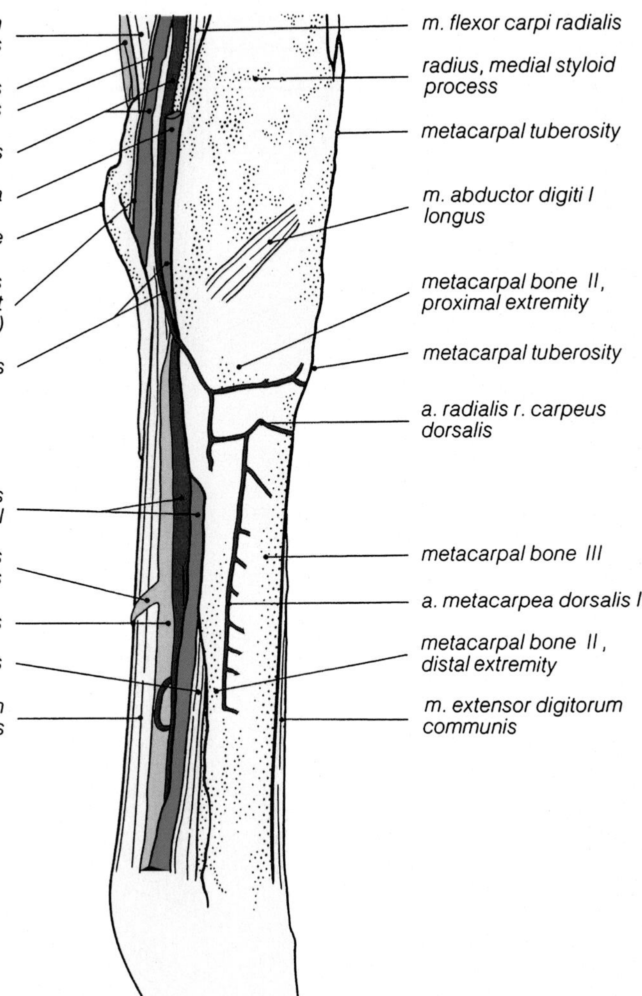

m. flexor digitorum superficialis
n. ulnaris
n. medianus
a.v. mediana r. palmaris
v. cephalica
accessory carpal bone
n. palmaris lateralis (n. medianus et n. ulnaris)
a.v. radialis
a.v. digitalis palmaris communis II
n. palmaris medialis r. communicans
n. palmaris medialis
m. interosseus
m. flexor digitorum superficialis
m. flexor carpi radialis
radius, medial styloid process
metacarpal tuberosity
m. abductor digiti I longus
metacarpal bone II, proximal extremity
metacarpal tuberosity
a. radialis r. carpeus dorsalis
metacarpal bone III
a. metacarpea dorsalis II
metacarpal bone II, distal extremity
m. extensor digitorum communis

Fig. 3.36 Structures of the left carpus and proximal metacarpus: medial view. The specimen is that shown in Figs. 3.30–3.35. The arteries in this dissection are shown more clearly in Fig. 3.40.

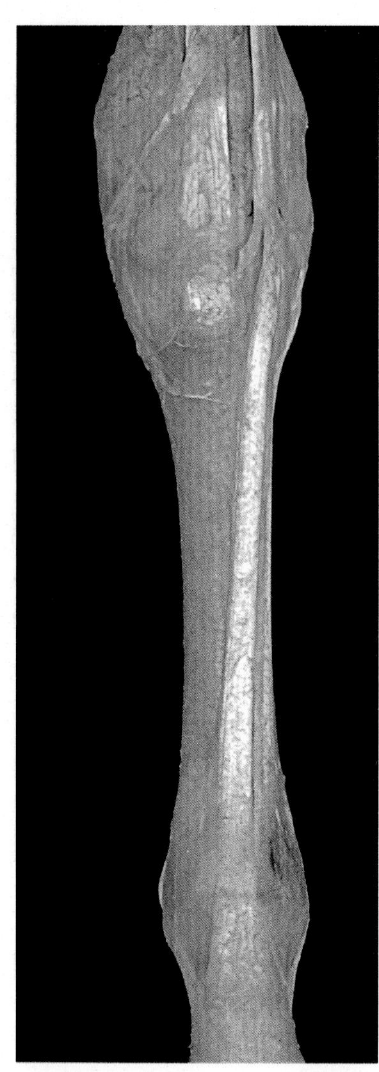

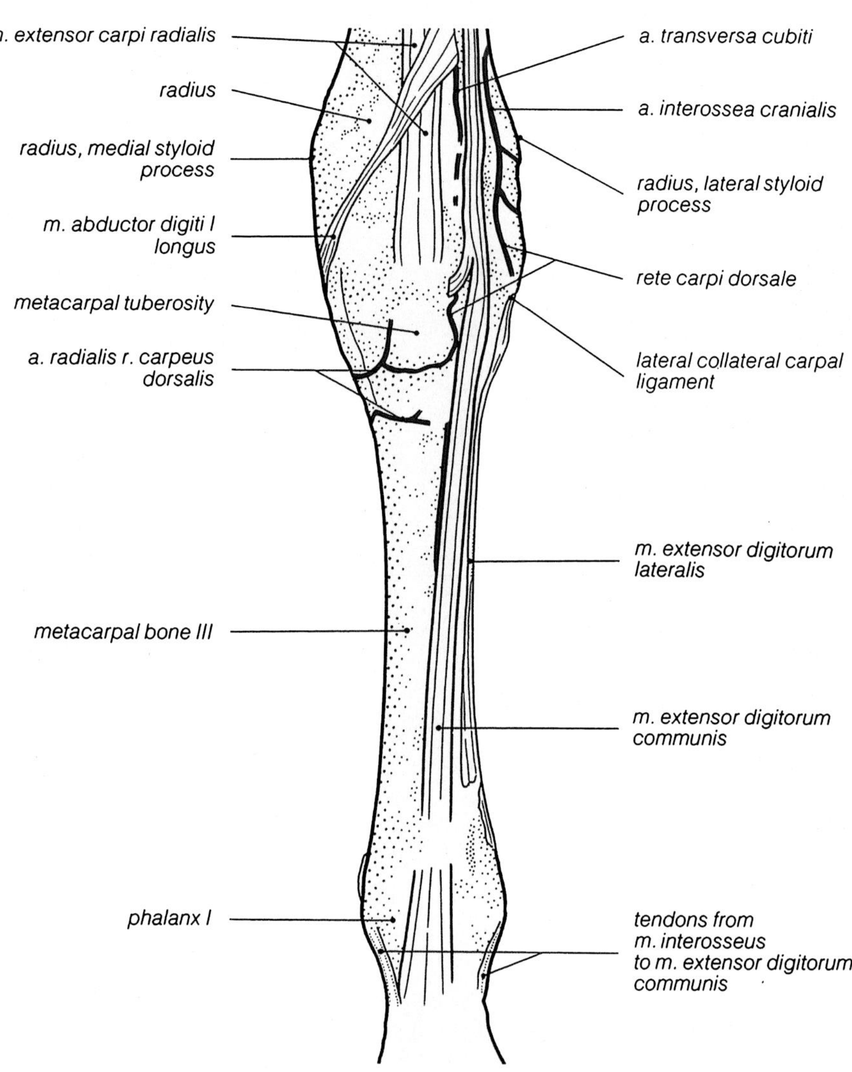
m. extensor carpi radialis
radius
radius, medial styloid process
m. abductor digiti I longus
metacarpal tuberosity
a. radialis r. carpeus dorsalis
metacarpal bone III
phalanx I
a. transversa cubiti
a. interossea cranialis
radius, lateral styloid process
rete carpi dorsale
lateral collateral carpal ligament
m. extensor digitorum lateralis
m. extensor digitorum communis
tendons from m. interosseus to m. extensor digitorum communis

Fig. 3.37 Muscles and arteries of the left carpus and metacarpus: dorsal view. This specimen is also shown in Figs. 3.38–3.40. The dissection shows the three major arteries contributing to the dorsal arterial network on the carpus. The disposition of the synovial tendon sheaths of the carpus is shown in Fig. 3.33.

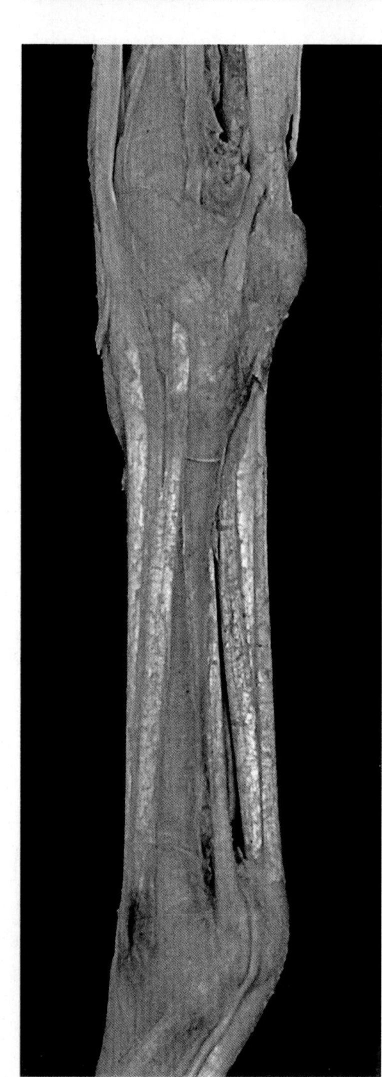

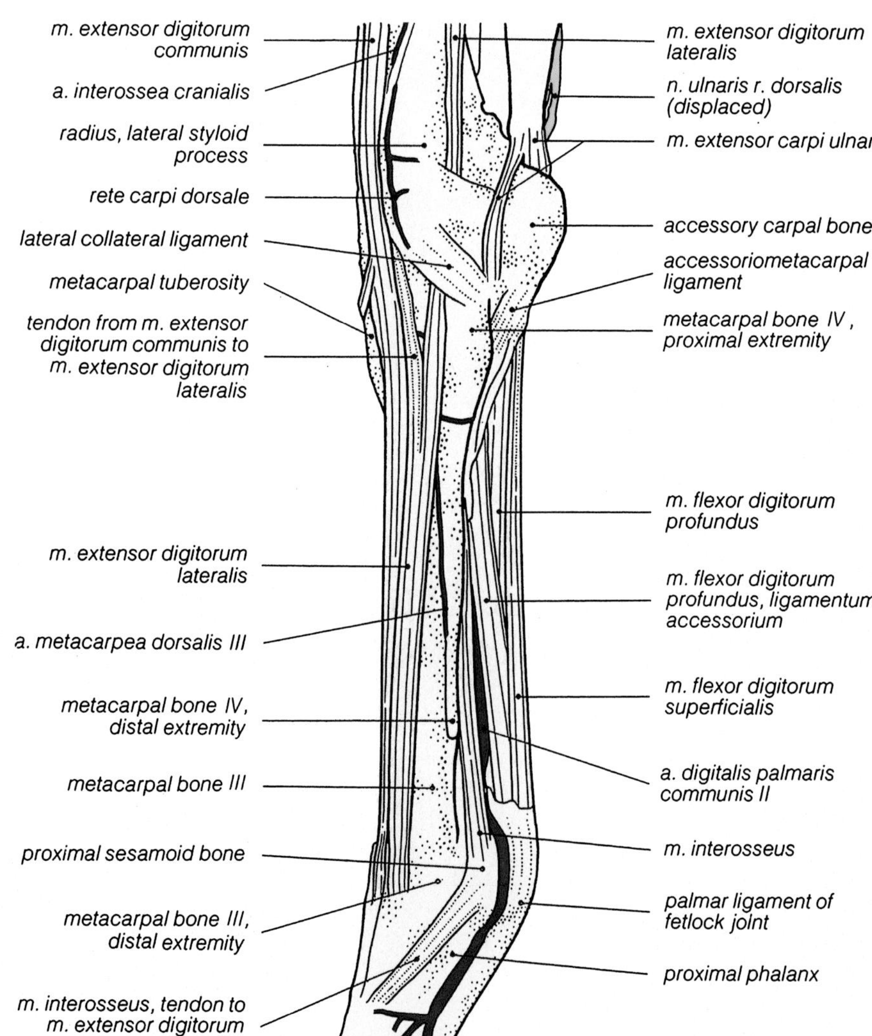
m. extensor digitorum communis
a. interossea cranialis
radius, lateral styloid process
rete carpi dorsale
lateral collateral ligament
metacarpal tuberosity
tendon from m. extensor digitorum communis to m. extensor digitorum lateralis
m. extensor digitorum lateralis
a. metacarpea dorsalis III
metacarpal bone IV, distal extremity
metacarpal bone III
proximal sesamoid bone
metacarpal bone III, distal extremity
m. interosseus, tendon to m. extensor digitorum communis
m. extensor digitorum lateralis
n. ulnaris r. dorsalis (displaced)
m. extensor carpi ulnaris
accessory carpal bone
accessoriometacarpal ligament
metacarpal bone IV, proximal extremity
m. flexor digitorum profundus
m. flexor digitorum profundus, ligamentum accessorium
m. flexor digitorum superficialis
a. digitalis palmaris communis II
m. interosseus
palmar ligament of fetlock joint
proximal phalanx

Fig. 3.38 Muscles and arteries of the left carpus and metacarpus: lateral view. The veins, nerves and superficial tissues have been removed to display the muscles of the region. The arteries have been preserved to provide reference points for the positions of other superficial structures that have been removed (compare with Fig. 3.34).

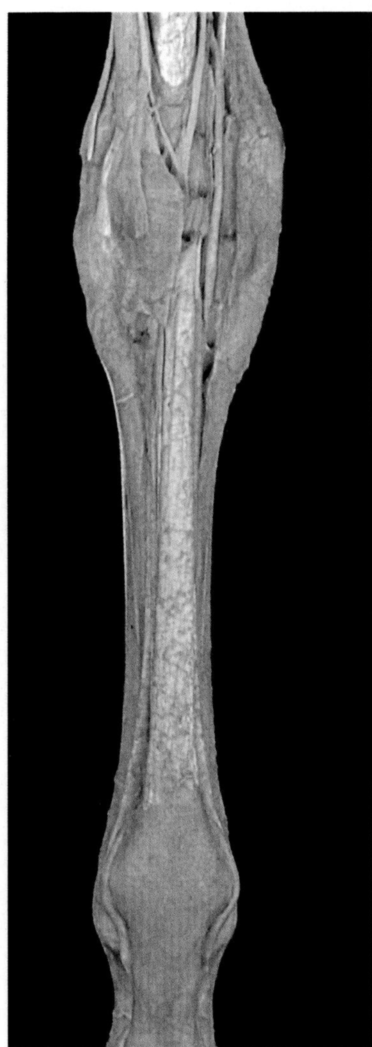

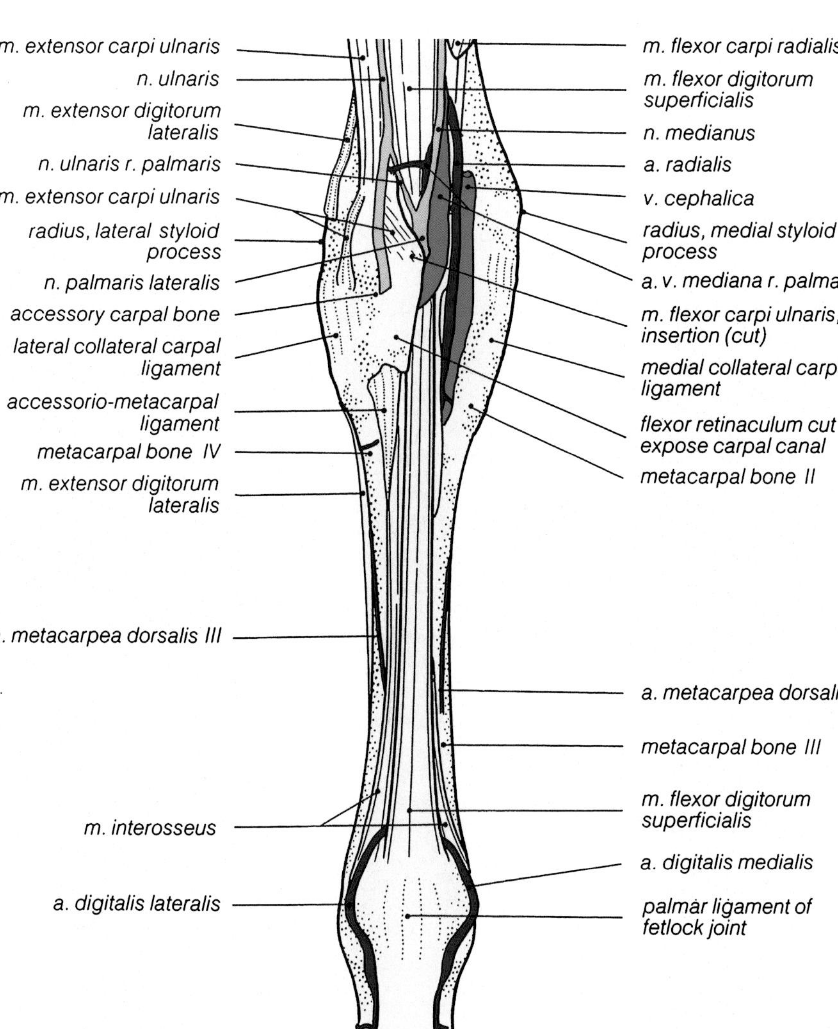
m. extensor carpi ulnaris
n. ulnaris
m. extensor digitorum lateralis
n. ulnaris r. palmaris
m. extensor carpi ulnaris
radius, lateral styloid process
n. palmaris lateralis
accessory carpal bone
lateral collateral carpal ligament
accessorio-metacarpal ligament
metacarpal bone IV
m. extensor digitorum lateralis
a. metacarpea dorsalis III
m. interosseus
a. digitalis lateralis
m. flexor carpi radialis
m. flexor digitorum superficialis
n. medianus
a. radialis
v. cephalica
radius, medial styloid process
a. v. mediana r. palmaris
m. flexor carpi ulnaris, insertion (cut)
medial collateral carpal ligament
flexor retinaculum cut to expose carpal canal
metacarpal bone II
a. metacarpea dorsalis II
metacarpal bone III
m. flexor digitorum superficialis
a. digitalis medialis
palmar ligament of fetlock joint

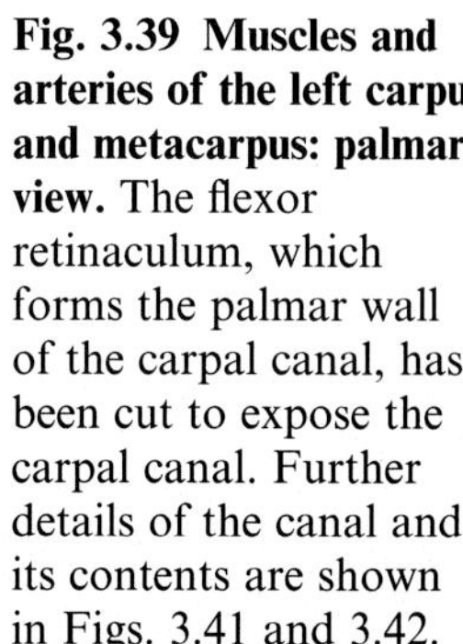
Fig. 3.39 Muscles and arteries of the left carpus and metacarpus: palmar view. The flexor retinaculum, which forms the palmar wall of the carpal canal, has been cut to expose the carpal canal. Further details of the canal and its contents are shown in Figs. 3.41 and 3.42.

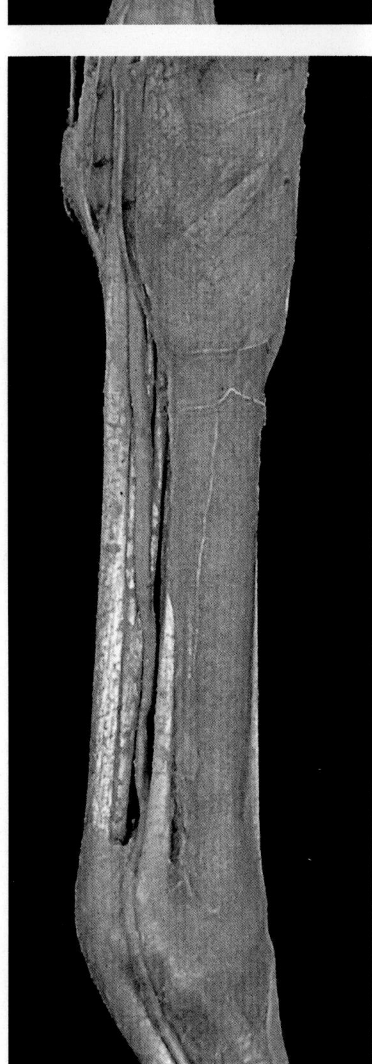

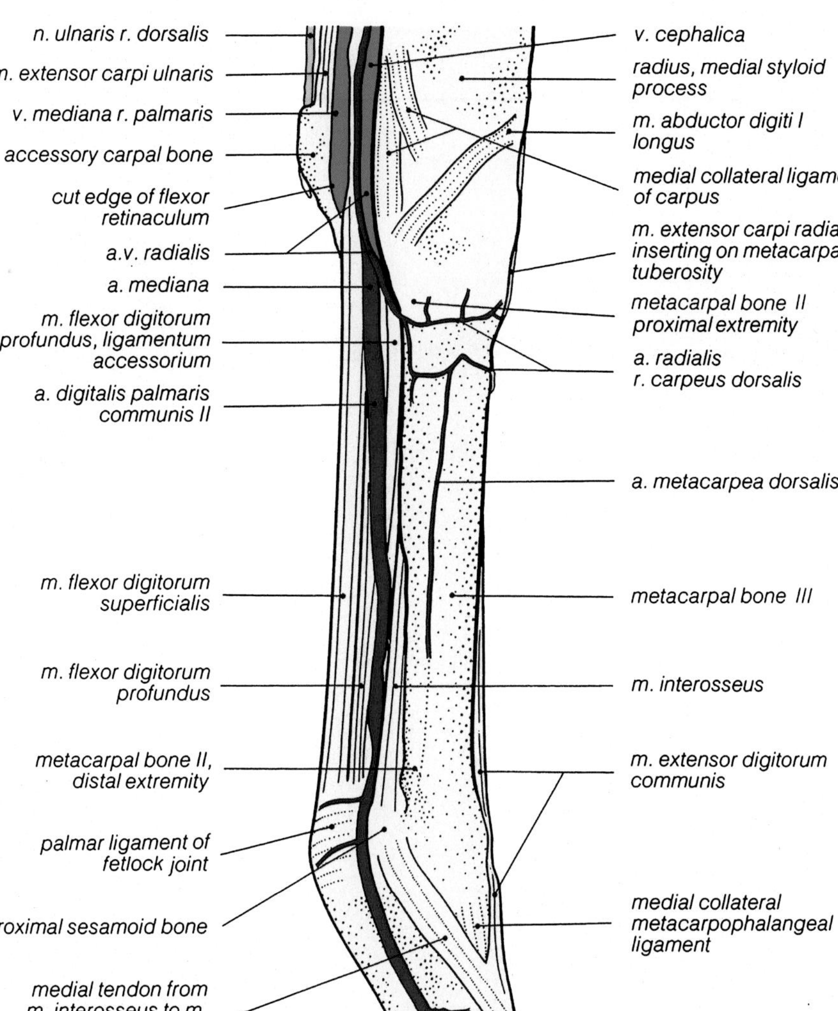
n. ulnaris r. dorsalis
m. extensor carpi ulnaris
v. mediana r. palmaris
accessory carpal bone
cut edge of flexor retinaculum
a.v. radialis
a. mediana
m. flexor digitorum profundus, ligamentum accessorium
a. digitalis palmaris communis II
m. flexor digitorum superficialis
m. flexor digitorum profundus
metacarpal bone II, distal extremity
palmar ligament of fetlock joint
proximal sesamoid bone
medial tendon from m. interosseus to m. extensor digitorum communis
v. cephalica
radius, medial styloid process
m. abductor digiti I longus
medial collateral ligament of carpus
m. extensor carpi radialis inserting on metacarpal tuberosity
metacarpal bone II proximal extremity
a. radialis r. carpeus dorsalis
a. metacarpea dorsalis II
metacarpal bone III
m. interosseus
m. extensor digitorum communis
medial collateral metacarpophalangeal ligament

Fig. 3.40 Muscles and arteries of the left carpus and metacarpus: medial view. This dissection is also shown in Figs. 3.37–3.39.

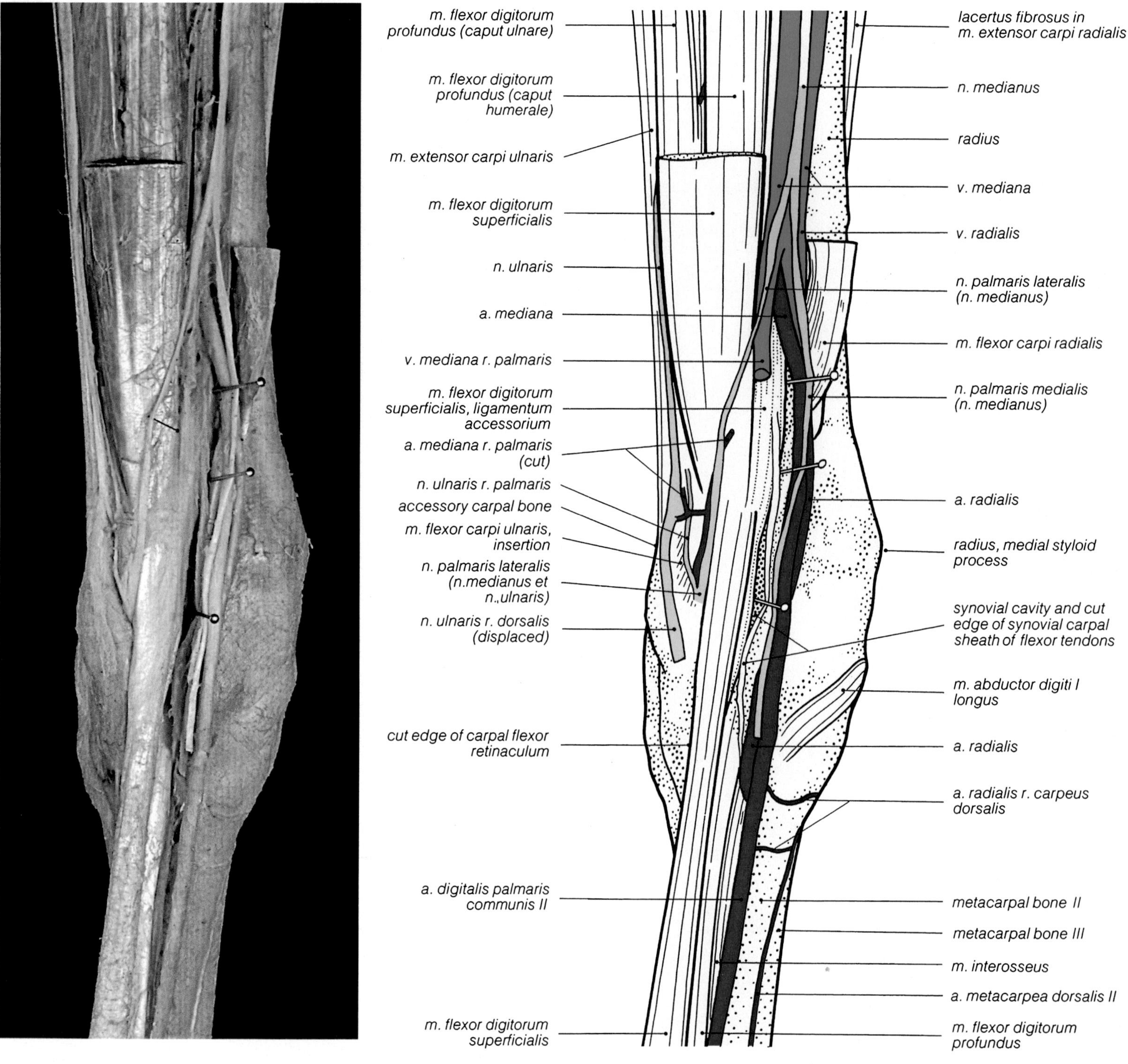
m. flexor digitorum profundus (caput ulnare)
m. flexor digitorum profundus (caput humerale)
m. extensor carpi ulnaris
m. flexor digitorum superficialis
n. ulnaris
a. mediana
v. mediana r. palmaris
m. flexor digitorum superficialis, ligamentum accessorium
a. mediana r. palmaris (cut)
n. ulnaris r. palmaris
accessory carpal bone
m. flexor carpi ulnaris, insertion
n. palmaris lateralis (n.medianus et n.,ulnaris)
n. ulnaris r. dorsalis (displaced)
cut edge of carpal flexor retinaculum
a. digitalis palmaris communis II
m. flexor digitorum superficialis
lacertus fibrosus in m. extensor carpi radialis
n. medianus
radius
v. mediana
v. radialis
n. palmaris lateralis (n. medianus)
m. flexor carpi radialis
n. palmaris medialis (n. medianus)
a. radialis
radius, medial styloid process
synovial cavity and cut edge of synovial carpal sheath of flexor tendons
m. abductor digiti I longus
a. radialis
a. radialis r. carpeus dorsalis
metacarpal bone II
metacarpal bone III
m. interosseus
a. metacarpea dorsalis II
m. flexor digitorum profundus

Fig. 3.41 The left carpal canal and its contents: oblique caudomedial view (1). After opening the carpal canal as shown in Fig. 3.39 the more superficial contents have been displaced medially to show the deeper flexor tendons. The lateral palmar nerve and the radial artery do not run through the carpal canal but traverse the flexor retinaculum.

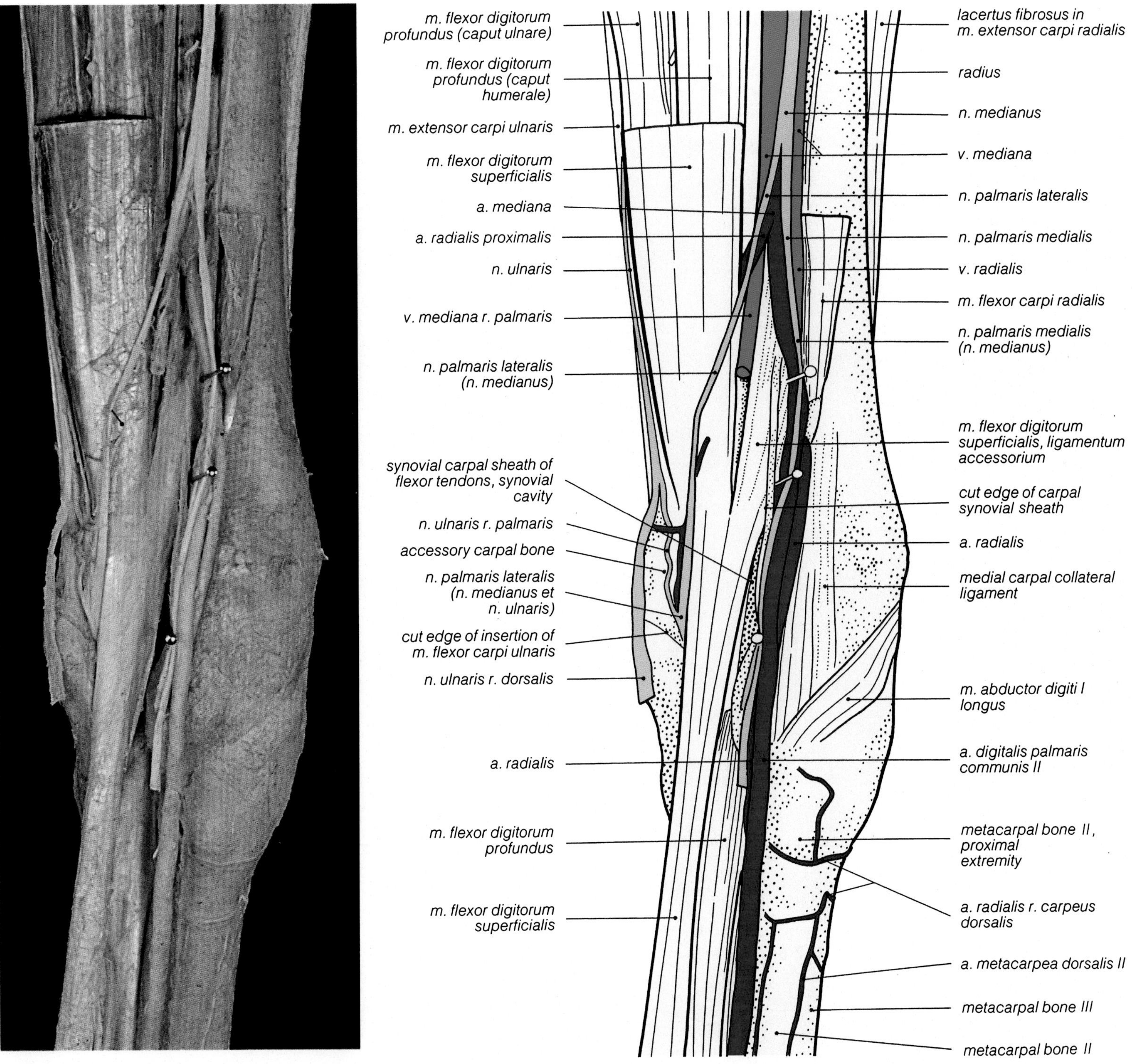
m. flexor digitorum profundus (caput ulnare)
m. flexor digitorum profundus (caput humerale)
m. extensor carpi ulnaris
m. flexor digitorum superficialis
a. mediana
a. radialis proximalis
n. ulnaris
v. mediana r. palmaris
n. palmaris lateralis (n. medianus)
synovial carpal sheath of flexor tendons, synovial cavity
n. ulnaris r. palmaris
accessory carpal bone
n. palmaris lateralis (n. medianus et n. ulnaris)
cut edge of insertion of m. flexor carpi ulnaris
n. ulnaris r. dorsalis
a. radialis
m. flexor digitorum profundus
m. flexor digitorum superficialis
lacertus fibrosus in m. extensor carpi radialis
radius
n. medianus
v. mediana
n. palmaris lateralis
n. palmaris medialis
v. radialis
m. flexor carpi radialis
n. palmaris medialis (n. medianus)
m. flexor digitorum superficialis, ligamentum accessorium
cut edge of carpal synovial sheath
a. radialis
medial carpal collateral ligament
m. abductor digiti I longus
a. digitalis palmaris communis II
metacarpal bone II, proximal extremity
a. radialis r. carpeus dorsalis
a. metacarpea dorsalis II
metacarpal bone III
metacarpal bone II

Fig. 3.42 The left carpal canal and its contents: oblique caudomedial view (2). The tendon of the superficial digital flexor muscle has been pulled out of the carpal canal to display its accessory, or check, ligament arising from the caudal surface of the radius. The accessory ligament of the deep digital flexor tendon is shown in Figs. 3.34 and 3.38.

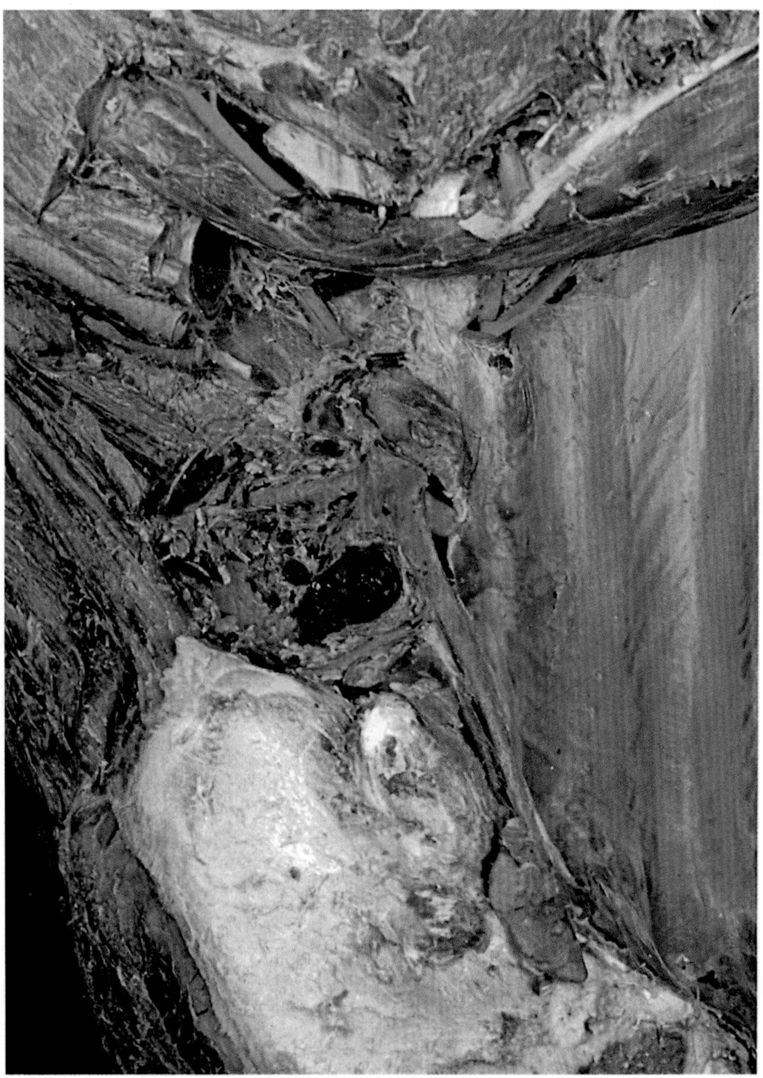

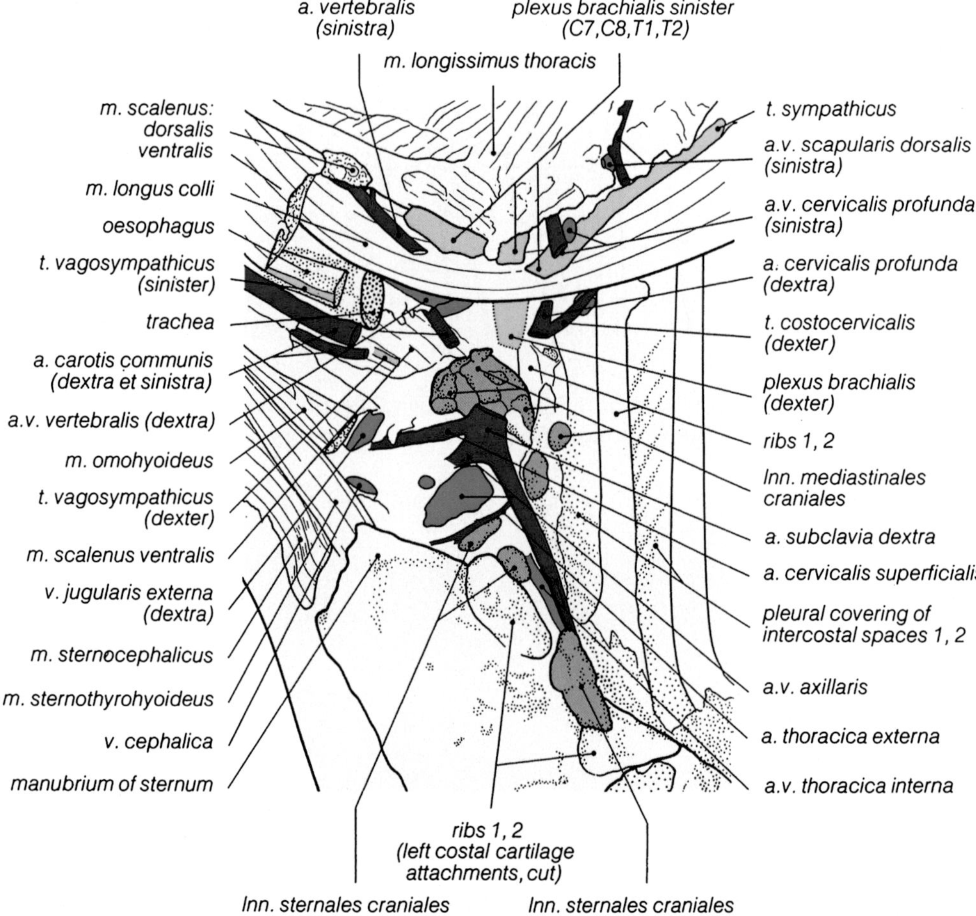
a. vertebralis (sinistra)
plexus brachialis sinister (C7,C8,T1,T2)
m. longissimus thoracis
m. scalenus: dorsalis ventralis
m. longus colli
oesophagus
t. vagosympathicus (sinister)
trachea
a. carotis communis (dextra et sinistra)
a.v. vertebralis (dextra)
m. omohyoideus
t. vagosympathicus (dexter)
m. scalenus ventralis
v. jugularis externa (dextra)
m. sternocephalicus
m. sternothyrohyoideus
v. cephalica
manubrium of sternum
t. sympathicus
a.v. scapularis dorsalis (sinistra)
a.v. cervicalis profunda (sinistra)
a. cervicalis profunda (dextra)
t. costocervicalis (dexter)
plexus brachialis (dexter)
ribs 1, 2
lnn. mediastinales craniales
a. subclavia dextra
a. cervicalis superficialis
pleural covering of intercostal spaces 1, 2
a.v. axillaris
a. thoracica externa
a.v. thoracica interna
ribs 1, 2 (left costal cartilage attachments, cut)
lnn. sternales craniales
lnn. sternales craniales

Fig. 3.43 Structures at the thoracic inlet of a young foal: right side in medial view. The left thoracic wall and the thoracic viscera have been removed. The caudal cervical and cranial thoracic regions of the right side are displayed. The subsequent dissections of this specimen (Figs.3.44–3.51) show the right forelimb, dissected from its medial aspect while still attached to the trunk.

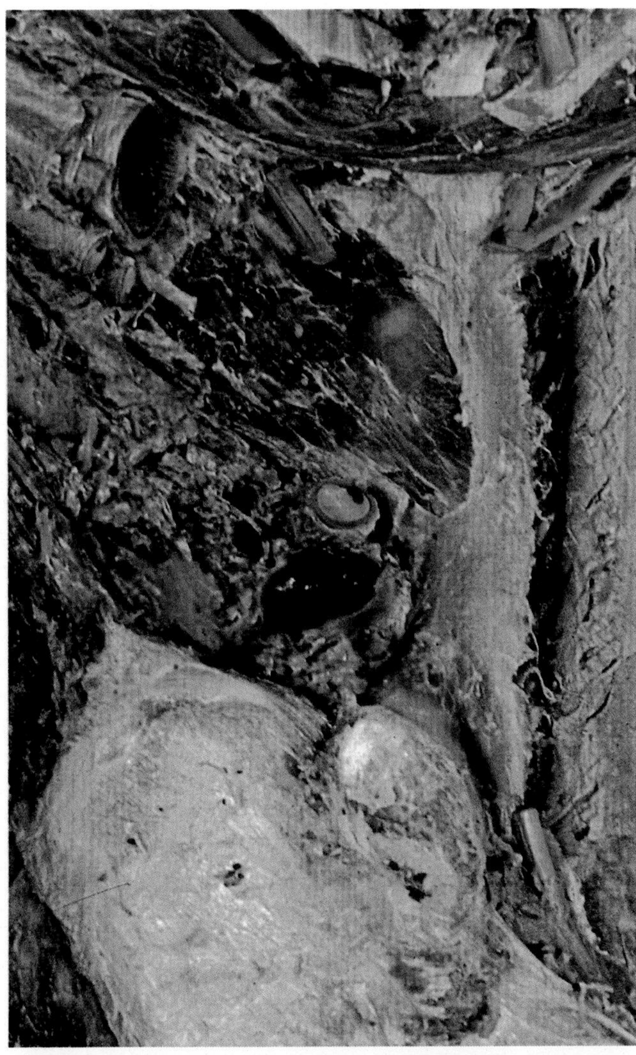

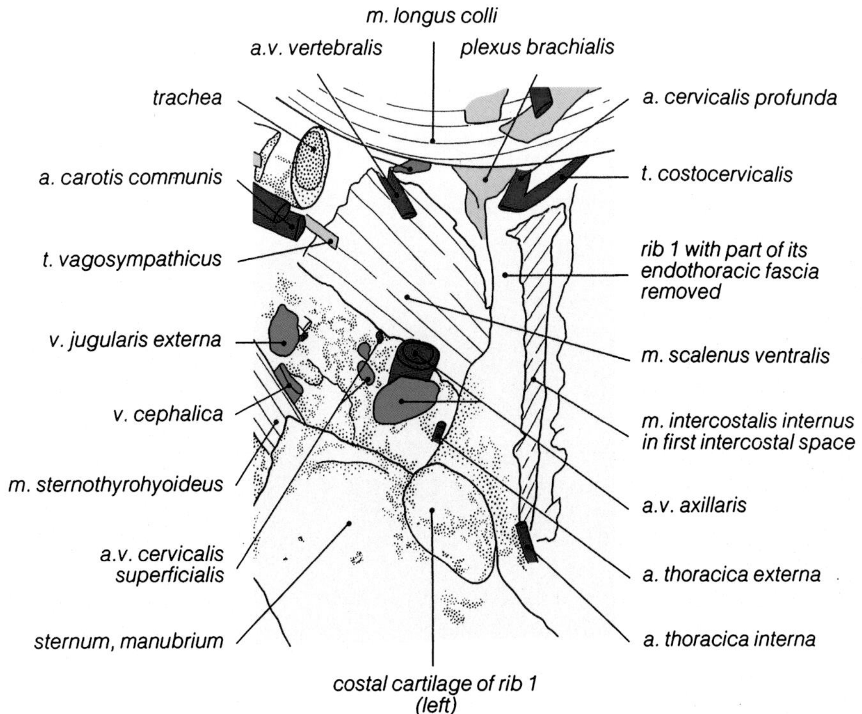
m. longus colli
a.v. vertebralis
plexus brachialis
trachea
a. cervicalis profunda
a. carotis communis
t. costocervicalis
t. vagosympathicus
rib 1 with part of its endothoracic fascia removed
v. jugularis externa
m. scalenus ventralis
v. cephalica
m. intercostalis internus in first intercostal space
m. sternothyrohyoideus
a.v. axillaris
a.v. cervicalis superficialis
a. thoracica externa
sternum, manubrium
a. thoracica interna
costal cartilage of rib 1 (left)

Fig. 3.44 Right brachial plexus and axillary vessels of the foal: medial view (1). The structures lying medial to the insertion of the ventral scalenus muscle have been removed to show how the muscle separates the brachial plexus from the axillary vessels at the cranial border of the first rib.

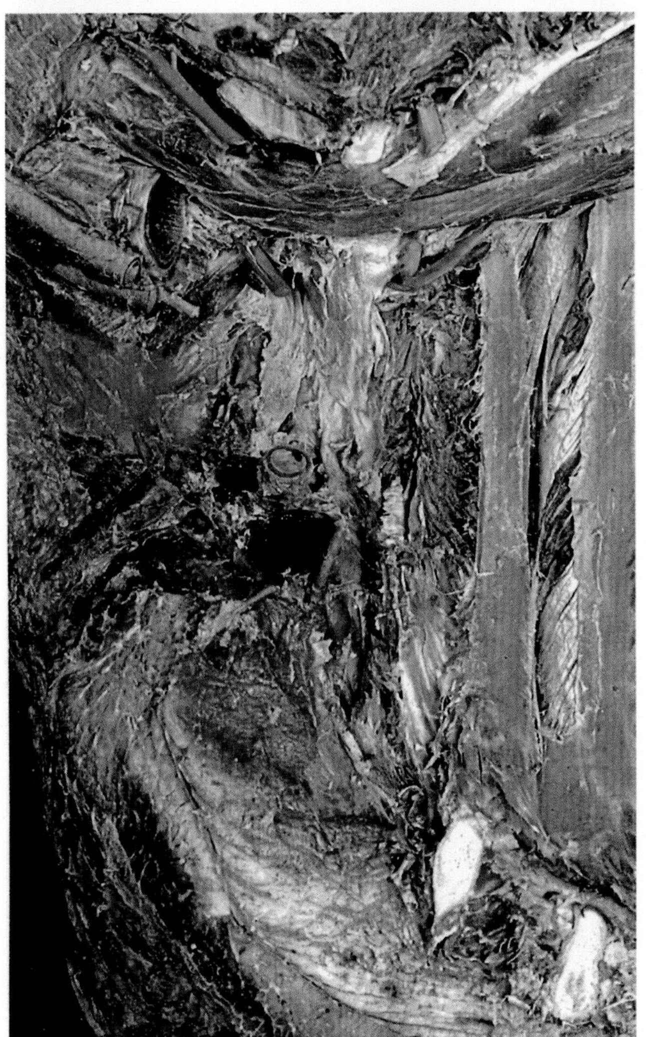

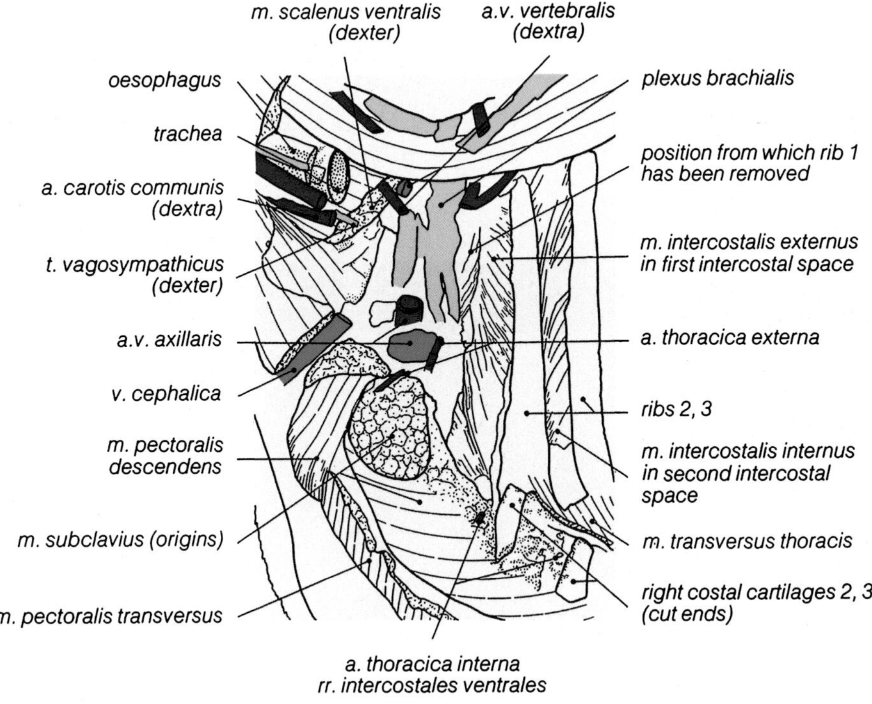
m. scalenus ventralis (dexter)
a.v. vertebralis (dextra)
oesophagus
plexus brachialis
trachea
position from which rib 1 has been removed
a. carotis communis (dextra)
m. intercostalis externus in first intercostal space
t. vagosympathicus (dexter)
a.v. axillaris
a. thoracica externa
v. cephalica
ribs 2, 3
m. pectoralis descendens
m. intercostalis internus in second intercostal space
m. subclavius (origins)
m. transversus thoracis
m. pectoralis transversus
right costal cartilages 2, 3 (cut ends)
a. thoracica interna
rr. intercostales ventrales

Fig. 3.45 Right brachial plexus and axillary vessels of the foal: medial view (2). The sternum and the right first rib have now been removed, revealing the origins of the subclavius muscle and the nerves arising from the brachial plexus.

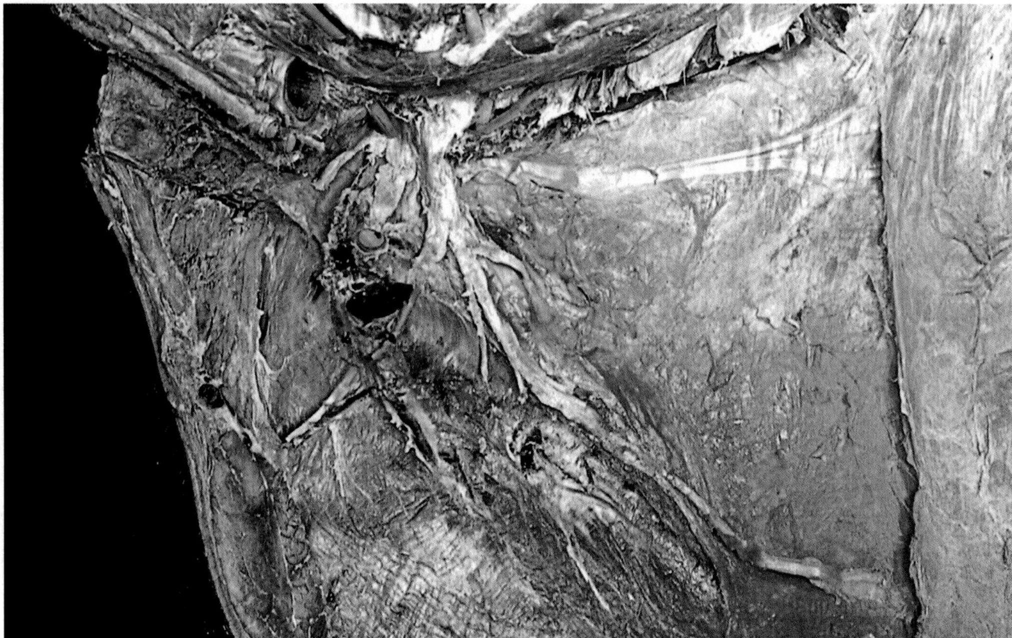

Fig. 3.46 Structures of the right axilla in the foal: medial view (1). The first five ribs and the ventral serrate muscle have been removed to reveal the right axilla. The subclavius muscle has also been cut away.

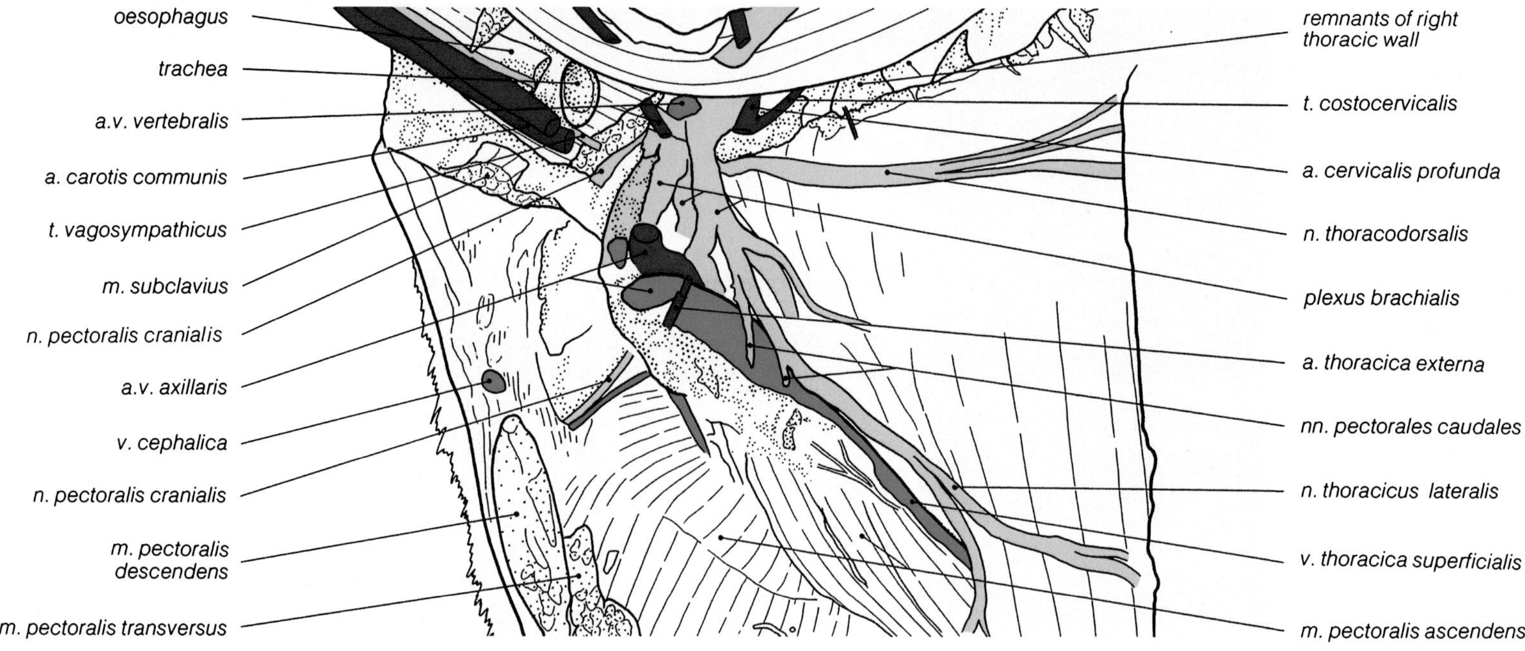
oesophagus
trachea
a.v. vertebralis
a. carotis communis
t. vagosympathicus
m. subclavius
n. pectoralis cranialis
a.v. axillaris
v. cephalica
n. pectoralis cranialis
m. pectoralis descendens
m. pectoralis transversus
remnants of right thoracic wall
t. costocervicalis
a. cervicalis profunda
n. thoracodorsalis
plexus brachialis
a. thoracica externa
nn. pectorales caudales
n. thoracicus lateralis
v. thoracica superficialis
m. pectoralis ascendens

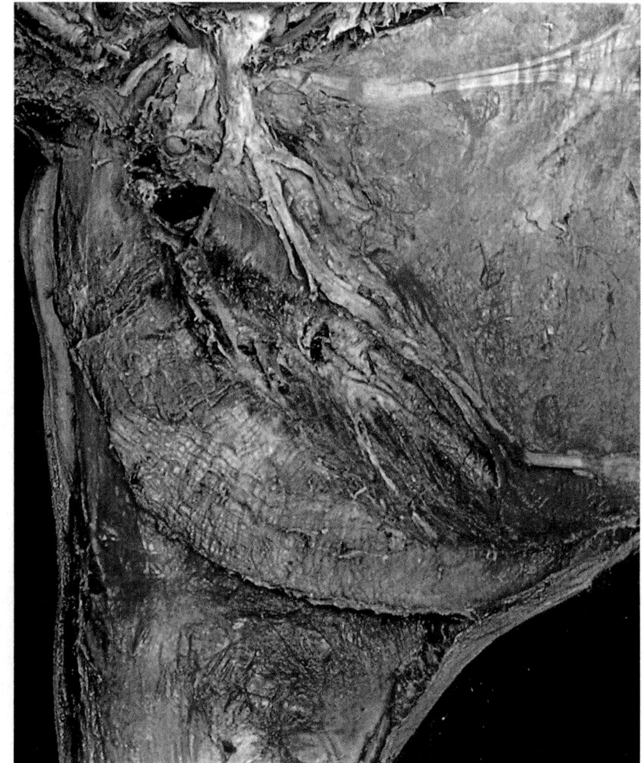

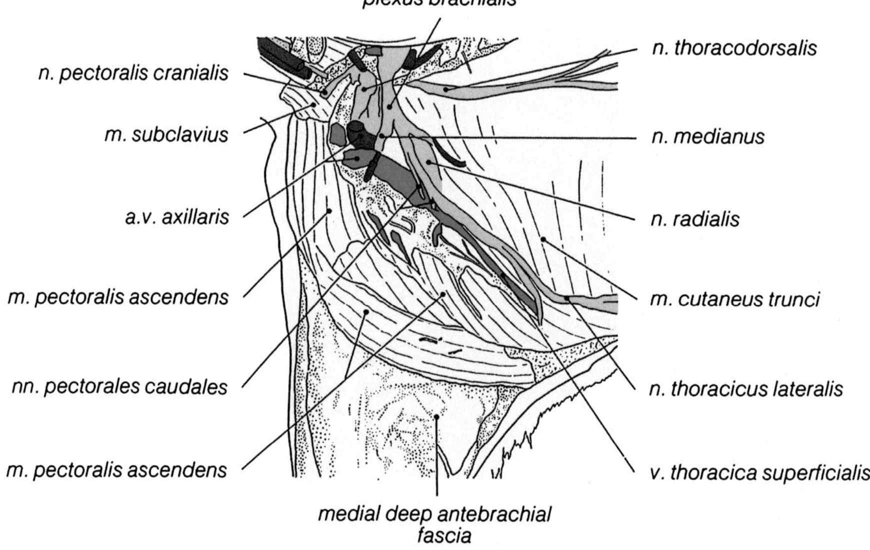
plexus brachialis
n. pectoralis cranialis
m. subclavius
a.v. axillaris
m. pectoralis ascendens
nn. pectorales caudales
m. pectoralis ascendens
medial deep antebrachial fascia
n. thoracodorsalis
n. medianus
n. radialis
m. cutaneus trunci
n. thoracicus lateralis
v. thoracica superficialis

Fig. 3.47 Structures of the right axilla in the foal: medial view (2). The superficial pectoral muscles have been removed.

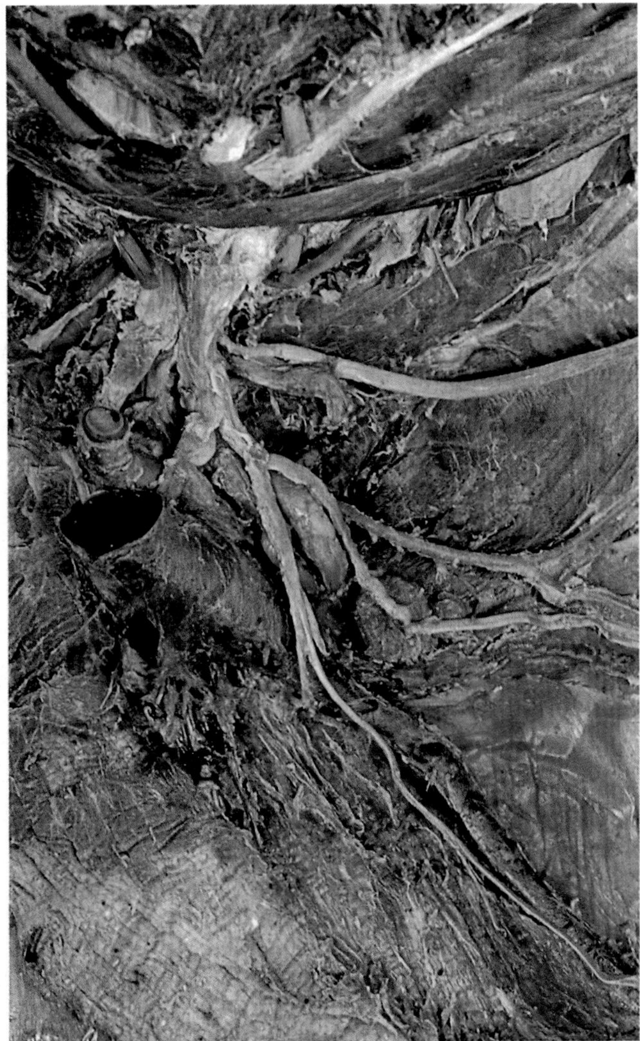

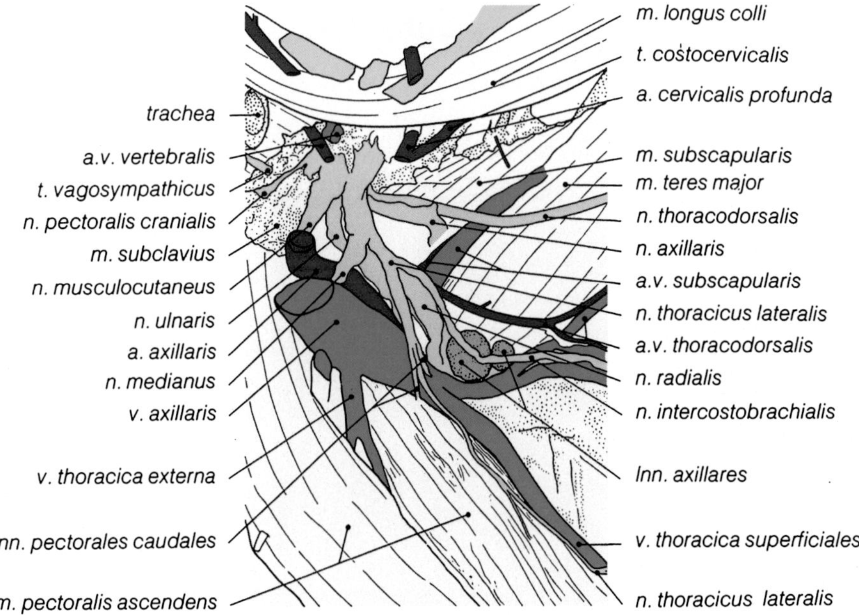
trachea
a.v. vertebralis
t. vagosympathicus
n. pectoralis cranialis
m. subclavius
n. musculocutaneus
n. ulnaris
a. axillaris
n. medianus
v. axillaris
v. thoracica externa
nn. pectorales caudales
m. pectoralis ascendens
m. longus colli
t. costocervicalis
a. cervicalis profunda
m. subscapularis
m. teres major
n. thoracodorsalis
n. axillaris
a.v. subscapularis
n. thoracicus lateralis
a.v. thoracodorsalis
n. radialis
n. intercostobrachialis
lnn. axillares
v. thoracica superficiales
n. thoracicus lateralis

Fig. 3.48 Structures of the right axilla in the foal: medial view (3). Further dissection reveals the vessels and nerves of the region more fully and shows the axillary lymph nodes.

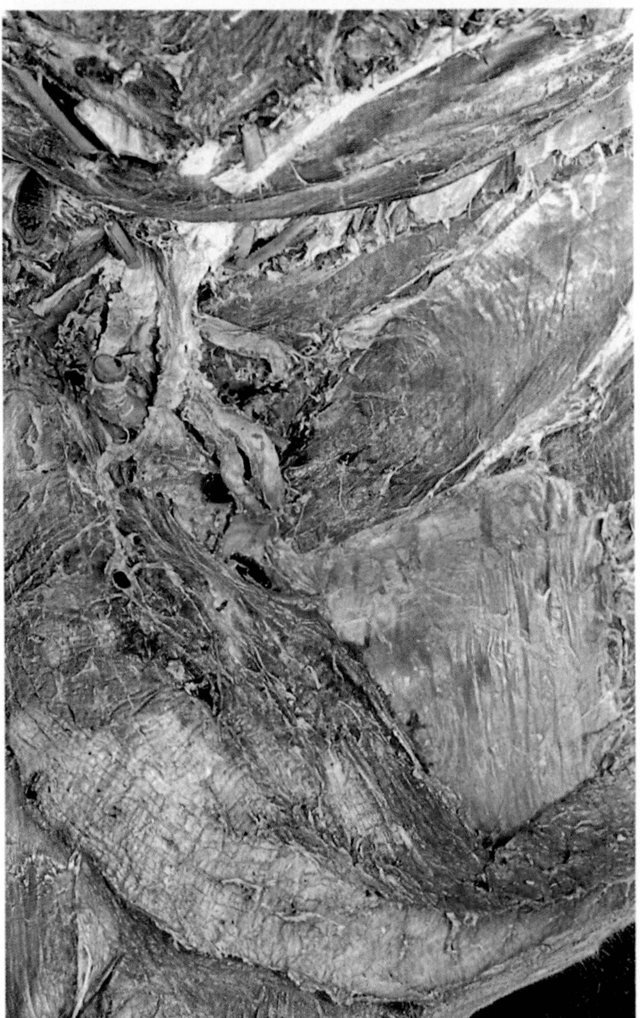

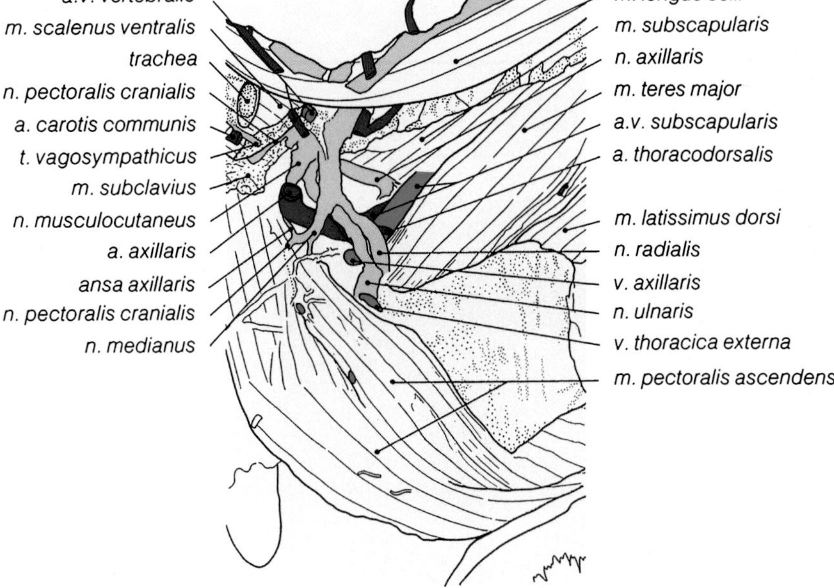
a.v. vertebralis
m. scalenus ventralis
trachea
n. pectoralis cranialis
a. carotis communis
t. vagosympathicus
m. subclavius
n. musculocutaneus
a. axillaris
ansa axillaris
n. pectoralis cranialis
n. medianus
m. longus colli
m. subscapularis
n. axillaris
m. teres major
a.v. subscapularis
a. thoracodorsalis
m. latissimus dorsi
n. radialis
v. axillaris
n. ulnaris
v. thoracica externa
m. pectoralis ascendens

Fig. 3.49 Structures of the right axilla in the foal: medial view (4). The axillary vein has been shortened to reveal the axillary loop formed by musculocutaneous and median nerves. The removal of the thoracodorsal and lateral thoracic vessels and nerves reveals more clearly the muscles of the axilla.

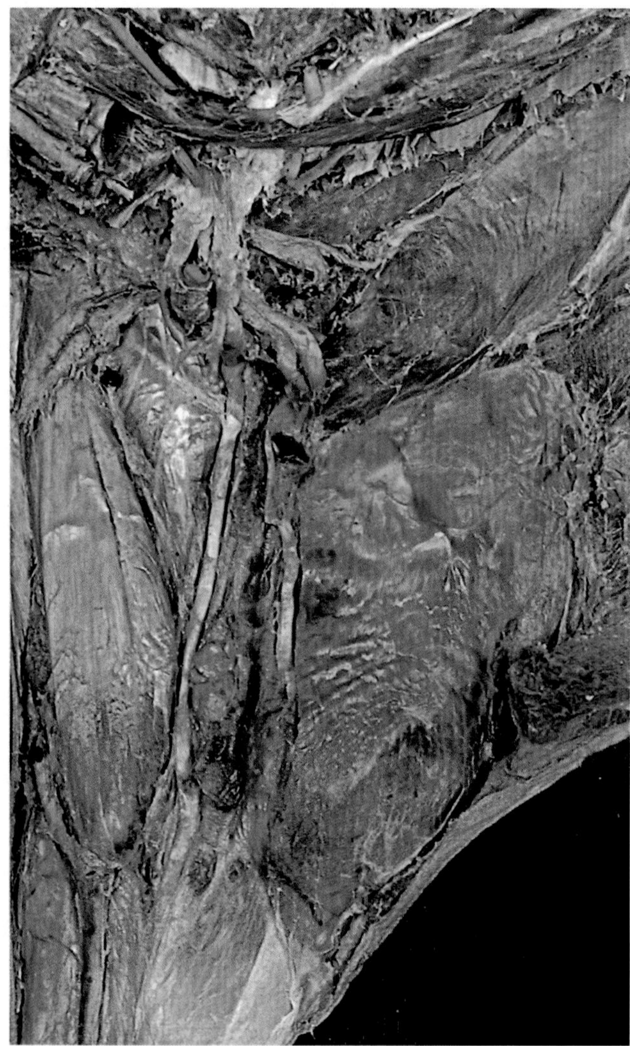

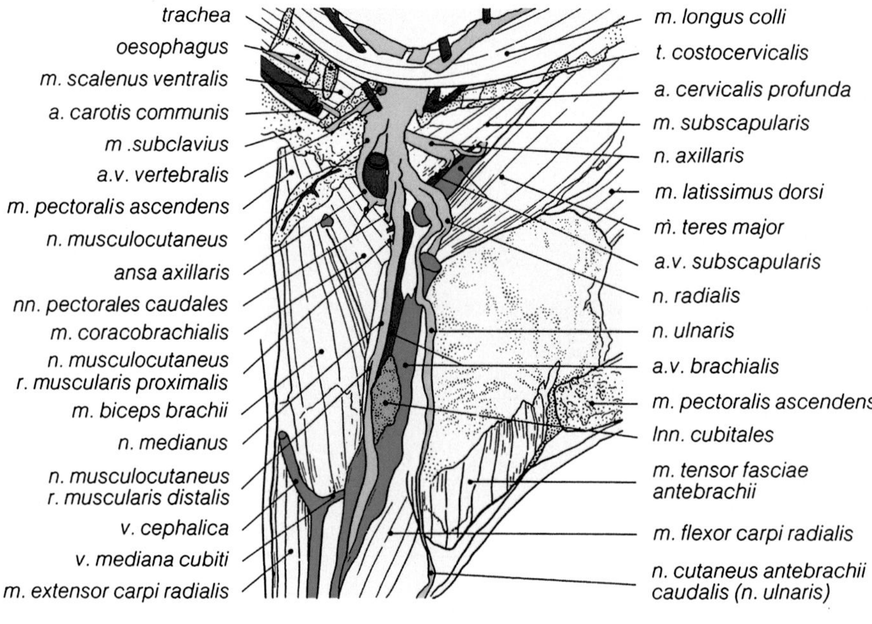
trachea
oesophagus
m. scalenus ventralis
a. carotis communis
m .subclavius
a.v. vertebralis
m. pectoralis ascendens
n. musculocutaneus
ansa axillaris
nn. pectorales caudales
m. coracobrachialis
n. musculocutaneus
r. muscularis proximalis
m. biceps brachii
n. medianus
n. musculocutaneus
r. muscularis distalis
v. cephalica
v. mediana cubiti
m. extensor carpi radialis
m. longus colli
t. costocervicalis
a. cervicalis profunda
m. subscapularis
n. axillaris
m. latissimus dorsi
m. teres major
a.v. subscapularis
n. radialis
n. ulnaris
a.v. brachialis
m. pectoralis ascendens
lnn. cubitales
m. tensor fasciae
antebrachii
m. flexor carpi radialis
n. cutaneus antebrachii
caudalis (n. ulnaris)

Fig. 3.50 Structures of the right axilla and brachial region of the foal: medial view. The ascending pectoral muscle has been removed.

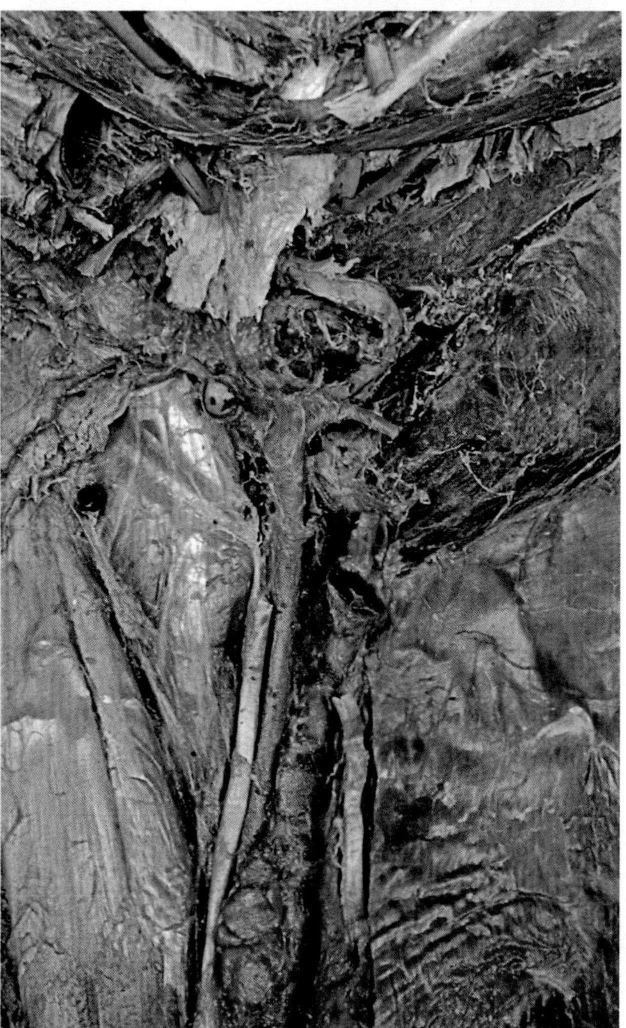

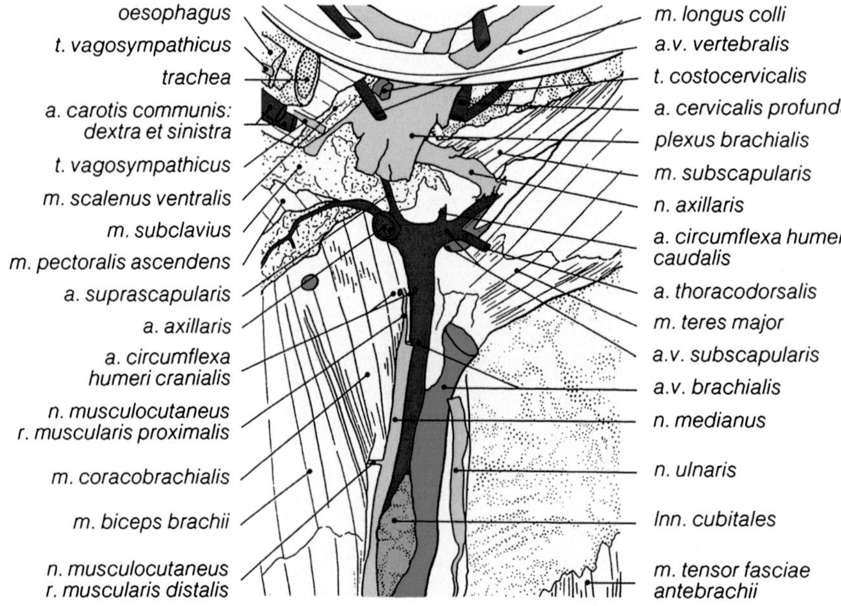
oesophagus
t. vagosympathicus
trachea
a. carotis communis:
dextra et sinistra
t. vagosympathicus
m. scalenus ventralis
m. subclavius
m. pectoralis ascendens
a. suprascapularis
a. axillaris
a. circumflexa
humeri cranialis
n. musculocutaneus
r. muscularis proximalis
m. coracobrachialis
m. biceps brachii
n. musculocutaneus
r. muscularis distalis
m. longus colli
a.v. vertebralis
t. costocervicalis
a. cervicalis profunda
plexus brachialis
m. subscapularis
n. axillaris
a. circumflexa humeri
caudalis
a. thoracodorsalis
m. teres major
a.v. subscapularis
a.v. brachialis
n. medianus
n. ulnaris
lnn. cubitales
m. tensor fasciae
antebrachii

Fig. 3.51 The right axillary artery in the foal: medial view. The nerves of the brachial plexus have been removed from around the axillary artery to show its branches and the brachial artery.

4. THE THORAX

Clinical importance of the thorax

The thorax contains two major organs that are of considerable importance in clinical medicine in the horse – the lungs and the heart – but the nostril is the point at which physical abnormalities of the respiratory tract such as blood, excess mucus, or a purulent nasal discharge, are seen. The real test in clinical diagnosis is to ascertain whether this abnormality is coming from the upper or lower respiratory tract and from which component part of either.

Other physical abnormalities of respiration are most commonly detected by watching (abnormal excursions of the thoracic walls) or listening (coughing, roaring or rales) to the breathing and it is usually these that will necessitate further, more detailed, examination of the respiratory tract. One of the most common findings is dyspnoea (difficult breathing) which is seen in 'heaves' (pulmonary emphysema); typically, the affected horse has a second expiratory effort. The respiratory tract includes a variety of clinically important components such as the nasal cavity, nasopharynx, larynx, and guttural pouches, as well as trachea and lungs. Examination of the mucous membranes of the eye and the mouth (paleness, blue discolouration, abnormal capillary refill time) may suggest general abnormalities of the cardiovascular system such as anaemia or hypoxia.

The arterial pulse will give information on the heart and circulation. This can be taken from several arteries, including the transverse facial, facial, digital, brachial, femoral and the external carotid. Also, the aorta can be palpated *per rectum*. In the horse there is also a jugular pulse, which can be seen from the thoracic inlet to halfway up the neck when the horse is in the normal standing position.

The area of the chest available for clinical examination is limited by the presence of the forelimb, thoracic musculature and the decreasing thickness of the lung in its caudal parts within the chest. The effective area for listening is bounded caudally by a line that runs from the 18th rib to the middle of the thorax at rib 13, to shoulder level at rib 11, and finishes at the point of the elbow. For both organ systems, further evaluation is carried out using auscultation, percussion, MRI scanning (upper respiratory tract and sinuses), endoscopy, radiography (mainly in foals due to size limitations and X-ray power required in adults) and laboratory-based evaluations. A wide variety of diagnostic techniques can be applied to the thorax. Lung biopsy is not widely used; less invasive techniques have replaced it and pneumothorax sometimes followed its use. If it is necessary to perform lung biopsy, the ventral half of intercostal spaces 7–10 can be used. Endoscopy is widely used for the collection of samples from all levels of the respiratory tract. Tracheal and broncho-alveolar lavage (BAL) can be used to obtain samples for microbiology and cytology from as low as the 4–5th generations of the bronchial tree, using sterile saline. Tracheal aspirates can be drawn directly from the trachea by inserting a sterile needle between the tracheal cartilages. Thoracocentesis (removal of fluid from the chest) uses intercostal spaces 6–9 on either side of the chest, with spaces 7–8 being the best. The site is just above the costochondral junction. The caudal part of the intercostal space is used, as the intercostal artery, vein, lymphatics and nerve lie in the rostral part. During this procedure, care is needed to avoid the superficial thoracic vein. Pleural fluid can be collected for cytology and bacteriology.

There are many examples of infectious respiratory disease including, in former times, the bacterial zoonosis, glanders. Strangles, associated with streptococcal infection (*S.equi* subspecies *equi*) is one of the most serious disorders, localising in the lymph nodes of the respiratory tract and causing purulent discharges and abscesses. False strangles is similar and is caused by *S. zooepidemicus*. Other bacterial infections of the respiratory tract include pneumonia associated with *Rhodococcus equi,* particularly in foals and young horses where there may be up to an 80% mortality. This disease can also lead to a severe arthritis with antigen/antibody complexes in the joints of young horses. A second category of pulmonary disease is associated with parasites including parasitic pneumonia caused by the migration of *P.equorum* and also lungworms such as *Dictyocaulus arnfeldii* (commonly picked up from donkeys, which are carriers of the infestation) and, occasionally, pulmonary hydatidosis. There are several severe viral infections of the equine respiratory tract. One of the most important is equine influenza. Equine herpes virus may cause upper and lower tract disease, specific laryngitis, pharyngitis and abortion. Other important viral diseases include rhinovirus infections, equine viral arteritis, African horse sickness and equine infectious anaemia (swamp fever). Pulmonary oedema, acute respiratory distress syndrome and aspiration pneumonia are also not unknown.

Non-infectious respiratory disease is also important. Epistaxis (nosebleed) occurs in approximately 5% of racehorses after galloping. Exercise-induced pulmonary haemorrhage occurs after exercise. Reversible airway obstruction occurs with an asthma-type equivalent which can also be found on summer pastures. Chronic obstructive pulmonary diseases (now called RAO – recurrent airway obstruction, COPD, 'heaves') are caused by allergy (hypersensitivity) to dust allergens. Occasionally the horse may suffer from amyloidosis, pulmonary effusions (these can be checked by thoracocentesis) and pneumothorax, which can be alleviated by inserting a cathether high in the 13th intercostal space and aspirating the air. As well as abnormalities of the heart, the equine thorax may also suffer damage to great vessels as in equine viral arteritis, thrombophlebitis, or *purpura haemorrhagica*. Arterial rupture and aneurysm (particularly of the internal carotid artery) have been known to follow damage to the arteries from migrating nematode larvae.

Equine cardiology is an important subject, with auscultation as the most important clinical technique. In addition, an electrocardiogram (ECG) or 12-lead ECG can be used for the diagnosis and assessment of the severity of valvular, pericardial, myocardial and great vessel disease. Up to 4 heart sounds may be heard in normal horses. The first, which marks systole, is the closure of the atrioventricular (A-V) valves and opening of the semi-lunar aortic and pulmonary valves. The left atrioventricular valves are best heard in the left 5th intercostal space, midway between the level of the point of the shoulder and the point of the elbow. The right A-V valves are best heard in the right 4th intercostal space, midway between the level of the point of the shoulder and the point of the elbow. The second sound, which marks diastole, is caused by the closure of the semilunar valves and the opening of the atrioventricular valves. The aortic valves can be heard in the left 4th intercostal space at the level of the point of the shoulder. The pulmonary valves are heard on the right side in the 4th intercostal space, midway between the level of the point of the shoulder and the point of the elbow. The third heart sound occurs early in diastole and is heard in only one-third of horses. It marks the point at which the blood decelerates, at the end of rapid ventricular filling. The fourth sound, audible in most horses, is the atrial contraction in late diastole.

There are various cardiac complaints in the horse. Congestive heart failure can be left-sided or right-sided. Pericarditis, pericardial effusions, and myocarditis (ionophore toxicity) occur. Aortic root rupture results in sudden death with massive haemorrhage into the thoracic cavity. Many abnormal sounds may be heard in the examination of the heart. They include cardiac murmurs which can indicate stenosis of valves, incompetence of valves, shunts, and pre-systolic and systolic murmurs. Ectopic beats also occur in some horses. Disorders of cardiac rhythms include sinus arrhythmia, sinus tachycardia, ventricular tachycardia, atrial fibrillation, ventricular fibrillation, atrio-ventricular block and sino-atrial block. Congenital heart defects do occur rarely in foals. These include ventral septal defects, persistent *ductus arteriosus*, patent *foramen ovale*, myocarditis and fibrocarditis.

Clinical considerations for the spine in the thoracic region are dealt with in the section on the spine in Chapter 8 (p. 269).

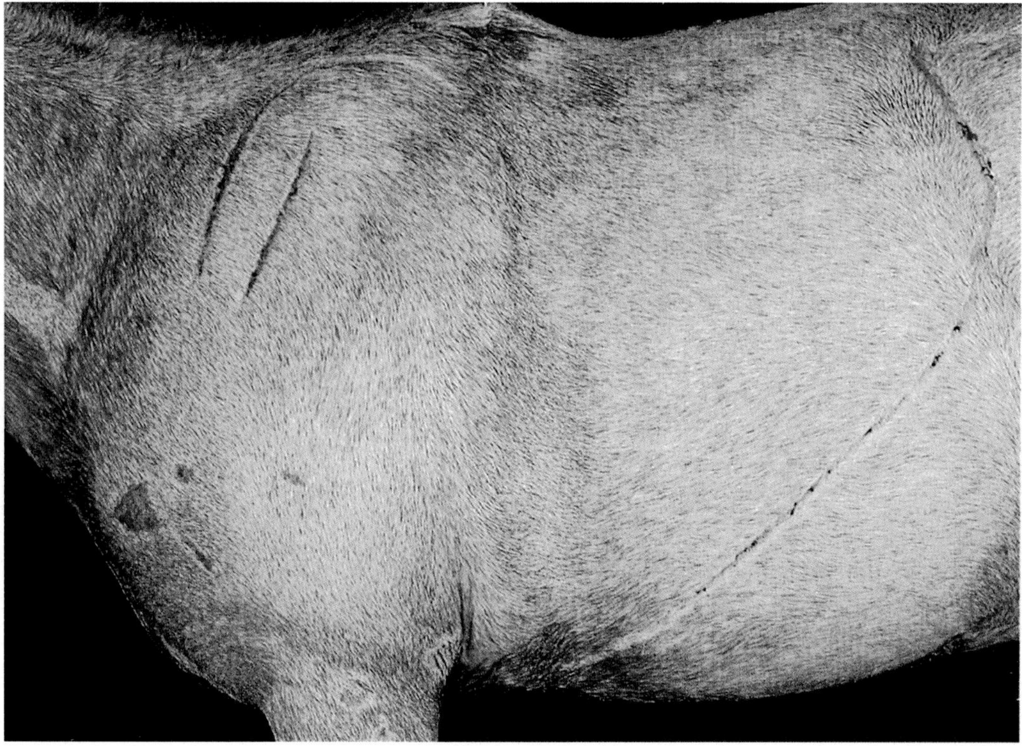

Fig. 4.1 Surface features of the neck, shoulder and thorax: left lateral view. The hair over the palpable surface features was shaved before embalming commenced. Rib 18 was small and not clearly palpable. The surface projections of the thoracic and cervical vertebrae, cupola of the diaphragm and diaphragmatic line of pleural reflection are based on the dissections shown in Figs. 4.17 and 4.22.

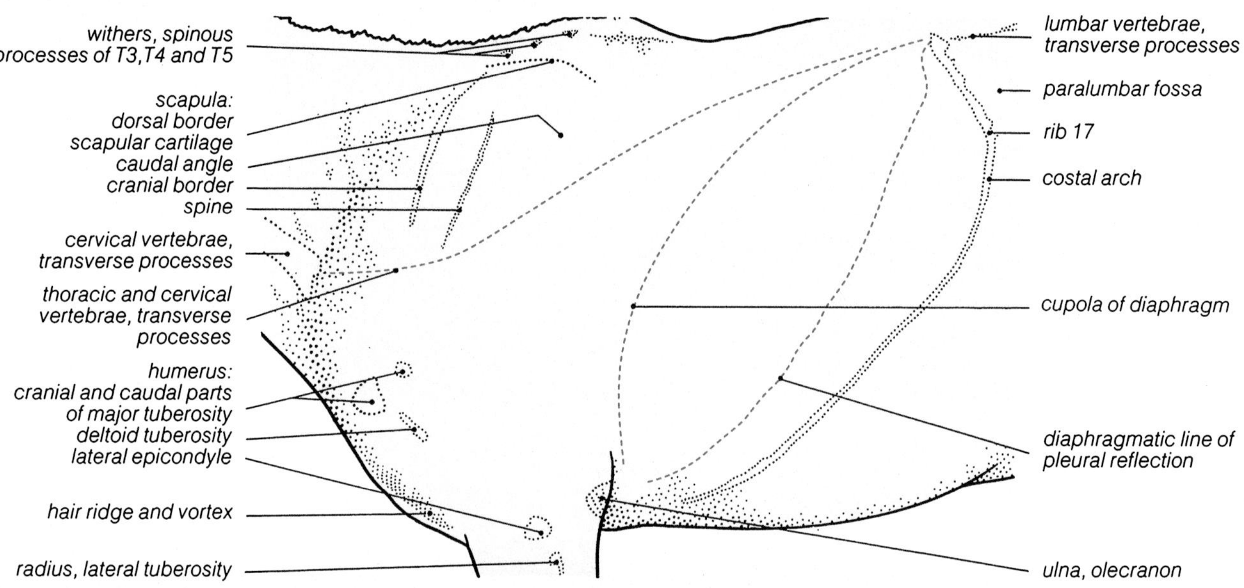
withers, spinous processes of T3,T4 and T5
scapula:
dorsal border
scapular cartilage
caudal angle
cranial border
spine
cervical vertebrae, transverse processes
thoracic and cervical vertebrae, transverse processes
humerus:
cranial and caudal parts of major tuberosity
deltoid tuberosity
lateral epicondyle
hair ridge and vortex
radius, lateral tuberosity
lumbar vertebrae, transverse processes
paralumbar fossa
rib 17
costal arch
cupola of diaphragm
diaphragmatic line of pleural reflection
ulna, olecranon

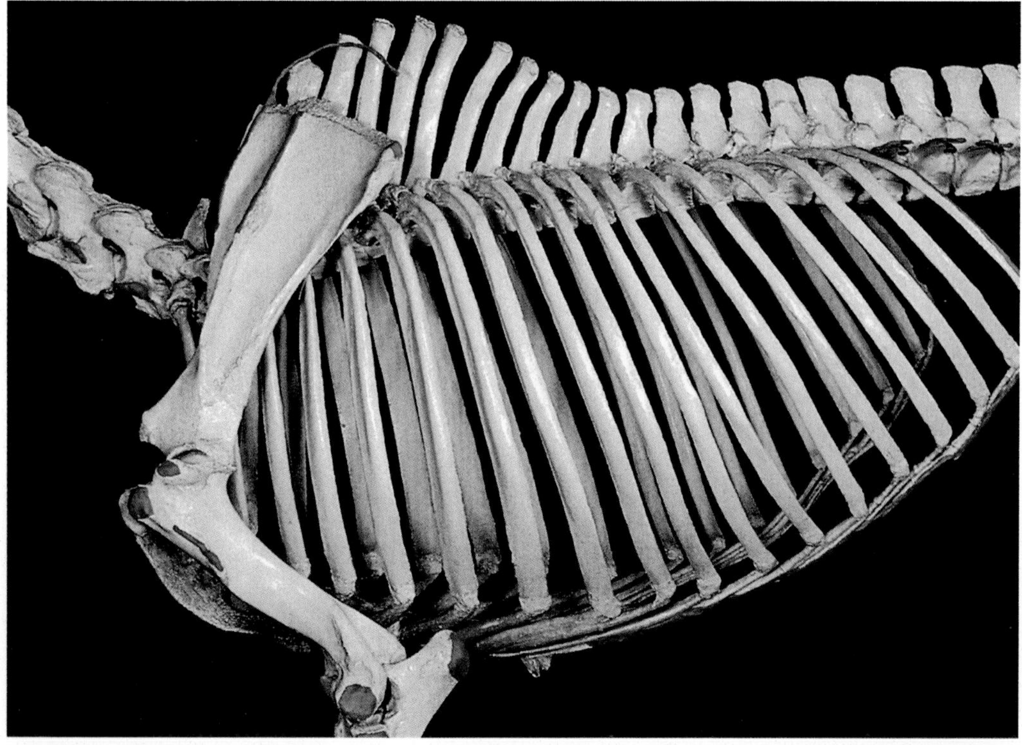

Fig. 4.2 Skeleton of proximal forelimb and thorax: left lateral view. The palpable features shown in Fig. 4.1 are coloured red except for the spinous processes at the withers. Note that in this articulated skeleton rib 18 is large. In the dissected specimen this rib was small (see Fig. 4.9) and the last distinctly palpable rib was rib 17.

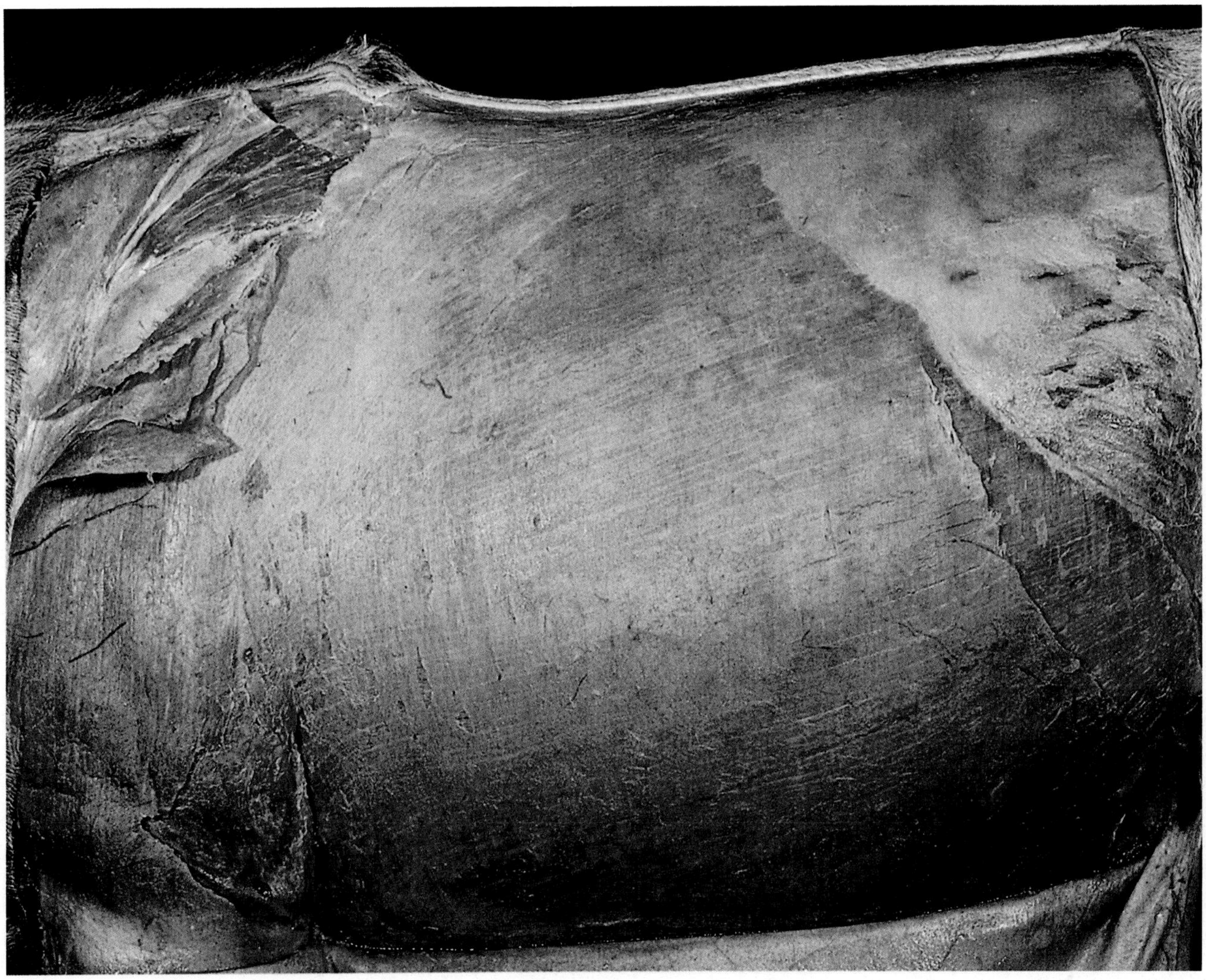

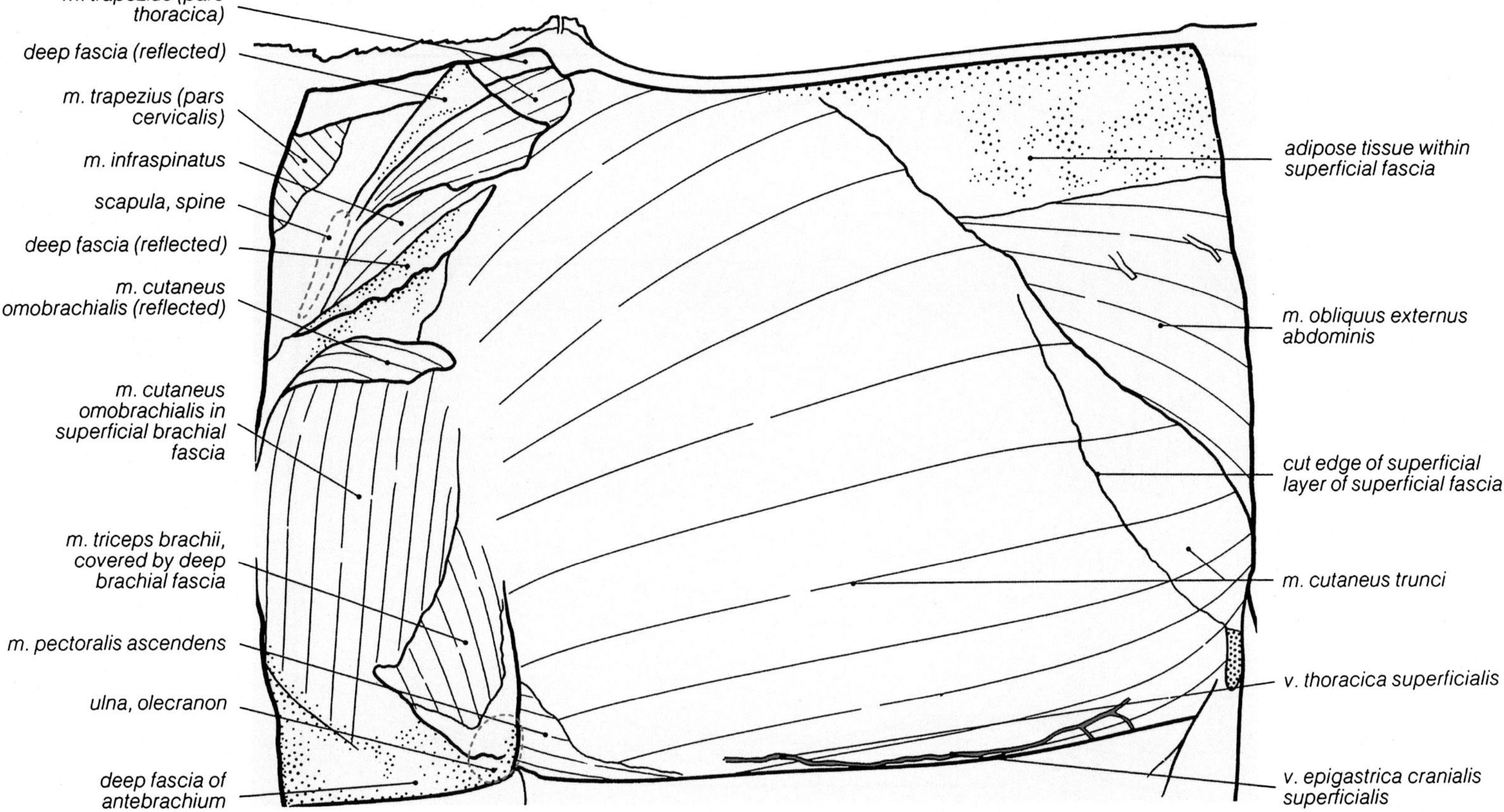
m. trapezius (pars thoracica)
deep fascia (reflected)
m. trapezius (pars cervicalis)
m. infraspinatus
scapula, spine
deep fascia (reflected)
m. cutaneus omobrachialis (reflected)
m. cutaneus omobrachialis in superficial brachial fascia
m. triceps brachii, covered by deep brachial fascia
m. pectoralis ascendens
ulna, olecranon
deep fascia of antebrachium
adipose tissue within superficial fascia
m. obliquus externus abdominis
cut edge of superficial layer of superficial fascia
m. cutaneus trunci
v. thoracica superficialis
v. epigastrica cranialis superficialis

Fig. 4.3 The cutaneous muscles and superficial fascia of the trunk: left lateral view. The skin has been carefully removed to display the cutaneous muscles which lie just beneath the dermis, within the superficial fascia. An earlier stage of the dissection is shown in Fig. 5.3.

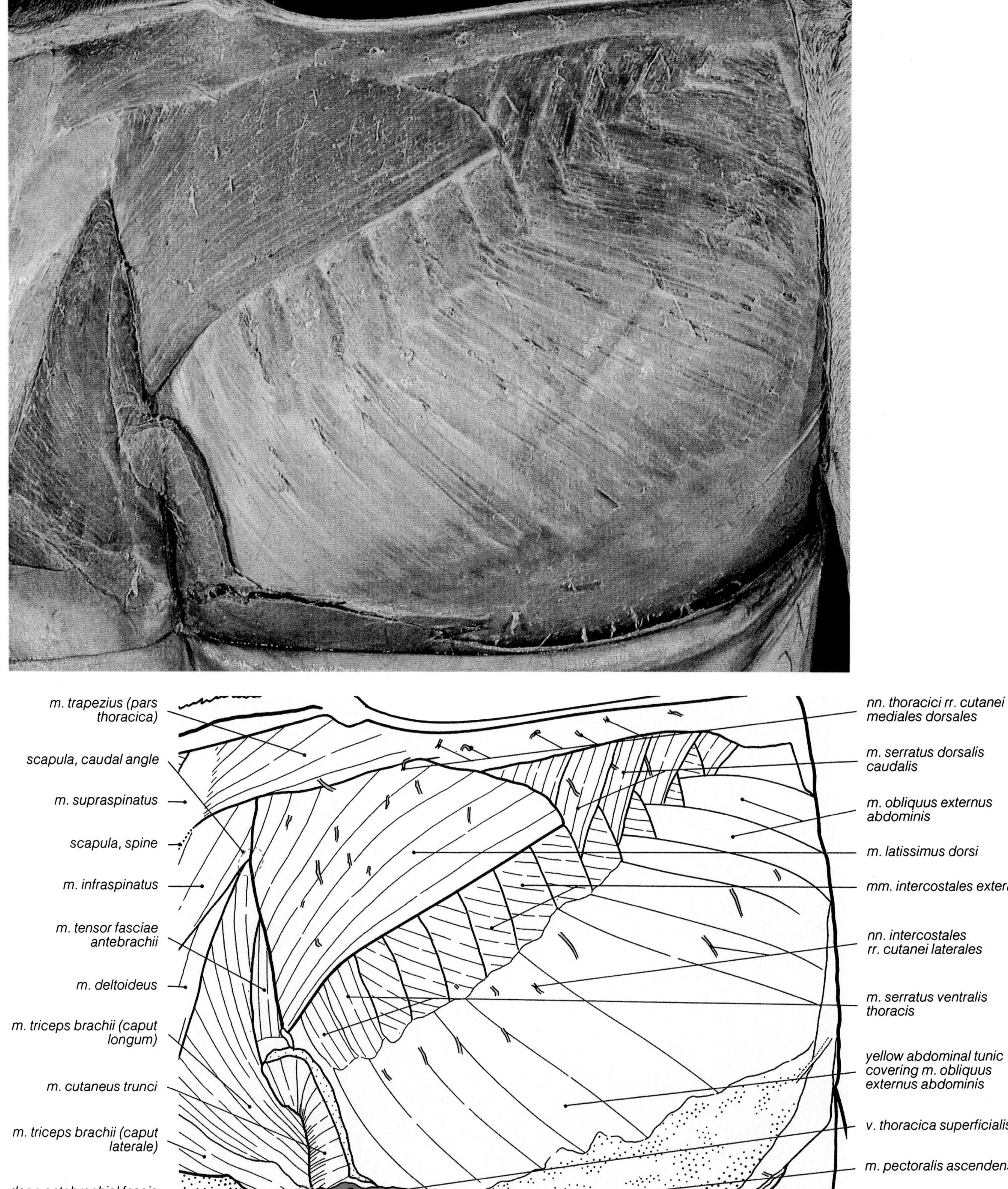
m. trapezius (pars thoracica)
scapula, caudal angle
m. supraspinatus
scapula, spine
m. infraspinatus
m. tensor fasciae antebrachii
m. deltoideus
m. triceps brachii (caput longum)
m. cutaneus trunci
m. triceps brachii (caput laterale)
deep antebrachial fascia
olecranon
nn. thoracici rr. cutanei mediales dorsales
m. serratus dorsalis caudalis
m. obliquus externus abdominis
m. latissimus dorsi
mm. intercostales externi
nn. intercostales rr. cutanei laterales
m. serratus ventralis thoracis
yellow abdominal tunic covering m. obliquus externus abdominis
v. thoracica superficialis
m. pectoralis ascendens
nn. intercostales rr. cutanei ventrales

Fig. 4.4 Superficial structures of the shoulder and thorax: left lateral view. The superficial fascia, including the cutaneous muscles, has been removed. The deep fascia has also been removed from the muscles of the scapular and brachial regions.

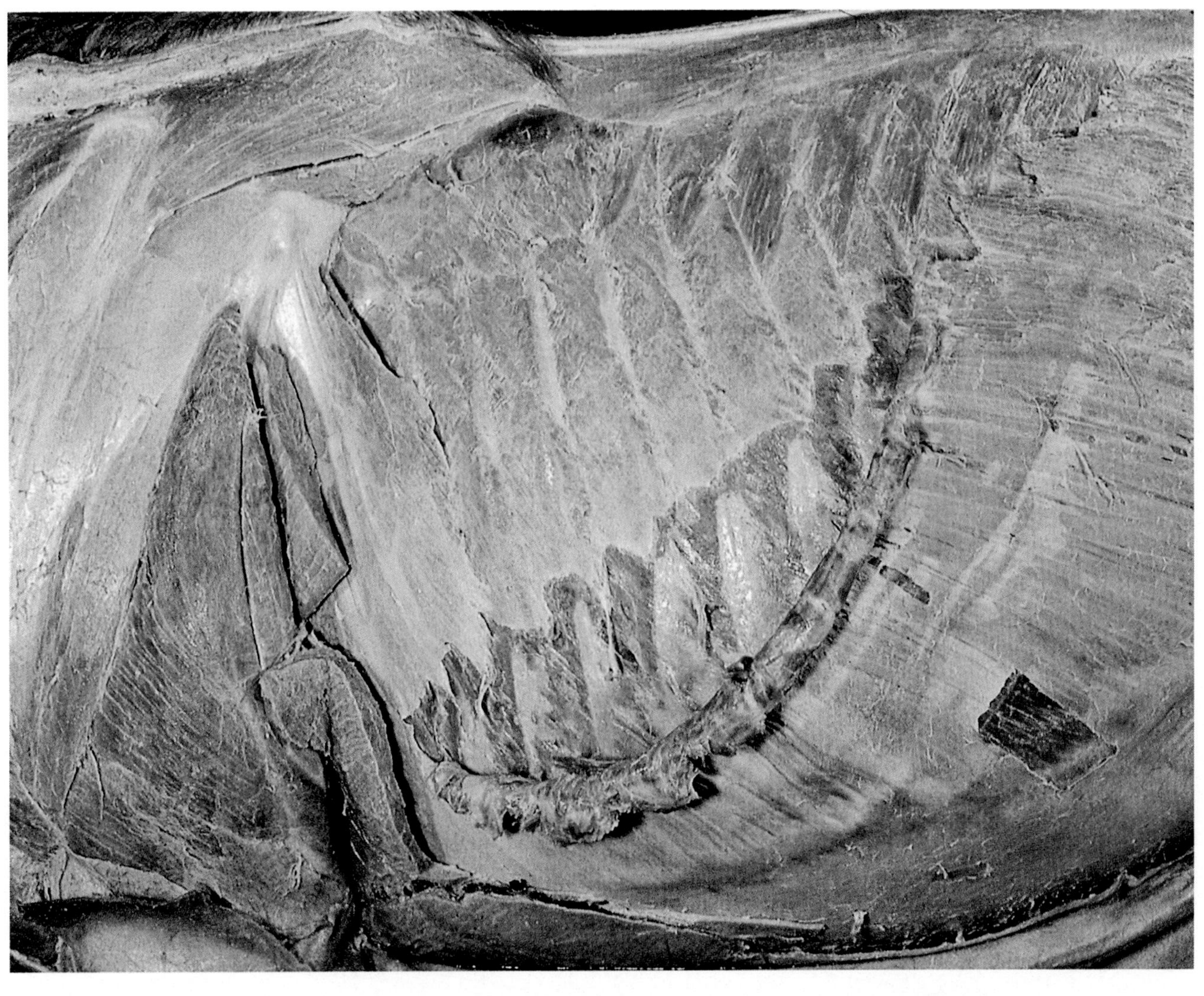

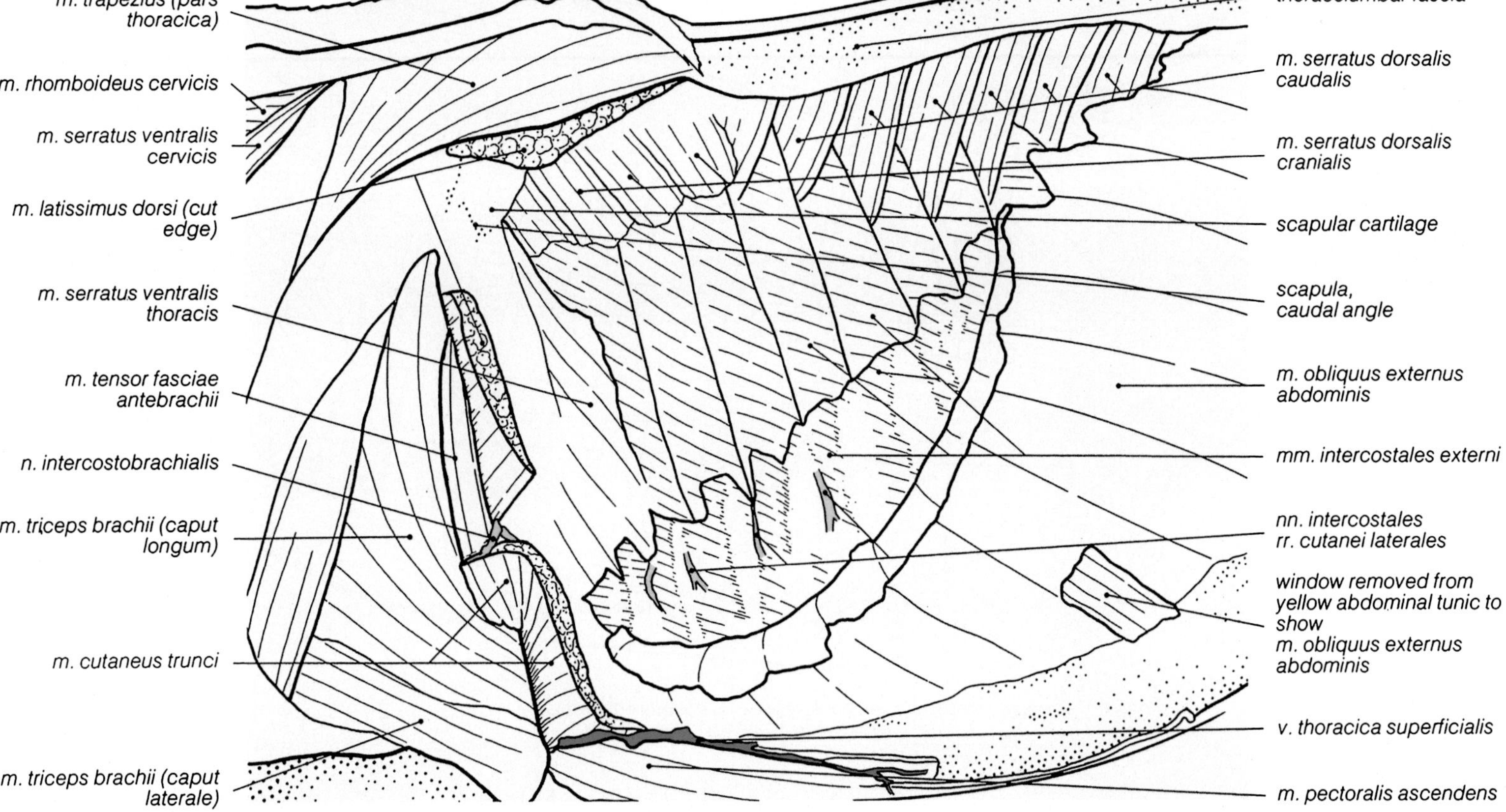
m. trapezius (pars thoracica)
m. rhomboideus cervicis
m. serratus ventralis cervicis
m. latissimus dorsi (cut edge)
m. serratus ventralis thoracis
m. tensor fasciae antebrachii
n. intercostobrachialis
m. triceps brachii (caput longum)
m. cutaneus trunci
m. triceps brachii (caput laterale)
thoracolumbar fascia
m. serratus dorsalis caudalis
m. serratus dorsalis cranialis
scapular cartilage
scapula, caudal angle
m. obliquus externus abdominis
mm. intercostales externi
nn. intercostales rr. cutanei laterales
window removed from yellow abdominal tunic to show m. obliquus externus abdominis
v. thoracica superficialis
m. pectoralis ascendens

Fig. 4.5 The thoracic wall after removal of the latissimus dorsi muscle: left lateral view. The origins of the external oblique abdominal muscle from the ribs have been cut; the elastic deep fascia (yellow abdominal tunic) has rolled the muscle ventrally to show the external intercostal muscles that lie beneath the oblique muscle.

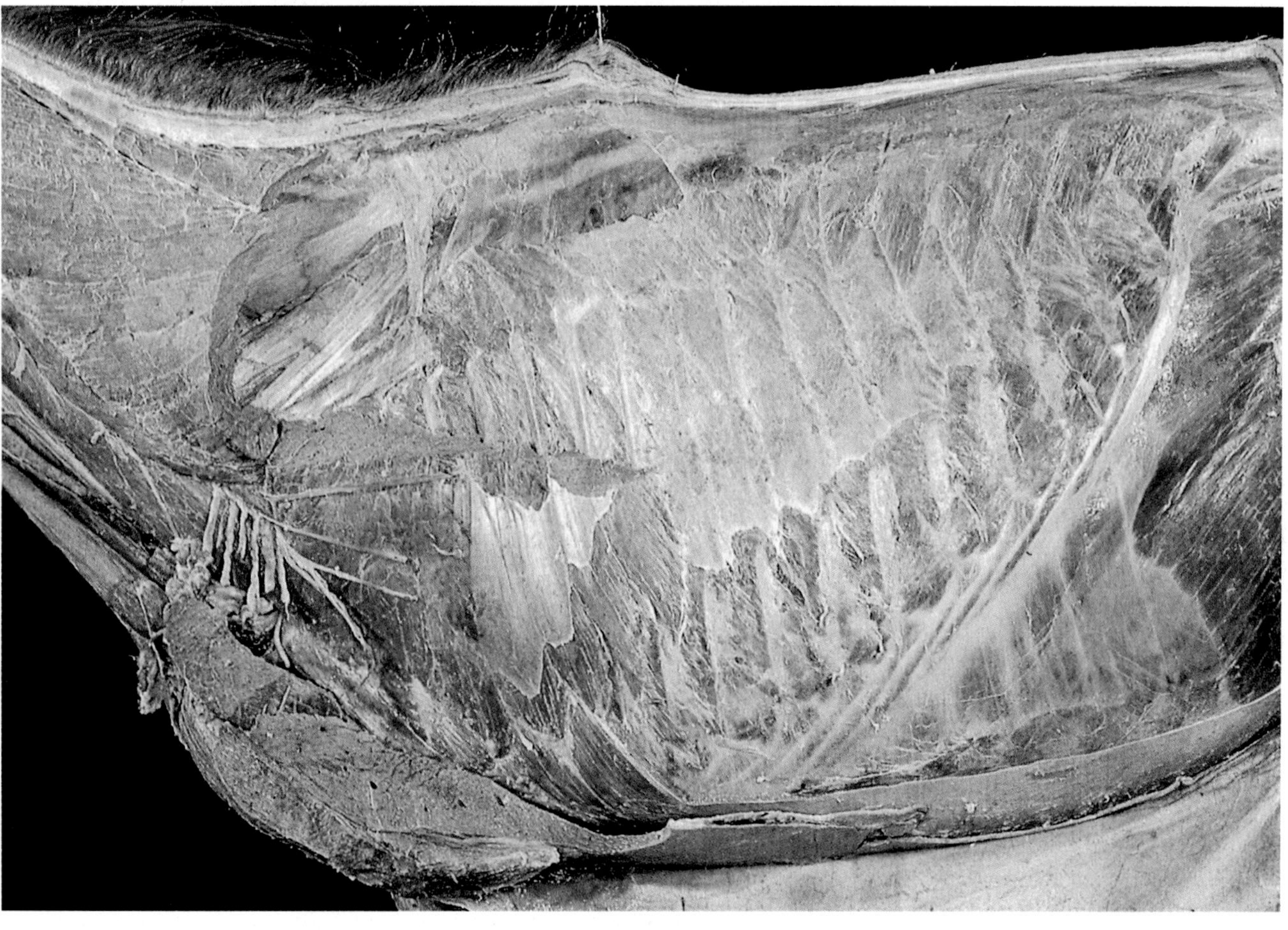

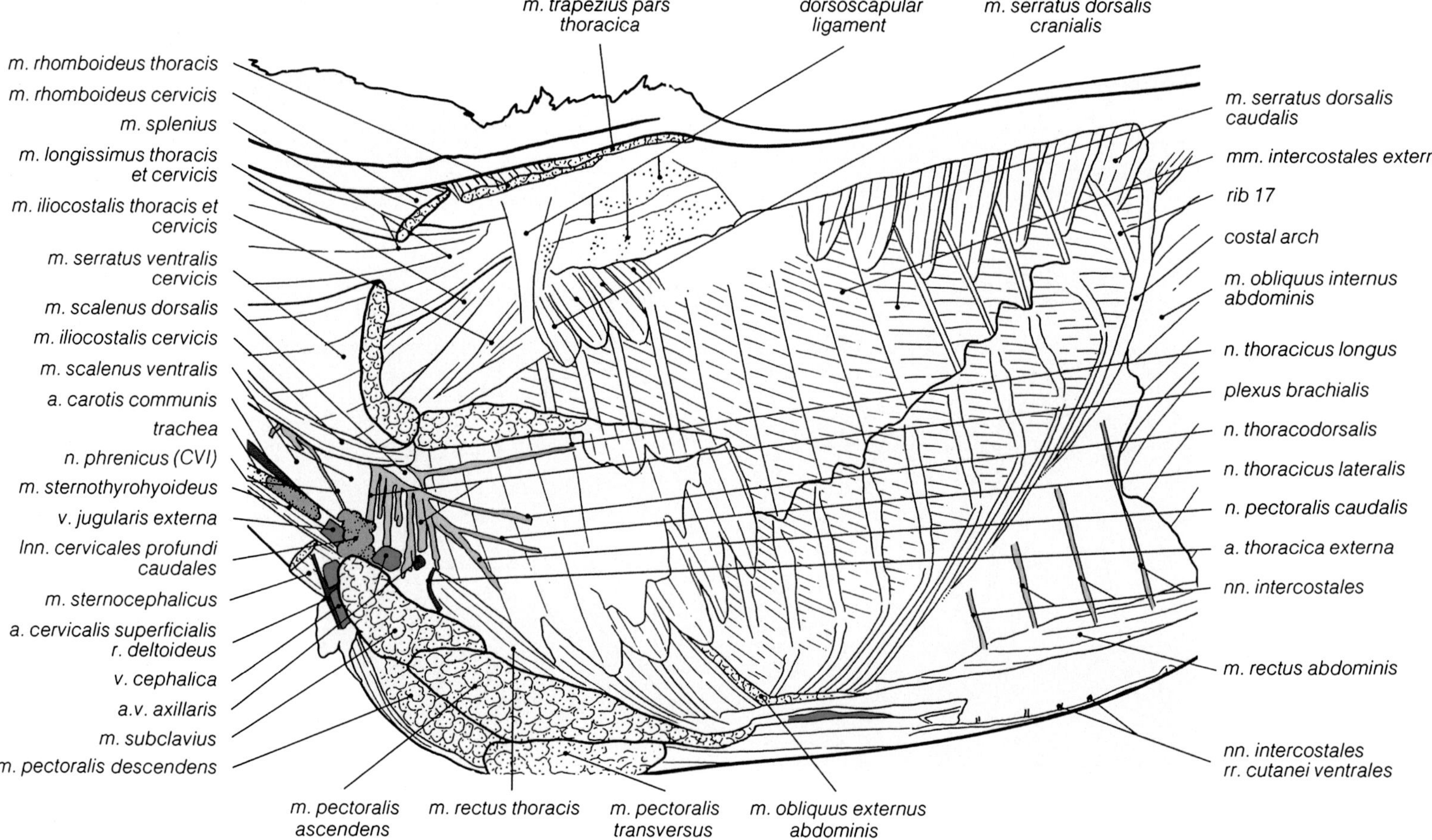
m. trapezius pars thoracica
dorsoscapular ligament
m. serratus dorsalis cranialis
m. rhomboideus thoracis
m. rhomboideus cervicis
m. splenius
m. longissimus thoracis et cervicis
m. iliocostalis thoracis et cervicis
m. serratus ventralis cervicis
m. scalenus dorsalis
m. iliocostalis cervicis
m. scalenus ventralis
a. carotis communis
trachea
n. phrenicus (CVI)
m. sternothyrohyoideus
v. jugularis externa
lnn. cervicales profundi caudales
m. sternocephalicus
a. cervicalis superficialis r. deltoideus
v. cephalica
a.v. axillaris
m. subclavius
m. pectoralis descendens
m. serratus dorsalis caudalis
mm. intercostales externi
rib 17
costal arch
m. obliquus internus abdominis
n. thoracicus longus
plexus brachialis
n. thoracodorsalis
n. thoracicus lateralis
n. pectoralis caudalis
a. thoracica externa
nn. intercostales
m. rectus abdominis
nn. intercostales rr. cutanei ventrales
m. pectoralis ascendens
m. rectus thoracis
m. pectoralis transversus
m. obliquus externus abdominis

Fig. 4.6 The thoracic wall after removal of the forelimb: left lateral view. The cut surfaces of the muscles joining the scapula and humerus to the trunk have been left in place. The external oblique abdominal muscle has been partially removed to show the caudal ribs more clearly.

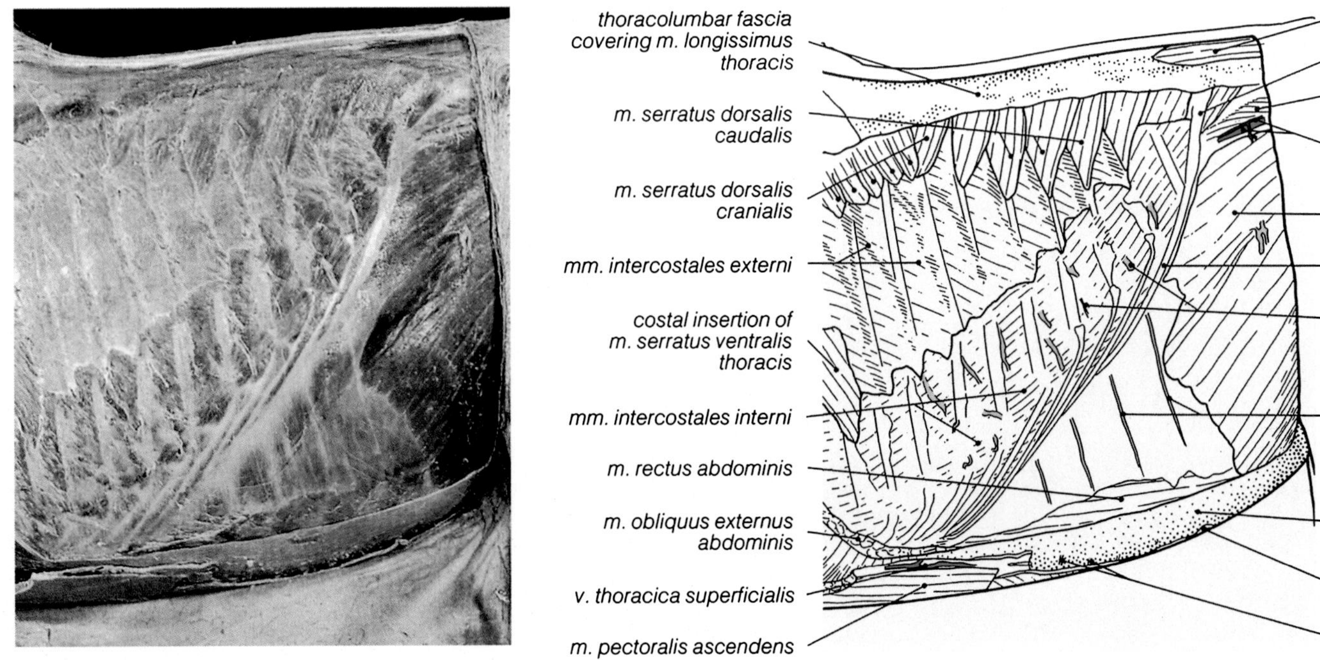
thoracolumbar fascia covering m. longissimus thoracis
m. serratus dorsalis caudalis
m. serratus dorsalis cranialis
mm. intercostales externi
costal insertion of m. serratus ventralis thoracis
mm. intercostales interni
m. rectus abdominis
m. obliquus externus abdominis
v. thoracica superficialis
m. pectoralis ascendens
m. gluteus medius
rib 18
m. retractor costae
a.v. ilium circumflexa profunda
m. obliquus internus abdominis
costal arch
nn. intercostales (XIV,XV) rr. cutanei laterales
nn. intercostales (XIV,XV) running between m. obliquus internus abdominis and m. transversus abdominis
yellow abdominal tunic covering m. obliquus externus abdominis
m. cutaneus trunci
nn. intercostales rr. cutanei ventrales

Fig. 4.7 The caudal ribs and costal arch:left lateral view. The external oblique abdominal muscle has been removed. This is part of the dissection shown in Fig. 4.6.

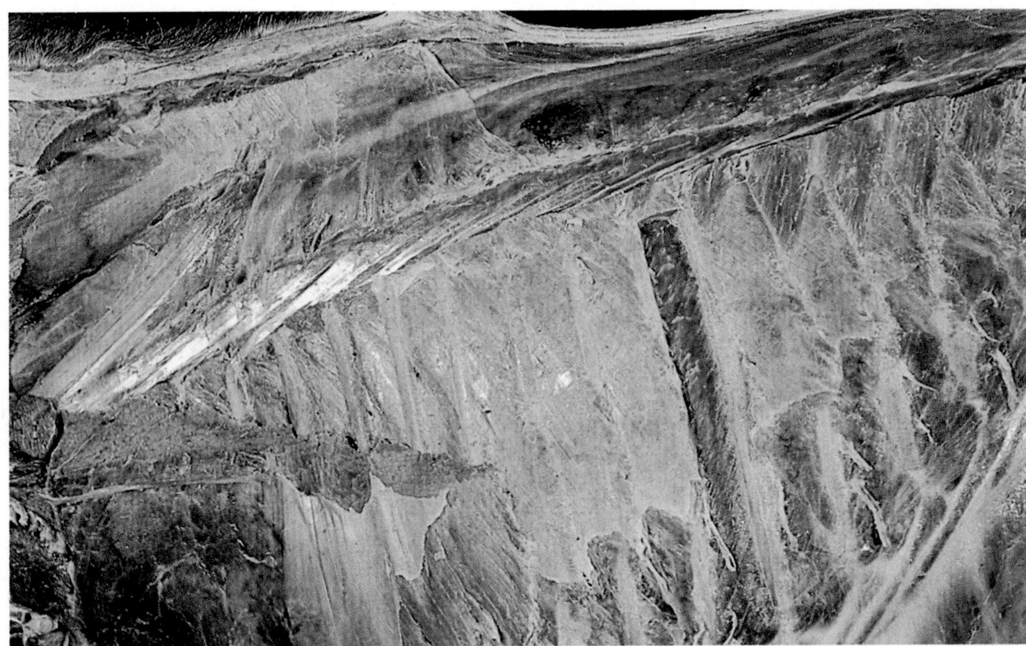

Fig. 4.8 Muscles and nerves of the thoracic wall:left lateral view. The cranial dorsal serrate muscle and its origin from the superficial part of the dorsoscapular ligament have been resected. One of the external intercostal muscles has been removed.

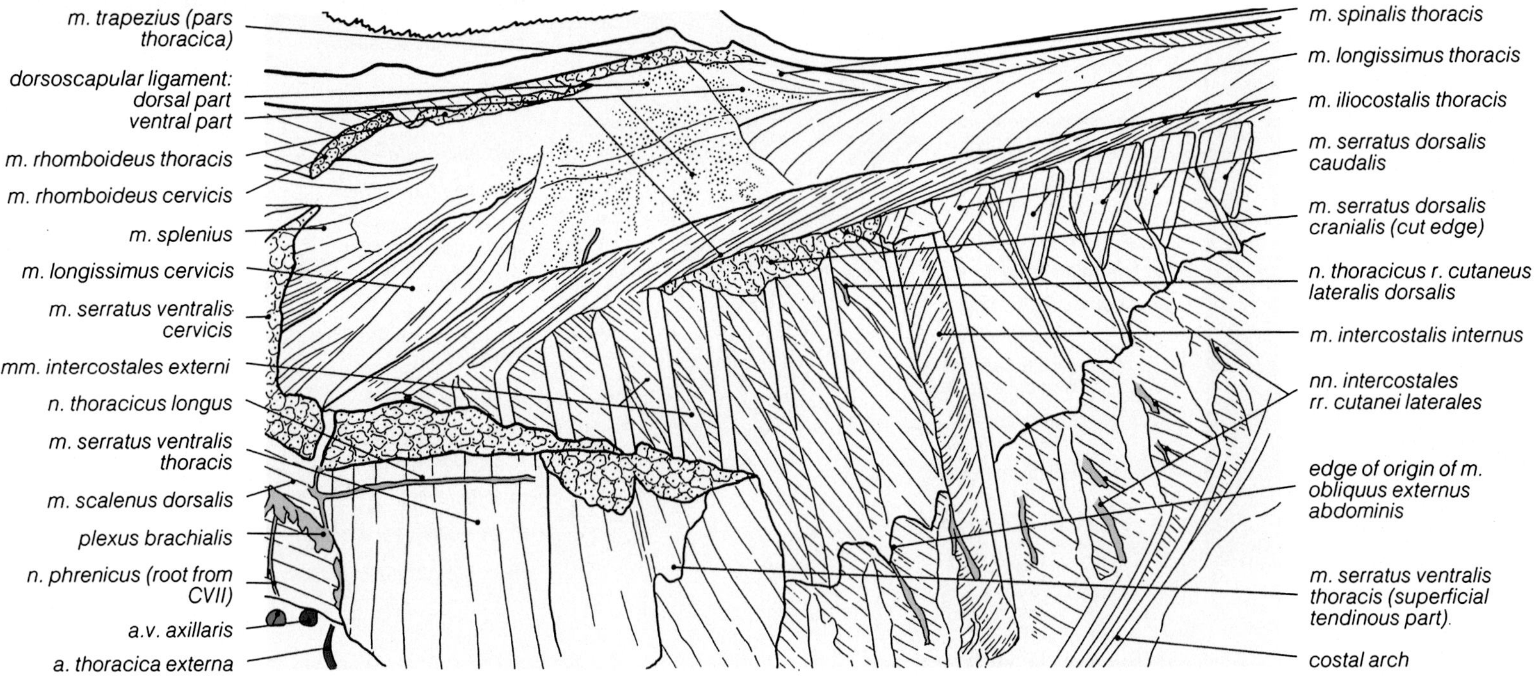
m. trapezius (pars thoracica)
dorsoscapular ligament: dorsal part
ventral part
m. rhomboideus thoracis
m. rhomboideus cervicis
m. splenius
m. longissimus cervicis
m. serratus ventralis cervicis
mm. intercostales externi
n. thoracicus longus
m. serratus ventralis thoracis
m. scalenus dorsalis
plexus brachialis
n. phrenicus (root from CVII)
a.v. axillaris
a. thoracica externa
m. spinalis thoracis
m. longissimus thoracis
m. iliocostalis thoracis
m. serratus dorsalis caudalis
m. serratus dorsalis cranialis (cut edge)
n. thoracicus r. cutaneus lateralis dorsalis
m. intercostalis internus
nn. intercostales rr. cutanei laterales
edge of origin of m. obliquus externus abdominis
m. serratus ventralis thoracis (superficial tendinous part)
costal arch

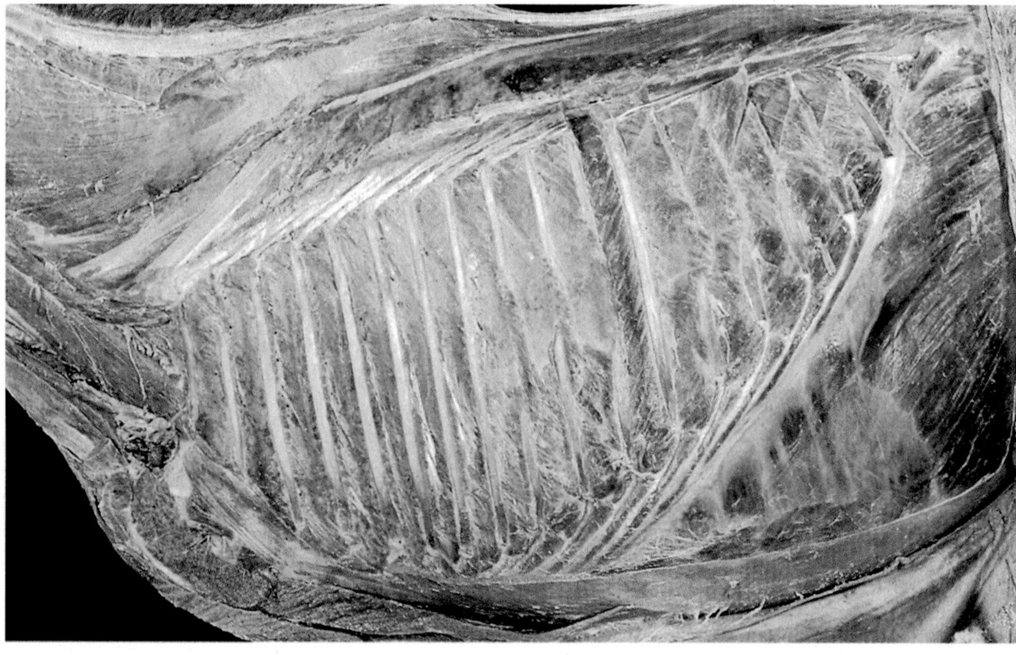

Fig. 4.9 The rib cage: superficial structures in left lateral view. The muscles of the forelimb have now been cut away to reveal the full extent of the rib cage. The external intercostal muscle in the eleventh intercostal space has been removed to show the internal intercostal muscle. The eighteenth rib in this specimen was very small; see Fig. 4.2.

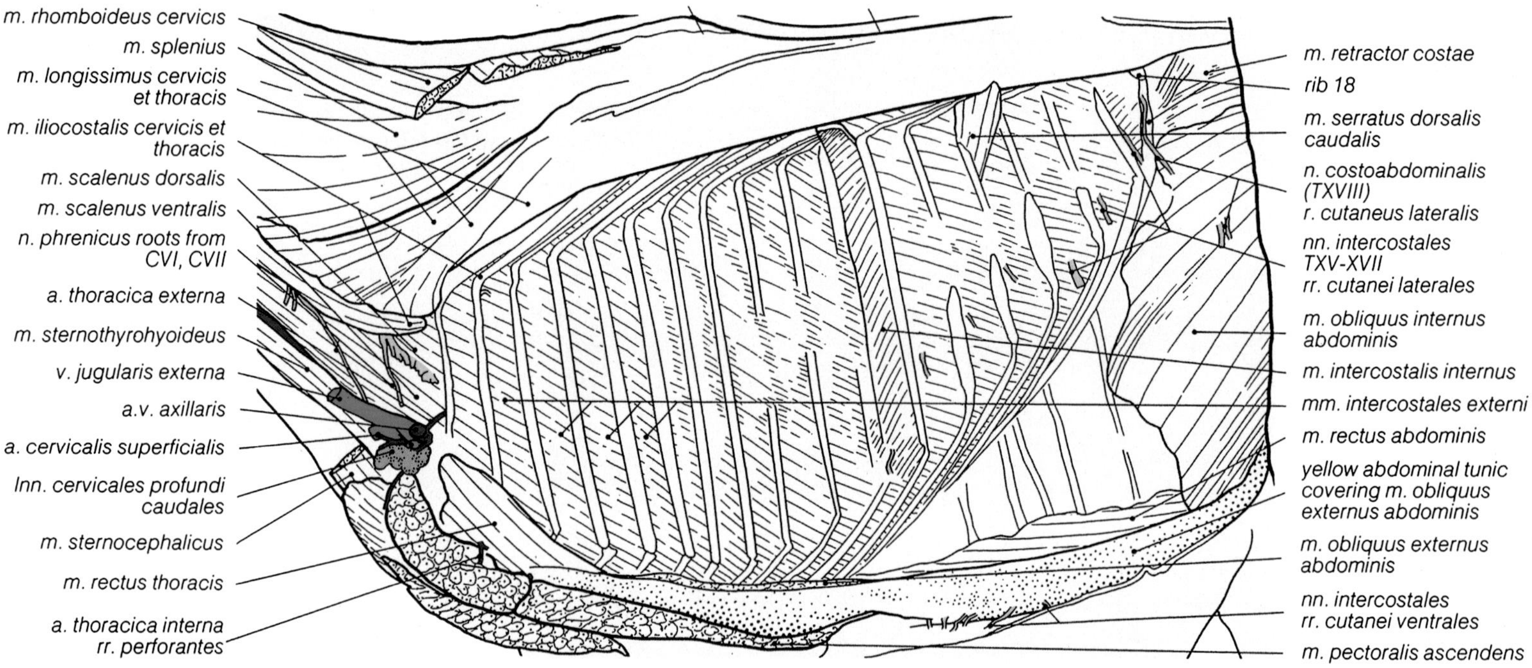

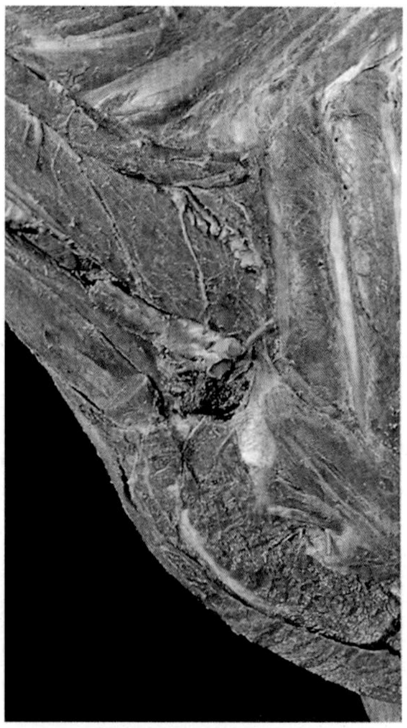

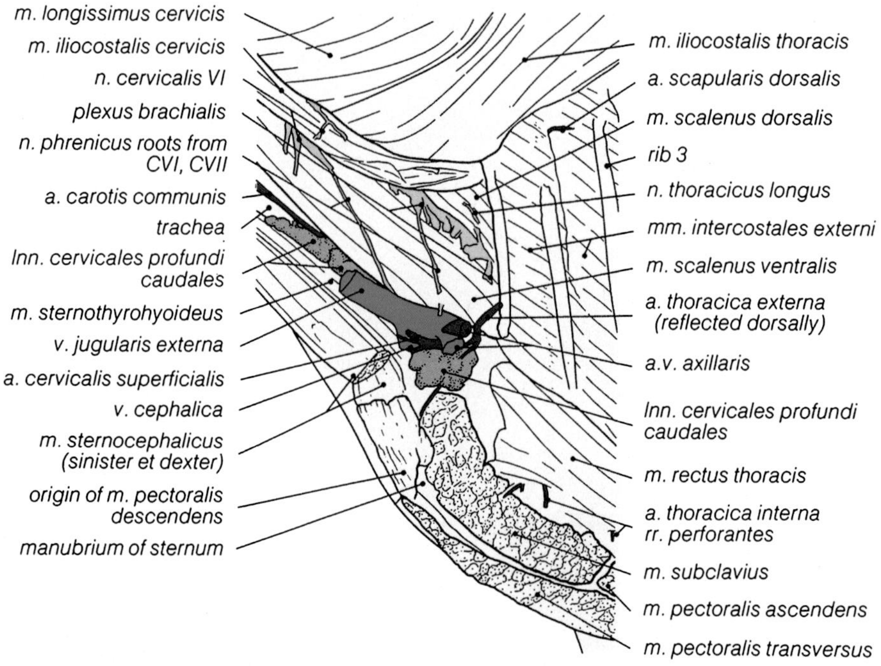

m. rhomboideus cervicis
m. splenius
m. longissimus cervicis et thoracis
m. iliocostalis cervicis et thoracis
m. scalenus dorsalis
m. scalenus ventralis
n. phrenicus roots from CVI, CVII
a. thoracica externa
m. sternothyrohyoideus
v. jugularis externa
a.v. axillaris
a. cervicalis superficialis
lnn. cervicales profundi caudales
m. sternocephalicus
m. rectus thoracis
a. thoracica interna rr. perforantes
m. retractor costae
rib 18
m. serratus dorsalis caudalis
n. costoabdominalis (TXVIII)
r. cutaneus lateralis
nn. intercostales TXV-XVII
rr. cutanei laterales
m. obliquus internus abdominis
m. intercostalis internus
mm. intercostales externi
m. rectus abdominis
yellow abdominal tunic covering m. obliquus externus abdominis
m. obliquus externus abdominis
nn. intercostales
rr. cutanei ventrales
m. pectoralis ascendens

m. longissimus cervicis
m. iliocostalis cervicis
n. cervicalis VI
plexus brachialis
n. phrenicus roots from CVI, CVII
a. carotis communis
trachea
lnn. cervicales profundi caudales
m. sternothyrohyoideus
v. jugularis externa
a. cervicalis superficialis
v. cephalica
m. sternocephalicus (sinister et dexter)
origin of m. pectoralis descendens
manubrium of sternum
m. iliocostalis thoracis
a. scapularis dorsalis
m. scalenus dorsalis
rib 3
n. thoracicus longus
mm. intercostales externi
m. scalenus ventralis
a. thoracica externa (reflected dorsally)
a.v. axillaris
lnn. cervicales profundi caudales
m. rectus thoracis
a. thoracica interna rr. perforantes
m. subclavius
m. pectoralis ascendens
m. pectoralis transversus

Fig. 4.10 The thoracic inlet: superficial structures in left lateral view. This is a closer view of a part of the specimen shown in Fig. 4.9.

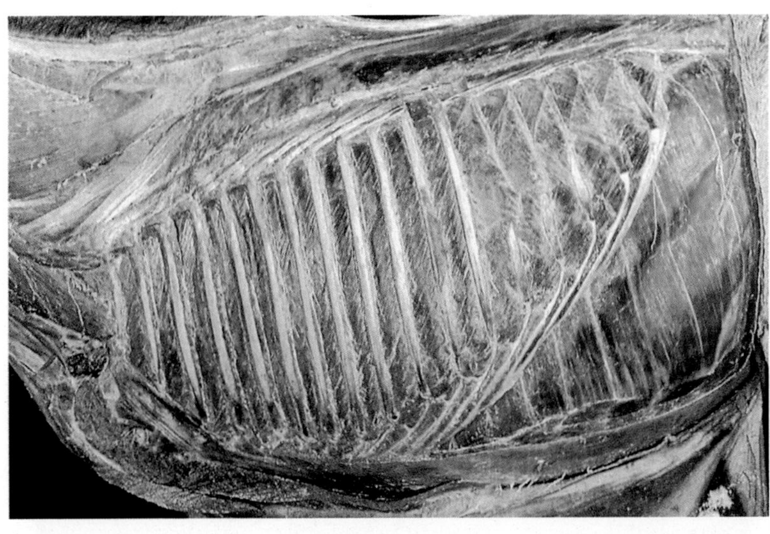

Fig. 4.11 The rib cage: deeper structures in left lateral view. The external intercostal muscles have been removed from the first eleven intercostal spaces. The structures within these spaces are shown in Figs.4.12 and 4.13. The internal oblique abdominal muscle has also been removed. Dorsally, the iliocostalis muscle has been removed from two intercostal spaces.

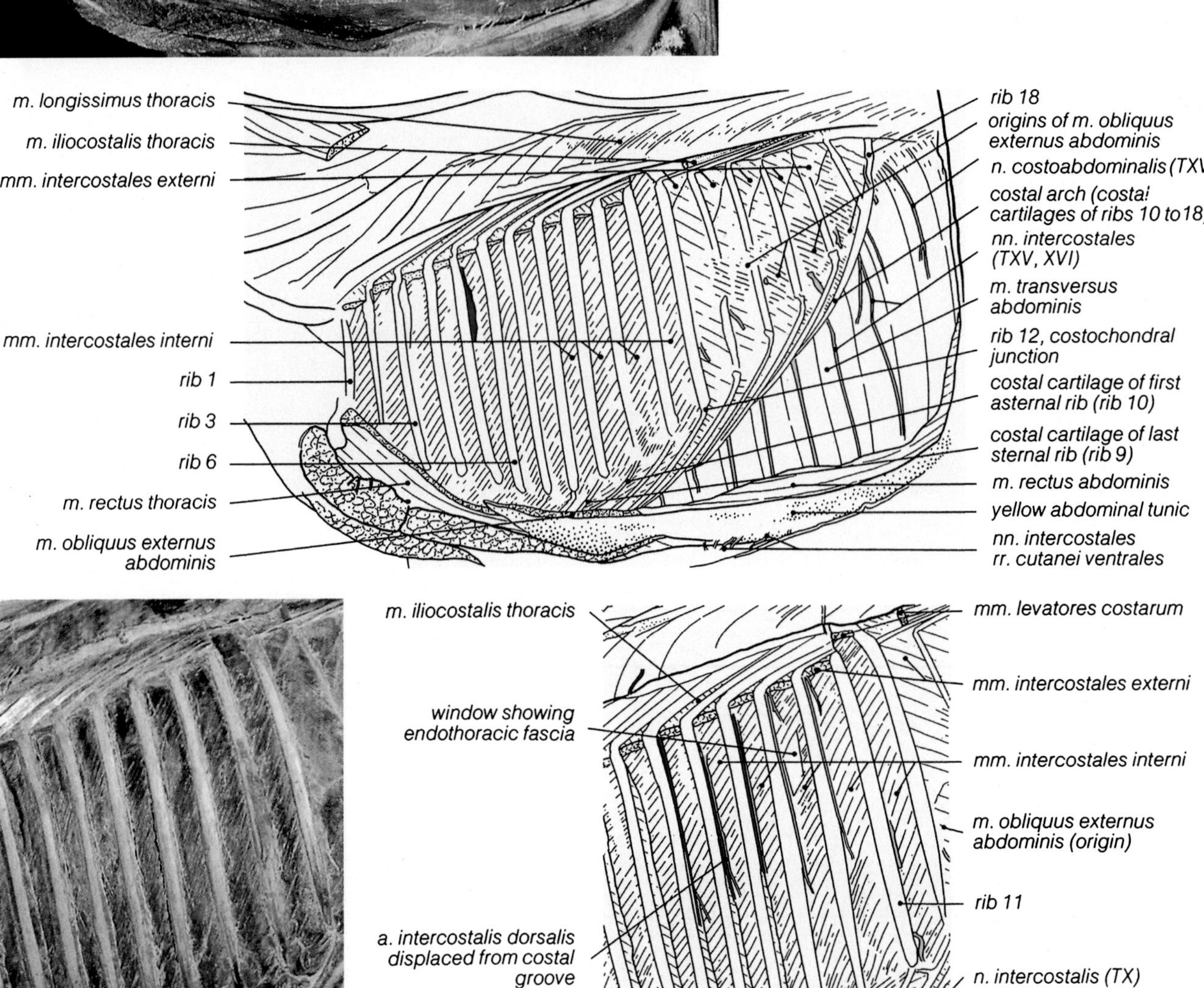
m. longissimus thoracis
m. iliocostalis thoracis
mm. intercostales externi
mm. intercostales interni
rib 1
rib 3
rib 6
m. rectus thoracis
m. obliquus externus abdominis
rib 18
origins of m. obliquus externus abdominis
n. costoabdominalis (TXVIII)
costal arch (costal cartilages of ribs 10 to 18)
nn. intercostales (TXV, XVI)
m. transversus abdominis
rib 12, costochondral junction
costal cartilage of first asternal rib (rib 10)
costal cartilage of last sternal rib (rib 9)
m. rectus abdominis
yellow abdominal tunic
nn. intercostales rr. cutanei ventrales

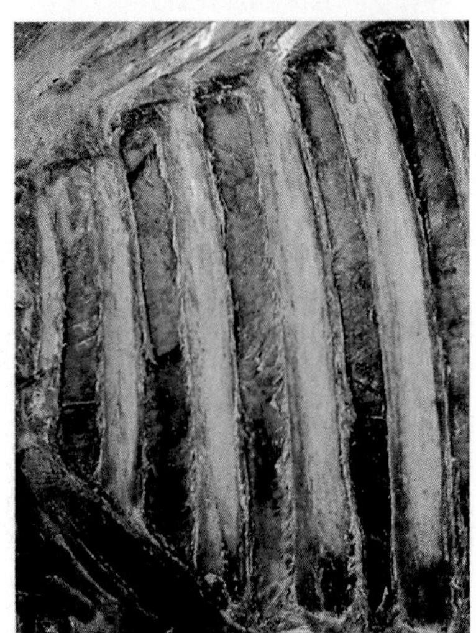

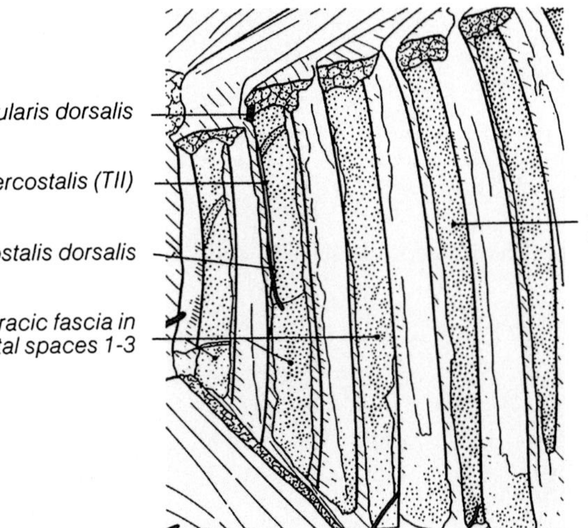
m. iliocostalis thoracis
window showing endothoracic fascia
a. intercostalis dorsalis displaced from costal groove
rib 5, costochondral junction
mm. levatores costarum
mm. intercostales externi
mm. intercostales interni
m. obliquus externus abdominis (origin)
rib 11
n. intercostalis (TX)
m. obliquus externus abdominis

Fig. 4.12 Structures of the intercostal spaces: left lateral view. This is a closer view of a part of the specimen shown in Fig. 4.11. The intercostal vessels and nerves have been displaced from the costal groove. A window has been cut in the 9th internal intercostal muscle.

a. scapularis dorsalis
n. intercostalis (TII)
a. intercostalis dorsalis
endothoracic fascia in intercostal spaces 1-3
left lung exposed in intercostal space 4

Fig. 4.13 The endothoracic fascia of the intercostal spaces: left lateral view. The intercostal muscles have been removed. The endothoracic fascia remains intact in the first three intercostal spaces.

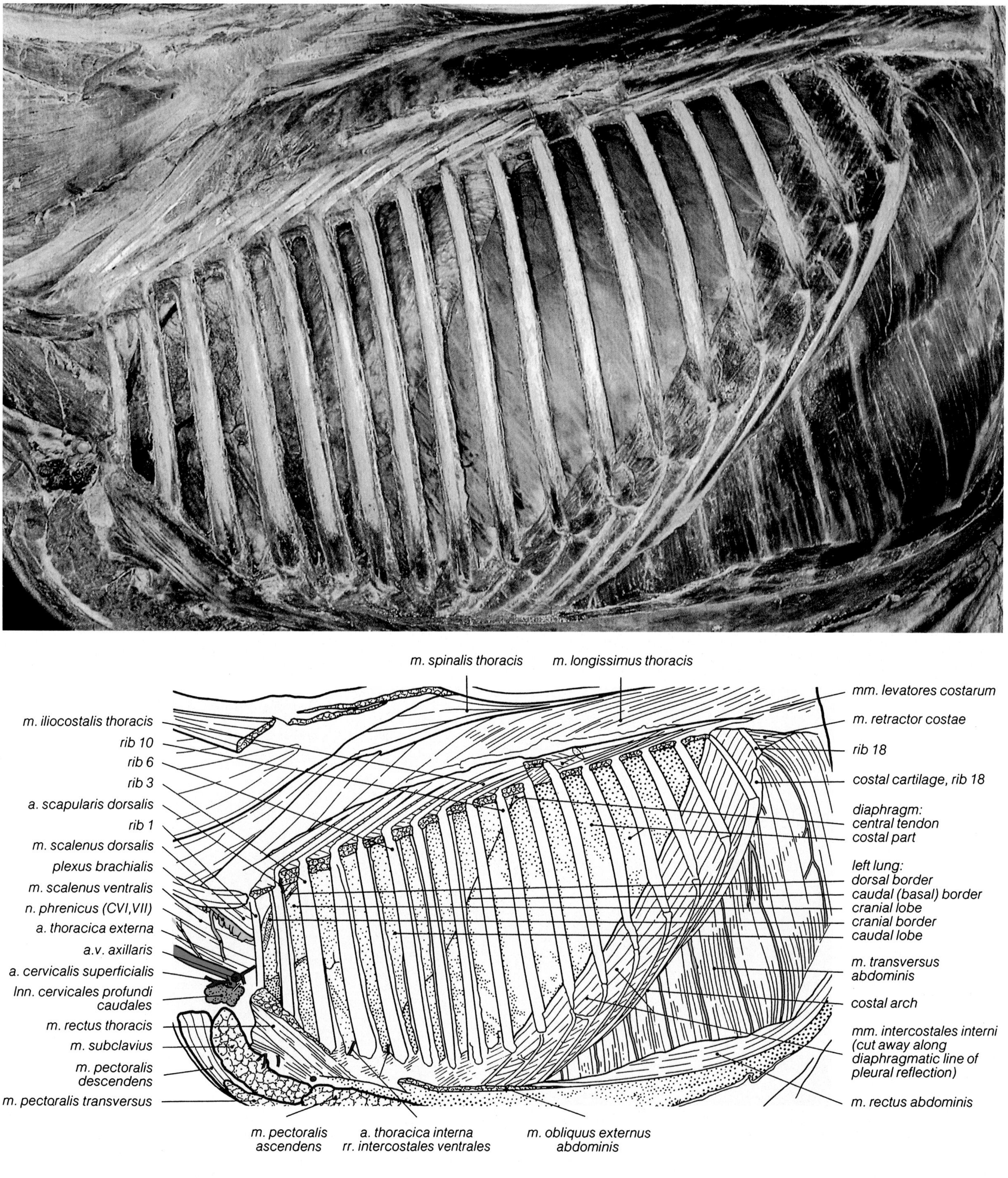

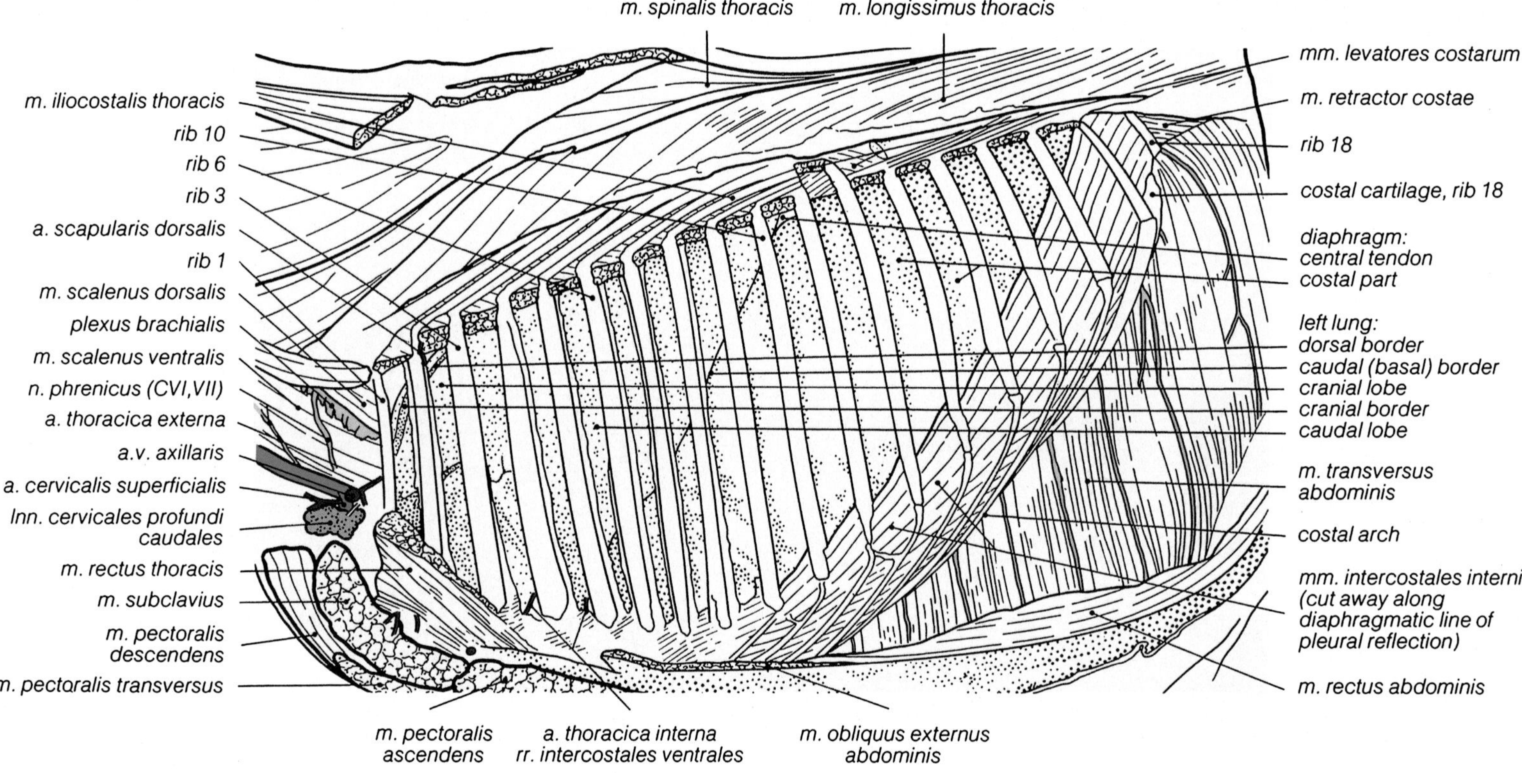
m. spinalis thoracis
m. longissimus thoracis
m. iliocostalis thoracis
rib 10
rib 6
rib 3
a. scapularis dorsalis
rib 1
m. scalenus dorsalis
plexus brachialis
m. scalenus ventralis
n. phrenicus (CVI,VII)
a. thoracica externa
a.v. axillaris
a. cervicalis superficialis
lnn. cervicales profundi caudales
m. rectus thoracis
m. subclavius
m. pectoralis descendens
m. pectoralis transversus
m. pectoralis ascendens
a. thoracica interna
rr. intercostales ventrales
m. obliquus externus abdominis
mm. levatores costarum
m. retractor costae
rib 18
costal cartilage, rib 18
diaphragm:
central tendon
costal part
left lung:
dorsal border
caudal (basal) border
cranial lobe
cranial border
caudal lobe
m. transversus abdominis
costal arch
mm. intercostales interni (cut away along diaphragmatic line of pleural reflection)
m. rectus abdominis

Fig. 4.14 The topography of the thorax: left lateral view. The intercostal muscles, endothoracic fascia and pleura of the intercostal spaces have been removed to show the ribs and the thoracic viscera.

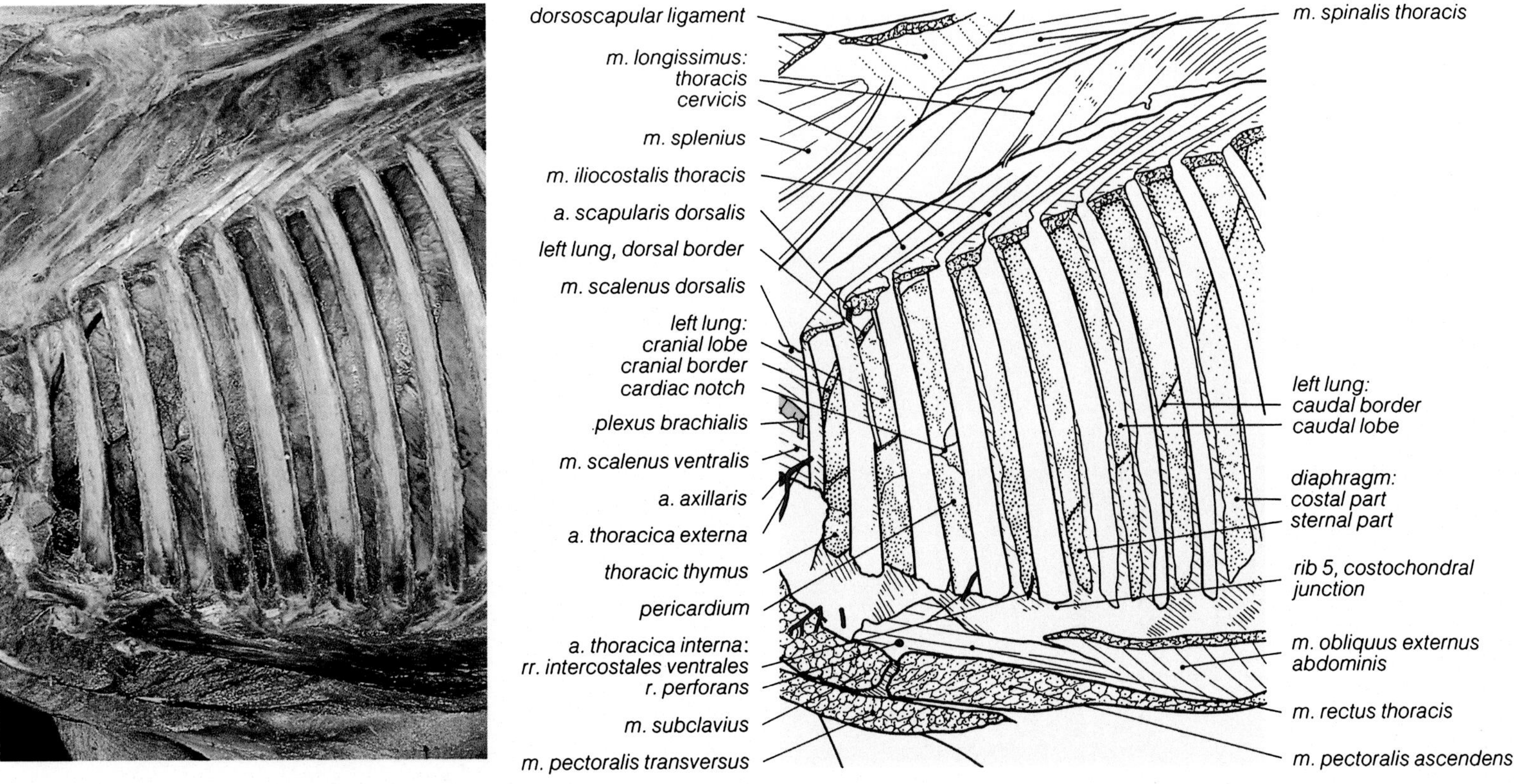

dorsoscapular ligament
m. longissimus:
thoracis
cervicis
m. splenius
m. iliocostalis thoracis
a. scapularis dorsalis
left lung, dorsal border
m. scalenus dorsalis
left lung:
cranial lobe
cranial border
cardiac notch
plexus brachialis
m. scalenus ventralis
a. axillaris
a. thoracica externa
thoracic thymus
pericardium
a. thoracica interna:
rr. intercostales ventrales
r. perforans
m. subclavius
m. pectoralis transversus
m. spinalis thoracis
left lung:
caudal border
caudal lobe
diaphragm:
costal part
sternal part
rib 5, costochondral junction
m. obliquus externus abdominis
m. rectus thoracis
m. pectoralis ascendens

Fig. 4.15 Thoracic viscera and ribs *in situ*, with the rib cage intact: left lateral view. This is a part of the specimen shown in Fig. 4.14. In this yearling horse, the thoracic thymus was still large; this structure regresses after the first year of life.

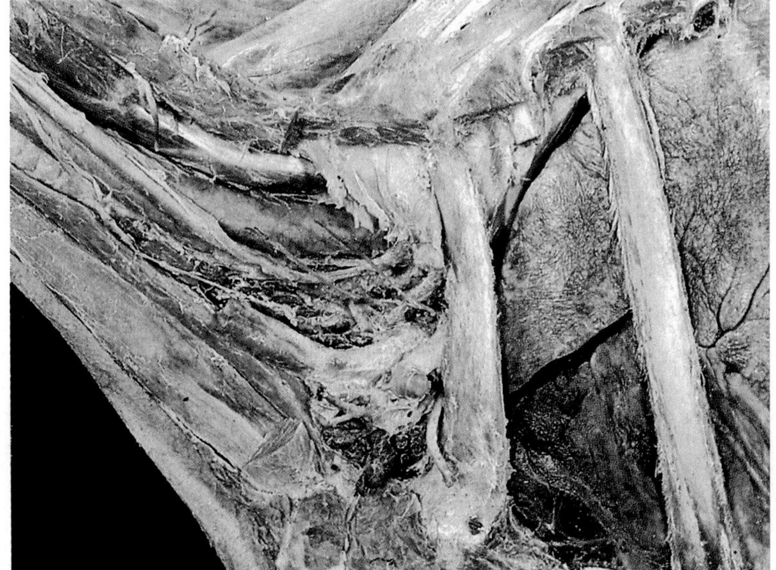

Fig. 4.16 The thoracic inlet: deeper structures: left lateral view. This is a closer view of a part of the dissection shown in Fig. 4.17. The dorsal and ventral scalenus muscles have been removed.

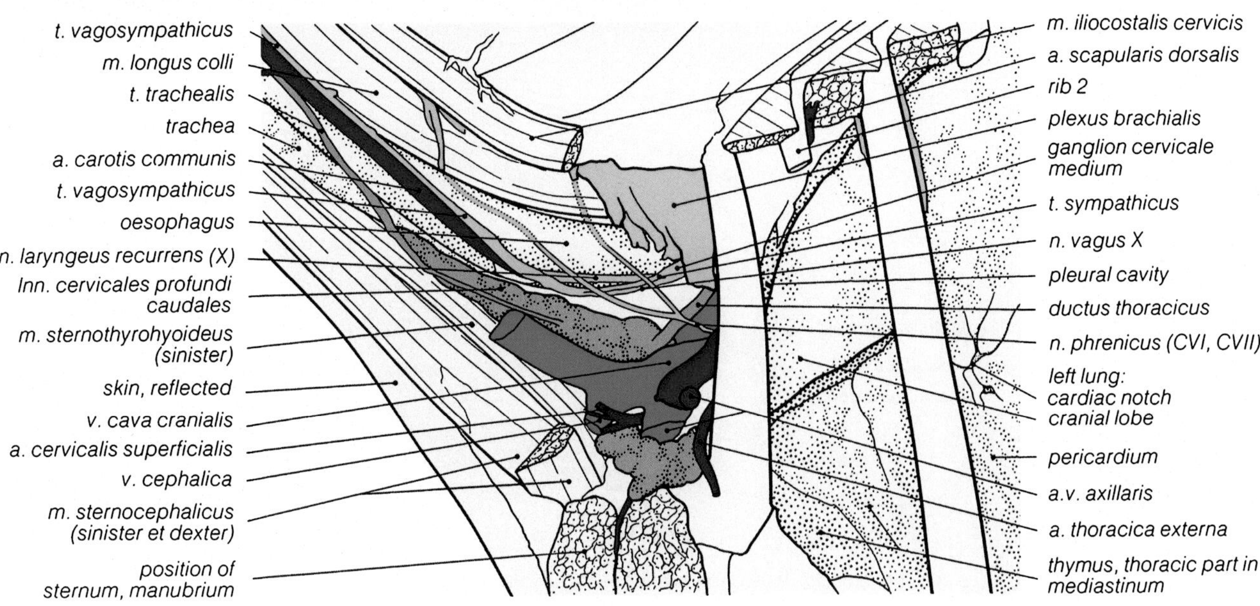

t. vagosympathicus
m. longus colli
t. trachealis
trachea
a. carotis communis
t. vagosympathicus
oesophagus
n. laryngeus recurrens (X)
lnn. cervicales profundi caudales
m. sternothyrohyoideus (sinister)
skin, reflected
v. cava cranialis
a. cervicalis superficialis
v. cephalica
m. sternocephalicus (sinister et dexter)
position of sternum, manubrium
m. iliocostalis cervicis
a. scapularis dorsalis
rib 2
plexus brachialis
ganglion cervicale medium
t. sympathicus
n. vagus X
pleural cavity
ductus thoracicus
n. phrenicus (CVI, CVII)
left lung:
cardiac notch
cranial lobe
pericardium
a.v. axillaris
a. thoracica externa
thymus, thoracic part in mediastinum

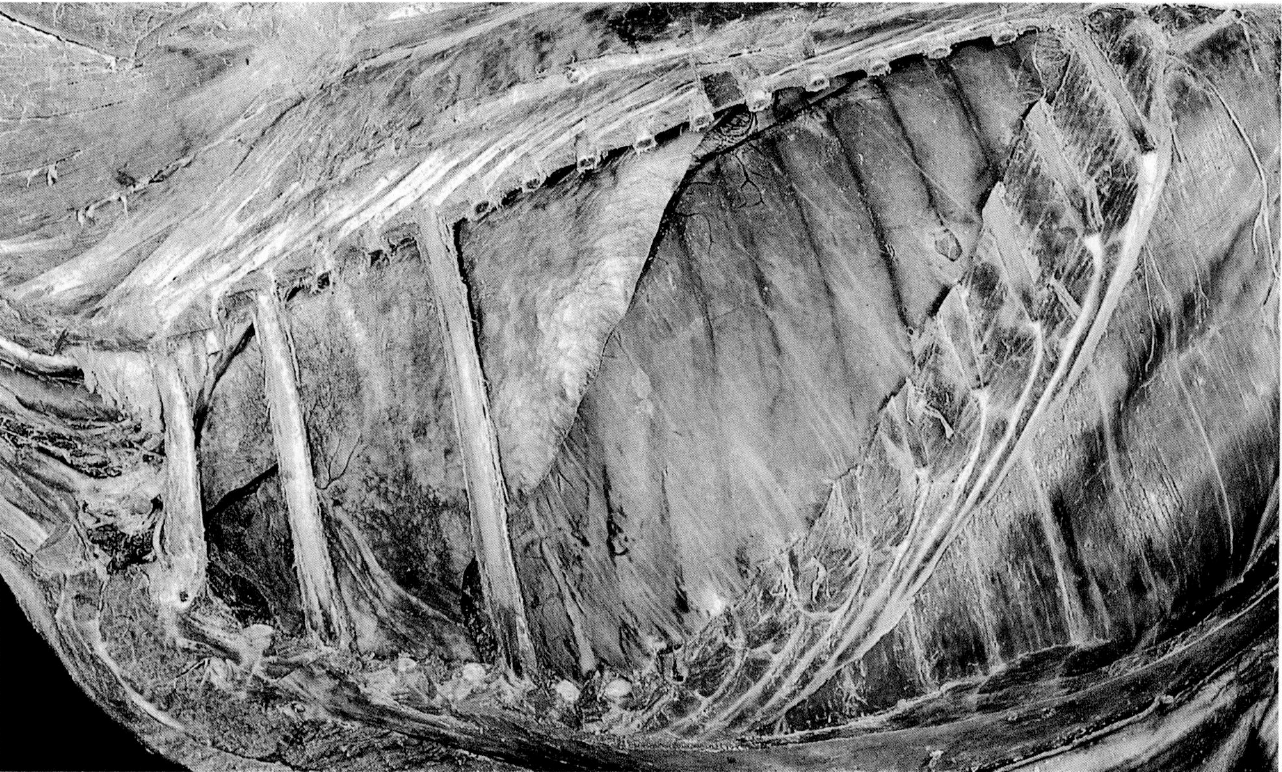

Fig. 4.17 Thoracic viscera *in situ*: left lateral view. Ribs 1, 3 and 6 have been left in place to show the costal relationships of the viscera. The lungs have been fixed in a contracted position. In life, the caudal, or basal, border lies more caudally, as shown by the broken blue line: its position varies with the respiratory movements.

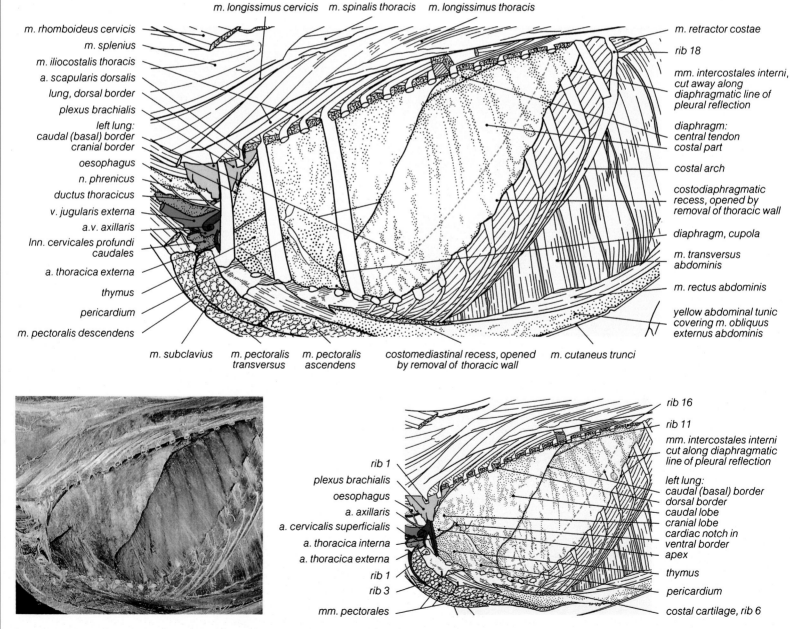

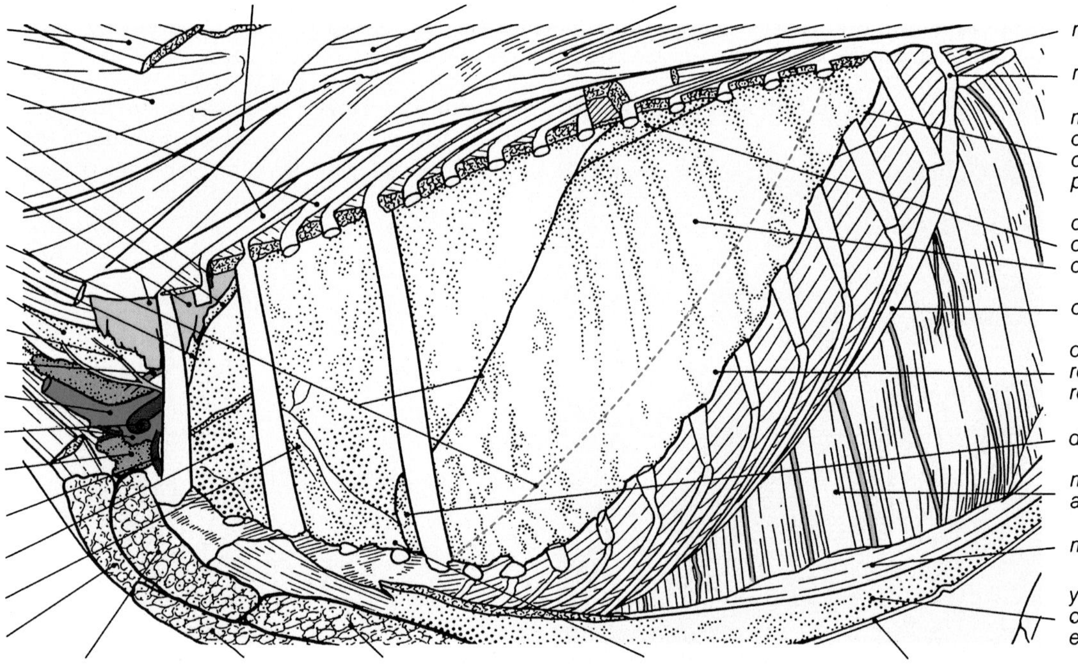

m. longissimus cervicis
m. spinalis thoracis
m. longissimus thoracis
m. rhomboideus cervicis
m. splenius
m. iliocostalis thoracis
a. scapularis dorsalis
lung, dorsal border
plexus brachialis
left lung:
caudal (basal) border
cranial border
oesophagus
n. phrenicus
ductus thoracicus
v. jugularis externa
a.v. axillaris
lnn. cervicales profundi caudales
a. thoracica externa
thymus
pericardium
m. pectoralis descendens
m. subclavius
m. pectoralis transversus
m. pectoralis ascendens
costomediastinal recess, opened by removal of thoracic wall
m. cutaneus trunci
m. retractor costae
rib 18
mm. intercostales interni, cut away along diaphragmatic line of pleural reflection
diaphragm:
central tendon
costal part
costal arch
costodiaphragmatic recess, opened by removal of thoracic wall
diaphragm, cupola
m. transversus abdominis
m. rectus abdominis
yellow abdominal tunic covering m. obliquus externus abdominis

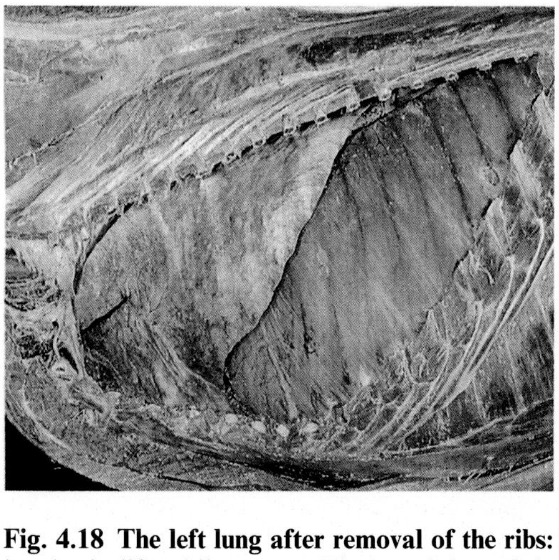

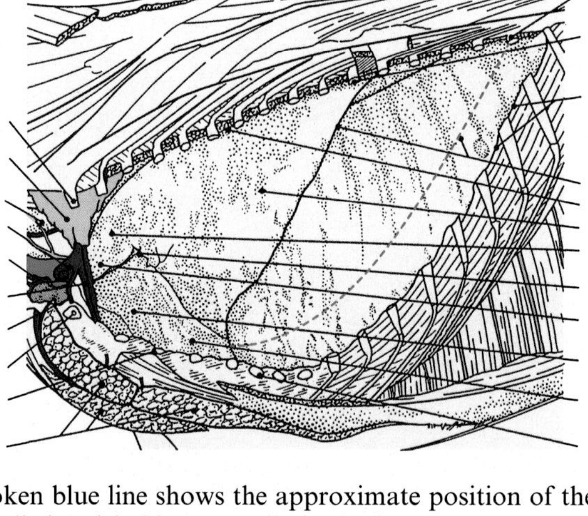

rib 16
rib 11
mm. intercostales interni cut along diaphragmatic line of pleural reflection
left lung:
caudal (basal) border
dorsal border
caudal lobe
cranial lobe
cardiac notch in ventral border
apex
thymus
pericardium
costal cartilage, rib 6
rib 1
plexus brachialis
oesophagus
a. axillaris
a. cervicalis superficialis
a. thoracica interna
a. thoracica externa
rib 1
rib 3
mm. pectorales

Fig. 4.18 The left lung after removal of the ribs: left lateral view. The broken blue line shows the approximate position of the caudal, or basal, border in life while at rest. The two lobes of the left lung are not clearly distinguishable externally in the horse.

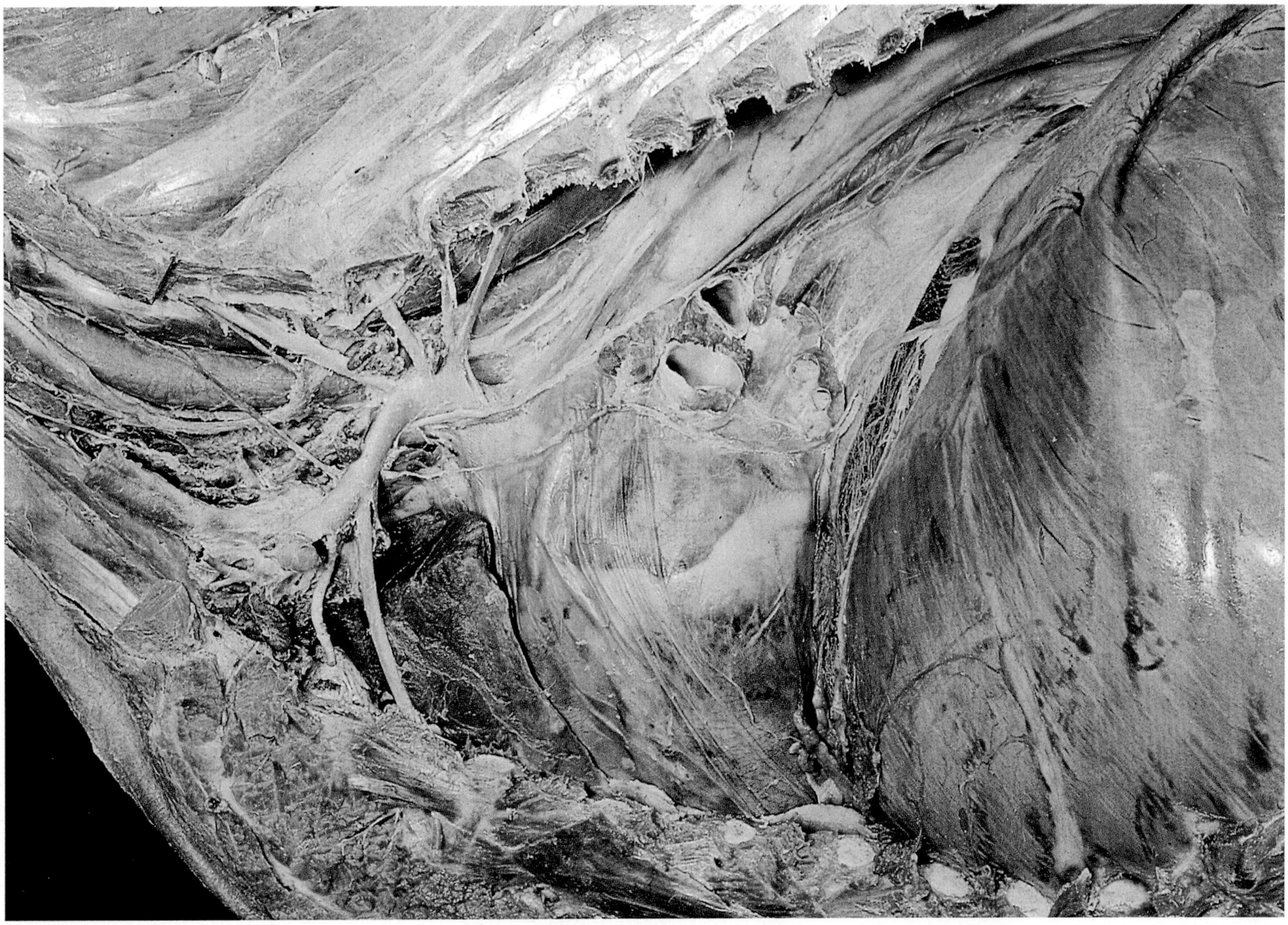

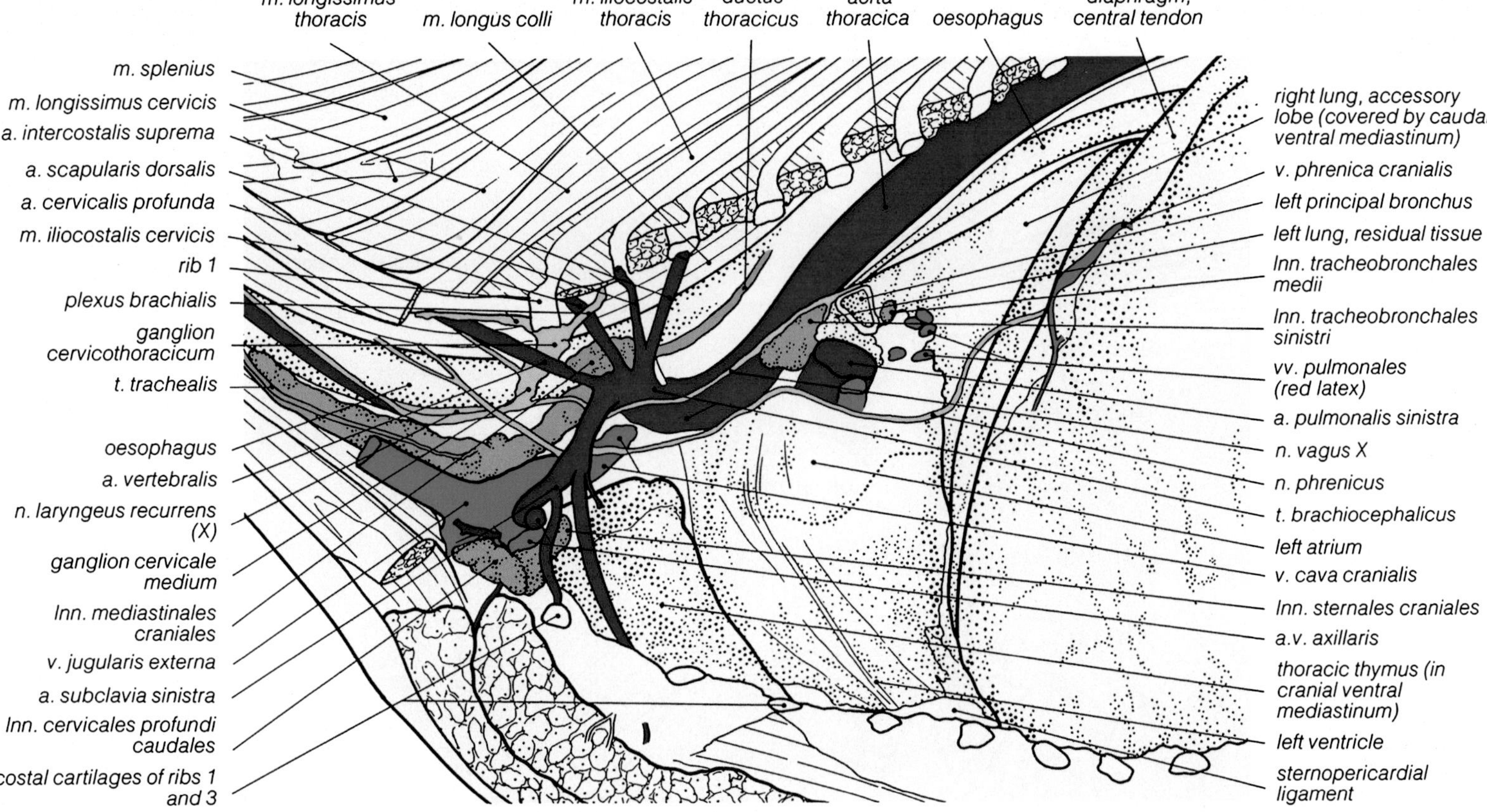
m. longissimus thoracis
m. longus colli
m. iliocostalis thoracis
ductus thoracicus
aorta thoracica
oesophagus
diaphragm, central tendon
m. splenius
m. longissimus cervicis
a. intercostalis suprema
a. scapularis dorsalis
a. cervicalis profunda
m. iliocostalis cervicis
rib 1
plexus brachialis
ganglion cervicothoracicum
t. trachealis
oesophagus
a. vertebralis
n. laryngeus recurrens (X)
ganglion cervicale medium
lnn. mediastinales craniales
v. jugularis externa
a. subclavia sinistra
lnn. cervicales profundi caudales
costal cartilages of ribs 1 and 3
right lung, accessory lobe (covered by caudal ventral mediastinum)
v. phrenica cranialis
left principal bronchus
left lung, residual tissue
lnn. tracheobronchales medii
lnn. tracheobronchales sinistri
vv. pulmonales (red latex)
a. pulmonalis sinistra
n. vagus X
n. phrenicus
t. brachiocephalicus
left atrium
v. cava cranialis
lnn. sternales craniales
a.v. axillaris
thoracic thymus (in cranial ventral mediastinum)
left ventricle
sternopericardial ligament

Fig. 4.19 The mediastinum after removal of the left lung: left lateral view. The lung has been removed at its hilus, leaving only a small remnant of lung tissue between the cut ends of its pulmonary artery and principal bronchus. The pulmonary veins have been filled with red latex injected into the right common carotid artery; it has filled the left ventricle, penetrated the left atrium (see Fig. 4.25) and so entered the pulmonary veins. Further details of the structures in this dissection are shown in Fig. 4.20 (see also Fig. 4.21).

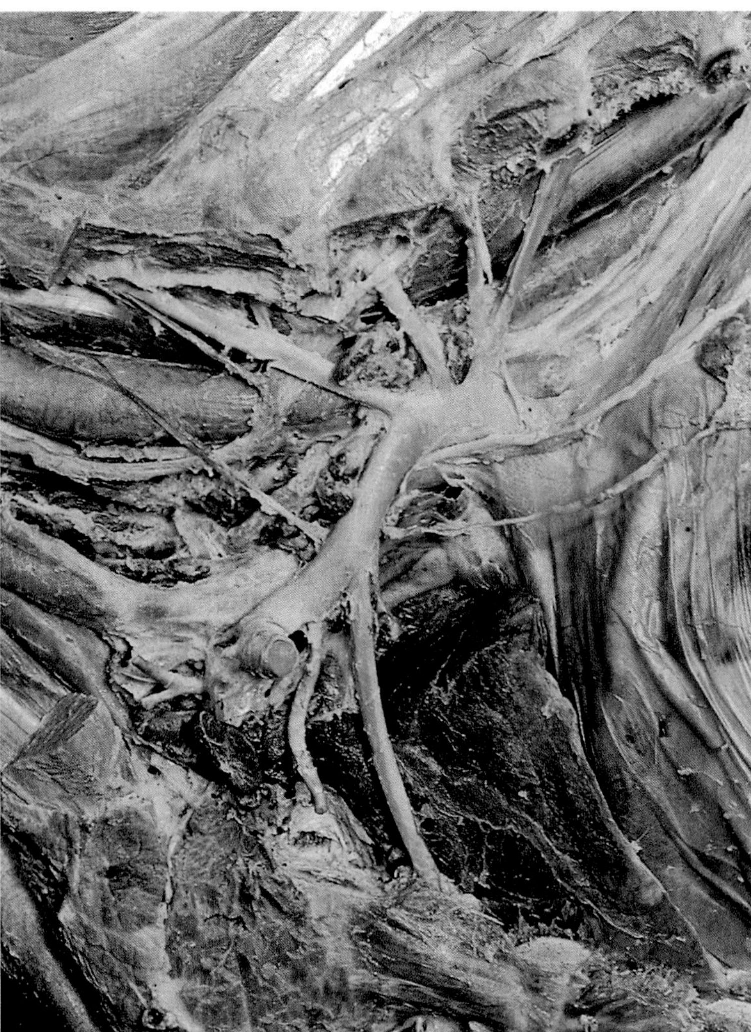

Fig. 4.20 Vessels and nerves of the cranial mediastinum: left lateral view. This is a closer view of a part of the dissection shown in Fig. 4.19. A further stage in the dissection of this region is shown in Fig. 4.24.

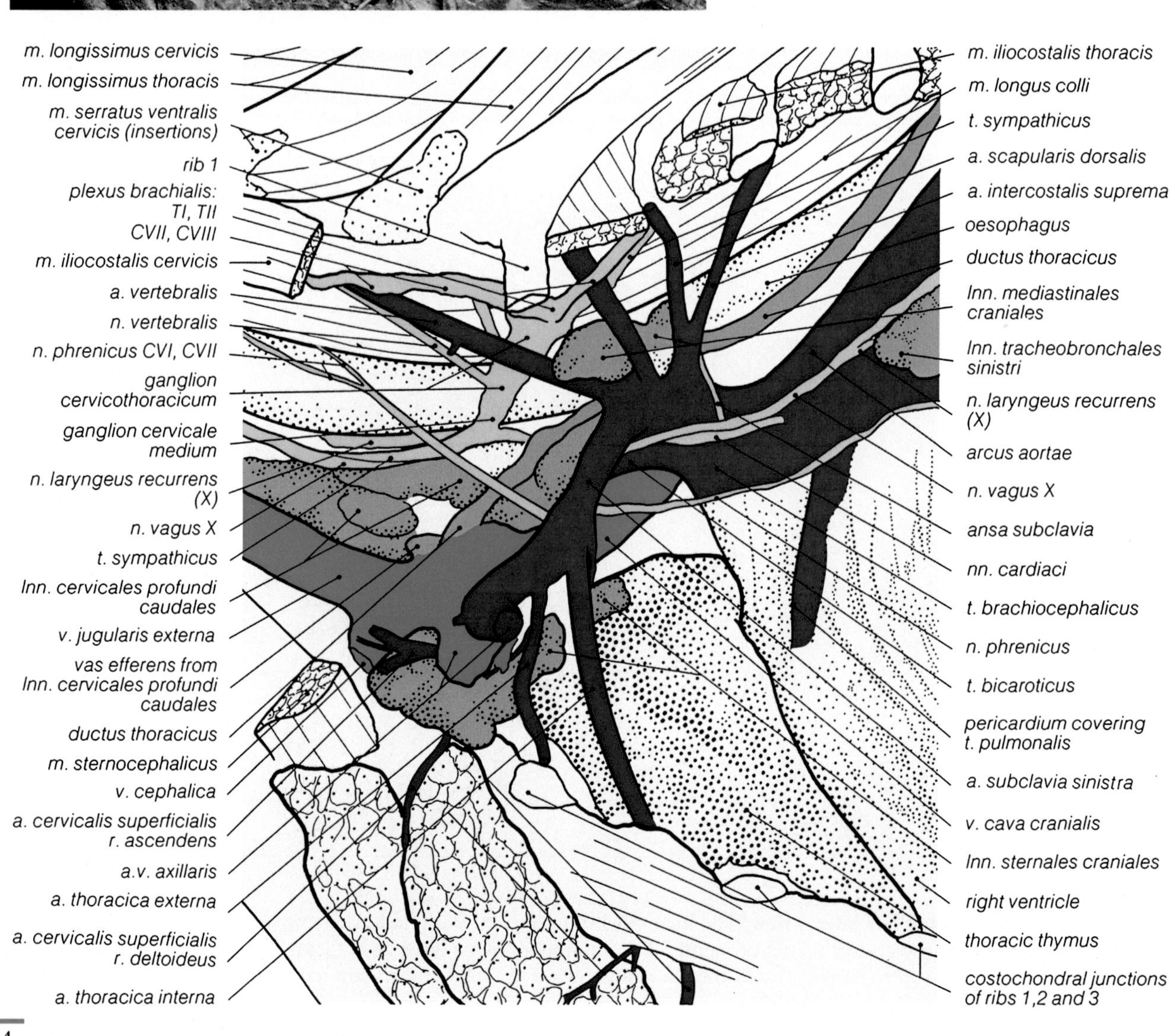
m. longissimus cervicis
m. longissimus thoracis
m. serratus ventralis cervicis (insertions)
rib 1
plexus brachialis: TI, TII CVII, CVIII
m. iliocostalis cervicis
a. vertebralis
n. vertebralis
n. phrenicus CVI, CVII
ganglion cervicothoracicum
ganglion cervicale medium
n. laryngeus recurrens (X)
n. vagus X
t. sympathicus
lnn. cervicales profundi caudales
v. jugularis externa
vas efferens from lnn. cervicales profundi caudales
ductus thoracicus
m. sternocephalicus
v. cephalica
a. cervicalis superficialis r. ascendens
a.v. axillaris
a. thoracica externa
a. cervicalis superficialis r. deltoideus
a. thoracica interna
m. iliocostalis thoracis
m. longus colli
t. sympathicus
a. scapularis dorsalis
a. intercostalis suprema
oesophagus
ductus thoracicus
lnn. mediastinales craniales
lnn. tracheobronchales sinistri
n. laryngeus recurrens (X)
arcus aortae
n. vagus X
ansa subclavia
nn. cardiaci
t. brachiocephalicus
n. phrenicus
t. bicaroticus
pericardium covering t. pulmonalis
a. subclavia sinistra
v. cava cranialis
lnn. sternales craniales
right ventricle
thoracic thymus
costochondral junctions of ribs 1,2 and 3

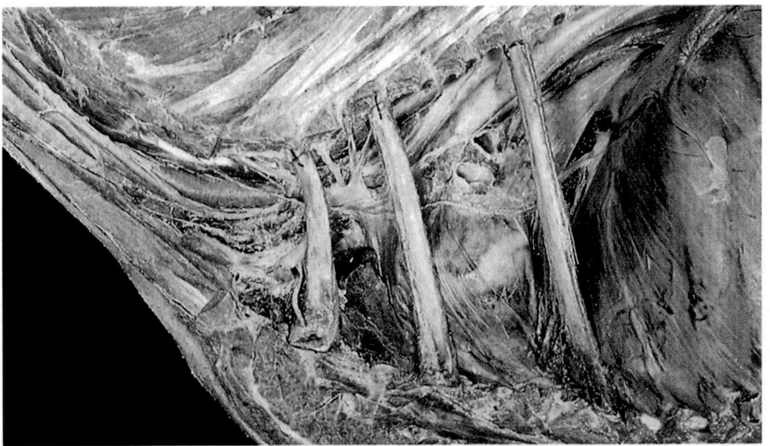

Fig. 4.21 Thoracic vessels and nerves in relation to the ribs: left lateral view. Three ribs have been pinned back into place, after dissection of the thoracic vessels and nerves, to facilitate location of these structures in relationship to the ribs. See also Fig. 4.19.

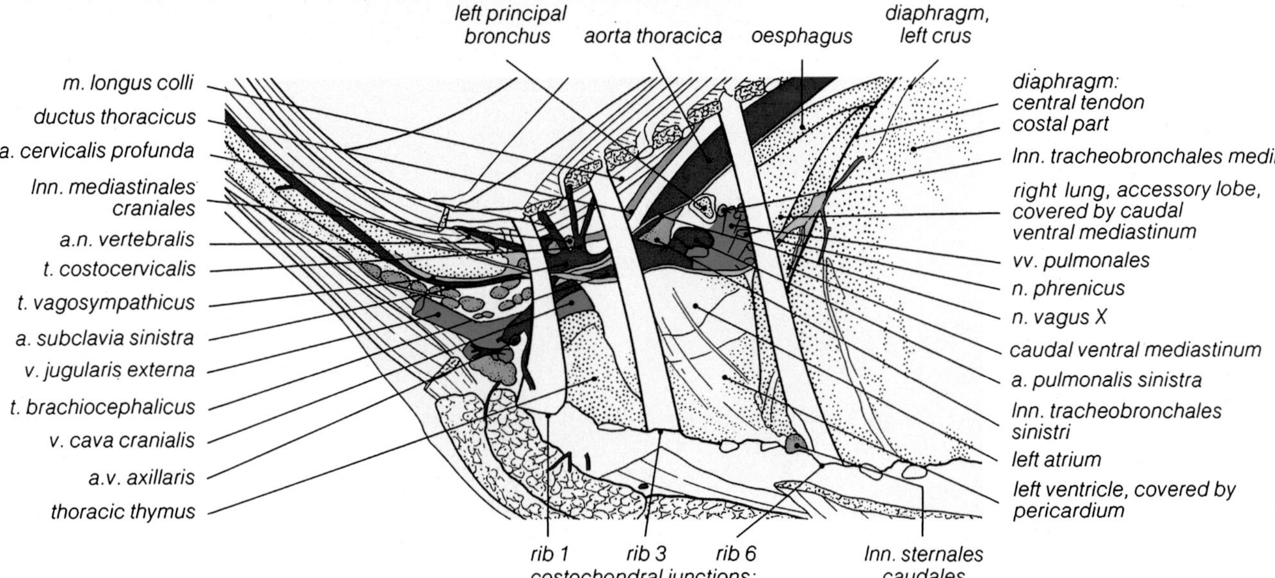
left principal bronchus
aorta thoracica
oesphagus
diaphragm, left crus
m. longus colli
ductus thoracicus
a. cervicalis profunda
lnn. mediastinales craniales
a.n. vertebralis
t. costocervicalis
t. vagosympathicus
a. subclavia sinistra
v. jugularis externa
t. brachiocephalicus
v. cava cranialis
a.v. axillaris
thoracic thymus
diaphragm: central tendon
costal part
lnn. tracheobronchales medii
right lung, accessory lobe, covered by caudal ventral mediastinum
vv. pulmonales
n. phrenicus
n. vagus X
caudal ventral mediastinum
a. pulmonalis sinistra
lnn. tracheobronchales sinistri
left atrium
left ventricle, covered by pericardium
rib 1
rib 3
rib 6
costochondral junctions:
lnn. sternales caudales

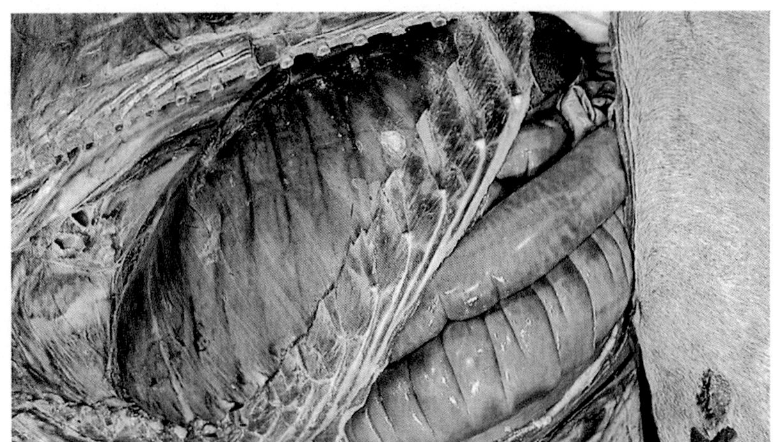

Fig. 4.22 The diaphragm and costal arch: left lateral view. The ribs and the internal intercostal muscles have been cut along the diaphragmatic line of pleural reflection to show the caudal extent of the pleural cavity. The costal attachments of the diaphragm are slightly more caudal, as shown in Fig. 5.15.

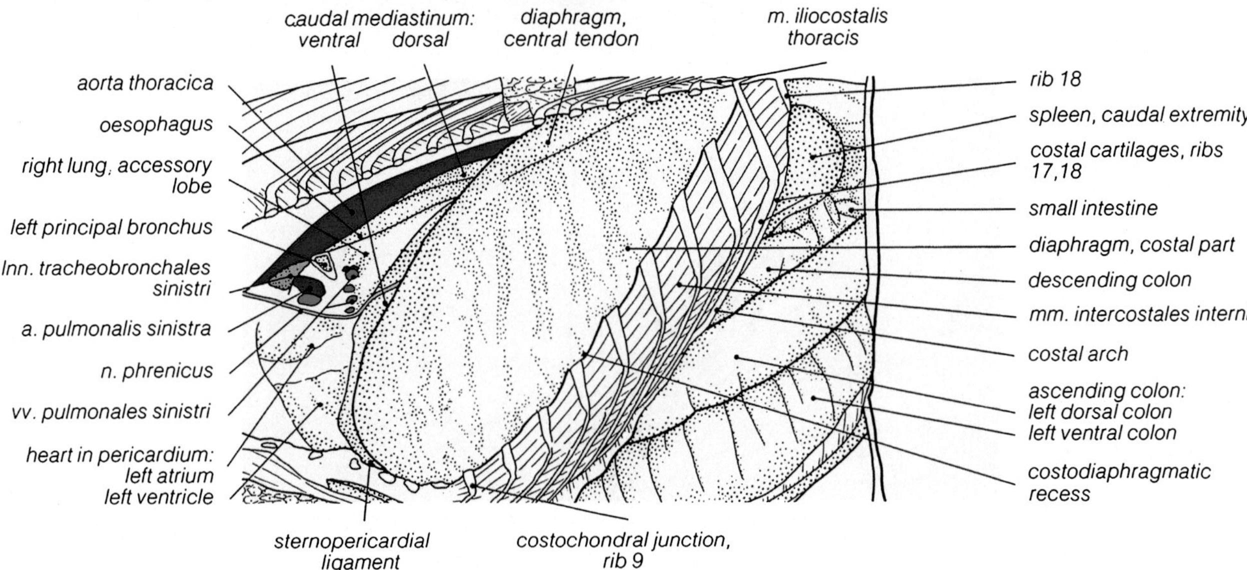
caudal mediastinum: ventral dorsal
diaphragm, central tendon
m. iliocostalis thoracis
aorta thoracica
oesophagus
right lung, accessory lobe
left principal bronchus
lnn. tracheobronchales sinistri
a. pulmonalis sinistra
n. phrenicus
vv. pulmonales sinistri
heart in pericardium: left atrium
left ventricle
rib 18
spleen, caudal extremity
costal cartilages, ribs 17,18
small intestine
diaphragm, costal part
descending colon
mm. intercostales interni
costal arch
ascending colon: left dorsal colon
left ventral colon
costodiaphragmatic recess
sternopericardial ligament
costochondral junction, rib 9

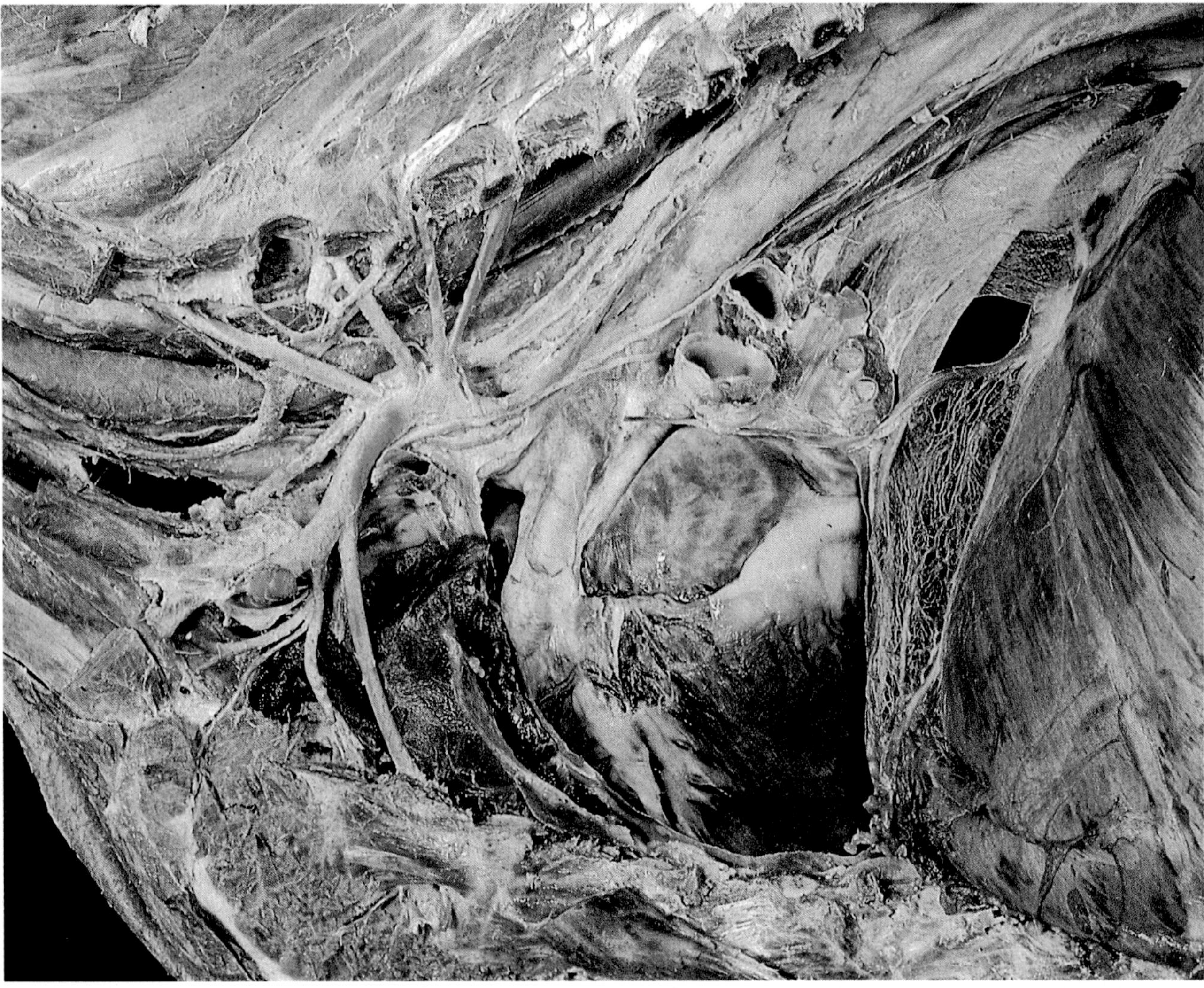

Fig. 4.23 The heart, great vessels and nerves of the thorax: left lateral view. The pericardium has been removed to display the left aspect of the heart. The head of the first rib has been removed to reveal the cervicothoracic (stellate) ganglion. The fragile ventral caudal mediastinum has been damaged during dissection.

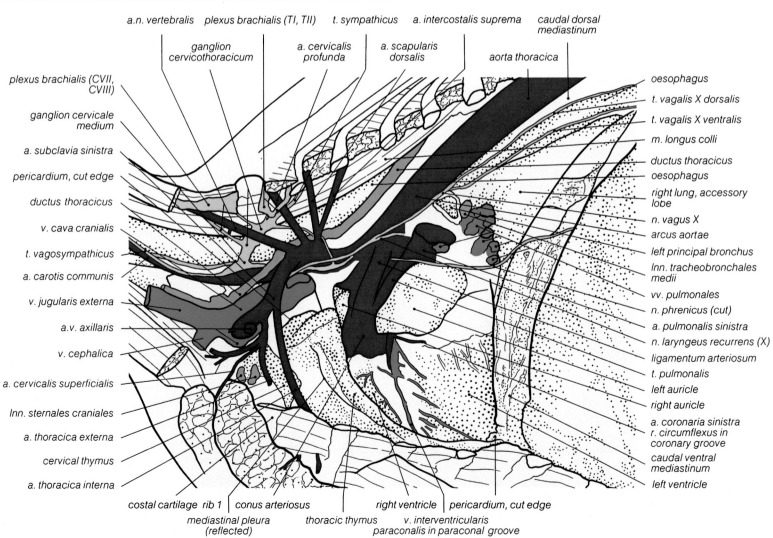

a.n. vertebralis
plexus brachialis (TI, TII)
t. sympathicus
a. intercostalis suprema
caudal dorsal mediastinum
ganglion cervicothoracicum
a. cervicalis profunda
a. scapularis dorsalis
aorta thoracica
plexus brachialis (CVII, CVIII)
ganglion cervicale medium
a. subclavia sinistra
pericardium, cut edge
ductus thoracicus
v. cava cranialis
t. vagosympathicus
a. carotis communis
v. jugularis externa
a.v. axillaris
v. cephalica
a. cervicalis superficialis
lnn. sternales craniales
a. thoracica externa
cervical thymus
a. thoracica interna
oesophagus
t. vagalis X dorsalis
t. vagalis X ventralis
m. longus colli
ductus thoracicus
oesophagus
right lung, accessory lobe
n. vagus X
arcus aortae
left principal bronchus
lnn. tracheobronchales medii
vv. pulmonales
n. phrenicus (cut)
a. pulmonalis sinistra
n. laryngeus recurrens (X)
ligamentum arteriosum
t. pulmonalis
left auricle
right auricle
a. coronaria sinistra r. circumflexus in coronary groove
caudal ventral mediastinum
left ventricle
costal cartilage rib 1
conus arteriosus
right ventricle
pericardium, cut edge
mediastinal pleura (reflected)
thoracic thymus
v. interventricularis paraconalis in paraconal groove

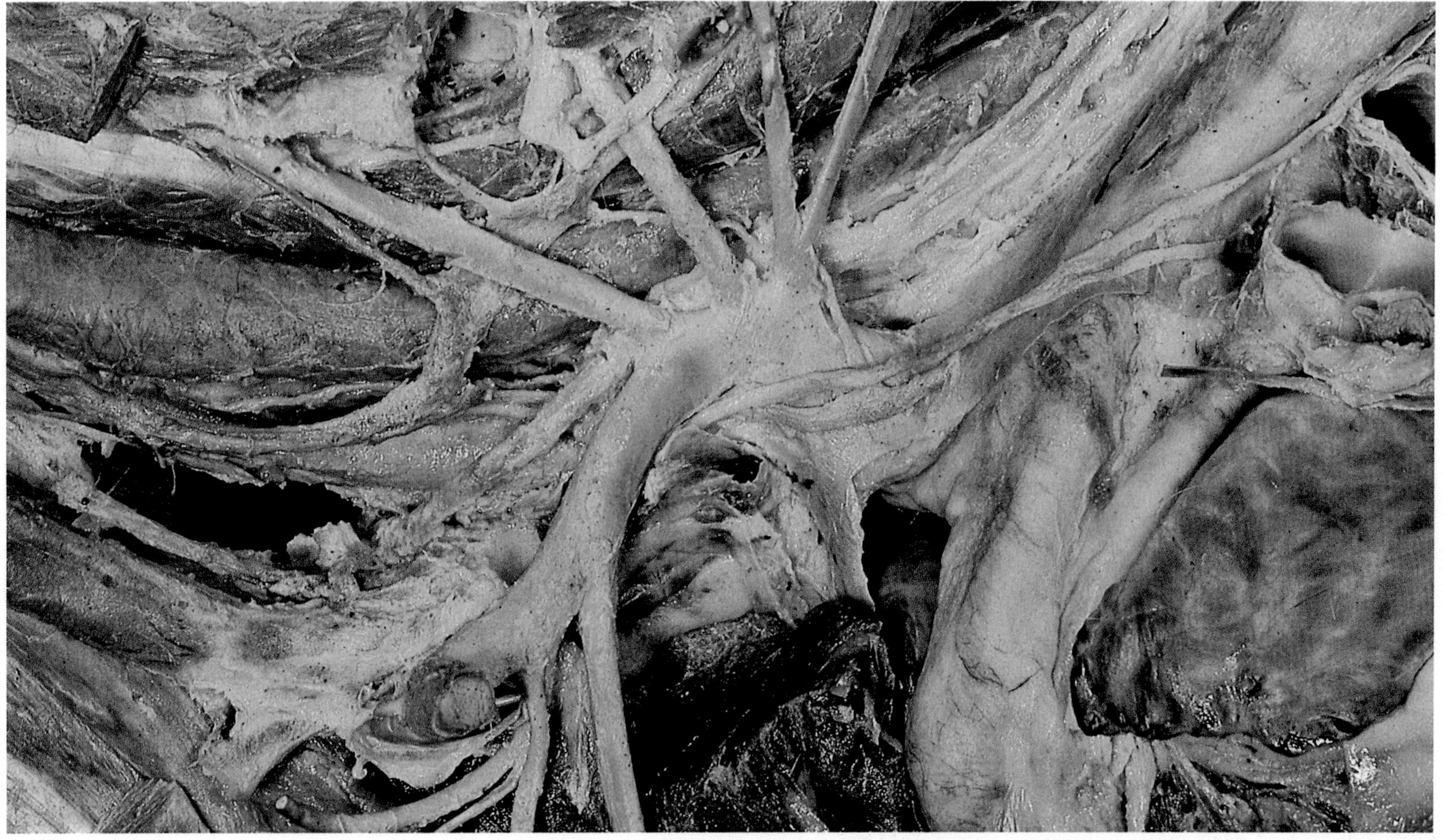

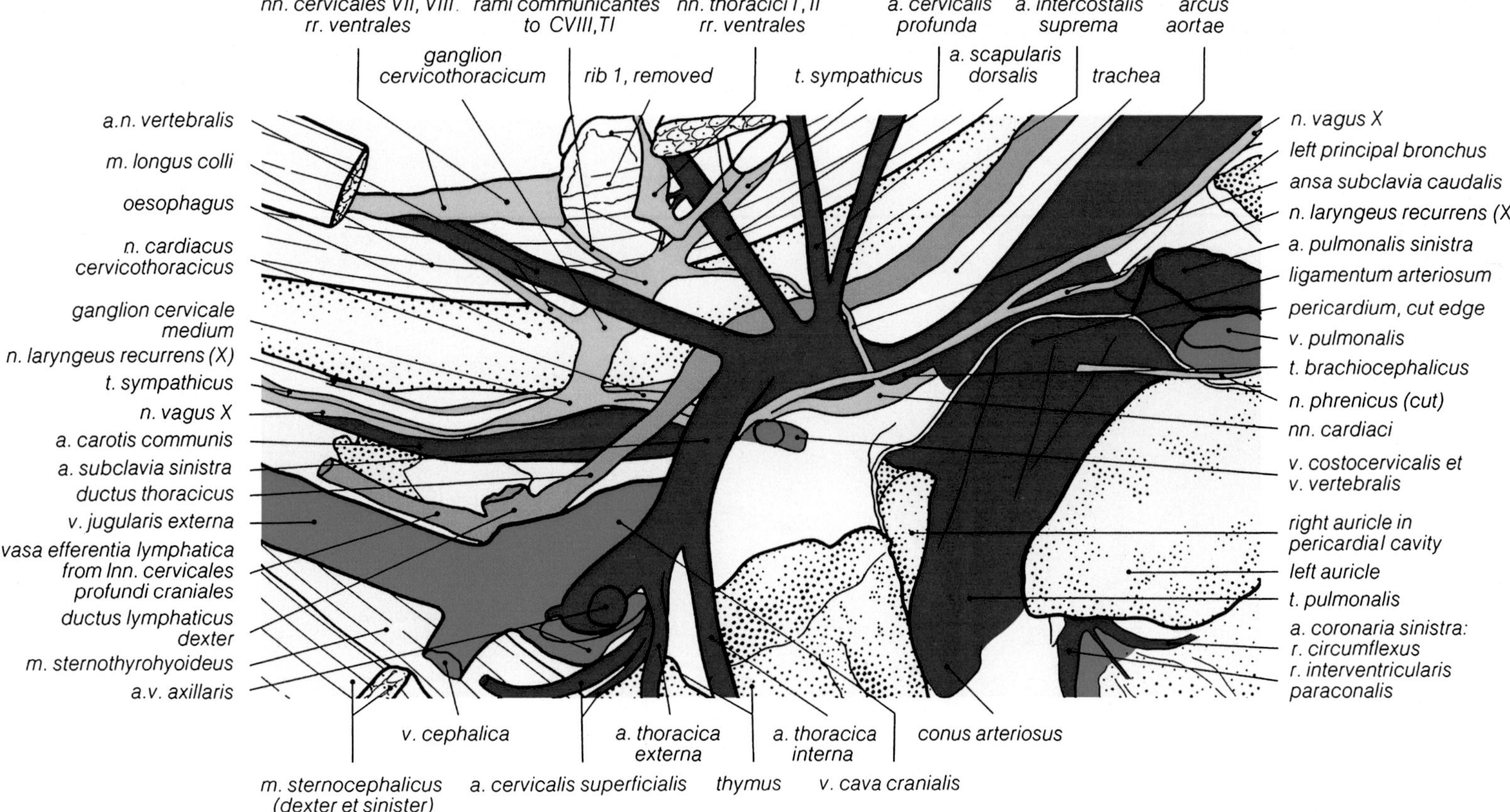
nn. cervicales VII, VIII. rr. ventrales
rami communicantes to CVIII,TI
nn. thoracici I, II rr. ventrales
a. cervicalis profunda
a. intercostalis suprema
arcus aortae
ganglion cervicothoracicum
rib 1, removed
t. sympathicus
a. scapularis dorsalis
trachea
a.n. vertebralis
m. longus colli
oesophagus
n. cardiacus cervicothoracicus
ganglion cervicale medium
n. laryngeus recurrens (X)
t. sympathicus
n. vagus X
a. carotis communis
a. subclavia sinistra
ductus thoracicus
v. jugularis externa
vasa efferentia lymphatica from lnn. cervicales profundi craniales
ductus lymphaticus dexter
m. sternothyrohyoideus
a.v. axillaris
n. vagus X
left principal bronchus
ansa subclavia caudalis
n. laryngeus recurrens (X)
a. pulmonalis sinistra
ligamentum arteriosum
pericardium, cut edge
v. pulmonalis
t. brachiocephalicus
n. phrenicus (cut)
nn. cardiaci
v. costocervicalis et v. vertebralis
right auricle in pericardial cavity
left auricle
t. pulmonalis
a. coronaria sinistra:
r. circumflexus
r. interventricularis paraconalis
v. cephalica
a. thoracica externa
a. thoracica interna
conus arteriosus
m. sternocephalicus (dexter et sinister)
a. cervicalis superficialis
thymus
v. cava cranialis

Fig. 4.24 Vessels and nerves of the cranial mediastinum: left lateral view. This is a closer view of a part of the specimen shown in Fig. 4.23. The phrenic nerve has been cut short: its position is shown in Fig. 4.20.

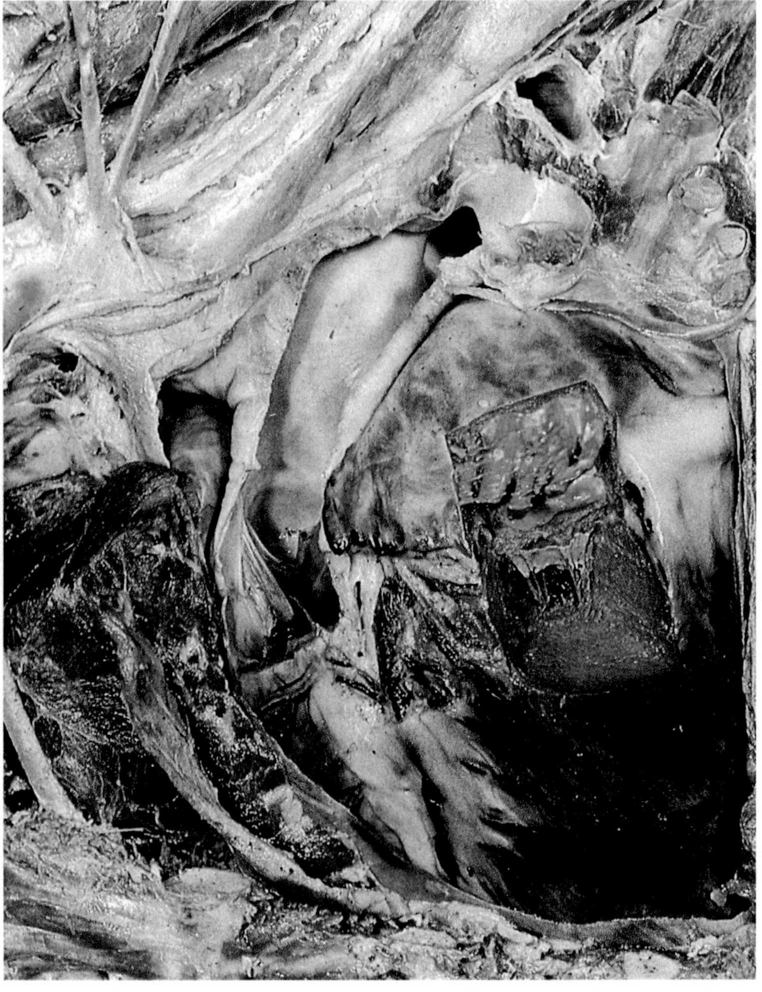

Fig. 4.25 Positions of the left atrioventricular and pulmonary heart valves: left lateral view. A window has been cut in the walls of the left atrium and left ventricle to show the left atrioventricular valve. Note that red latex injected into the right common carotid artery has entered the left ventricle, passed through the atrioventricular valve and filled the left atrium and the pulmonary veins. The pulmonary trunk and conus arteriosus have been opened: red latex has not traversed the pulmonary capillaries.

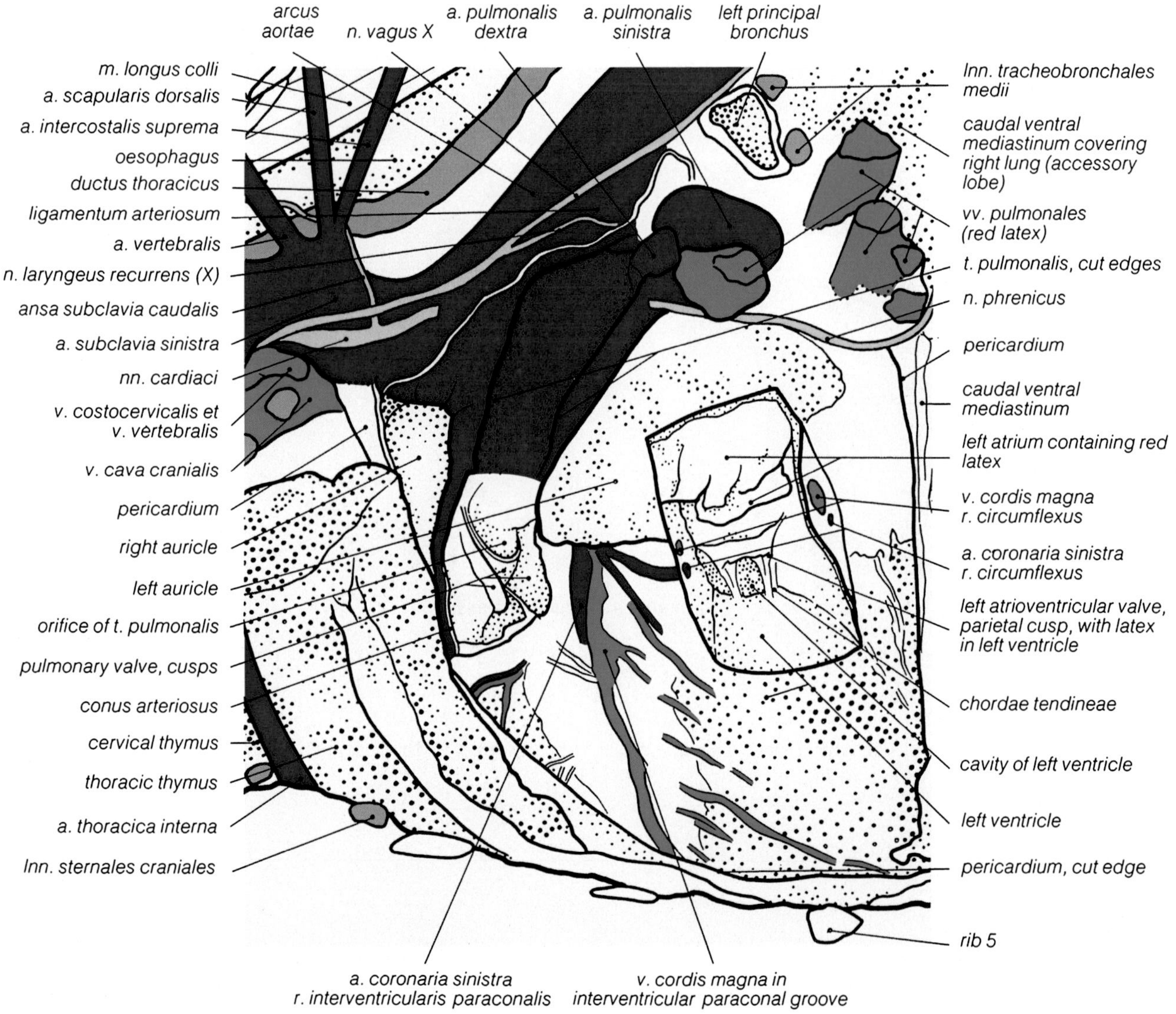

arcus aortae
n. vagus X
a. pulmonalis dextra
a. pulmonalis sinistra
left principal bronchus
m. longus colli
a. scapularis dorsalis
a. intercostalis suprema
oesophagus
ductus thoracicus
ligamentum arteriosum
a. vertebralis
n. laryngeus recurrens (X)
ansa subclavia caudalis
a. subclavia sinistra
nn. cardiaci
v. costocervicalis et v. vertebralis
v. cava cranialis
pericardium
right auricle
left auricle
orifice of t. pulmonalis
pulmonary valve, cusps
conus arteriosus
cervical thymus
thoracic thymus
a. thoracica interna
lnn. sternales craniales
lnn. tracheobronchales medii
caudal ventral mediastinum covering right lung (accessory lobe)
vv. pulmonales (red latex)
t. pulmonalis, cut edges
n. phrenicus
pericardium
caudal ventral mediastinum
left atrium containing red latex
v. cordis magna r. circumflexus
a. coronaria sinistra r. circumflexus
left atrioventricular valve, parietal cusp, with latex in left ventricle
chordae tendineae
cavity of left ventricle
left ventricle
pericardium, cut edge
rib 5
a. coronaria sinistra r. interventricularis paraconalis
v. cordis magna in interventricular paraconal groove

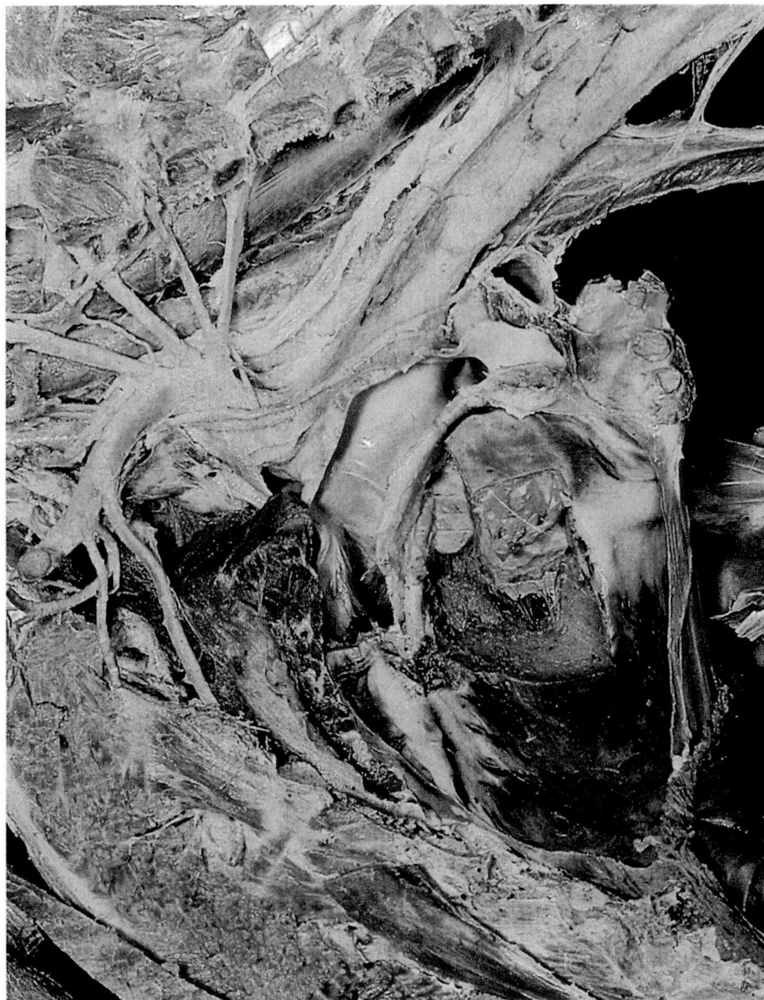

Fig. 4.26 Positions of the aortic and pulmonary valves: left lateral view. The cranial part of the left atrium has been removed to show the aortic valve lying caudodorsal to the pulmonary valve at the level of the fourth rib.

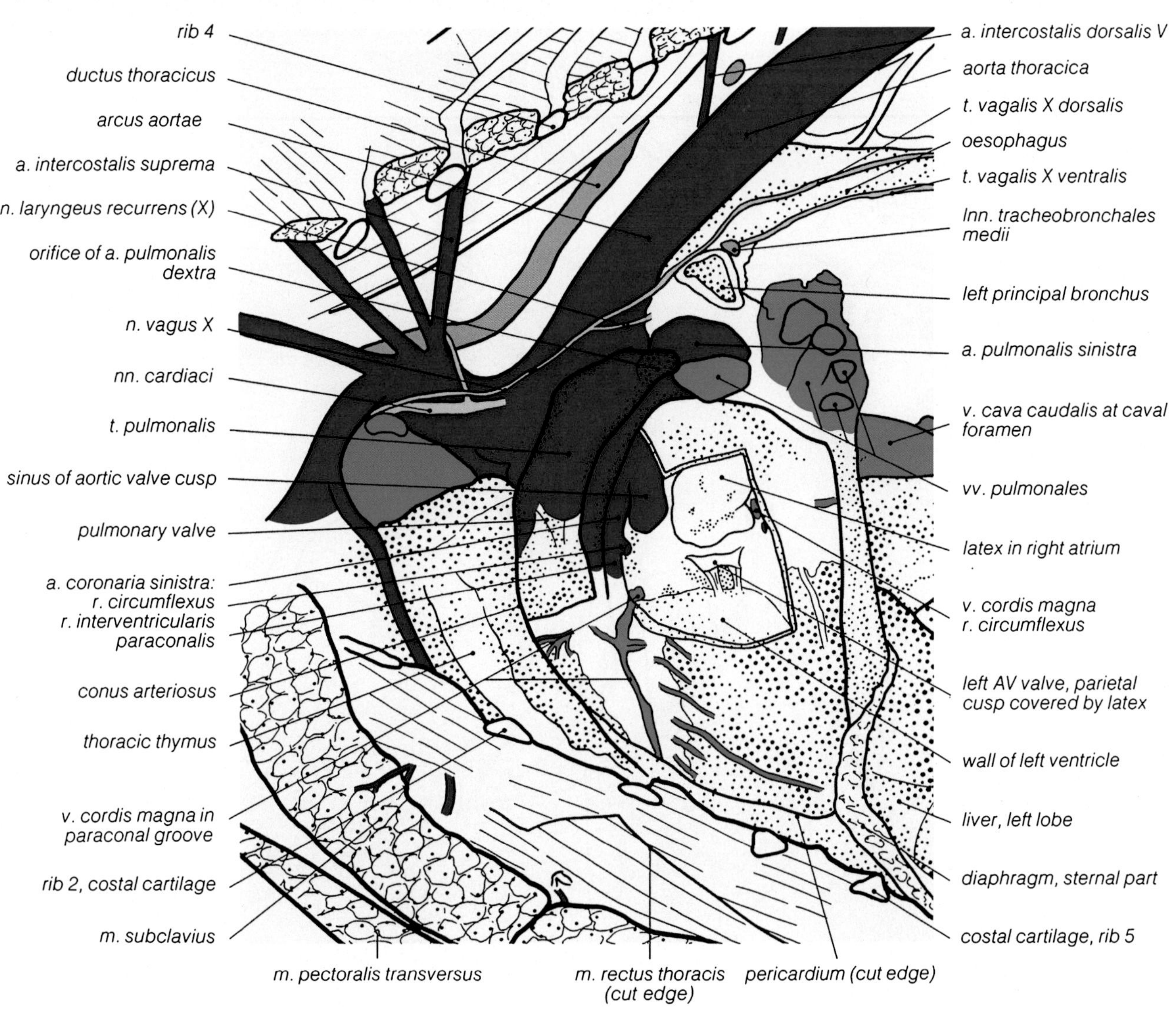
rib 4
ductus thoracicus
arcus aortae
a. intercostalis suprema
n. laryngeus recurrens (X)
orifice of a. pulmonalis dextra
n. vagus X
nn. cardiaci
t. pulmonalis
sinus of aortic valve cusp
pulmonary valve
a. coronaria sinistra:
r. circumflexus
r. interventricularis paraconalis
conus arteriosus
thoracic thymus
v. cordis magna in paraconal groove
rib 2, costal cartilage
m. subclavius
m. pectoralis transversus
m. rectus thoracis (cut edge)
pericardium (cut edge)
a. intercostalis dorsalis V
aorta thoracica
t. vagalis X dorsalis
oesophagus
t. vagalis X ventralis
lnn. tracheobronchales medii
left principal bronchus
a. pulmonalis sinistra
v. cava caudalis at caval foramen
vv. pulmonales
latex in right atrium
v. cordis magna
r. circumflexus
left AV valve, parietal cusp covered by latex
wall of left ventricle
liver, left lobe
diaphragm, sternal part
costal cartilage, rib 5

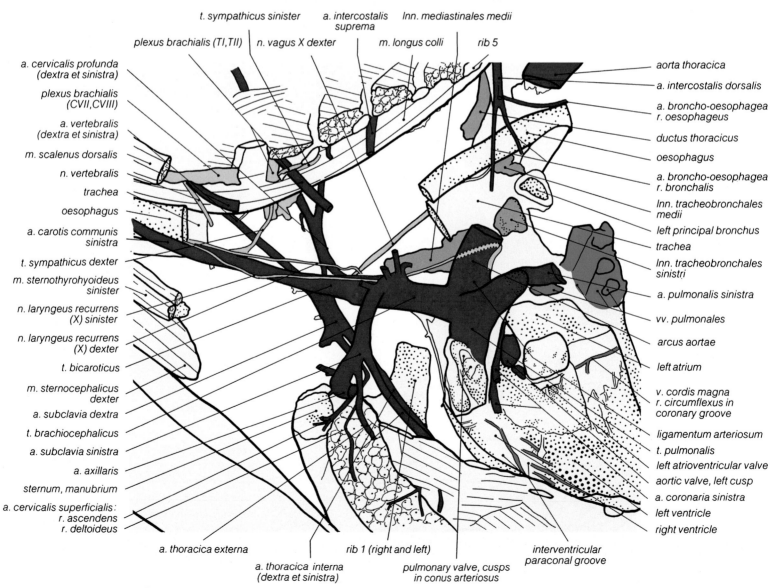

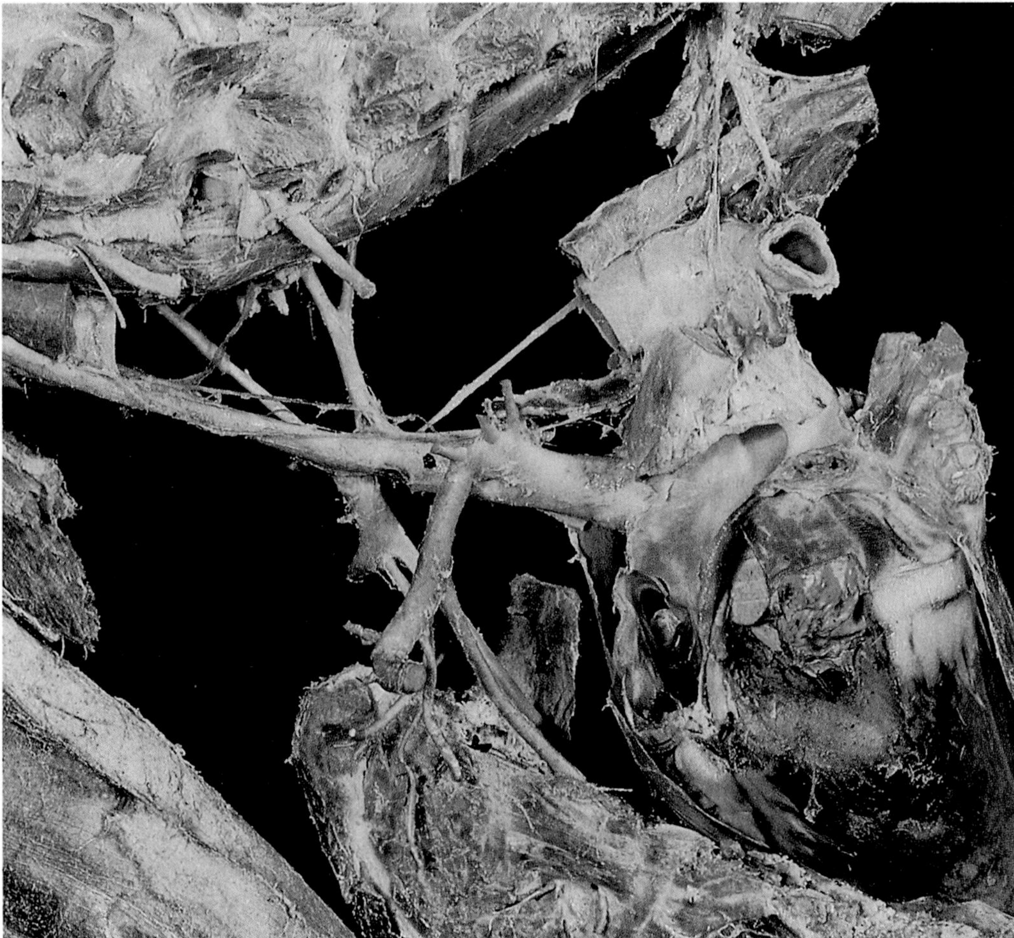
t. sympathicus sinister
a. intercostalis suprema
lnn. mediastinales medii
plexus brachialis (TI,TII)
n. vagus X dexter
m. longus colli
rib 5
a. cervicalis profunda (dextra et sinistra)
plexus brachialis (CVII,CVIII)
a. vertebralis (dextra et sinistra)
m. scalenus dorsalis
n. vertebralis
trachea
oesophagus
a. carotis communis sinistra
t. sympathicus dexter
m. sternothyrohyoideus sinister
n. laryngeus recurrens (X) sinister
n. laryngeus recurrens (X) dexter
t. bicaroticus
m. sternocephalicus dexter
a. subclavia dextra
t. brachiocephalicus
a. subclavia sinistra
a. axillaris
sternum, manubrium
a. cervicalis superficialis:
r. ascendens
r. deltoideus
a. thoracica externa
a. thoracica interna (dextra et sinistra)
rib 1 (right and left)
pulmonary valve, cusps in conus arteriosus
interventricular paraconal groove
aorta thoracica
a. intercostalis dorsalis
a. broncho-oesophagea r. oesophageus
ductus thoracicus
oesophagus
a. broncho-oesophagea r. bronchalis
lnn. tracheobronchales medii
left principal bronchus
trachea
lnn. tracheobronchales sinistri
a. pulmonalis sinistra
vv. pulmonales
arcus aortae
left atrium
v. cordis magna r. circumflexus in coronary groove
ligamentum arteriosum
t. pulmonalis
left atrioventricular valve
aortic valve, left cusp
a. coronaria sinistra
left ventricle
right ventricle

Fig. 4.27 The heart, arteries and recurrent laryngeal nerves: left lateral view. Both left and right sides of the rib cage have been removed and the topographical relationships of the thoracic structures are considerably disturbed. The oesophagus and trachea have been partially resected and the veins have been removed. The right side of this specimen is shown in Fig. 4.40.

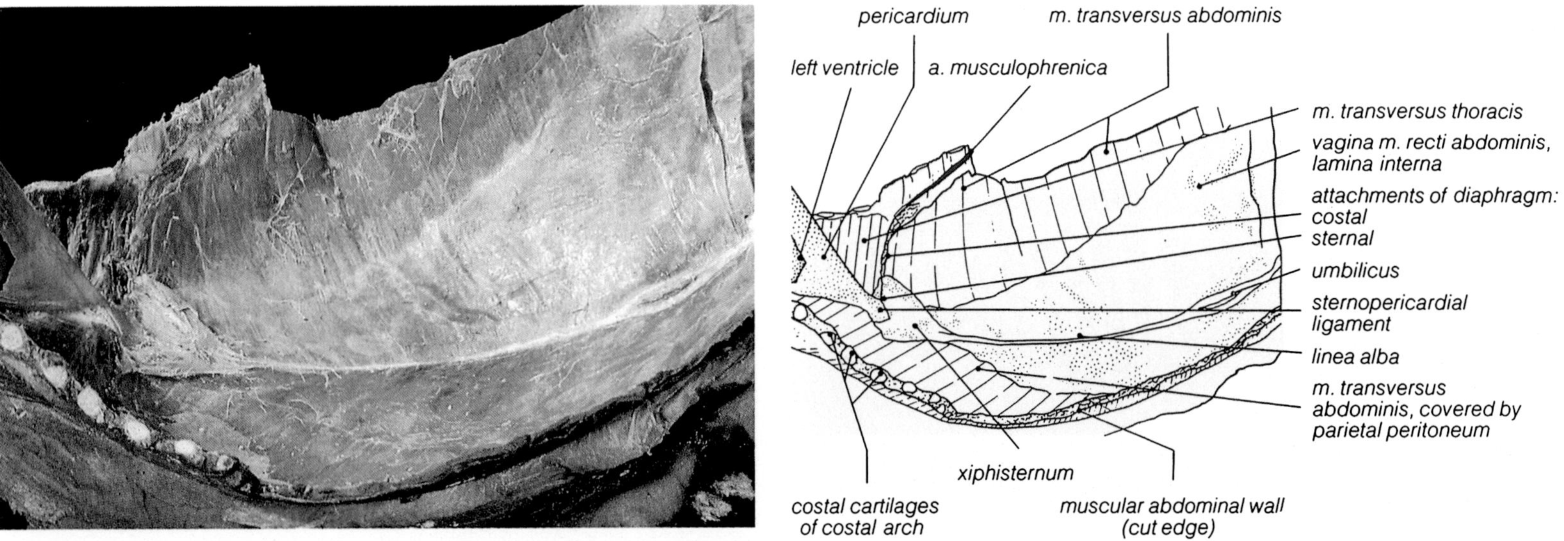
pericardium
m. transversus abdominis
left ventricle
a. musculophrenica
m. transversus thoracis
vagina m. recti abdominis, lamina interna
attachments of diaphragm: costal
sternal
umbilicus
sternopericardial ligament
linea alba
m. transversus abdominis, covered by parietal peritoneum
xiphisternum
costal cartilages of costal arch
muscular abdominal wall (cut edge)

Fig. 4.28 The sternopericardial ligament and abdominal floor: left dorsolateral view. The abdominal viscera and the diaphragm have been removed.

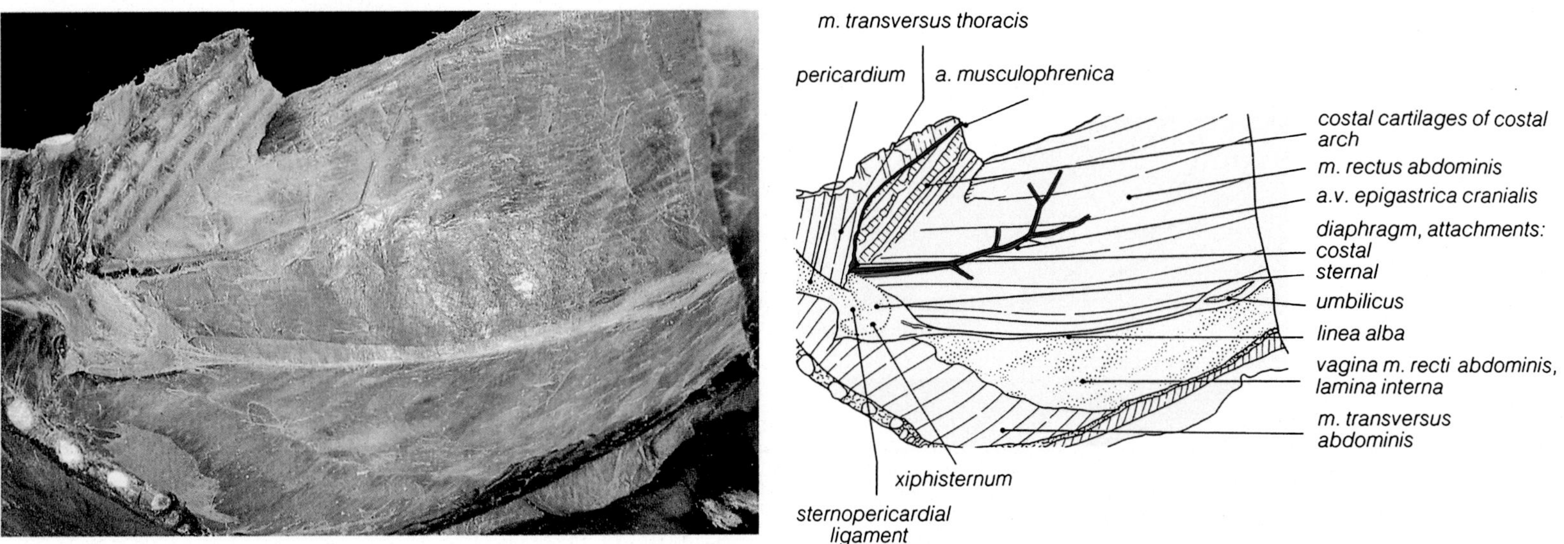
m. transversus thoracis
pericardium
a. musculophrenica
costal cartilages of costal arch
m. rectus abdominis
a.v. epigastrica cranialis
diaphragm, attachments: costal
sternal
umbilicus
linea alba
vagina m. recti abdominis, lamina interna
m. transversus abdominis
xiphisternum
sternopericardial ligament

Fig. 4.29 The terminal branches of the internal thoracic artery and abdominal floor: left dorsolateral view. The transverse abdominal muscle has been removed on the right side to display the cranial epigastric vessels.

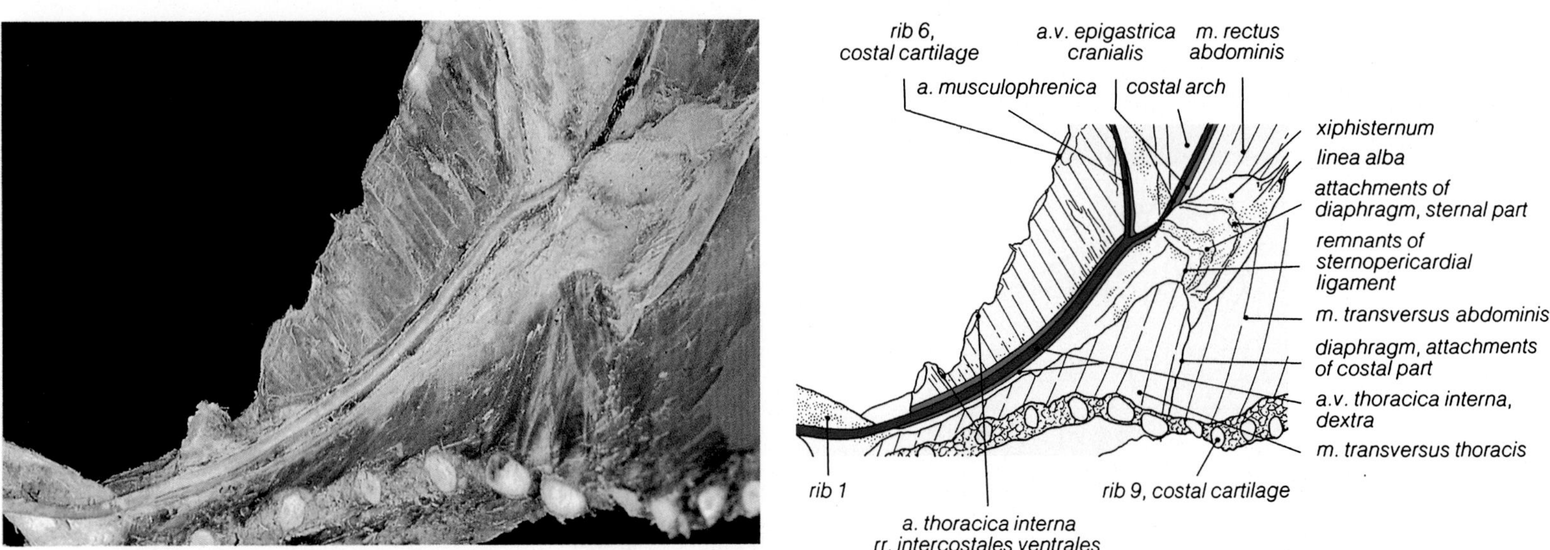
rib 6, costal cartilage
a.v. epigastrica cranialis
m. rectus abdominis
a. musculophrenica
costal arch
xiphisternum
linea alba
attachments of diaphragm, sternal part
remnants of sternopericardial ligament
m. transversus abdominis
diaphragm, attachments of costal part
a.v. thoracica interna, dextra
m. transversus thoracis
rib 1
rib 9, costal cartilage
a. thoracica interna rr. intercostales ventrales

Fig. 4.30 The thoracic floor: left dorsolateral view. After removal of the thoracic viscera and diaphragm, the right transverse thoracic muscle has been dissected to show the course of the internal thoracic vessels. The left internal thoracic vessels, running ventral to the transverse thoracic and abdominal muscles, have not been exposed.

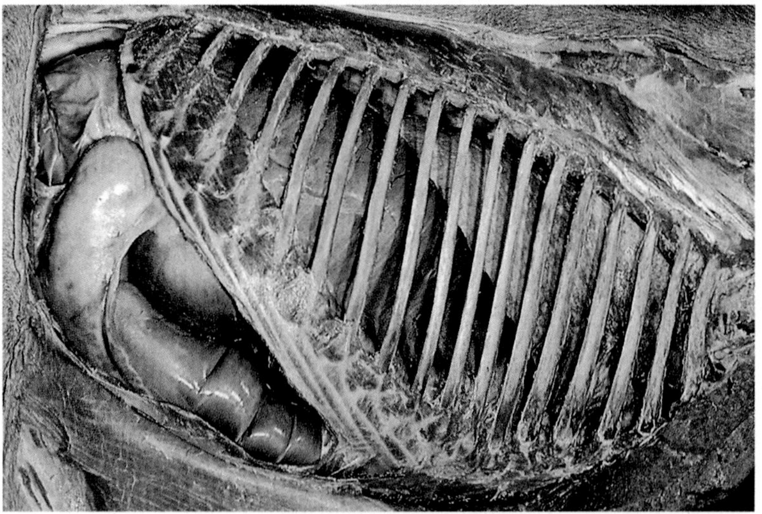

Fig. 4.31 The topography of the thorax: right lateral view. The iliocostalis and longissimus muscles have been partly cut away to show the angles of the ribs. It should be remembered that in life the first five ribs are covered by the forelimb; the olecranon lies adjacent to the costochondral junction of the fifth rib in normal level standing (see Figs. 4.2, 4.3 and 4.4).

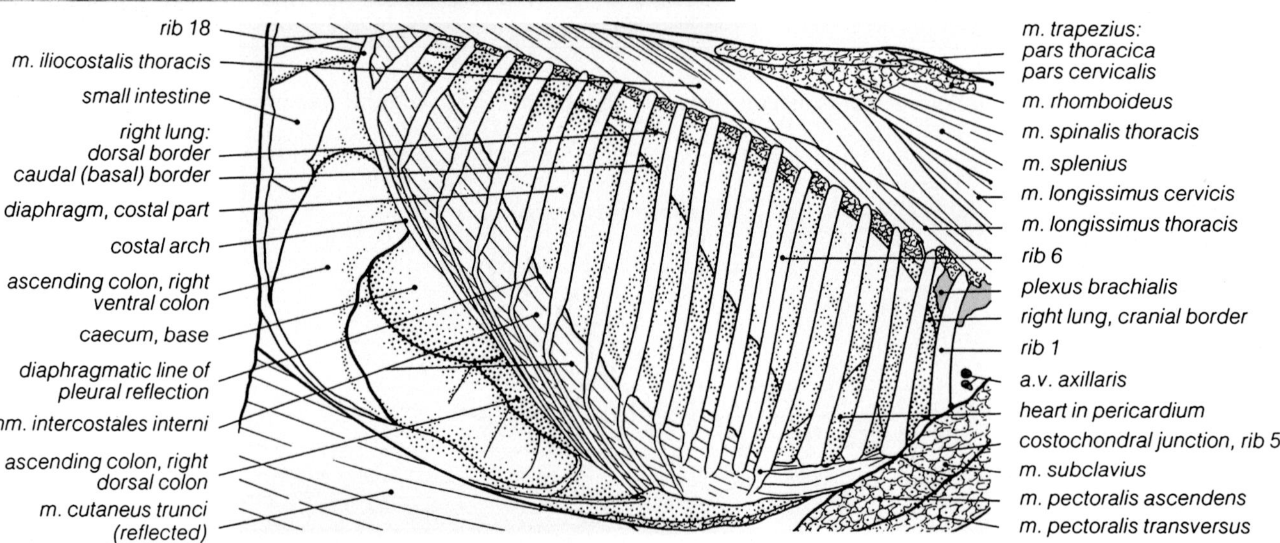
rib 18
m. iliocostalis thoracis
small intestine
right lung:
dorsal border
caudal (basal) border
diaphragm, costal part
costal arch
ascending colon, right ventral colon
caecum, base
diaphragmatic line of pleural reflection
mm. intercostales interni
ascending colon, right dorsal colon
m. cutaneus trunci (reflected)
m. trapezius:
pars thoracica
pars cervicalis
m. rhomboideus
m. spinalis thoracis
m. splenius
m. longissimus cervicis
m. longissimus thoracis
rib 6
plexus brachialis
right lung, cranial border
rib 1
a.v. axillaris
heart in pericardium
costochondral junction, rib 5
m. subclavius
m. pectoralis ascendens
m. pectoralis transversus

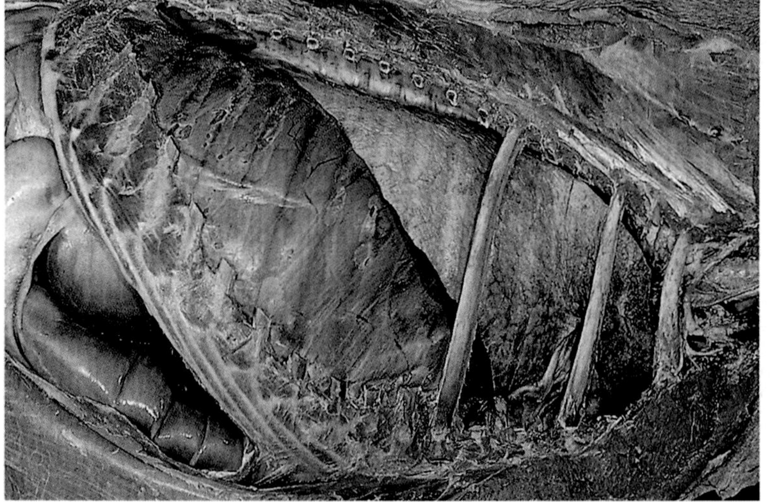

Fig. 4.32 Thoracic viscera *in situ*: right lateral view. This view corresponds with that shown in Fig. 4.17 for the left thorax. The caudal, or basal, border of the lung is much more cranial after fixation than it is in life; the broken blue line shows its approximate position in life when at rest.

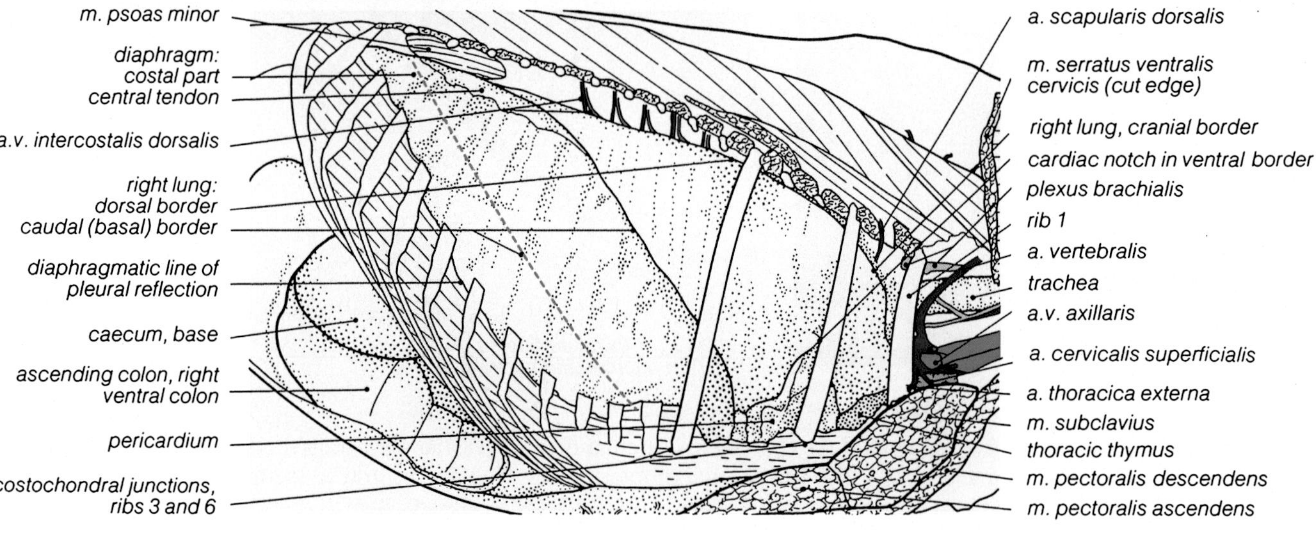
m. psoas minor
diaphragm:
costal part
central tendon
a.v. intercostalis dorsalis
right lung:
dorsal border
caudal (basal) border
diaphragmatic line of pleural reflection
caecum, base
ascending colon, right ventral colon
pericardium
costochondral junctions, ribs 3 and 6
a. scapularis dorsalis
m. serratus ventralis cervicis (cut edge)
right lung, cranial border
cardiac notch in ventral border
plexus brachialis
rib 1
a. vertebralis
trachea
a.v. axillaris
a. cervicalis superficialis
a. thoracica externa
m. subclavius
thoracic thymus
m. pectoralis descendens
m. pectoralis ascendens

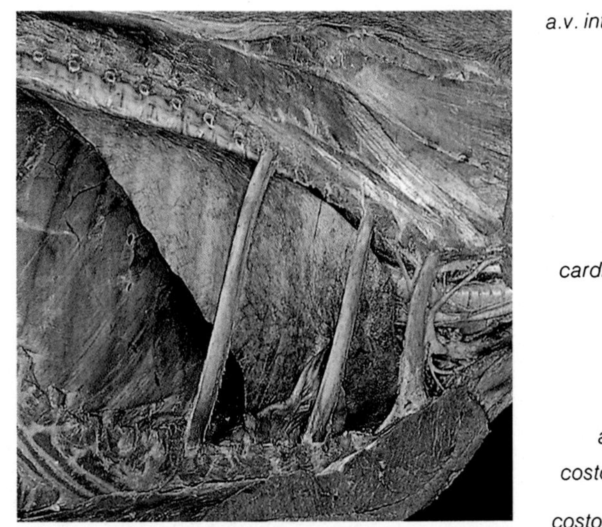

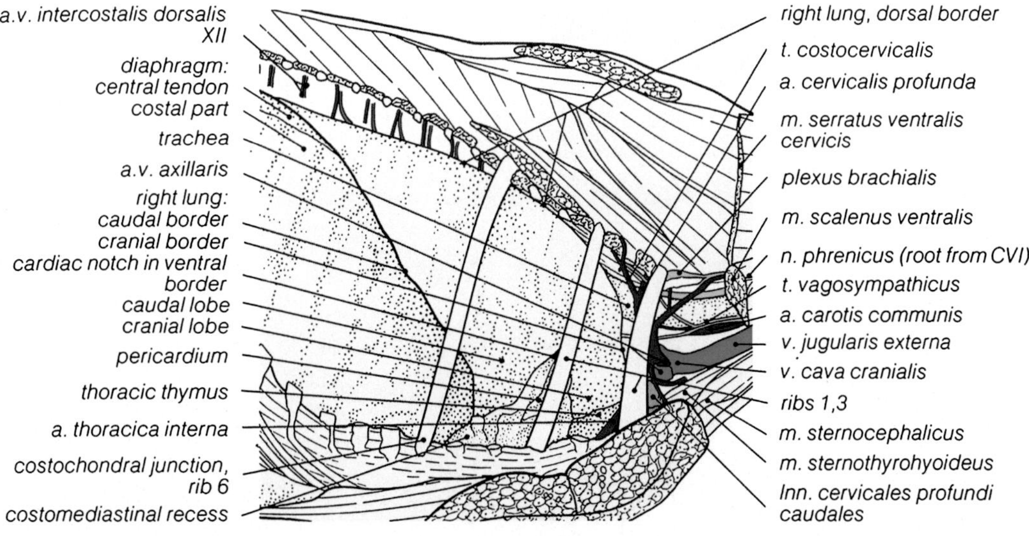

a.v. intercostalis dorsalis XII
diaphragm: central tendon
costal part
trachea
a.v. axillaris
right lung: caudal border
cranial border
cardiac notch in ventral border
caudal lobe
cranial lobe
pericardium
thoracic thymus
a. thoracica interna
costochondral junction, rib 6
costomediastinal recess
right lung, dorsal border
t. costocervicalis
a. cervicalis profunda
m. serratus ventralis cervicis
plexus brachialis
m. scalenus ventralis
n. phrenicus (root from CVI)
t. vagosympathicus
a. carotis communis
v. jugularis externa
v. cava cranialis
ribs 1,3
m. sternocephalicus
m. sternothyrohyoideus
lnn. cervicales profundi caudales

Fig. 4.33 The right lung and thoracic inlet: right lateral view. Three ribs have been left in place to mark the positions of the viscera in relation to the rib cage. Further details of the thoracic inlet are shown in Fig. 4.34. The two visible lobes of the lung are not clearly demarcated by an external groove in the horse. The accessory lobe of the right lung is seen from the left side in Fig. 4.19; it lies to the left of the caudal vena cava (Fig. 4.39) within the right pleural cavity.

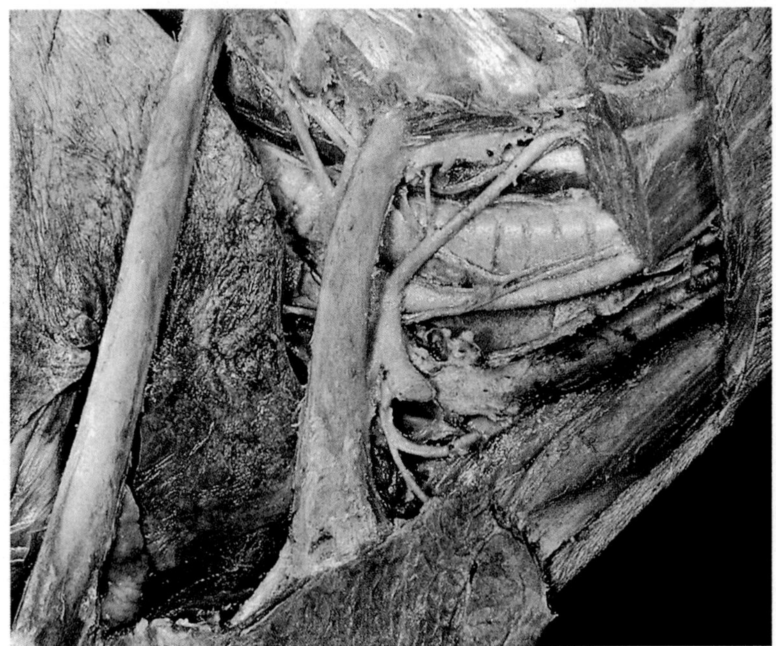

Fig. 4.34 The thoracic inlet: right lateral view. This is a closer view of a part of the specimen shown in Fig. 4.33. The phrenic nerve has been cut just cranial to the subclavian artery.

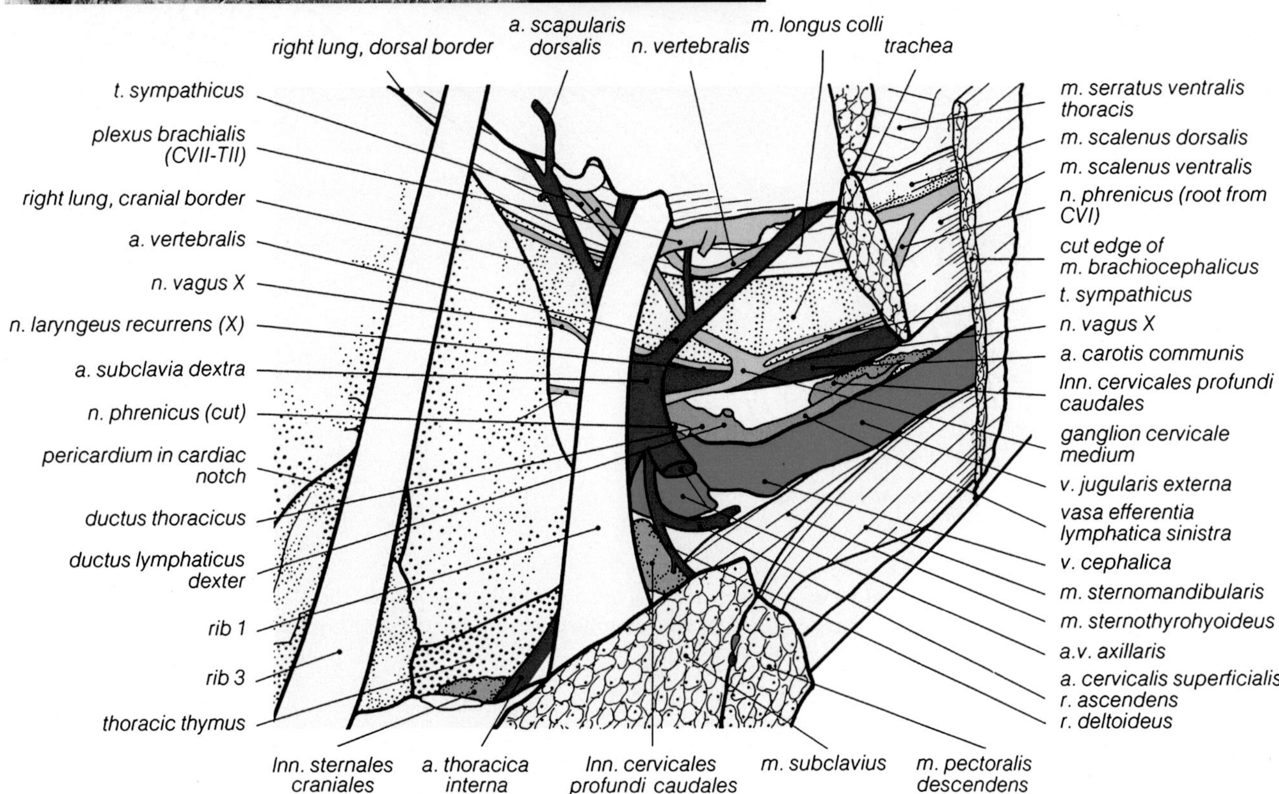

right lung, dorsal border
a. scapularis dorsalis
n. vertebralis
m. longus colli
trachea
t. sympathicus
plexus brachialis (CVII-TII)
right lung, cranial border
a. vertebralis
n. vagus X
n. laryngeus recurrens (X)
a. subclavia dextra
n. phrenicus (cut)
pericardium in cardiac notch
ductus thoracicus
ductus lymphaticus dexter
rib 1
rib 3
thoracic thymus
m. serratus ventralis thoracis
m. scalenus dorsalis
m. scalenus ventralis
n. phrenicus (root from CVI)
cut edge of m. brachiocephalicus
t. sympathicus
n. vagus X
a. carotis communis
lnn. cervicales profundi caudales
ganglion cervicale medium
v. jugularis externa
vasa efferentia lymphatica sinistra
v. cephalica
m. sternomandibularis
m. sternothyrohyoideus
a.v. axillaris
a. cervicalis superficialis
r. ascendens
r. deltoideus
lnn. sternales craniales
a. thoracica interna
lnn. cervicales profundi caudales
m. subclavius
m. pectoralis descendens

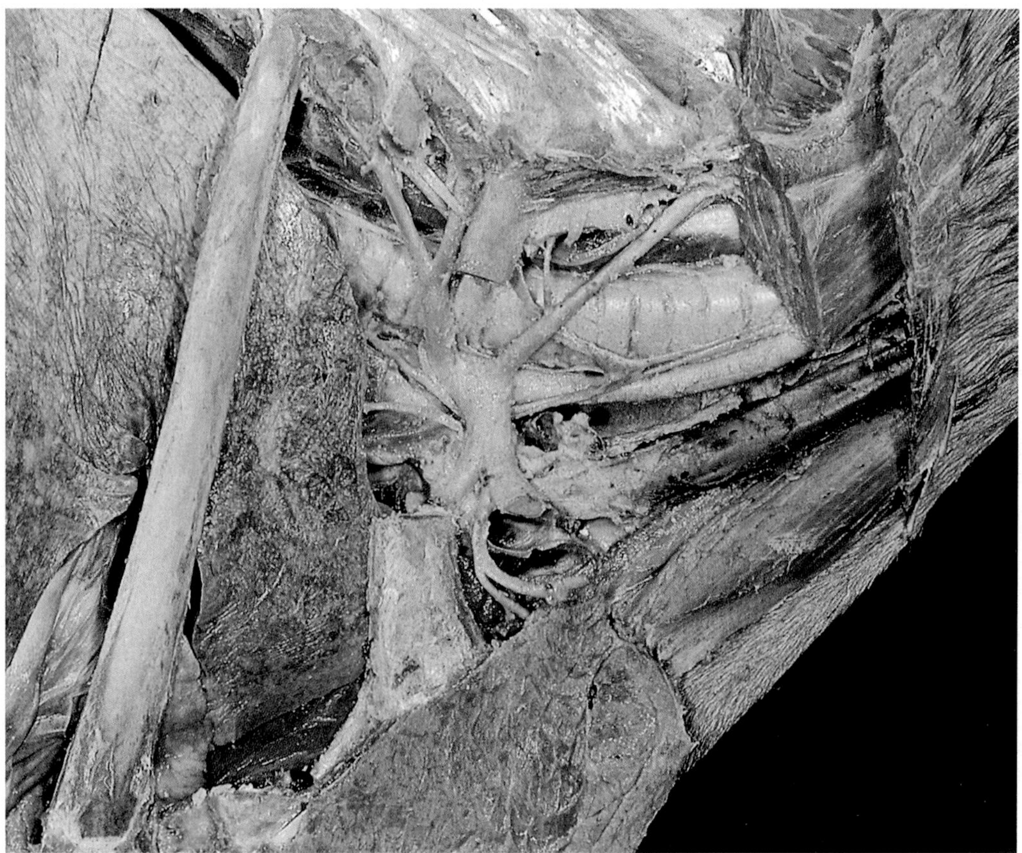

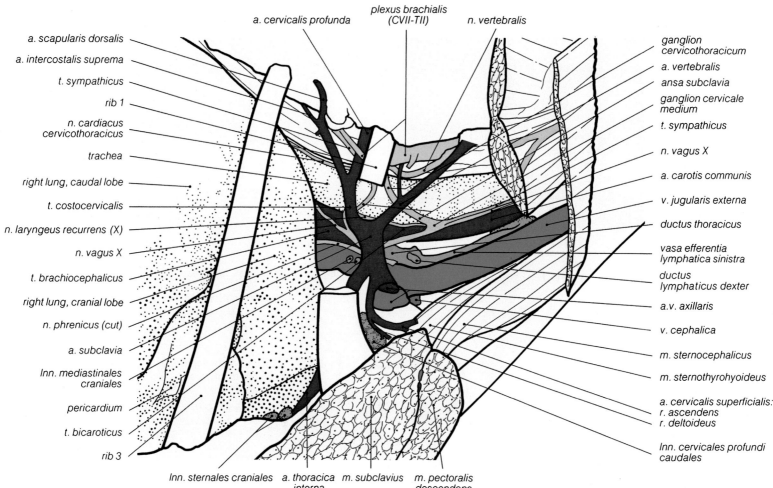

a. cervicalis profunda
plexus brachialis (CVII-TII)
n. vertebralis
a. scapularis dorsalis
a. intercostalis suprema
t. sympathicus
rib 1
n. cardiacus cervicothoracicus
trachea
right lung, caudal lobe
t. costocervicalis
n. laryngeus recurrens (X)
n. vagus X
t. brachiocephalicus
right lung, cranial lobe
n. phrenicus (cut)
a. subclavia
lnn. mediastinales craniales
pericardium
t. bicaroticus
rib 3
lnn. sternales craniales
a. thoracica interna
m. subclavius
m. pectoralis descendens
ganglion cervicothoracicum
a. vertebralis
ansa subclavia
ganglion cervicale medium
t. sympathicus
n. vagus X
a. carotis communis
v. jugularis externa
ductus thoracicus
vasa efferentia lymphatica sinistra
ductus lymphaticus dexter
a.v. axillaris
v. cephalica
m. sternocephalicus
m. sternothyrohyoideus
a. cervicalis superficialis:
r. ascendens
r. deltoideus
lnn. cervicales profundi caudales

Fig. 4.35 Nerves and vessels of the cranial mediastinum: right lateral view. The first rib has been partially resected to show the recurrent laryngeal nerve looping round the right costocervical trunk. The most dorsal part of the first rib remains covering the cervicothoracic (stellate) ganglion and obscuring its connections with other nerves.

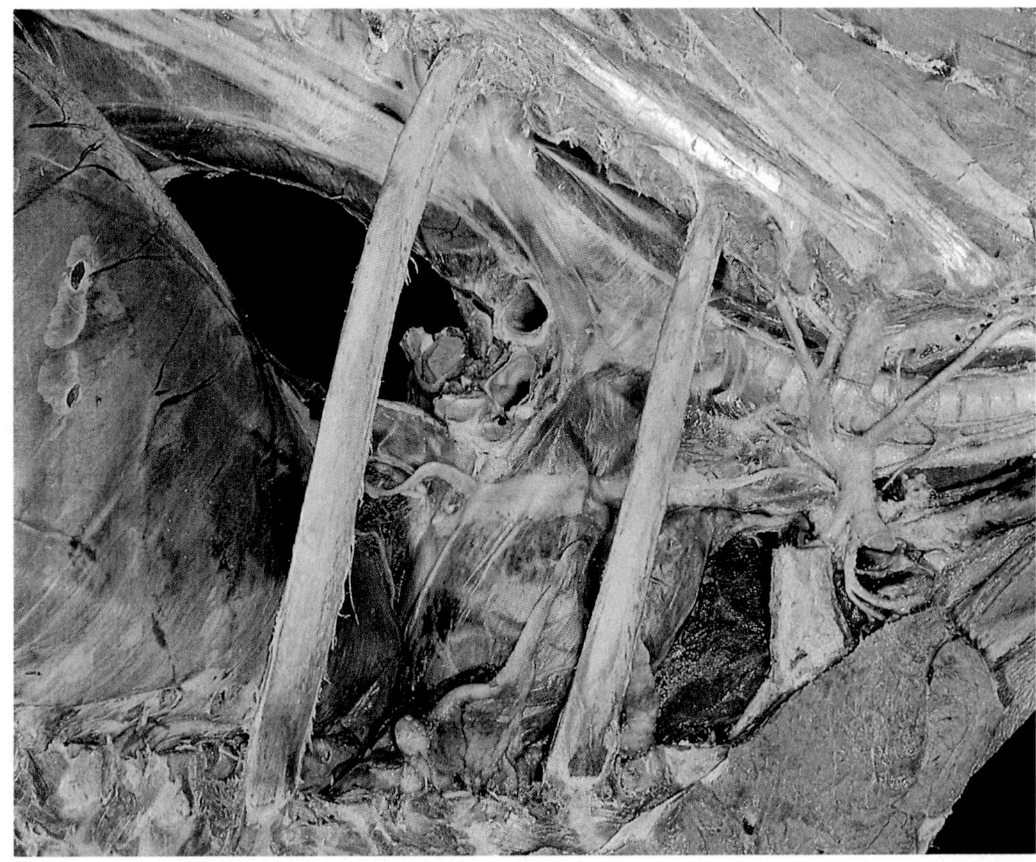

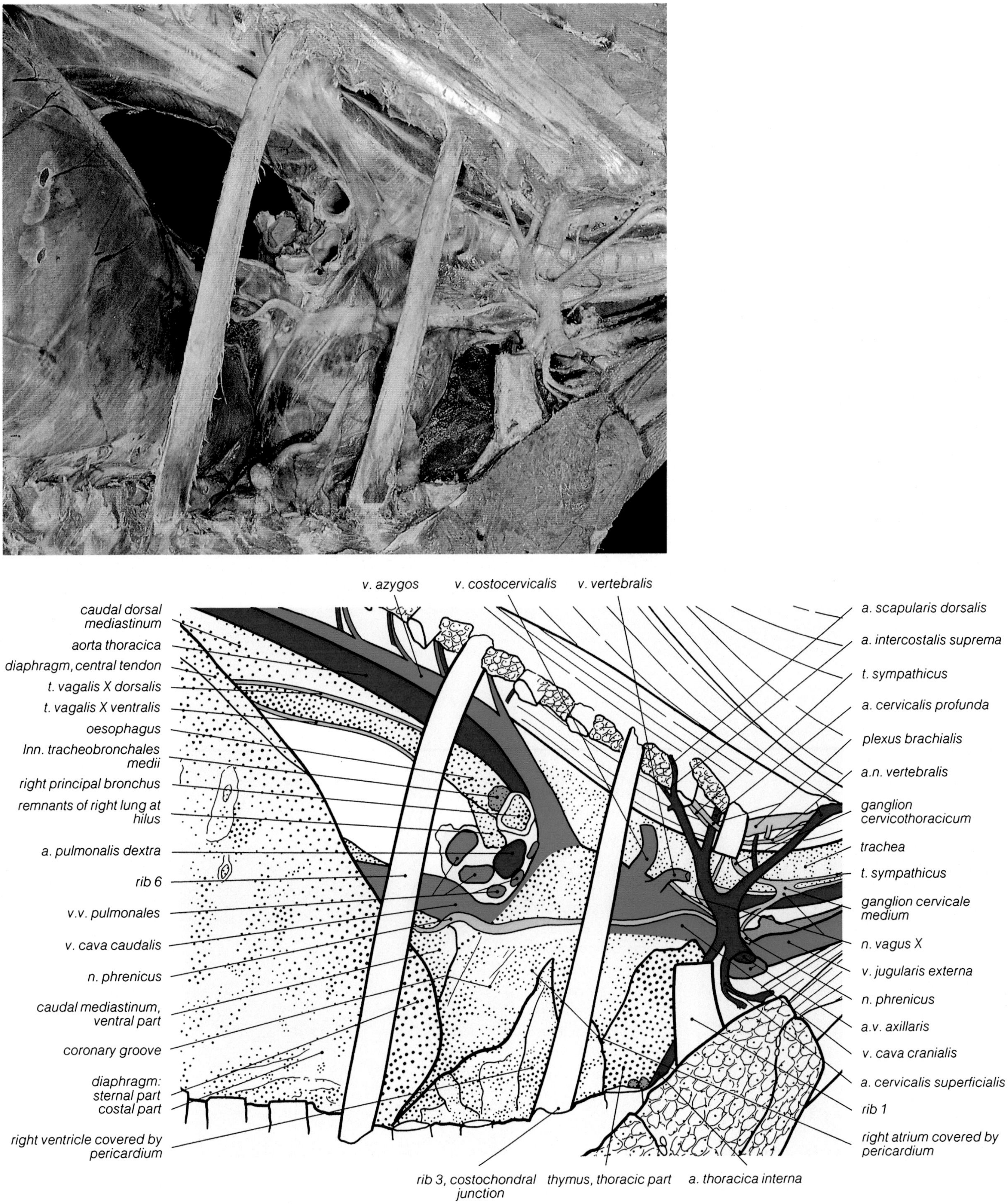

v. azygos
v. costocervicalis
v. vertebralis
caudal dorsal mediastinum
aorta thoracica
diaphragm, central tendon
t. vagalis X dorsalis
t. vagalis X ventralis
oesophagus
lnn. tracheobronchales medii
right principal bronchus
remnants of right lung at hilus
a. pulmonalis dextra
rib 6
v.v. pulmonales
v. cava caudalis
n. phrenicus
caudal mediastinum, ventral part
coronary groove
diaphragm: sternal part
costal part
right ventricle covered by pericardium
rib 3, costochondral junction
thymus, thoracic part
a. thoracica interna
a. scapularis dorsalis
a. intercostalis suprema
t. sympathicus
a. cervicalis profunda
plexus brachialis
a.n. vertebralis
ganglion cervicothoracicum
trachea
t. sympathicus
ganglion cervicale medium
n. vagus X
v. jugularis externa
n. phrenicus
a.v. axillaris
v. cava cranialis
a. cervicalis superficialis
rib 1
right atrium covered by pericardium

Fig. 4.36 The mediastinum after removal of the right lung: right lateral view. In removing the right lung, that part of the ventral mediastinum lying dorsal to the caudal vena cava has been torn: the left thorax has already been dissected, and this part of the mediastinum appears as a large black space.

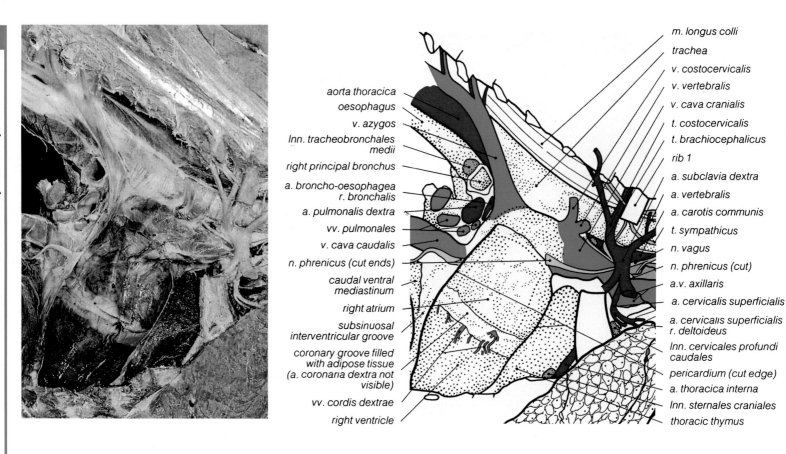

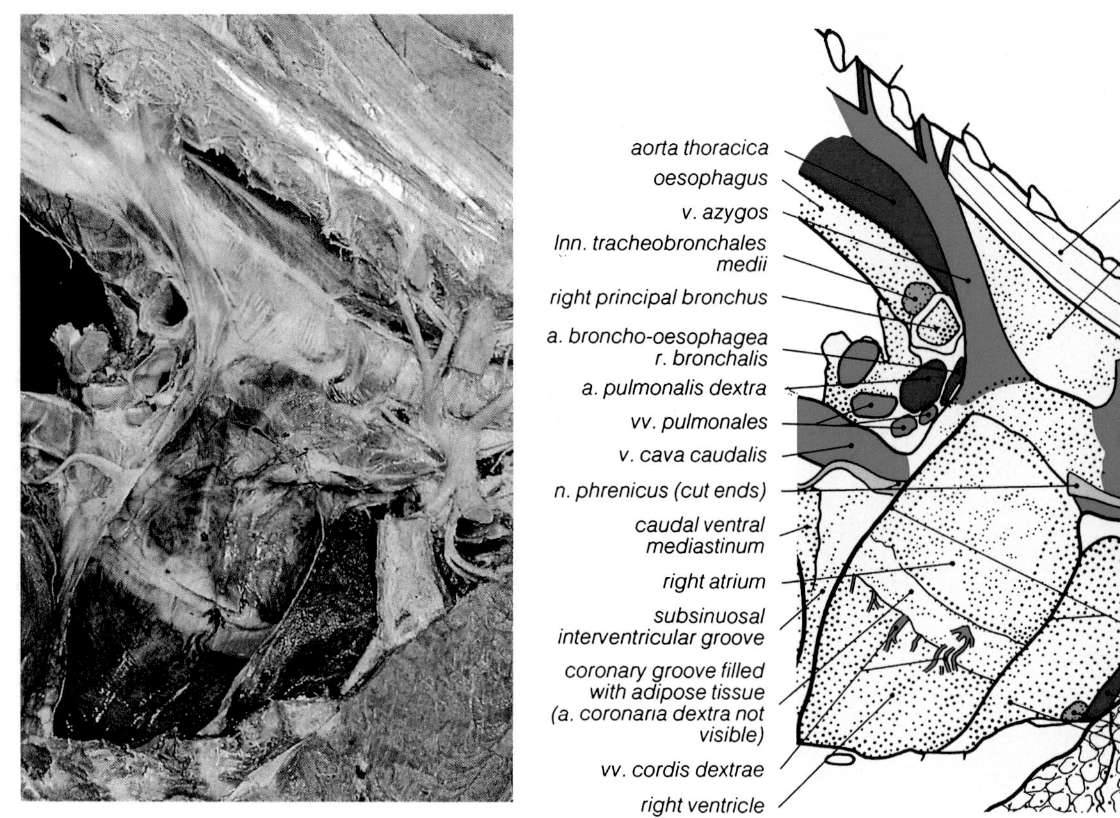
aorta thoracica
oesophagus
v. azygos
lnn. tracheobronchales medii
right principal bronchus
a. broncho-oesophagea r. bronchalis
a. pulmonalis dextra
vv. pulmonales
v. cava caudalis
n. phrenicus (cut ends)
caudal ventral mediastinum
right atrium
subsinuosal interventricular groove
coronary groove filled with adipose tissue (a. coronaria dextra not visible)
vv. cordis dextrae
right ventricle
m. longus colli
trachea
v. costocervicalis
v. vertebralis
v. cava cranialis
t. costocervicalis
t. brachiocephalicus
rib 1
a. subclavia dextra
a. vertebralis
a. carotis communis
t. sympathicus
n. vagus
n. phrenicus (cut)
a.v. axillaris
a. cervicalis superficialis
a. cervicalis superficialis r. deltoideus
lnn. cervicales profundi caudales
pericardium (cut edge)
a. thoracica interna
lnn. sternales craniales
thoracic thymus

Fig. 4.37 The heart and great vessels: right lateral view. The pericardium has been cut away to show the atrium and ventricle within the pericardial cavity. The dotted line shows where an incision has been made in the atrial wall to expose the cavity of the right atrium as in Fig. 4.38. Note the position of the subsinuosal groove (see Fig. 4.40).

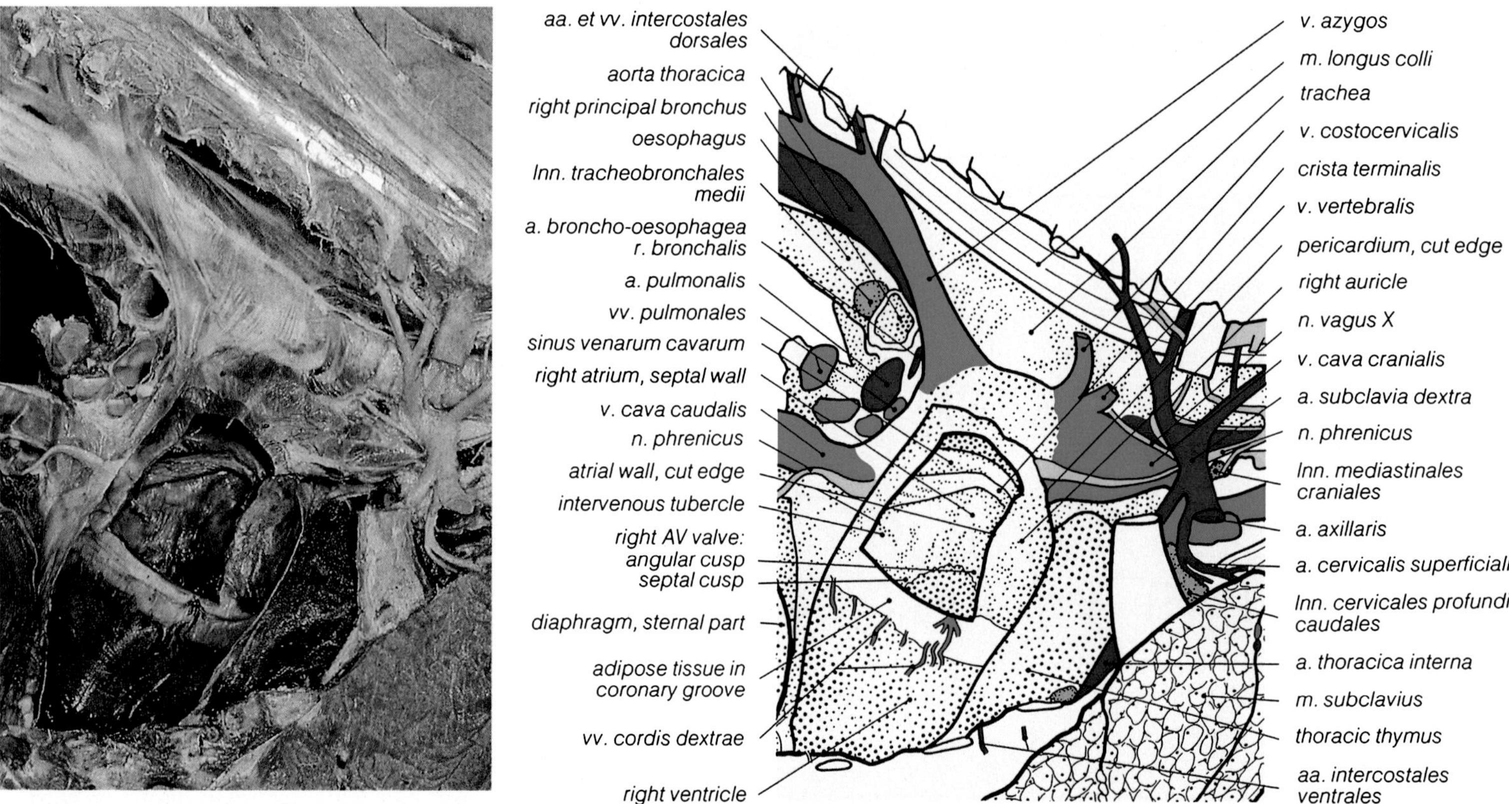
aa. et vv. intercostales dorsales
aorta thoracica
right principal bronchus
oesophagus
lnn. tracheobronchales medii
a. broncho-oesophagea r. bronchalis
a. pulmonalis
vv. pulmonales
sinus venarum cavarum
right atrium, septal wall
v. cava caudalis
n. phrenicus
atrial wall, cut edge
intervenous tubercle
right AV valve:
angular cusp
septal cusp
diaphragm, sternal part
adipose tissue in coronary groove
vv. cordis dextrae
right ventricle
v. azygos
m. longus colli
trachea
v. costocervicalis
crista terminalis
v. vertebralis
pericardium, cut edge
right auricle
n. vagus X
v. cava cranialis
a. subclavia dextra
n. phrenicus
lnn. mediastinales craniales
a. axillaris
a. cervicalis superficialis
lnn. cervicales profundi caudales
a. thoracica interna
m. subclavius
thoracic thymus
aa. intercostales ventrales

Fig. 4.38 The cavity of the right atrium and the right atrioventricular valve: right lateral view (1). The wall of the right atrium has been partly removed to show the position of the right atrioventricular valve (compare with Figs. 4.37 and 4.39).

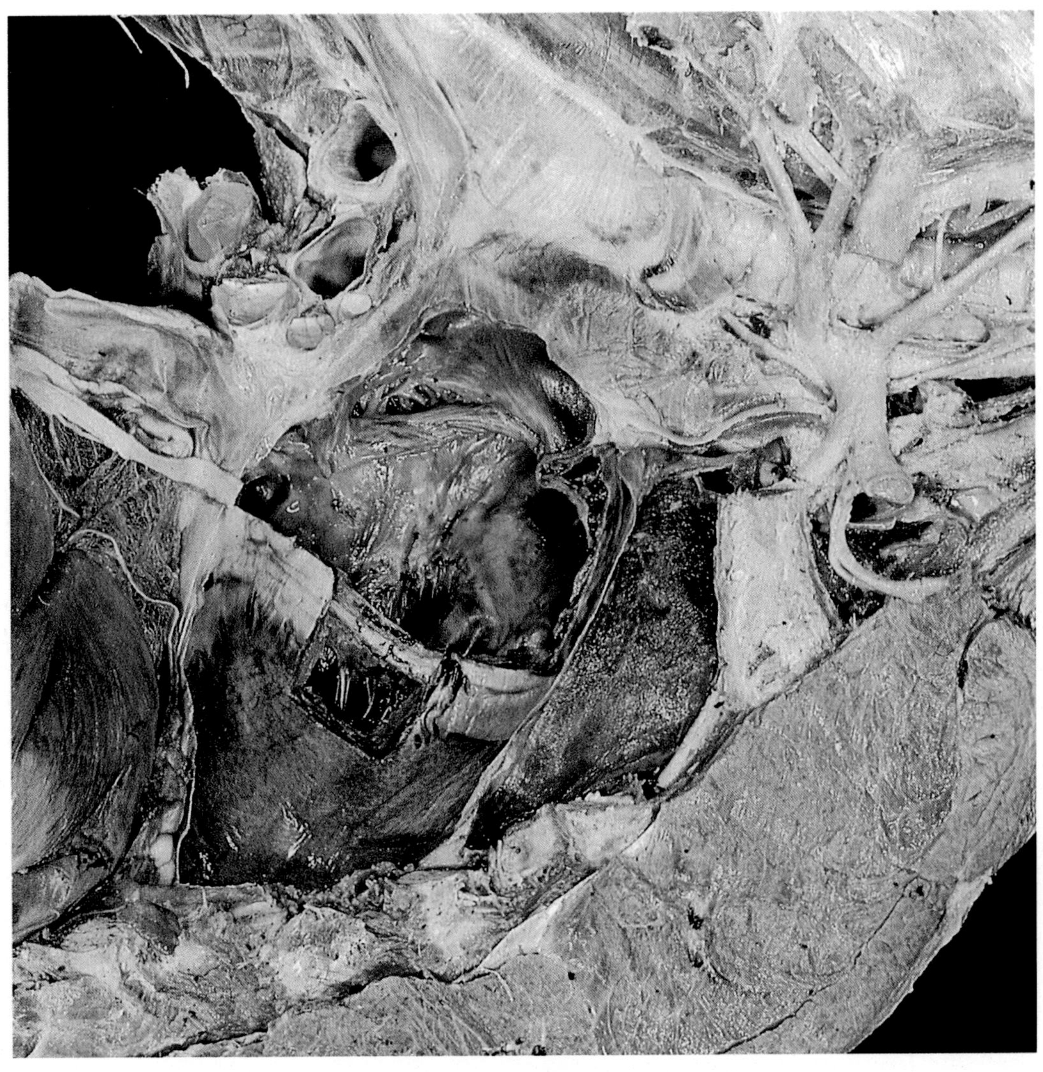

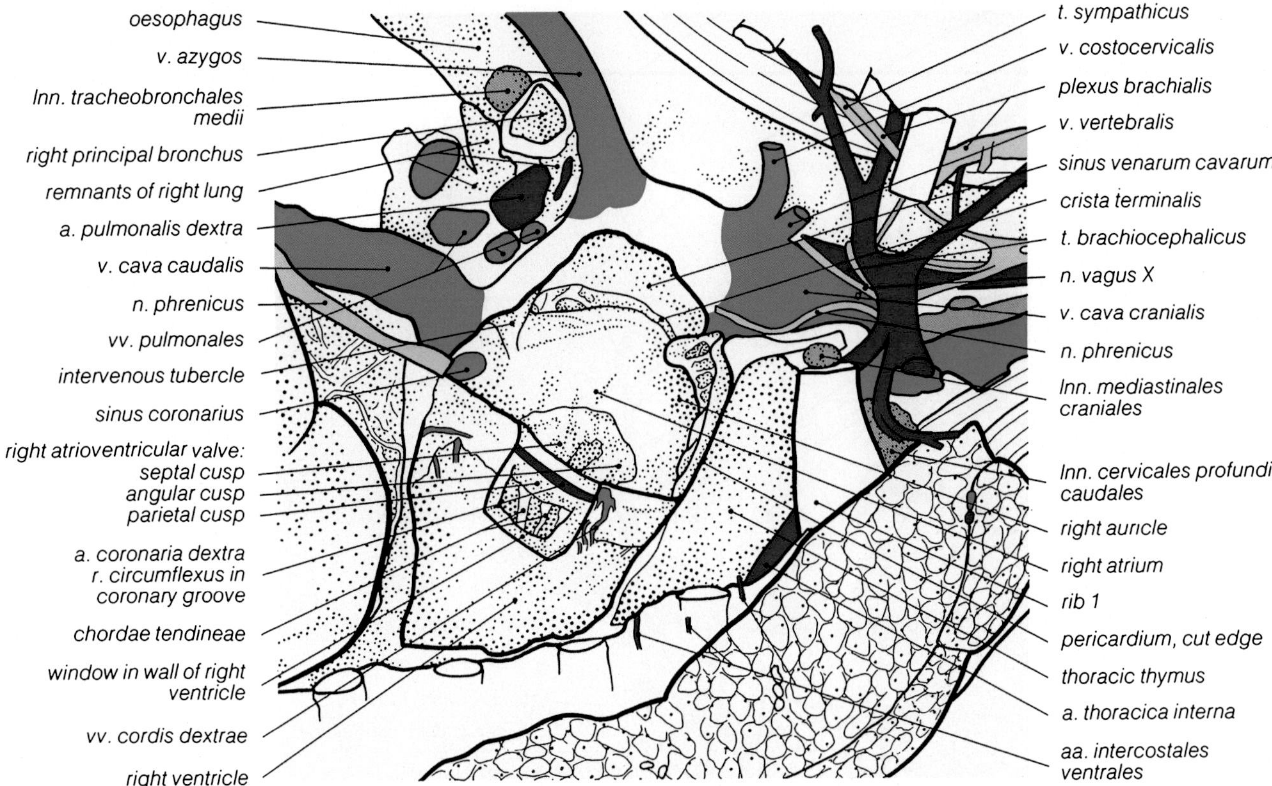
oesophagus
v. azygos
lnn. tracheobronchales medii
right principal bronchus
remnants of right lung
a. pulmonalis dextra
v. cava caudalis
n. phrenicus
vv. pulmonales
intervenous tubercle
sinus coronarius
right atrioventricular valve:
septal cusp
angular cusp
parietal cusp
a. coronaria dextra r. circumflexus in coronary groove
chordae tendineae
window in wall of right ventricle
vv. cordis dextrae
right ventricle
t. sympathicus
v. costocervicalis
plexus brachialis
v. vertebralis
sinus venarum cavarum
crista terminalis
t. brachiocephalicus
n. vagus X
v. cava cranialis
n. phrenicus
lnn. mediastinales craniales
lnn. cervicales profundi caudales
right auricle
right atrium
rib 1
pericardium, cut edge
thoracic thymus
a. thoracica interna
aa. intercostales ventrales

Fig. 4.39 The cavity of the right atrium and the right atrioventricular valve: right lateral view (2). The window cut in the wall of the right atrium in Figs. 4.37 and 4.38 has been enlarged to show the auricle and the coronary sinus. A window has been cut in the wall of the right ventricle to show the parietal cusp of the right atrioventricular (tricuspid) valve.

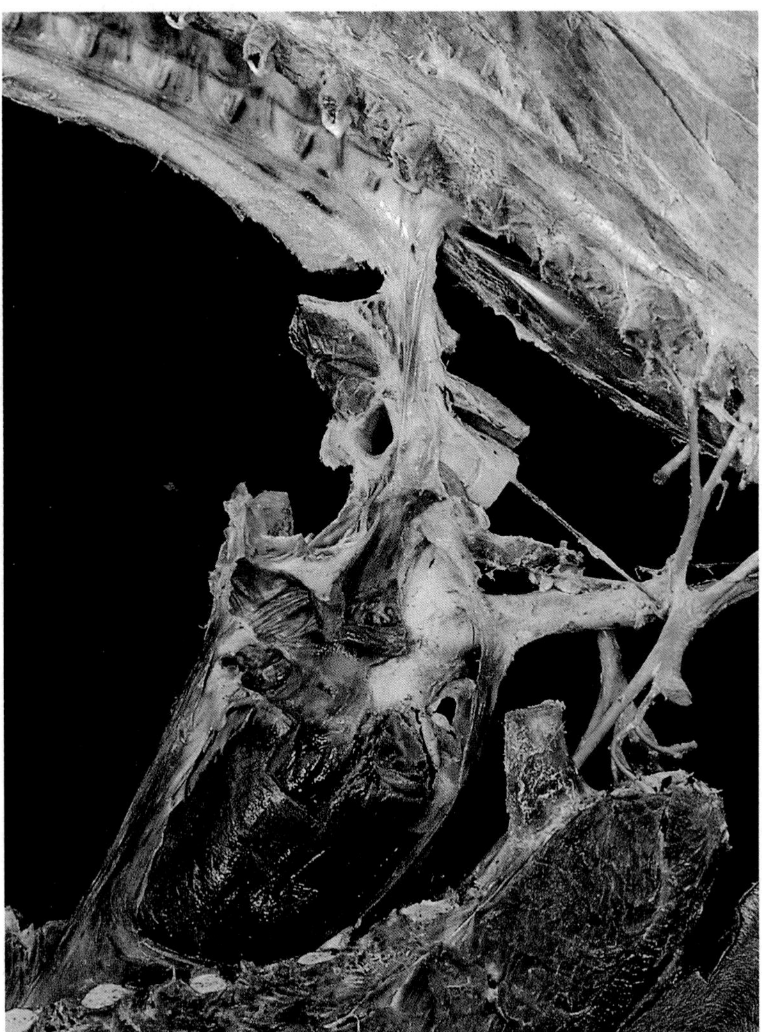

Fig. 4.40 The heart, arteries and recurrent laryngeal nerves: right lateral view. The specimen is at the same stage of dissection as that shown in Fig. 4.27. A large part of the medial wall of the right atrium, and its auricle, have been removed to show the aortic arch and the origin of the right coronary artery. Only the first part of this artery has been filled with red latex. Removal of the rib cage while in the standing position has greatly altered topographical relationships of the heart (see Figs. 4.36 and 4.37). Note the position of the subsinuosal groove: this is usually represented as being much more lateral than is, in fact, topographically correct.

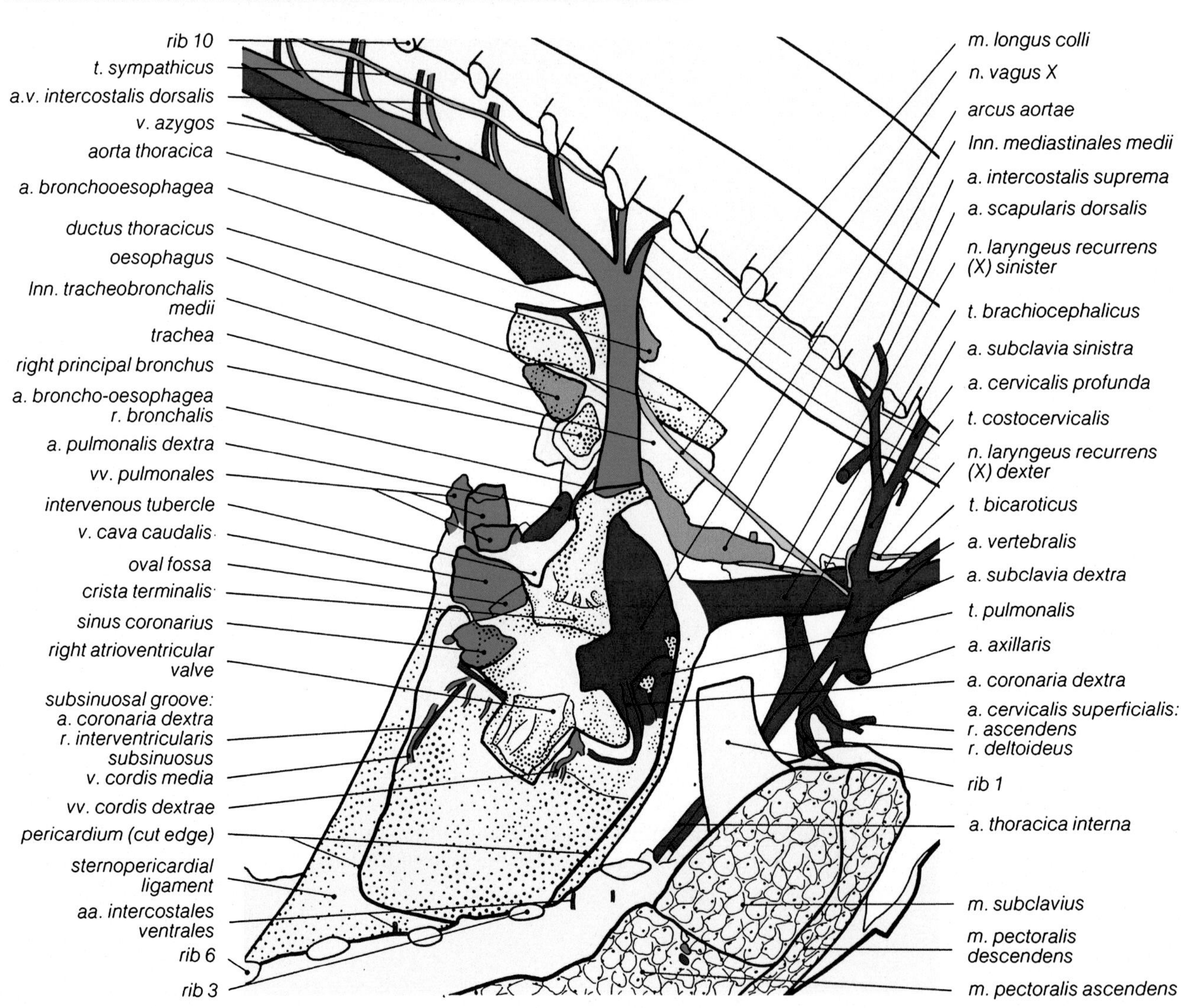

rib 10
t. sympathicus
a.v. intercostalis dorsalis
v. azygos
aorta thoracica
a. bronchooesophagea
ductus thoracicus
oesophagus
lnn. tracheobronchalis medii
trachea
right principal bronchus
a. broncho-oesophagea r. bronchalis
a. pulmonalis dextra
vv. pulmonales
intervenous tubercle
v. cava caudalis
oval fossa
crista terminalis
sinus coronarius
right atrioventricular valve
subsinuosal groove: a. coronaria dextra r. interventricularis subsinuosus
v. cordis media
vv. cordis dextrae
pericardium (cut edge)
sternopericardial ligament
aa. intercostales ventrales
rib 6
rib 3
m. longus colli
n. vagus X
arcus aortae
lnn. mediastinales medii
a. intercostalis suprema
a. scapularis dorsalis
n. laryngeus recurrens (X) sinister
t. brachiocephalicus
a. subclavia sinistra
a. cervicalis profunda
t. costocervicalis
n. laryngeus recurrens (X) dexter
t. bicaroticus
a. vertebralis
a. subclavia dextra
t. pulmonalis
a. axillaris
a. coronaria dextra
a. cervicalis superficialis: r. ascendens r. deltoideus
rib 1
a. thoracica interna
m. subclavius
m. pectoralis descendens
m. pectoralis ascendens

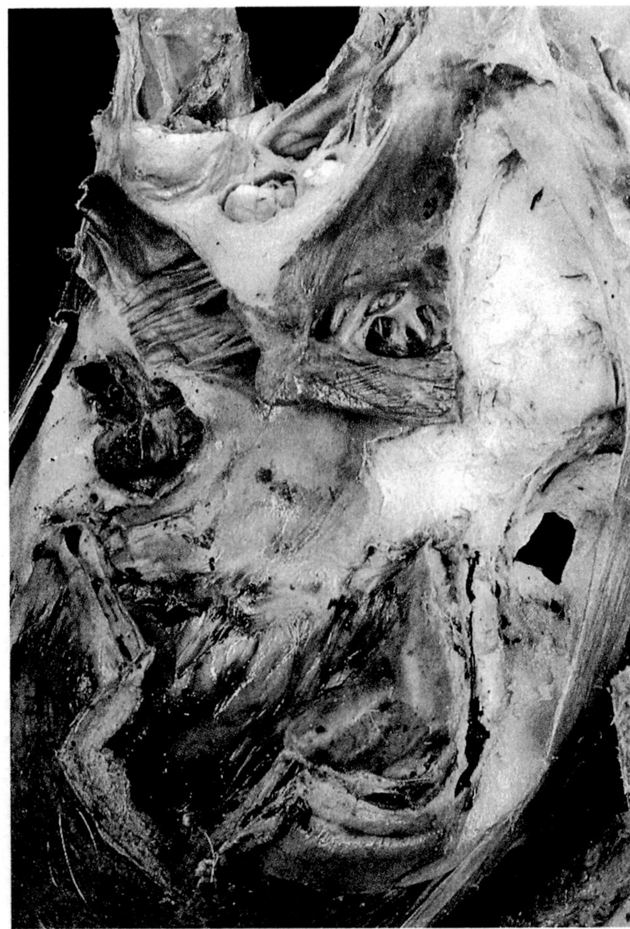

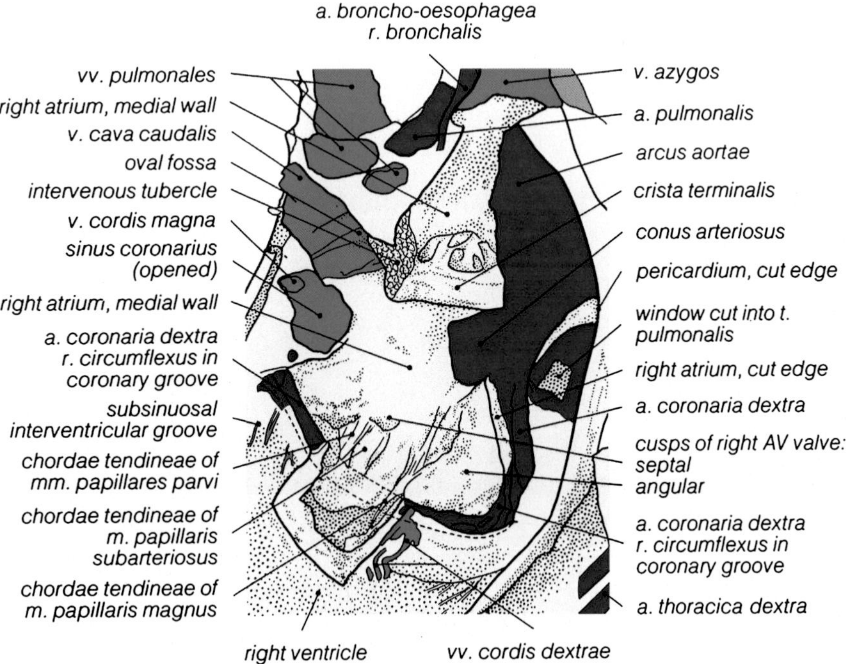
a. broncho-oesophagea
r. bronchalis
vv. pulmonales
right atrium, medial wall
v. cava caudalis
oval fossa
intervenous tubercle
v. cordis magna
sinus coronarius (opened)
right atrium, medial wall
a. coronaria dextra
r. circumflexus in coronary groove
subsinuosal interventricular groove
chordae tendineae of mm. papillares parvi
chordae tendineae of m. papillaris subarteriosus
chordae tendineae of m. papillaris magnus
right ventricle
vv. cordis dextrae
v. azygos
a. pulmonalis
arcus aortae
crista terminalis
conus arteriosus
pericardium, cut edge
window cut into t. pulmonalis
right atrium, cut edge
a. coronaria dextra
cusps of right AV valve:
septal
angular
a. coronaria dextra
r. circumflexus in coronary groove
a. thoracica dextra

Fig. 4.41 The right atrioventricular valve: right lateral view. This is a slightly more dorsal view of a part of the specimen shown in Fig. 4.40. The right coronary artery is shown passing to the right of the pulmonary trunk, and entering the coronary groove. Here it is not filled with latex, and its lumen has been opened when incising the groove. Broken lines show where a part of the artery was cut away after displaying the lumen of the right ventricle (Fig. 4.39). The parietal cusp of the right atrioventricular valve is not visible, it is shown in Fig. 4.39.

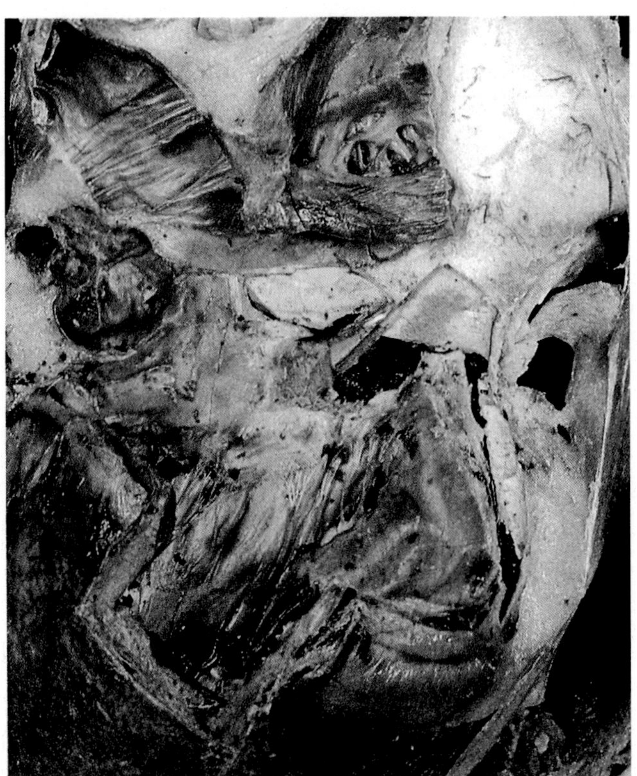

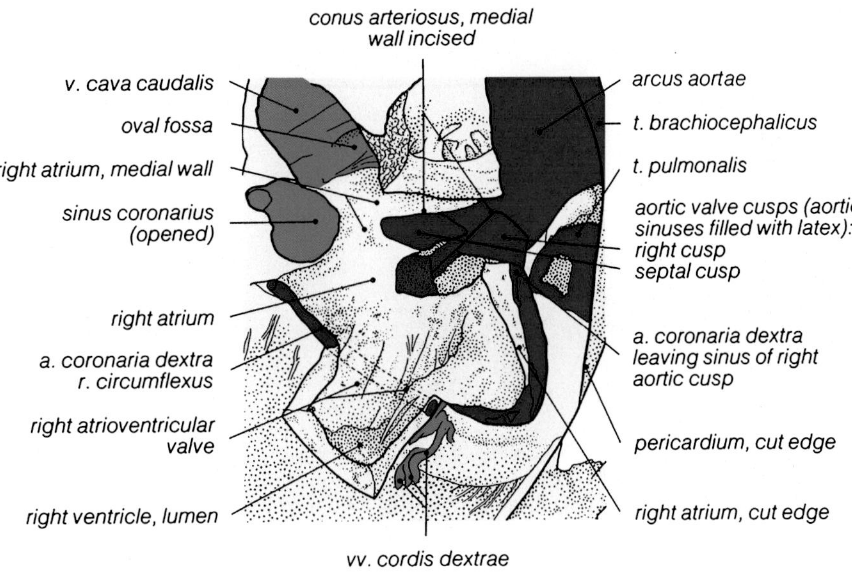
conus arteriosus, medial wall incised
v. cava caudalis
oval fossa
right atrium, medial wall
sinus coronarius (opened)
right atrium
a. coronaria dextra
r. circumflexus
right atrioventricular valve
right ventricle, lumen
vv. cordis dextrae
arcus aortae
t. brachiocephalicus
t. pulmonalis
aortic valve cusps (aortic sinuses filled with latex):
right cusp
septal cusp
a. coronaria dextra leaving sinus of right aortic cusp
pericardium, cut edge
right atrium, cut edge

Fig. 4.42 The aortic valve, in right lateral view. Part of the medial wall of the right atrium has been removed, and a window has been cut in the wall of the conus arteriosus to show two cusps of the aortic valve. The third left cusp is shown in Fig. 4.26 as is the left coronary artery.

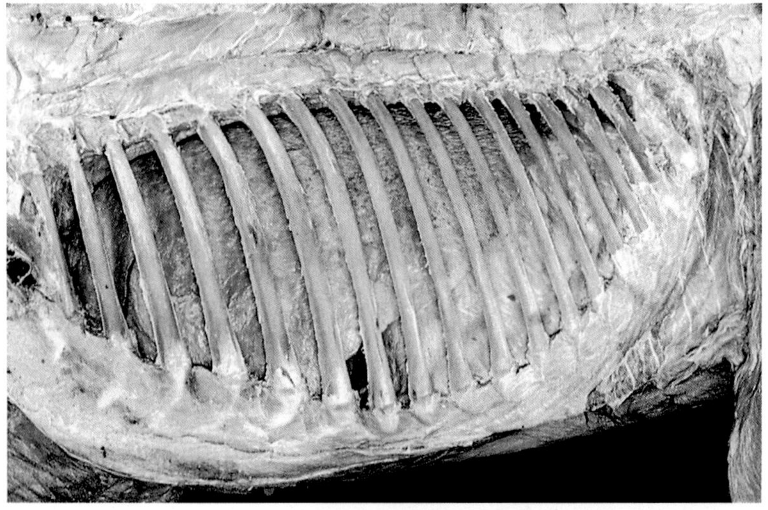

Fig. 4.43 The rib cage of a new-born foal: left lateral view. The intercostal structures have been removed to show the extent of the left pleural cavity and the relationships of the viscera to the ribs. The corresponding view in the adult horse is shown in Fig. 4.14.

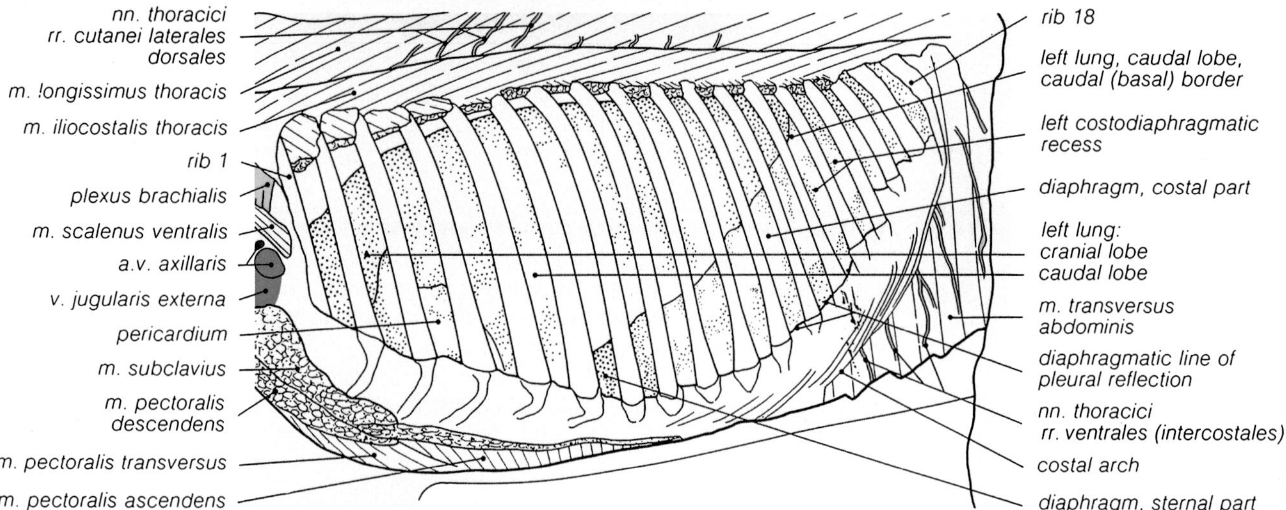
nn. thoracici
rr. cutanei laterales dorsales
m. longissimus thoracis
m. iliocostalis thoracis
rib 1
plexus brachialis
m. scalenus ventralis
a.v. axillaris
v. jugularis externa
pericardium
m. subclavius
m. pectoralis descendens
m. pectoralis transversus
m. pectoralis ascendens
rib 18
left lung, caudal lobe, caudal (basal) border
left costodiaphragmatic recess
diaphragm, costal part
left lung:
cranial lobe
caudal lobe
m. transversus abdominis
diaphragmatic line of pleural reflection
nn. thoracici
rr. ventrales (intercostales)
costal arch
diaphragm, sternal part

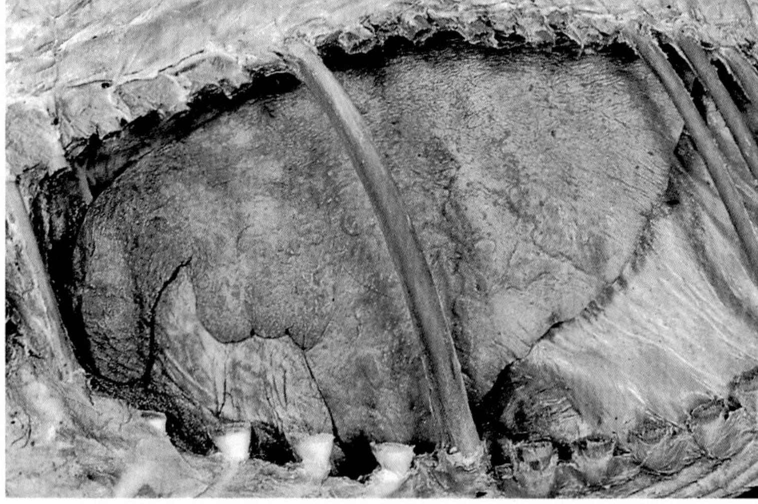

Fig. 4.44 The left lung of the new-born foal: left lateral view. Ribs 2–5 and 7–11 inclusive have been removed, leaving their costal cartilages, to show the topography of the left lung.

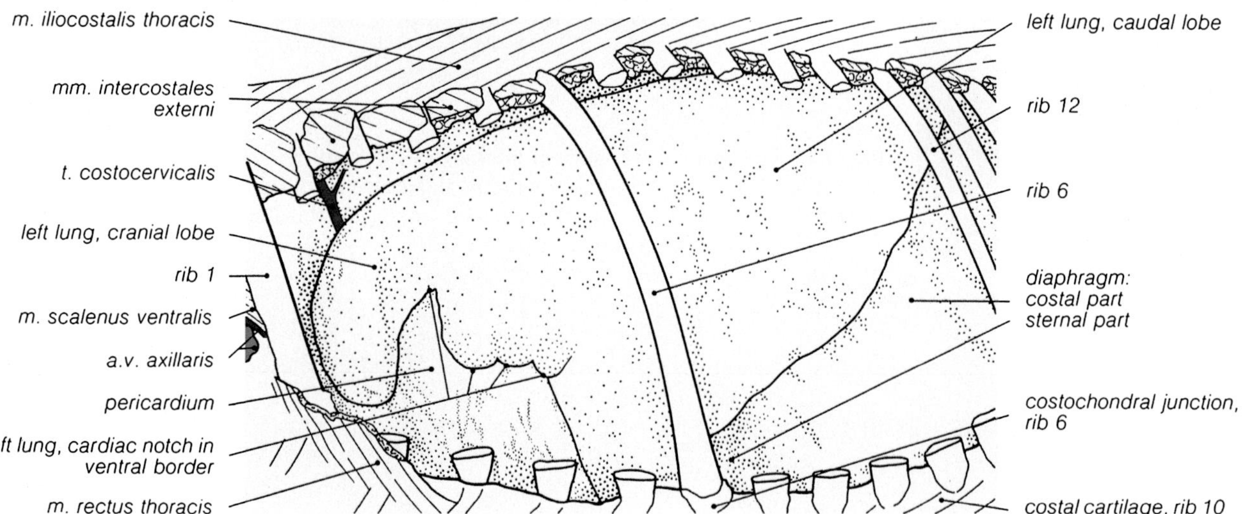
m. iliocostalis thoracis
mm. intercostales externi
t. costocervicalis
left lung, cranial lobe
rib 1
m. scalenus ventralis
a.v. axillaris
pericardium
left lung, cardiac notch in ventral border
m. rectus thoracis
left lung, caudal lobe
rib 12
rib 6
diaphragm:
costal part
sternal part
costochondral junction, rib 6
costal cartilage, rib 10

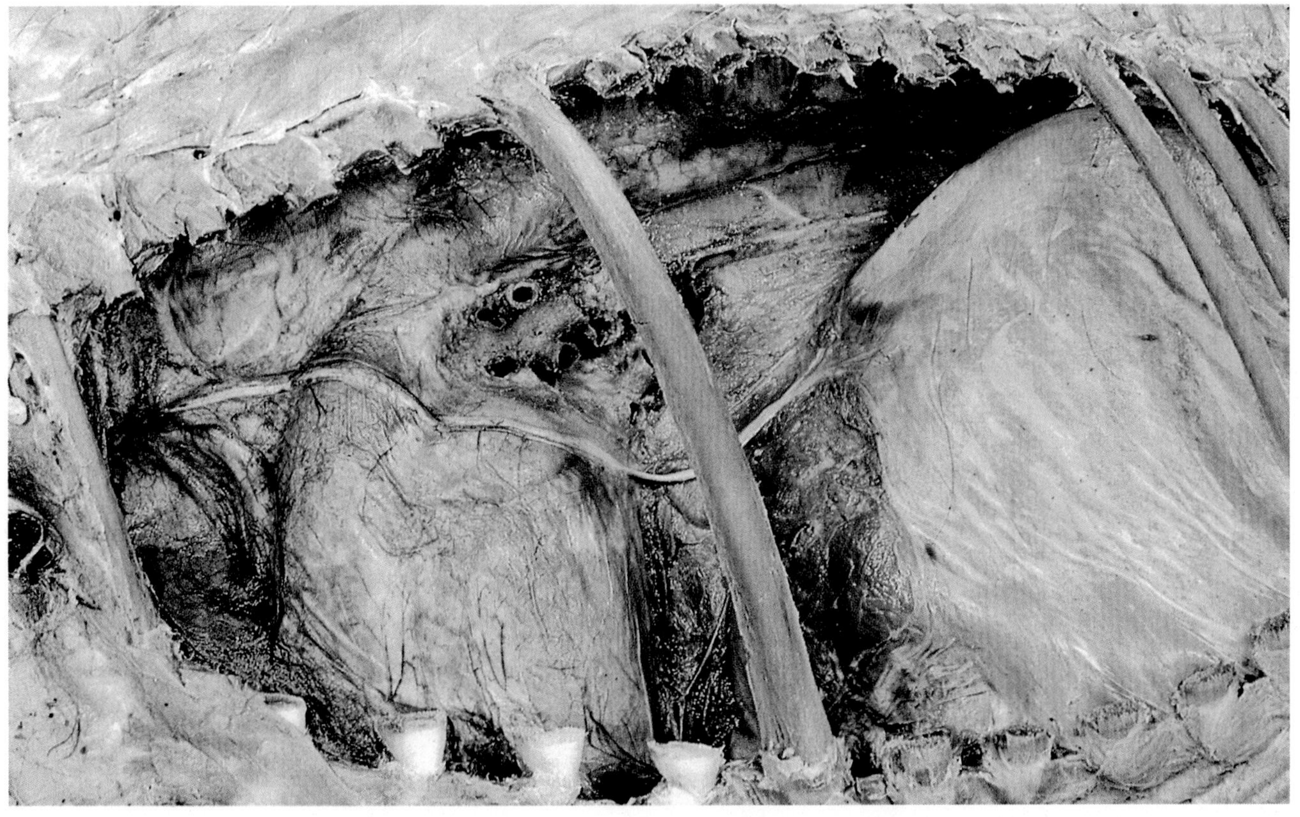

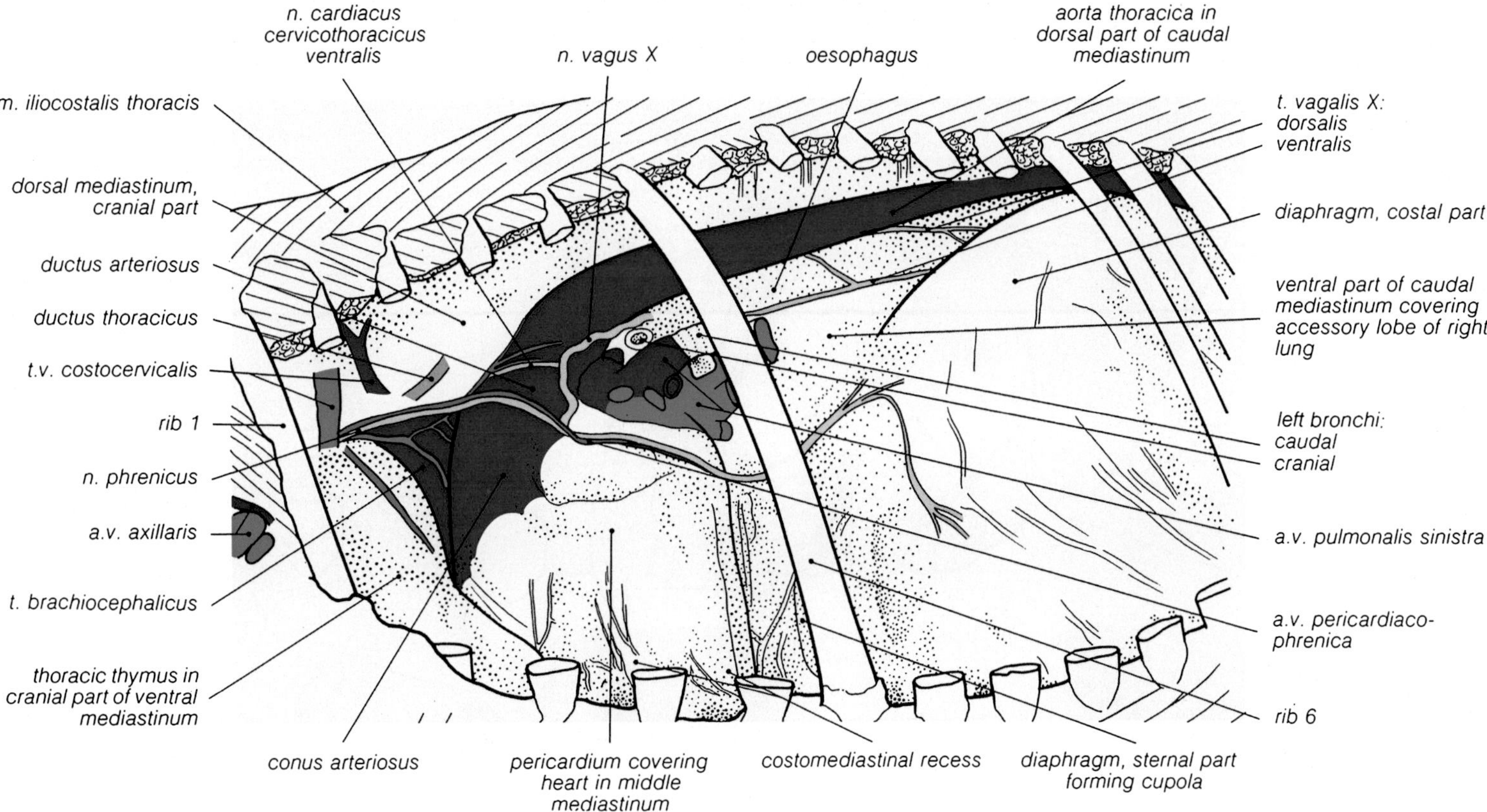
n. cardiacus cervicothoracicus ventralis
n. vagus X
oesophagus
aorta thoracica in dorsal part of caudal mediastinum
m. iliocostalis thoracis
t. vagalis X:
dorsalis
ventralis
dorsal mediastinum, cranial part
diaphragm, costal part
ductus arteriosus
ventral part of caudal mediastinum covering accessory lobe of right lung
ductus thoracicus
t.v. costocervicalis
rib 1
left bronchi:
caudal
cranial
n. phrenicus
a.v. axillaris
a.v. pulmonalis sinistra
t. brachiocephalicus
a.v. pericardiaco-phrenica
thoracic thymus in cranial part of ventral mediastinum
rib 6
conus arteriosus
pericardium covering heart in middle mediastinum
costomediastinal recess
diaphragm, sternal part forming cupola

Fig. 4.45 The mediastinum of the new-born foal: left lateral view. Removal of the left lung exposes the mediastinum, which divides left and right pleural cavities. No attempt has yet been made to dissect out the contents of the mediastinum. The structures lying in the mediastinum are shown, after dissection, in Fig. 4.46.

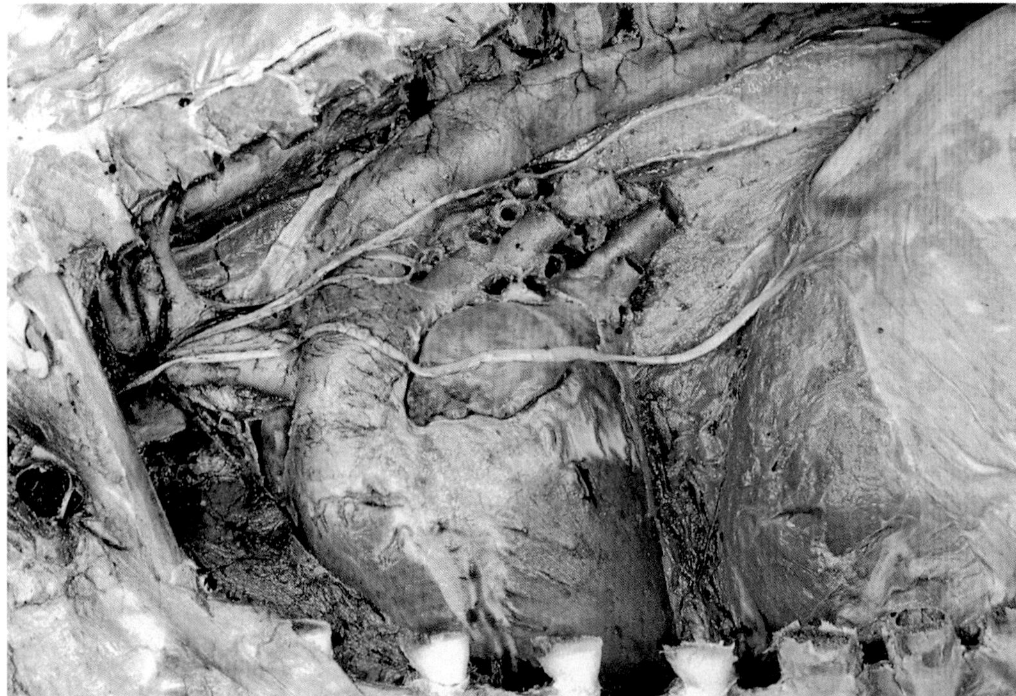
a.v. intercostalis dorsalis V
m. longus colli
ductus thoracicus
ductus arteriosus
oesophagus
arcus aortae
t.v. costocervicalis
a.v. cervicalis profunda
nn. cardiaci cervicothoracici
n. vagus X
nn. cardiaci
n. phrenicus
t. brachiocephalicus
v. cava cranialis
pericardial cavity
conus arteriosus
right auricle
rib 1
right ventricle
pericardium, cut edge
thoracic thymus
rib 6
aorta thoracica
vasa vasorum
t. vagalis X dorsalis
oesophagus
t. vagalis X ventralis
lnn. tracheobronchales: medii sinistri
principal bronchus to left lung
a.v. pulmonalis
nn. cardiaci
n. vagus X, r. cardiacus
n. cardiacus cervicothoracicus
n. laryngeus recurrens (X)
left atrium
left ventricle
pericardium, cut edge
a. coronaria sinistra r. circumflexus r. interventricularis paraconalis
v. interventricularis paraconalis

Fig. 4.46 Vessels and nerves of the mediastinum of the new-born foal: left lateral view. This dissection should be compared with that in Fig. 4.45, in which the correct topographical relationships of the structures are preserved.

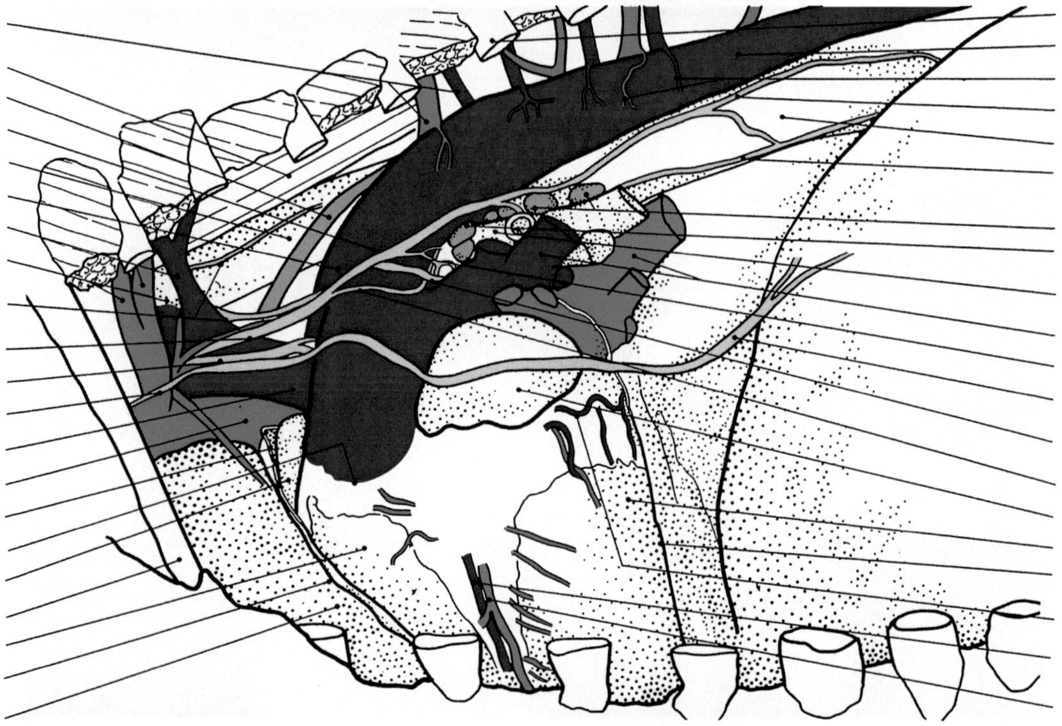

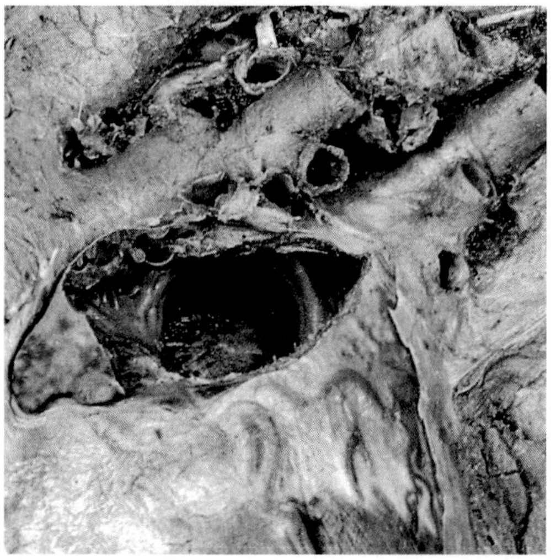

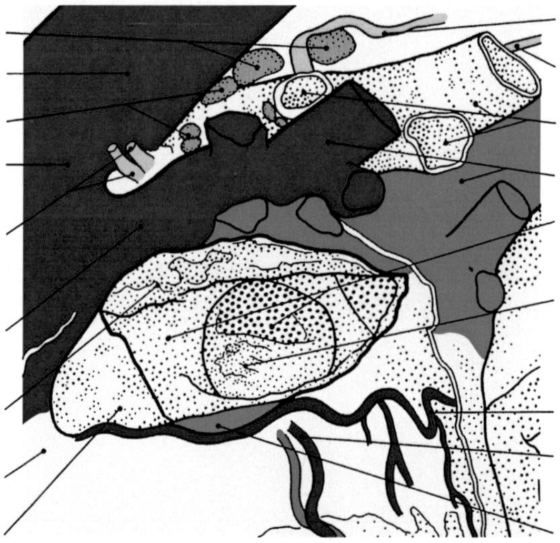

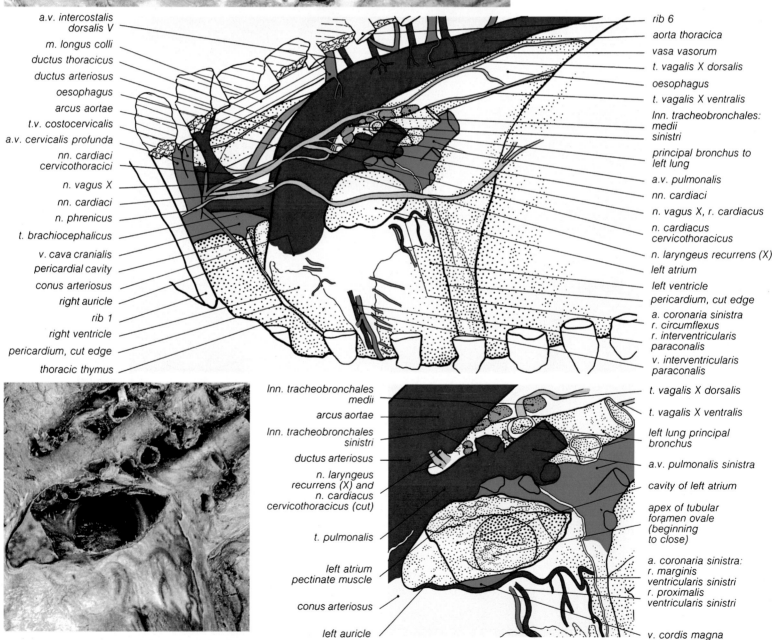

lnn. tracheobronchales medii
arcus aortae
lnn. tracheobronchales sinistri
ductus arteriosus
n. laryngeus recurrens (X) and n. cardiacus cervicothoracicus (cut)
t. pulmonalis
left atrium pectinate muscle
conus arteriosus
left auricle
t. vagalis X dorsalis
t. vagalis X ventralis
left lung principal bronchus
a.v. pulmonalis sinistra
cavity of left atrium
apex of tubular foramen ovale (beginning to close)
a. coronaria sinistra: r. marginis ventricularis sinistri r. proximalis ventricularis sinistri
v. cordis magna

Fig. 4.47 The cavity of the left atrium of the new-born foal: left lateral view. The vessels and nerves of the mediastinum have been removed, and the lateral wall of the atrium has been partially excised. The tubular foramen ovale, which in foetal life is a communication between caudal vena cava and left atrium, is already closing in this new-born foal. Anatomical closure is usually complete at 2 weeks of age in the foal.

5. THE ABDOMEN

Clinical importance of the abdomen

The equine clinician spends a large amount of time attending to medical and surgical conditions of the equine abdomen. This is principally due to the occurrence of colic (abdominal pain) which can arise from any of the abdominal organs. Colic is believed to be the single most important clinical cause of death in the horse. It is also the most common acute emergency. Approximately 90% of cases may respond to medical treatment, particularly pain relief, supportive therapy and prevention of dehydration.

Diagnostic techniques used in the examination of the abdomen include palpation, auscultation, percussion and rectal examination. Radiography is useful in foals and endoscopy is useful for investigation of stomach disorders, particularly gastric ulceration. Ultrasonography is particularly useful in cases of intussusception and for viewing colonic displacements. The ultimate diagnostic techniques are laparoscopy and laparotomy (surgical opening of the abdomen). For laparotomy, the horse is usually placed in dorsal recumbency and surgery will involve a midline incision. In this way most of the small intestine can be exteriorised but not the rostral 1 metre and the last 15–20 cm. The apex and part of the body of the caecum can be lifted out. In addition, the left ventral colon, left dorsal colon and parts of the right dorsal colon and right ventral colon can be lifted out. As in a rectal examination, identification of the various parts of the large bowel is fundamental in cases of displacement or distortion. The major help in this is the presence of the taeniae in the wall of the large intestine; the caecum and the right and left ventral colon all have 4, the pelvic flexure 1, the left dorsal colon 1, and the right dorsal colon has 3 taeniae.

One of the key factors in problems of the digestive system is the inability of the horse to vomit. Once inside the digestive tract, the ingesta (no matter how indigestible or toxic) is there to stay. It is, however, the peculiar anatomy and disposition of the large intestine which especially predisposes to colic. Special features in this respect are the four components of the large colon (two dorsal and two ventral parts) of different calibres and weights; the flexures (particularly the pelvic flexure); the blind-ending sac of the caecum; the long small intestine, which is freely movable; and the considerable narrowing of the lumen from the large colon to the small colon. The left ventral and left dorsal colon are freely movable. The left colon can become displaced to the lateral surface of the caecum, next to the body wall. The pelvic flexure may be displaced forward to the sternum, lateral to the caecum. The left colon can also be displaced to a position between the dorsal body wall and the suspensory ligament of the spleen.

Diet, management, and the presence of particularly virulent parasitic infestations of the gut around the branches of the cranial mesenteric arteries are significant factors in the occurence of colic. Intestinal parasites are less of a common problem these days, thanks to the effective endoparasiticides and better management. Colic can be classified as mild, moderate or severe abdominal pain. It is usually associated with an obstruction to the passage of contents, caused by a failure of gut motility. This causes a rise in intra-abdominal tension, and pain results from the tensions in the mesenteries. Ischaemia of the affected bowel is followed by gut stasis, irritation of the mucosal surfaces and eventually necrosis and inflammation. Several sorts of colic are described. The details are beyond the scope of this introduction but they include spasmodic, impactive, flatulent, obstructive, non-strangulation infarction, enteritis and idiopathic cases.

Displacements of organs, particularly large bowel displacements and torsions, can occur in several sorts of colic. Spasmodic colic may be responsible for 40% of cases and may be associated with increased vagal tone. The condition of 'grass sickness' (equine dysautonomia) in horses is essentially an impaired motility of the gut, resulting in spasmodic colic. Impactive colic is often the result of abnormal feeding, including coarse feed, and failure of a proper fresh water supply. Poor dentition leading to poor mastication, lack of regular worm treatments and failure to remove foreign bodies from the diet, can contribute. Inactivity (i.e. following box rest for orthopaedic conditions) can also contribute to the problem.

The transverse colon is often the site of impaction with enteroliths and faeces and, in the foal, with meconium. Enteroliths are caused by the precipitation of magnesium and ammonium phosphate crystals around a nucleus such as a stone, nail or other foreign body. As they increase in size they are particularly prone to getting stuck in the small intestine and transverse colon. Impaction is very common in the caecum and in the pelvic flexure of the colon. Caecal impaction, if severe, may be followed by caecal perforation. Pelvic flexure impaction is often caused by a combination of coarse roughage, sand and gas. The stomach can become impacted with corn and bedding, and the duodenum can be impacted with coarse ingesta.

Flatulent colic is a result of excessive production of gas associated with fermentation of the feed (usually of poor quality). Excessive gas production can be detected by listening for a 'ping' when simultaneous percussion and auscultation is carried out. It can be relieved by caecal trocarisation in which a trocar and a cannula are inserted into the caecum though the right paralumbar fossa.

Obstructive more colic and infarction is usually a result of nematode parasites. The 4th and 5th stages of *Strongylus vulgaris* damage the blood supply by migrating through the walls of the cranial mesenteric artery. The resultant thrombi cause intra-vascular occlusion of the vessels and ischaemia. The ileum may become thickened (hypertrophic) in response to persistent parasitic infestation.

A particular form of obstruction occurs with sand (picked up with the food) and also with the ingestion of foreign materials (e.g. plastic bags). Idiopathic colic (where there is at present no known cause) may, perhaps, include colitis X. Colitis can also result from prolonged drug therapy (e.g. right dorsal colitis with phenylbutazone therapy). In addition, strangulation of the bowel can occur and also torsion. Both will cause impaction and obstruction. Small intestinal volvulus occurs when a segment of the small intestine rotates around the long axis of its mesentery. A 180 degree rotation of the jejunum may also occur, and frequently the ileum is involved because of its fixed attachment at the ileo-caeco-colic junction. Large bowel volvulus involves a rotation of the dorsal and ventral parts of the colon on their horizontal axes and this also frequently involves the caecum.

Enteritis is not common in the horse but there is, on occasion, an acute severe enteritis in horses associated with clostridial infections. It causes an acute colic and is often diagnosed only at surgery or post-mortem examination. There are up to 10 parasites that may live in the large bowel and cause irritation which may lead to diarrhoea. Severe diarrhoea, with irritation and constant straining, may lead to intussusception. Sudden dietary changes and parasitic infestation are usually a cause of this condition. There is also a real possibility of salmonellosis in any horse that is stressed or has been subjected to surgery. Several other conditions may also cause acute enteritis such as Potomac horse fever in certain parts of the world. Chronic inflammatory bowel disease can also occur. It usually involves internal parasites but also may involve strangles, *Rhodococcus equi* or even

M. paratuberculosis. A naso-gastric (stomach) tube can be used to deliver large volumes of oral rehydration therapy.

Dysfunctions of the liver can be investigated by percutaneous liver biopsy in the right 12–13th intercostal space, with sedation and local anaesthesia. It should be carried out between lines drawn from the tuber coxae to the point of the shoulder and to the point of the olecranon. The liver normally lies deep to intercostal spaces 10–14 but may atrophy considerably with age. Liver disease is quite common in the horse, probably as a result of eating plants of the genus *Senecio,* particularly ragwort. It is often associated with damage to the bile ducts. It causes weight loss, and investigations should include analysis of liver enzymes and liver function tests. In severe cases, hepatic encephalopathy can occur; nervous signs result from circulating waste products. Complete liver failure is quite rare, as there is a huge functional reserve in the equine liver, and over 70% has to be damaged before this will occur.

The horse is particularly prone to peritonitis, probably because of the fragility of the gut. It can be primary or secondary, diffuse or localized. It is usually acute and diffuse and follows gastro-intestinal disease. Haemoperitoneum follows migration of strongyle larvae through the cranial mesenteric vessels, or foaling or rupture of the spleen or liver following traumatic accidents.

Uroperitoneum may result from rupture of the bladder. In a foal, during the first week of life, this must be differentiated from other types of colic which are caused by distension. If an accumulation of peritoneal fluid is suspected, abdominocentesis can be performed. Needles are used to drain fluid from a site about 5 cm caudal to the xiphoid cartilage in the right paramedian position (this avoids penetrating the spleen). Abdominal ultrasound can be used. (The normal approach for paracentesis of the abdomen is midline through the *linea alba* at the most dependent area.)

External hernias are protrusions of an organ or part of an organ through a normal opening in the wall of the cavity. Umbilical, inguinal and perineal are the usual types. In young animals the congenital hernias can be left if small or surgically repaired if large. Most inguinal hernias fall into this group. Umbilical hernias occur in about 2% of thoroughbred horses, are more common in females than in males, and have a strong hereditary component. Diaphragmatic hernias are internal hernias. They can occur as congenital defects but are more likely as a result of trauma, as when a horse is trapped over a gate or fence or jump, resulting in an increase in intra-abdominal pressure. If abdominal contents pass through one of the normal openings in the diaphragm (caval, oesophageal or aortic hiatuses) colic may result.

It is also possible to have an internal herniation of abdominal viscera through the epiploic foramen. Through this foramen, the greater peritoneal cavity communicates with the lesser cavity or omental bursa. It lies in the right dorsal quadrant of the abdomen, situated on the ventral surface of the liver, dorsal to the portal fissure. Dorsal to the foramen lie the caudate process of the liver, hepatic portal vein, gastro-pancreatic fold and the caudal vena cava. Ventrally, there are relations to the right lobe of the pancreas, the gastro-pancreatic fold and the portal vein. Rostrally, lies the hepato-duodenal ligament. Caudally, lie the pancreas and mesoduodenum. There is no real age association for this internal hernia, but there are suggestions that the condition may be more common in the horse that crib bites or wind sucks (8 times more likely). In old horses, this foramen may be 10 cm long, mainly due to the atrophy of the right lobe of the liver. This atrophy may predispose to internal herniation. In these animals there is the possibility of a segment of small intestine passing through the foramen. The intestine may enter the omental bursa from right to left, or may slip through the foramen from left to right. The amount of intestine that slips through varies from several centimetres to all of the small intestine.

All the boundaries of the abdomen may have ruptures which do not traverse the natural openings but traverse defects in the walls or membranes. Complex internal ruptures may occur, as when the gastro-splenic ligament is torn and the distal jejunum goes from a caudal to a cranial direction. Mesocolic rupture may occur during parturition, involving the mesentery of the small colon. It is a complication of rectal prolapse often accompanied by prolapse of bladder, uterus, vagina and intestine or any combination thereof.

Abdominal abscesses usually involve the mesenteric lymph nodes and are associated with the usual pus-forming bacteria of the horse – streptococci, *E.coli*, salmonella or *Rhodococcus equi*. Abdominal neoplasia is rare. Alimentary lymphoma is seen infrequently, but lipomas are a common cause of colic, especially in grey horses. Intestinal or other alimentary melanomas are also common in grey horses.

Clinical considerations for the spine in the abdominal region are dealt with in the section on the spine in Chapter 8 (p. 269).

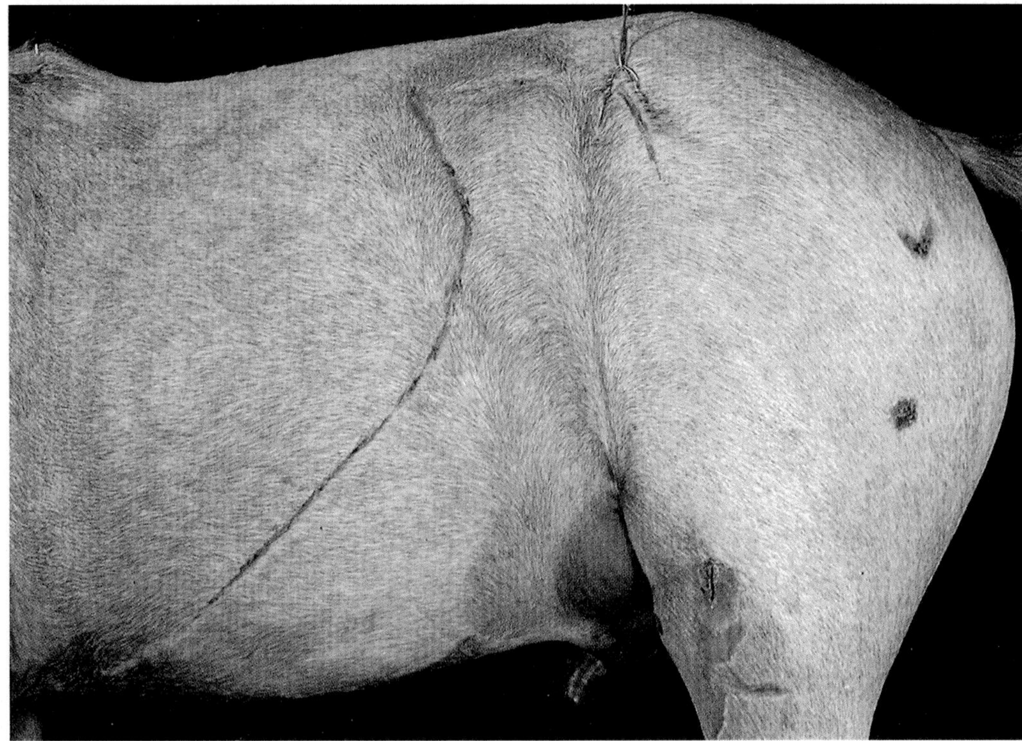

Fig. 5.1 Surface features of the abdomen: left lateral view. The hair has been shaved over the palpable bony prominences. The umbilicus lies in the median plane, just cranial to the prepuce, and its position in the female is shown in Fig. 5.55.

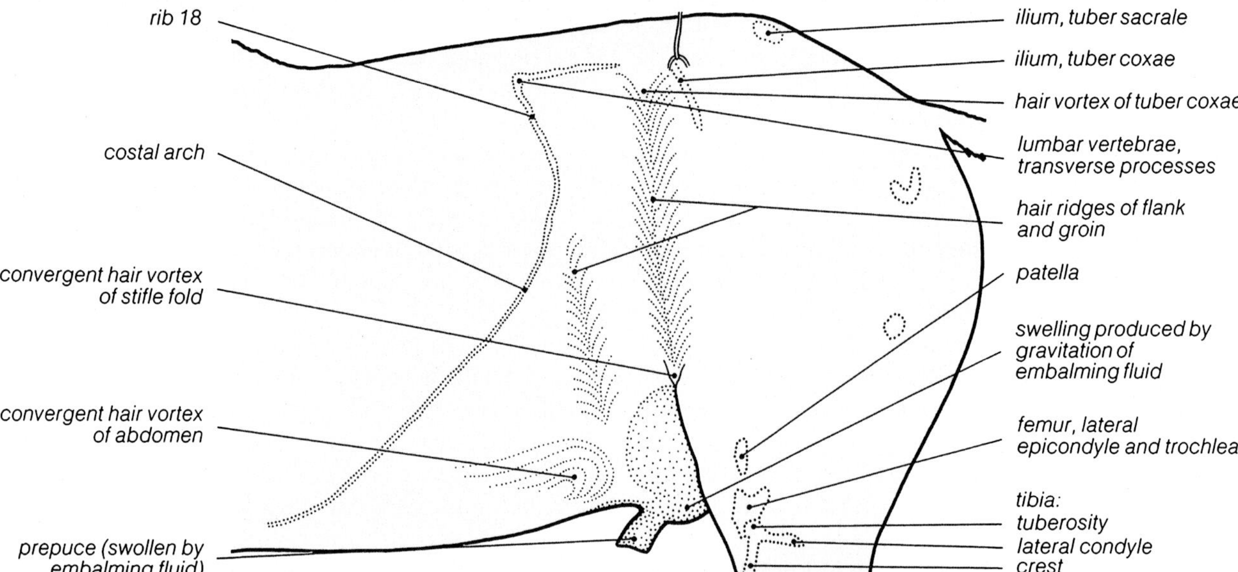
rib 18
costal arch
convergent hair vortex of stifle fold
convergent hair vortex of abdomen
prepuce (swollen by embalming fluid)
ilium, tuber sacrale
ilium, tuber coxae
hair vortex of tuber coxae
lumbar vertebrae, transverse processes
hair ridges of flank and groin
patella
swelling produced by gravitation of embalming fluid
femur, lateral epicondyle and trochlea
tibia:
tuberosity
lateral condyle
crest

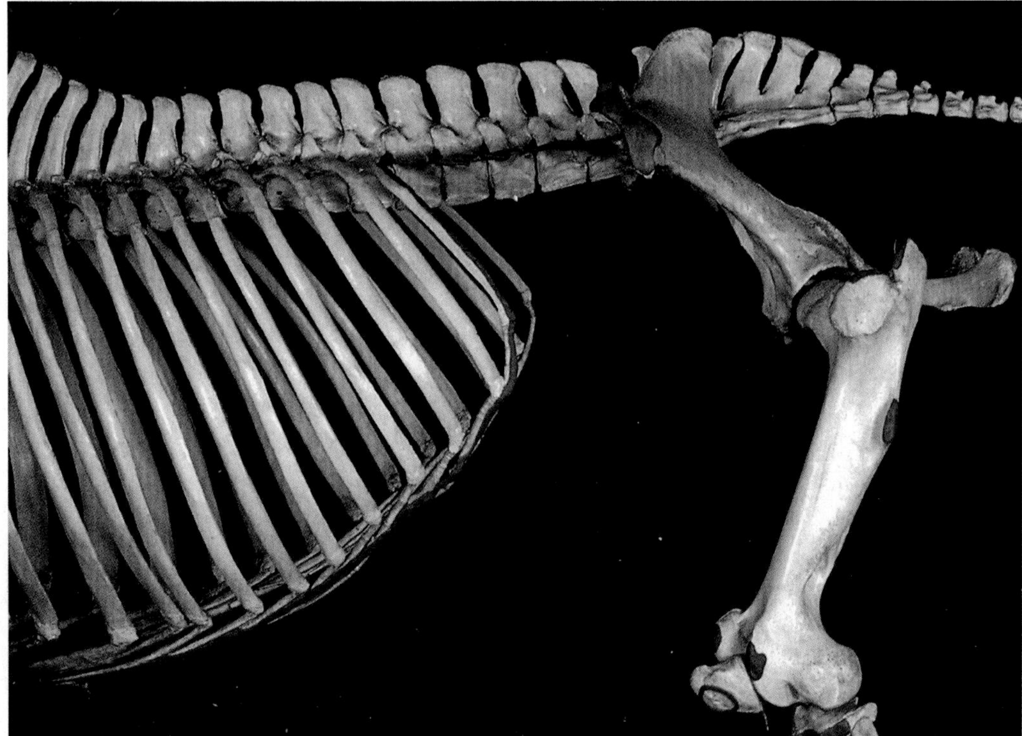

Fig. 5.2 Bones related to the abdomen: left lateral view. The palpable bony prominences shown in Fig. 5.1 are coloured red, except for the tuber sacrale.

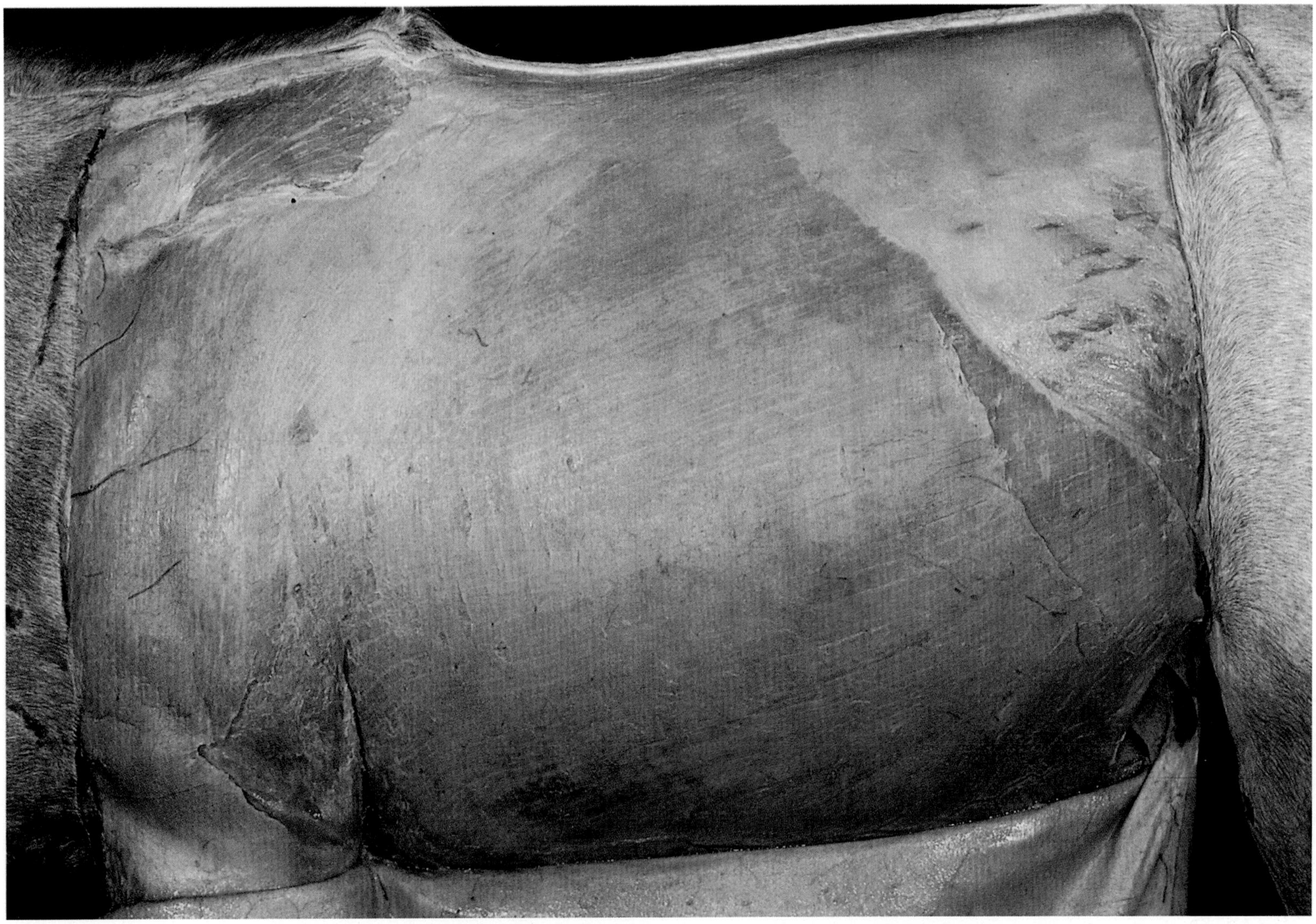

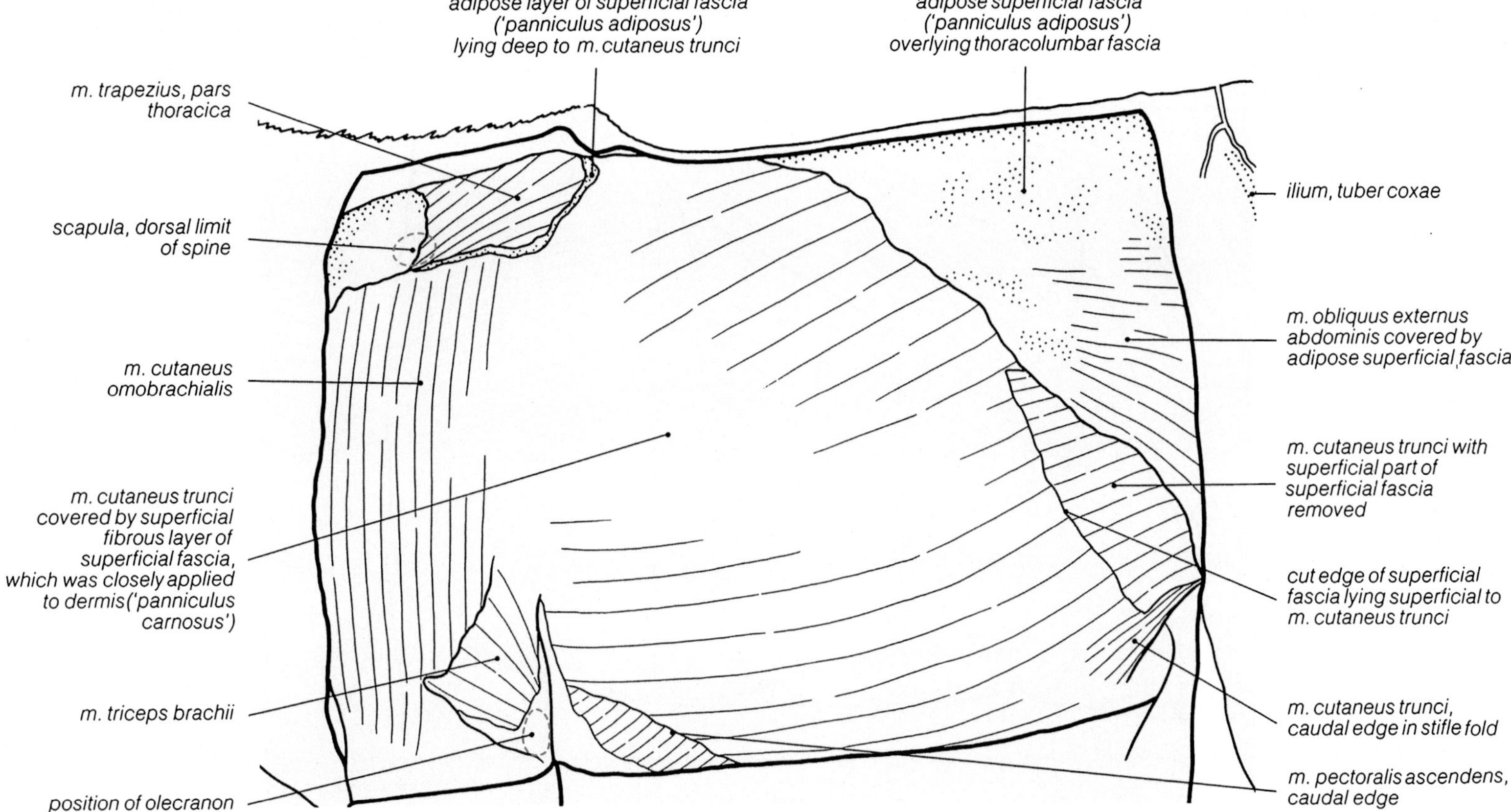
adipose layer of superficial fascia ('panniculus adiposus') lying deep to m. cutaneus trunci
adipose superficial fascia ('panniculus adiposus') overlying thoracolumbar fascia
m. trapezius, pars thoracica
ilium, tuber coxae
scapula, dorsal limit of spine
m. obliquus externus abdominis covered by adipose superficial fascia
m. cutaneus omobrachialis
m. cutaneus trunci with superficial part of superficial fascia removed
m. cutaneus trunci covered by superficial fibrous layer of superficial fascia, which was closely applied to dermis('panniculus carnosus')
cut edge of superficial fascia lying superficial to m. cutaneus trunci
m. triceps brachii
m. cutaneus trunci, caudal edge in stifle fold
position of olecranon
m. pectoralis ascendens, caudal edge

Fig. 5.3 The cutaneous muscle of the trunk: left lateral view. The muscle lies in the superficial fascia; superficially it is closely adherent to the dermis and forms the 'panniculus carnosus'. Deep to it, the superficial fascia contains extensive fat deposits ('panniculus adiposus'). The cutaneous nerves are shown in Figs. 5.4 and 5.10. See also Fig. 5.9.

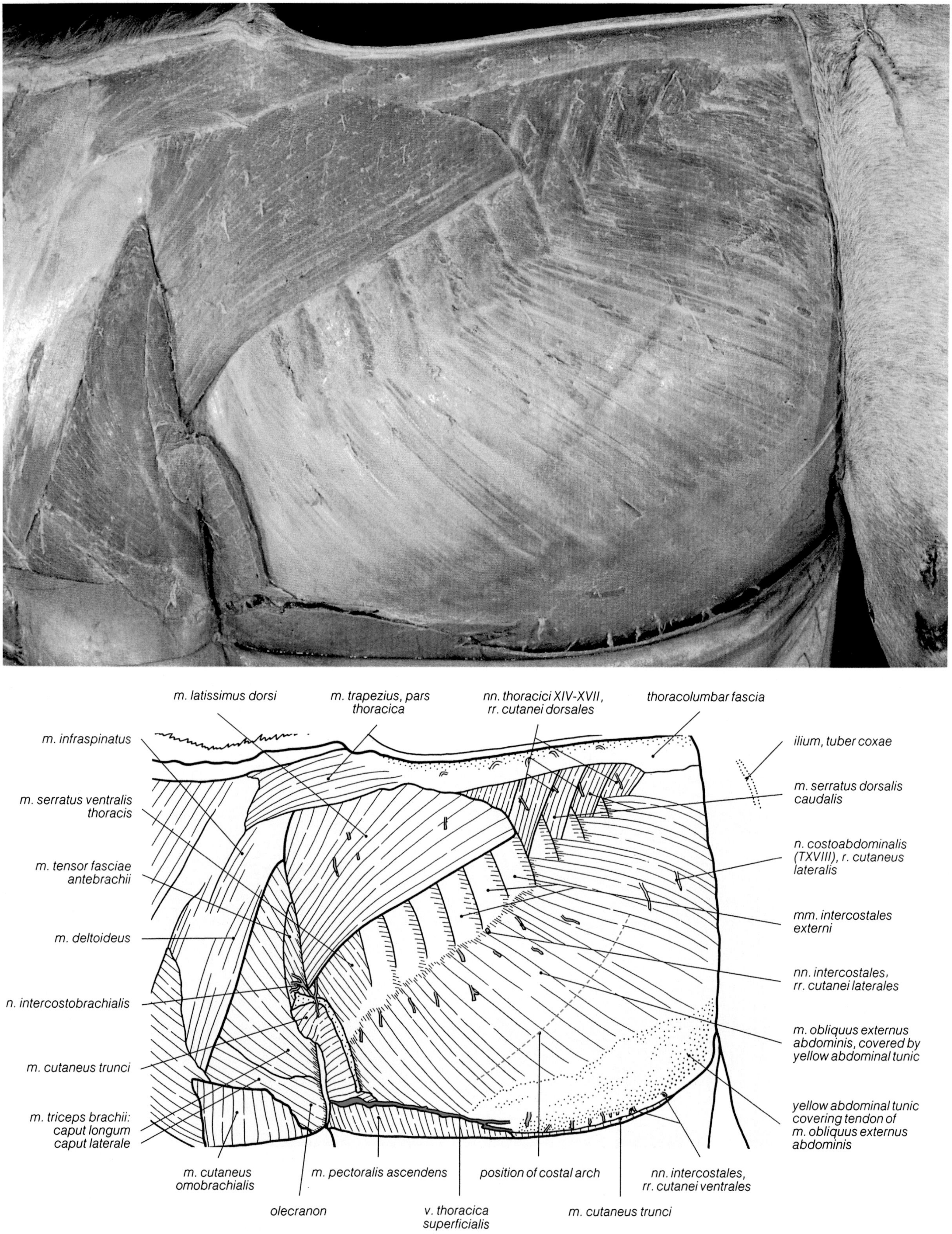

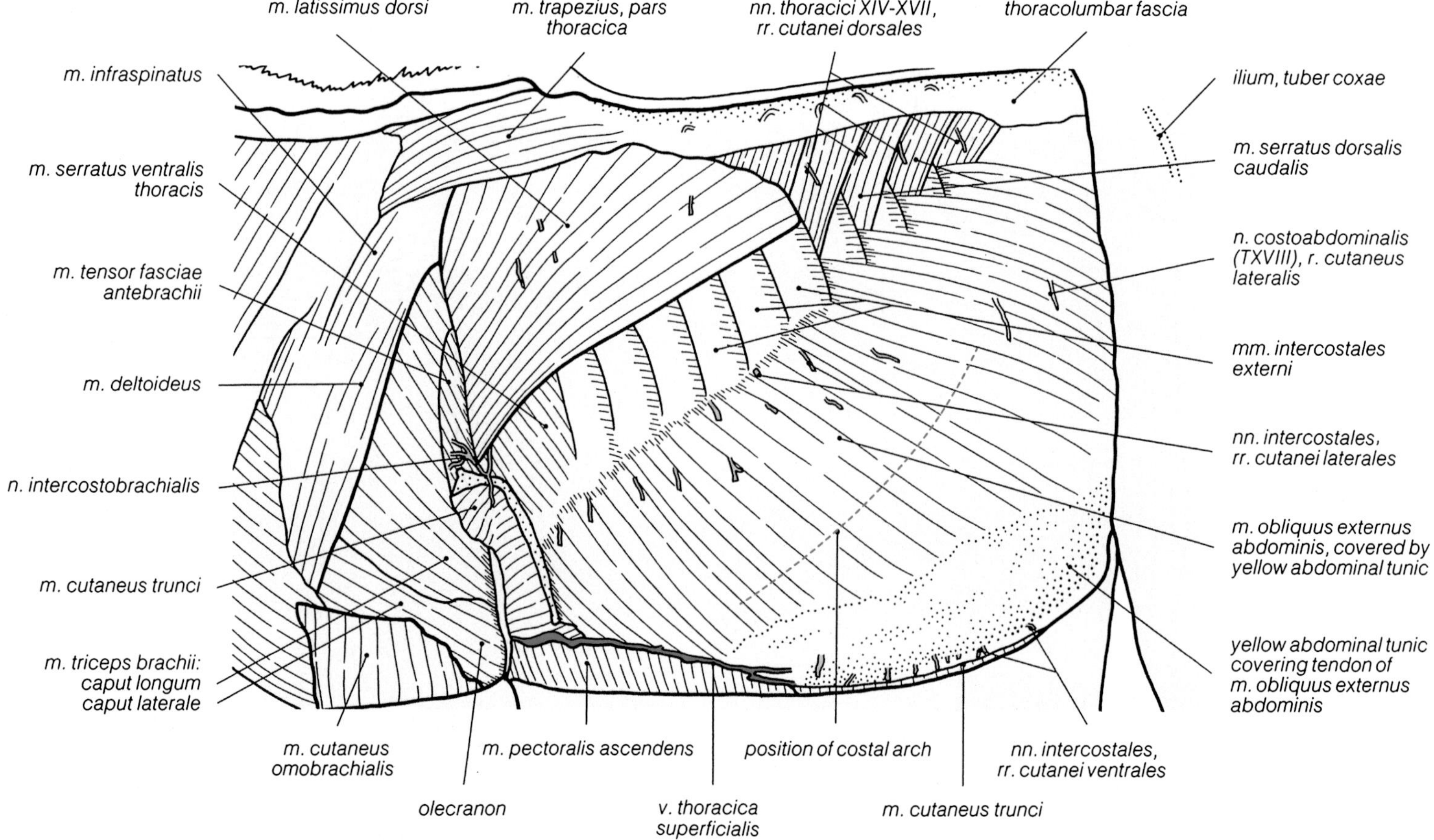
m. latissimus dorsi
m. trapezius, pars thoracica
nn. thoracici XIV-XVII, rr. cutanei dorsales
thoracolumbar fascia
m. infraspinatus
ilium, tuber coxae
m. serratus ventralis thoracis
m. serratus dorsalis caudalis
m. tensor fasciae antebrachii
n. costoabdominalis (TXVIII), r. cutaneus lateralis
mm. intercostales externi
m. deltoideus
nn. intercostales, rr. cutanei laterales
n. intercostobrachialis
m. obliquus externus abdominis, covered by yellow abdominal tunic
m. cutaneus trunci
yellow abdominal tunic covering tendon of m. obliquus externus abdominis
m. triceps brachii: caput longum caput laterale
m. cutaneus omobrachialis
m. pectoralis ascendens
position of costal arch
nn. intercostales, rr. cutanei ventrales
olecranon
v. thoracica superficialis
m. cutaneus trunci

Fig. 5.4 The external oblique abdominal muscle and cutaneous nerves of the thoracic and abdominal wall: left lateral view. The cutaneous muscles have been removed. Further details of the nerves are shown in Fig. 5.10.

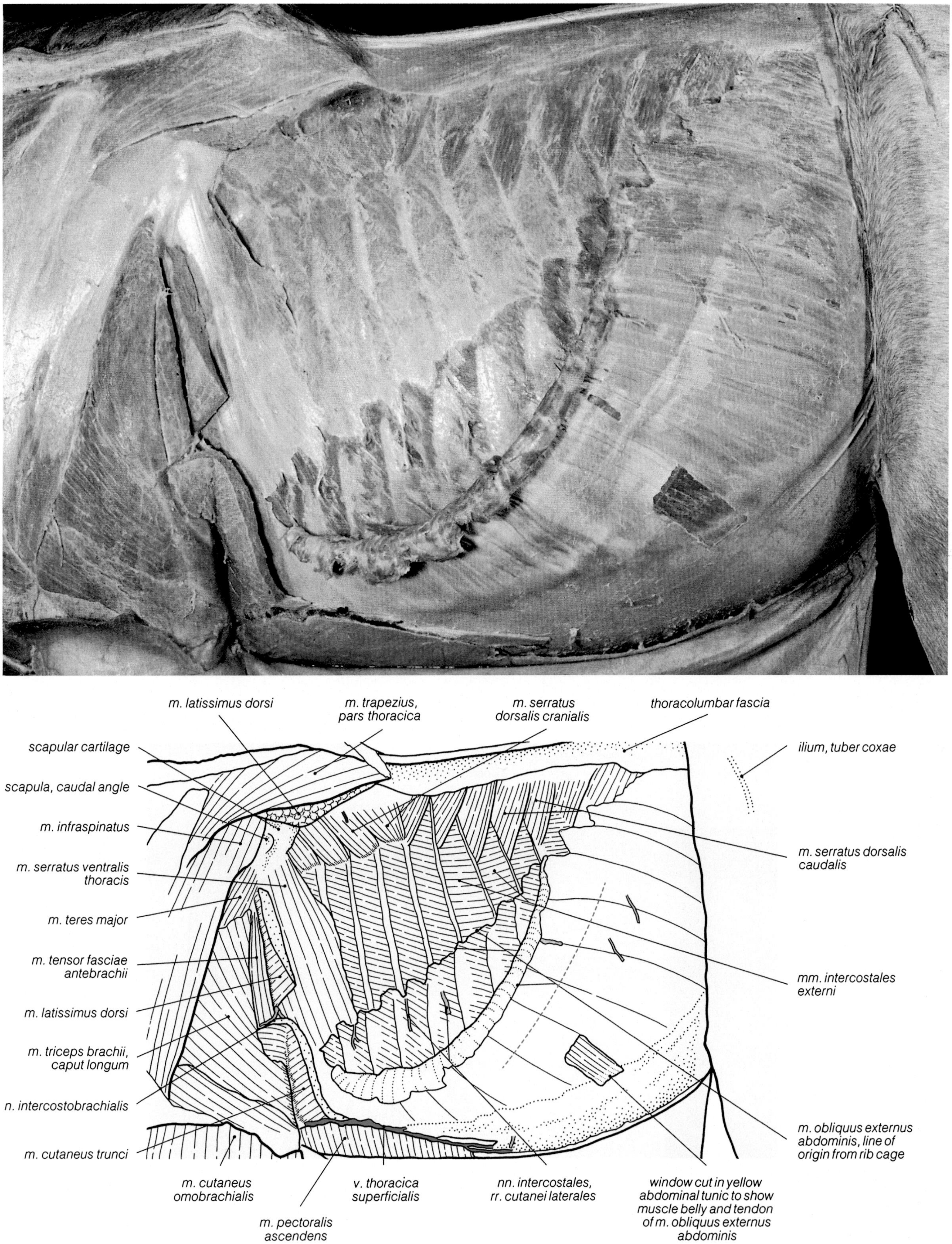

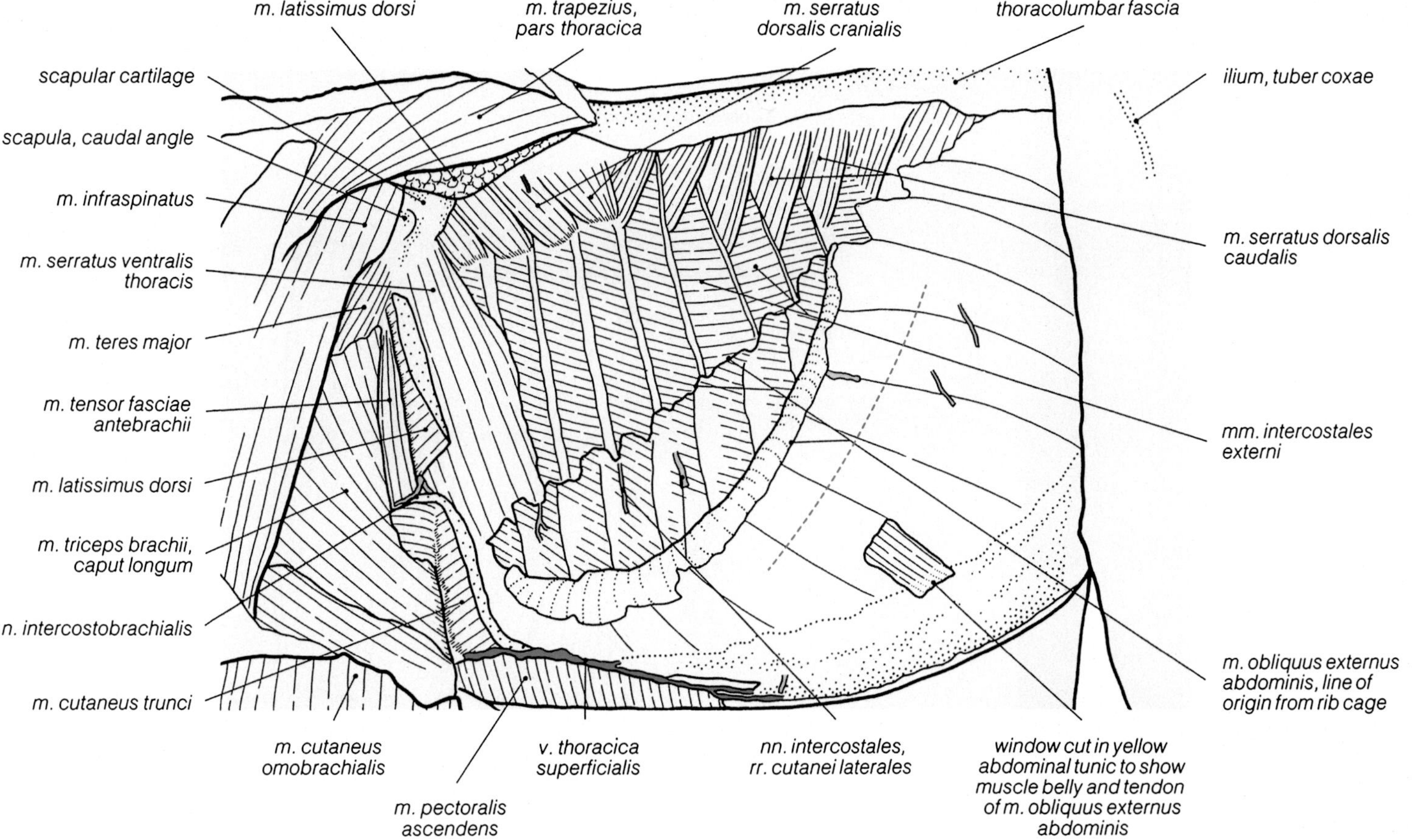
m. latissimus dorsi
m. trapezius, pars thoracica
m. serratus dorsalis cranialis
thoracolumbar fascia
scapular cartilage
ilium, tuber coxae
scapula, caudal angle
m. infraspinatus
m. serratus ventralis thoracis
m. serratus dorsalis caudalis
m. teres major
m. tensor fasciae antebrachii
mm. intercostales externi
m. latissimus dorsi
m. triceps brachii, caput longum
n. intercostobrachialis
m. obliquus externus abdominis, line of origin from rib cage
m. cutaneus trunci
m. cutaneus omobrachialis
v. thoracica superficialis
nn. intercostales, rr. cutanei laterales
window cut in yellow abdominal tunic to show muscle belly and tendon of m. obliquus externus abdominis
m. pectoralis ascendens

Fig. 5.5 The external oblique abdominal muscle and yellow abdominal tunic: left lateral view. The latissimus dorsi muscle has been excised. The origins of the external oblique muscle have been severed; the curling of the muscle that results is due to the outer elastic fascia of the yellow abdominal tunic.

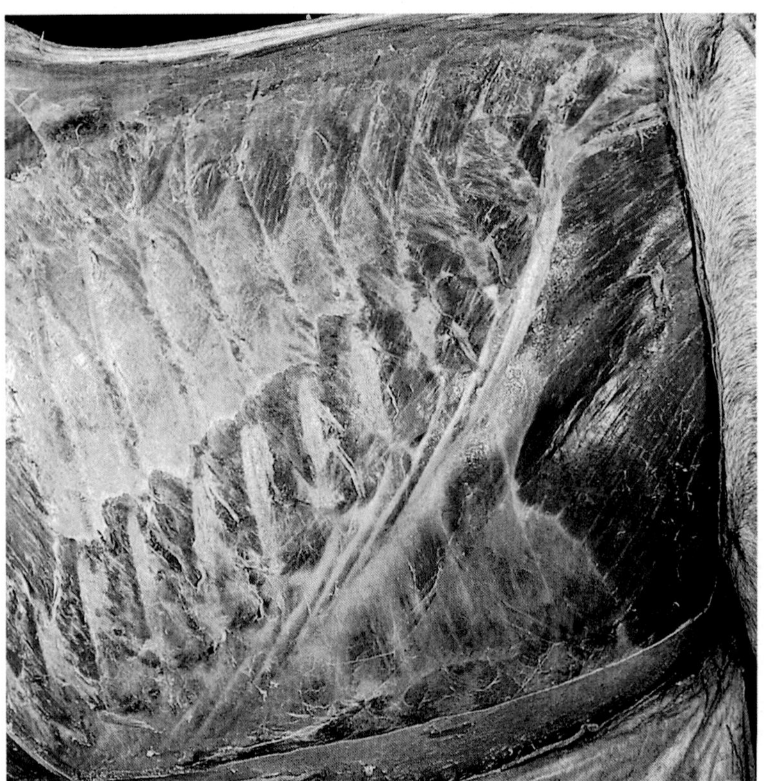

Fig. 5.6 The internal oblique abdominal muscle: left lateral view. The origin of this muscle from the tuber coxae is shown in Fig. 5.11. The ventral parts of the ventral branches of the intercostal nerves (and also the lumbar nerves; see Fig. 5.7) run between the transverse and the internal oblique muscles.

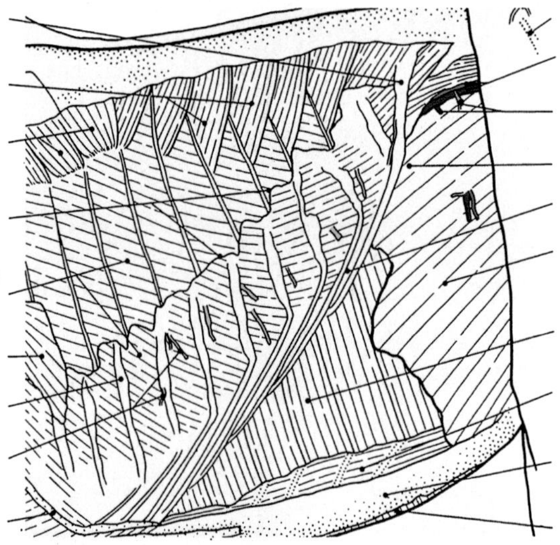

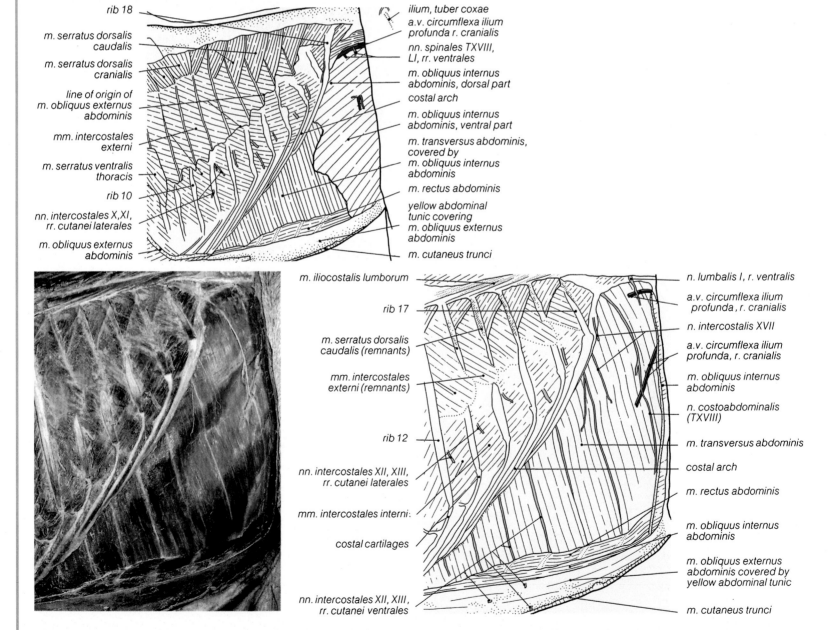

rib 18
m. serratus dorsalis caudalis
m. serratus dorsalis cranialis
line of origin of m. obliquus externus abdominis
mm. intercostales externi
m. serratus ventralis thoracis
rib 10
nn. intercostales X,XI, rr. cutanei laterales
m. obliquus externus abdominis
ilium, tuber coxae
a.v. circumflexa ilium profunda r. cranialis
nn. spinales TXVIII, LI, rr. ventrales
m. obliquus internus abdominis, dorsal part
costal arch
m. obliquus internus abdominis, ventral part
m. transversus abdominis, covered by m. obliquus internus abdominis
m. rectus abdominis
yellow abdominal tunic covering m. obliquus externus abdominis
m. cutaneus trunci

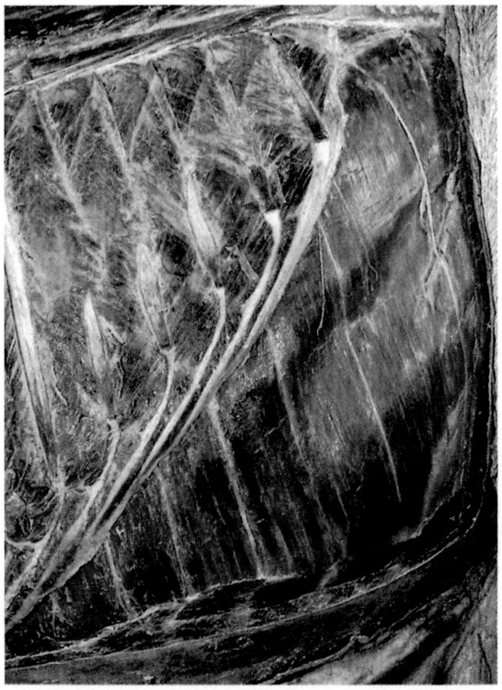

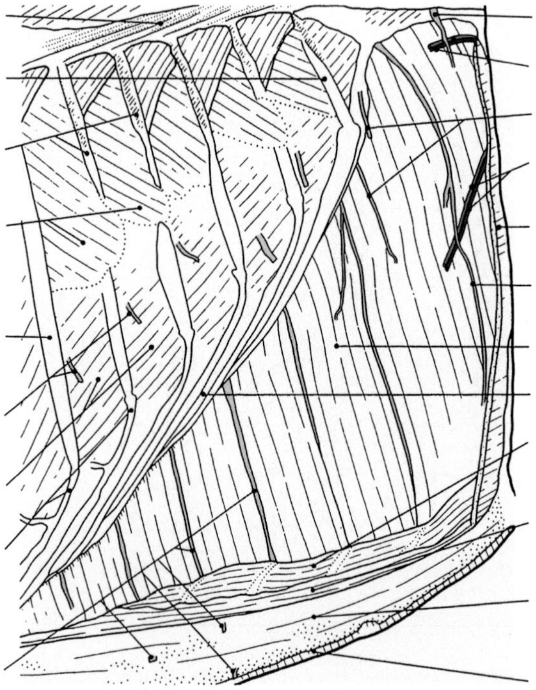

m. iliocostalis lumborum
rib 17
m. serratus dorsalis caudalis (remnants)
mm. intercostales externi (remnants)
rib 12
nn. intercostales XII, XIII, rr. cutanei laterales
mm. intercostales interni
costal cartilages
nn. intercostales XII, XIII, rr. cutanei ventrales
n. lumbalis I, r. ventralis
a.v. circumflexa ilium profunda, r. cranialis
n. intercostalis XVII
a.v. circumflexa ilium profunda, r. cranialis
m. obliquus internus abdominis
n. costoabdominalis (TXVIII)
m. transversus abdominis
costal arch
m. rectus abdominis
m. obliquus internus abdominis
m. obliquus externus abdominis covered by yellow abdominal tunic
m. cutaneus trunci

Fig. 5.7 The transverse abdominal muscle: left lateral view. The 18th rib in this specimen was very small (see Fig. 5.15 and compare with Fig. 5.43). The more caudal part of the origin of this muscle is seen in Fig. 5.12.

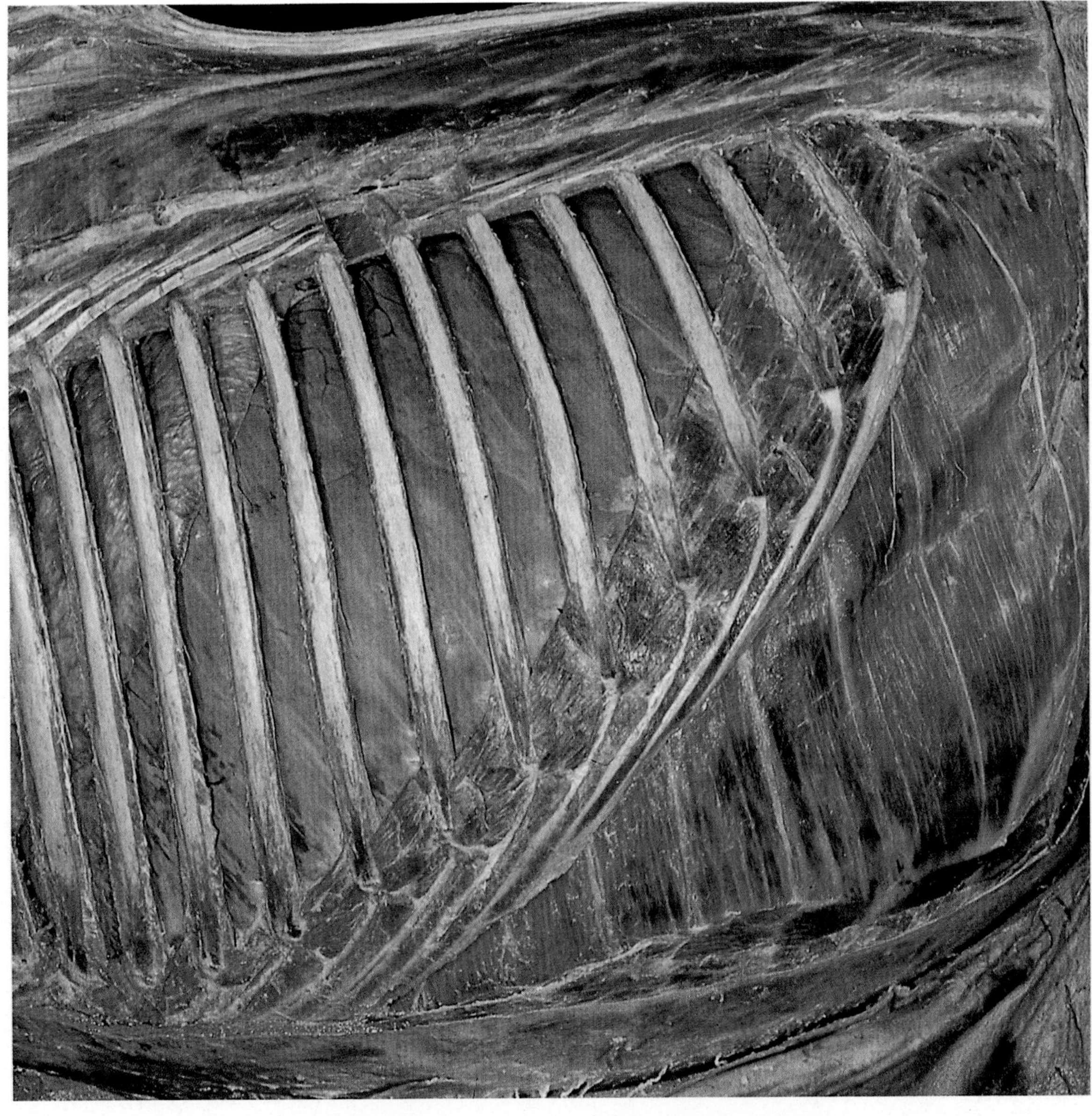

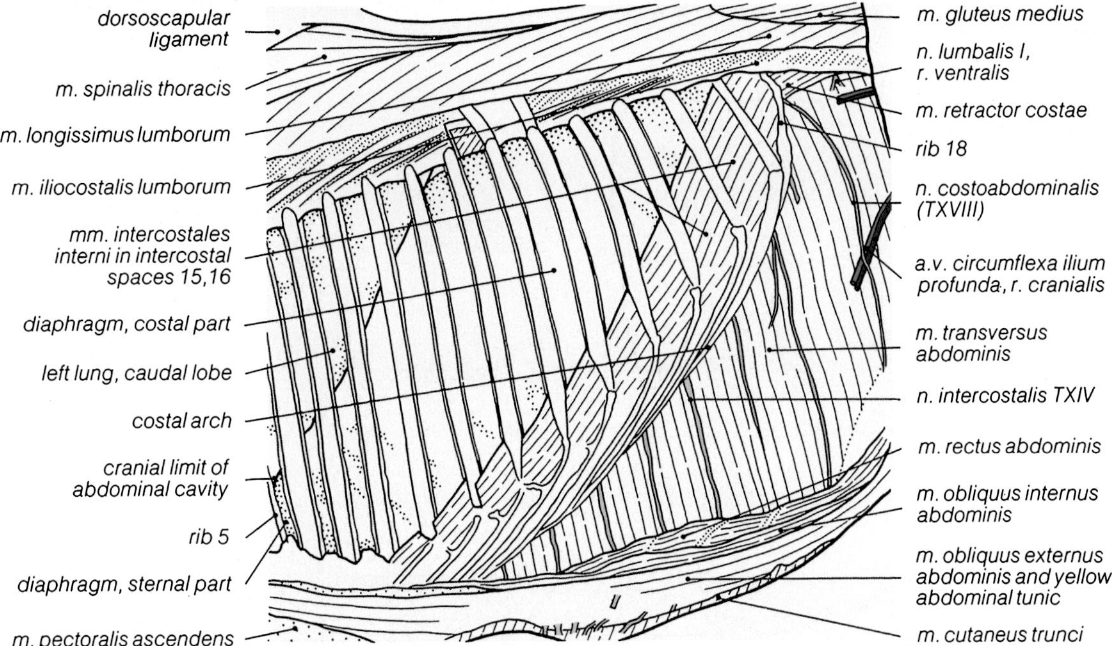
dorsoscapular ligament
m. spinalis thoracis
m. longissimus lumborum
m. iliocostalis lumborum
mm. intercostales interni in intercostal spaces 15,16
diaphragm, costal part
left lung, caudal lobe
costal arch
cranial limit of abdominal cavity
rib 5
diaphragm, sternal part
m. pectoralis ascendens
m. gluteus medius
n. lumbalis I, r. ventralis
m. retractor costae
rib 18
n. costoabdominalis (TXVIII)
a.v. circumflexa ilium profunda, r. cranialis
m. transversus abdominis
n. intercostalis TXIV
m. rectus abdominis
m. obliquus internus abdominis
m. obliquus externus abdominis and yellow abdominal tunic
m. cutaneus trunci

Fig. 5.8 The transverse abdominal muscle and diaphragm: left lateral view. This dissection shows the extent of the abdominal cavity in relationship to the rib cage. A view of the superficial viscera on the left side is shown in Fig. 5.14.

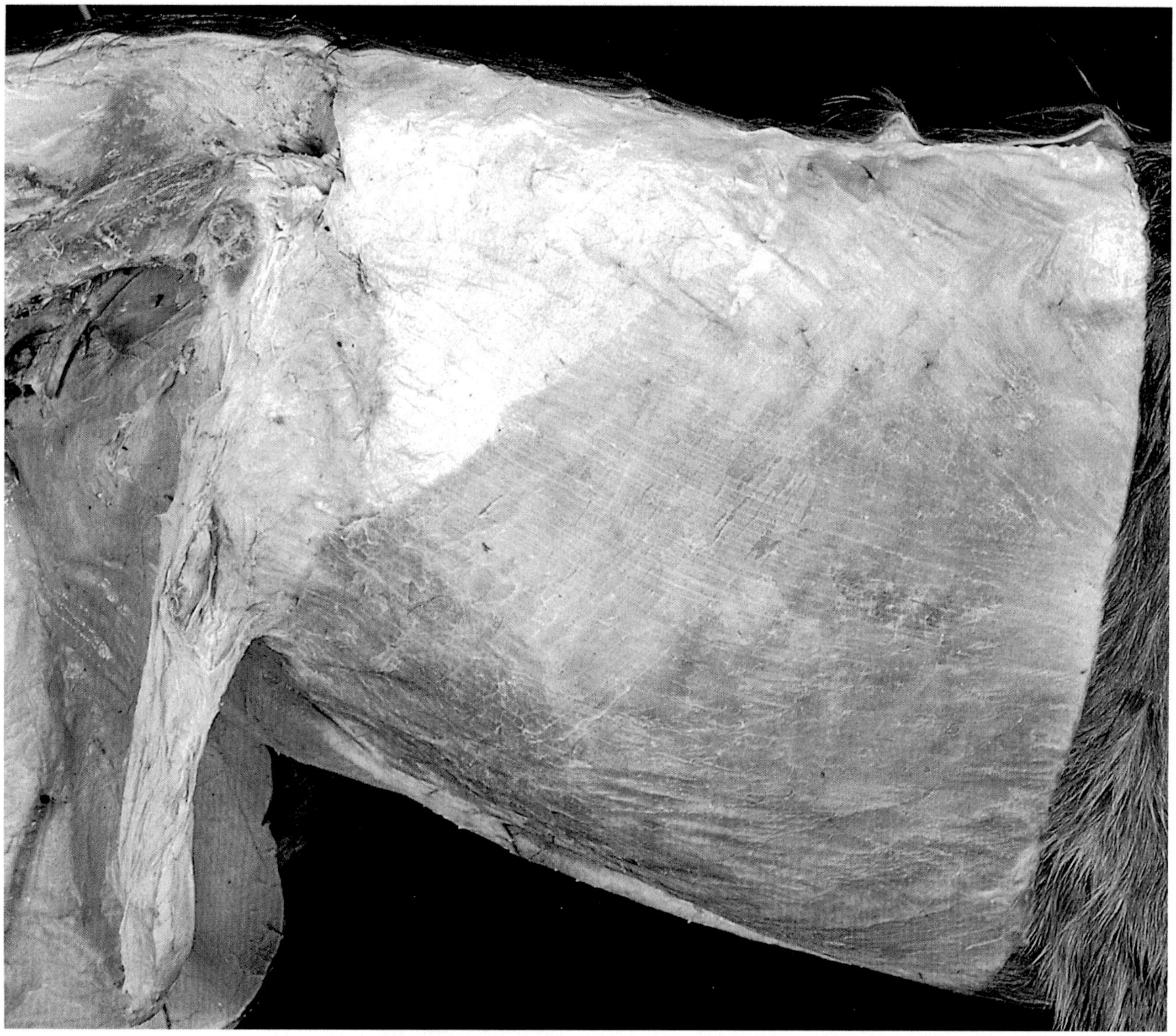

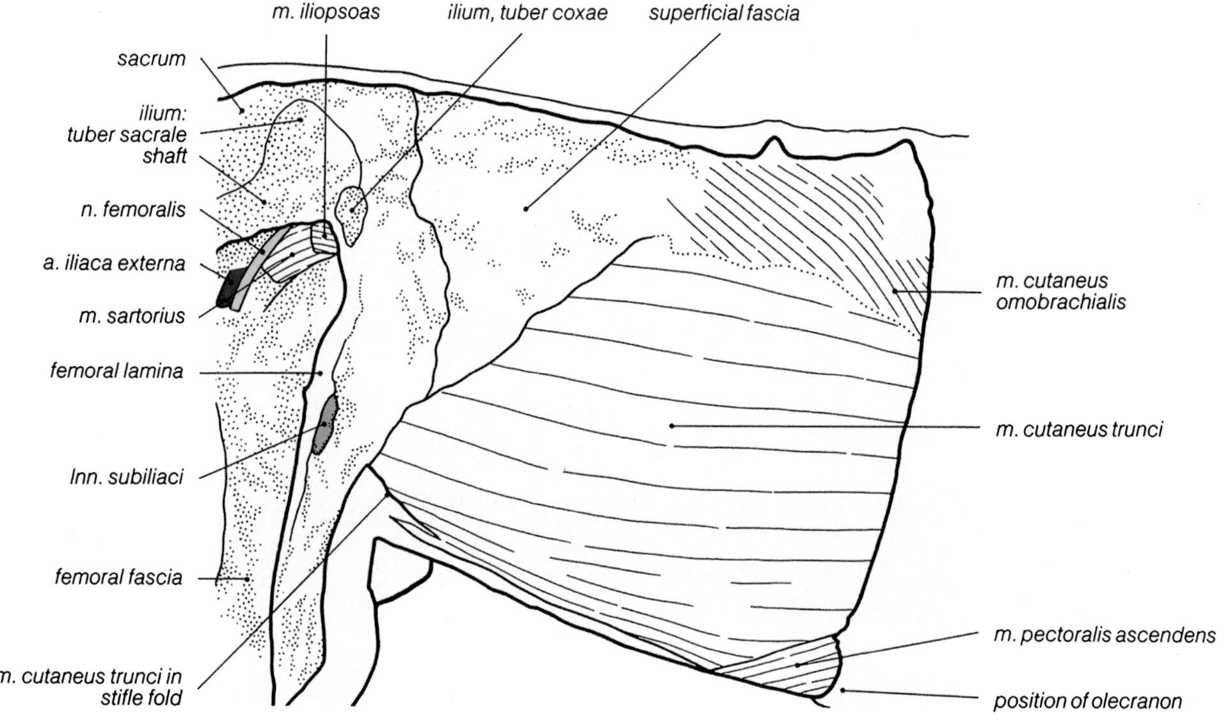
m. iliopsoas
ilium, tuber coxae
superficial fascia
sacrum
ilium:
tuber sacrale
shaft
n. femoralis
a. iliaca externa
m. sartorius
femoral lamina
lnn. subiliaci
femoral fascia
m. cutaneus trunci in
stifle fold
m. cutaneus
omobrachialis
m. cutaneus trunci
m. pectoralis ascendens
position of olecranon

Fig. 5.9 The cutaneous muscle of the trunk in a new-born female foal: right lateral view. The right hindlimb has been removed but the femoral fascia on its medial aspect has been preserved. The femoral lamina, joining the femoral fascia to the deep fascia of the abdominal wall, has also been preserved (see Fig. 5.10). The ilium has been coloured red. Further dissections of the abdominal wall in this specimen are shown in Figs.5.10–5.12.

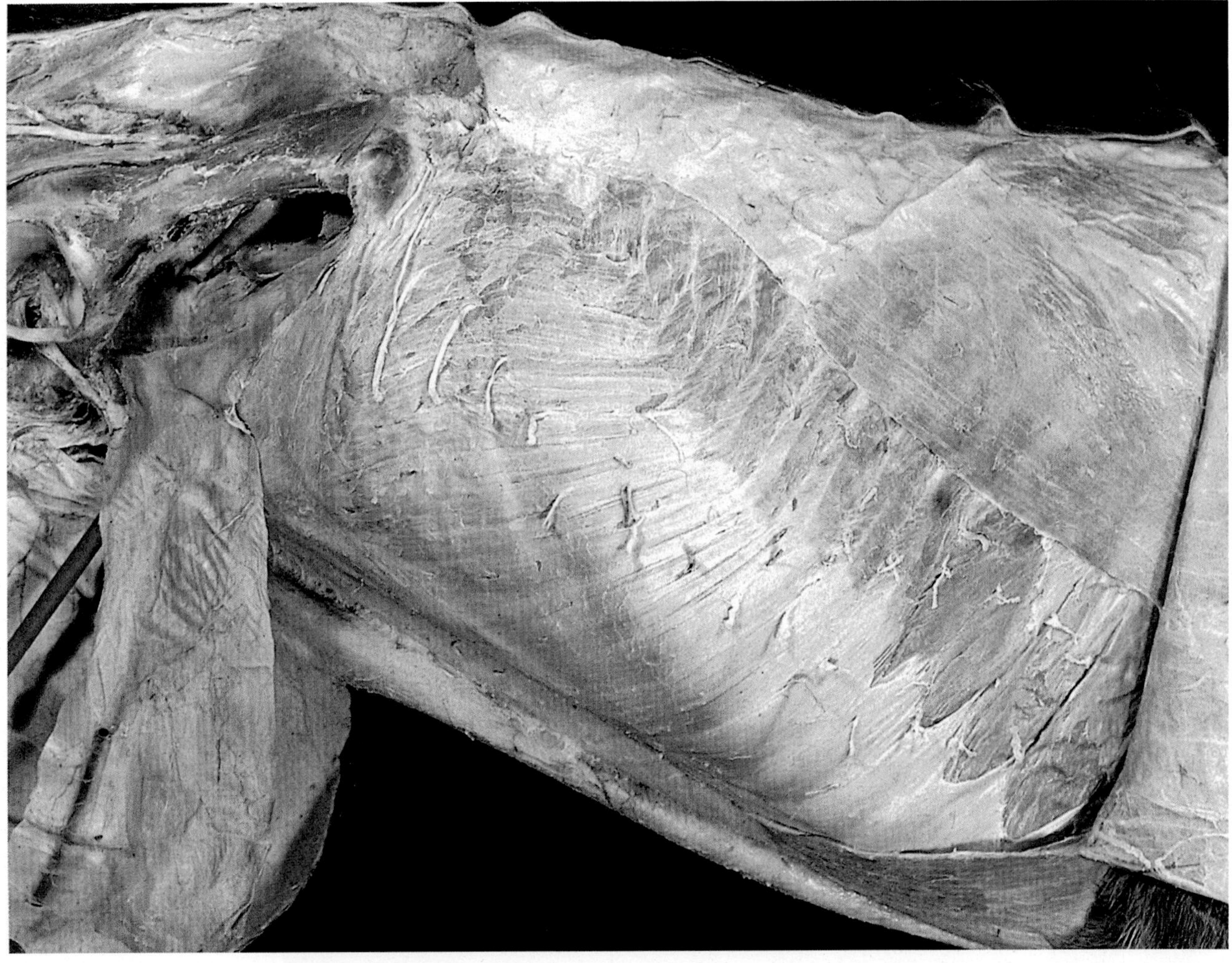

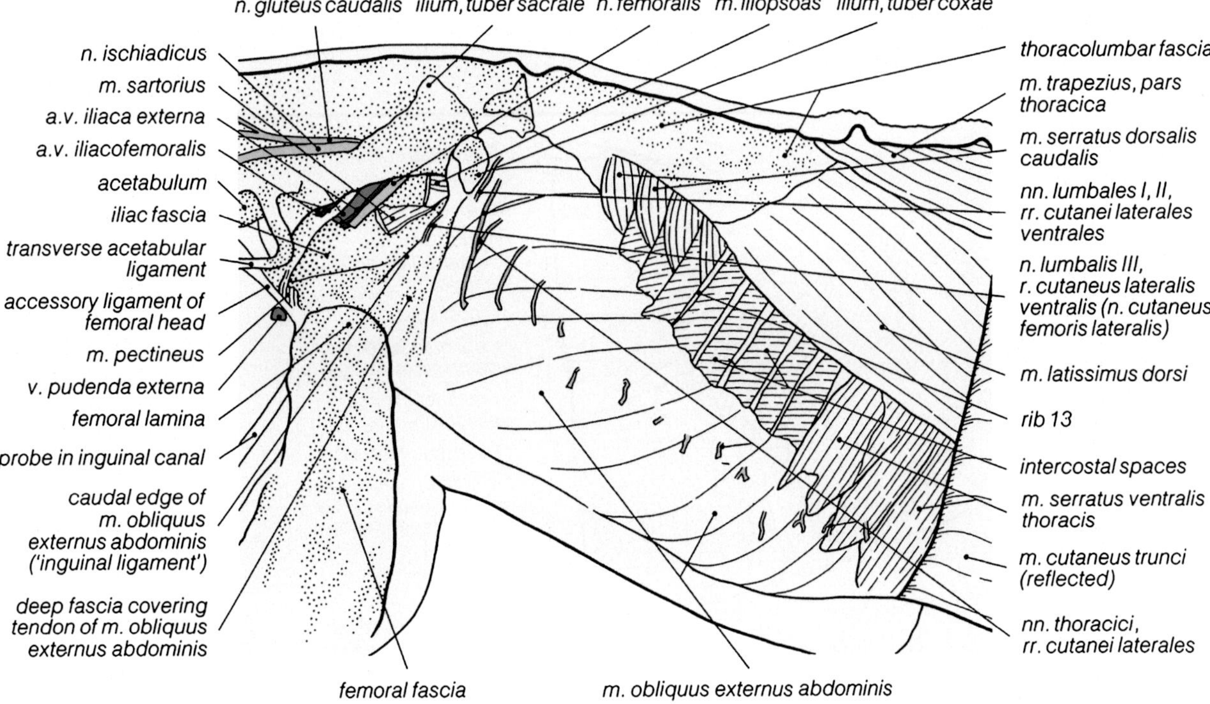
n. gluteus caudalis
ilium, tuber sacrale
n. femoralis
m. iliopsoas
ilium, tuber coxae
n. ischiadicus
m. sartorius
a.v. iliaca externa
a.v. iliacofemoralis
acetabulum
iliac fascia
transverse acetabular ligament
accessory ligament of femoral head
m. pectineus
v. pudenda externa
femoral lamina
probe in inguinal canal
caudal edge of m. obliquus externus abdominis ('inguinal ligament')
deep fascia covering tendon of m. obliquus externus abdominis
femoral fascia
m. obliquus externus abdominis
thoracolumbar fascia
m. trapezius, pars thoracica
m. serratus dorsalis caudalis
nn. lumbales I, II, rr. cutanei laterales ventrales
n. lumbalis III, r. cutaneus lateralis ventralis (n. cutaneus femoris lateralis)
m. latissimus dorsi
rib 13
intercostal spaces
m. serratus ventralis thoracis
m. cutaneus trunci (reflected)
nn. thoracici, rr. cutanei laterales

Fig. 5.10 The external oblique abdominal muscle of the foal: right lateral view. The cutaneous muscle has been reflected cranially. The superficial fascia has been removed from the femoral lamina to show its attachments to the deep abdominal and femoral fasciae.

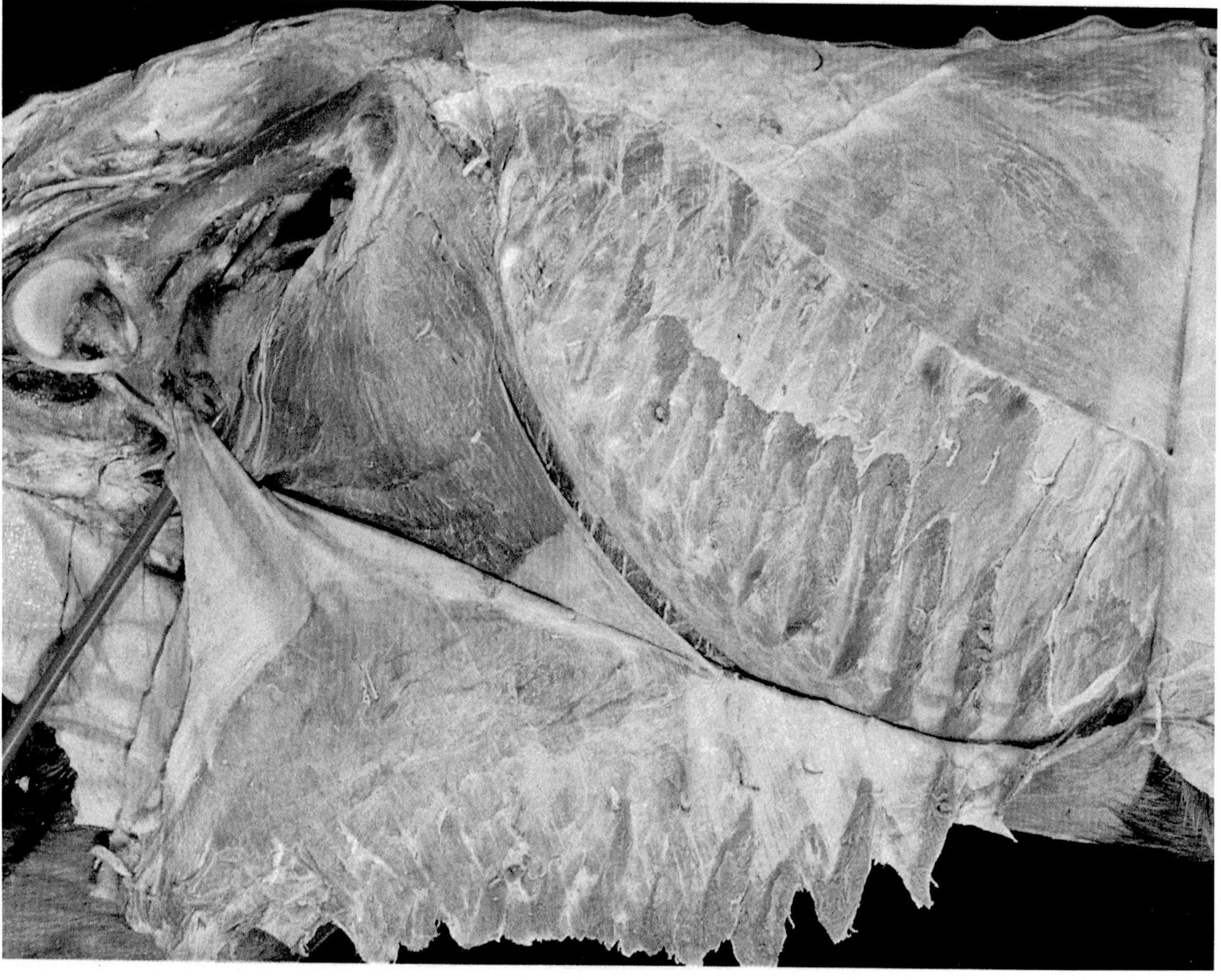

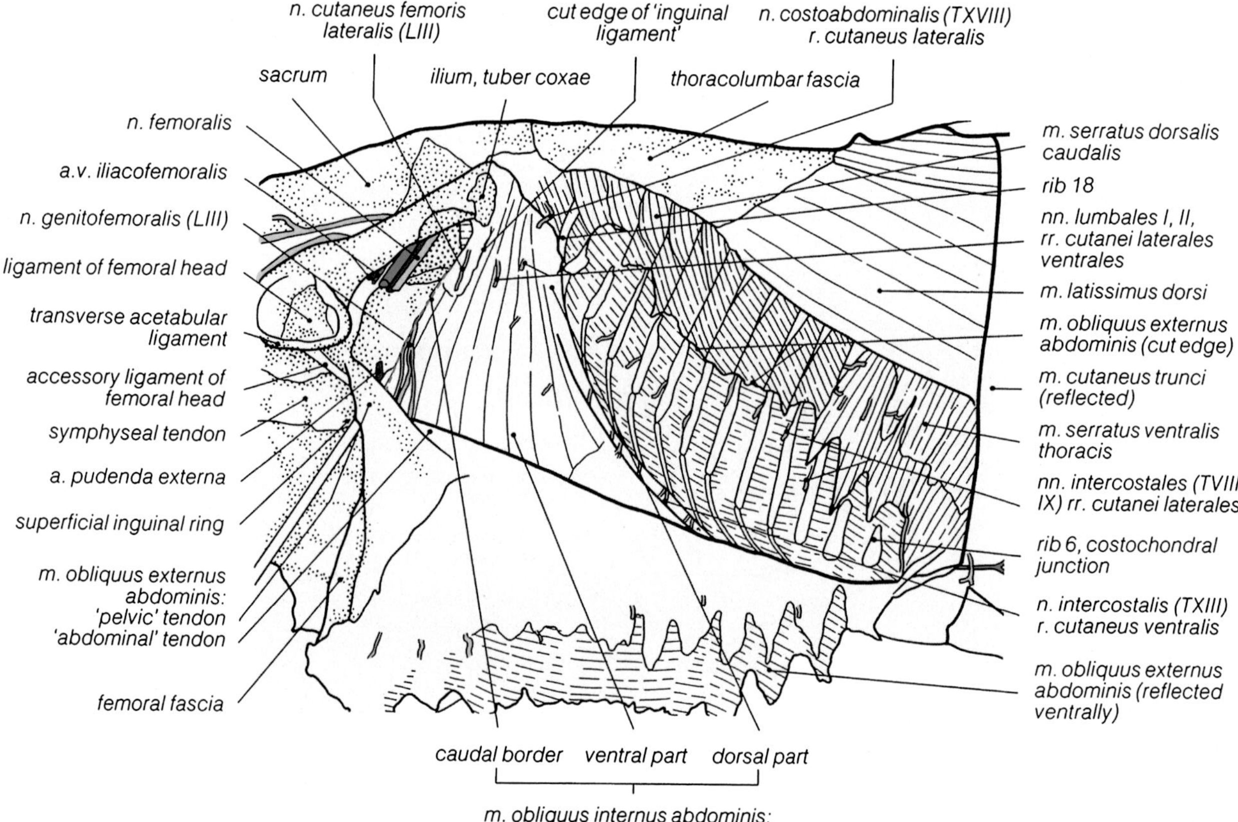
n. cutaneus femoris lateralis (LIII)
cut edge of 'inguinal ligament'
n. costoabdominalis (TXVIII) r. cutaneus lateralis
sacrum
ilium, tuber coxae
thoracolumbar fascia
n. femoralis
a.v. iliacofemoralis
n. genitofemoralis (LIII)
ligament of femoral head
transverse acetabular ligament
accessory ligament of femoral head
symphyseal tendon
a. pudenda externa
superficial inguinal ring
m. obliquus externus abdominis: 'pelvic' tendon 'abdominal' tendon
femoral fascia
m. serratus dorsalis caudalis
rib 18
nn. lumbales I, II, rr. cutanei laterales ventrales
m. latissimus dorsi
m. obliquus externus abdominis (cut edge)
m. cutaneus trunci (reflected)
m. serratus ventralis thoracis
nn. intercostales (TVIII, IX) rr. cutanei laterales
rib 6, costochondral junction
n. intercostalis (TXIII) r. cutaneus ventralis
m. obliquus externus abdominis (reflected ventrally)
caudal border
ventral part
dorsal part
m. obliquus internus abdominis:

Fig. 5.11 The internal oblique abdominal muscle of the foal: right lateral view. The external oblique muscle has been reflected ventrally and it can be seen that the red probe has passed through the superficial inguinal ring. The caudal border of the internal oblique muscle, marked by a broken blue line, is the cranial boundary of the deep inguinal ring.

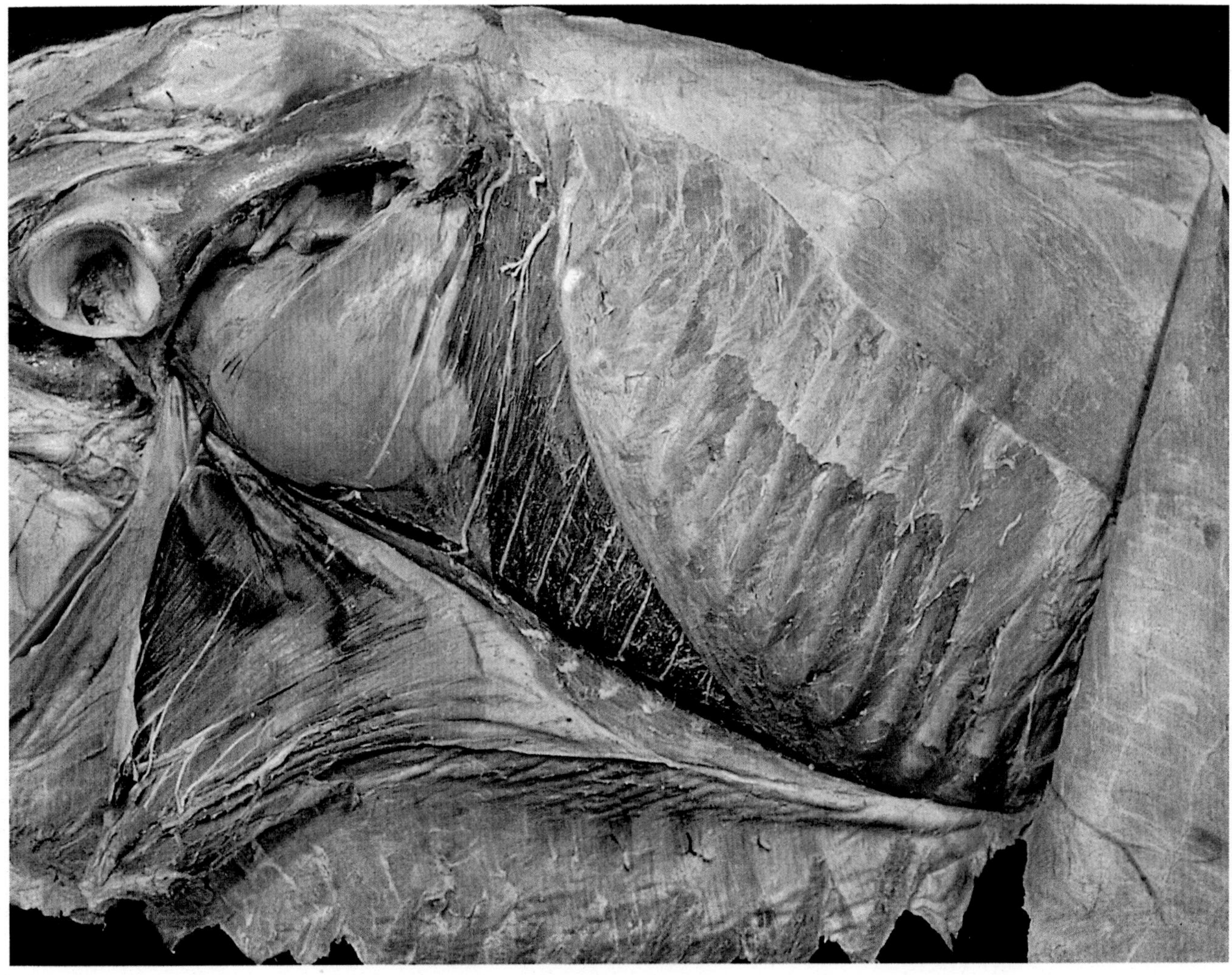

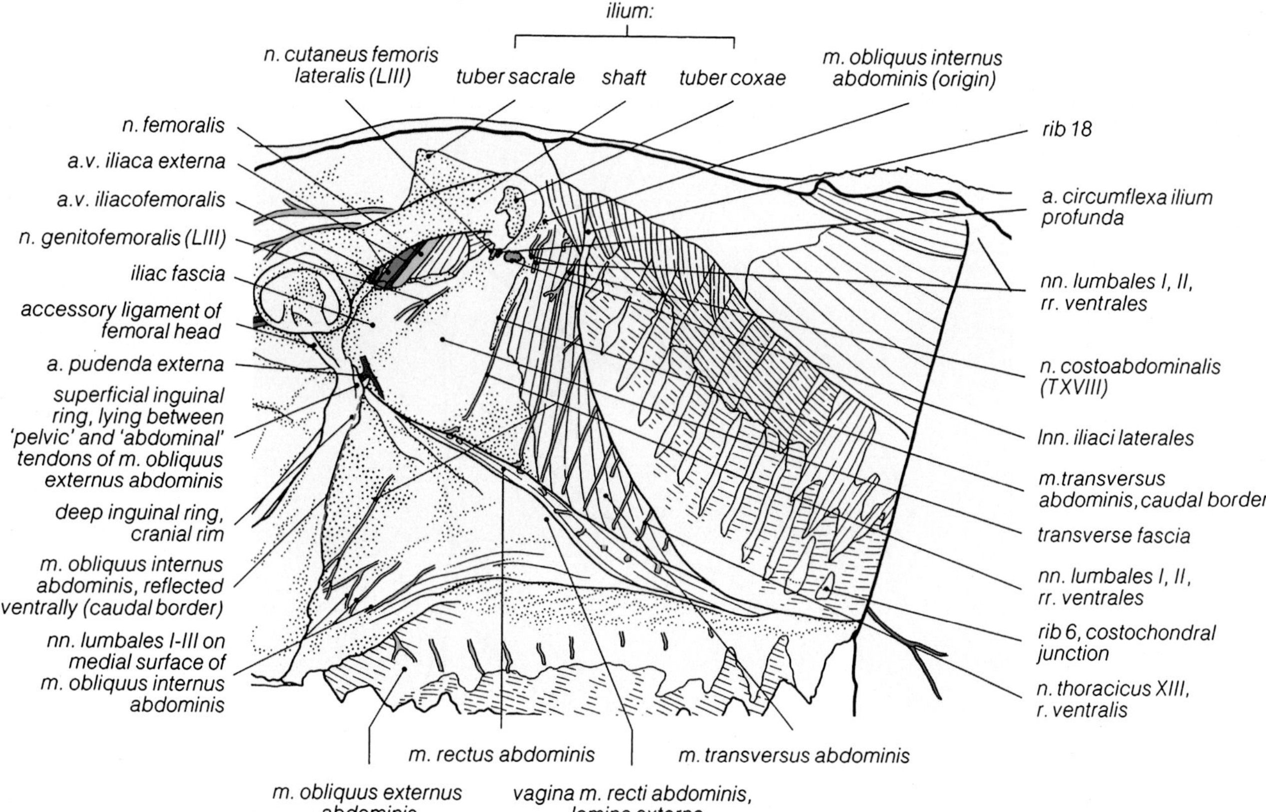
ilium:
n. cutaneus femoris lateralis (LIII)
tuber sacrale
shaft
tuber coxae
m. obliquus internus abdominis (origin)
n. femoralis
a.v. iliaca externa
a.v. iliacofemoralis
n. genitofemoralis (LIII)
iliac fascia
accessory ligament of femoral head
a. pudenda externa
superficial inguinal ring, lying between 'pelvic' and 'abdominal' tendons of m. obliquus externus abdominis
deep inguinal ring, cranial rim
m. obliquus internus abdominis, reflected ventrally (caudal border)
nn. lumbales I-III on medial surface of m. obliquus internus abdominis
rib 18
a. circumflexa ilium profunda
nn. lumbales I, II, rr. ventrales
n. costoabdominalis (TXVIII)
lnn. iliaci laterales
m.transversus abdominis, caudal border
transverse fascia
nn. lumbales I, II, rr. ventrales
rib 6, costochondral junction
n. thoracicus XIII, r. ventralis
m. rectus abdominis
m. transversus abdominis
m. obliquus externus abdominis
vagina m. recti abdominis, lamina externa

Fig. 5.12 The transverse abdominal muscle of the foal: right lateral view. The internal oblique muscle has been reflected ventrally to display the transverse abdominal muscle. The transverse fascia of the caudal part of the abdomen is not covered by the transverse muscle. The red probe lies in the inguinal canal, and its tip occupies the deep inguinal ring, caudal to the internal oblique abdominal muscle. The two principal parts of the ventral ramus of the third lumbar nerve are shown: the more dorsal (lateral cutaneous femoral) is the last of the lateral cutaneous spinal nerve series. The more ventral (genitofemoral) is the last of the medial cutaneous spinal nerve series.

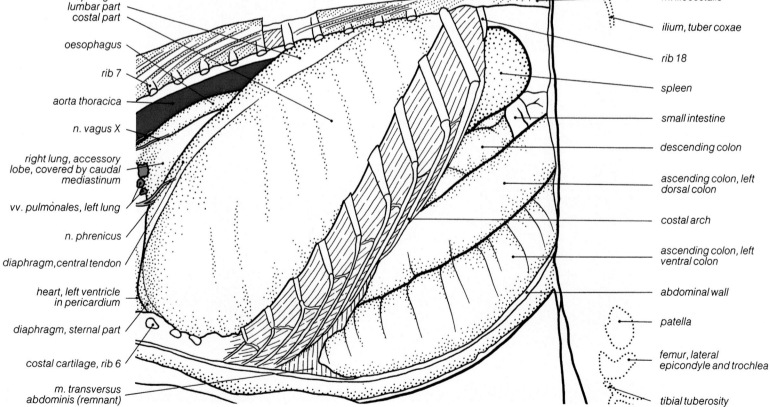

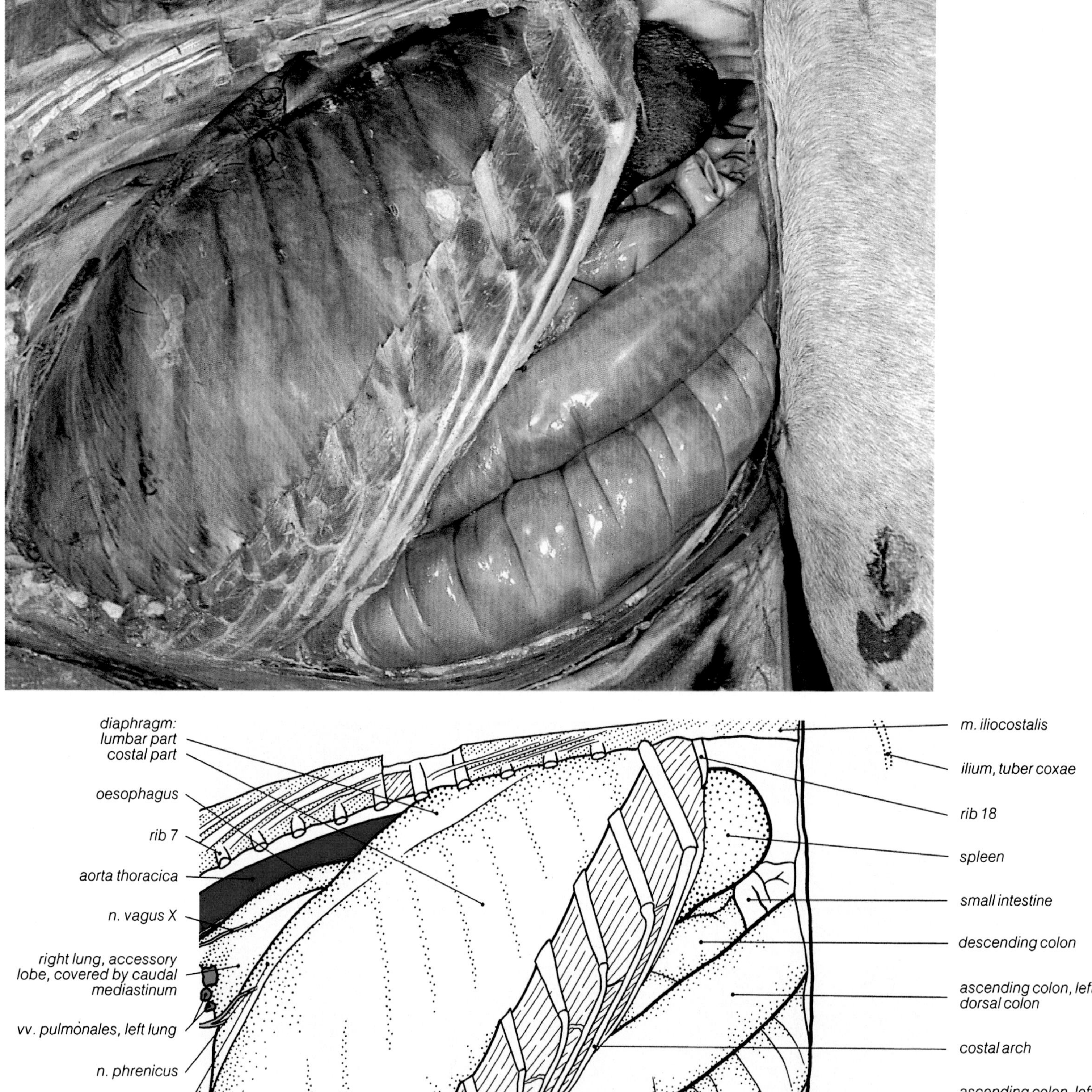
diaphragm:
lumbar part
costal part
oesophagus
rib 7
aorta thoracica
n. vagus X
right lung, accessory lobe, covered by caudal mediastinum
vv. pulmonales, left lung
n. phrenicus
diaphragm, central tendon
heart, left ventricle in pericardium
diaphragm, sternal part
costal cartilage, rib 6
m. transversus abdominis (remnant)
m. iliocostalis
ilium, tuber coxae
rib 18
spleen
small intestine
descending colon
ascending colon, left dorsal colon
costal arch
ascending colon, left ventral colon
abdominal wall
patella
femur, lateral epicondyle and trochlea
tibial tuberosity

Fig. 5.13 Abdominal viscera caudal to the costal arch: left lateral view. The ascending colon has been inflated to imitate its condition in life. In this specimen the spleen extends caudal to the costal arch to a greater extent than usual, but note that rib 18 is small (compare with Fig. 5.43). This young horse was bled out under chloral hydrate anaesthesia.

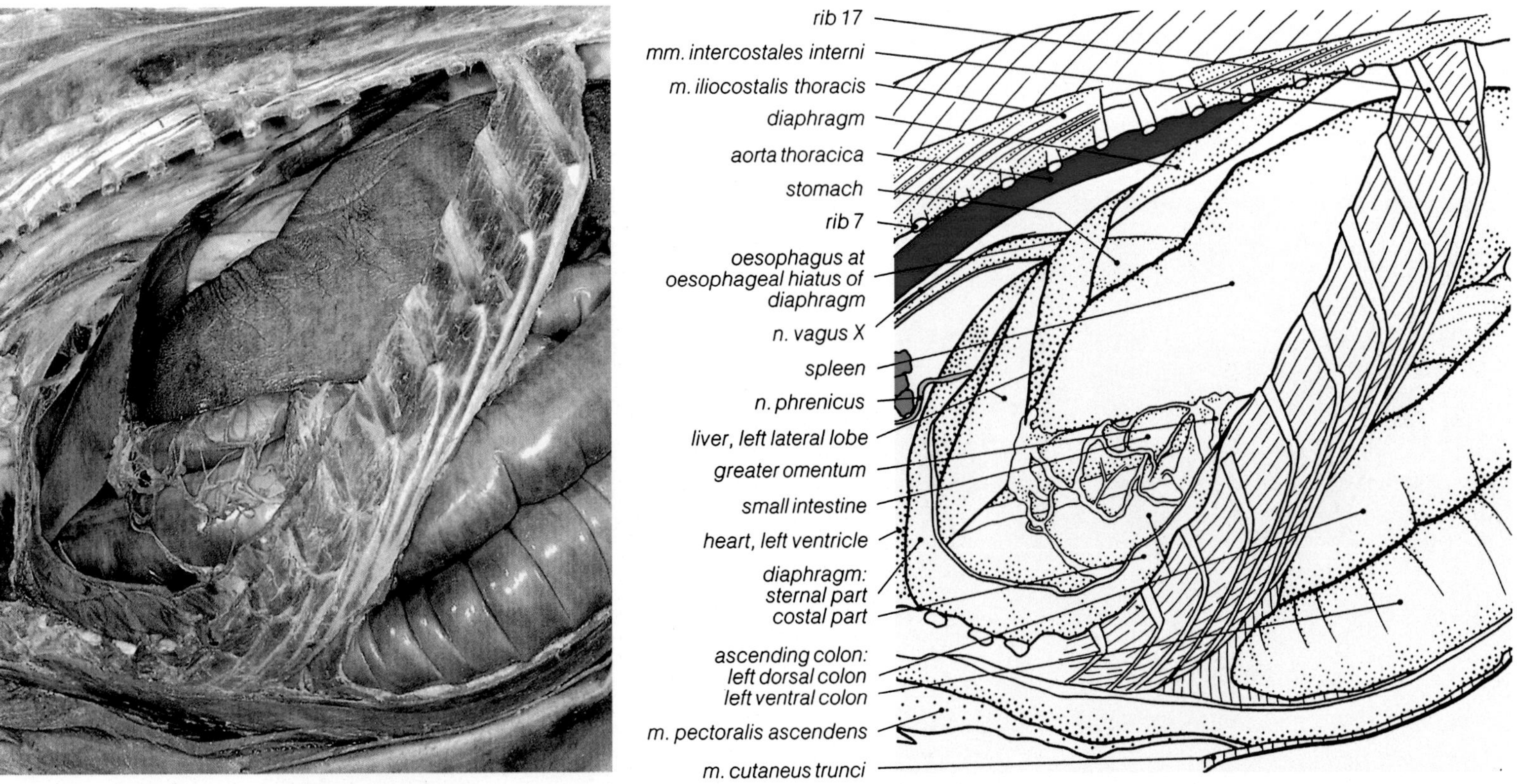
rib 17
mm. intercostales interni
m. iliocostalis thoracis
diaphragm
aorta thoracica
stomach
rib 7
oesophagus at
oesophageal hiatus of
diaphragm
n. vagus X
spleen
n. phrenicus
liver, left lateral lobe
greater omentum
small intestine
heart, left ventricle
diaphragm:
sternal part
costal part
ascending colon:
left dorsal colon
left ventral colon
m. pectoralis ascendens
m. cutaneus trunci

Fig. 5.14 Abdominal viscera after partial removal of the left body wall and diaphragm: left lateral view. The ascending colon has been inflated to imitate its condition in life. See also Figs.5.43, 5.49 and 5.52.

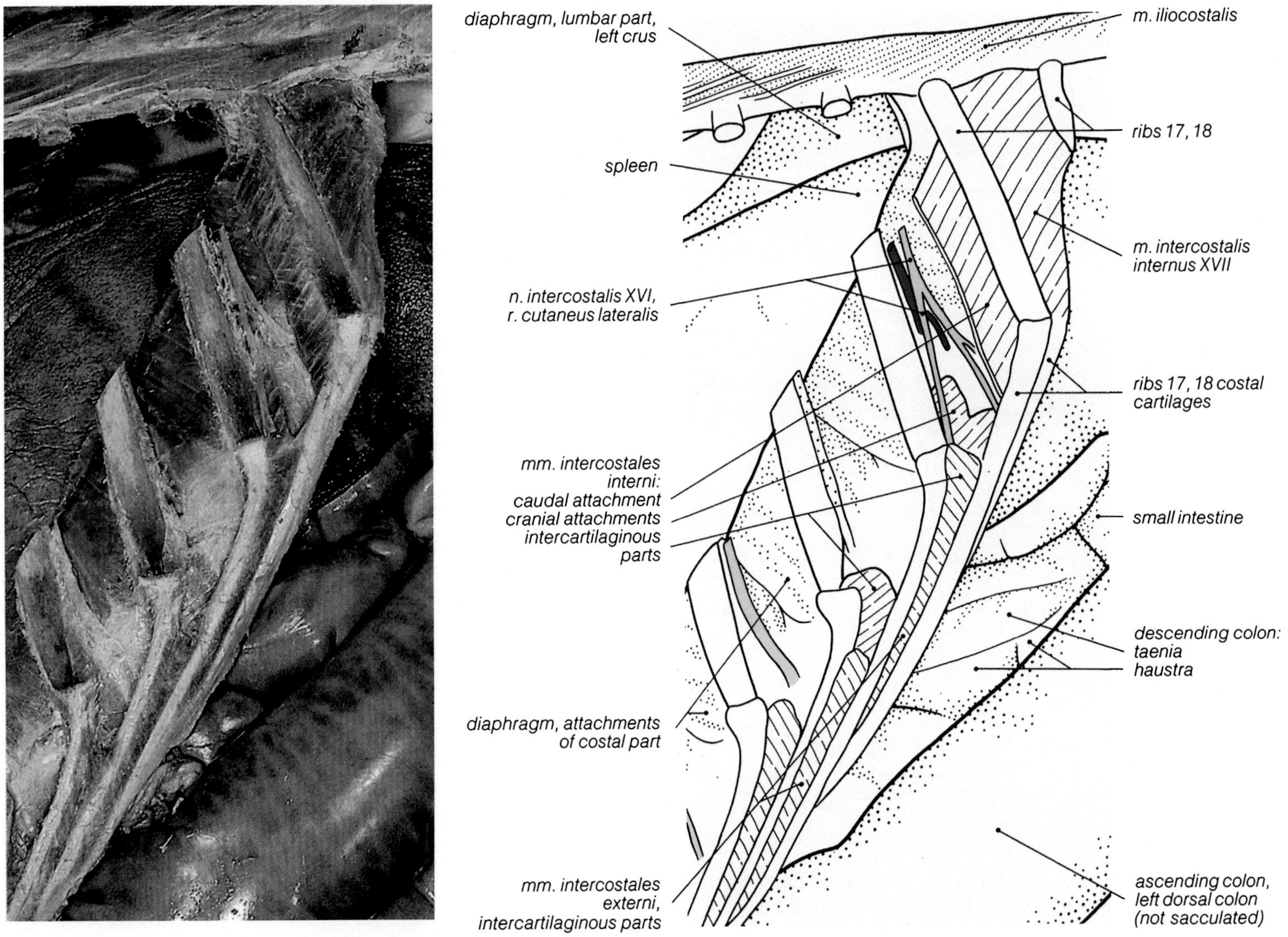

diaphragm, lumbar part,
left crus
m. iliocostalis
ribs 17, 18
spleen
m. intercostalis
internus XVII
n. intercostalis XVI,
r. cutaneus lateralis
ribs 17, 18 costal
cartilages
mm. intercostales
interni:
caudal attachment
cranial attachments
intercartilaginous
parts
small intestine
descending colon:
taenia
haustra
diaphragm, attachments
of costal part
mm. intercostales
externi,
intercartilaginous parts
ascending colon,
left dorsal colon
(not sacculated)

Fig. 5.15 The costal arch and attachments of the diaphragm: left lateral view. The last two internal intercostal muscles, and the intercartilaginous parts of the intercostal muscles, have been retained. In this specimen, the very small rib 18 is a floating rib, but its costal cartilage is recognizable in the costal arch.

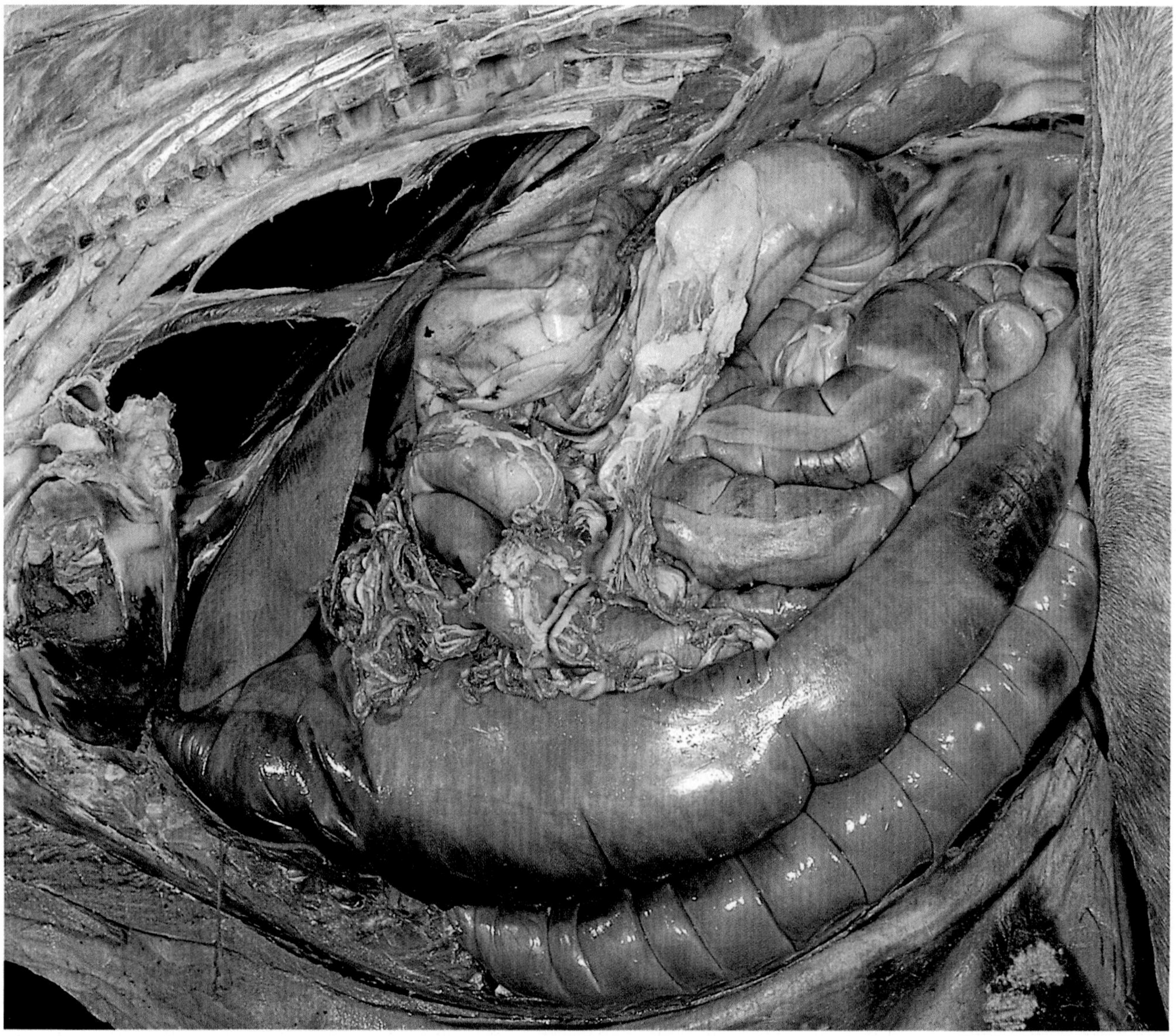

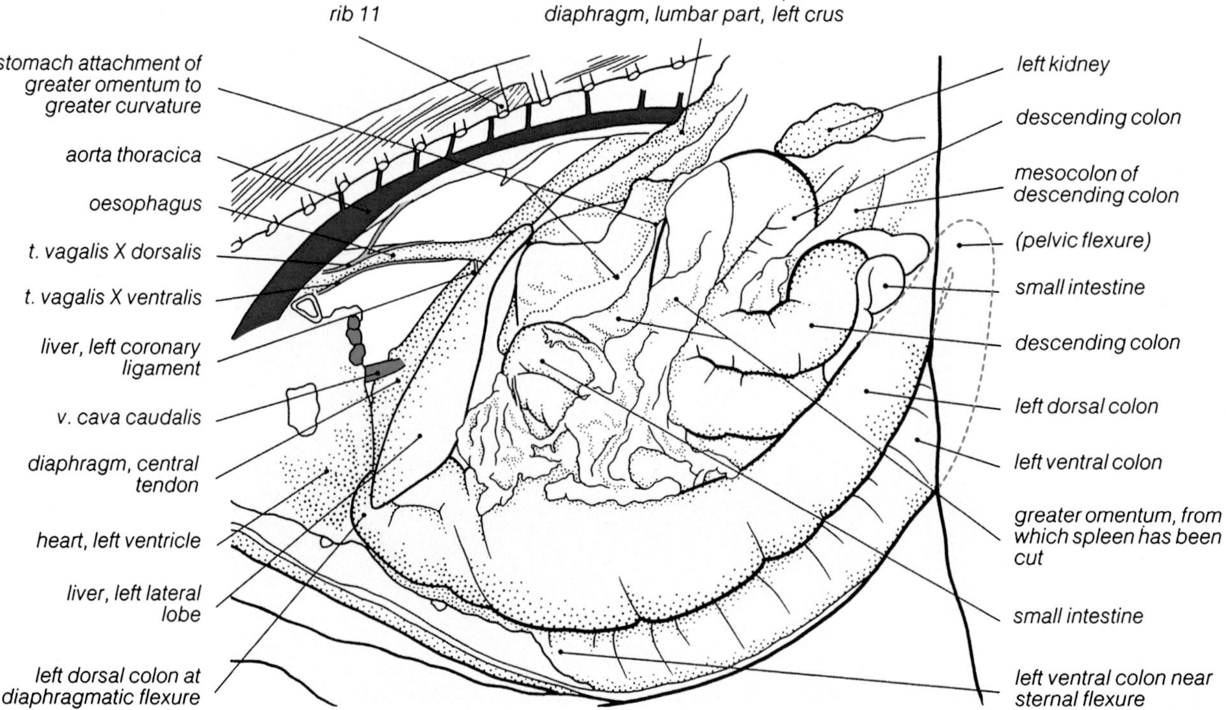
rib 11
diaphragm, lumbar part, left crus
stomach attachment of greater omentum to greater curvature
aorta thoracica
oesophagus
t. vagalis X dorsalis
t. vagalis X ventralis
liver, left coronary ligament
v. cava caudalis
diaphragm, central tendon
heart, left ventricle
liver, left lateral lobe
left dorsal colon at diaphragmatic flexure
left kidney
descending colon
mesocolon of descending colon
(pelvic flexure)
small intestine
descending colon
left dorsal colon
left ventral colon
greater omentum, from which spleen has been cut
small intestine
left ventral colon near sternal flexure

Fig. 5.16 Abdominal viscera after removal of the spleen: left lateral view (1). The costal arch has been resected. The right lung was removed in dissecting the right thorax and abdomen. The broken blue line indicates how the pelvic flexure of the ascending colon is formed (see Figs. 5.24 and 5.32). A closer view of this specimen is shown in Fig. 5.17. See also Fig. 5.50.

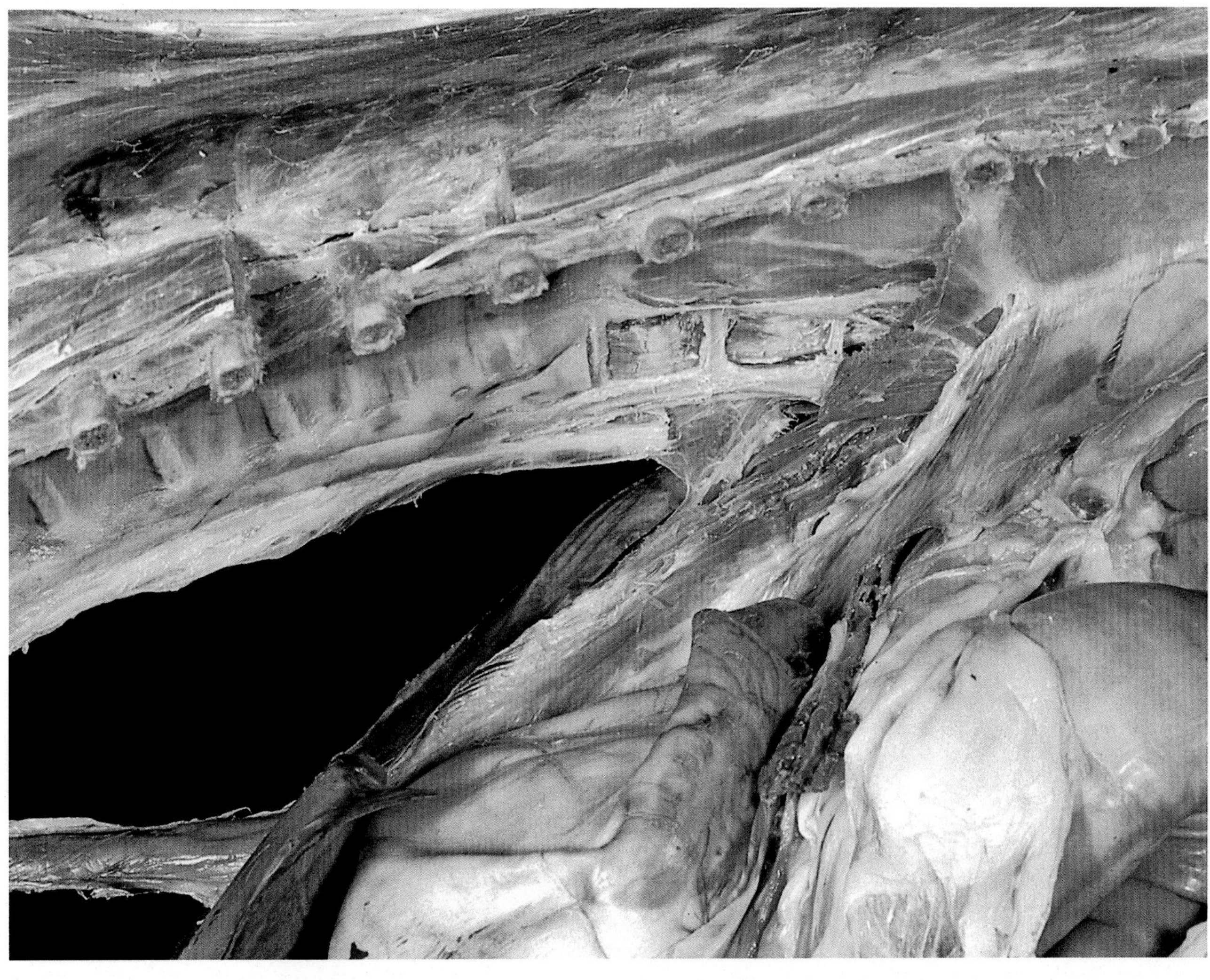

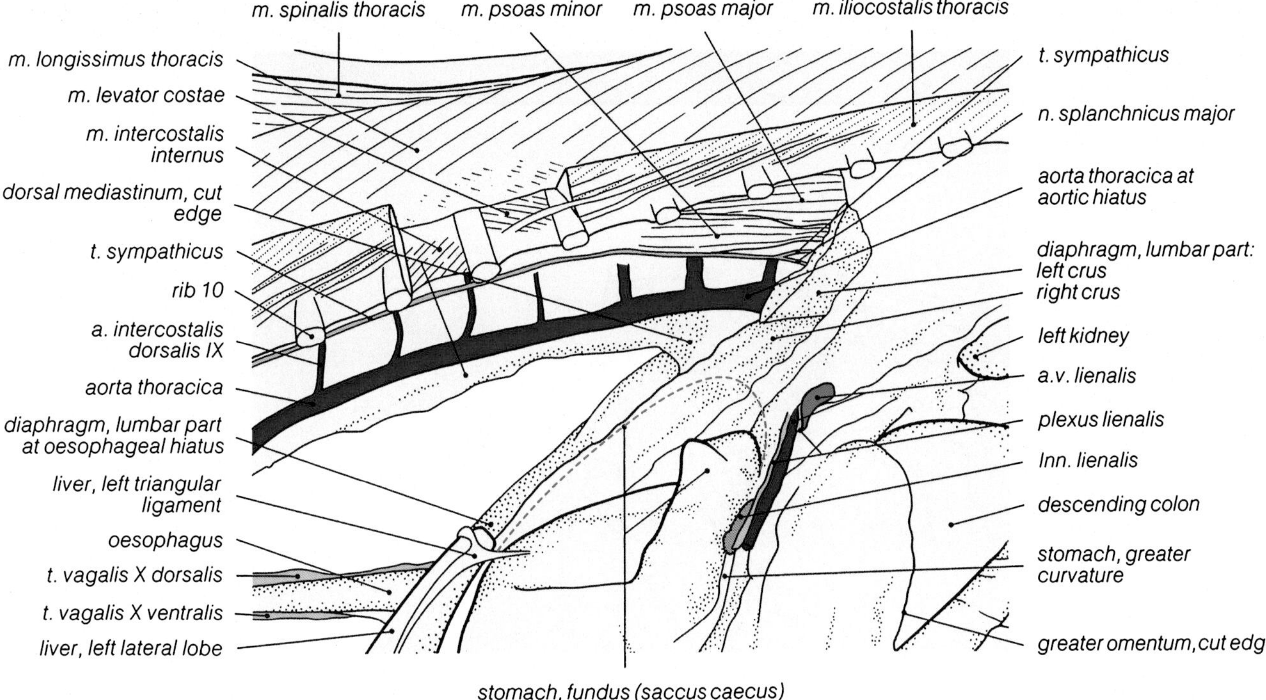
m. spinalis thoracis
m. psoas minor
m. psoas major
m. iliocostalis thoracis
m. longissimus thoracis
m. levator costae
m. intercostalis internus
dorsal mediastinum, cut edge
t. sympathicus
rib 10
a. intercostalis dorsalis IX
aorta thoracica
diaphragm, lumbar part at oesophageal hiatus
liver, left triangular ligament
oesophagus
t. vagalis X dorsalis
t. vagalis X ventralis
liver, left lateral lobe
t. sympathicus
n. splanchnicus major
aorta thoracica at aortic hiatus
diaphragm, lumbar part: left crus
right crus
left kidney
a.v. lienalis
plexus lienalis
lnn. lienalis
descending colon
stomach, greater curvature
greater omentum, cut edge
stomach, fundus (saccus caecus)

Fig. 5.17 Abdominal viscera after removal of the spleen: left lateral view (2). The fundus, or saccus caecus, of the stomach is collapsed; its position when distended is shown by a broken blue line. Further dissections of the aortic hiatus and adjacent structures are shown in Figs. 5.19 and 5.20.

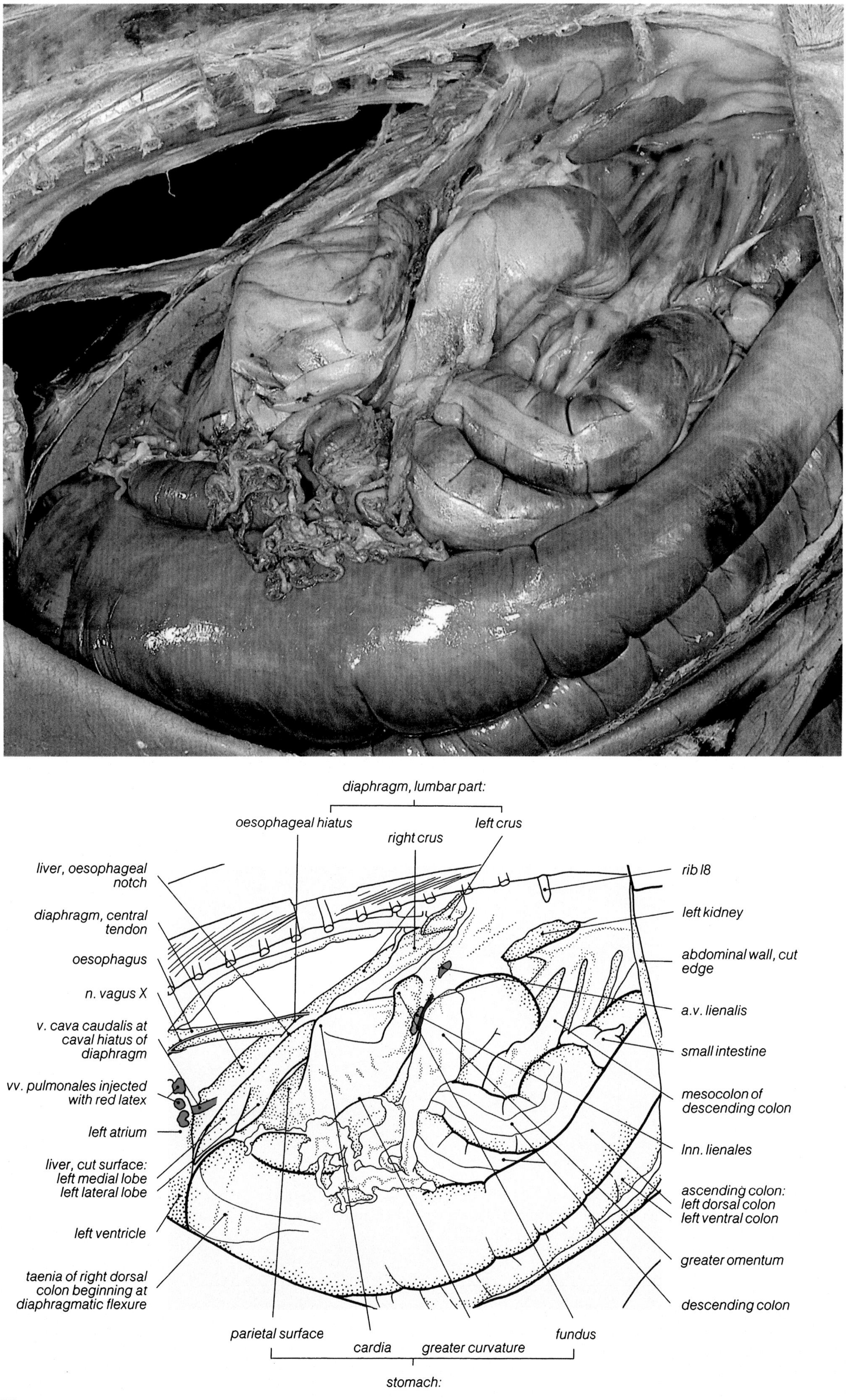

Fig. 5.18 Abdominal viscera after partial removal of the liver: left lateral view. The left side of the liver has been cut away by a sagittal incision to the left of the median plane.

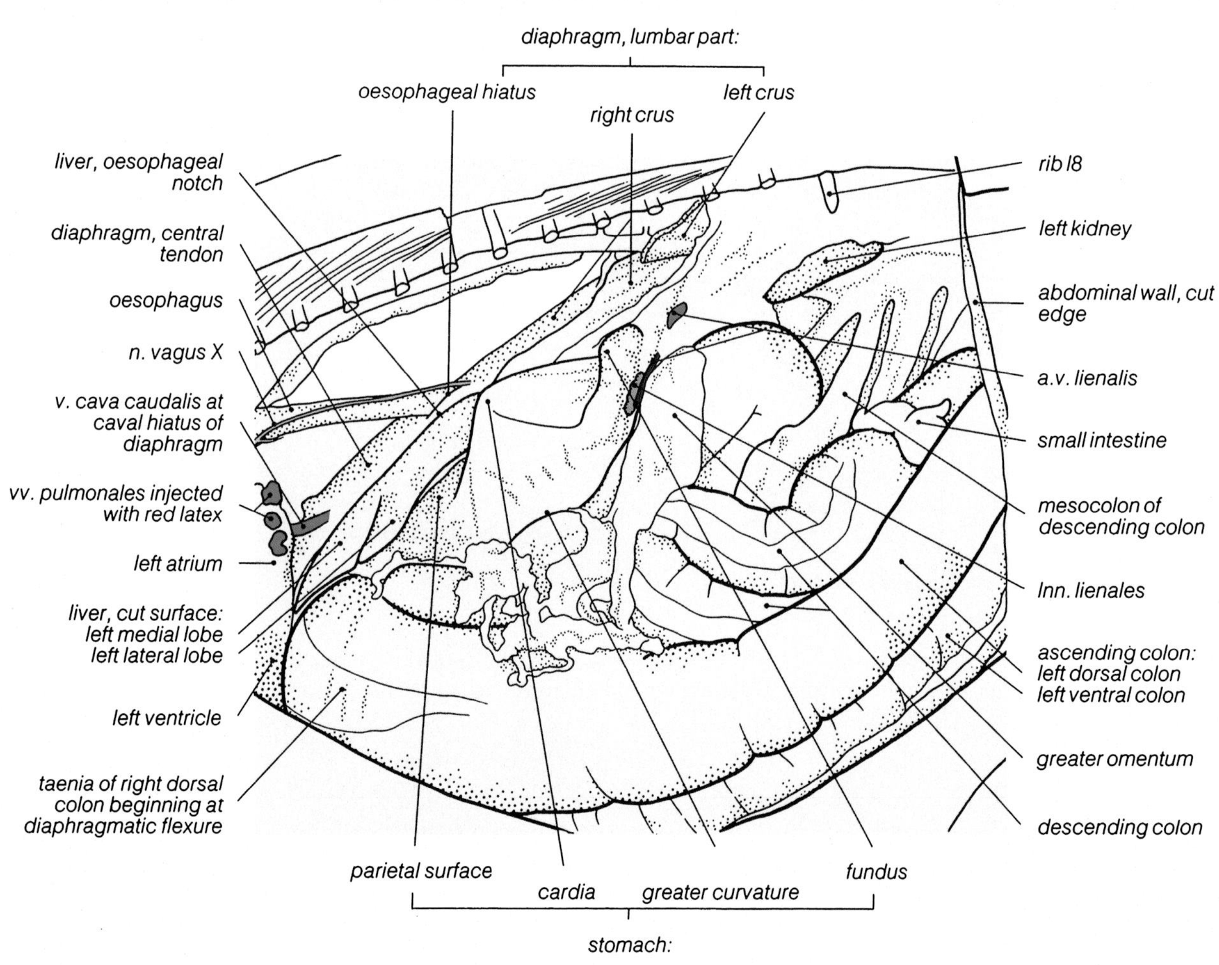
diaphragm, lumbar part:
oesophageal hiatus
right crus
left crus
liver, oesophageal notch
diaphragm, central tendon
oesophagus
n. vagus X
v. cava caudalis at caval hiatus of diaphragm
vv. pulmonales injected with red latex
left atrium
liver, cut surface: left medial lobe left lateral lobe
left ventricle
taenia of right dorsal colon beginning at diaphragmatic flexure
rib 18
left kidney
abdominal wall, cut edge
a.v. lienalis
small intestine
mesocolon of descending colon
lnn. lienales
ascending colon: left dorsal colon left ventral colon
greater omentum
descending colon
parietal surface
cardia
greater curvature
fundus
stomach:

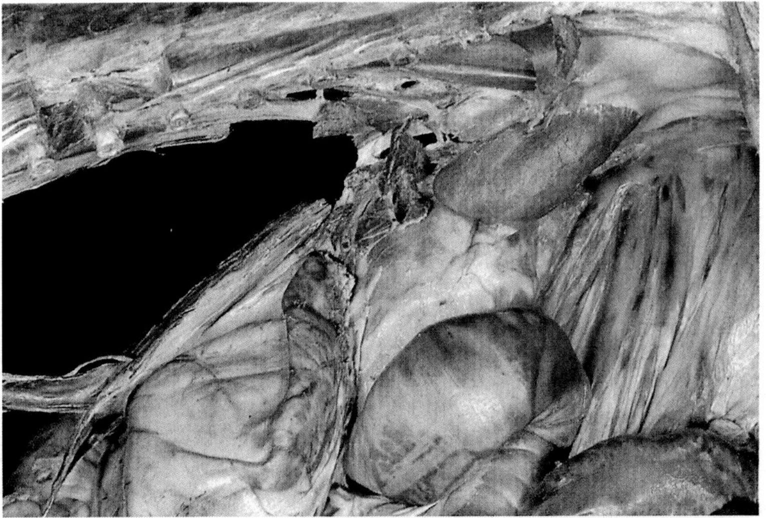

Fig. 5.19 The aortic hiatus and related structures: left lateral view. The left and right diaphragmatic crura, which surround the aortic hiatus, have been cut. The left kidney has been displaced ventrally to reveal the structures immediately caudal to the aortic hiatus.

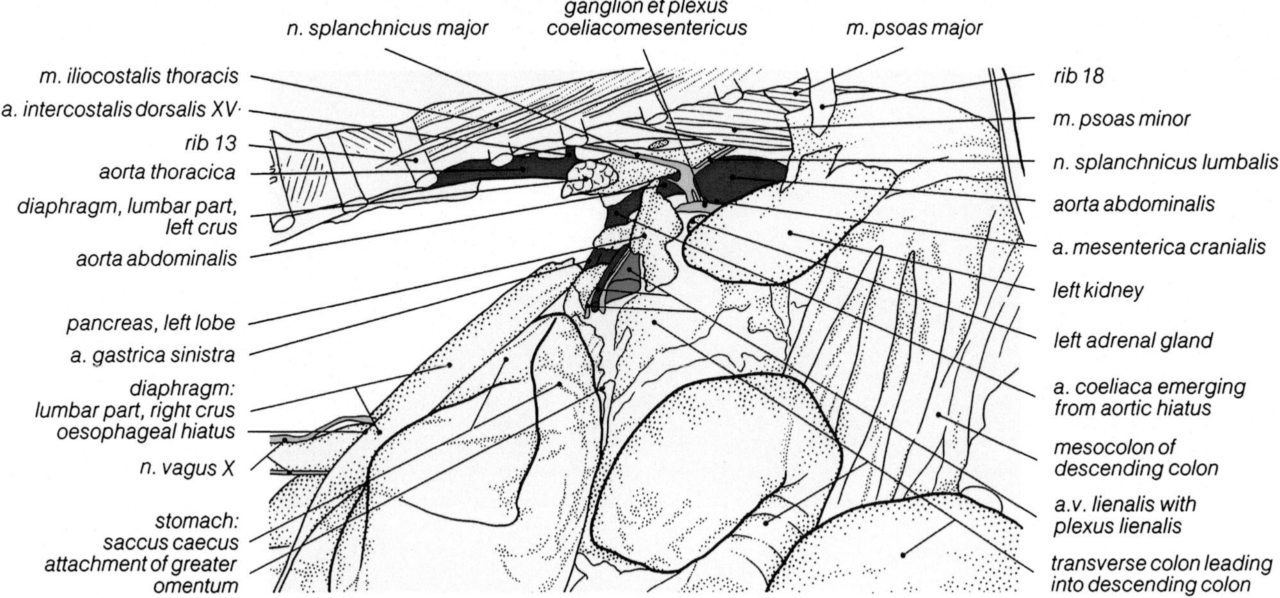
n. splanchnicus major
ganglion et plexus coeliacomesentericus
m. psoas major
m. iliocostalis thoracis
a. intercostalis dorsalis XV
rib 13
aorta thoracica
diaphragm, lumbar part, left crus
aorta abdominalis
pancreas, left lobe
a. gastrica sinistra
diaphragm: lumbar part, right crus
oesophageal hiatus
n. vagus X
stomach: saccus caecus
attachment of greater omentum
rib 18
m. psoas minor
n. splanchnicus lumbalis
aorta abdominalis
a. mesenterica cranialis
left kidney
left adrenal gland
a. coeliaca emerging from aortic hiatus
mesocolon of descending colon
a.v. lienalis with plexus lienalis
transverse colon leading into descending colon

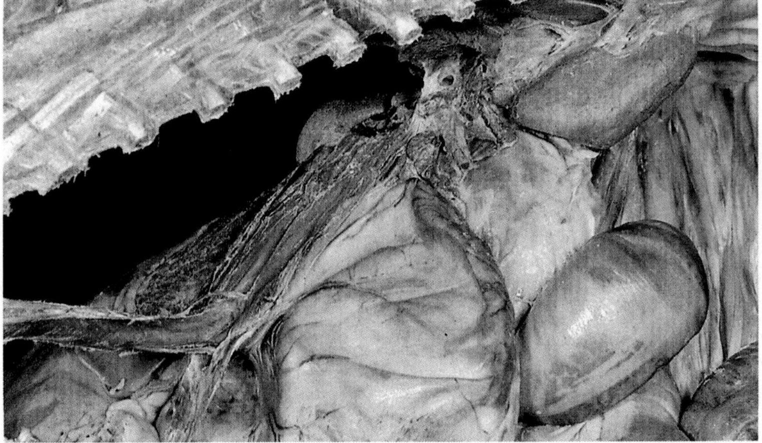

Fig. 5.20 The aortic and oesophageal hiatuses: left craniolateral view. This is a more cranial view of the specimen at a slightly later stage of dissection than that shown in Fig. 5.19. A right lateral view of the specimen, at this stage of dissection, is shown in Fig. 5.37.

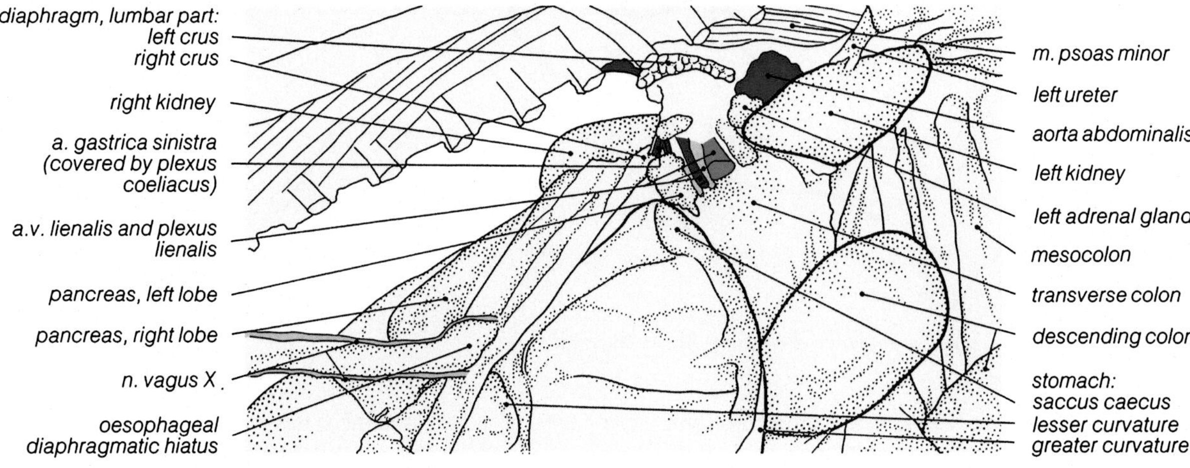
diaphragm, lumbar part:
left crus
right crus
right kidney
a. gastrica sinistra (covered by plexus coeliacus)
a.v. lienalis and plexus lienalis
pancreas, left lobe
pancreas, right lobe
n. vagus X
oesophageal diaphragmatic hiatus
m. psoas minor
left ureter
aorta abdominalis
left kidney
left adrenal gland
mesocolon
transverse colon
descending colon
stomach:
saccus caecus
lesser curvature
greater curvature

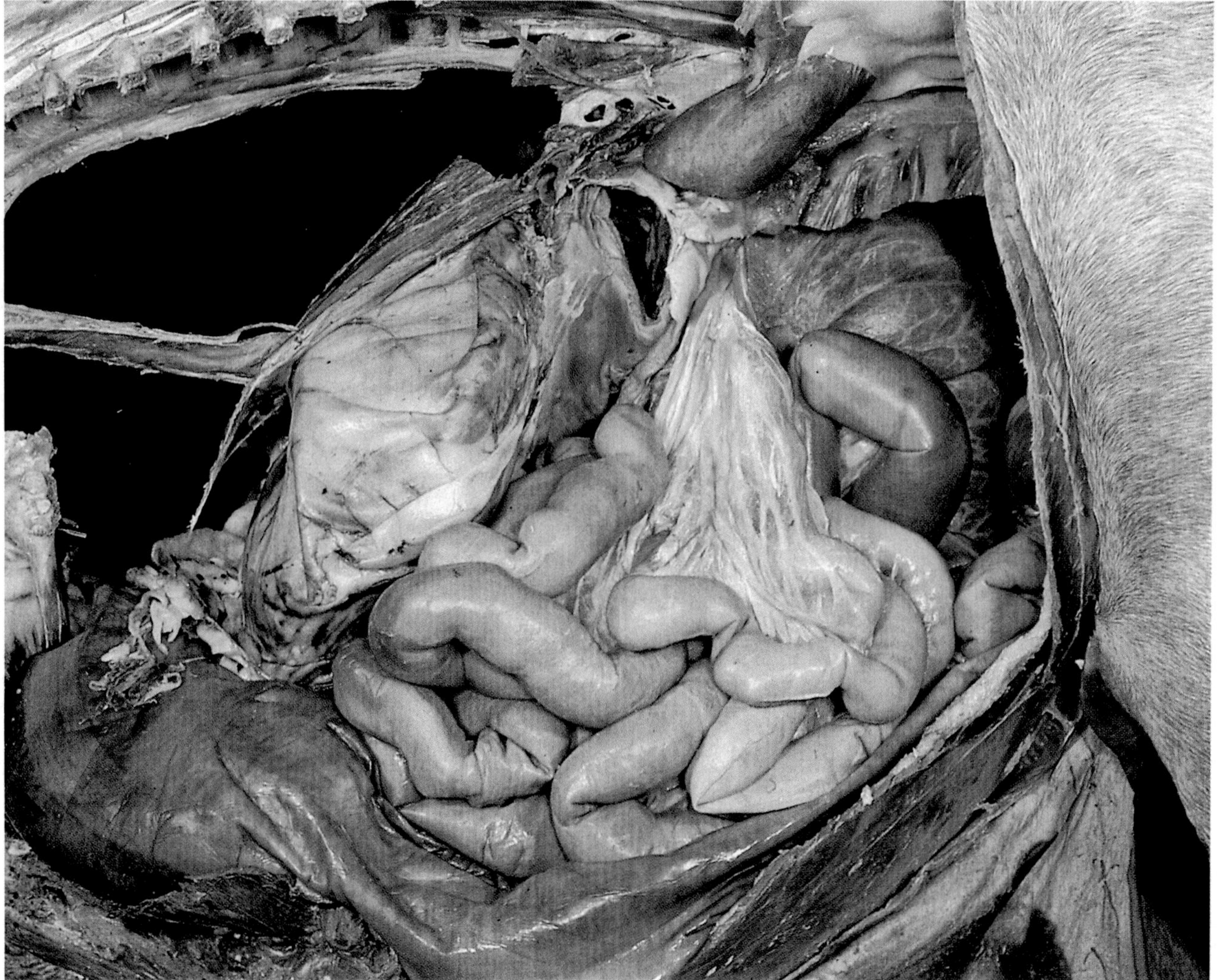

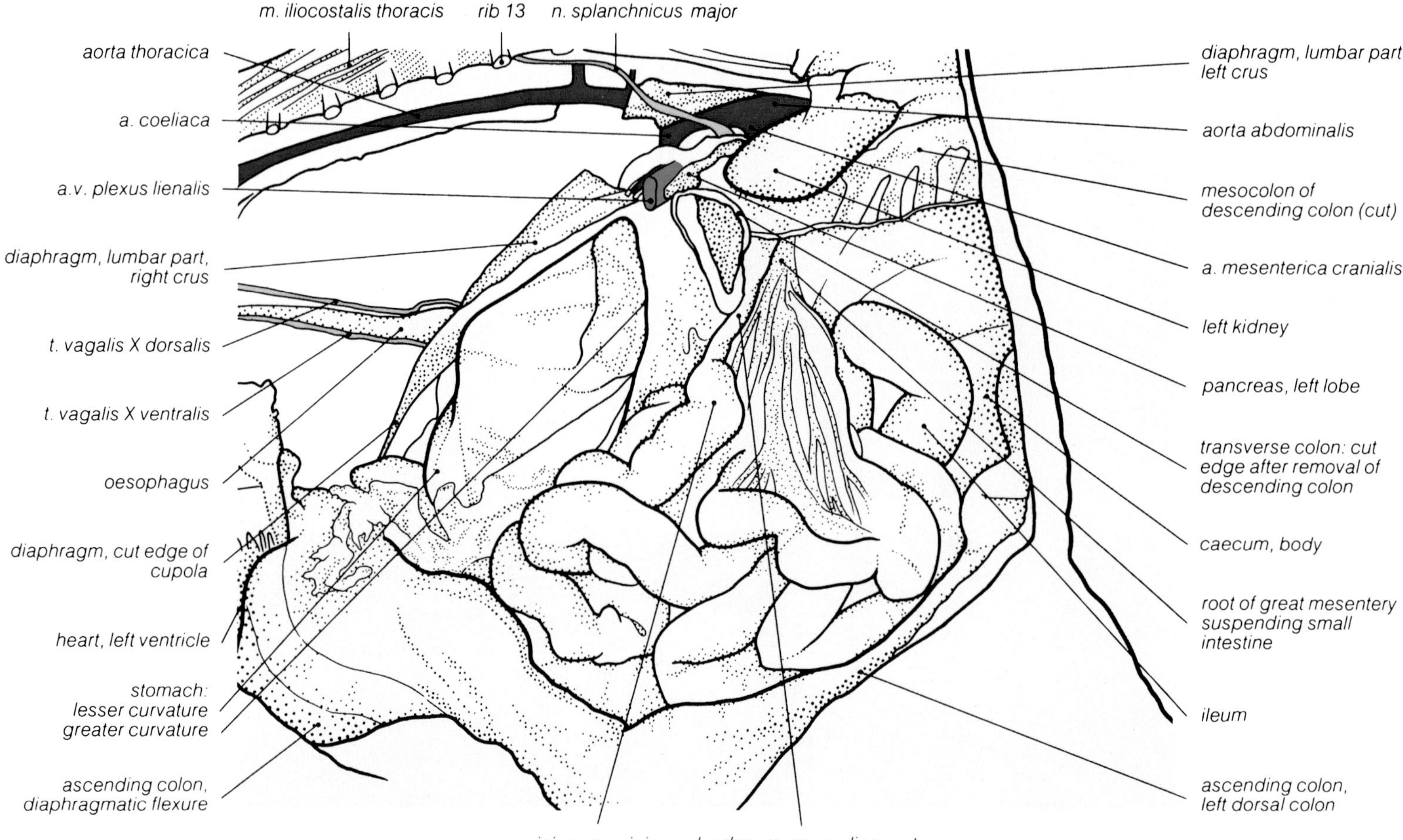
m. iliocostalis thoracis
rib 13
n. splanchnicus major
aorta thoracica
a. coeliaca
a.v. plexus lienalis
diaphragm, lumbar part, right crus
t. vagalis X dorsalis
t. vagalis X ventralis
oesophagus
diaphragm, cut edge of cupola
heart, left ventricle
stomach:
lesser curvature
greater curvature
ascending colon, diaphragmatic flexure
jejunum, origin
duodenum, ascending part
diaphragm, lumbar part, left crus
aorta abdominalis
mesocolon of descending colon (cut)
a. mesenterica cranialis
left kidney
pancreas, left lobe
transverse colon: cut edge after removal of descending colon
caecum, body
root of great mesentery suspending small intestine
ileum
ascending colon, left dorsal colon

Fig. 5.21 The small intestine: left lateral view (1). The very long descending colon (measuring 300 cm in this specimen) has been removed to reveal the small intestine lying medial to it and the root of the great mesentery.

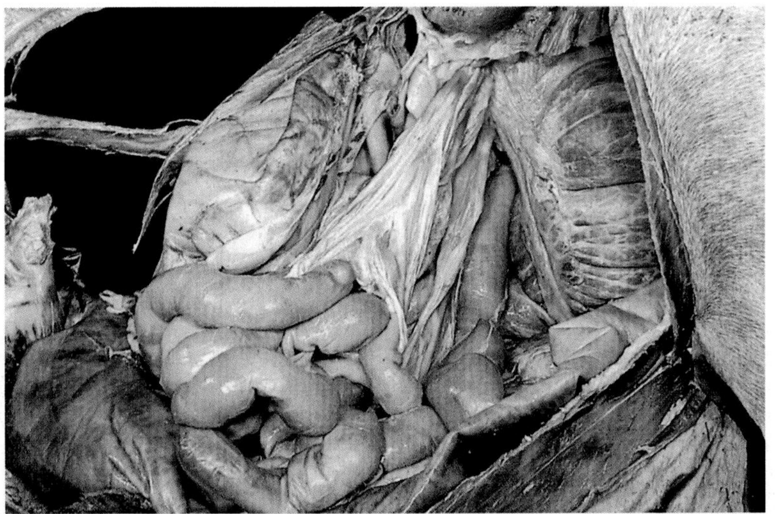

Fig. 5.22 The small intestine: left lateral view (2). The mass of the small intestine has been displaced cranially to reveal the terminal part of the ileum near its junction with the caecum. The root of the great mesentery of the small intestine lies between the transverse parts of colon (cranially) and duodenum (caudally).

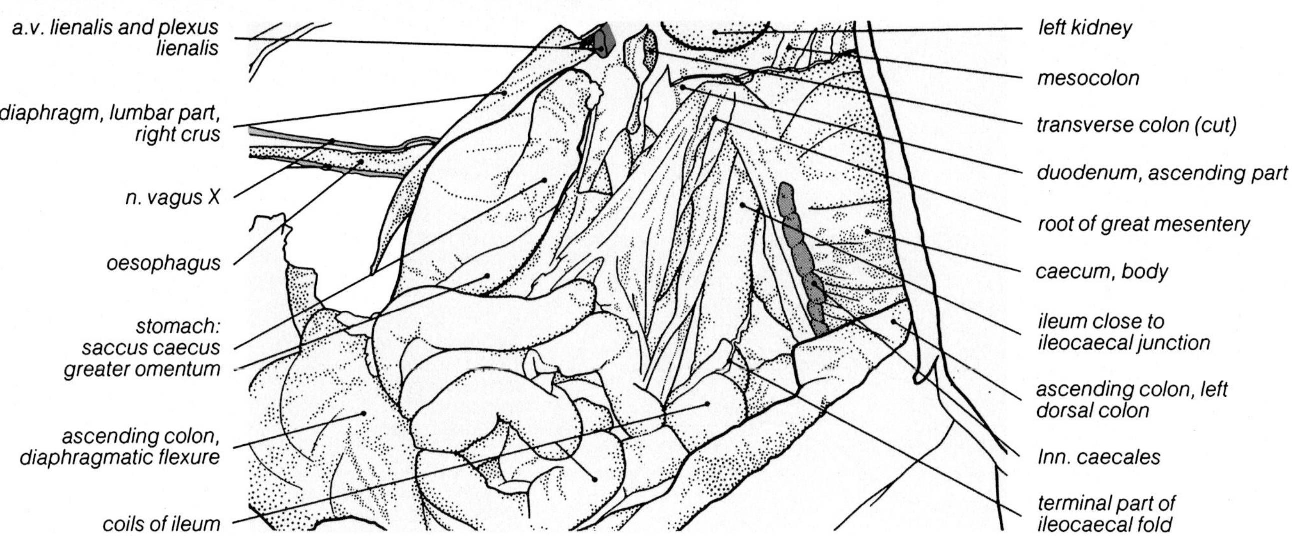
a.v. lienalis and plexus lienalis
diaphragm, lumbar part, right crus
n. vagus X
oesophagus
stomach: saccus caecus
greater omentum
ascending colon, diaphragmatic flexure
coils of ileum
left kidney
mesocolon
transverse colon (cut)
duodenum, ascending part
root of great mesentery
caecum, body
ileum close to ileocaecal junction
ascending colon, left dorsal colon
lnn. caecales
terminal part of ileocaecal fold

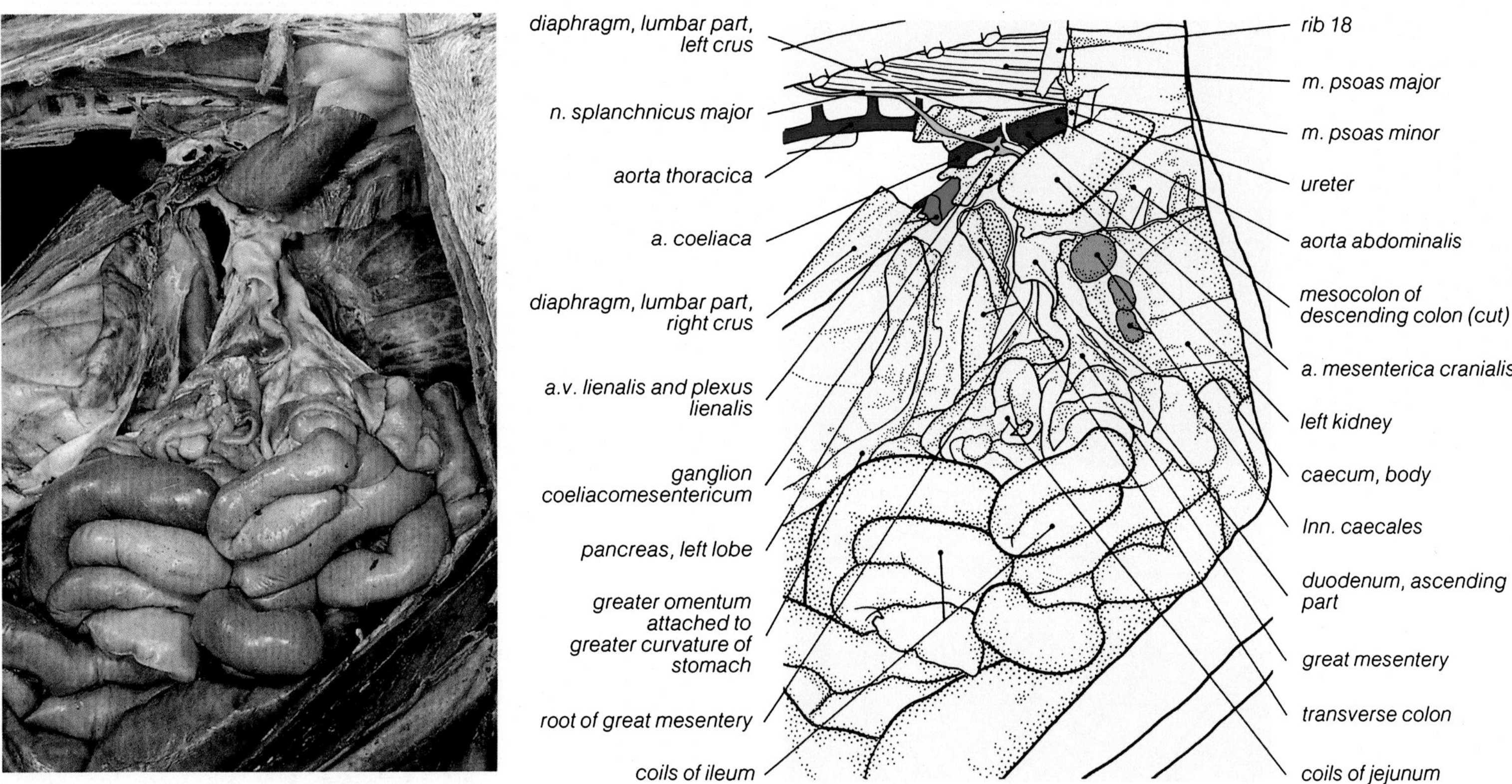
diaphragm, lumbar part, left crus
n. splanchnicus major
aorta thoracica
a. coeliaca
diaphragm, lumbar part, right crus
a.v. lienalis and plexus lienalis
ganglion coeliacomesentericum
pancreas, left lobe
greater omentum attached to greater curvature of stomach
root of great mesentery
coils of ileum
rib 18
m. psoas major
m. psoas minor
ureter
aorta abdominalis
mesocolon of descending colon (cut)
a. mesenterica cranialis
left kidney
caecum, body
lnn. caecales
duodenum, ascending part
great mesentery
transverse colon
coils of jejunum

Fig. 5.23 The small intestine: left lateral view (3). The coils of the small intestine have been rearranged to show more clearly the transition of the ascending duodenum into the jejunum and the relation of the root of the great mesentery to the duodenum and transverse colon. Note that the ileum is considered to be that part of the small intestine which is filled with ingesta and the jejunum that part which contains very little ingesta.

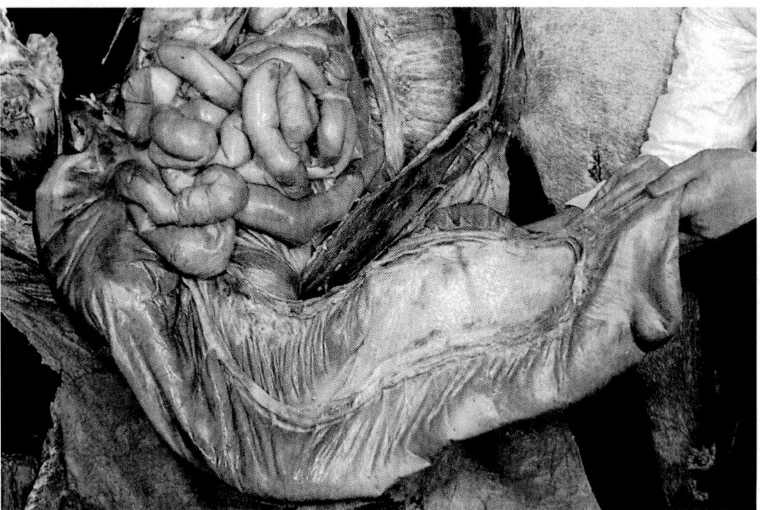

Fig. 5.24 The loop of the ascending colon: left lateral view. The pelvic flexure has been pulled outside the abdomen, displaying the entire left side of the colonic loop and the diaphragmatic and sternal flexures. The normal topographical positions of those parts are shown in Figs. 5.14 and 5.32.

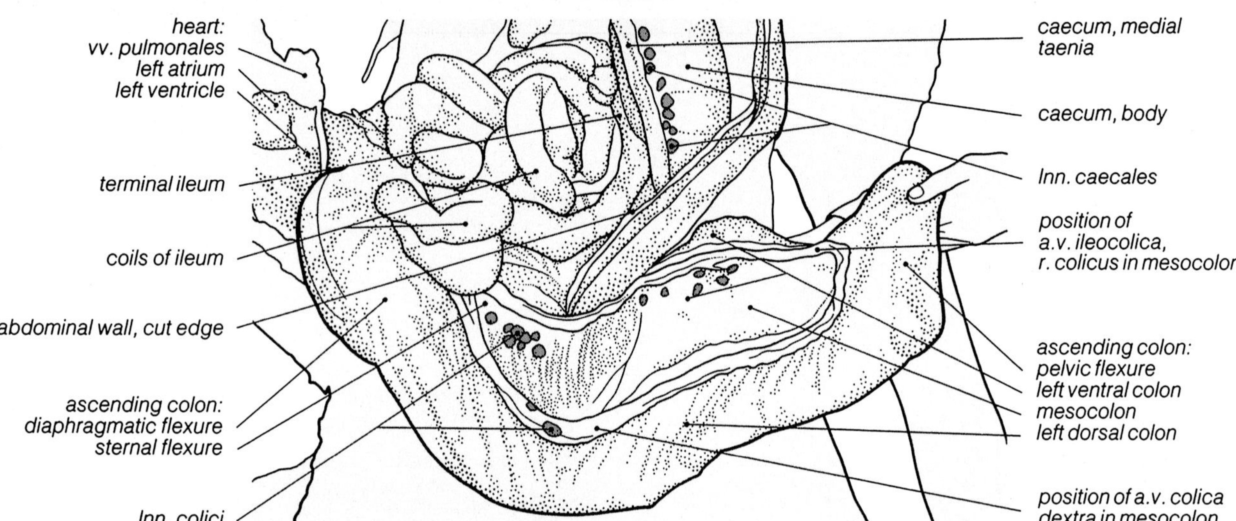
heart:
vv. pulmonales
left atrium
left ventricle
terminal ileum
coils of ileum
abdominal wall, cut edge
ascending colon:
diaphragmatic flexure
sternal flexure
lnn. colici
caecum, medial taenia
caecum, body
lnn. caecales
position of
a.v. ileocolica,
r. colicus in mesocolon
ascending colon:
pelvic flexure
left ventral colon
mesocolon
left dorsal colon
position of a.v. colica dextra in mesocolon

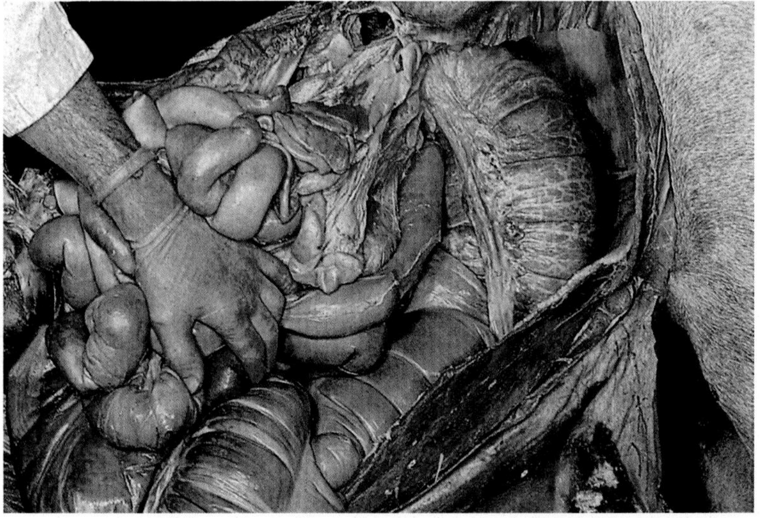

Fig. 5.25 The caecum: left lateral view. The loop of the ascending colon has been removed from the abdomen (see Fig. 5.24). The coils of the small intestine have now been displaced cranially to show the position of the apex of the caecum on the floor of the abdomen.

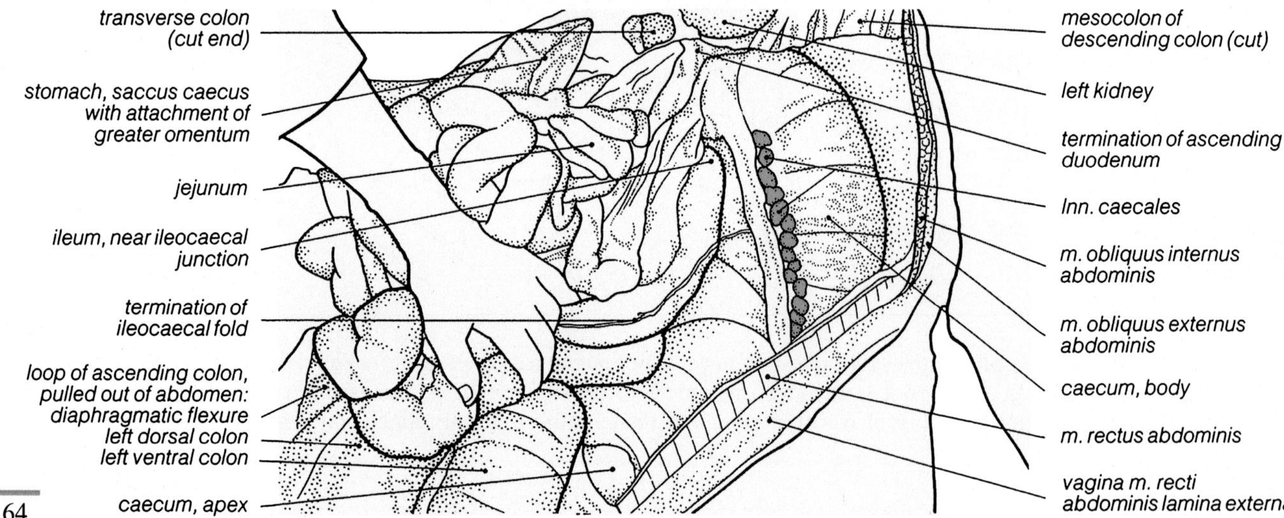
transverse colon (cut end)
stomach, saccus caecus with attachment of greater omentum
jejunum
ileum, near ileocaecal junction
termination of ileocaecal fold
loop of ascending colon, pulled out of abdomen:
diaphragmatic flexure
left dorsal colon
left ventral colon
caecum, apex
mesocolon of descending colon (cut)
left kidney
termination of ascending duodenum
lnn. caecales
m. obliquus internus abdominis
m. obliquus externus abdominis
caecum, body
m. rectus abdominis
vagina m. recti abdominis lamina externa

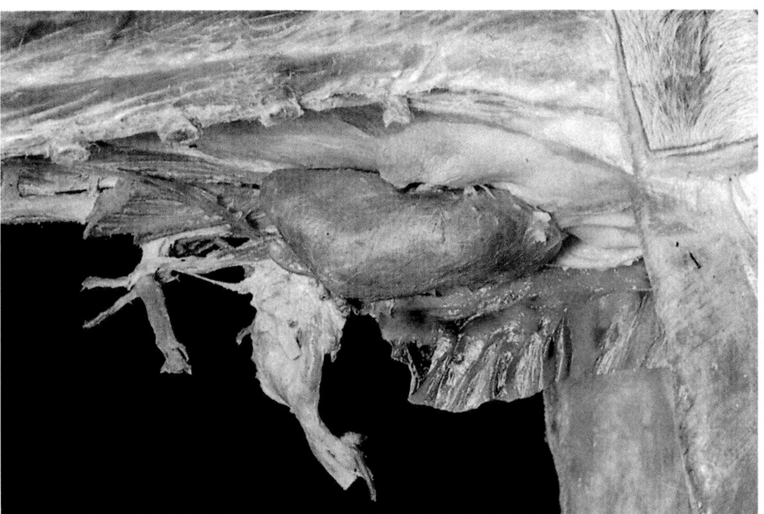

Fig. 5.26 Roots of the coeliac and cranial mesenteric arteries: left lateral view. The abdominal parts of the digestive tract have now been removed and the left kidney pinned to the abdominal roof. The roots of the coeliac and cranial mesenteric arteries, and the vessels arising from them, are ensheathed by a plexus of sympathetic nerves derived from the coeliac and cranial mesenteric ganglia. These nerves have not been removed: they obscure the details of the arterial branchings. The root of the cranial mesenteric artery is enlarged by a parasitic infestation (see Fig. 5.28) and this enlargement (verminous aneurysm) is more clearly seen on the right side (Fig. 5.42).

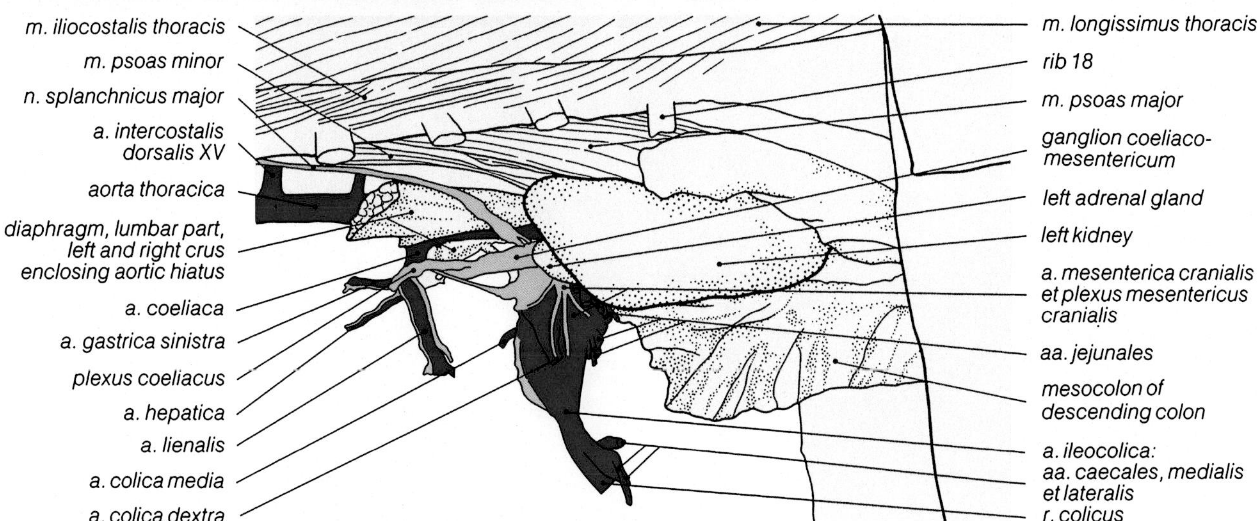
m. iliocostalis thoracis
m. psoas minor
n. splanchnicus major
a. intercostalis dorsalis XV
aorta thoracica
diaphragm, lumbar part, left and right crus enclosing aortic hiatus
a. coeliaca
a. gastrica sinistra
plexus coeliacus
a. hepatica
a. lienalis
a. colica media
a. colica dextra
m. longissimus thoracis
rib 18
m. psoas major
ganglion coeliaco-mesentericum
left adrenal gland
left kidney
a. mesenterica cranialis et plexus mesentericus cranialis
aa. jejunales
mesocolon of descending colon
a. ileocolica:
aa. caecales, medialis et lateralis
r. colicus

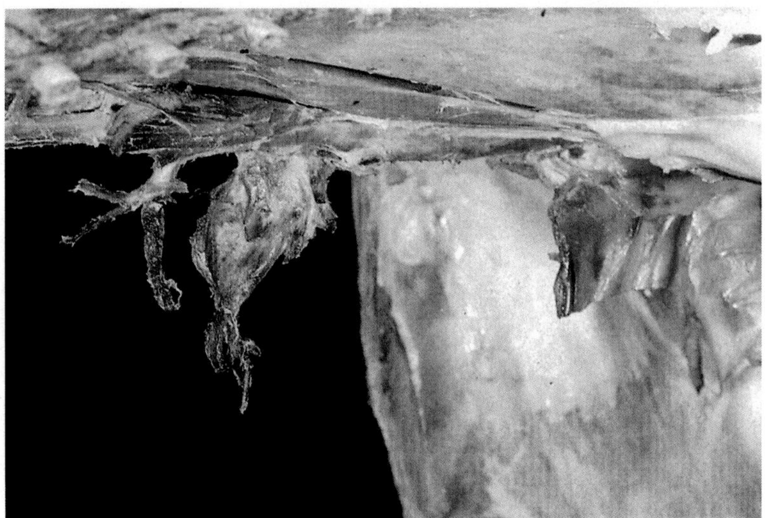

Fig. 5.27 Roots of the cranial and caudal mesenteric arteries: left lateral view. Removal of the left kidney exposes the origin of the renal artery and the caudal mesenteric artery has been dissected within the mesocolon.

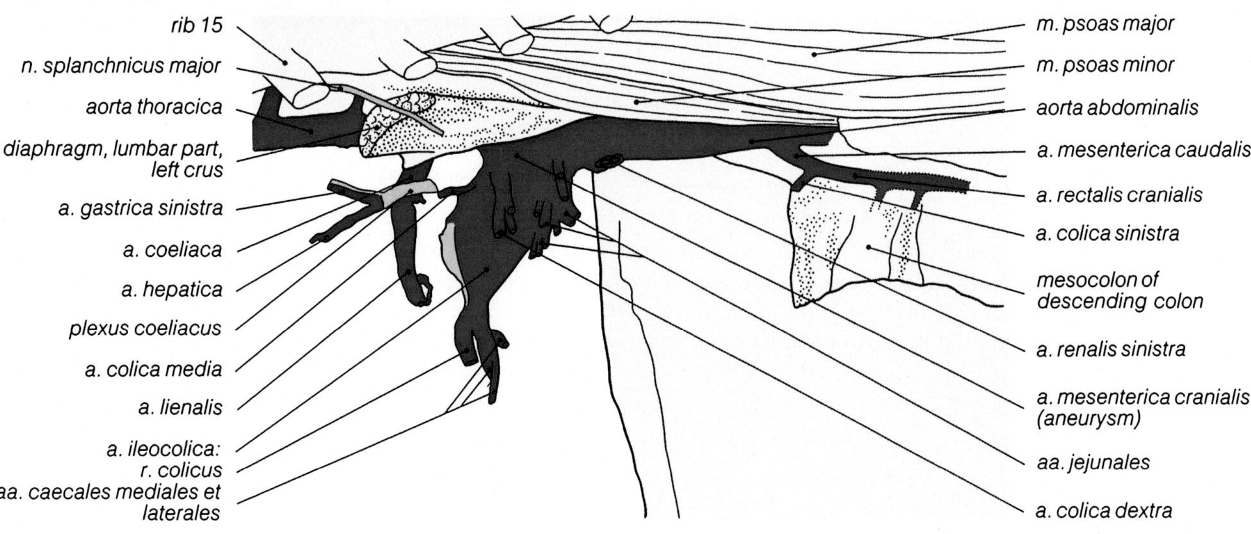
rib 15
n. splanchnicus major
aorta thoracica
diaphragm, lumbar part, left crus
a. gastrica sinistra
a. coeliaca
a. hepatica
plexus coeliacus
a. colica media
a. lienalis
a. ileocolica:
r. colicus
aa. caecales mediales et laterales
m. psoas major
m. psoas minor
aorta abdominalis
a. mesenterica caudalis
a. rectalis cranialis
a. colica sinistra
mesocolon of descending colon
a. renalis sinistra
a. mesenterica cranialis (aneurysm)
aa. jejunales
a. colica dextra

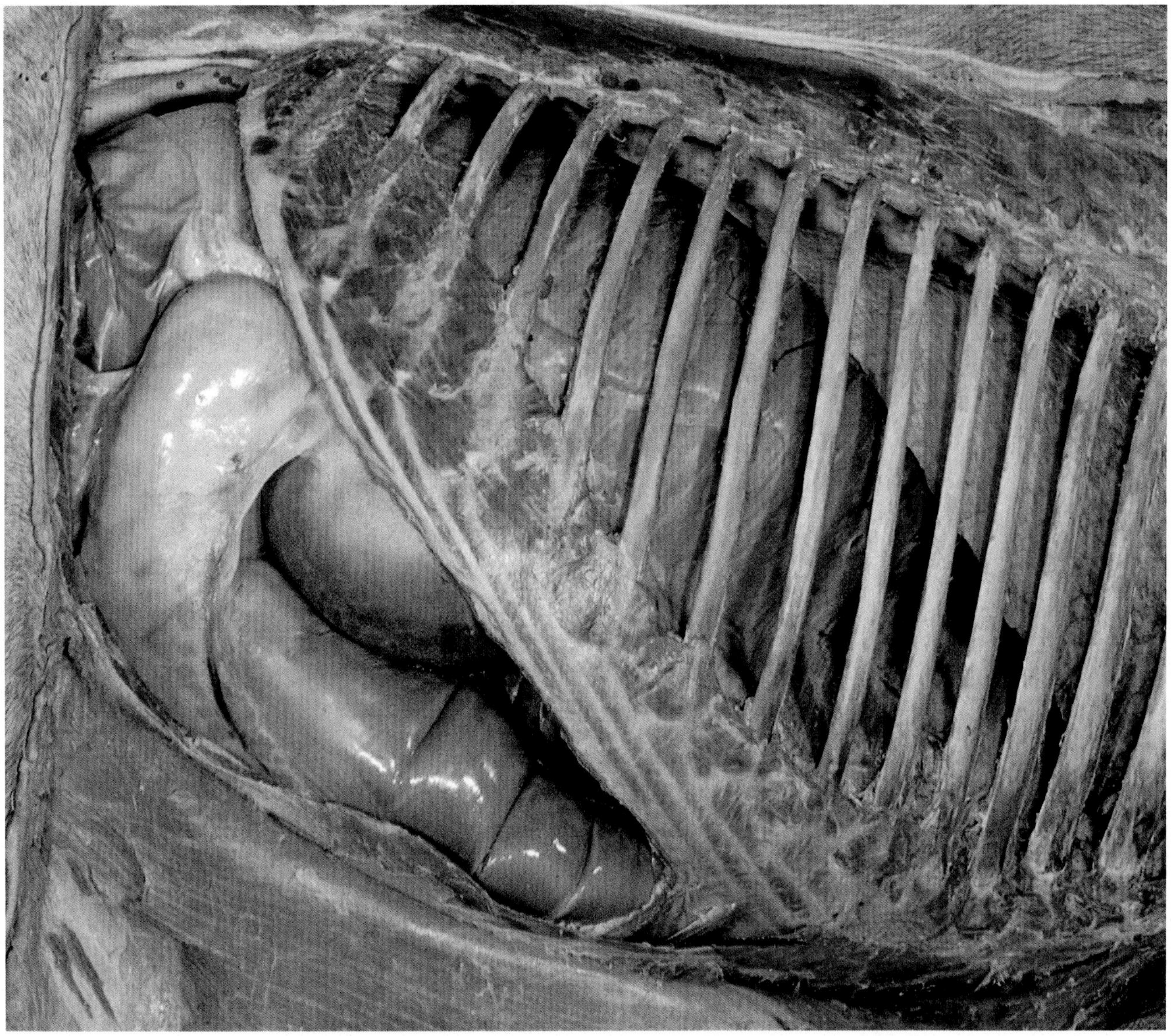

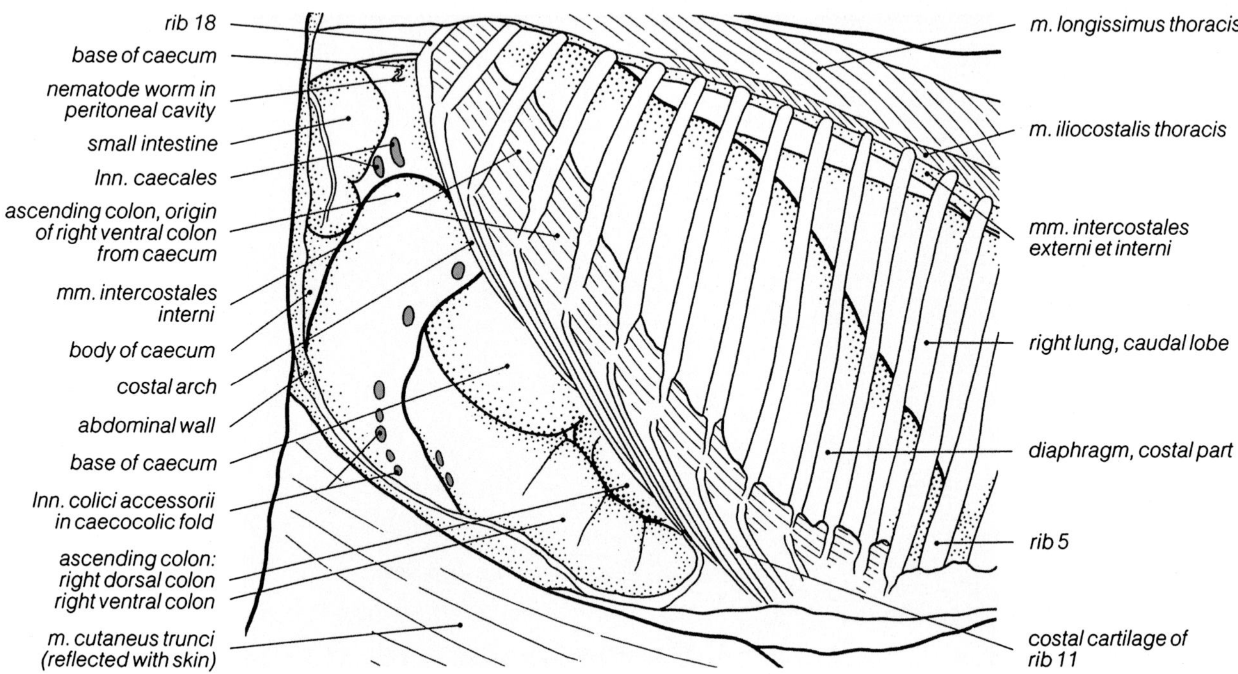
rib 18
base of caecum
nematode worm in peritoneal cavity
small intestine
lnn. caecales
ascending colon, origin of right ventral colon from caecum
mm. intercostales interni
body of caecum
costal arch
abdominal wall
base of caecum
lnn. colici accessorii in caecocolic fold
ascending colon: right dorsal colon right ventral colon
m. cutaneus trunci (reflected with skin)
m. longissimus thoracis
m. iliocostalis thoracis
mm. intercostales externi et interni
right lung, caudal lobe
diaphragm, costal part
rib 5
costal cartilage of rib 11

Fig. 5.28 Abdominal viscera caudal to the costal arch: right lateral view. The abdominal wall has been removed but the diaphragm and rib cage have been retained. The large intestine has been moderately inflated to imitate the condition found in life. Nematode worms (*Strongylus spp.*) are frequently found in the peritoneal cavity during dissection of young horses carrying a heavy intestinal worm burden. See also Fig. 5.42.

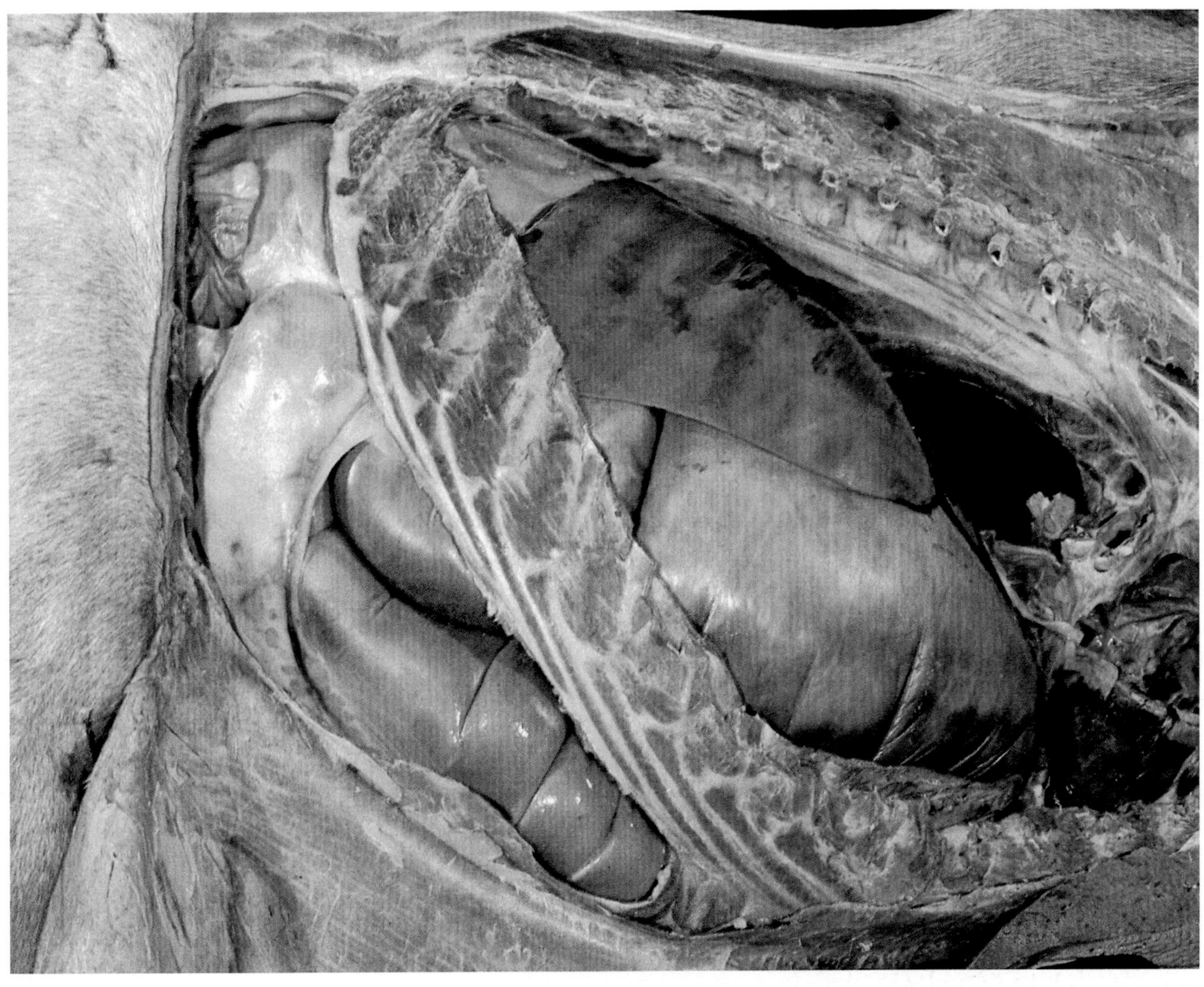

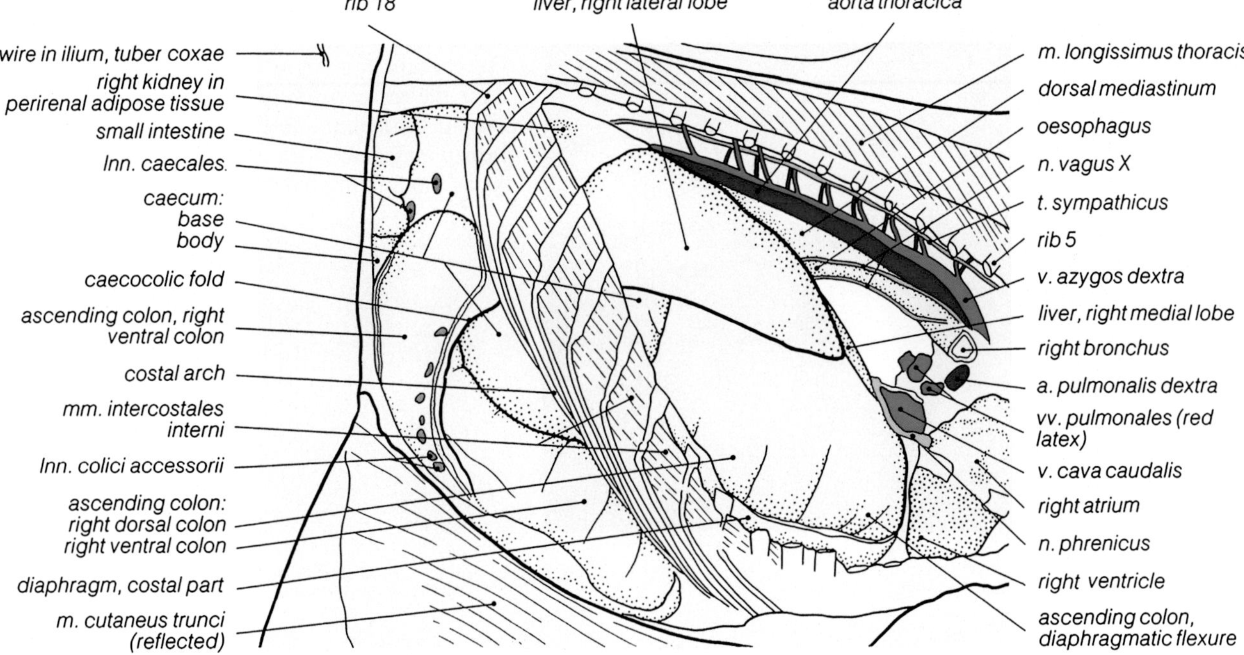
rib 18
liver, right lateral lobe
aorta thoracica
wire in ilium, tuber coxae
right kidney in perirenal adipose tissue
small intestine
lnn. caecales.
caecum: base
body
caecocolic fold
ascending colon, right ventral colon
costal arch
mm. intercostales interni
lnn. colici accessorii
ascending colon: right dorsal colon
right ventral colon
diaphragm, costal part
m. cutaneus trunci (reflected)
m. longissimus thoracis
dorsal mediastinum
oesophagus
n. vagus X
t. sympathicus
rib 5
v. azygos dextra
liver, right medial lobe
right bronchus
a. pulmonalis dextra
vv. pulmonales (red latex)
v. cava caudalis
right atrium
n. phrenicus
right ventricle
ascending colon, diaphragmatic flexure

Fig. 5.29 Abdominal viscera, after partial removal of the right body wall and diaphragm: right lateral view. The right lung and the fragile ventral mediastinum have been removed during dissection of the thorax. See also Figs. 5.44 and 5.46.

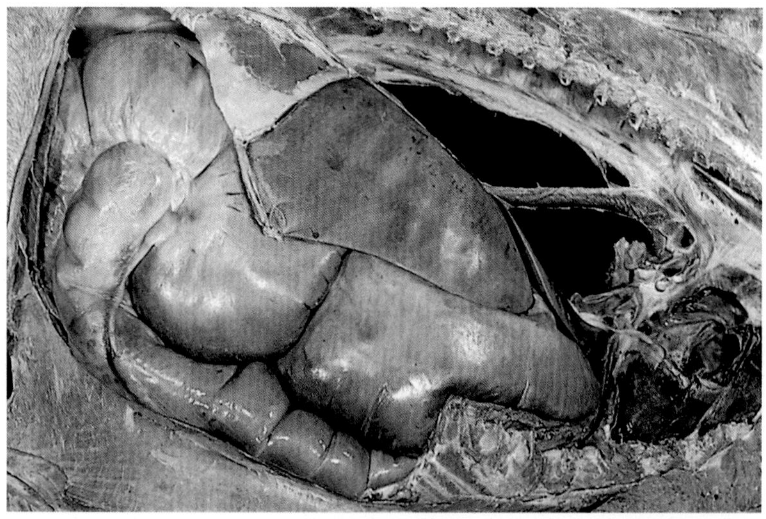

Fig. 5.30 Abdominal viscera: right lateral view. The costal arch has been removed; note that rib 18 is small in this specimen. The dorsal mediastinum has been removed and part of the longissimus muscle has been resected. Further details of this stage of the dissection are shown in Figs. 5.31–5.33. The liver of the horse lacks a gall bladder and therefore the term quadrate lobe has been avoided; this lobe has been called the right medial lobe.

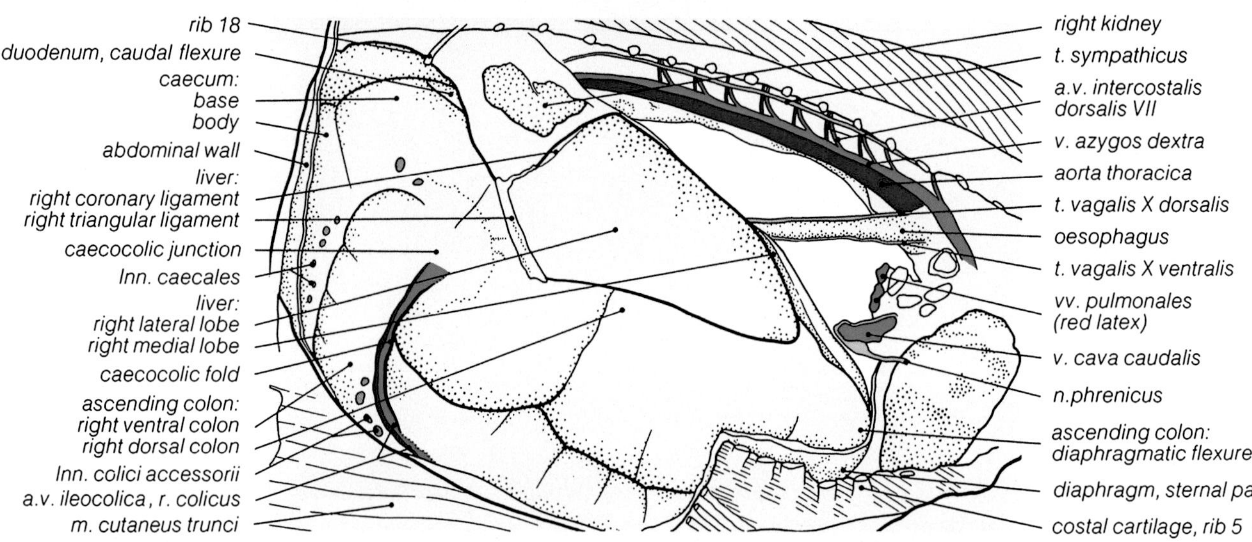
rib 18
duodenum, caudal flexure
caecum:
base
body
abdominal wall
liver:
right coronary ligament
right triangular ligament
caecocolic junction
lnn. caecales
liver:
right lateral lobe
right medial lobe
caecocolic fold
ascending colon:
right ventral colon
right dorsal colon
lnn. colici accessorii
a.v. ileocolica, r. colicus
m. cutaneus trunci
right kidney
t. sympathicus
a.v. intercostalis dorsalis VII
v. azygos dextra
aorta thoracica
t. vagalis X dorsalis
oesophagus
t. vagalis X ventralis
vv. pulmonales (red latex)
v. cava caudalis
n.phrenicus
ascending colon:
diaphragmatic flexure
diaphragm, sternal part
costal cartilage, rib 5

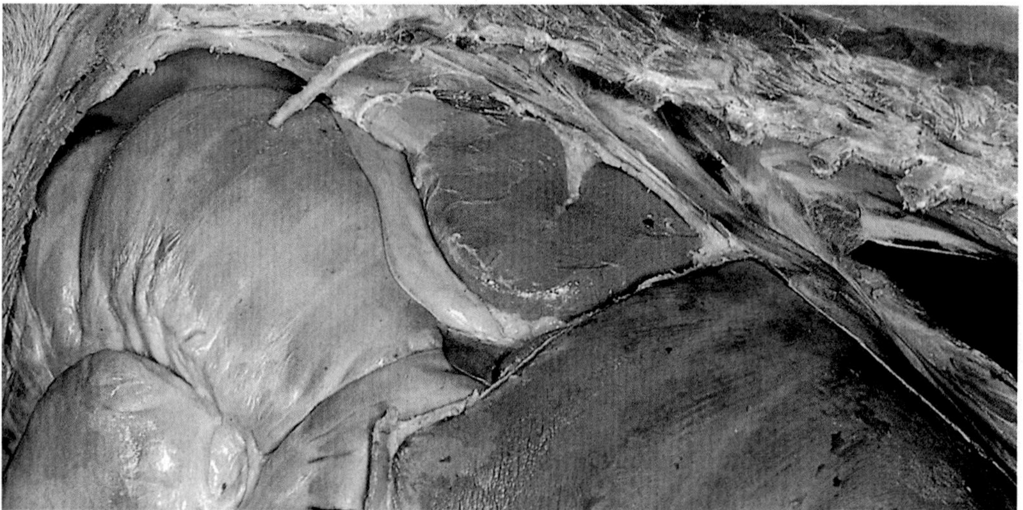

Fig. 5.31 The right kidney: right lateral view. The caecum and colon have been inflated to show the relationship of the right kidney to the last rib, duodenum, liver and caecum. The right kidney may extend, caudal to the costal arch, as far as the first lumbar transverse process.

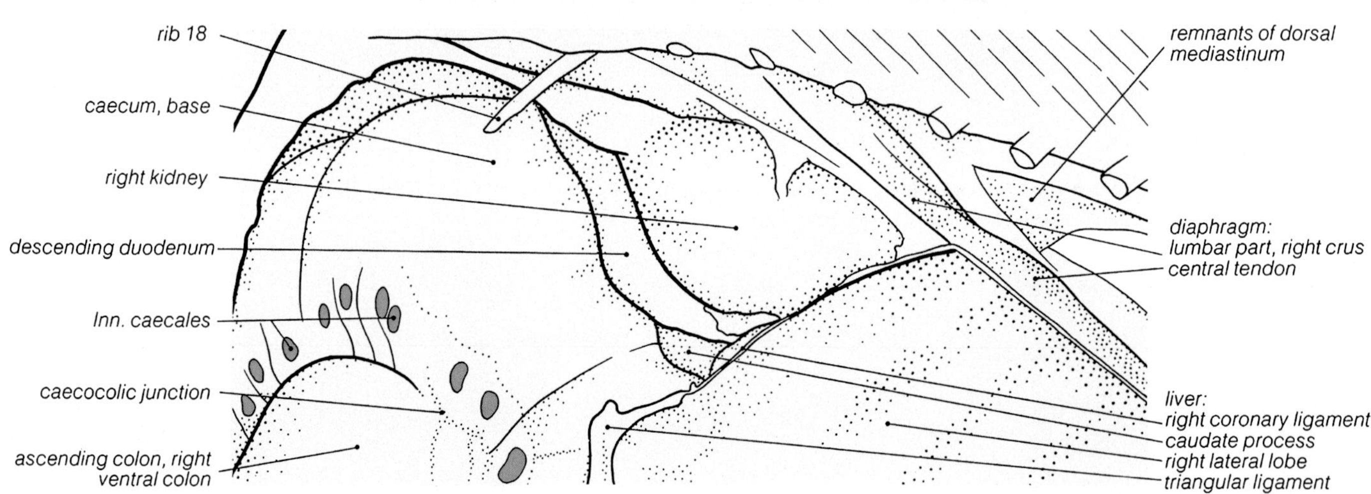
rib 18
caecum, base
right kidney
descending duodenum
lnn. caecales
caecocolic junction
ascending colon, right ventral colon
remnants of dorsal mediastinum
diaphragm:
lumbar part, right crus
central tendon
liver:
right coronary ligament
caudate process
right lateral lobe
triangular ligament

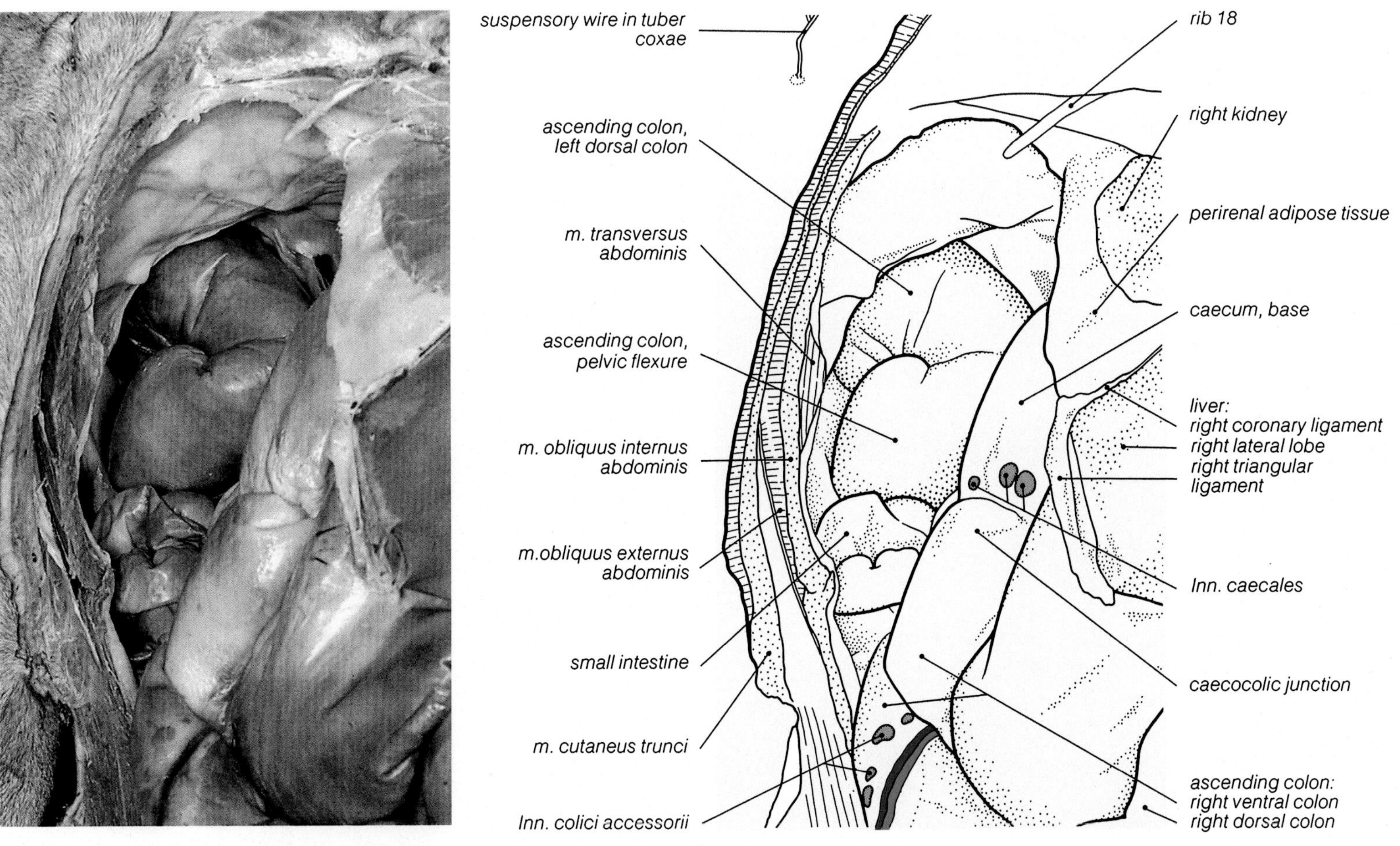
suspensory wire in tuber coxae
ascending colon, left dorsal colon
m. transversus abdominis
ascending colon, pelvic flexure
m. obliquus internus abdominis
m.obliquus externus abdominis
small intestine
m. cutaneus trunci
lnn. colici accessorii
rib 18
right kidney
perirenal adipose tissue
caecum, base
liver:
right coronary ligament
right lateral lobe
right triangular ligament
lnn. caecales
caecocolic junction
ascending colon:
right ventral colon
right dorsal colon

Fig. 5.32 The pelvic flexure: right lateral view. The large intestine has been deflated and the caecum has been displaced cranially (compare with Fig. 5.30) to show the pelvic flexure of the ascending ('large') colon. The position of this flexure varies greatly, but it usually lies close to, or even within, the pelvic cavity (see also Fig. 5.16).

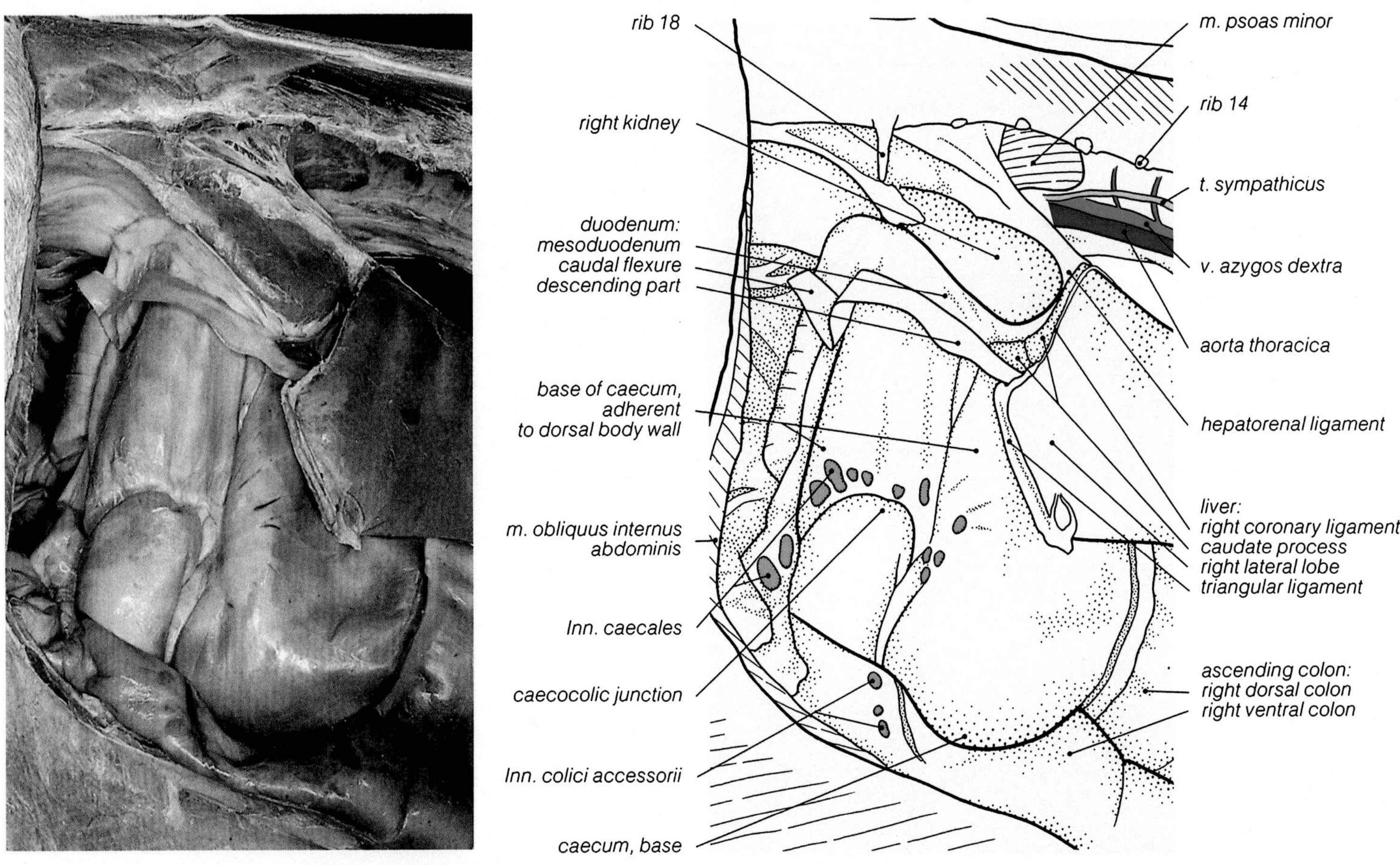
rib 18
right kidney
duodenum:
mesoduodenum
caudal flexure
descending part
base of caecum, adherent to dorsal body wall
m. obliquus internus abdominis
lnn. caecales
caecocolic junction
lnn. colici accessorii
caecum, base
m. psoas minor
rib 14
t. sympathicus
v. azygos dextra
aorta thoracica
hepatorenal ligament
liver:
right coronary ligament
caudate process
right lateral lobe
triangular ligament
ascending colon:
right dorsal colon
right ventral colon

Fig. 5.33 The caudal flexure of the duodenum: right lateral view. The caecum and colon have been deflated to display the course of the duodenum around the right kidney and caecal base more completely. In the duodenum, the rate of passage of ingesta is rapid and the organ rarely, if ever, appears tubular. The full extent of the duodenum is seen (in right lateral view) in Fig. 5.34 and the ascending duodenum in Fig. 5.23.

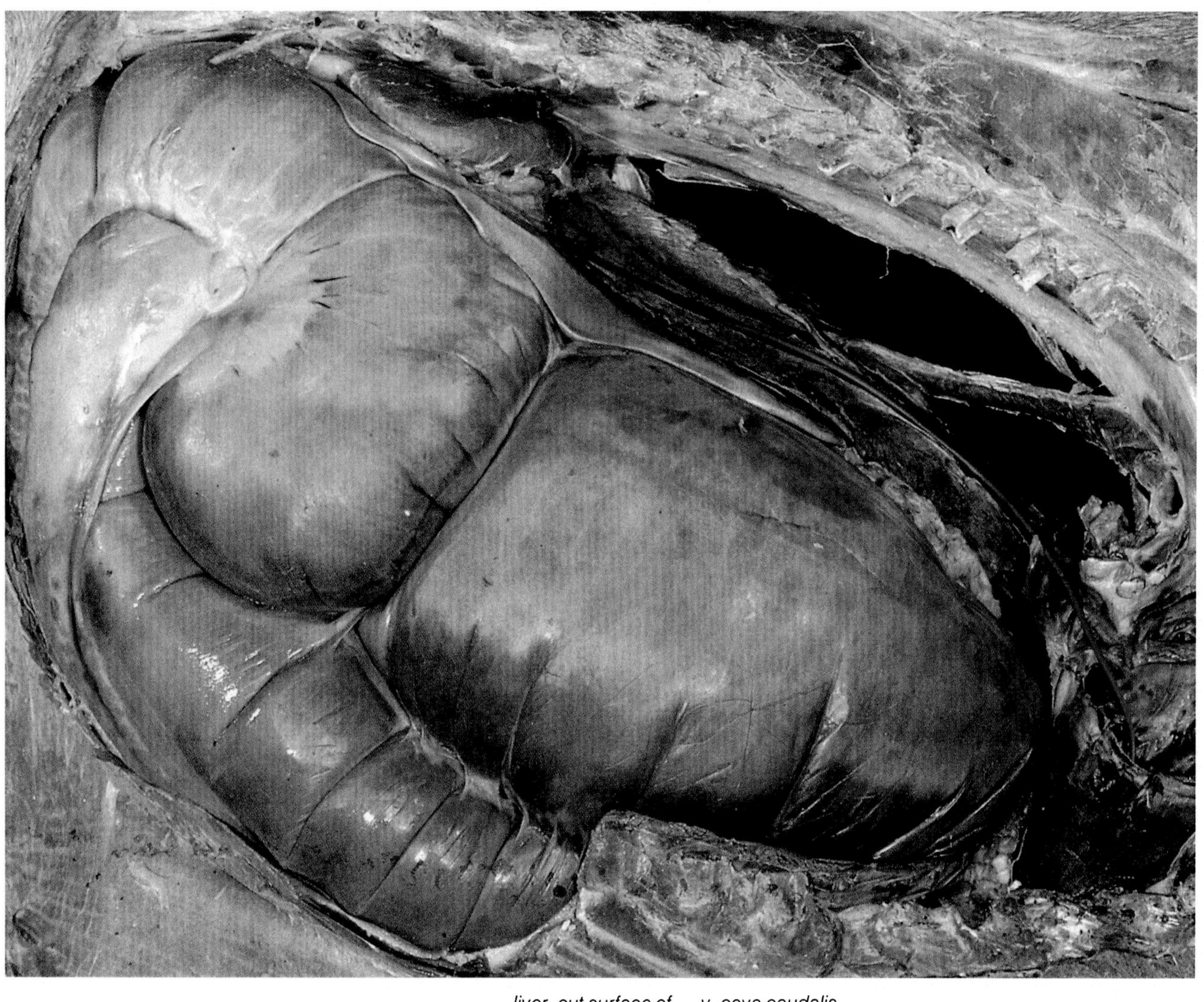

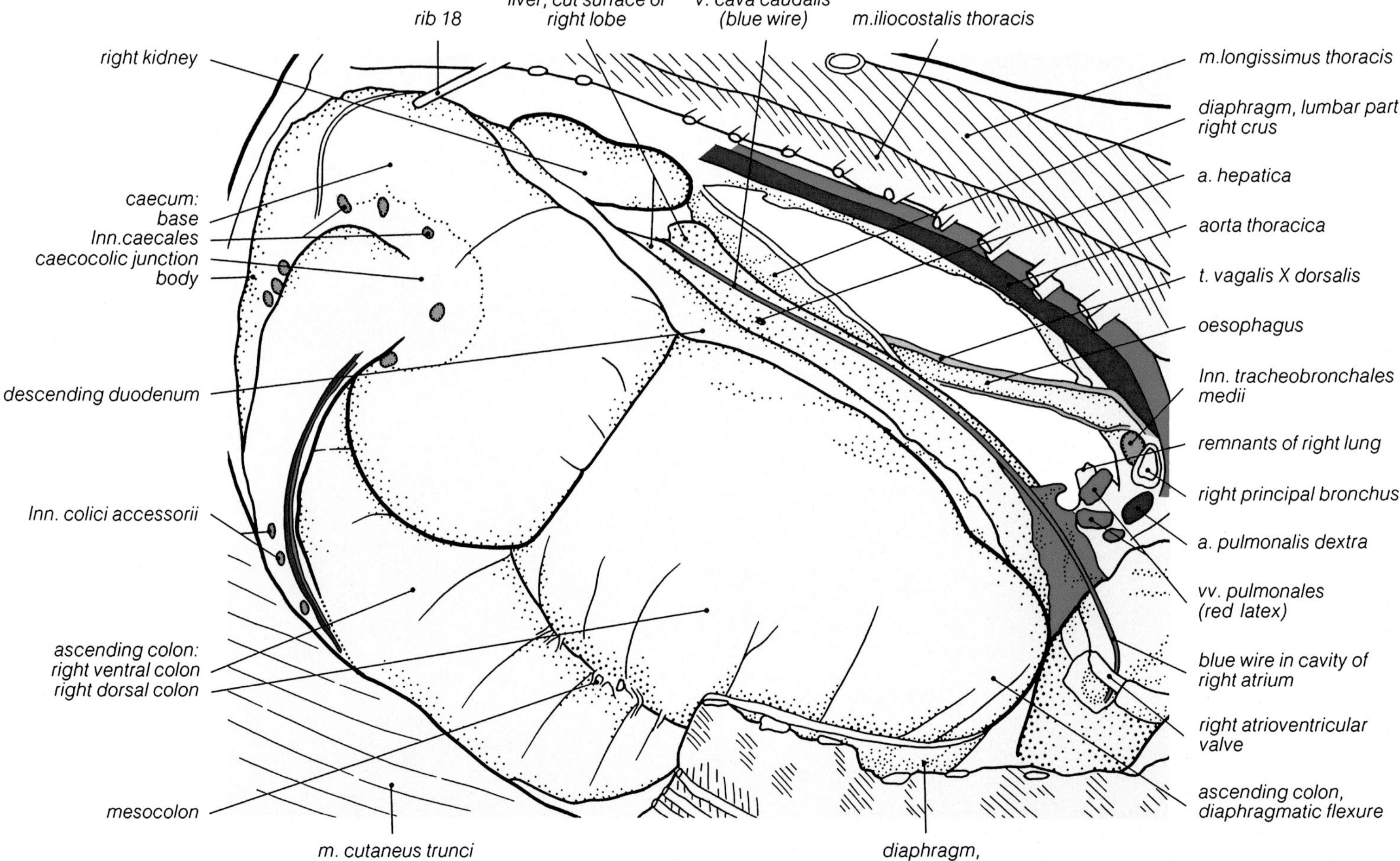
rib 18
liver, cut surface of right lobe
v. cava caudalis (blue wire)
m.iliocostalis thoracis
right kidney
caecum: base
lnn.caecales
caecocolic junction
body
descending duodenum
lnn. colici accessorii
ascending colon: right ventral colon
right dorsal colon
mesocolon
m. cutaneus trunci
diaphragm, sternal part
m.longissimus thoracis
diaphragm, lumbar part, right crus
a. hepatica
aorta thoracica
t. vagalis X dorsalis
oesophagus
lnn. tracheobronchales medii
remnants of right lung
right principal bronchus
a. pulmonalis dextra
vv. pulmonales (red latex)
blue wire in cavity of right atrium
right atrioventricular valve
ascending colon, diaphragmatic flexure

Fig. 5.34 Abdominal viscera after partial removal of the liver: right lateral view. The liver has been removed after making a sagittal incision along the line of the caudal vena cava. A blue wire has been laid in this vein and at its cranial end the wire traverses the right atrium and enters the right ventricle. The large intestine has been inflated. See also Fig. 5.47.

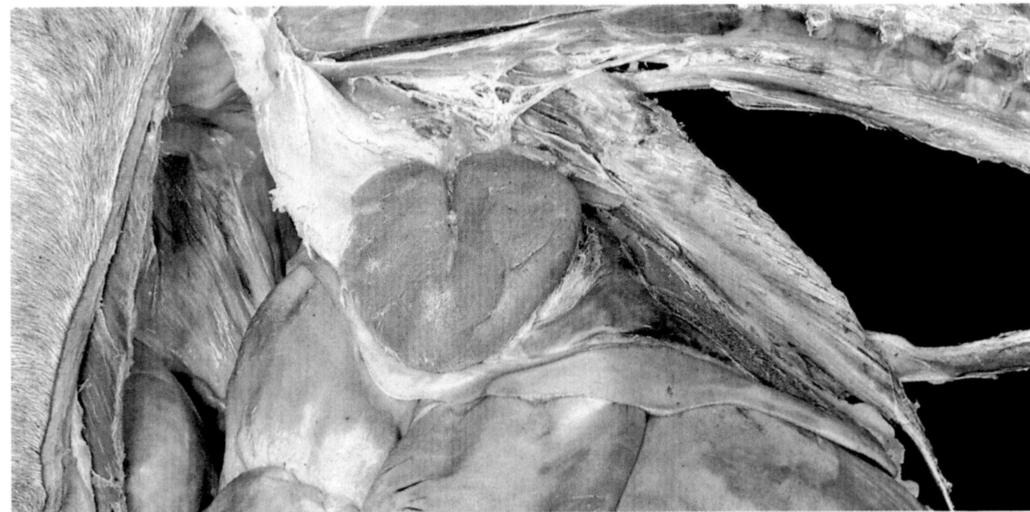

Fig. 5.35 Relationship of the pancreas: right lateral view. The large intestine has been deflated to show the dorsal surface of the pancreas. During removal of the liver the caudal vena cava was cut near its entry into the hepatic portal sulcus and the portal vein and hepatic artery were cut close to the hepatic porta.

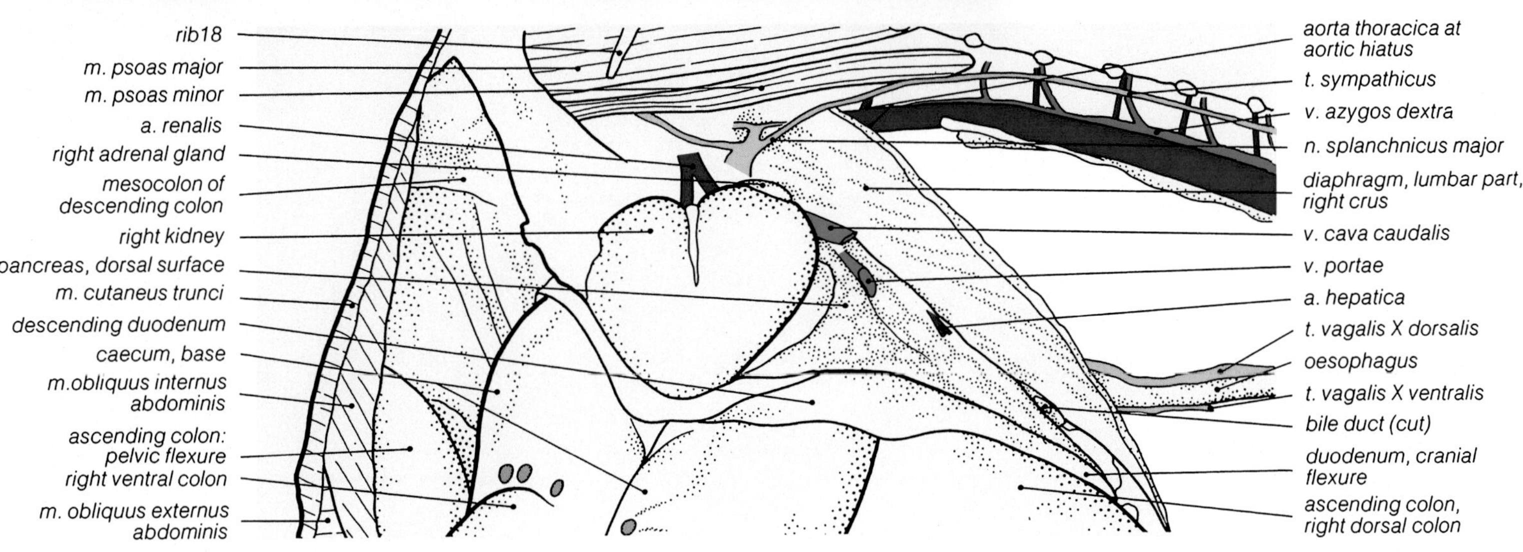
rib18
m. psoas major
m. psoas minor
a. renalis
right adrenal gland
mesocolon of descending colon
right kidney
pancreas, dorsal surface
m. cutaneus trunci
descending duodenum
caecum, base
m.obliquus internus abdominis
ascending colon: pelvic flexure
right ventral colon
m. obliquus externus abdominis
aorta thoracica at aortic hiatus
t. sympathicus
v. azygos dextra
n. splanchnicus major
diaphragm, lumbar part, right crus
v. cava caudalis
v. portae
a. hepatica
t. vagalis X dorsalis
oesophagus
t. vagalis X ventralis
bile duct (cut)
duodenum, cranial flexure
ascending colon, right dorsal colon

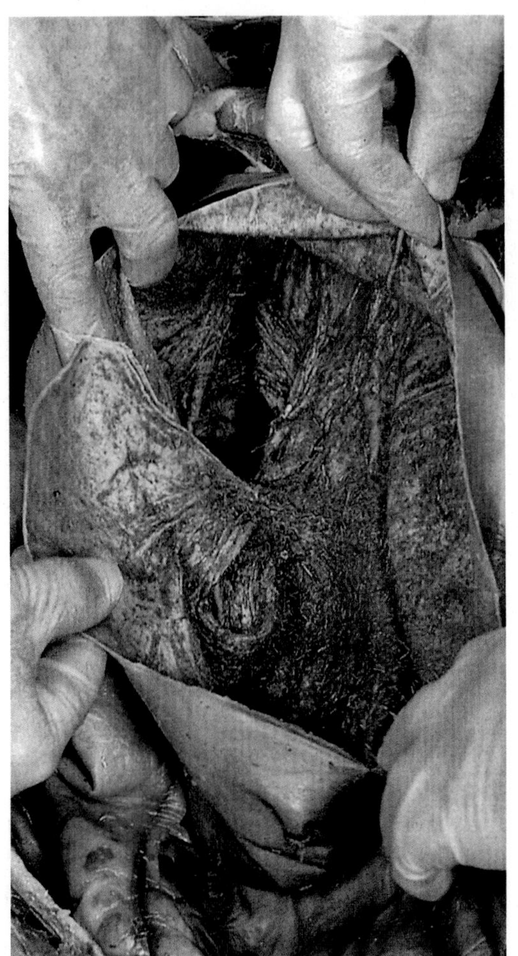

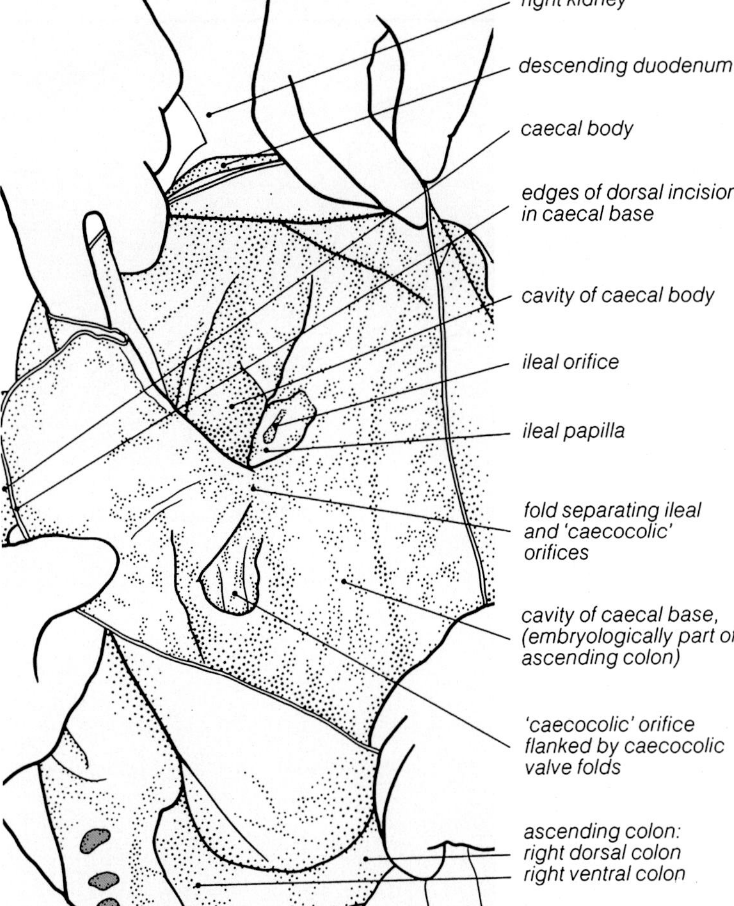
right kidney
descending duodenum
caecal body
edges of dorsal incision in caecal base
cavity of caecal body
ileal orifice
ileal papilla
fold separating ileal and 'caecocolic' orifices
cavity of caecal base, (embryologically part of ascending colon)
'caecocolic' orifice flanked by caecocolic valve folds
ascending colon: right dorsal colon right ventral colon
lnn. colici accessorii

Fig. 5.36 The ileal and 'caecocolic' orifices of the caecum: craniodorsal view. A sagittal incision has been made in the craniodorsal wall (greater curvature) of the caecal base (see Fig. 5.34) and the contents have been removed to expose the two orifices in the ventral wall (lesser curvature). Embryological studies show that the ileal orifice marks the true junction between caecum and colon; the 'caecocolic' orifice is, in fact, a constriction in the initial part of the colon.

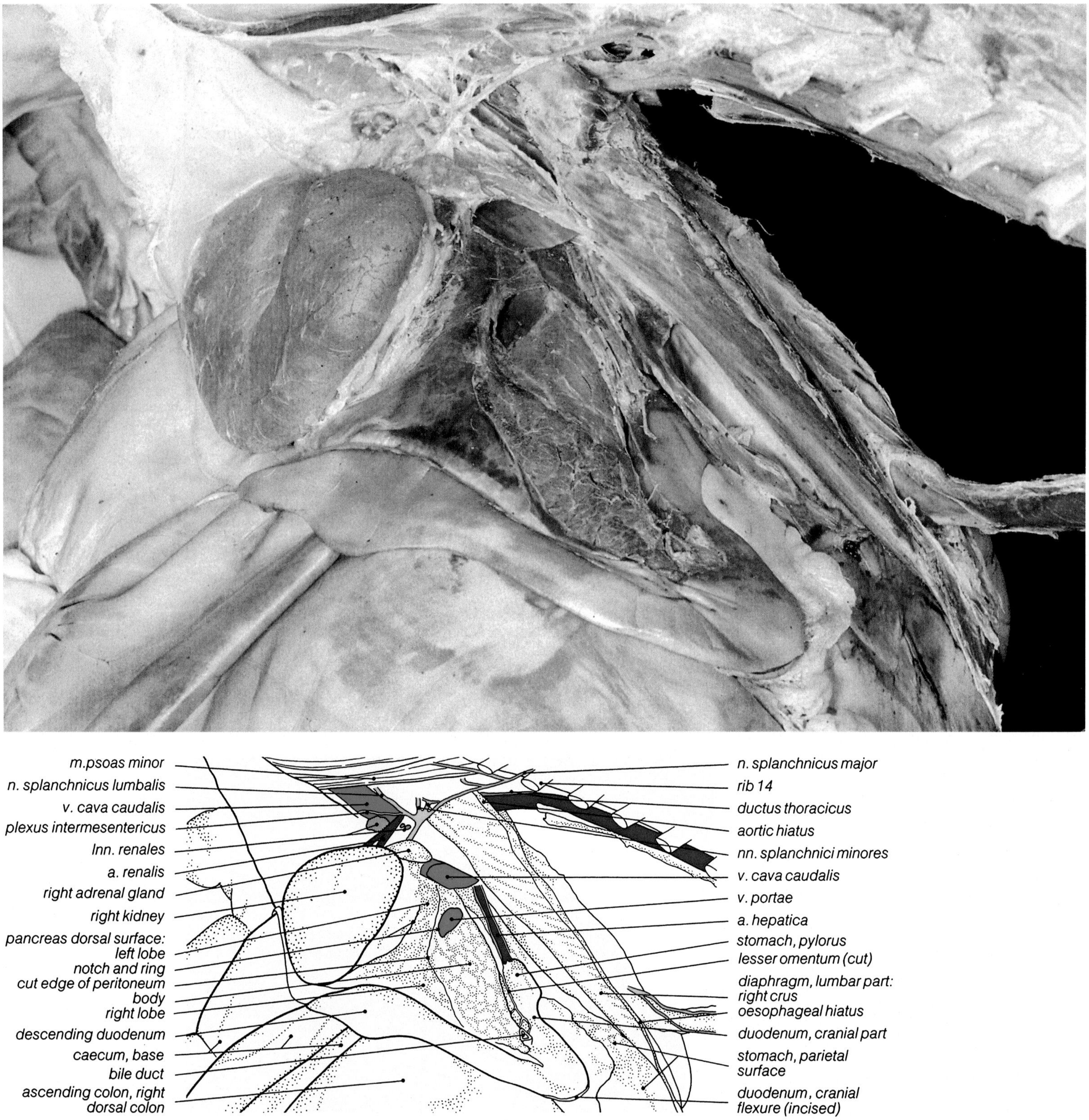

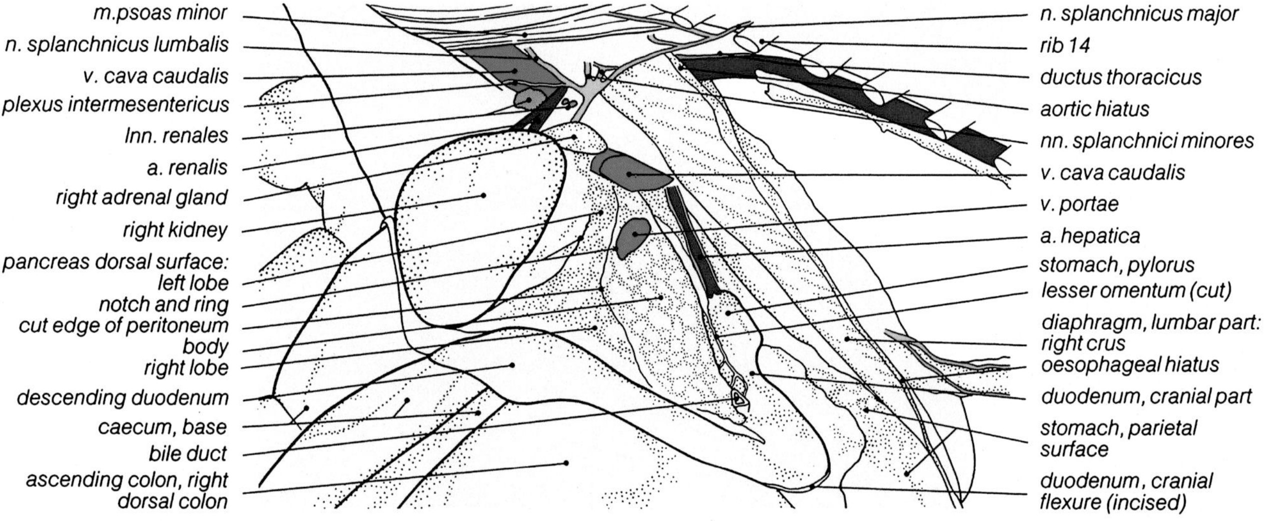
m.psoas minor
n. splanchnicus lumbalis
v. cava caudalis
plexus intermesentericus
lnn. renales
a. renalis
right adrenal gland
right kidney
pancreas dorsal surface:
left lobe
notch and ring
cut edge of peritoneum
body
right lobe
descending duodenum
caecum, base
bile duct
ascending colon, right dorsal colon
n. splanchnicus major
rib 14
ductus thoracicus
aortic hiatus
nn. splanchnici minores
v. cava caudalis
v. portae
a. hepatica
stomach, pylorus
lesser omentum (cut)
diaphragm, lumbar part:
right crus
oesophageal hiatus
duodenum, cranial part
stomach, parietal surface
duodenum, cranial flexure (incised)

Fig. 5.37 Relationships of the pancreas: right craniolateral view. The specimen is at a similar stage of dissection to that shown in Fig. 5.35, but this view shows the dorsal surface of the organ, and its relationship to the stomach, more clearly. The pancreatic duct, which leaves the gland near the bile duct, is not distinguishable (see Fig. 5.38).

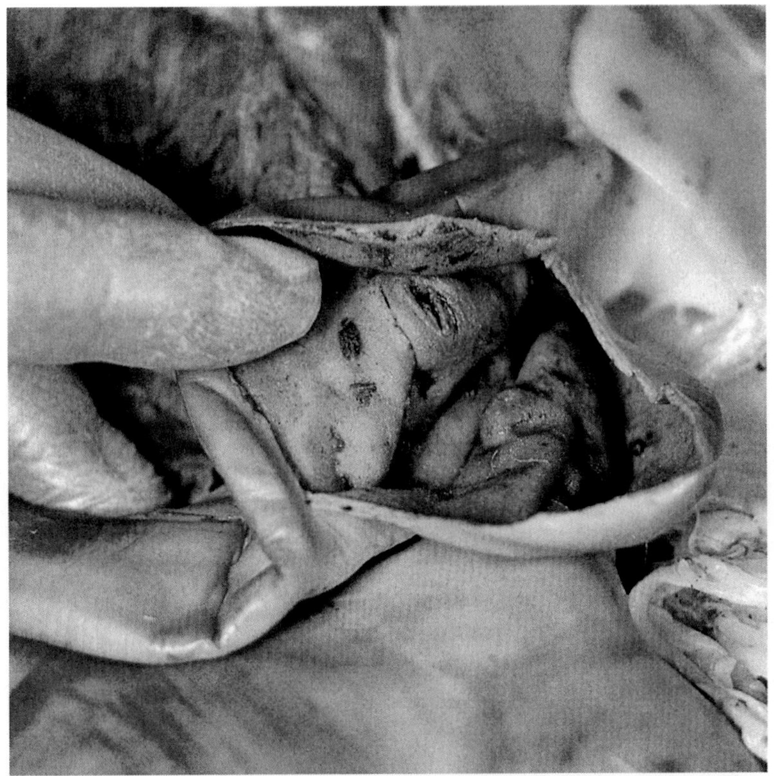

Fig. 5.38 The duodenal papillae: right lateral view. The cranial flexure of the duodenum has been incised (see Fig. 5.37) and opened to reveal the major papilla (bile duct and pancreatic duct) and the minor papilla (accessory pancreatic duct; see Fig. 5.39).

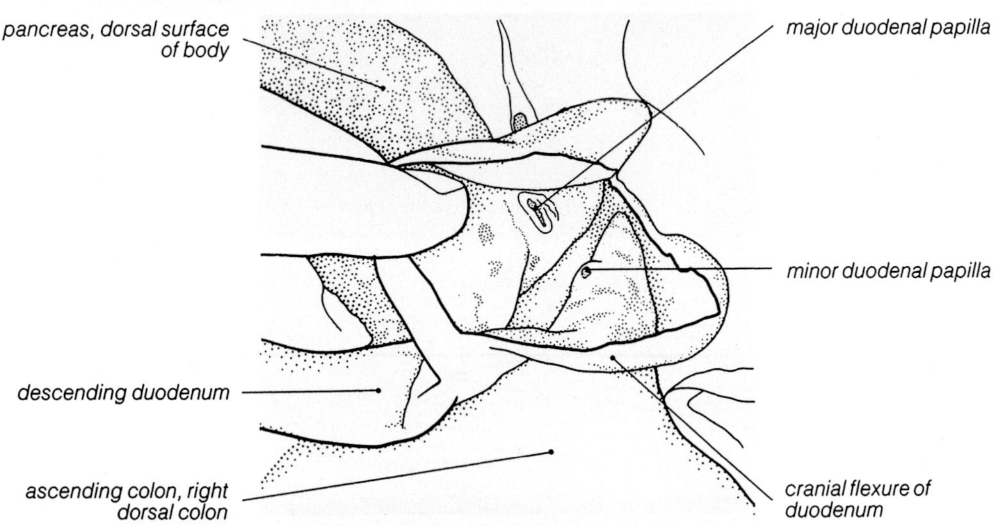
pancreas, dorsal surface of body
major duodenal papilla
minor duodenal papilla
descending duodenum
ascending colon, right dorsal colon
cranial flexure of duodenum

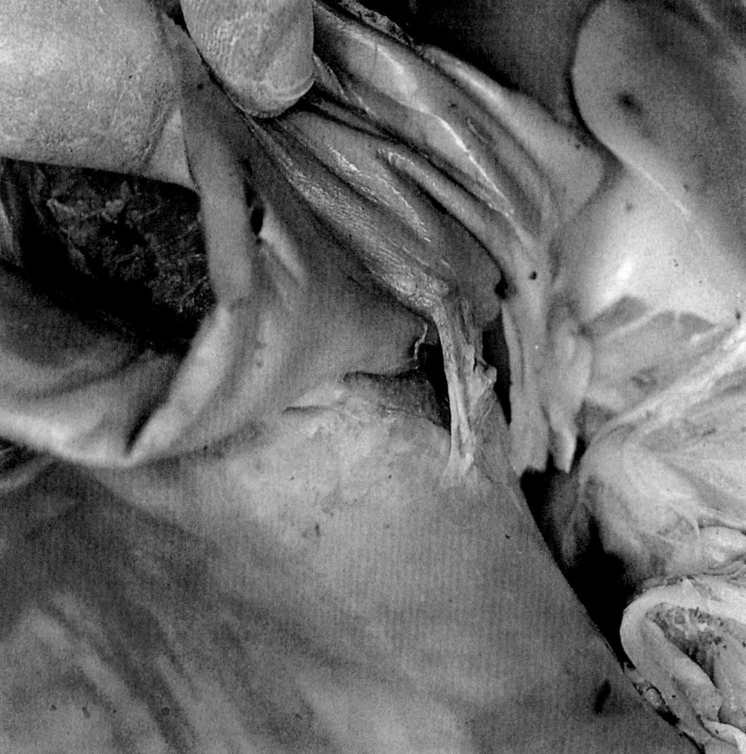

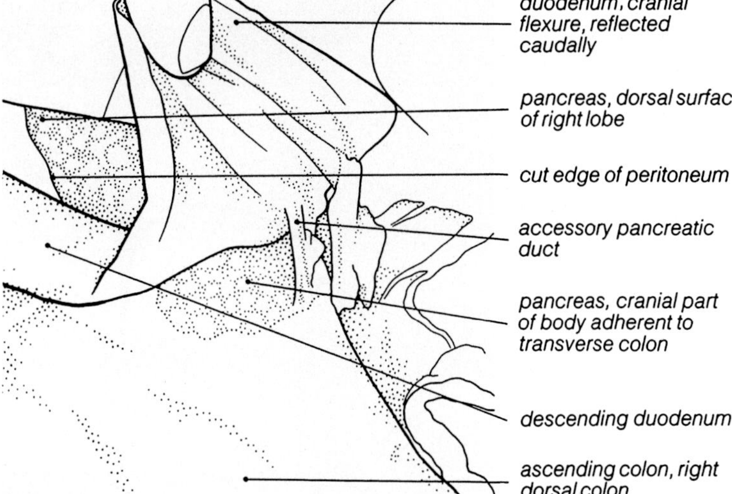
duodenum, cranial flexure, reflected caudally
pancreas, dorsal surface of right lobe
cut edge of peritoneum
accessory pancreatic duct
pancreas, cranial part of body adherent to transverse colon
descending duodenum
ascending colon, right dorsal colon

Fig. 5.39 The accessory pancreatic duct: right lateral view. The cranial flexure of the duodenum has been reflected caudally to expose the transverse colon, the body of the pancreas attached to it, and the accessory pancreatic duct. Although this duct lies ventral to the pancreatic duct, it is derived embryologically from the dorsal pancreatic duct.

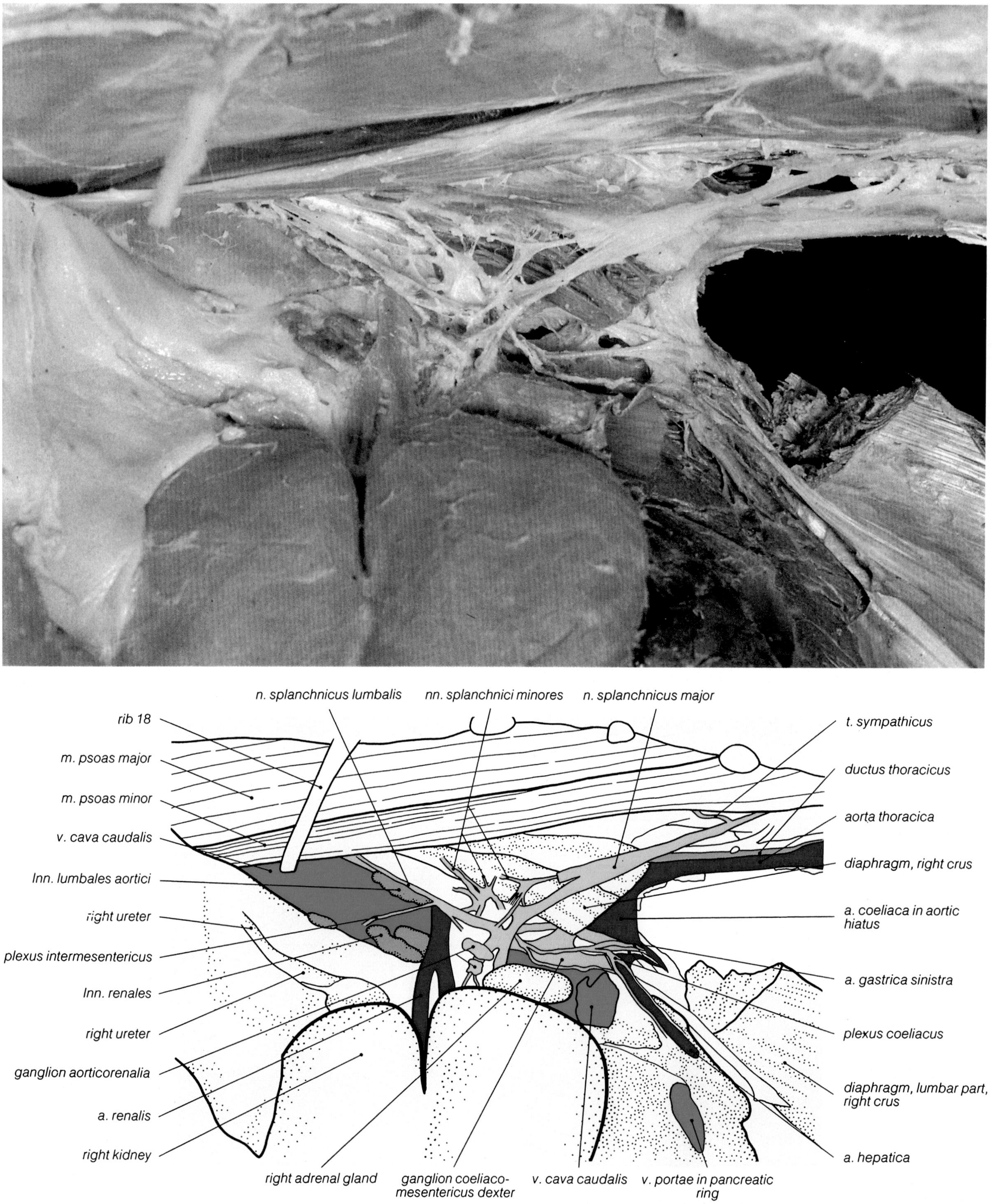

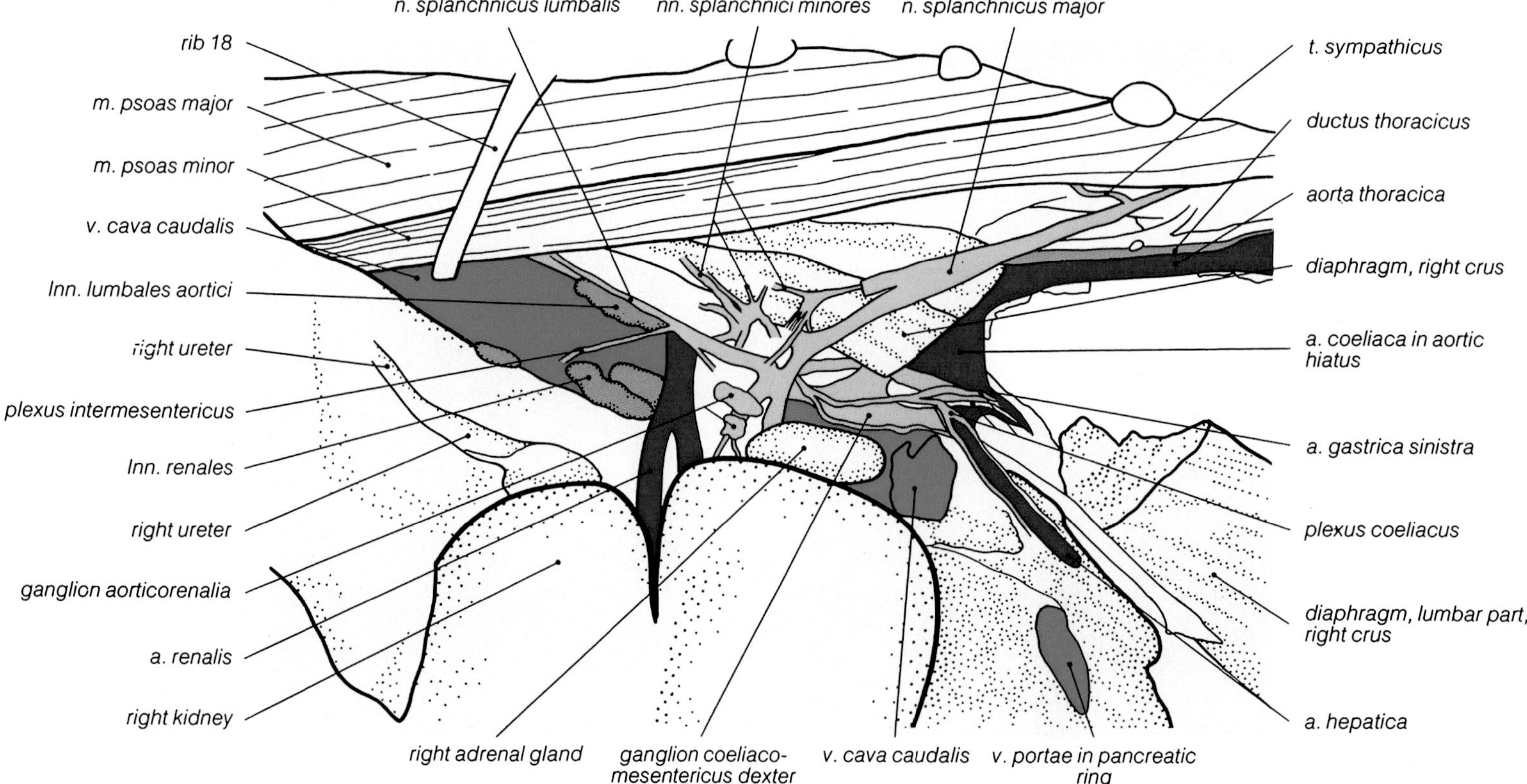
n. splanchnicus lumbalis
nn. splanchnici minores
n. splanchnicus major
rib 18
m. psoas major
m. psoas minor
v. cava caudalis
lnn. lumbales aortici
right ureter
plexus intermesentericus
lnn. renales
right ureter
ganglion aorticorenalia
a. renalis
right kidney
t. sympathicus
ductus thoracicus
aorta thoracica
diaphragm, right crus
a. coeliaca in aortic hiatus
a. gastrica sinistra
plexus coeliacus
diaphragm, lumbar part, right crus
a. hepatica
right adrenal gland
ganglion coeliaco-mesentericus dexter
v. cava caudalis
v. portae in pancreatic ring

Fig. 5.40 The aortic hiatus and adjacent structures: right lateral view (1). Part of the right diaphragmatic crus has been removed to display the coeliac artery arising from the aorta in the aortic hiatus. Dissection of the specimen in the standing position causes the kidney and adjacent structures to drop ventrally after cutting the diaphragmatic crus.

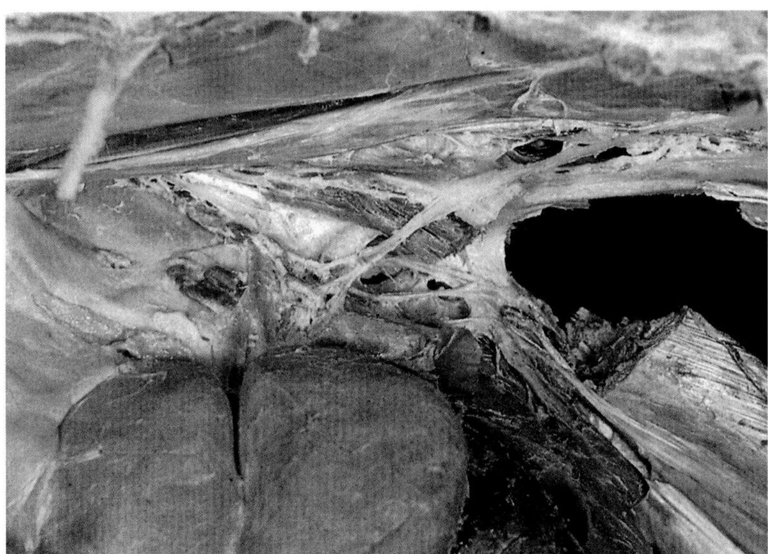

Fig. 5.41 The aortic hiatus and adjacent structures: right lateral view (2). Further dissection reveals the origins of the cranial mesenteric and renal arteries just caudal to the aortic hiatus. See also Fig. 5.42.

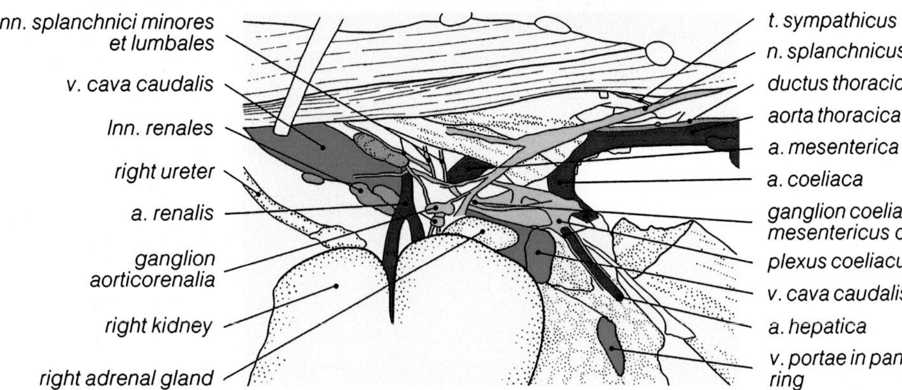
nn. splanchnici minores et lumbales
v. cava caudalis
lnn. renales
right ureter
a. renalis
ganglion aorticorenalia
right kidney
right adrenal gland
t. sympathicus
n. splanchnicus major
ductus thoracicus
aorta thoracica
a. mesenterica cranialis
a. coeliaca
ganglion coeliaco-mesentericus dexter
plexus coeliacus
v. cava caudalis
a. hepatica
v. portae in pancreatic ring

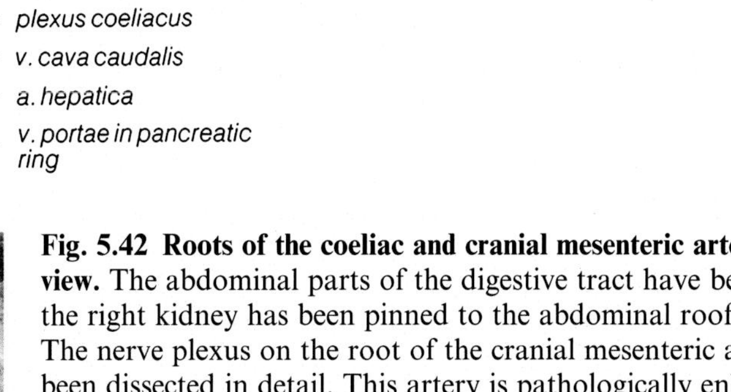

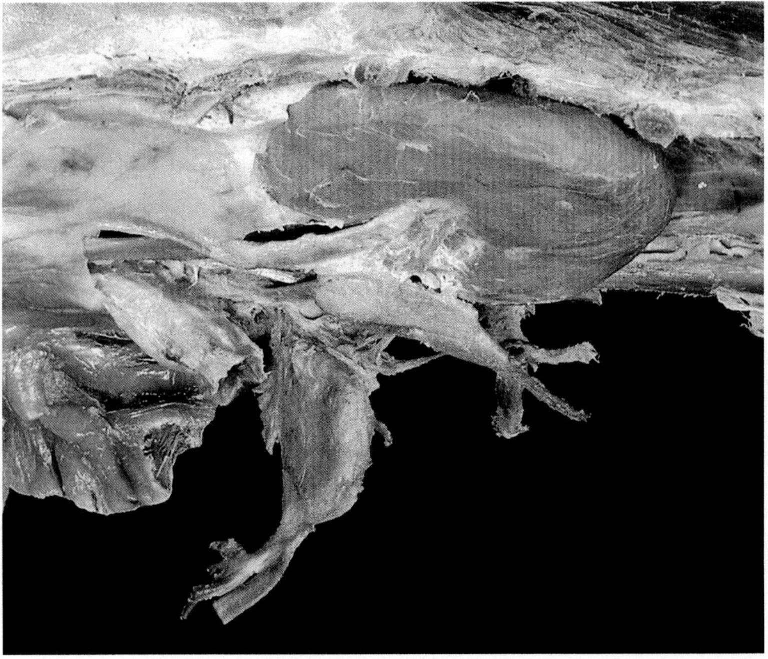

Fig. 5.42 Roots of the coeliac and cranial mesenteric arteries: right lateral view. The abdominal parts of the digestive tract have been removed and the right kidney has been pinned to the abdominal roof (see Fig. 5.41). The nerve plexus on the root of the cranial mesenteric artery has not been dissected in detail. This artery is pathologically enlarged by nematode worms (*Strongylus spp*). The left lateral view of this specimen is shown in Fig. 5.26.

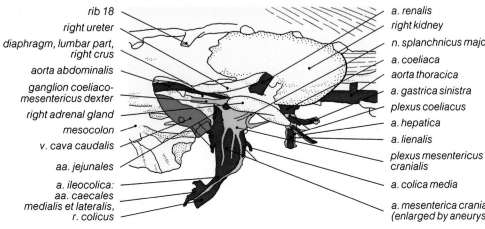

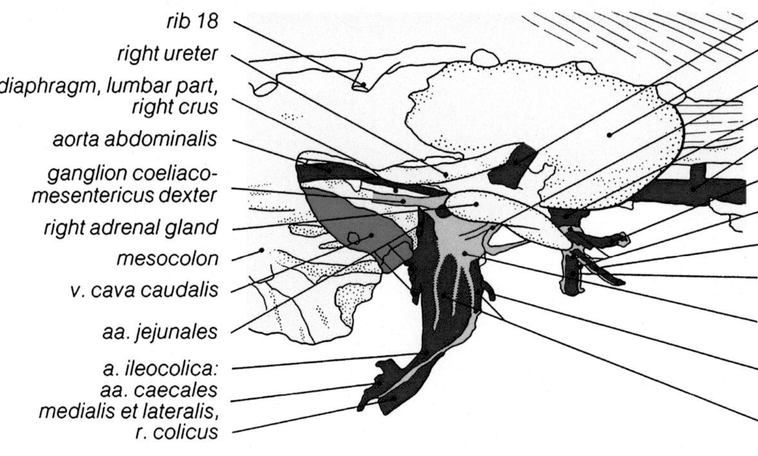
rib 18
right ureter
diaphragm, lumbar part, right crus
aorta abdominalis
ganglion coeliaco-mesentericus dexter
right adrenal gland
mesocolon
v. cava caudalis
aa. jejunales
a. ileocolica: aa. caecales medialis et lateralis, r. colicus
a. renalis
right kidney
n. splanchnicus major
a. coeliaca
aorta thoracica
a. gastrica sinistra
plexus coeliacus
a. hepatica
a. lienalis
plexus mesentericus cranialis
a. colica media
a. mesenterica cranialis (enlarged by aneurysm)

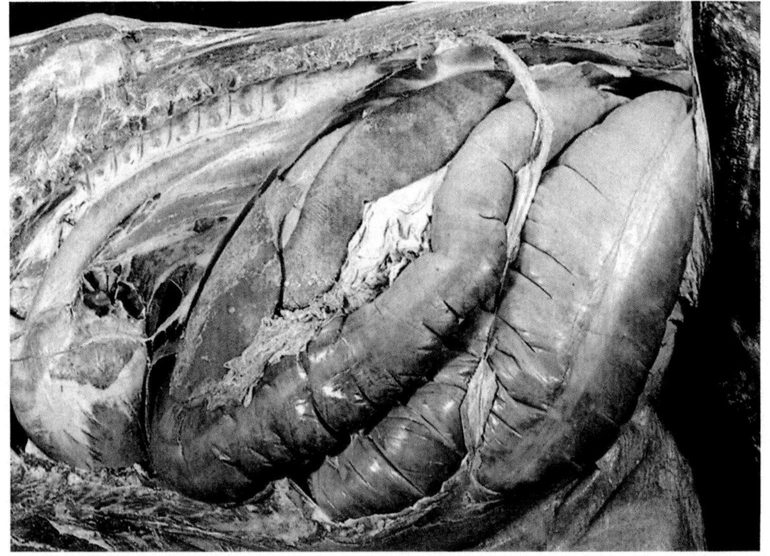

Fig. 5.43 Abdominal viscera of a non-pregnant mare: left lateral view. The thoracic and abdominal walls have been removed and the left lung has been excised. The colon has been moderately inflated to resemble its size in life. Note that the spleen does not extend caudal to the costal arch in this specimen.

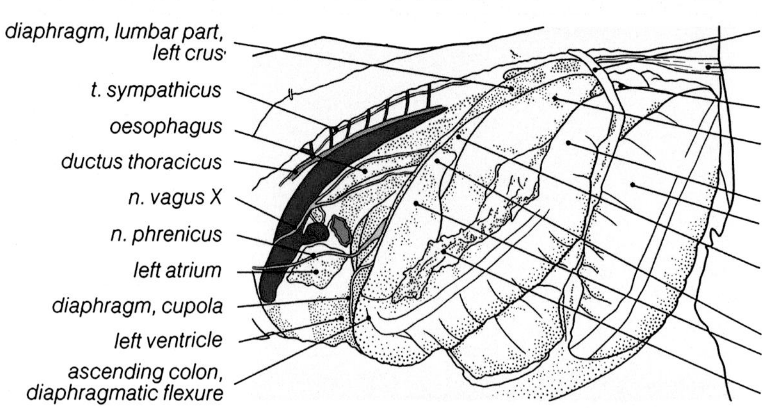

diaphragm, lumbar part, left crus
t. sympathicus
oesophagus
ductus thoracicus
n. vagus X
n. phrenicus
left atrium
diaphragm, cupola
left ventricle
ascending colon, diaphragmatic flexure
rib 18
m. psoas major
left kidney
spleen
ascending colon:
left dorsal colon
left ventral colon
stomach, greater curvature
liver:
left triangular ligament
left lobe
greater omentum

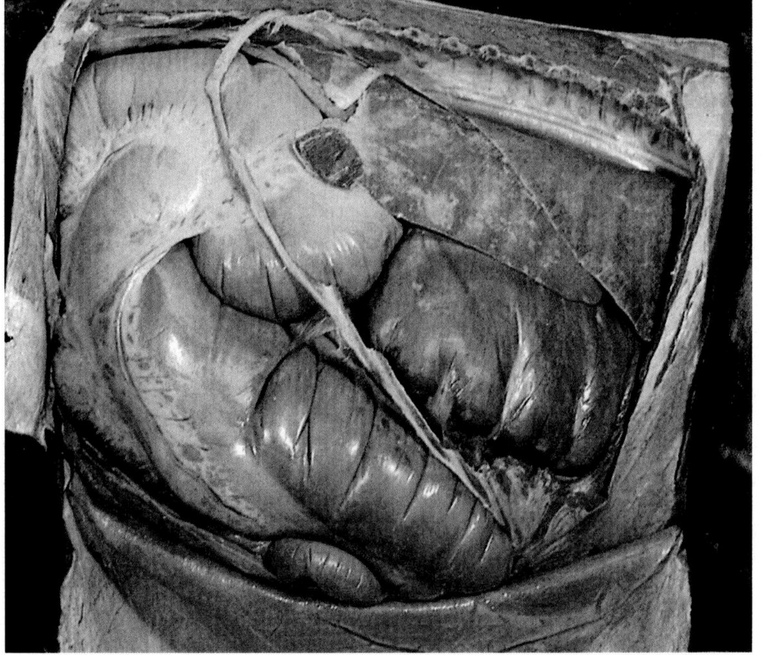

Fig. 5.44 Abdominal viscera of a non-pregnant mare: right lateral view. The abdominal and thoracic walls have been removed and the diaphragm has been excised. The caecum and colon have been moderately inflated to resemble their size in life.

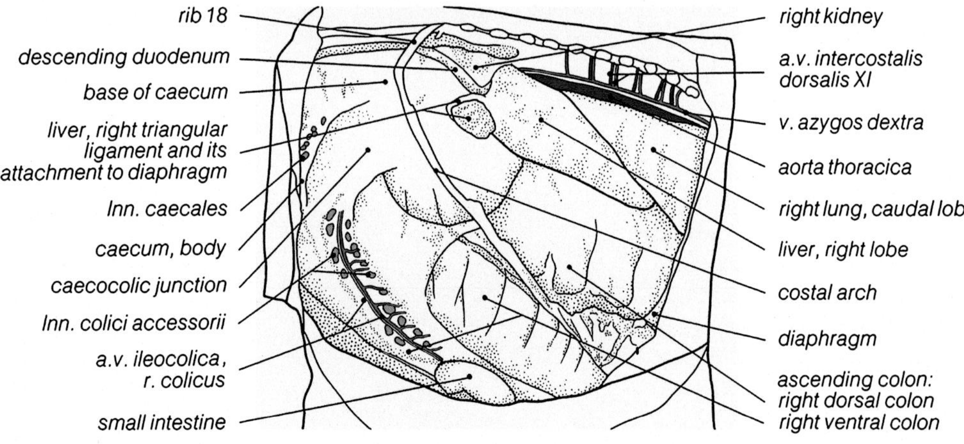

rib 18
descending duodenum
base of caecum
liver, right triangular ligament and its attachment to diaphragm
lnn. caecales
caecum, body
caecocolic junction
lnn. colici accessorii
a.v. ileocolica, r. colicus
small intestine
right kidney
a.v. intercostalis dorsalis XI
v. azygos dextra
aorta thoracica
right lung, caudal lobe
liver, right lobe
costal arch
diaphragm
ascending colon:
right dorsal colon
right ventral colon

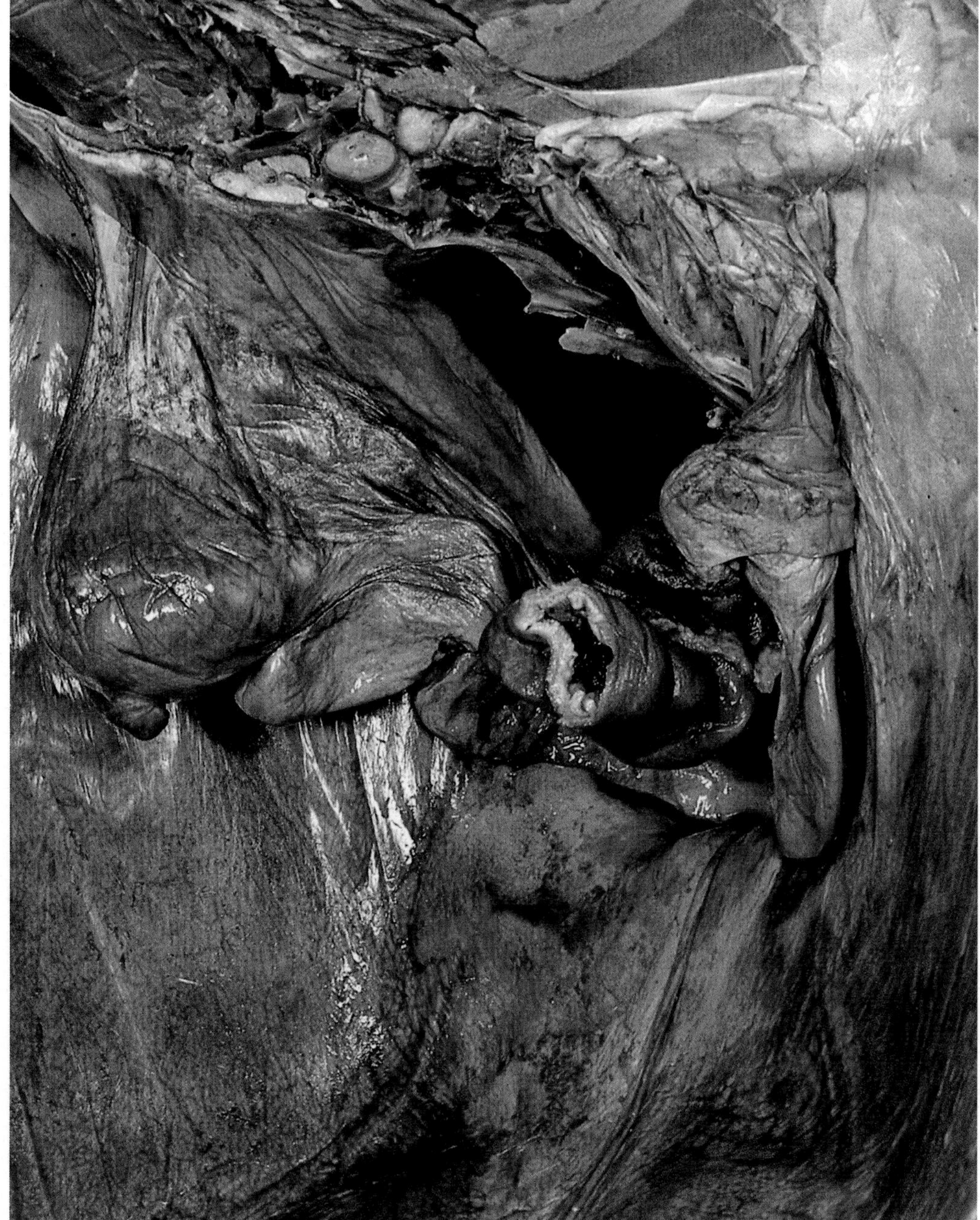

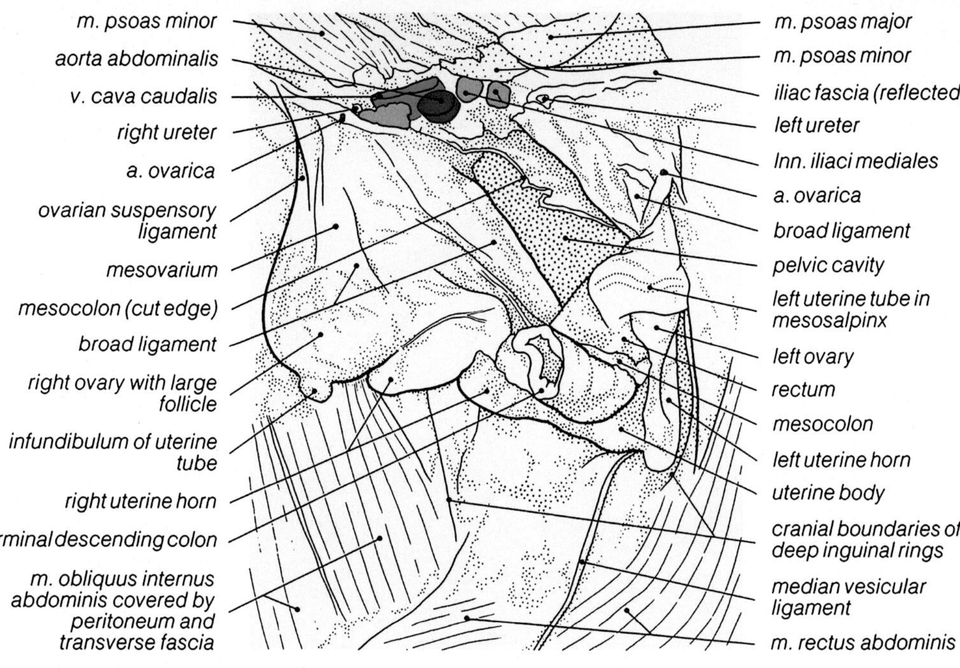
m. psoas minor
aorta abdominalis
v. cava caudalis
right ureter
a. ovarica
ovarian suspensory ligament
mesovarium
mesocolon (cut edge)
broad ligament
right ovary with large follicle
infundibulum of uterine tube
right uterine horn
terminal descending colon
m. obliquus internus abdominis covered by peritoneum and transverse fascia
m. psoas major
m. psoas minor
iliac fascia (reflected)
left ureter
lnn. iliaci mediales
a. ovarica
broad ligament
pelvic cavity
left uterine tube in mesosalpinx
left ovary
rectum
mesocolon
left uterine horn
uterine body
cranial boundaries of deep inguinal rings
median vesicular ligament
m. rectus abdominis

Fig. 5.45 The female tract in the abdomen of a yearling mare: left craniolateral view. The abdominal wall has been removed and the digestive organs excised after cutting the descending colon close to its transition into the rectum. The empty urinary bladder lies entirely within the pelvis.

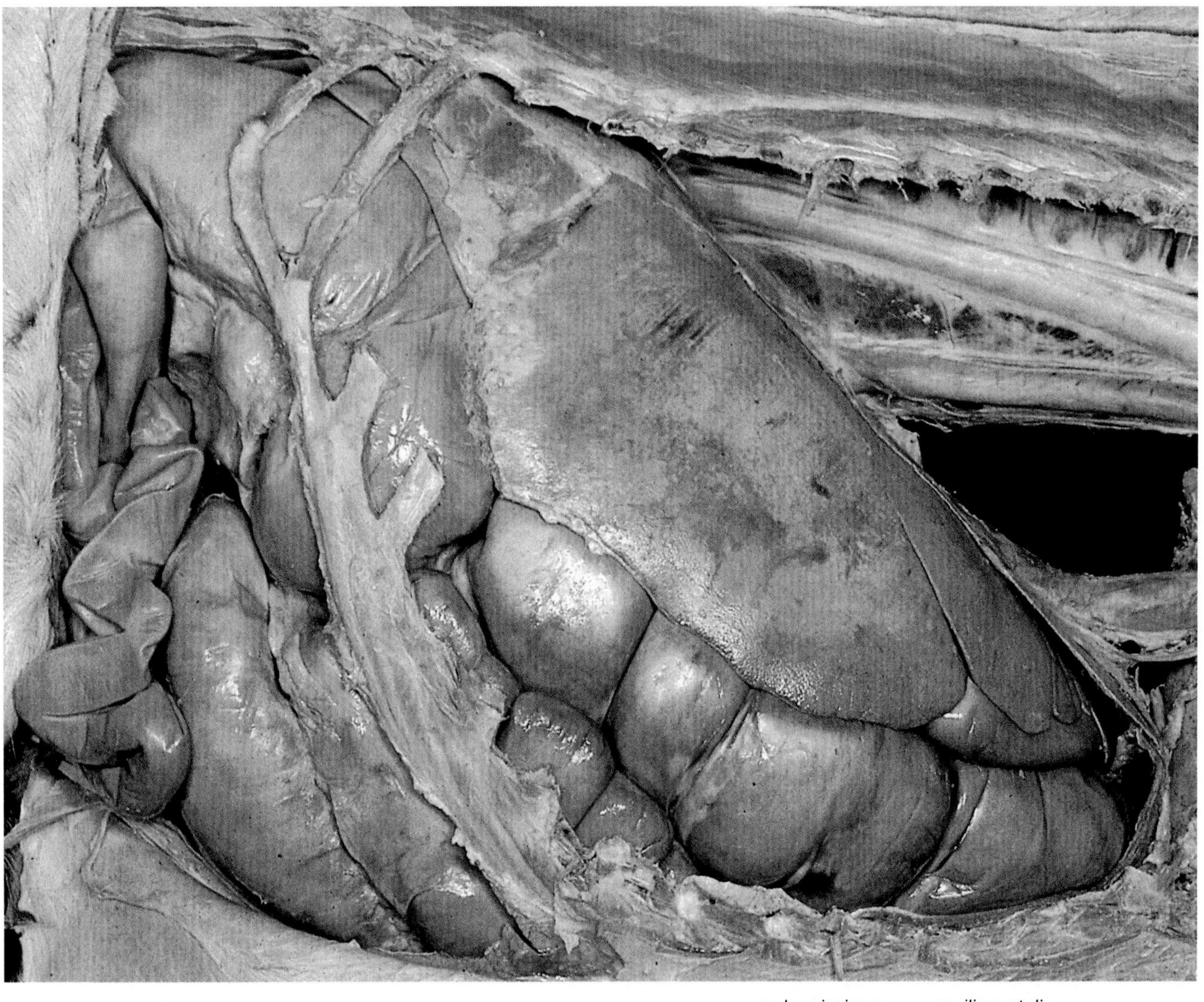

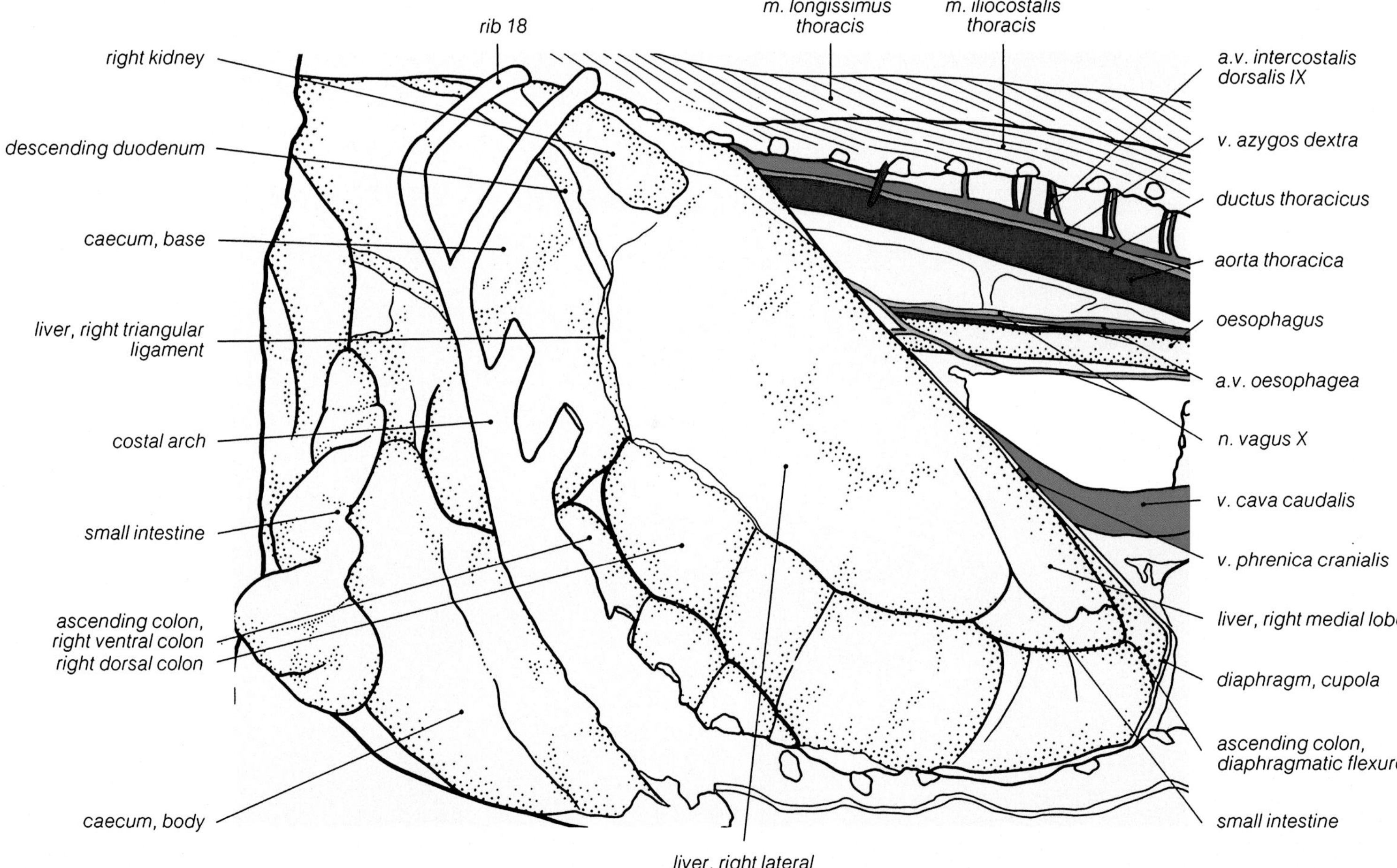
right kidney
descending duodenum
caecum, base
liver, right triangular ligament
costal arch
small intestine
ascending colon, right ventral colon
right dorsal colon
caecum, body
rib 18
m. longissimus thoracis
m. iliocostalis thoracis
a.v. intercostalis dorsalis IX
v. azygos dextra
ductus thoracicus
aorta thoracica
oesophagus
a.v. oesophagea
n. vagus X
v. cava caudalis
v. phrenica cranialis
liver, right medial lobe
diaphragm, cupola
ascending colon, diaphragmatic flexure
small intestine
liver, right lateral lobe

Fig. 5.46 The abdomen in early pregnancy (1): superficial right lateral view. This mare was over 8 years old, and was 3½ months pregnant at the time of death. The large intestine has been inflated to imitate its condition during life. Figs. 5.46–5.48 show right abdominal topography in this mare. The terminology used for the right lobe of the liver is dealt with in Figs. 5.30 and 5.53.

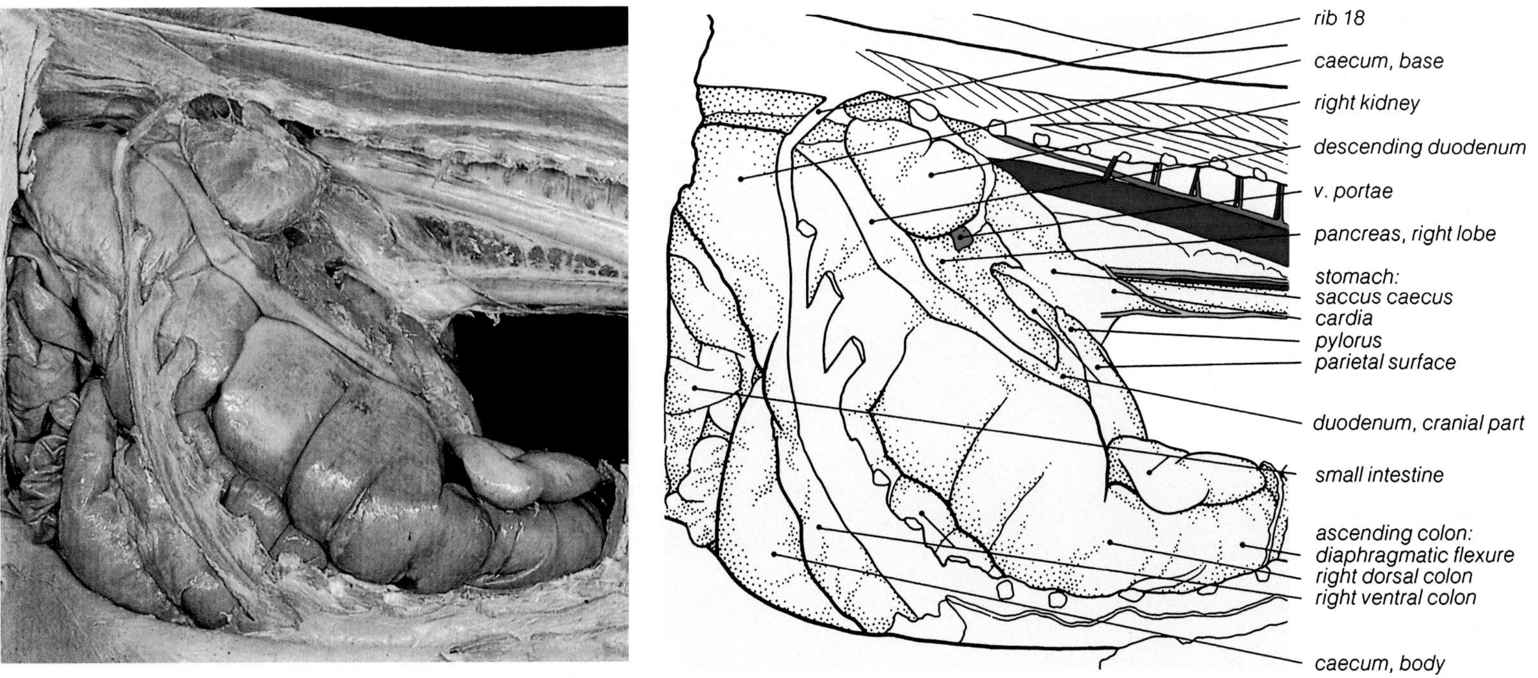
rib 18
caecum, base
right kidney
descending duodenum
v. portae
pancreas, right lobe
stomach:
saccus caecus
cardia
pylorus
parietal surface
duodenum, cranial part
small intestine
ascending colon:
diaphragmatic flexure
right dorsal colon
right ventral colon
caecum, body

Fig. 5.47 The abdomen in early pregancy (2), after removal of the liver: right lateral view. Compared with the non-pregnant abdomen, the small intestine tends to be displaced laterally and cranially from the confines of the loop of the colon. The pregnant uterus also displaces the caecal body laterally. The caudal vena cava has been removed with the liver.

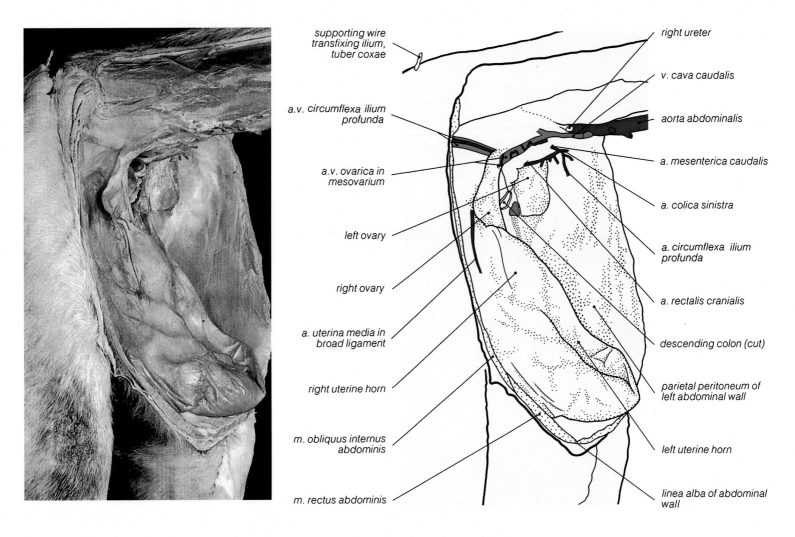

supporting wire transfixing ilium, tuber coxae
a.v. circumflexa ilium profunda
a.v. ovarica in mesovarium
left ovary
right ovary
a. uterina media in broad ligament
right uterine horn
m. obliquus internus abdominis
m. rectus abdominis
right ureter
v. cava caudalis
aorta abdominalis
a. mesenterica caudalis
a. colica sinistra
a. circumflexa ilium profunda
a. rectalis cranialis
descending colon (cut)
parietal peritoneum of left abdominal wall
left uterine horn
linea alba of abdominal wall

Fig. 5.48 The abdomen in early pregnancy (3): ovaries and uterus in right craniolateral view. The abdominal digestive organs have been removed to show the female reproductive tract which occupies the caudal abdomen. The fetus lay in the left horn and body of the uterus and was 20 cm in length from crown to rump. Further details of the reproductive organs are seen in Figs. 8.57–8.61. With advancing pregnancy, the uterus occupies a ventral position between the right and left parts of the loop of the ascending colon. The caecum is displaced to the right, and the small intestine and descending colon are displaced mainly to the left.

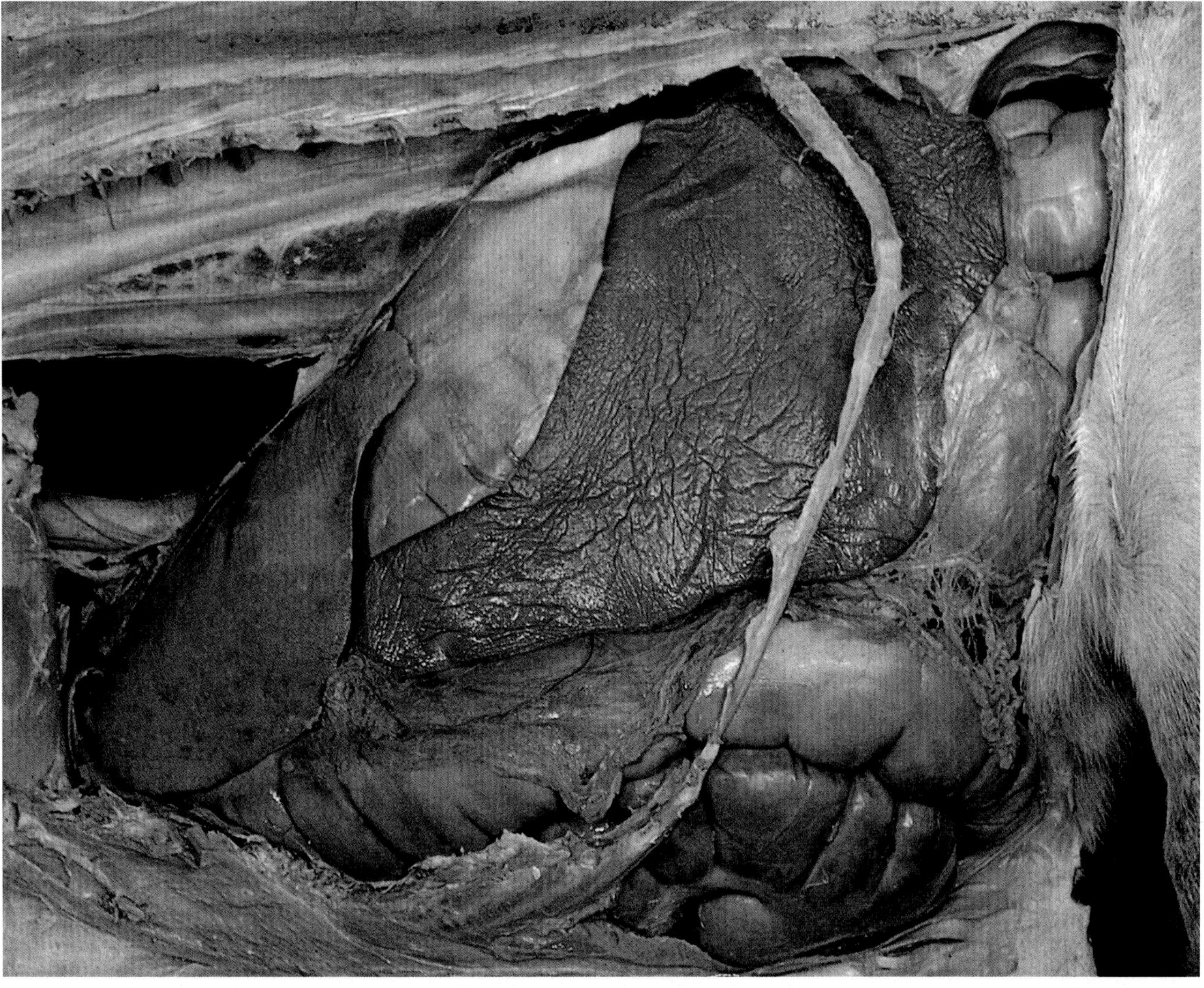

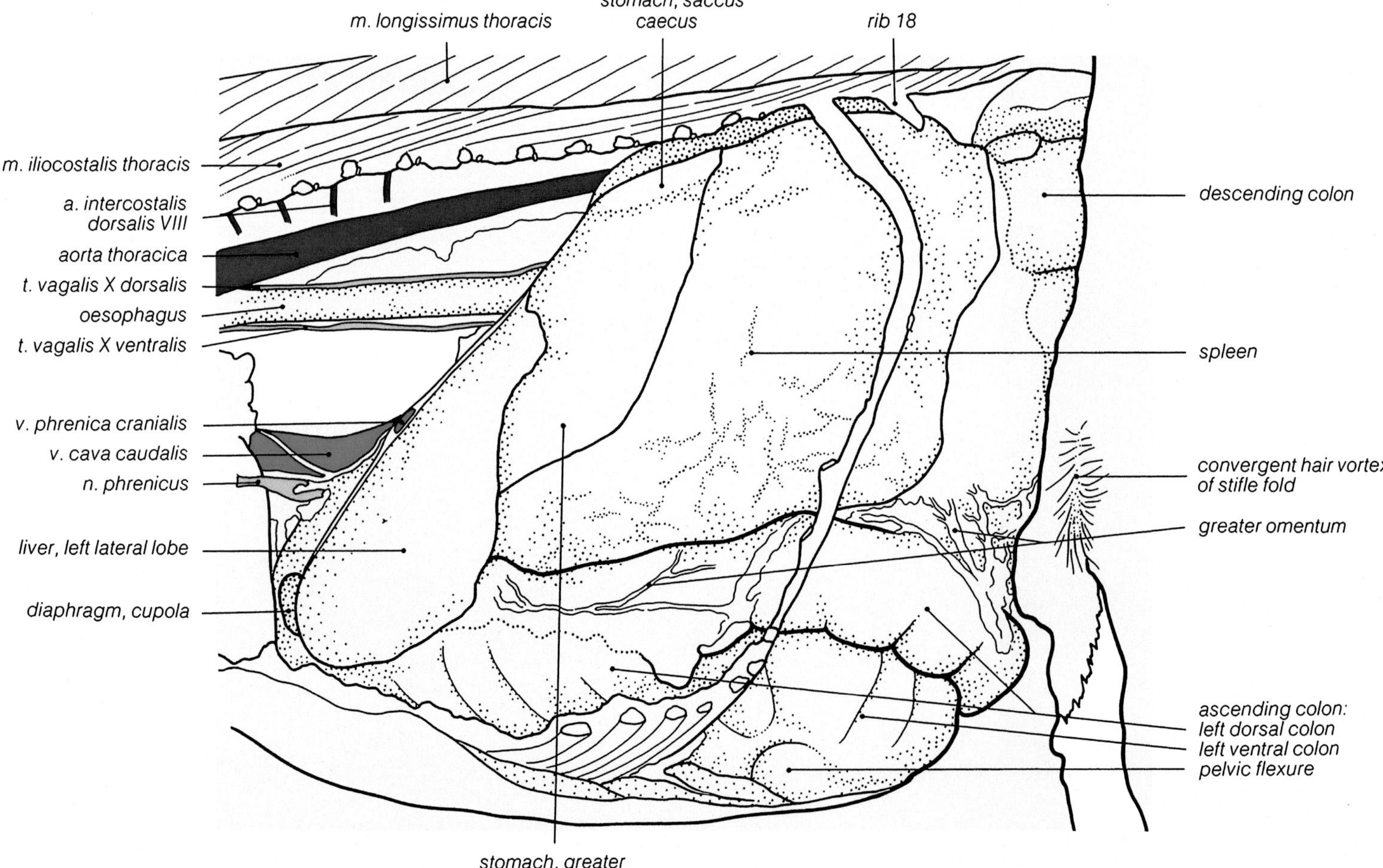
m. longissimus thoracis
stomach, saccus caecus
rib 18
m. iliocostalis thoracis
a. intercostalis dorsalis VIII
aorta thoracica
t. vagalis X dorsalis
oesophagus
t. vagalis X ventralis
v. phrenica cranialis
v. cava caudalis
n. phrenicus
liver, left lateral lobe
diaphragm, cupola
descending colon
spleen
convergent hair vortex of stifle fold
greater omentum
ascending colon:
left dorsal colon
left ventral colon
pelvic flexure
stomach, greater curvature

Fig. 5.49 The abdomen in early pregnancy (4): superficial left lateral view. The spleen extends rather more caudally than usual but this was also the case in the specimen shown in Fig. 5.13. The pelvic flexure of the ascending colonic loop lies more ventral and cranial than usual; this may be due to the enlargement of the pregnant uterus (see Fig. 5.51). Figs. 5.49–5.51 show the left abdominal topography in this mare.

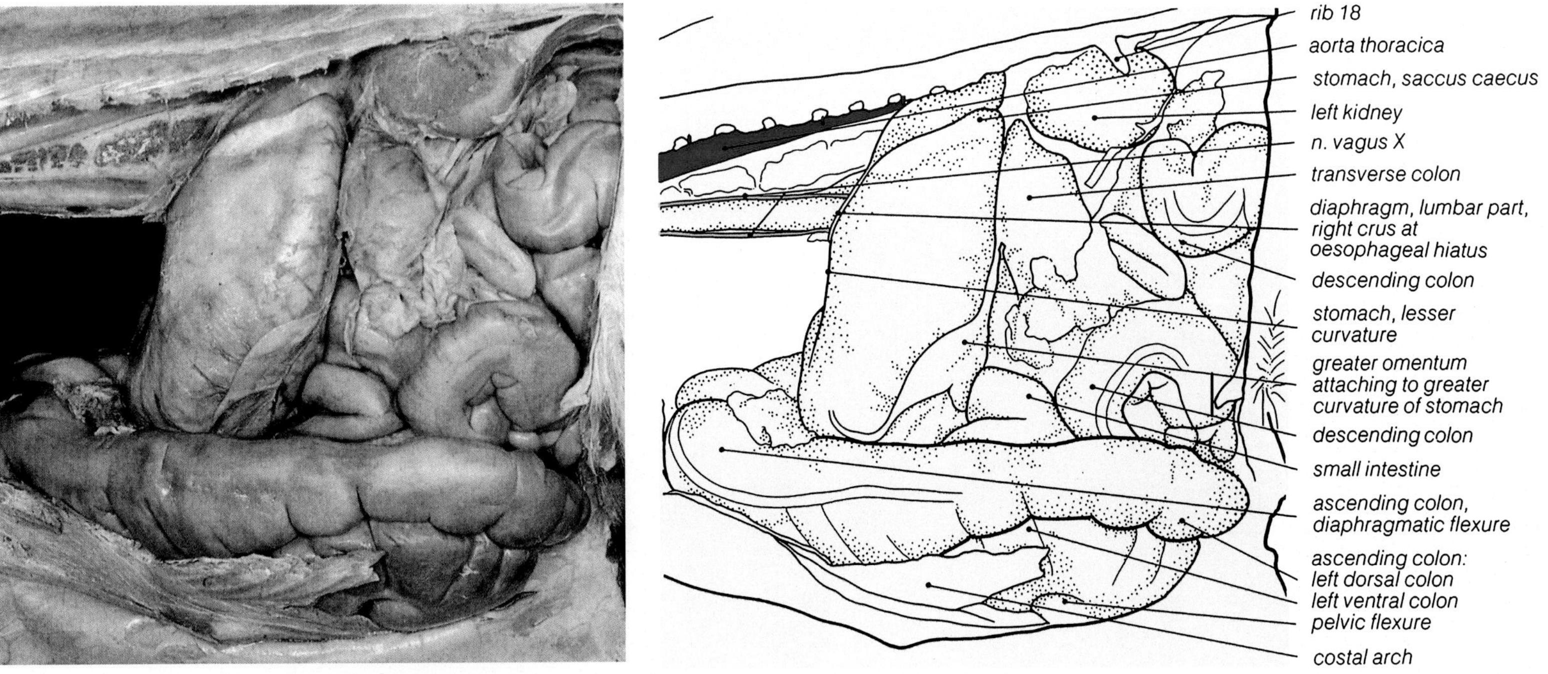
rib 18
aorta thoracica
stomach, saccus caecus
left kidney
n. vagus X
transverse colon
diaphragm, lumbar part, right crus at oesophageal hiatus
descending colon
stomach, lesser curvature
greater omentum attaching to greater curvature of stomach
descending colon
small intestine
ascending colon, diaphragmatic flexure
ascending colon: left dorsal colon
left ventral colon
pelvic flexure
costal arch

Fig. 5.50 The abdomen in early pregnancy (5), after removal of the spleen: left lateral view. The spleen develops in the dorsal mesogastrium and its removal necessitates removal of part of the greater omentum. The caudal vena cava has also been removed.

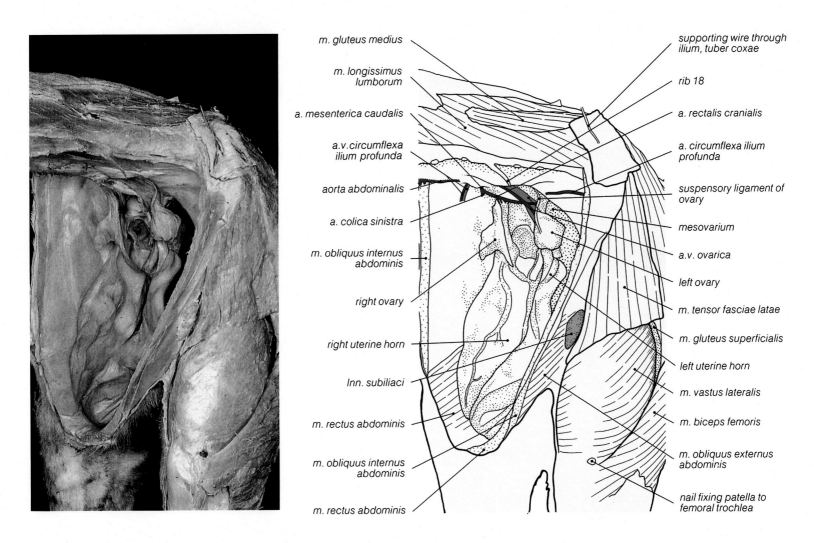

m. gluteus medius
m. longissimus lumborum
a. mesenterica caudalis
a.v. circumflexa ilium profunda
aorta abdominalis
a. colica sinistra
m. obliquus internus abdominis
right ovary
right uterine horn
lnn. subiliaci
m. rectus abdominis
m. obliquus internus abdominis
m. rectus abdominis
supporting wire through ilium, tuber coxae
rib 18
a. rectalis cranialis
a. circumflexa ilium profunda
suspensory ligament of ovary
mesovarium
a.v. ovarica
left ovary
m. tensor fasciae latae
m. gluteus superficialis
left uterine horn
m. vastus lateralis
m. biceps femoris
m. obliquus externus abdominis
nail fixing patella to femoral trochlea

Fig. 5.51 The abdomen in early pregnancy (6): ovaries and uterus in left craniolateral view. The right craniolateral view of this specimen is shown in Fig. 5.48.

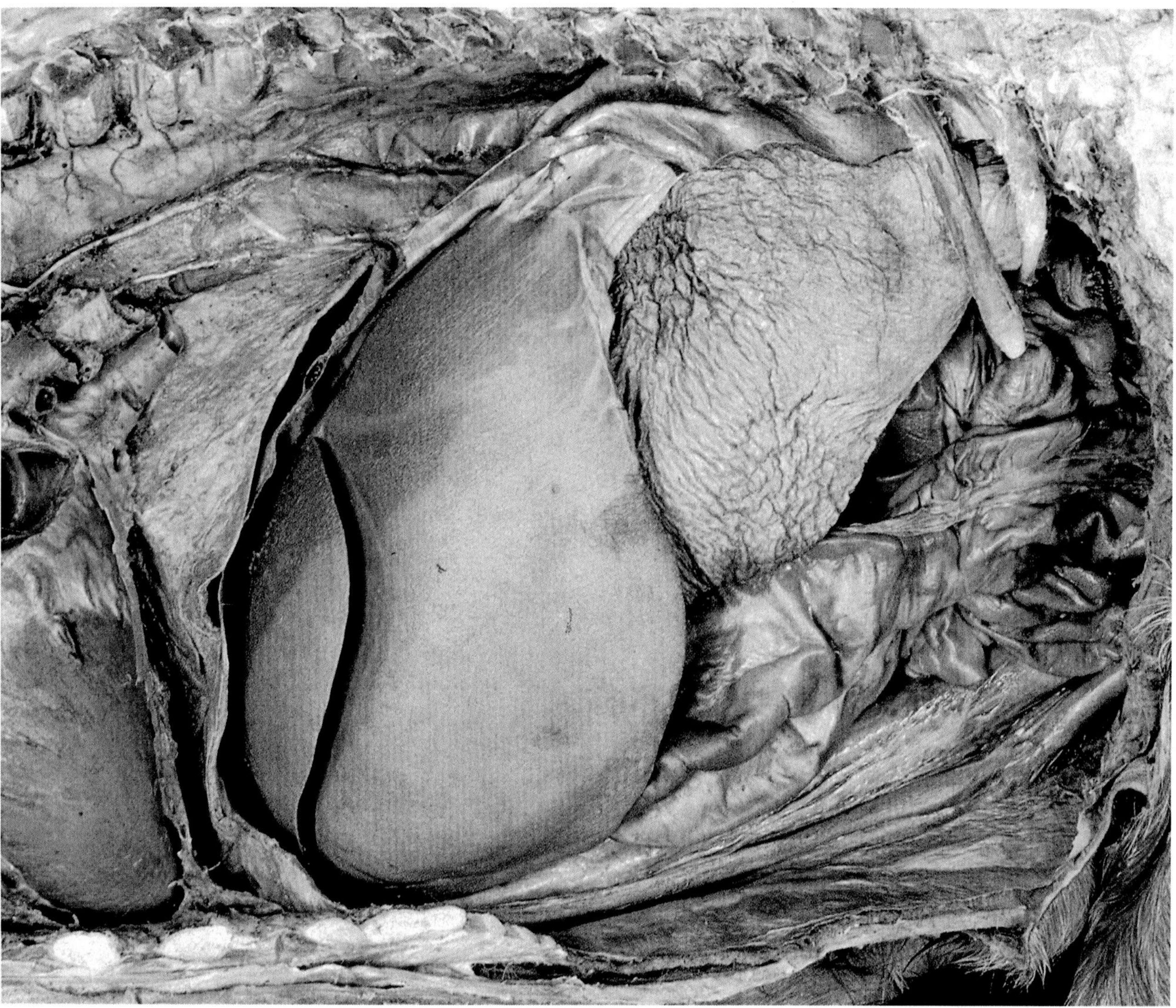

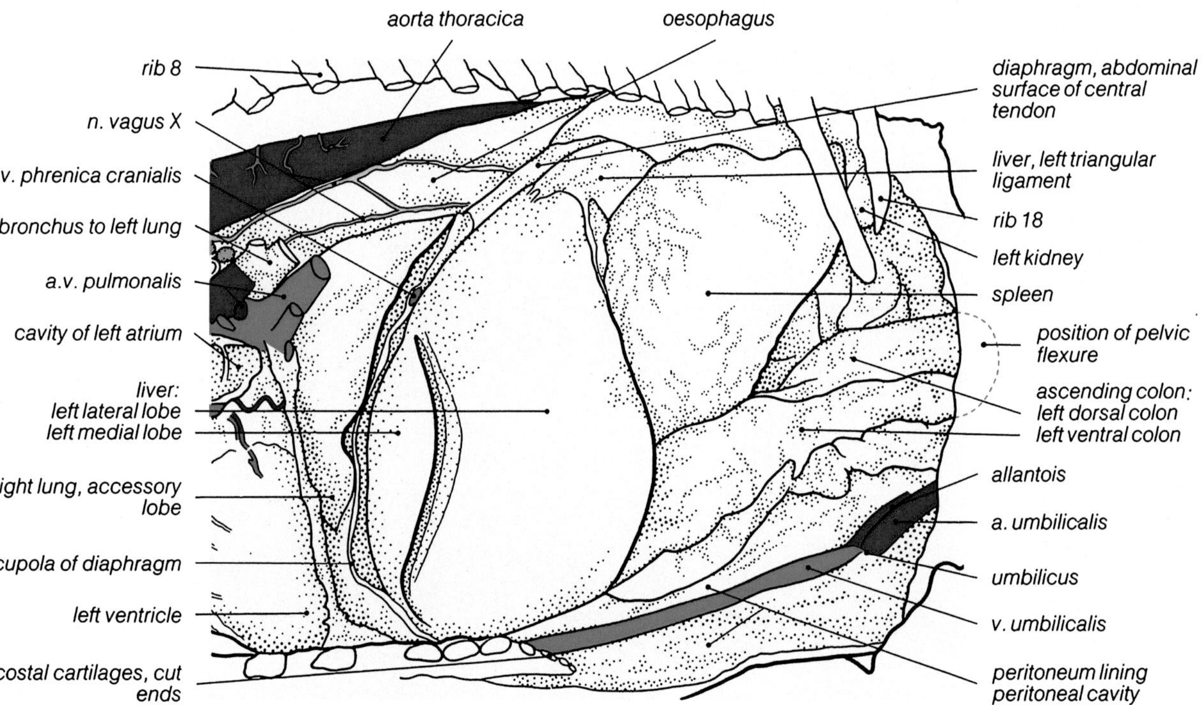
aorta thoracica
oesophagus
rib 8
n. vagus X
v. phrenica cranialis
bronchus to left lung
a.v. pulmonalis
cavity of left atrium
liver:
left lateral lobe
left medial lobe
right lung, accessory lobe
cupola of diaphragm
left ventricle
costal cartilages, cut ends
diaphragm, abdominal surface of central tendon
liver, left triangular ligament
rib 18
left kidney
spleen
position of pelvic flexure
ascending colon:
left dorsal colon
left ventral colon
allantois
a. umbilicalis
umbilicus
v. umbilicalis
peritoneum lining peritoneal cavity

Fig. 5.52 Abdominal viscera of the new-born foal: left lateral view. The colon has not been inflated. Compare the relative size and topographical position of the liver in this foal with that of the adult horse (Figs. 5.14, 5.43 and 5.49).

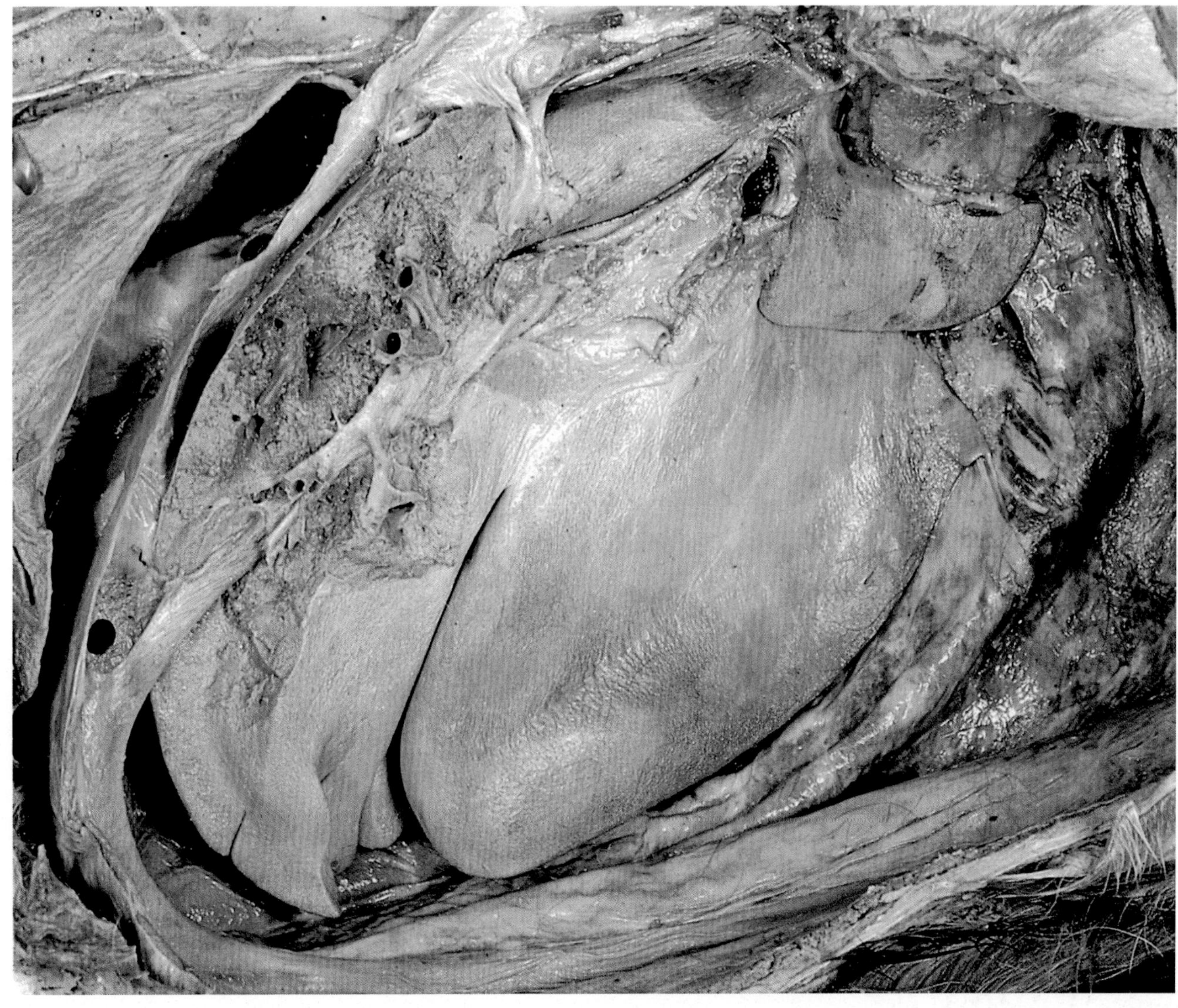

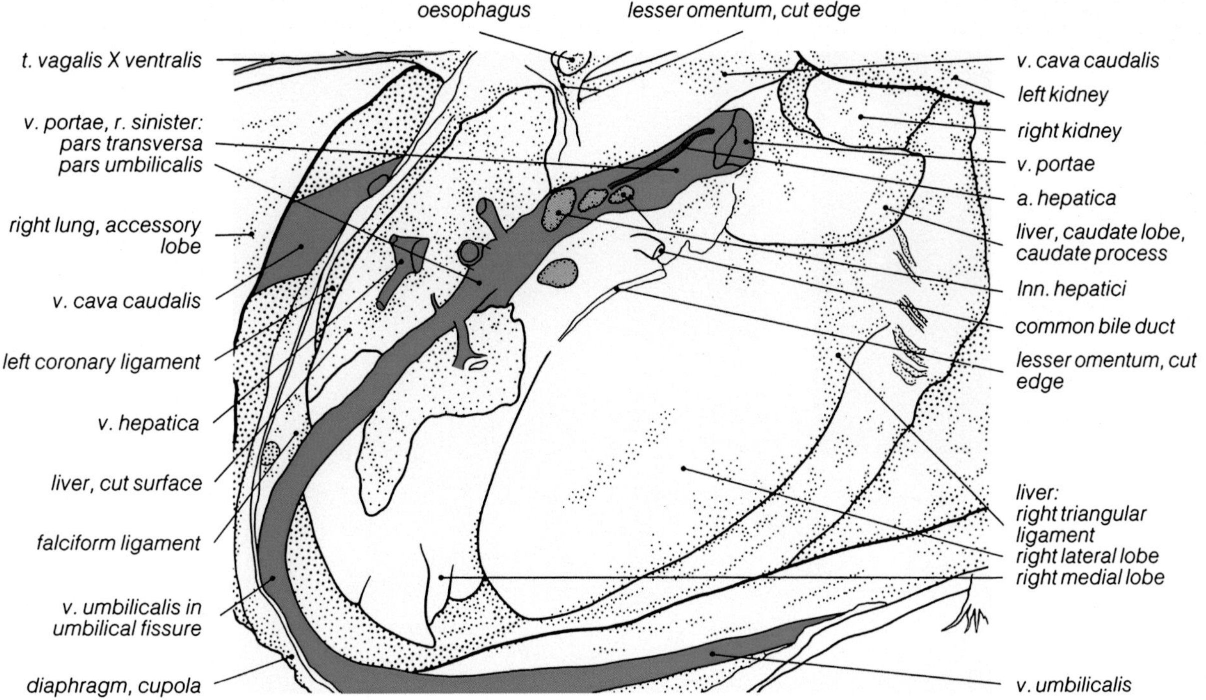
oesophagus
lesser omentum, cut edge
t. vagalis X ventralis
v. portae, r. sinister:
pars transversa
pars umbilicalis
right lung, accessory lobe
v. cava caudalis
left coronary ligament
v. hepatica
liver, cut surface
falciform ligament
v. umbilicalis in umbilical fissure
diaphragm, cupola
v. cava caudalis
left kidney
right kidney
v. portae
a. hepatica
liver, caudate lobe, caudate process
lnn. hepatici
common bile duct
lesser omentum, cut edge
liver:
right triangular ligament
right lateral lobe
right medial lobe
v. umbilicalis

Fig. 5.53 The portal and umbilical veins of the new-born foal: left lateral view. The stomach and intestine have been removed. The left lobe of the liver has been excised to expose the visceral surface of the right and caudate lobes. In the late fetal foal there is no clearly defined anatomical connection between the umbilical vein and the caudal vena cava; the 'ductus venosus' is absent. The umbilical vein, as in other mammals, drains into the left branch of the portal vein. Because there is no gall bladder in the horse, the term 'quadrate lobe' has been avoided; the lobe to the right of the umbilical vein has been considered as the right medial liver lobe, in conformity with zoological mammalian nomenclature.

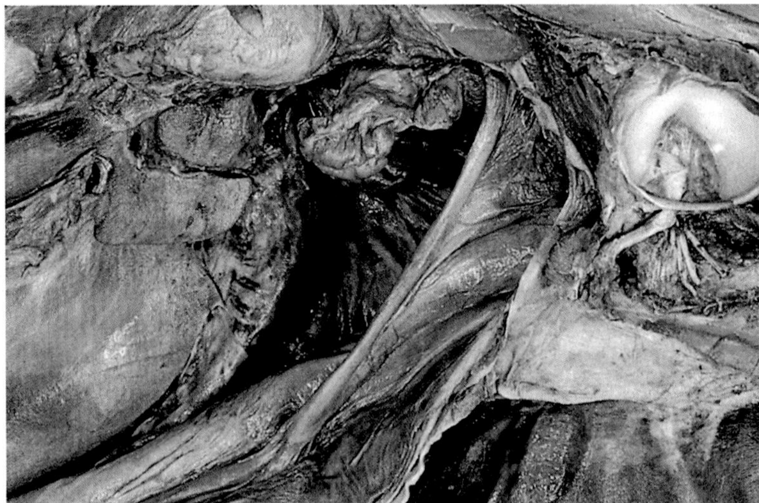

Fig. 5.54 The caudal abdomen of the new-born female foal: left lateral view. This is a more caudal view of the specimen at the stage of dissection shown in Fig. 5.53.

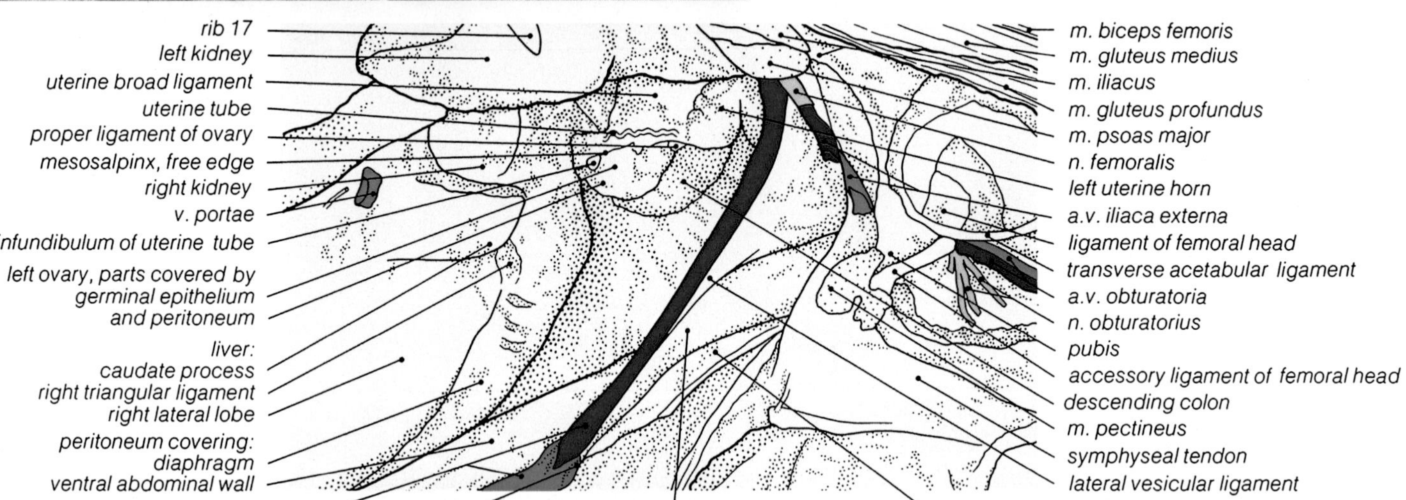
rib 17
left kidney
uterine broad ligament
uterine tube
proper ligament of ovary
mesosalpinx, free edge
right kidney
v. portae
infundibulum of uterine tube
left ovary, parts covered by germinal epithelium and peritoneum
liver:
caudate process
right triangular ligament
right lateral lobe
peritoneum covering:
diaphragm
ventral abdominal wall
a.v. umbilicalis
umbilicus
allantoic urinary bladder
median vesicular ligament
m. biceps femoris
m. gluteus medius
m. iliacus
m. gluteus profundus
m. psoas major
n. femoralis
left uterine horn
a.v. iliaca externa
ligament of femoral head
transverse acetabular ligament
a.v. obturatoria
n. obturatorius
pubis
accessory ligament of femoral head
descending colon
m. pectineus
symphyseal tendon
lateral vesicular ligament

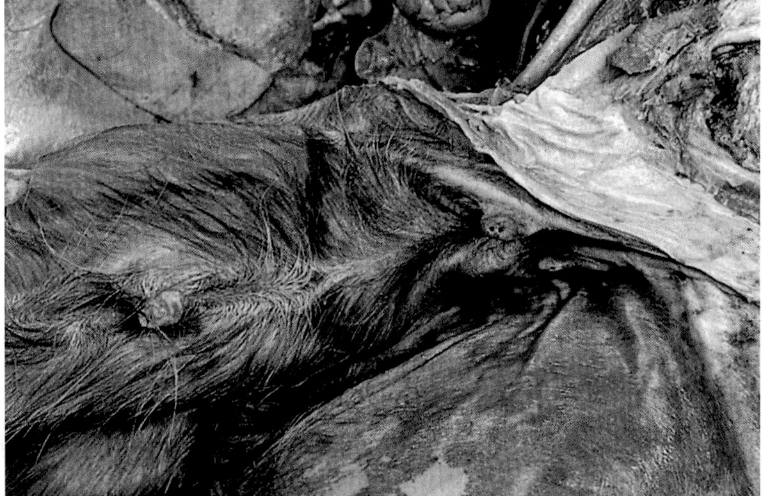

Fig. 5.55 Umbilicus and mammary glands of the new-born foal: ventral view. Part of the left side of the abdominal wall has been removed, as shown in Figs. 5.52–5.54. This figure is a ventral view of the specimen at the stage of dissection shown in Fig. 5.54.

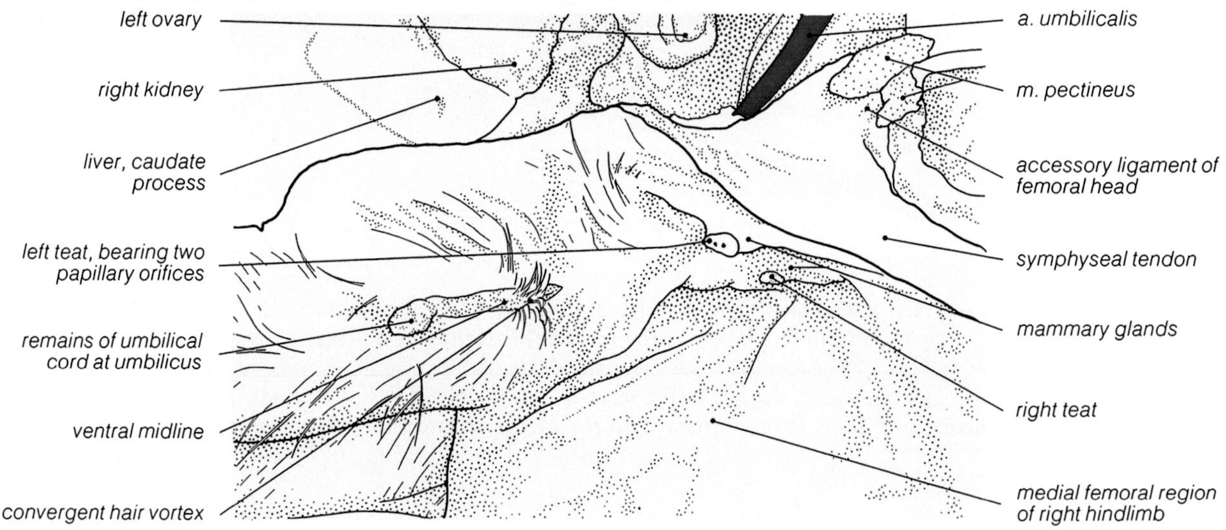
left ovary
right kidney
liver, caudate process
left teat, bearing two papillary orifices
remains of umbilical cord at umbilicus
ventral midline
convergent hair vortex
a. umbilicalis
m. pectineus
accessory ligament of femoral head
symphyseal tendon
mammary glands
right teat
medial femoral region of right hindlimb

6. THE HINDLIMB

Clinical importance of the hindlimb

The hindlimb can be examined clinically by radiography, by ultrasonography and MRI scanning, and by nerve blocks and anaesthesia of the joints. The major difference between the fore and hind limbs is that in the hindlimb the foot is not the major source of clinical lameness. Also, examination of a hindlimb has many more safety implications than examination of a forelimb. In foals and young horses, trauma and genetics in any combination are the major contributors to lameness problems.

'Epiphyseal fusion times' are not always a true indicator of growth plate closures. There are breed variations – generally the growth plates close earlier in the lighter breeds than the heavier breeds. In general, distal growth plates heal earlier than proximal ones. For the femur, the proximal growth plate fuses at 24–36 months and the distal at 24–30 months. For the tibia the corresponding values are 24–30 months and 17–24 months. The lateral malleolus of the tibia has a separate ossification centre, which is shown embryonically to be the distal epiphysis of the fibula. The separate ossification centre for the tibial tuberosity fuses to the epiphysis at 9–12 months of age and to the metaphysis at 30–36 months. The proximal end of the fibula ossifies soon after birth. Two or three separate ossification centres in the fibrous shaft may remain separate for many years. The proximal growth plate of metacarpal bone III is fused at birth and the distal plate fuses at 9–12 months. In foals, the most rapid growth period is from birth to 10 weeks. The activity of the growth plate determines bone length and, to some extent, bone shape. Abnormalities of endochondral ossification may affect bone length and also the axial alignment of the ends of the bones and the shapes of the joints. These effects are visible in the foal.

The hock has six tarsal bones – tibial (talus) and fibular (calcaneus), central, and tarsal bones I, II (fused) and III, IV. The epiphysis of the fibular tarsal bone is evident by 2 weeks and fuses between 24–36 months. Intra-articular fractures of the tarsus are not so common as in the carpus, because the hind limb is not so often involved in trauma.

The hip joint is one of the 'high motion' joints of the horse, all of these have large synovial spaces which can be entered with a needle. Therefore, anaesthesia of the joint can be used for diagnostic purposes, antibiotics and anti-inflammatory drugs can be administered, and samples can be taken for culture or cytology. The 'low motion' joints, for example the tarsus, have small synovial spaces and are bounded by a wealth of collagenous ligaments, tendons and joint capsules. They are therefore much less accessible clinically. Intra-articular analgesia of the coxo-femoral (hip) joint may be used as a diagnostic test. To reach the hip joint, which is not easily palpated because of the massive gluteal muscles, a needle is inserted between the cranial and caudal processes of the greater trochanter of the femur. The needle is directed in a slightly cranial, medial and distal direction to reach the joint. Coxo-femoral luxation does occur, but rarely, and attempts to reduce the dislocation are usually unsuccessful as it is difficult to keep the femoral head in place. Osteoarthritis of the hip joint is rare.

Fractures of the femur are relatively rare and little can be done to repair them. Fracture of the tibia is more common and requires 'Robert Jones type' fixation.

The stifle joint is the most common site of pathological problems in the hindlimb. Osteoarthritis is quite common in this joint. The femoral articular cartilage may be 3–4 cm thick and is the thickest in the equine joints. The medial femoral condyle is a common site for bone cysts. Patellar fracture does occur rarely and is usually the result of direct trauma, usually from a kick. *Osteochondrosis dissecans* is also fairly common in the stifle joint. The stifle joint relies on the particular anatomy of the femur for fixation in extension. The medial ridge of the femoral trochlea can act as a 'catch' for the patellar fibrocartilage and the medial patellar ligament, enabling the joint to be locked in extension. One of the most common injuries of the stifle is upward fixation of the patella, diagnosed by palpation and radiography. In this condition the patella does not spontaneously unlock when attempts are made to flex the joint. Problems may also occur when the lateral femoral trochlear ridge is hypoplastic and there is no ridge to hook over the patellar ligaments. It is often congenital and in that case it is often bilateral. The femoro-patellar joint communicates with the medial femoro-tibial joint and, in 25% of horses, also with the lateral femoro-tibial joint. In the other 75% of horses the lateral femoro-tibial joint is separate. The two synovial cavities of the femoro-tibial joint do not directly communicate with each other. The seat of lameness can be detected by anaesthesia of these synovial cavities. The femoro-patellar joint is approached for intra-articular analgesia by inserting a needle proximal to the tibial crest, lateral or medial to the middle patellar ligament, with the needle directed slightly proximal. The medial femoro-tibial joint is approached proximal to the tibia, with the needle inserted between the medial patellar ligament and the medial collateral ligaments. The lateral femoro-tibial joint is approached proximal to the tibia, with the needle inserted caudal to the long digital extensor tendon and cranial to the lateral collateral ligament. The femoro-tibial joint is the site of a wide variety of stifle injuries including those to the menisci, the articular cartilage, the collateral ligaments and the cruciate ligaments (commonly caused by twisting of the stifle). All of these can be investigated by arthroscopy under general anaesthesia.

There are four synovial sacs in the hock. The first is in the tarso-crural joint. The second is in the proximal intertarsal joints (this communicates with the sac of the first joint). The third is in the distal intertarsal joints (this communicates with the sac in the tarso-metatarsal joint) and finally there is the synovial sac of the tarso-metatarsal joint. The hock can be investigated using intra-articular analgesia. The proximal joint (tarso-crural) is entered by inserting a needle either side of the saphenous vein, just distal to the medial malleolus. The distal intertarsal joint can be found on the medial aspect of the hock, just distal to the proximal border of the medial branch (cunean) of the tendon of the cranial tibial muscle. The needle is inserted in a lateral direction, horizontally, between the third and central tarsal bones. The tarso-metatarsal joint is approached via a small depression proximal to the head of the lateral splint bone (metatarsal bone IV). A needle is inserted in a horizontal and slightly downward direction to a depth of approximately 2–3 cm.

Osteoarthritis of the small hock joints does occur. 'Bog spavin' is a descriptive term for synovial effusion of the tarso-crural joint. It is the result of a low-grade synovitis. The swelling appears in the proximo-medial part of the hock. It is not a major cause of persistent hindlimb lameness in the horse. *Osteochondrosis dissecans,* a degenerative condition of cartilage, also affects the hock, particularly the distal intermediate ridge of the tibia and the lateral trochlear ridges of the tibio-tarsal joint. The hock joint can also suffer from bacterial infection and inflammation, similar to gonitis of the stifle joint. This often results in extensive necrosis and ultimately joint collapse. Another important condition of the hock is fluid distension of the tarso-crural joint which occurs dorso-medially between the fibularis (peroneus) tertius muscle and the medial malleolus; dorso-medially between the medial malleolus and the deep digital flexor tendon; and caudo-laterally between the lateral malleolus and the tuber calcis. Tarso-crural dislocation (luxation) is a rare event which is virtually impossible to repair and is an indication for immediate euthanasia.

A considerable amount of clinical time is spent dealing with the problems associated with the muscles and tendons of the hindlimb. Rupture of the fibularis (peroneus) tertius muscle (which runs from the extensor fossa of the distal femur to the dorso-lateral aspect of metatarsal bone III, the calcaneus and tarsal bones III, IV) occurs when there is overextension of the hock joint, usually in racing. It is important, as this tendinous muscle is part of the hindlimb stay apparatus, which enables the hock and stifle to flex or extend in unison. 'Capped hock' is distension of the subcutaneous bursa overlying the superficial digital flexor tendon (SDFT) at the point of the hock. It is usually only of cosmetic significance. It results from trauma. 'Deep capped hock' is damage to the large synovial bursa underneath the tendon, resulting in swelling on both sides of the tendon. Traumatic injury to the semitendinosus muscle results in scarring with adhesions between the semitendinosus and semimembranosus muscles. Rupture of the gastrocnemius muscle can occur and tendinitis of the muscle is also a possibility. The muscles of the hindlimb that are injured most often are the major flexor muscles together with their tendon sheaths and suspensory ligaments. The SDFT is easily damaged and may be partially dislocated (sub-luxated) when the horse is in work. Most commonly, this occurs laterally but sometimes medially. The problem is made much worse when the tendon is also split. Surgical correction of this is generally unrewarding. There is also a specific condition known by the colloquial name of 'curb' which is desmitis (inflammation) of the SDFT. It is seen clinically as a swelling on the plantar aspect of the hock, approximately 10 cm distal to the point of the hock. 'False curb' is a swelling or enlargement on the proximal aspect of the splint bones (metatarsal bones II and IV). The extensor muscles and their tendon sheaths can also be damaged, but in these cases the injuries are not so severe, and conservative treatment is usually successful. Injuries to the suspensory apparatus also occur. Lesions confined to the proximal third of the metatarsus are usually referred to as proximal suspensory desmitis. Here there is localized oedema, swelling, heat, distension of the medial palmar vein and possibly pain. The condition may be mild, moderate or severe and can become chronic. More rarely there are avulsion ('tearing') fractures of the whole tendon and complete breakdown of the tendon. Sub-tarsal analgesia and ultrasonography can be used for diagnosis.

Fluid distension of the tarsal sheath of the deep flexor tendon is known as 'thoroughpin'. It is usually caused by trauma. The sheath begins approximately 5–7 cm proximal to the level of the medial malleolus and extends distally to the upper third of the metatarsus. Swellings can be found on either side of the common calcaneal tendon and cranial to the tendon.

The femoral nerve can be damaged by penetrating wounds of the caudal flank which result in abscesses. The nerve is also damaged rarely by tumours, aneurysms, and pressure during parturition. Since it innervates the quadriceps group, which flexes the hip and extends the stifle, forward movement is limited. The cranial gluteal nerve may be damaged by trauma; if this happens atrophy of the gluteal muscles may follow. The sciatic nerve can be damaged by systemic bacterial infections such as salmonellosis, but also by infectious processes extending from the sacrum and the pelvis. Damage will affect both tibial and fibular (peroneal) nerves.

Paralysis of the tibial nerve, which innervates the extensors of the tarsus and the flexors of the digits and stifle, is not uncommon. Diagnostic blocking can be achieved by injection 10 cm proximal to the tuber calcis on the caudo-medial aspect of the limb, in the space between the deep digital flexor tendon and the common calcaneal tendon. The nerve lies beneath the superficial fascia, about 1 cm deep, and the needle should be directed just cranial to the common calcaneal tendon, with care not to penetrate the skin on the lateral aspect.

The fibular (peroneal) nerve innervates the flexors of the tarsus and the extensors of the digit. It can be blocked 10 cm proximal to the point of the hock, in a groove between the long and lateral digital extensor muscles, just above the musculo-tendinous junction. This is proximal to the lateral malleolus of the tibia, on the lateral aspect of the thigh. The deep branch of the fibular (peroneal) nerve can be blocked 2–3 cm below the superficial fascia and the superficial branch 1–2 cm below the fascia.

Below the hock, the plantar nerves can be blocked between the deep digital flexor tendon and the suspensory ligament. The plantar metatarsal nerves can be ring-blocked on the proximal metatarsus. The plantar metatarsal nerves are blocked axial to the splint bones, abaxial to the suspensory ligament, and along the plantar cortex of metatarsal bone III.

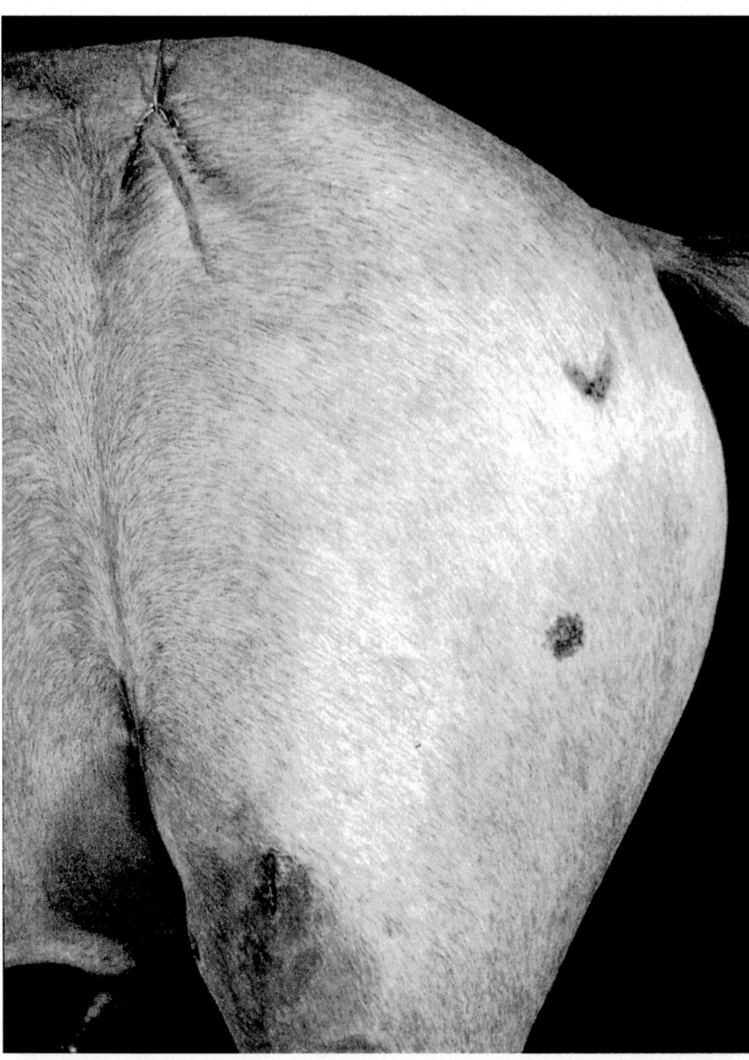

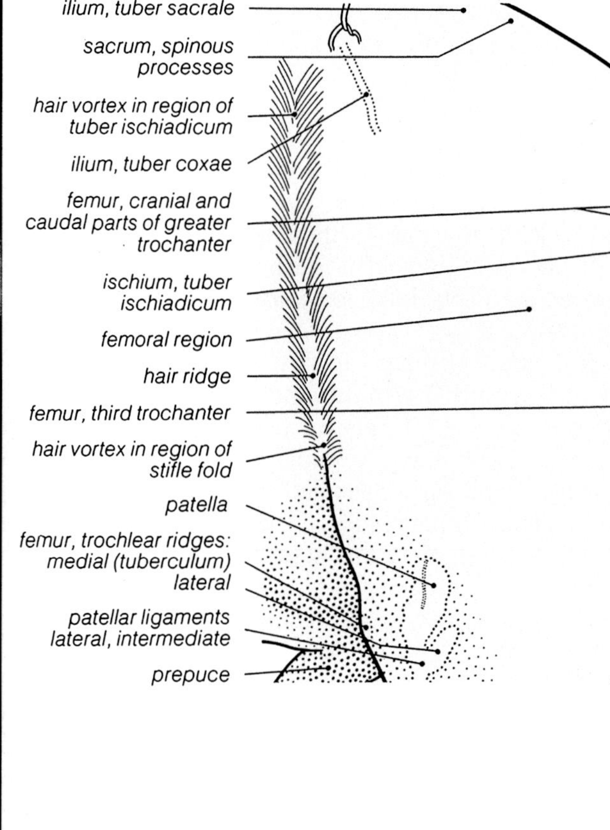
ilium, tuber sacrale
sacrum, spinous processes
hair vortex in region of tuber ischiadicum
ilium, tuber coxae
femur, cranial and caudal parts of greater trochanter
ischium, tuber ischiadicum
femoral region
hair ridge
femur, third trochanter
hair vortex in region of stifle fold
patella
femur, trochlear ridges: medial (tuberculum) lateral
patellar ligaments lateral, intermediate
prepuce

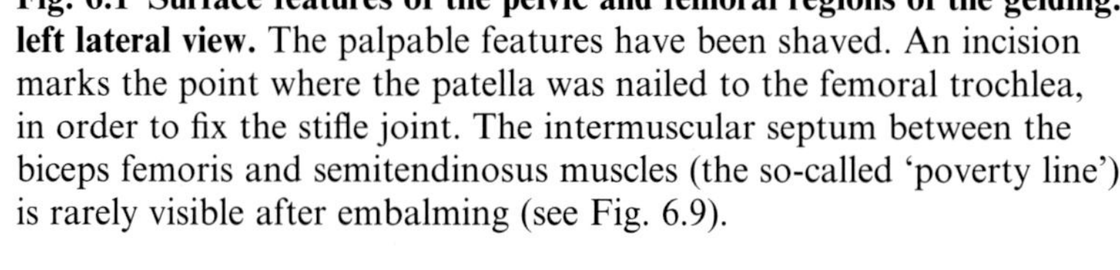
Fig. 6.1 Surface features of the pelvic and femoral regions of the gelding: left lateral view. The palpable features have been shaved. An incision marks the point where the patella was nailed to the femoral trochlea, in order to fix the stifle joint. The intermuscular septum between the biceps femoris and semitendinosus muscles (the so-called 'poverty line') is rarely visible after embalming (see Fig. 6.9).

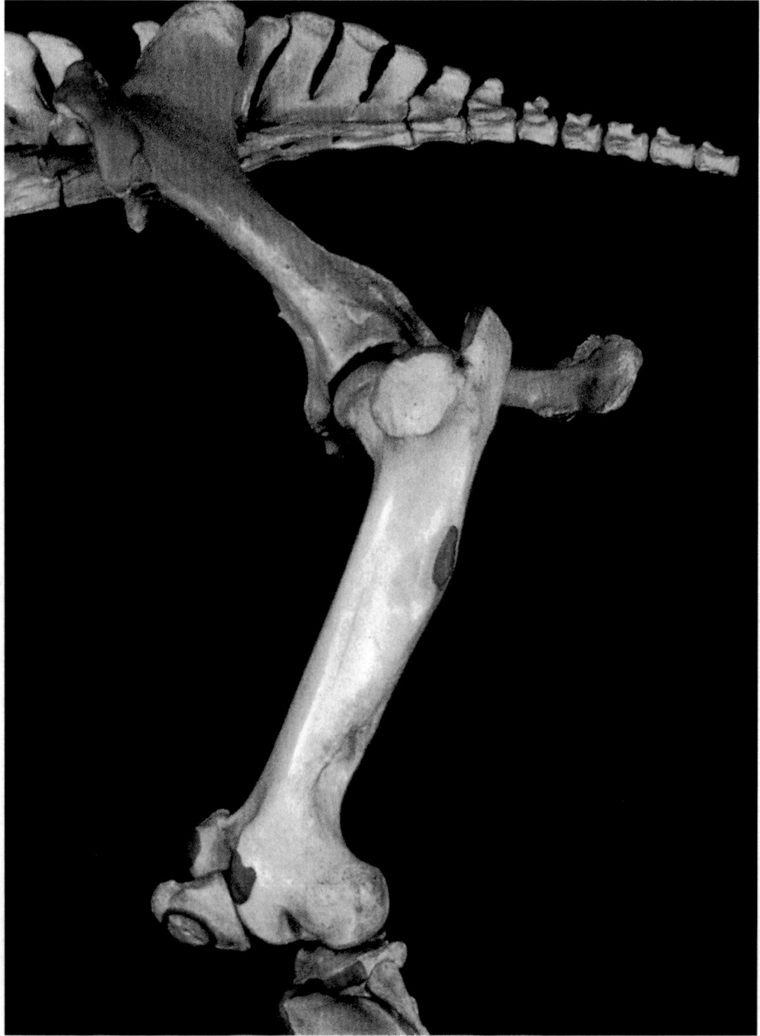

Fig. 6.2 Bones of the pelvic and femoral regions: left lateral view. The palpable bony features shown in Fig. 6.1 have been coloured red, except the tuber sacrale and the sacral spines. In this skeleton the patella has not been positioned so distally in the trochlea: in the embalmed horse the hindlimb was fully extended before nailing the patella to the trochlea.

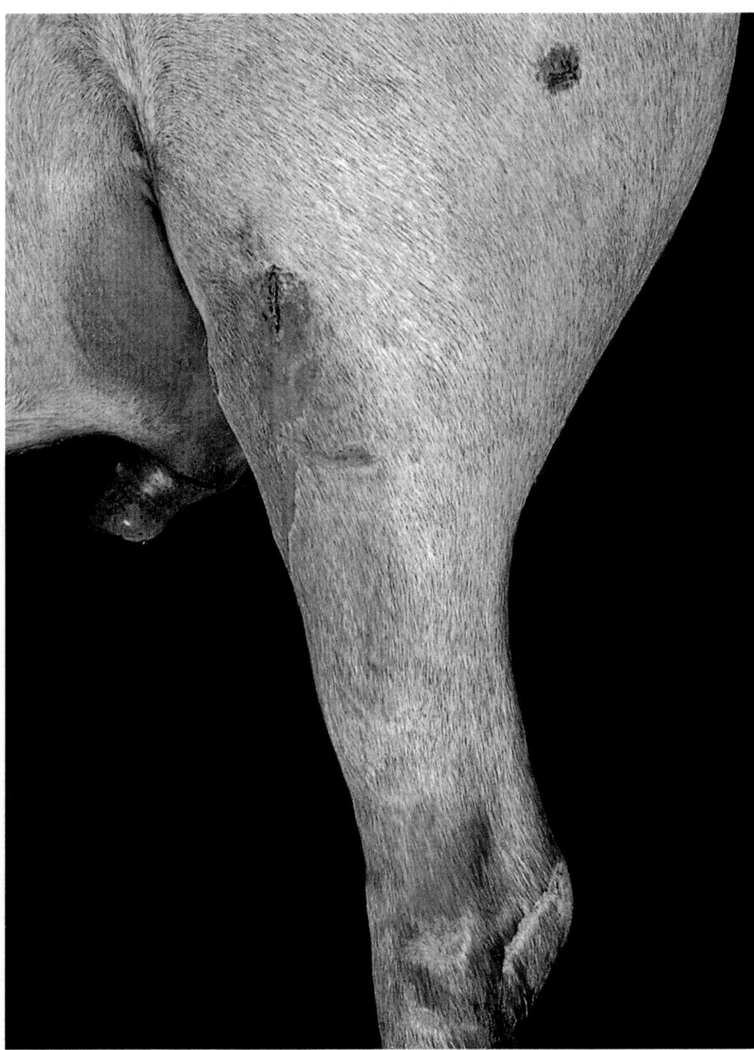

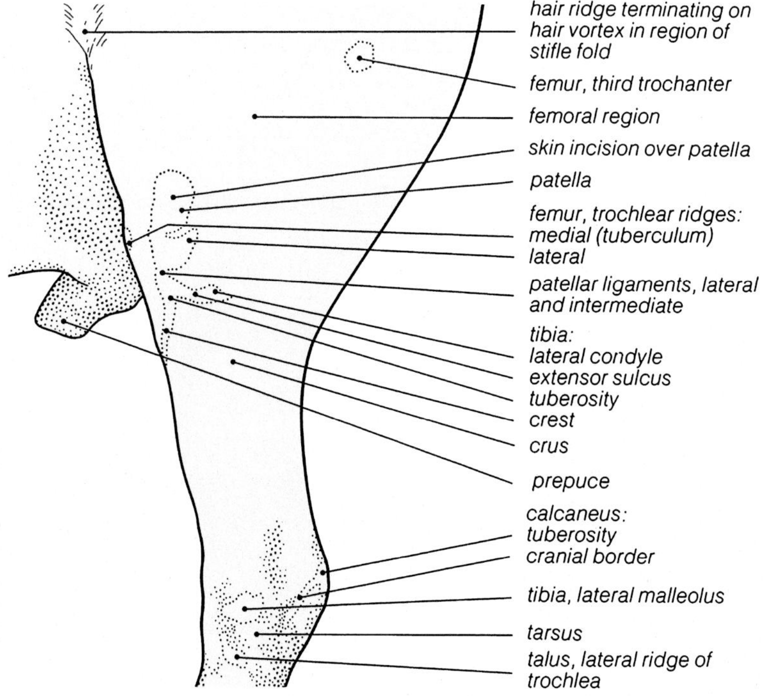
hair ridge terminating on hair vortex in region of stifle fold
femur, third trochanter
femoral region
skin incision over patella
patella
femur, trochlear ridges:
medial (tuberculum)
lateral
patellar ligaments, lateral and intermediate
tibia:
lateral condyle
extensor sulcus
tuberosity
crest
crus
prepuce
calcaneus:
tuberosity
cranial border
tibia, lateral malleolus
tarsus
talus, lateral ridge of trochlea

Fig. 6.3 Surface features of the femoral region, crus and tarsus: left lateral view. The palpable features have been shaved. The patella is also marked by the skin incision made for nailing it to the femoral trochlea.

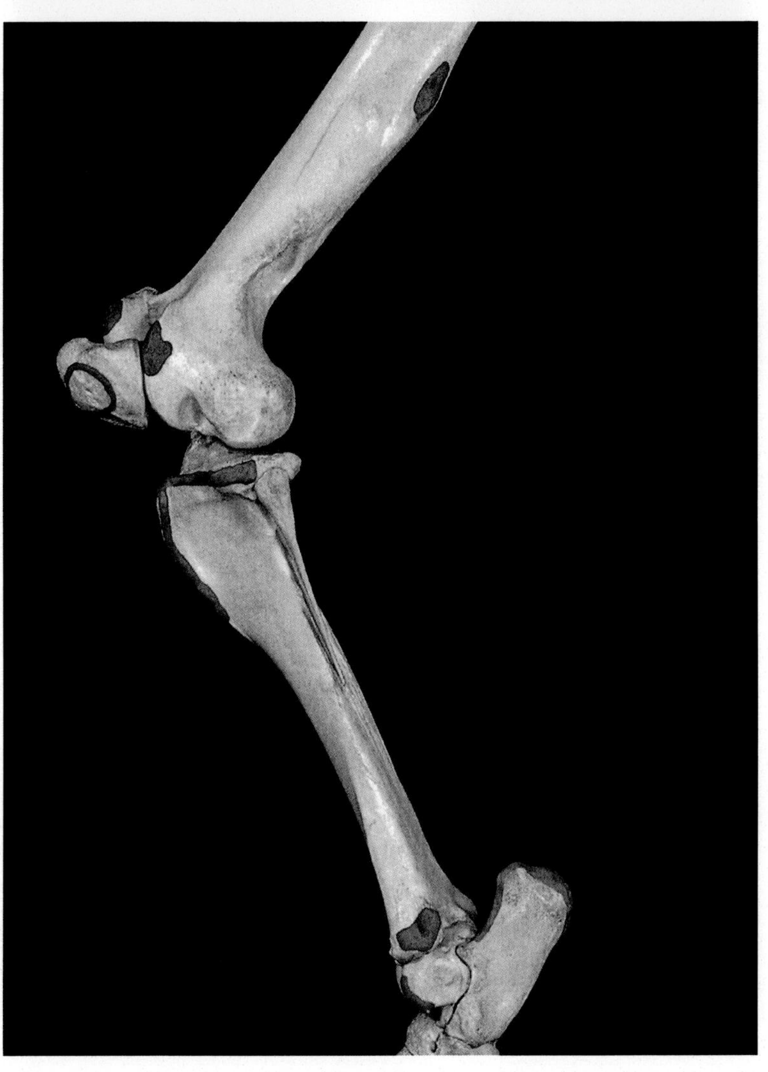

Fig. 6.4 Bones of the femoral region, crus and tarsus: left lateral view. The features shown in Fig. 6.3 have been coloured red. The bones of the pes are shown in Fig.7.36.

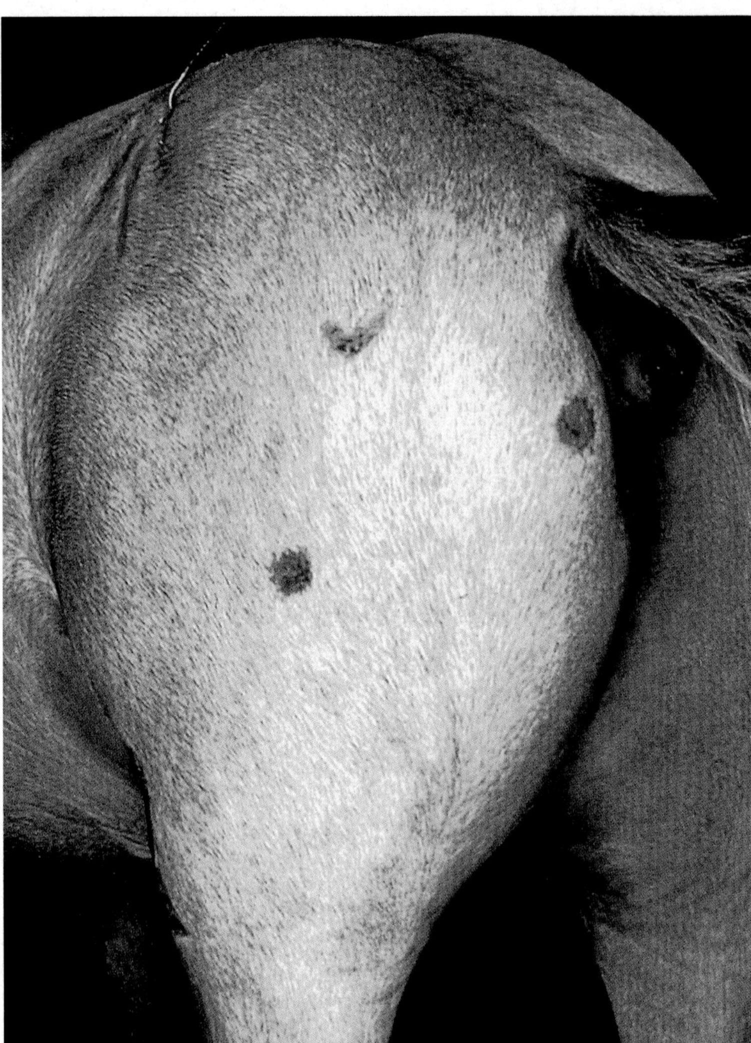

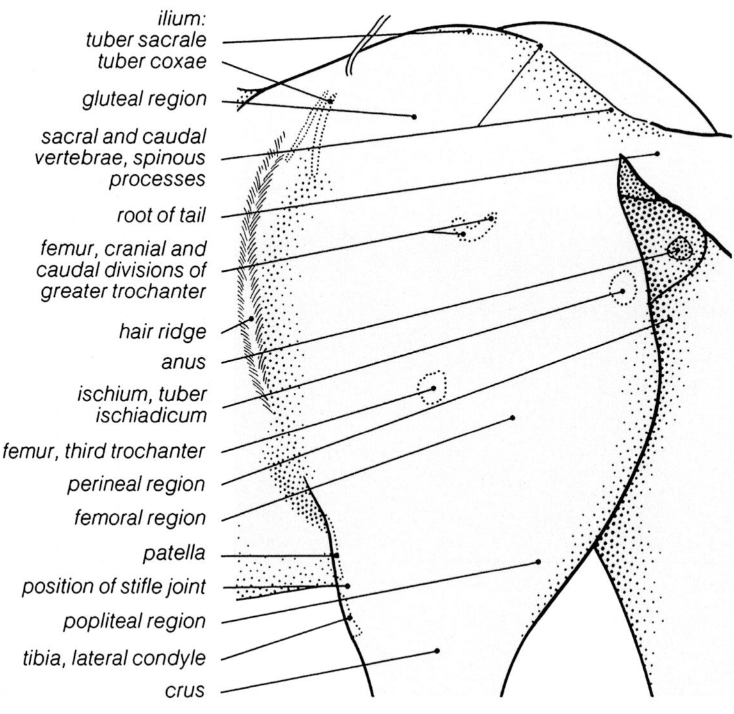
ilium:
tuber sacrale
tuber coxae
gluteal region
sacral and caudal vertebrae, spinous processes
root of tail
femur, cranial and caudal divisions of greater trochanter
hair ridge
anus
ischium, tuber ischiadicum
femur, third trochanter
perineal region
femoral region
patella
position of stifle joint
popliteal region
tibia, lateral condyle
crus

Fig. 6.5 Surface features of the pelvic and femoral regions: left caudolateral view. The palpable features have been shaved.

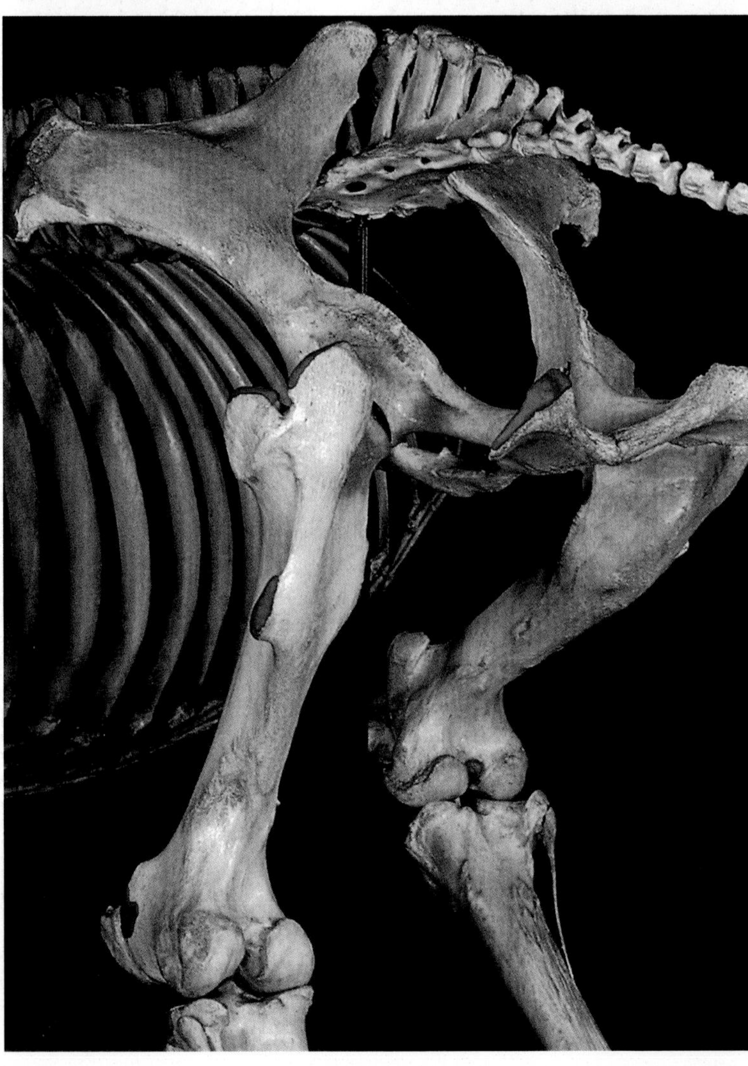

Fig. 6.6 Bones of the pelvic and femoral regions: left caudolateral view. The palpable bony features shown in Fig. 6.5 have been coloured red except for the tuber sacrale and the vertebral spinous processes.

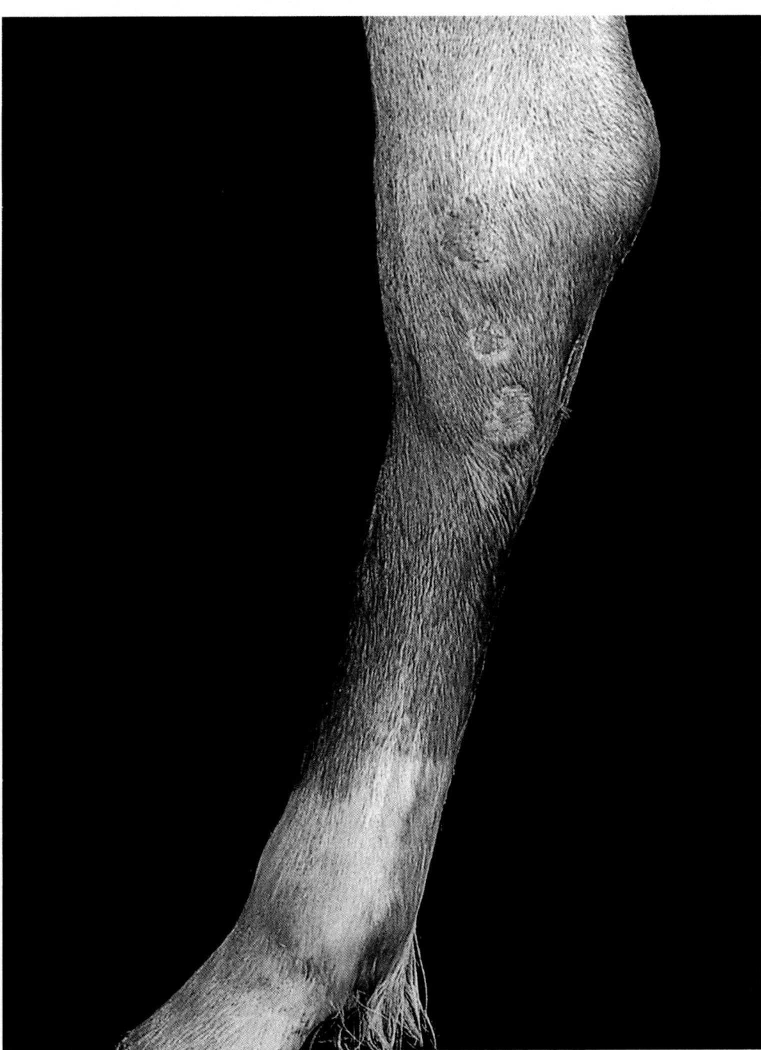

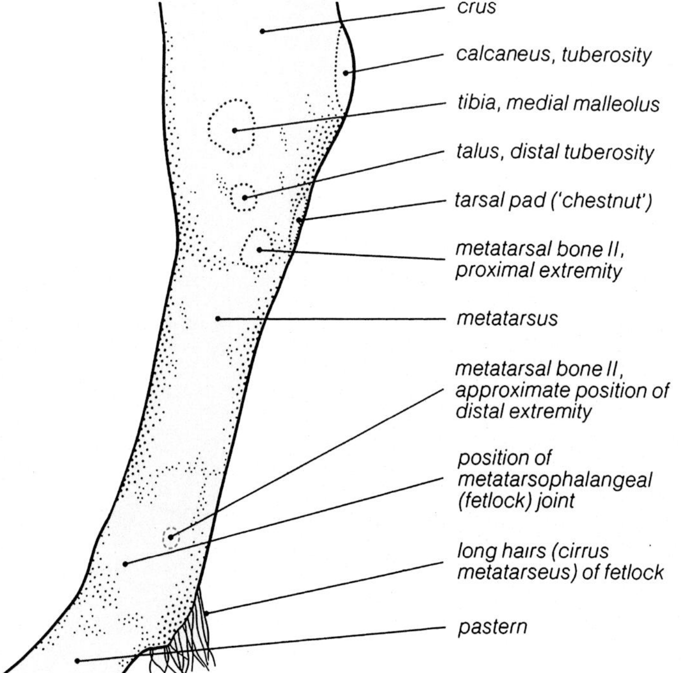
crus
calcaneus, tuberosity
tibia, medial malleolus
talus, distal tuberosity
tarsal pad ('chestnut')
metatarsal bone II, proximal extremity
metatarsus
metatarsal bone II, approximate position of distal extremity
position of metatarsophalangeal (fetlock) joint
long hairs (cirrus metatarseus) of fetlock
pastern

Fig. 6.7 Surface features of the right tarsus and metatarsus: medial view. The palpable features have been shaved. Further details of the pes are shown in Figs. 7.39 and 7.40.

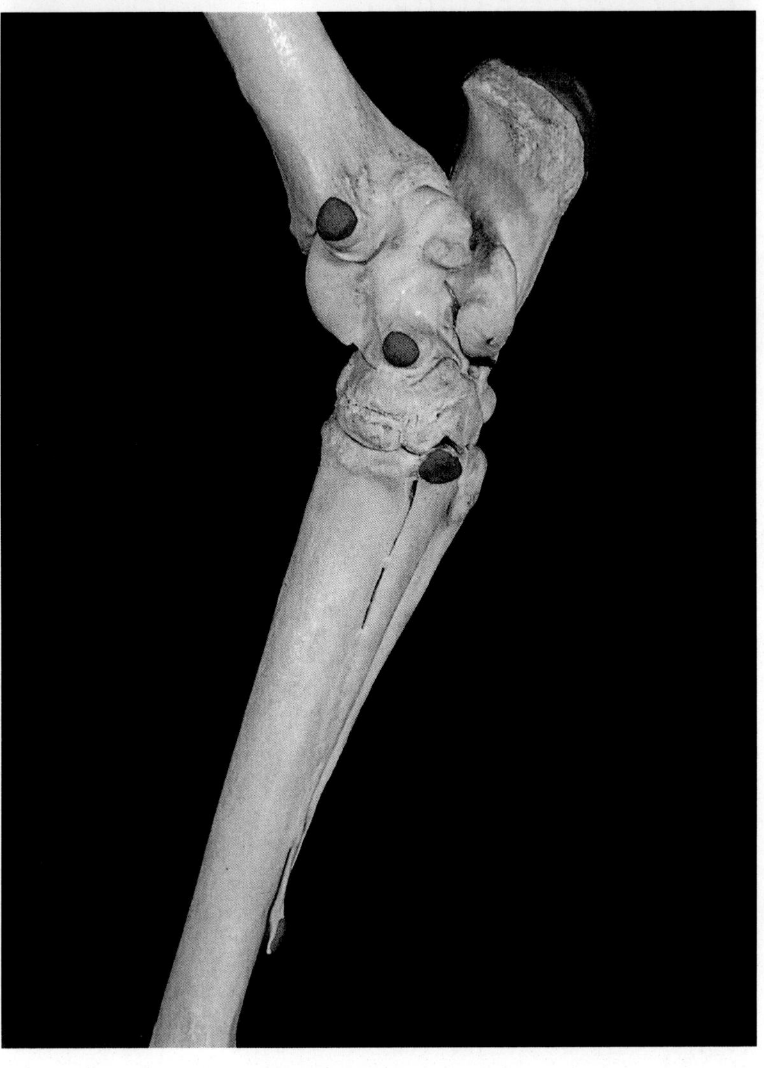

Fig. 6.8 Bones of the right tarsus and metatarsus in medial view. The palpable bony features shown in Fig. 6.7 have been coloured red. Further details of the pes are shown in Fig. 7.40.

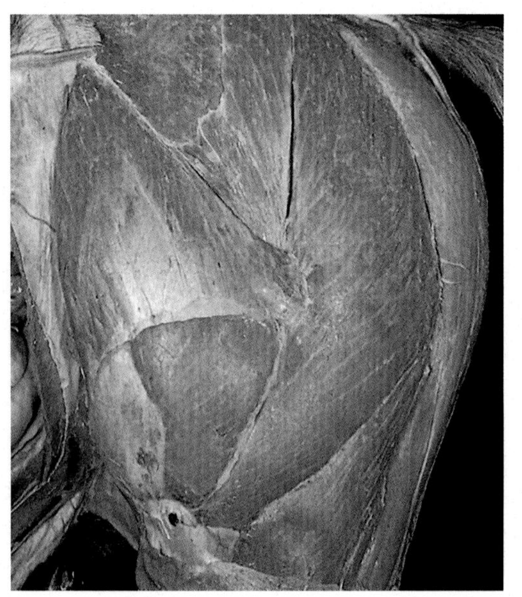

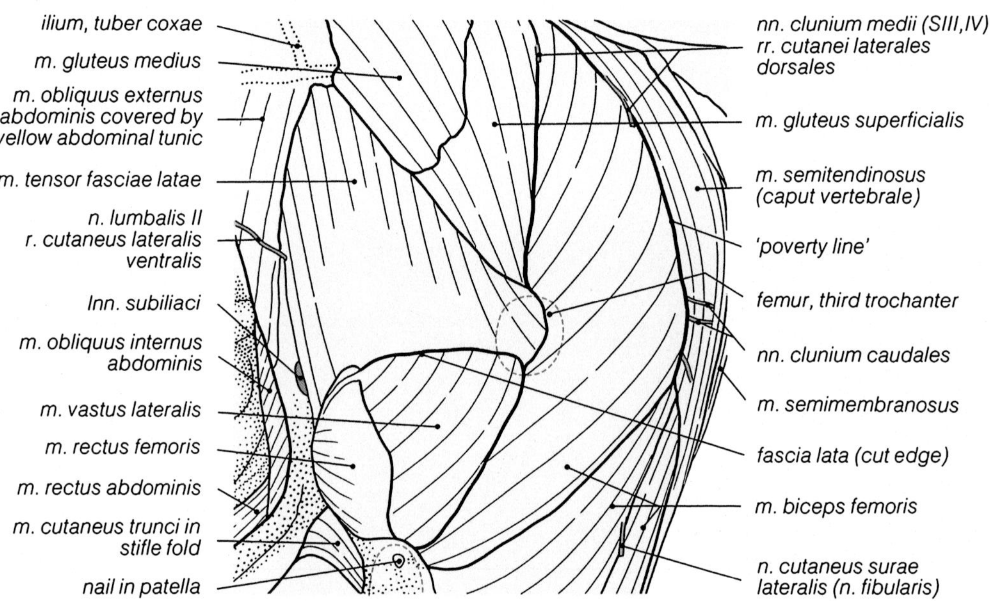
ilium, tuber coxae
m. gluteus medius
m. obliquus externus abdominis covered by yellow abdominal tunic
m. tensor fasciae latae
n. lumbalis II r. cutaneus lateralis ventralis
lnn. subiliaci
m. obliquus internus abdominis
m. vastus lateralis
m. rectus femoris
m. rectus abdominis
m. cutaneus trunci in stifle fold
nail in patella
nn. clunium medii (SIII,IV) rr. cutanei laterales dorsales
m. gluteus superficialis
m. semitendinosus (caput vertebrale)
'poverty line'
femur, third trochanter
nn. clunium caudales
m. semimembranosus
fascia lata (cut edge)
m. biceps femoris
n. cutaneus surae lateralis (n. fibularis)

Fig. 6.9 Superficial muscles of the pelvic and femoral regions: left lateral view. When cleared of connective tissue, the intermuscular groove between the biceps femoris and semitendinosus muscles ('poverty line') shows clearly. In the living animal, this groove is best seen if the horse is in a poor condition. The most dorsal and cranial part of the biceps femoris muscle may be considered to be part of the superficial gluteal muscle.

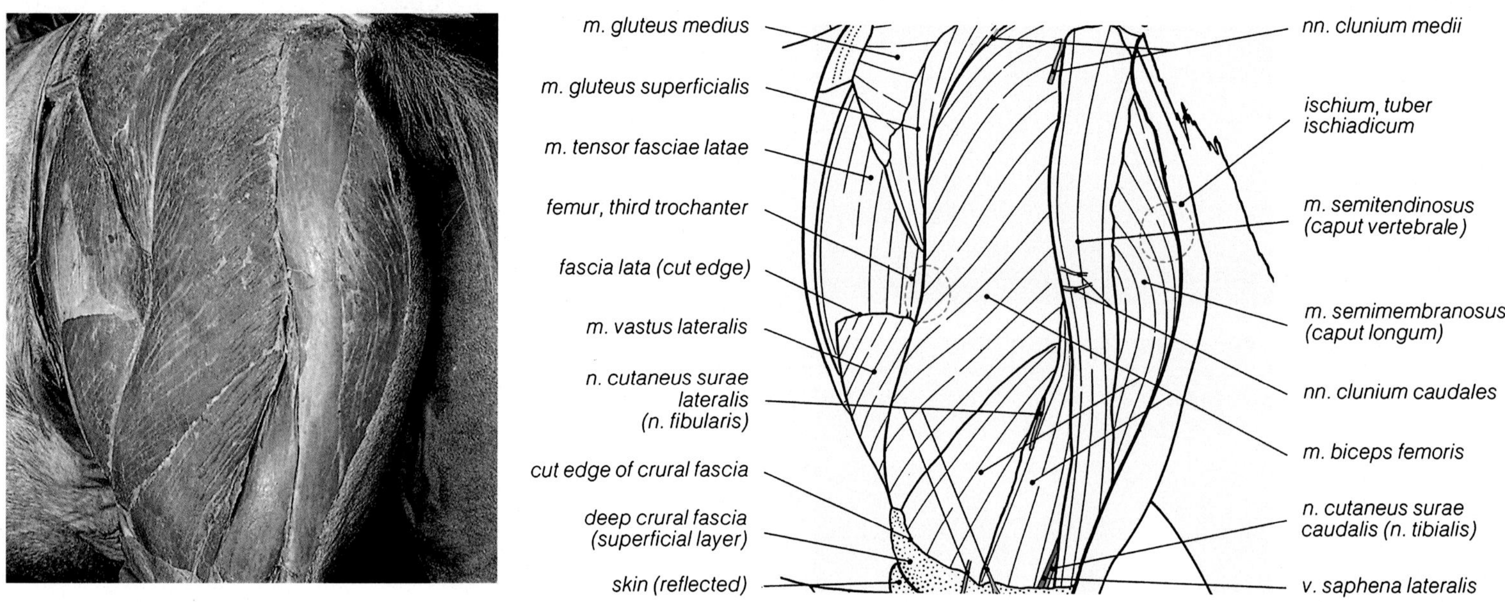
m. gluteus medius
m. gluteus superficialis
m. tensor fasciae latae
femur, third trochanter
fascia lata (cut edge)
m. vastus lateralis
n. cutaneus surae lateralis (n. fibularis)
cut edge of crural fascia
deep crural fascia (superficial layer)
skin (reflected)
nn. clunium medii
ischium, tuber ischiadicum
m. semitendinosus (caput vertebrale)
m. semimembranosus (caput longum)
nn. clunium caudales
m. biceps femoris
n. cutaneus surae caudalis (n. tibialis)
v. saphena lateralis

Fig. 6.10 Superficial muscles of the pelvic and femoral regions: right caudolateral view. In this figure and Fig. 6.9, the deep gluteal fascia and the fascia lata have been removed.

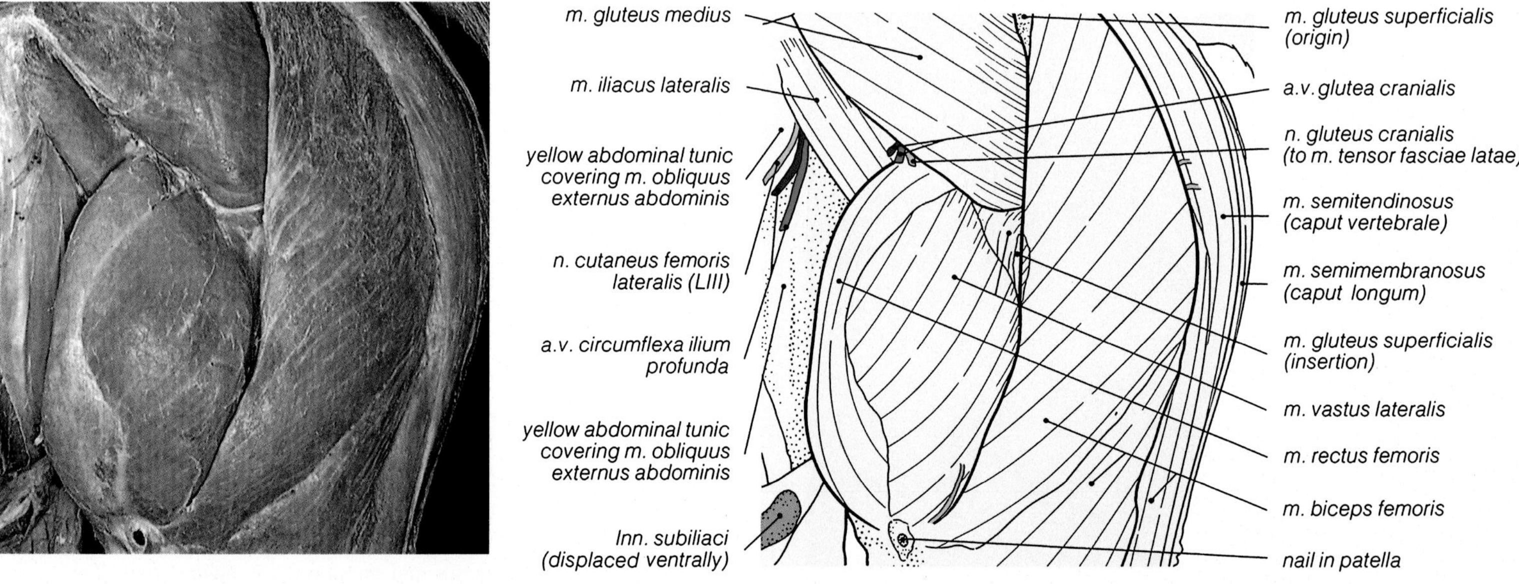
m. gluteus medius
m. iliacus lateralis
yellow abdominal tunic covering m. obliquus externus abdominis
n. cutaneus femoris lateralis (LIII)
a.v. circumflexa ilium profunda
yellow abdominal tunic covering m. obliquus externus abdominis
lnn. subiliaci (displaced ventrally)
m. gluteus superficialis (origin)
a.v. glutea cranialis
n. gluteus cranialis (to m. tensor fasciae latae)
m. semitendinosus (caput vertebrale)
m. semimembranosus (caput longum)
m. gluteus superficialis (insertion)
m. vastus lateralis
m. rectus femoris
m. biceps femoris
nail in patella

Fig. 6.11 Muscles of the pelvic and femoral regions: left lateral view. The superficial gluteal muscle and the tensor of the fascia lata have been removed.

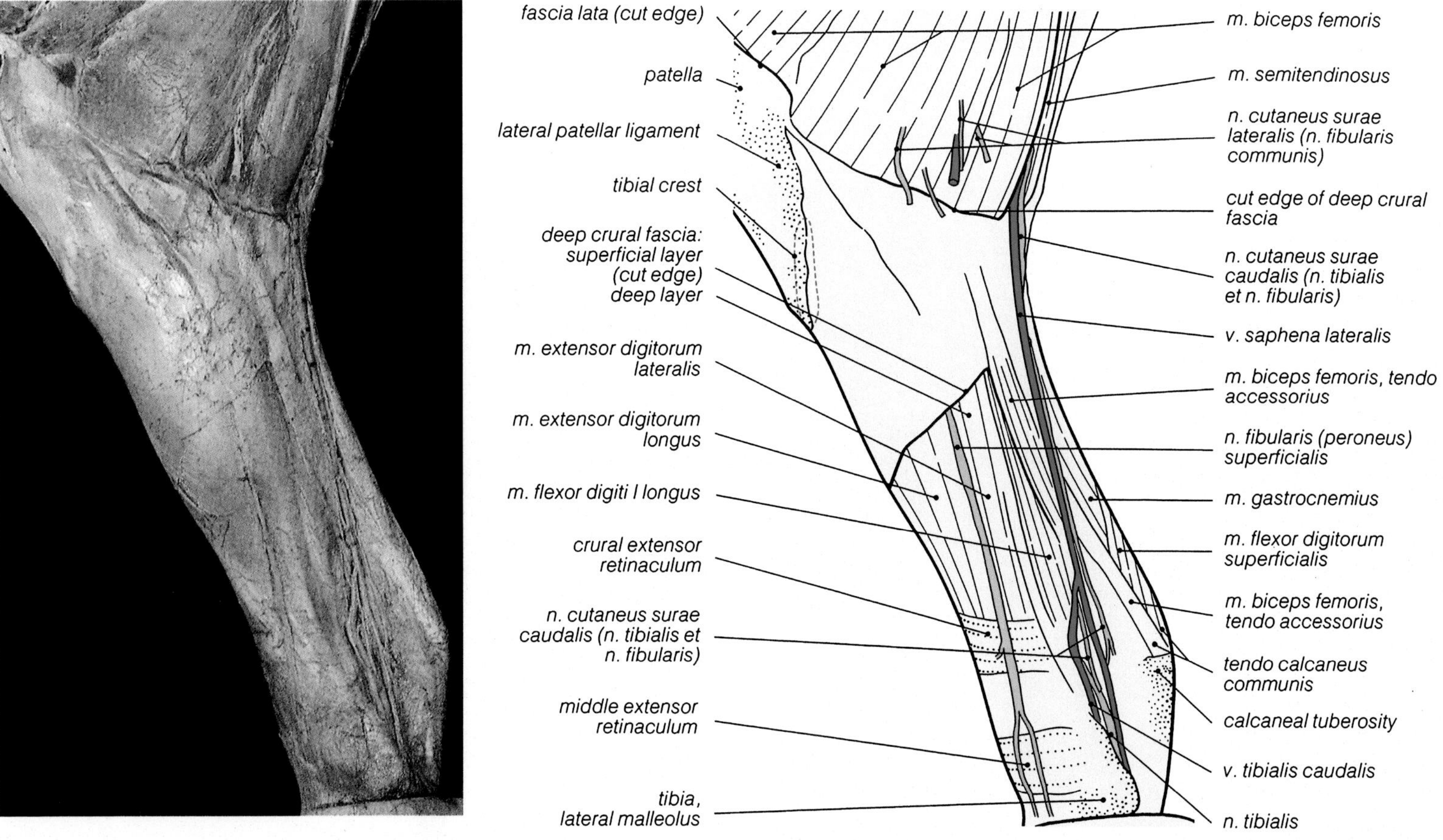
fascia lata (cut edge)
patella
lateral patellar ligament
tibial crest
deep crural fascia:
superficial layer
(cut edge)
deep layer
m. extensor digitorum lateralis
m. extensor digitorum longus
m. flexor digiti I longus
crural extensor retinaculum
n. cutaneus surae caudalis (n. tibialis et n. fibularis)
middle extensor retinaculum
tibia, lateral malleolus
m. biceps femoris
m. semitendinosus
n. cutaneus surae lateralis (n. fibularis communis)
cut edge of deep crural fascia
n. cutaneus surae caudalis (n. tibialis et n. fibularis)
v. saphena lateralis
m. biceps femoris, tendo accessorius
n. fibularis (peroneus) superficialis
m. gastrocnemius
m. flexor digitorum superficialis
m. biceps femoris, tendo accessorius
tendo calcaneus communis
calcaneal tuberosity
v. tibialis caudalis
n. tibialis

Fig. 6.12 Superficial structures of the left crus: left lateral view. Part of the most superficial layer of the deep crural fascia has been removed to display the superficial fibular (peroneal) nerve. The medial view of the region at this stage of dissection is shown in Fig. 6.13.

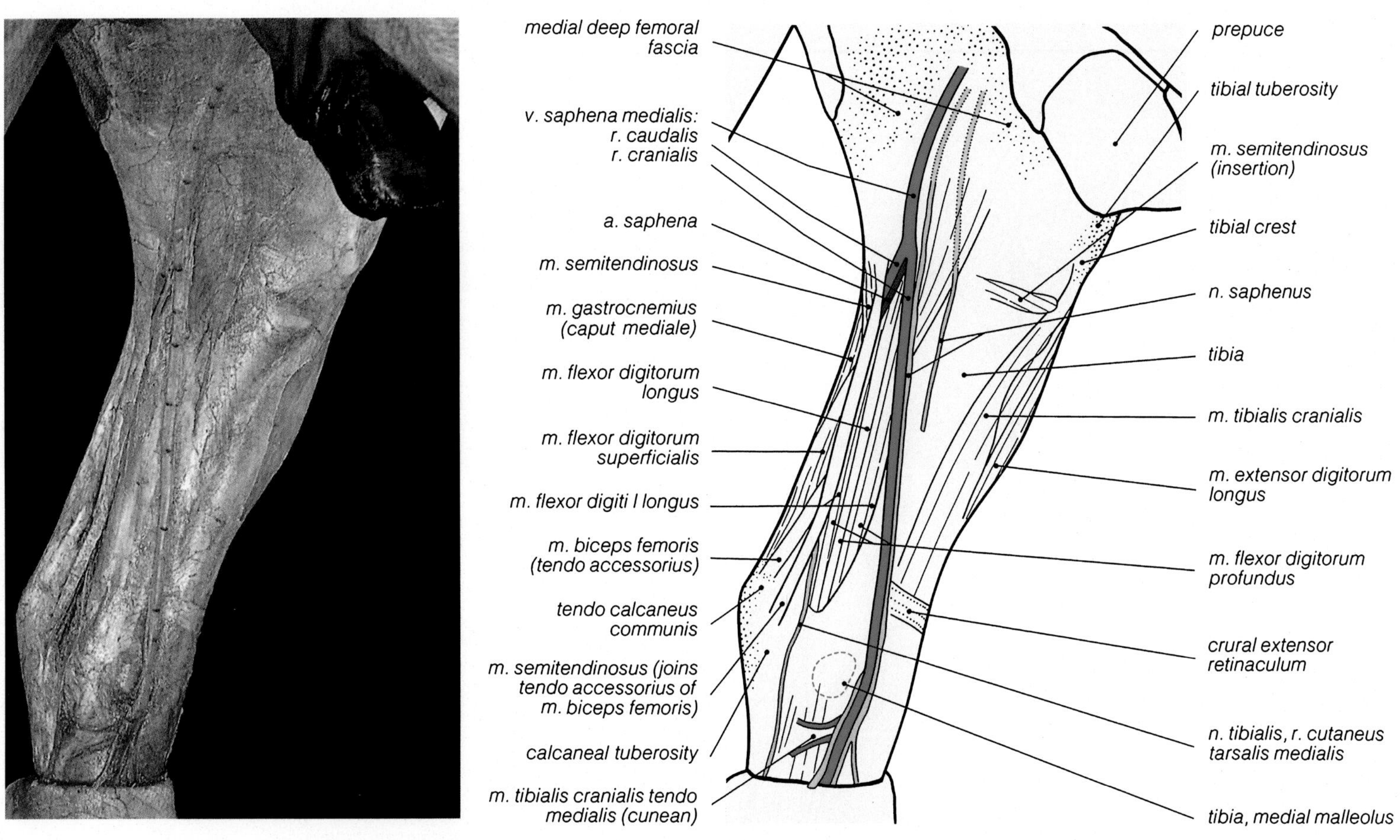
medial deep femoral fascia
v. saphena medialis:
r. caudalis
r. cranialis
a. saphena
m. semitendinosus
m. gastrocnemius (caput mediale)
m. flexor digitorum longus
m. flexor digitorum superficialis
m. flexor digiti I longus
m. biceps femoris (tendo accessorius)
tendo calcaneus communis
m. semitendinosus (joins tendo accessorius of m. biceps femoris)
calcaneal tuberosity
m. tibialis cranialis tendo medialis (cunean)
prepuce
tibial tuberosity
m. semitendinosus (insertion)
tibial crest
n. saphenus
tibia
m. tibialis cranialis
m. extensor digitorum longus
m. flexor digitorum profundus
crural extensor retinaculum
n. tibialis, r. cutaneus tarsalis medialis
tibia, medial malleolus

Fig. 6.13 Superficial structures of the left hindlimb: medial view. The skin and superficial fascia have been removed and the deep fascia overlying the cranial tibial and long digital extensor muscles has been excised. Further dissections of this region are shown in Figs. 6.28, 6.30 and 6.56.

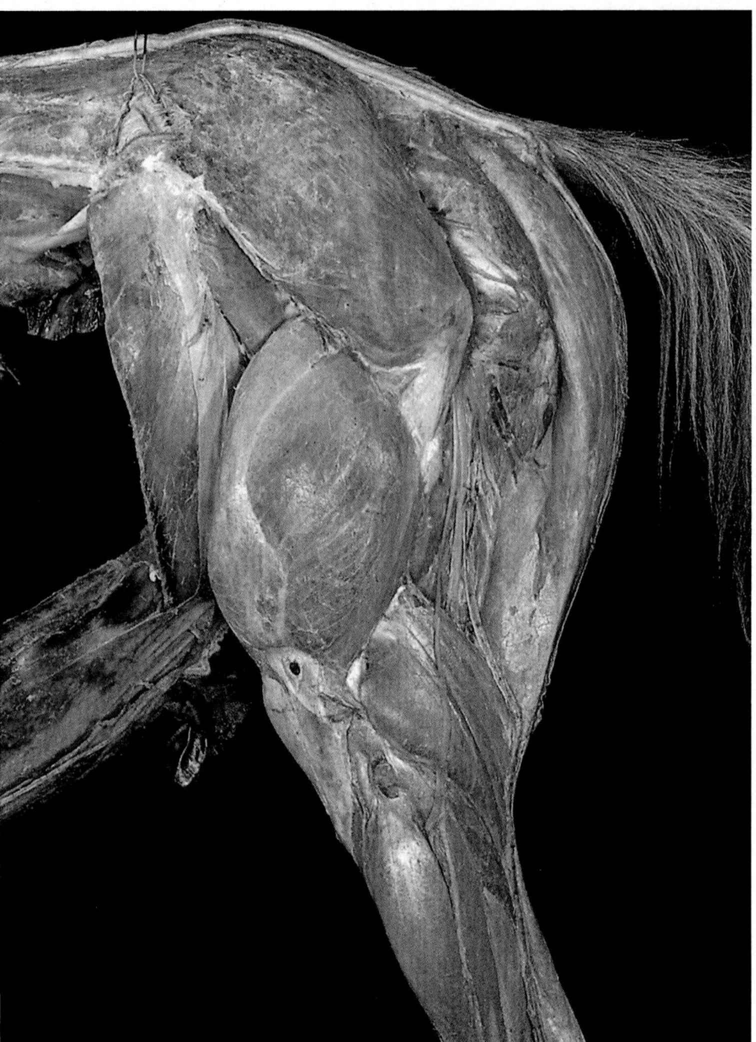

Fig. 6.14 Superficial structures of the left hindlimb: left lateral view. The biceps femoris muscle has been removed. Further details of the muscles, nerves and vessels are shown in Fig. 6.15.

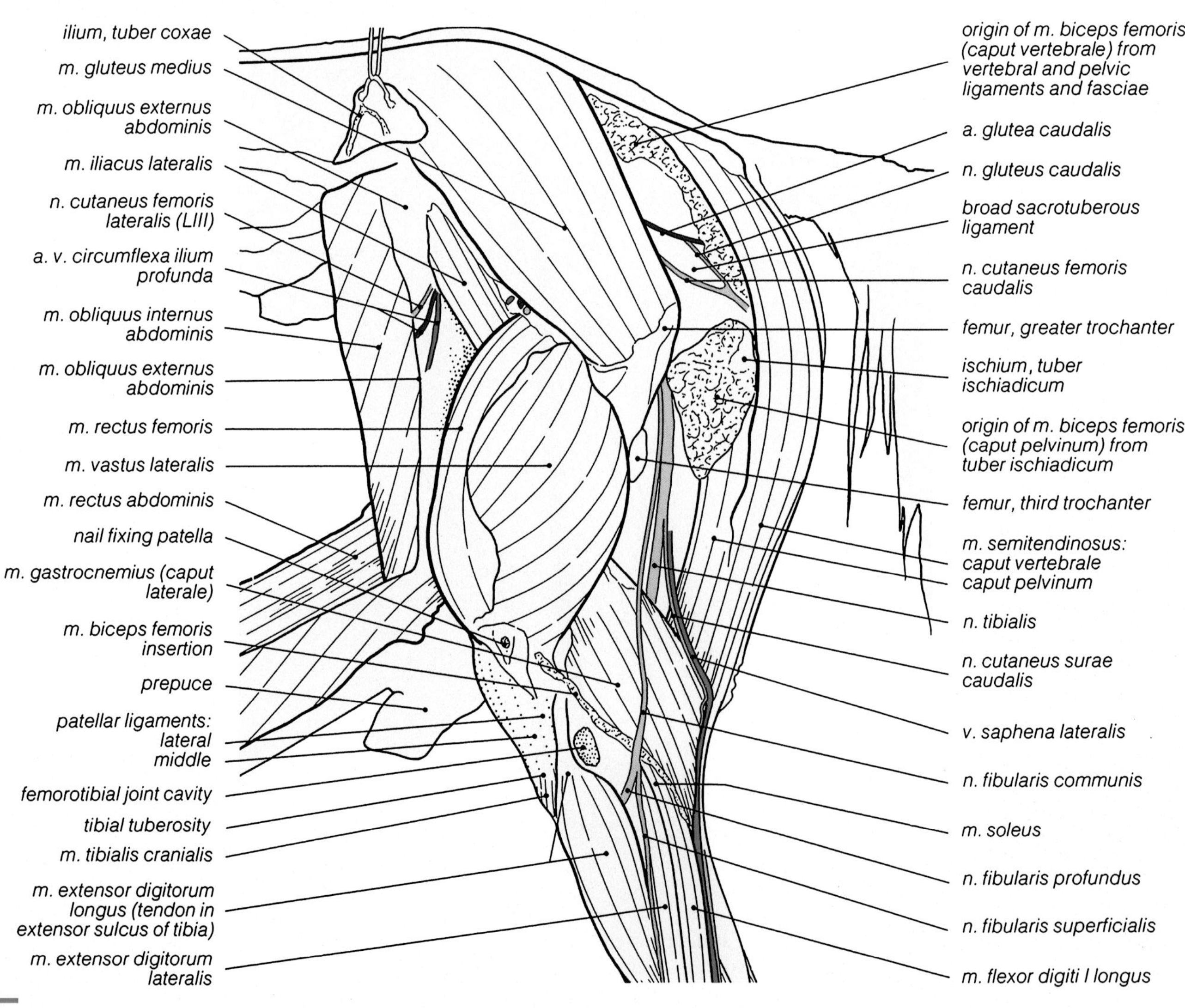
ilium, tuber coxae
m. gluteus medius
m. obliquus externus abdominis
m. iliacus lateralis
n. cutaneus femoris lateralis (LIII)
a. v. circumflexa ilium profunda
m. obliquus internus abdominis
m. obliquus externus abdominis
m. rectus femoris
m. vastus lateralis
m. rectus abdominis
nail fixing patella
m. gastrocnemius (caput laterale)
m. biceps femoris insertion
prepuce
patellar ligaments:
lateral
middle
femorotibial joint cavity
tibial tuberosity
m. tibialis cranialis
m. extensor digitorum longus (tendon in extensor sulcus of tibia)
m. extensor digitorum lateralis
origin of m. biceps femoris (caput vertebrale) from vertebral and pelvic ligaments and fasciae
a. glutea caudalis
n. gluteus caudalis
broad sacrotuberous ligament
n. cutaneus femoris caudalis
femur, greater trochanter
ischium, tuber ischiadicum
origin of m. biceps femoris (caput pelvinum) from tuber ischiadicum
femur, third trochanter
m. semitendinosus:
caput vertebrale
caput pelvinum
n. tibialis
n. cutaneus surae caudalis
v. saphena lateralis
n. fibularis communis
m. soleus
n. fibularis profundus
n. fibularis superficialis
m. flexor digiti I longus

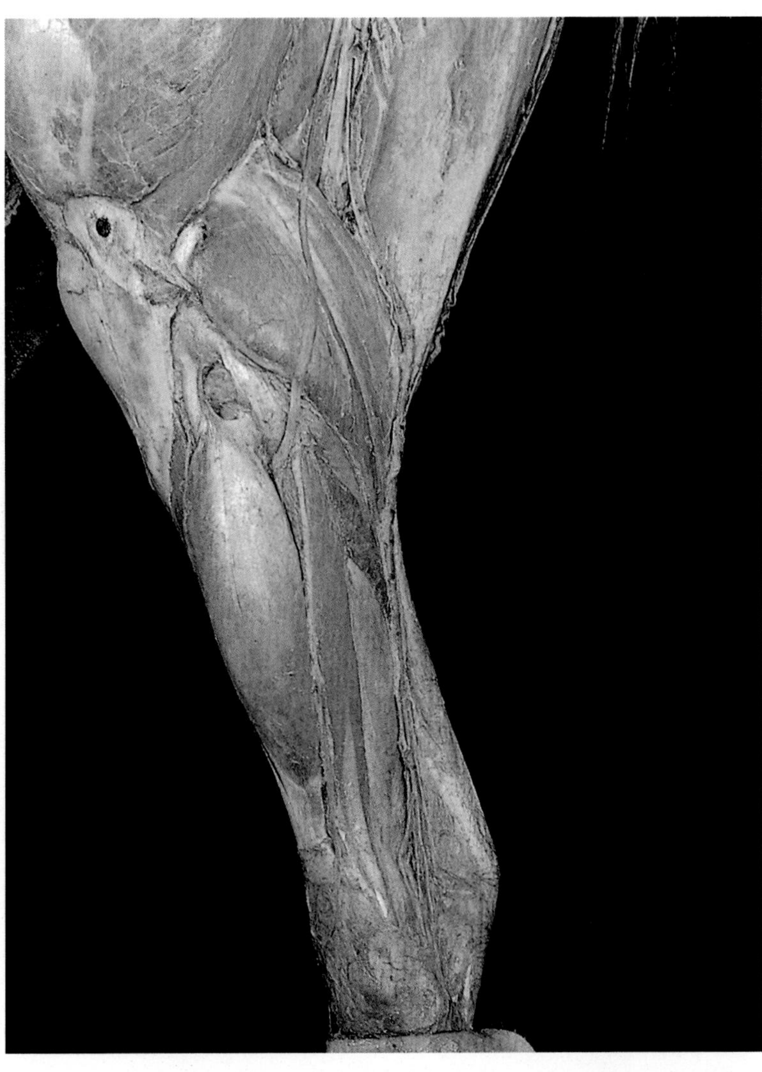

Fig. 6.15 The stifle and tarsal regions and crus: left lateral view. This is a closer view of a part of the dissection shown in Fig. 6.14.

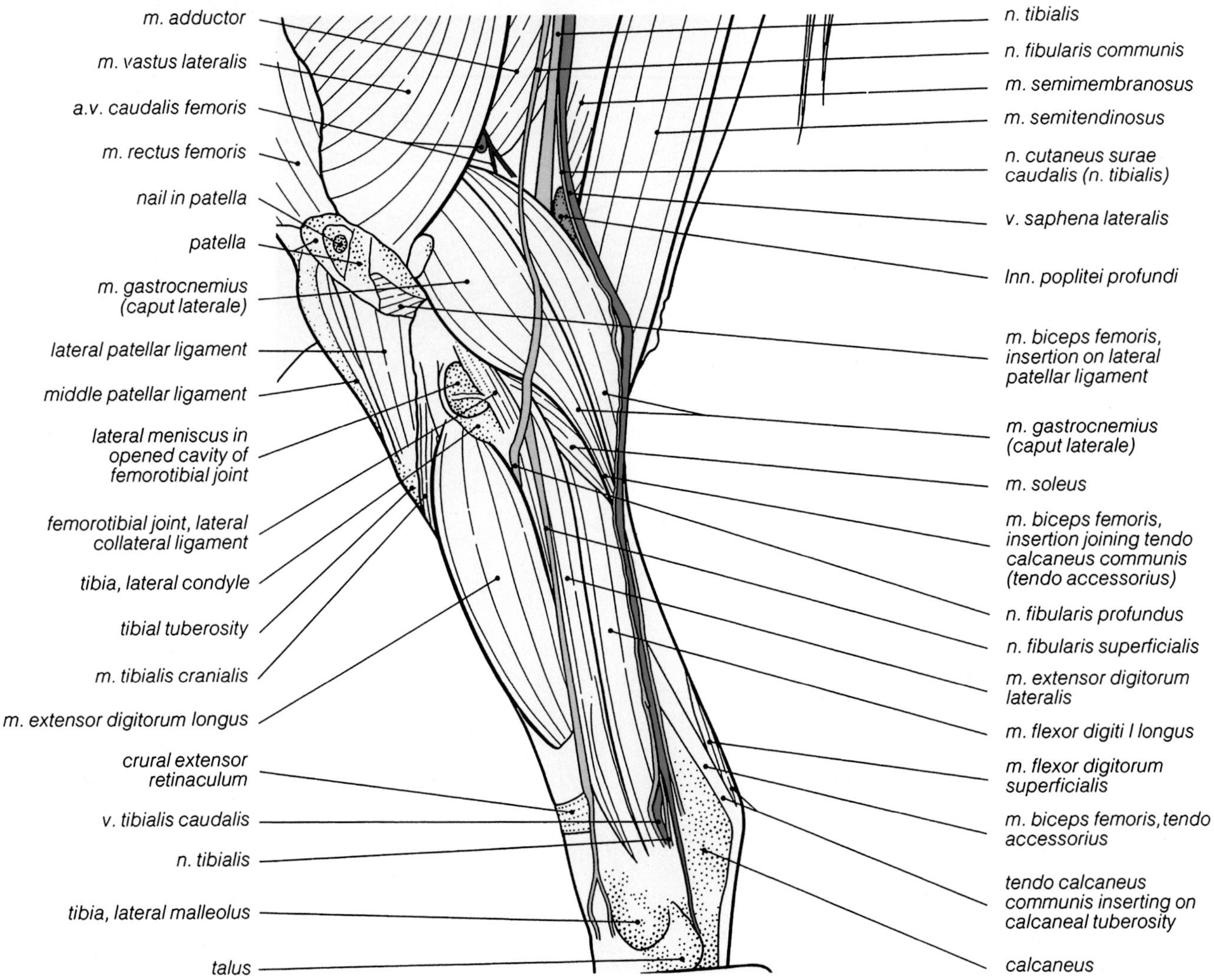

m. adductor
m. vastus lateralis
a.v. caudalis femoris
m. rectus femoris
nail in patella
patella
m. gastrocnemius (caput laterale)
lateral patellar ligament
middle patellar ligament
lateral meniscus in opened cavity of femorotibial joint
femorotibial joint, lateral collateral ligament
tibia, lateral condyle
tibial tuberosity
m. tibialis cranialis
m. extensor digitorum longus
crural extensor retinaculum
v. tibialis caudalis
n. tibialis
tibia, lateral malleolus
talus

n. tibialis
n. fibularis communis
m. semimembranosus
m. semitendinosus
n. cutaneus surae caudalis (n. tibialis)
v. saphena lateralis
lnn. poplitei profundi
m. biceps femoris, insertion on lateral patellar ligament
m. gastrocnemius (caput laterale)
m. soleus
m. biceps femoris, insertion joining tendo calcaneus communis (tendo accessorius)
n. fibularis profundus
n. fibularis superficialis
m. extensor digitorum lateralis
m. flexor digiti I longus
m. flexor digitorum superficialis
m. biceps femoris, tendo accessorius
tendo calcaneus communis inserting on calcaneal tuberosity
calcaneus

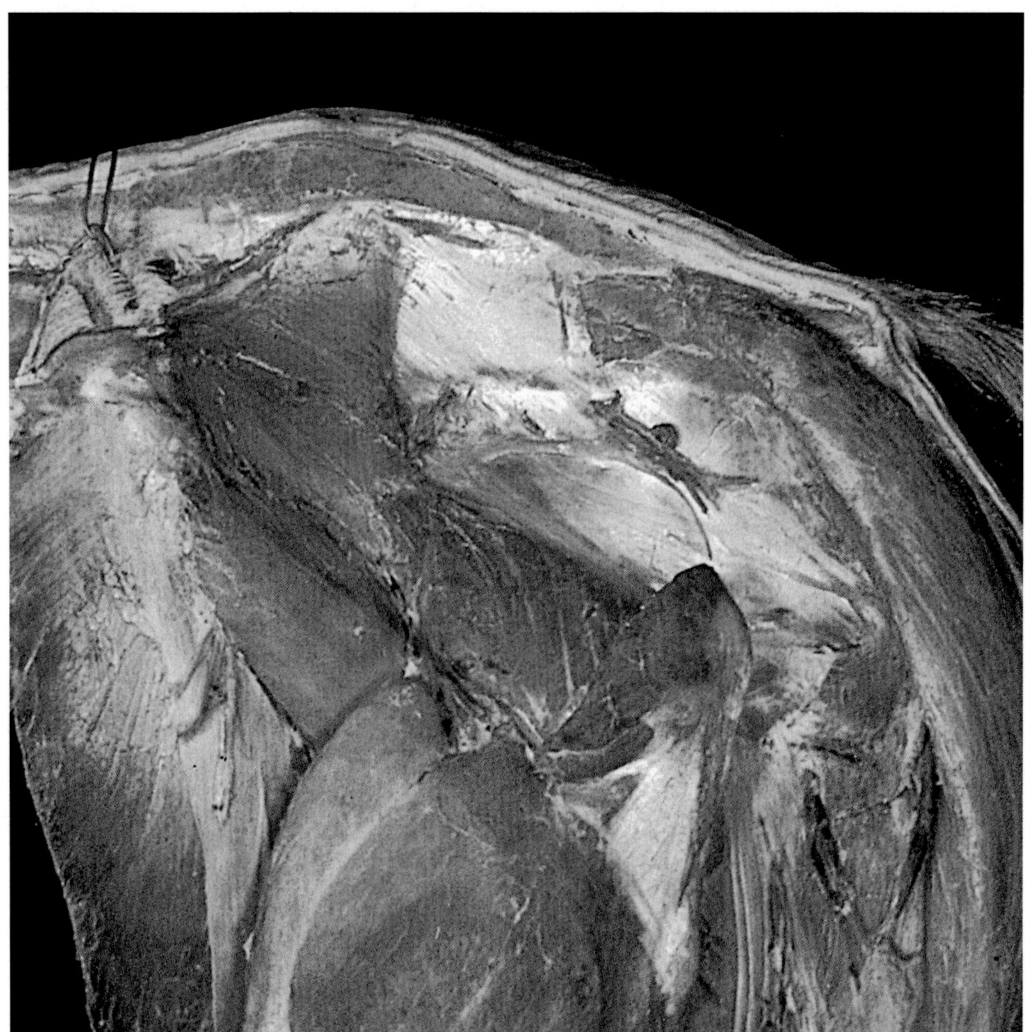

Fig. 6.16 The sciatic and gluteal nerves: left lateral view. The middle gluteal muscle has been removed.

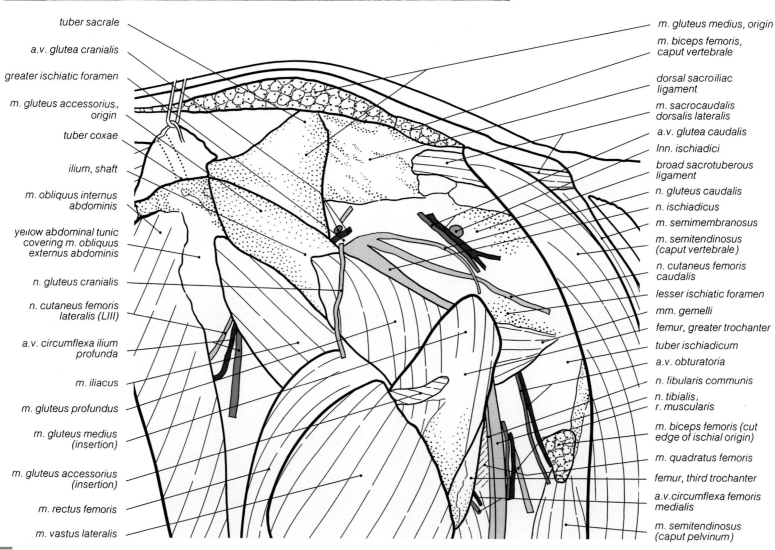

tuber sacrale
a.v. glutea cranialis
greater ischiatic foramen
m. gluteus accessorius, origin
tuber coxae
ilium, shaft
m. obliquus internus abdominis
yellow abdominal tunic covering m. obliquus externus abdominis
n. gluteus cranialis
n. cutaneus femoris lateralis (LIII)
a.v. circumflexa ilium profunda
m. iliacus
m. gluteus profundus
m. gluteus medius (insertion)
m. gluteus accessorius (insertion)
m. rectus femoris
m. vastus lateralis

m. gluteus medius, origin
m. biceps femoris, caput vertebrale
dorsal sacroiliac ligament
m. sacrocaudalis dorsalis lateralis
a.v. glutea caudalis
lnn. ischiadici
broad sacrotuberous ligament
n. gluteus caudalis
n. ischiadicus
m. semimembranosus
m. semitendinosus (caput vertebrale)
n. cutaneus femoris caudalis
lesser ischiatic foramen
mm. gemelli
femur, greater trochanter
tuber ischiadicum
a.v. obturatoria
n. fibularis communis
n. tibialis, r. muscularis
m. biceps femoris (cut edge of ischial origin)
m. quadratus femoris
femur, third trochanter
a.v. circumflexa femoris medialis
m. semitendinosus (caput pelvinum)

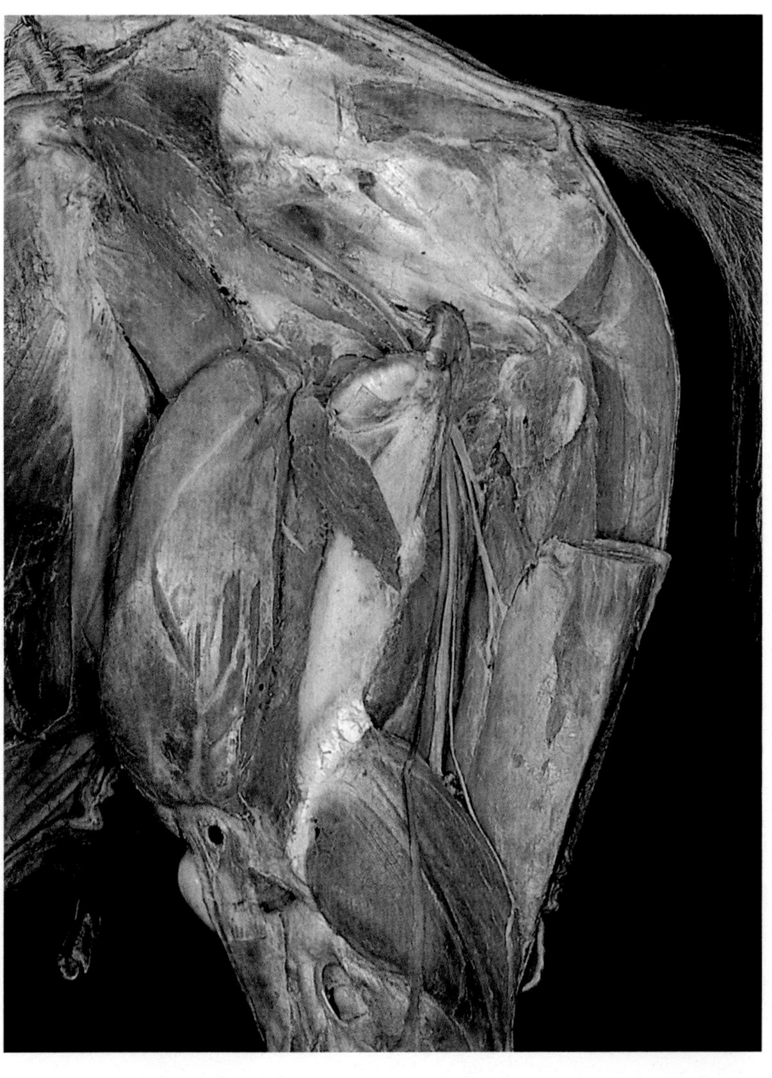

Fig. 6.17 The sciatic, fibular and tibial nerves in the pelvic and femoral regions: left lateral view. The middle and deep gluteal muscles have been removed and part of the semitendinosus muscle has been resected.

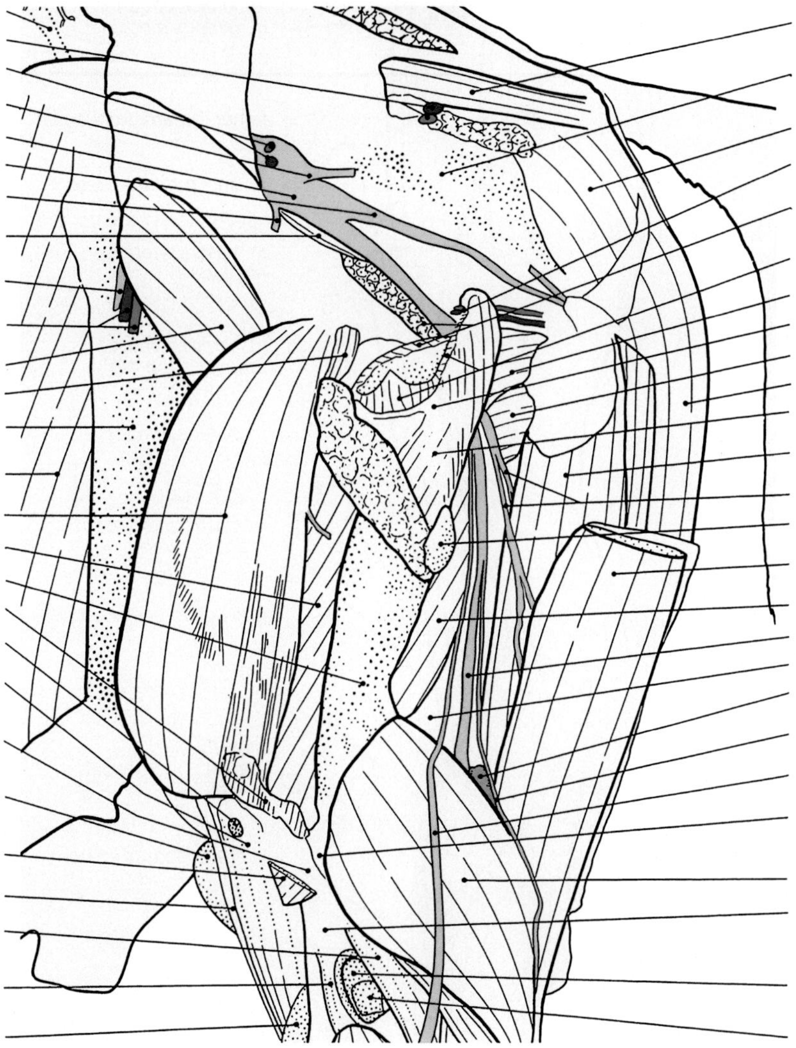

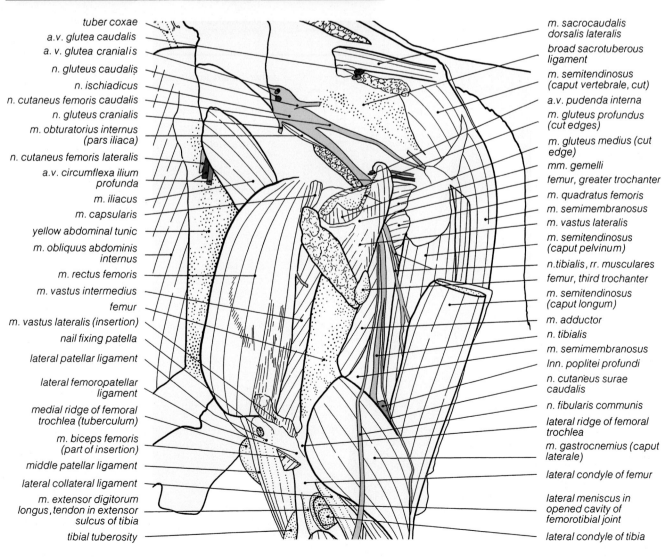

tuber coxae
a.v. glutea caudalis
a. v. glutea cranialis
n. gluteus caudalis
n. ischiadicus
n. cutaneus femoris caudalis
n. gluteus cranialis
m. obturatorius internus (pars iliaca)
n. cutaneus femoris lateralis
a.v. circumflexa ilium profunda
m. iliacus
m. capsularis
yellow abdominal tunic
m. obliquus abdominis internus
m. rectus femoris
m. vastus intermedius
femur
m. vastus lateralis (insertion)
nail fixing patella
lateral patellar ligament
lateral femoropatellar ligament
medial ridge of femoral trochlea (tuberculum)
m. biceps femoris (part of insertion)
middle patellar ligament
lateral collateral ligament
m. extensor digitorum longus, tendon in extensor sulcus of tibia
tibial tuberosity
m. sacrocaudalis dorsalis lateralis
broad sacrotuberous ligament
m. semitendinosus (caput vertebrale, cut)
a.v. pudenda interna
m. gluteus profundus (cut edges)
m. gluteus medius (cut edge)
mm. gemelli
femur, greater trochanter
m. quadratus femoris
m. semimembranosus
m. vastus lateralis
m. semitendinosus (caput pelvinum)
n.tibialis, rr. musculares
femur, third trochanter
m. semitendinosus (caput longum)
m. adductor
n. tibialis
m. semimembranosus
lnn. poplitei profundi
n. cutaneus surae caudalis
n. fibularis communis
lateral ridge of femoral trochlea
m. gastrocnemius (caput laterale)
lateral condyle of femur
lateral meniscus in opened cavity of femorotibial joint
lateral condyle of tibia

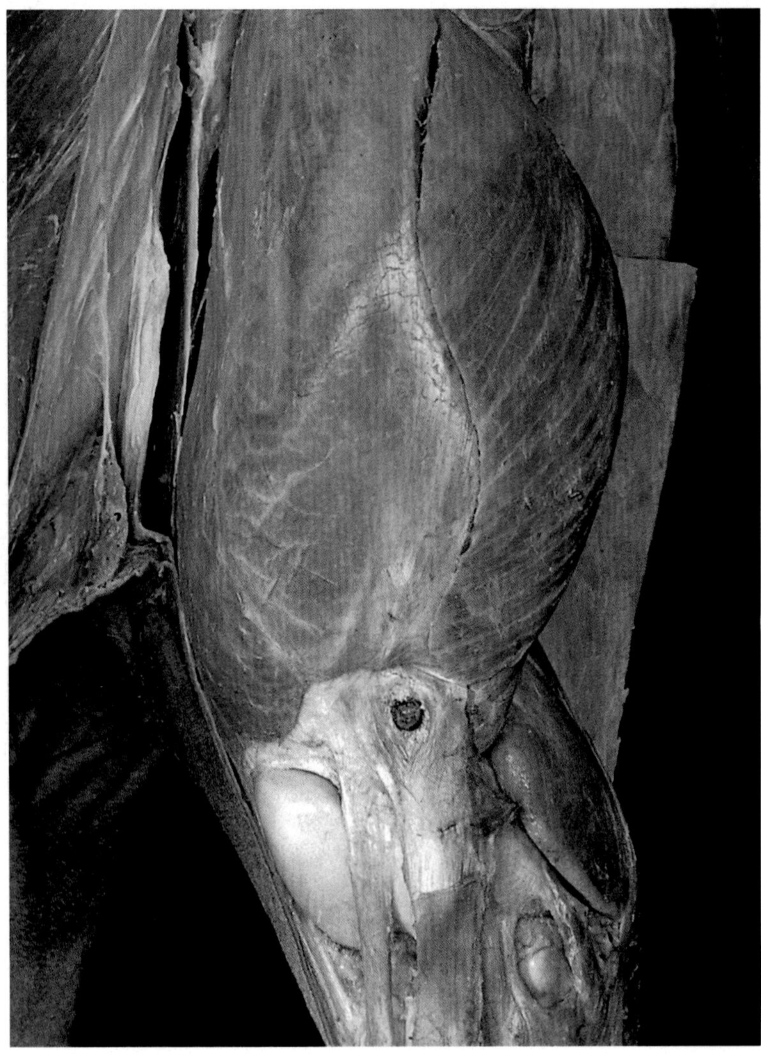

Fig. 6.18 The left quadriceps femoris muscle: cranial view. The lateral vastus muscle, which was removed (see Fig. 6.17), has been replaced to show the complete quadriceps femoris muscle with its sesamoid bone (patella) and tendons of insertion ('patellar ligaments'). The intermediate vastus muscle is shown in Fig. 6.20. Further details of the genual articulation (stifle joint) are shown in Fig. 6.19.

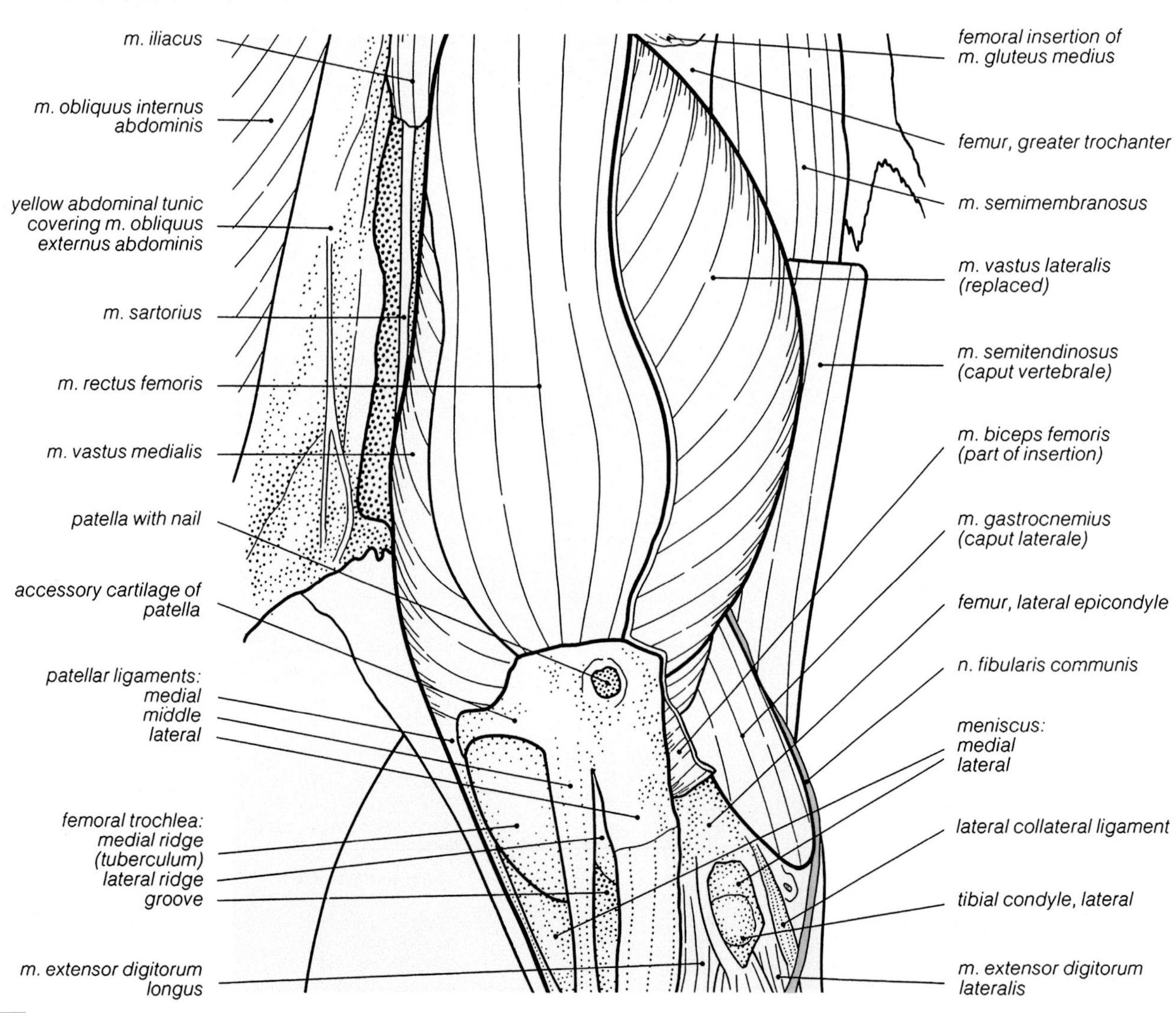
m. iliacus
m. obliquus internus abdominis
yellow abdominal tunic covering m. obliquus externus abdominis
m. sartorius
m. rectus femoris
m. vastus medialis
patella with nail
accessory cartilage of patella
patellar ligaments:
medial
middle
lateral
femoral trochlea:
medial ridge (tuberculum)
lateral ridge
groove
m. extensor digitorum longus
femoral insertion of m. gluteus medius
femur, greater trochanter
m. semimembranosus
m. vastus lateralis (replaced)
m. semitendinosus (caput vertebrale)
m. biceps femoris (part of insertion)
m. gastrocnemius (caput laterale)
femur, lateral epicondyle
n. fibularis communis
meniscus:
medial
lateral
lateral collateral ligament
tibial condyle, lateral
m. extensor digitorum lateralis

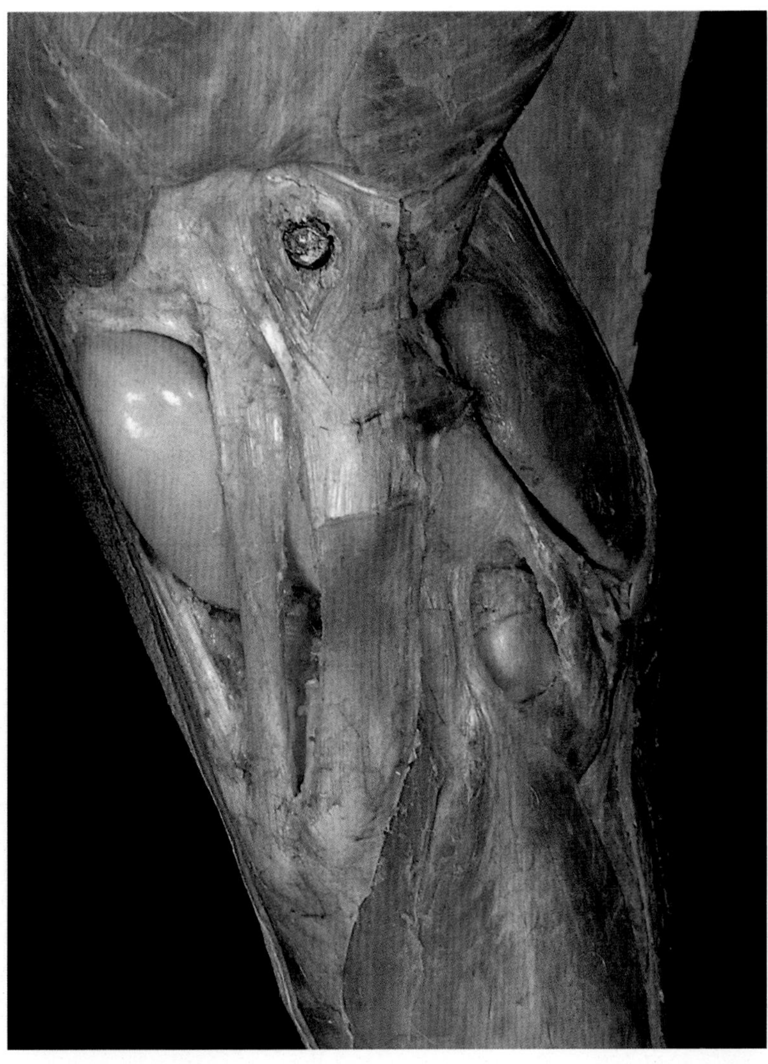

Fig. 6.19 The left stifle joint: cranial view. The femoropatellar joint was nailed and fixed, with the medial patellar ligament and patellar cartilage hooked over the tuberculum of the trochlea (stifle in the 'locked' position). During movement these are not so hooked and the patella moves freely in the trochlear groove.

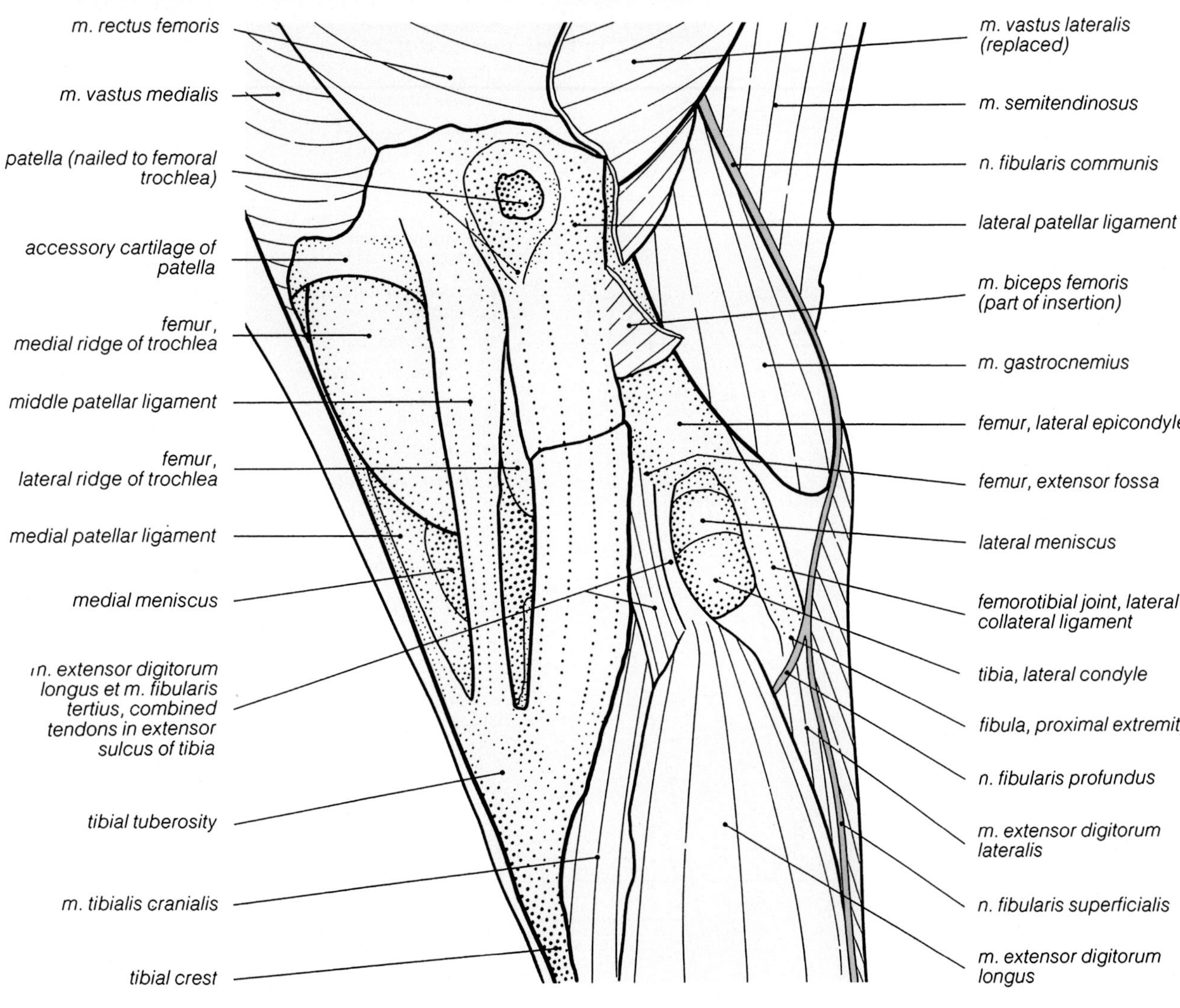
m. rectus femoris
m. vastus medialis
patella (nailed to femoral trochlea)
accessory cartilage of patella
femur, medial ridge of trochlea
middle patellar ligament
femur, lateral ridge of trochlea
medial patellar ligament
medial meniscus
m. extensor digitorum longus et m. fibularis tertius, combined tendons in extensor sulcus of tibia
tibial tuberosity
m. tibialis cranialis
tibial crest
m. vastus lateralis (replaced)
m. semitendinosus
n. fibularis communis
lateral patellar ligament
m. biceps femoris (part of insertion)
m. gastrocnemius
femur, lateral epicondyle
femur, extensor fossa
lateral meniscus
femorotibial joint, lateral collateral ligament
tibia, lateral condyle
fibula, proximal extremity
n. fibularis profundus
m. extensor digitorum lateralis
n. fibularis superficialis
m. extensor digitorum longus

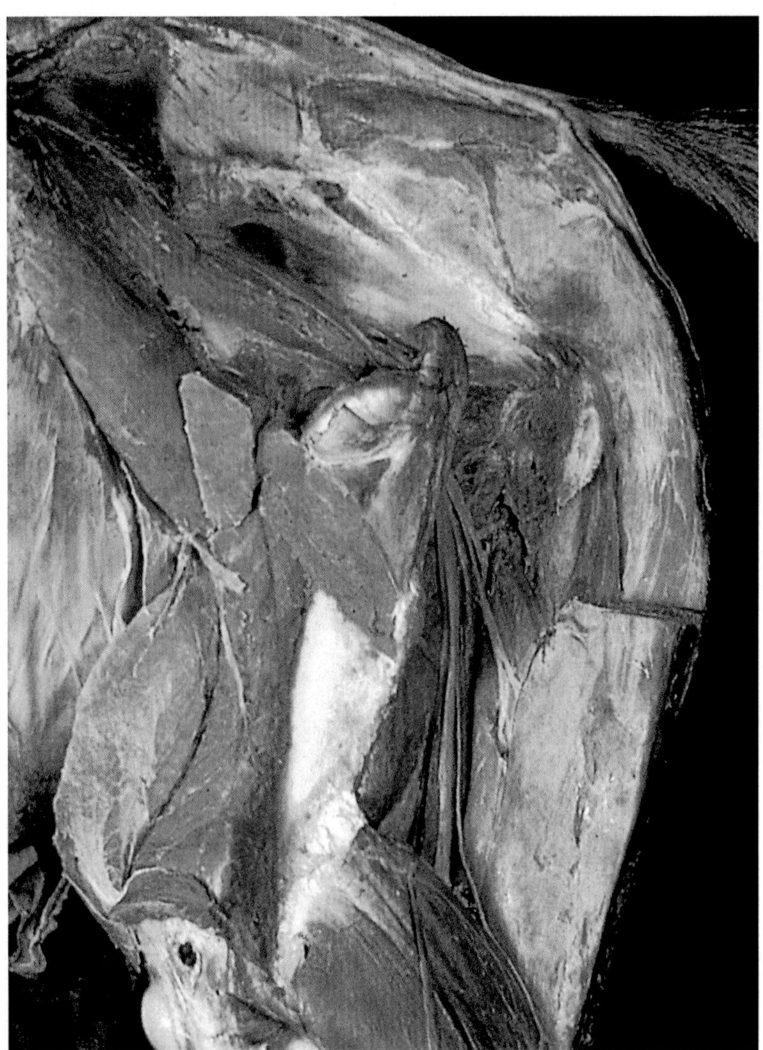

Fig. 6.20 The medial and intermediate vastus muscles and the femoral nerve: left lateral view. The lateral vastus and rectus femoris muscles have been partially resected.

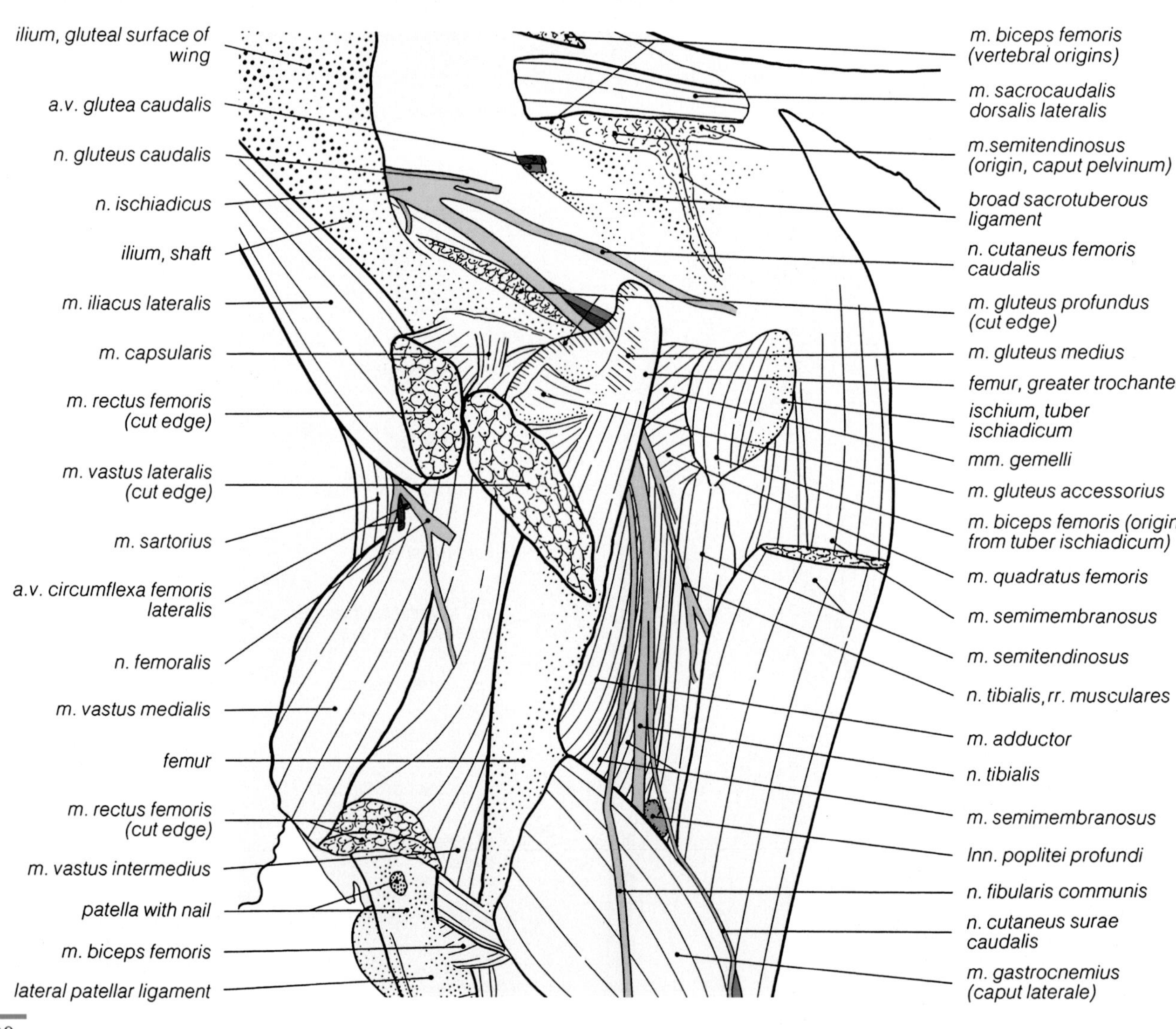
ilium, gluteal surface of wing
a.v. glutea caudalis
n. gluteus caudalis
n. ischiadicus
ilium, shaft
m. iliacus lateralis
m. capsularis
m. rectus femoris (cut edge)
m. vastus lateralis (cut edge)
m. sartorius
a.v. circumflexa femoris lateralis
n. femoralis
m. vastus medialis
femur
m. rectus femoris (cut edge)
m. vastus intermedius
patella with nail
m. biceps femoris
lateral patellar ligament
m. biceps femoris (vertebral origins)
m. sacrocaudalis dorsalis lateralis
m.semitendinosus (origin, caput pelvinum)
broad sacrotuberous ligament
n. cutaneus femoris caudalis
m. gluteus profundus (cut edge)
m. gluteus medius
femur, greater trochanter
ischium, tuber ischiadicum
mm. gemelli
m. gluteus accessorius
m. biceps femoris (origin from tuber ischiadicum)
m. quadratus femoris
m. semimembranosus
m. semitendinosus
n. tibialis, rr. musculares
m. adductor
n. tibialis
m. semimembranosus
lnn. poplitei profundi
n. fibularis communis
n. cutaneus surae caudalis
m. gastrocnemius (caput laterale)

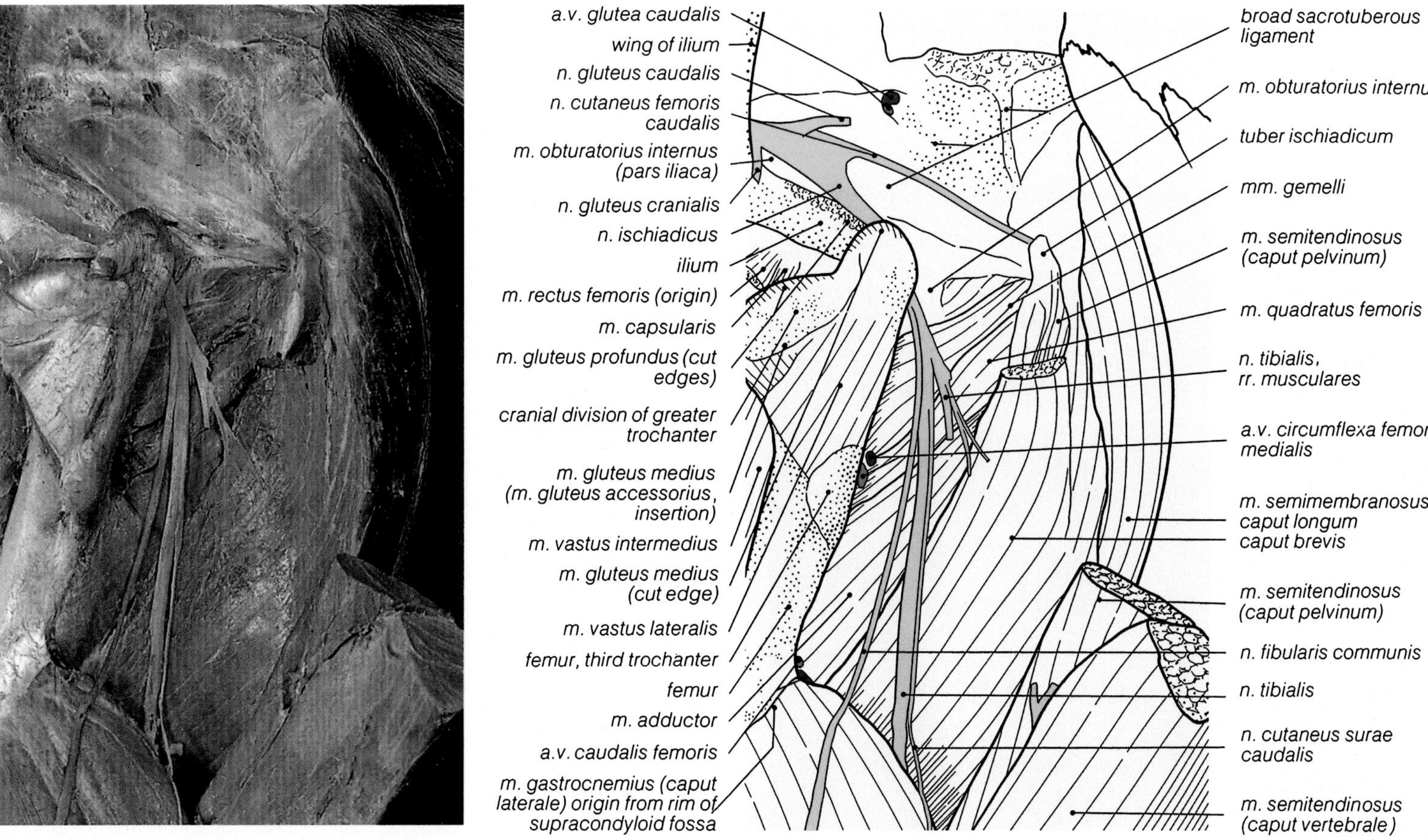
a.v. glutea caudalis
wing of ilium
n. gluteus caudalis
n. cutaneus femoris caudalis
m. obturatorius internus (pars iliaca)
n. gluteus cranialis
n. ischiadicus
ilium
m. rectus femoris (origin)
m. capsularis
m. gluteus profundus (cut edges)
cranial division of greater trochanter
m. gluteus medius (m. gluteus accessorius, insertion)
m. vastus intermedius
m. gluteus medius (cut edge)
m. vastus lateralis
femur, third trochanter
femur
m. adductor
a.v. caudalis femoris
m. gastrocnemius (caput laterale) origin from rim of supracondyloid fossa
broad sacrotuberous ligament
m. obturatorius internus
tuber ischiadicum
mm. gemelli
m. semitendinosus (caput pelvinum)
m. quadratus femoris
n. tibialis, rr. musculares
a.v. circumflexa femoris medialis
m. semimembranosus: caput longum caput brevis
m. semitendinosus (caput pelvinum)
n. fibularis communis
n. tibialis
n. cutaneus surae caudalis
m. semitendinosus (caput vertebrale)

Fig. 6.21 The medial muscles of the thigh: left lateral view. The pelvic head of the semitendinosus muscle has been transected and the muscle has been displaced caudally to show the two heads of the semimembranosus muscle.

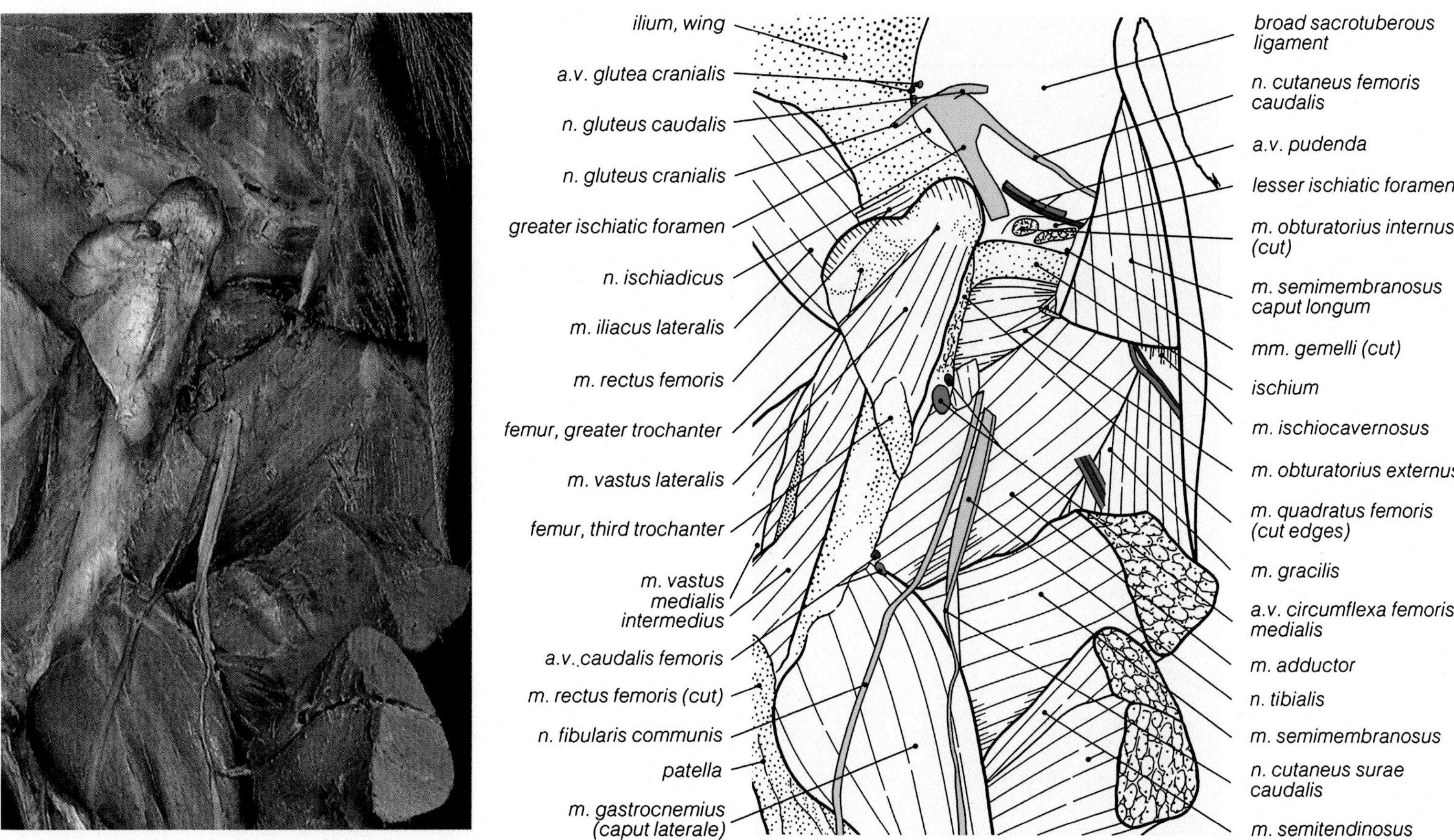
ilium, wing
a.v. glutea cranialis
n. gluteus caudalis
n. gluteus cranialis
greater ischiatic foramen
n. ischiadicus
m. iliacus lateralis
m. rectus femoris
femur, greater trochanter
m. vastus lateralis
femur, third trochanter
m. vastus medialis intermedius
a.v. caudalis femoris
m. rectus femoris (cut)
n. fibularis communis
patella
m. gastrocnemius (caput laterale)
broad sacrotuberous ligament
n. cutaneus femoris caudalis
a.v. pudenda
lesser ischiatic foramen
m. obturatorius internus (cut)
m. semimembranosus caput longum
mm. gemelli (cut)
ischium
m. ischiocavernosus
m. obturatorius externus
m. quadratus femoris (cut edges)
m. gracilis
a.v. circumflexa femoris medialis
m. adductor
n. tibialis
m. semimembranosus
n. cutaneus surae caudalis
m. semitendinosus

Fig. 6.22 The medial muscles of the thigh: left caudolateral view. The semimembranosus muscle has been transected and its distal part has been displaced caudally to show the adductor and gracilis muscles. The gemelli and quadratus femoris muscles have been resected to show the external obturator muscle. The tibial and fibular nerves have been cut.

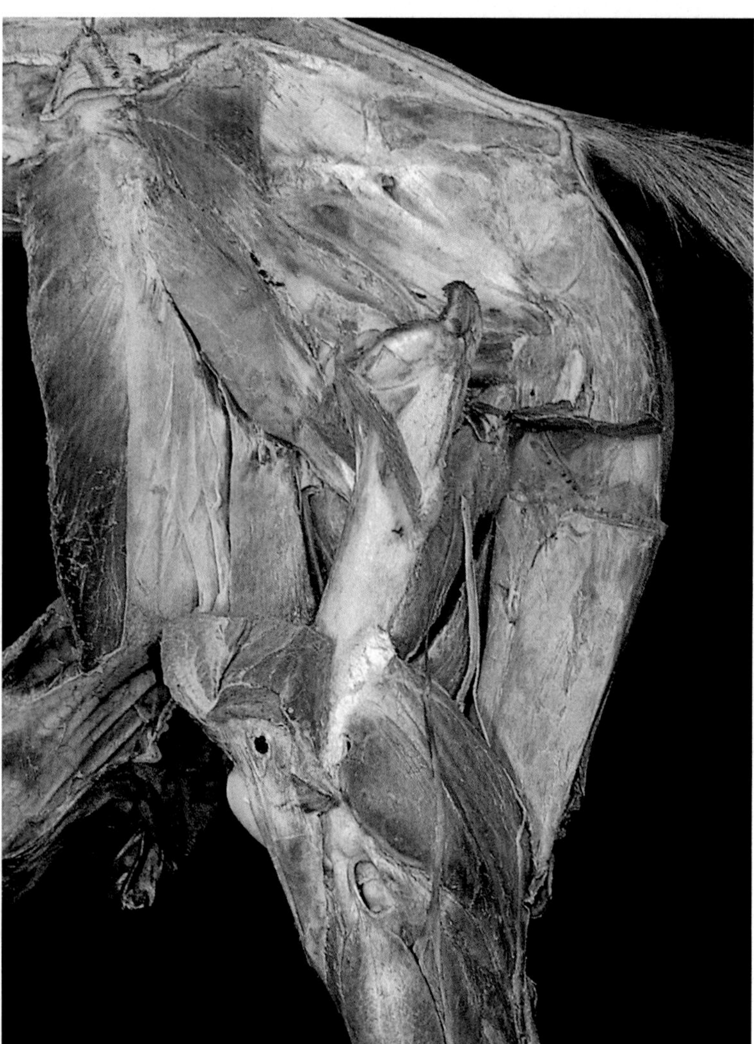

Fig. 6.23 The pelvis and femur and associated muscles: left lateral view. The medial parts of the quadriceps femoris muscle (medial and intermediate vastus muscles) have been resected. The bony pelvis and femur, together with the proximal tibia, are sufficiently visible to allow comparison with Figs. 6.1 and 6.2. Further details of this dissection are shown in Figs. 6.24 and 6.25.

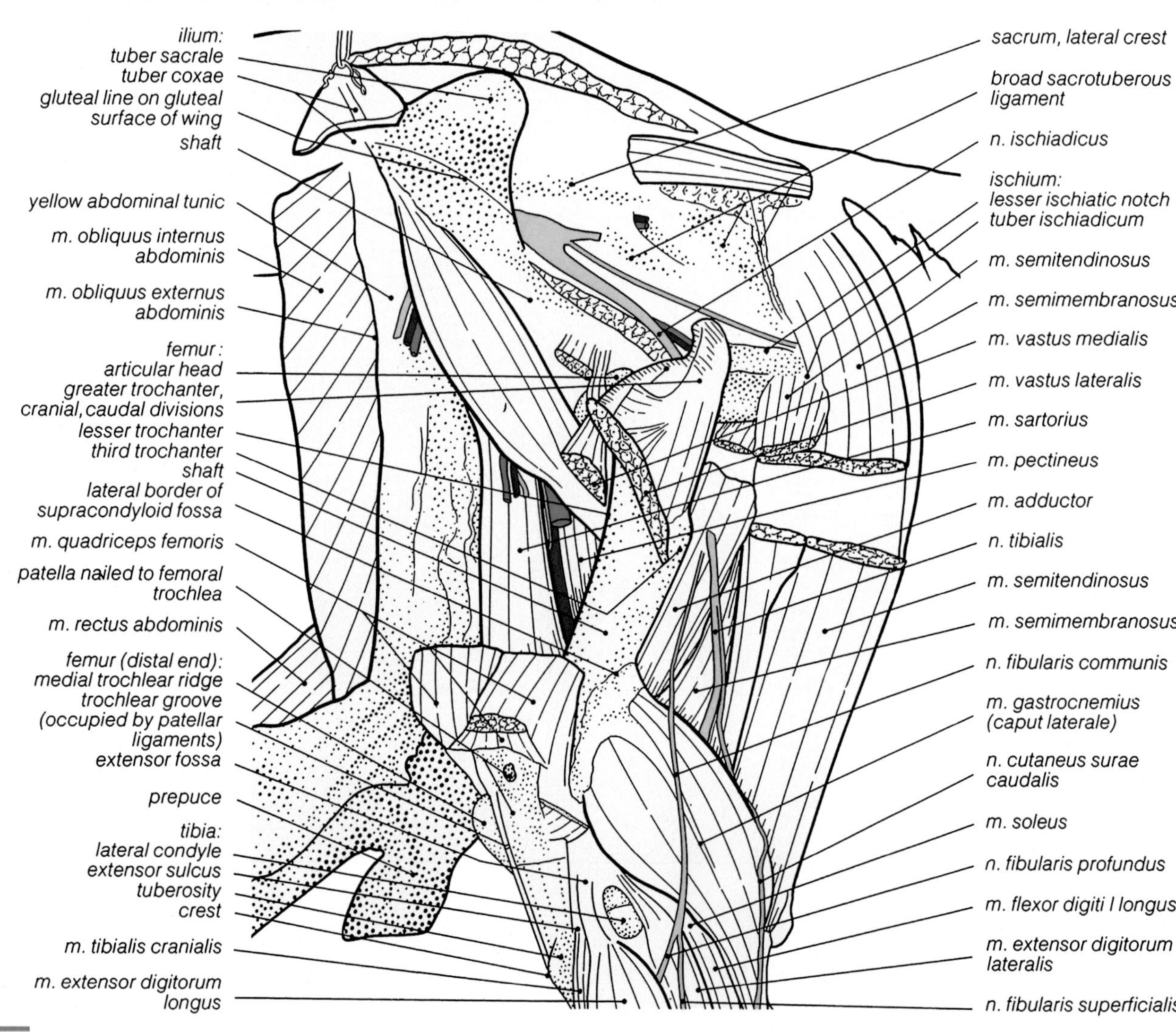
ilium:
tuber sacrale
tuber coxae
gluteal line on gluteal surface of wing
shaft
yellow abdominal tunic
m. obliquus internus abdominis
m. obliquus externus abdominis
femur:
articular head
greater trochanter, cranial, caudal divisions
lesser trochanter
third trochanter
shaft
lateral border of supracondyloid fossa
m. quadriceps femoris
patella nailed to femoral trochlea
m. rectus abdominis
femur (distal end):
medial trochlear ridge
trochlear groove (occupied by patellar ligaments)
extensor fossa
prepuce
tibia:
lateral condyle
extensor sulcus
tuberosity
crest
m. tibialis cranialis
m. extensor digitorum longus
sacrum, lateral crest
broad sacrotuberous ligament
n. ischiadicus
ischium:
lesser ischiatic notch
tuber ischiadicum
m. semitendinosus
m. semimembranosus
m. vastus medialis
m. vastus lateralis
m. sartorius
m. pectineus
m. adductor
n. tibialis
m. semitendinosus
m. semimembranosus
n. fibularis communis
m. gastrocnemius (caput laterale)
n. cutaneus surae caudalis
m. soleus
n. fibularis profundus
m. flexor digiti I longus
m. extensor digitorum lateralis
n. fibularis superficialis

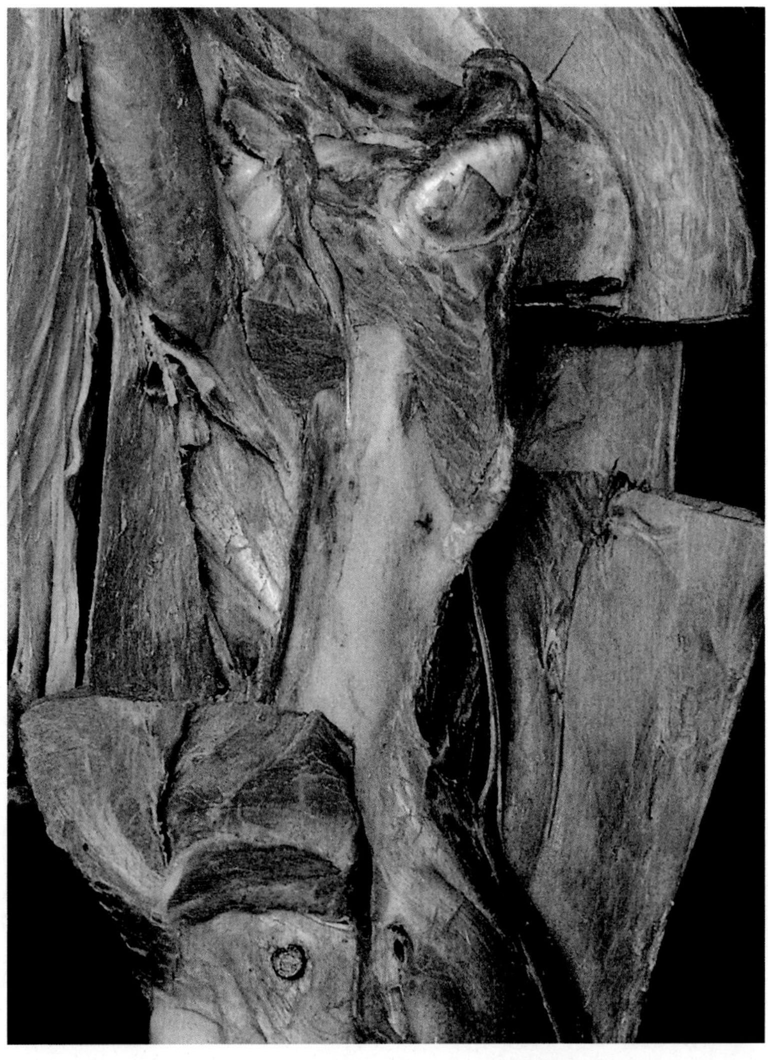

Fig. 6.24 The hip joint and medial muscles of the thigh: left craniolateral view. This is a closer view of the part of the dissection shown in Figs. 6.23 and 6.25, taken from a more cranial angle to show further details of the hip joint.

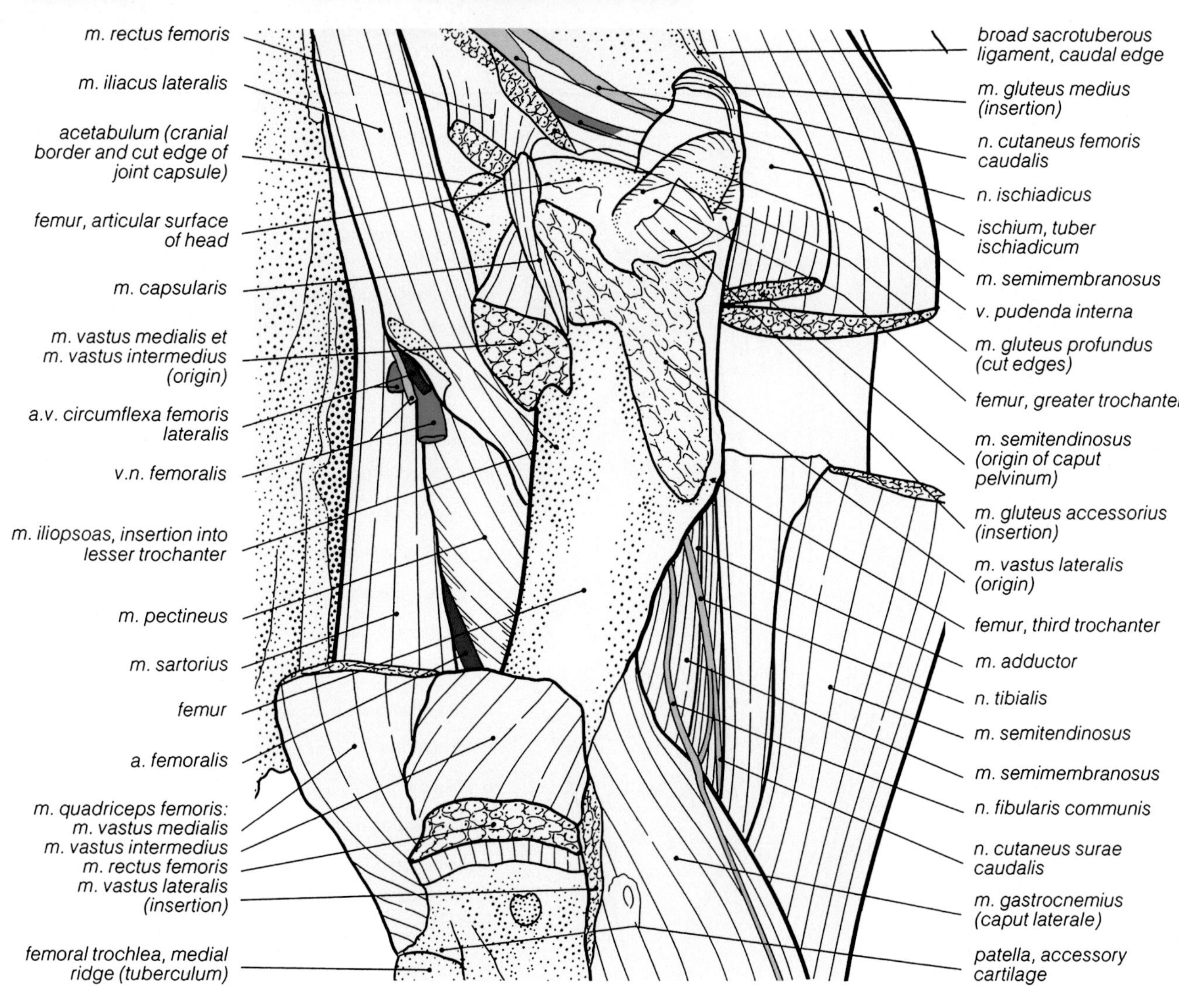
m. rectus femoris
m. iliacus lateralis
acetabulum (cranial border and cut edge of joint capsule)
femur, articular surface of head
m. capsularis
m. vastus medialis et m. vastus intermedius (origin)
a.v. circumflexa femoris lateralis
v.n. femoralis
m. iliopsoas, insertion into lesser trochanter
m. pectineus
m. sartorius
femur
a. femoralis
m. quadriceps femoris:
m. vastus medialis
m. vastus intermedius
m. rectus femoris
m. vastus lateralis (insertion)
femoral trochlea, medial ridge (tuberculum)
broad sacrotuberous ligament, caudal edge
m. gluteus medius (insertion)
n. cutaneus femoris caudalis
n. ischiadicus
ischium, tuber ischiadicum
m. semimembranosus
v. pudenda interna
m. gluteus profundus (cut edges)
femur, greater trochanter
m. semitendinosus (origin of caput pelvinum)
m. gluteus accessorius (insertion)
m. vastus lateralis (origin)
femur, third trochanter
m. adductor
n. tibialis
m. semitendinosus
m. semimembranosus
n. fibularis communis
n. cutaneus surae caudalis
m. gastrocnemius (caput laterale)
patella, accessory cartilage

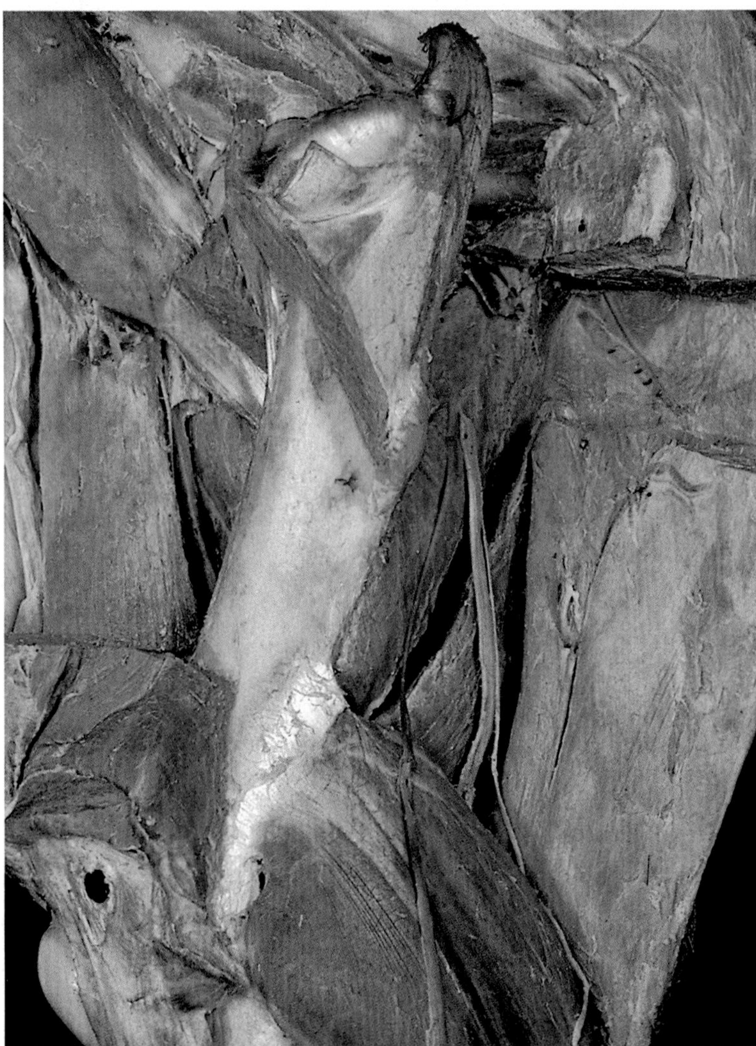

Fig. 6.25 The medial muscles of the thigh: left lateral view. This is a closer view of a part of the dissection shown in Fig. 6.23.

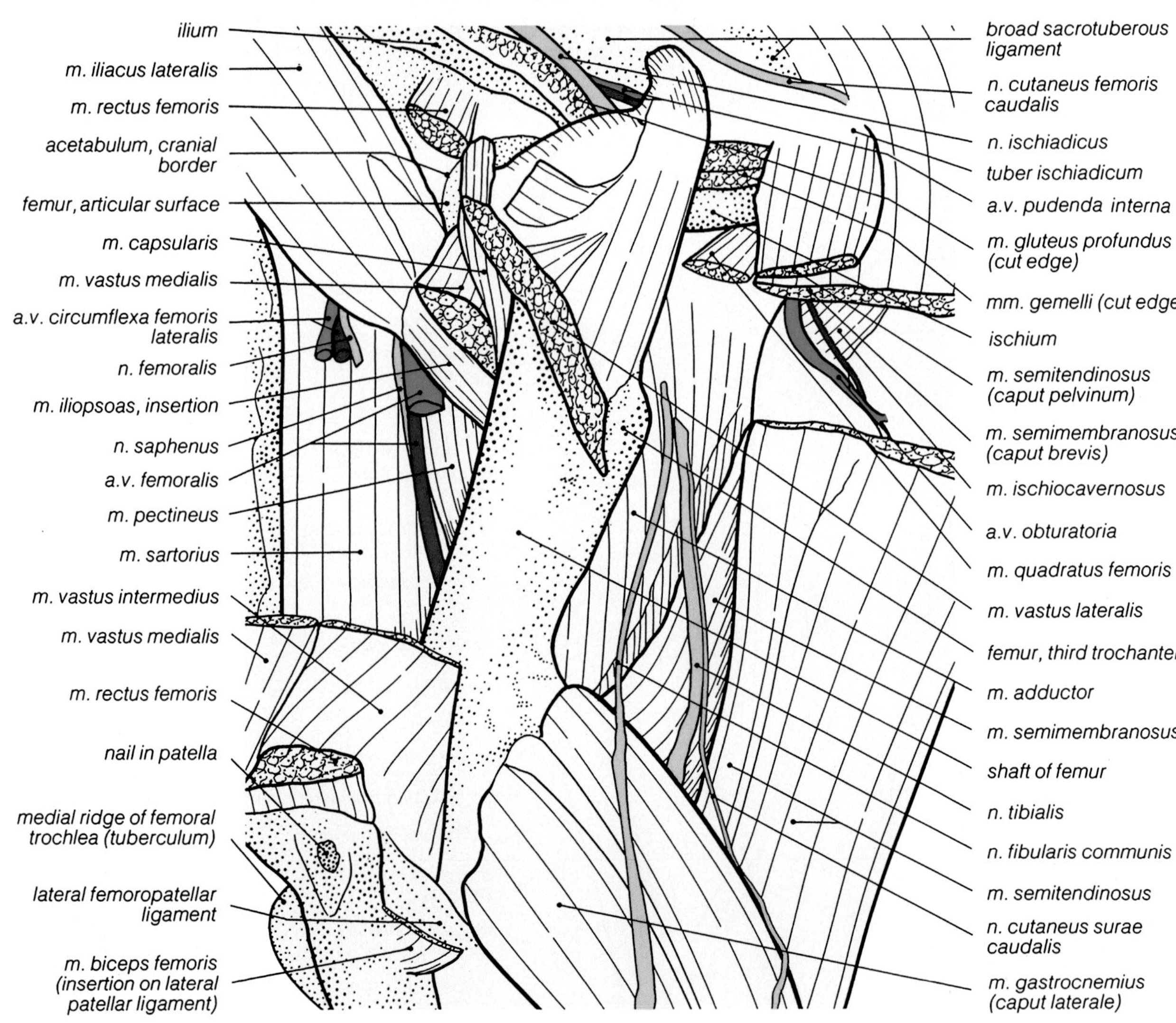
ilium
m. iliacus lateralis
m. rectus femoris
acetabulum, cranial border
femur, articular surface
m. capsularis
m. vastus medialis
a.v. circumflexa femoris lateralis
n. femoralis
m. iliopsoas, insertion
n. saphenus
a.v. femoralis
m. pectineus
m. sartorius
m. vastus intermedius
m. vastus medialis
m. rectus femoris
nail in patella
medial ridge of femoral trochlea (tuberculum)
lateral femoropatellar ligament
m. biceps femoris (insertion on lateral patellar ligament)
broad sacrotuberous ligament
n. cutaneus femoris caudalis
n. ischiadicus
tuber ischiadicum
a.v. pudenda interna
m. gluteus profundus (cut edge)
mm. gemelli (cut edge)
ischium
m. semitendinosus (caput pelvinum)
m. semimembranosus (caput brevis)
m. ischiocavernosus
a.v. obturatoria
m. quadratus femoris
m. vastus lateralis
femur, third trochanter
m. adductor
m. semimembranosus
shaft of femur
n. tibialis
n. fibularis communis
m. semitendinosus
n. cutaneus surae caudalis
m. gastrocnemius (caput laterale)

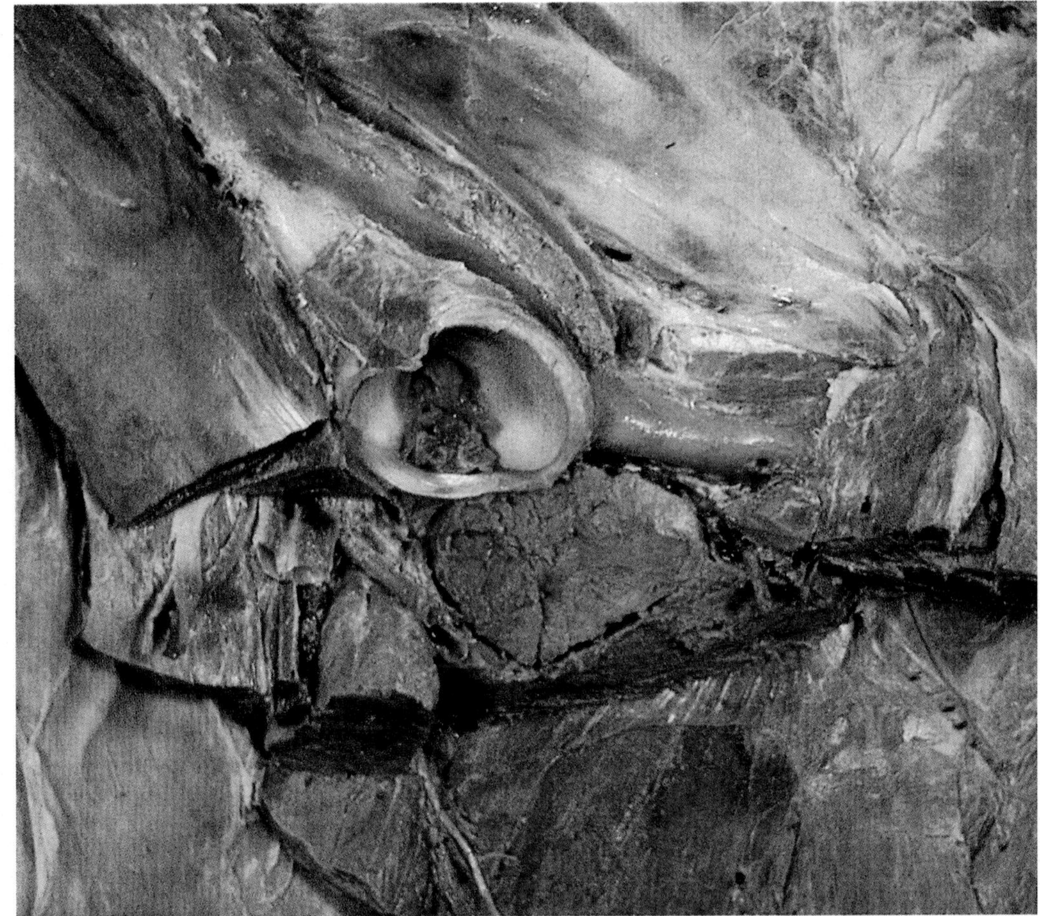

Fig. 6.26 The acetabulum and structures of the medial thigh: left lateral view. The hindlimb has been removed, and the cut ends of the muscles cleaned up to show their relationship to each other and to the vessels and nerves. Further dissections of this region are shown in Chapter 8, Figs. 8.17 and 8.18.

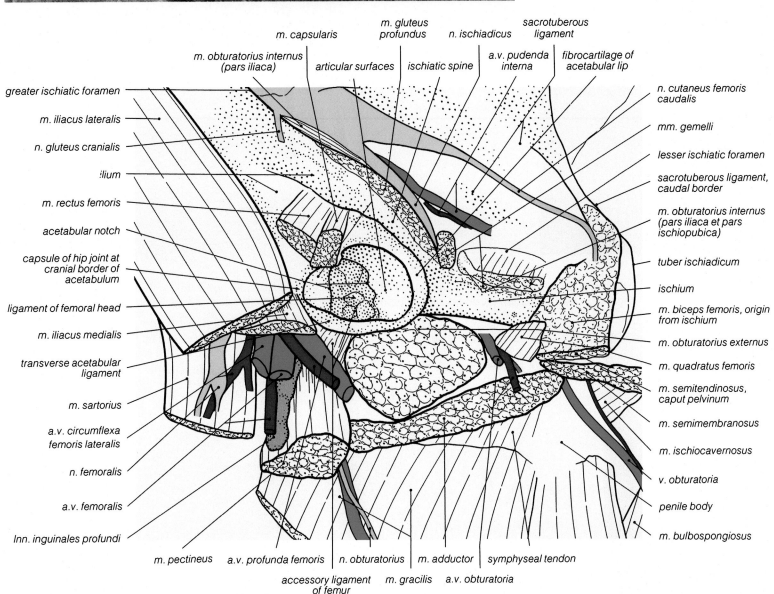

m. capsularis
m. gluteus profundus
n. ischiadicus
sacrotuberous ligament
m. obturatorius internus (pars iliaca)
articular surfaces
ischiatic spine
a.v. pudenda interna
fibrocartilage of acetabular lip
greater ischiatic foramen
m. iliacus lateralis
n. gluteus cranialis
ilium
m. rectus femoris
acetabular notch
capsule of hip joint at cranial border of acetabulum
ligament of femoral head
m. iliacus medialis
transverse acetabular ligament
m. sartorius
a.v. circumflexa femoris lateralis
n. femoralis
a.v. femoralis
lnn. inguinales profundi
n. cutaneus femoris caudalis
mm. gemelli
lesser ischiatic foramen
sacrotuberous ligament, caudal border
m. obturatorius internus (pars iliaca et pars ischiopubica)
tuber ischiadicum
ischium
m. biceps femoris, origin from ischium
m. obturatorius externus
m. quadratus femoris
m. semitendinosus, caput pelvinum
m. semimembranosus
m. ischiocavernosus
v. obturatoria
penile body
m. bulbospongiosus
m. pectineus
a.v. profunda femoris
n. obturatorius
m. adductor
symphyseal tendon
accessory ligament of femur
m. gracilis
a.v. obturatoria

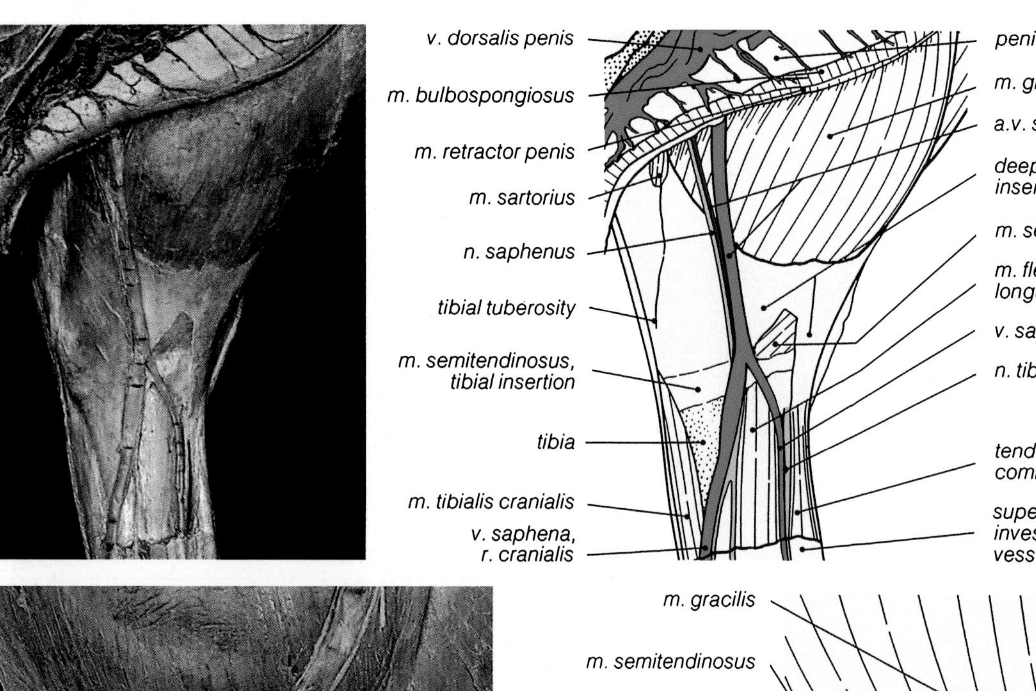
v. dorsalis penis
m. bulbospongiosus
m. retractor penis
m. sartorius
n. saphenus
tibial tuberosity
m. semitendinosus, tibial insertion
tibia
m. tibialis cranialis
v. saphena, r. cranialis
penile body
m. gracilis
a.v. saphena
deep crural fascia and insertion of m. gracilis
m. semitendinosus
m. flexor digitorum longus
v. saphena, r. caudalis
n. tibialis
tendo calcaneus communis
superficial crural fascia investing superficial vessels and nerves

Fig. 6.27 Superficial structures of the right femoral and crural regions in the gelding: medial view. A window cut in the deep crural fascia and tendon of the gracilis muscle shows the tibial insertion of the semitendinosus muscle.

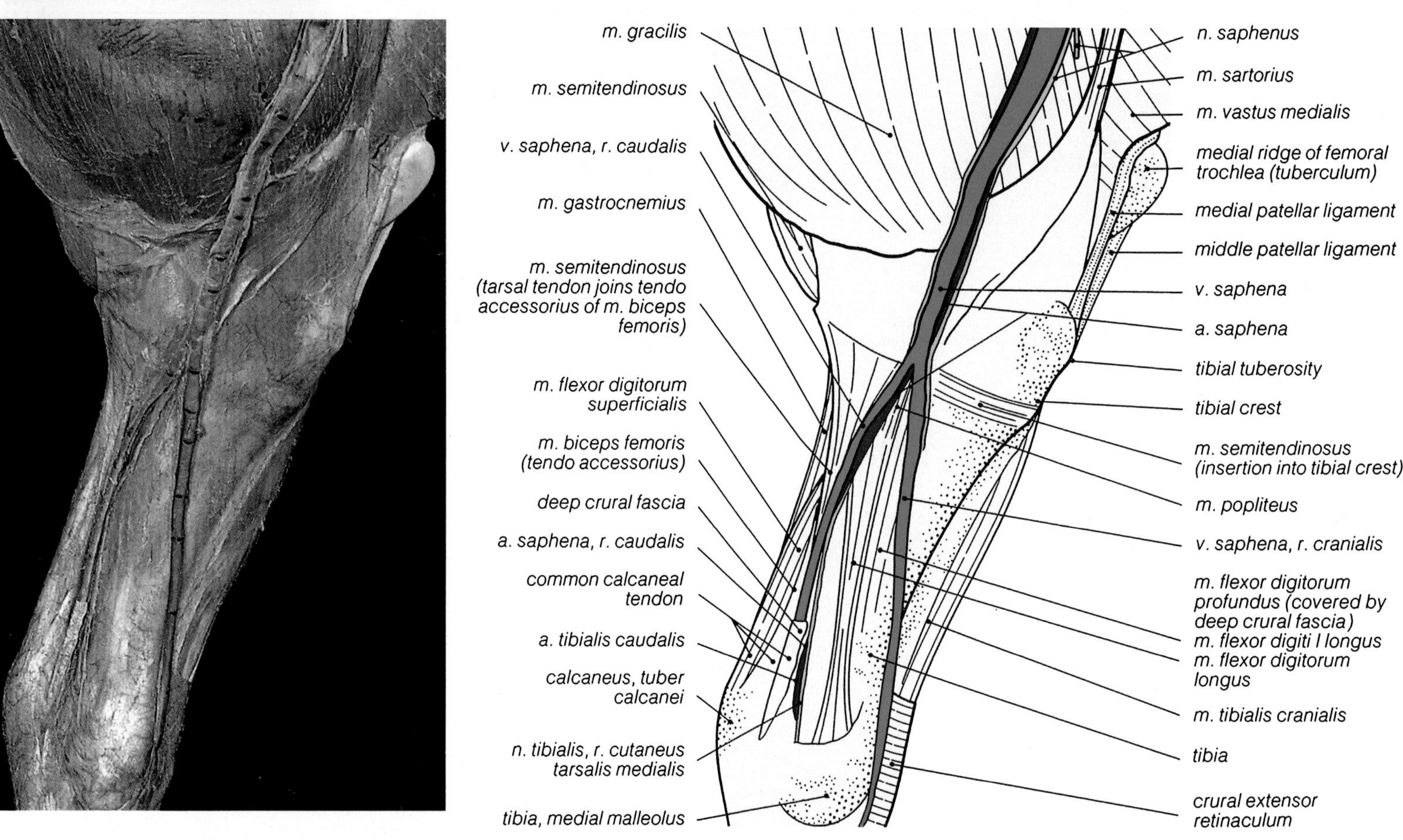
m. gracilis
m. semitendinosus
v. saphena, r. caudalis
m. gastrocnemius
m. semitendinosus (tarsal tendon joins tendo accessorius of m. biceps femoris)
m. flexor digitorum superficialis
m. biceps femoris (tendo accessorius)
deep crural fascia
a. saphena, r. caudalis
common calcaneal tendon
a. tibialis caudalis
calcaneus, tuber calcanei
n. tibialis, r. cutaneus tarsalis medialis
tibia, medial malleolus
n. saphenus
m. sartorius
m. vastus medialis
medial ridge of femoral trochlea (tuberculum)
medial patellar ligament
middle patellar ligament
v. saphena
a. saphena
tibial tuberosity
tibial crest
m. semitendinosus (insertion into tibial crest)
m. popliteus
v. saphena, r. cranialis
m. flexor digitorum profundus (covered by deep crural fascia)
m. flexor digiti I longus
m. flexor digitorum longus
m. tibialis cranialis
tibia
crural extensor retinaculum

Fig. 6.28 The left saphenous artery, vein and nerve: medial view. The superficial dissection of this region is shown in Fig. 6.13. The tarsal tendon of the semitendinosus muscle, which blends with the deep crural fascia, has been partly resected to show the caudal saphenous vein and the tibial nerve more clearly (see also Fig. 6.29).

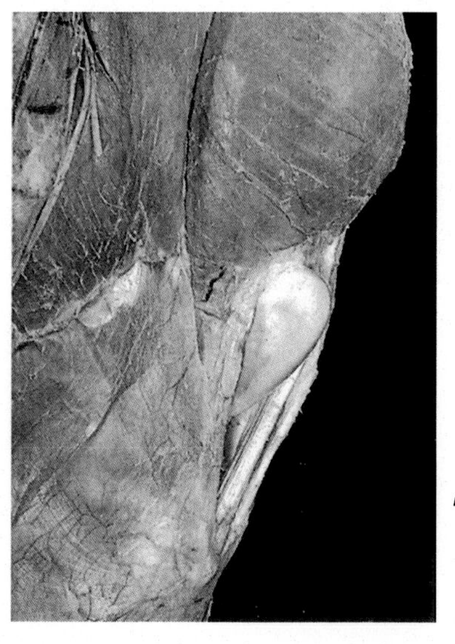

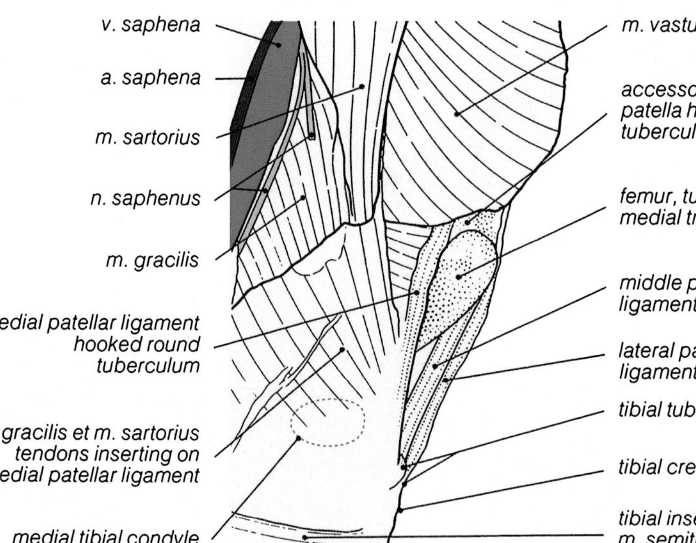
v. saphena
a. saphena
m. sartorius
n. saphenus
m. gracilis
medial patellar ligament hooked round tuberculum
m. gracilis et m. sartorius tendons inserting on medial patellar ligament
medial tibial condyle
m. vastus medialis
accessory cartilage of patella hooked over tuberculum
femur, tuberculum of medial trochlear ridge
middle patellar ligament
lateral patellar ligament
tibial tuberosity
tibial crest
tibial insertion of m. semitendinosus

Fig. 6.29 The stifle joint locked in extension: medial view. This is a closer view of a part of the dissection shown in Fig. 6.28. The genual (stifle) joint was fixed in full extension and shows the 'patellar locking mechanism' in action.

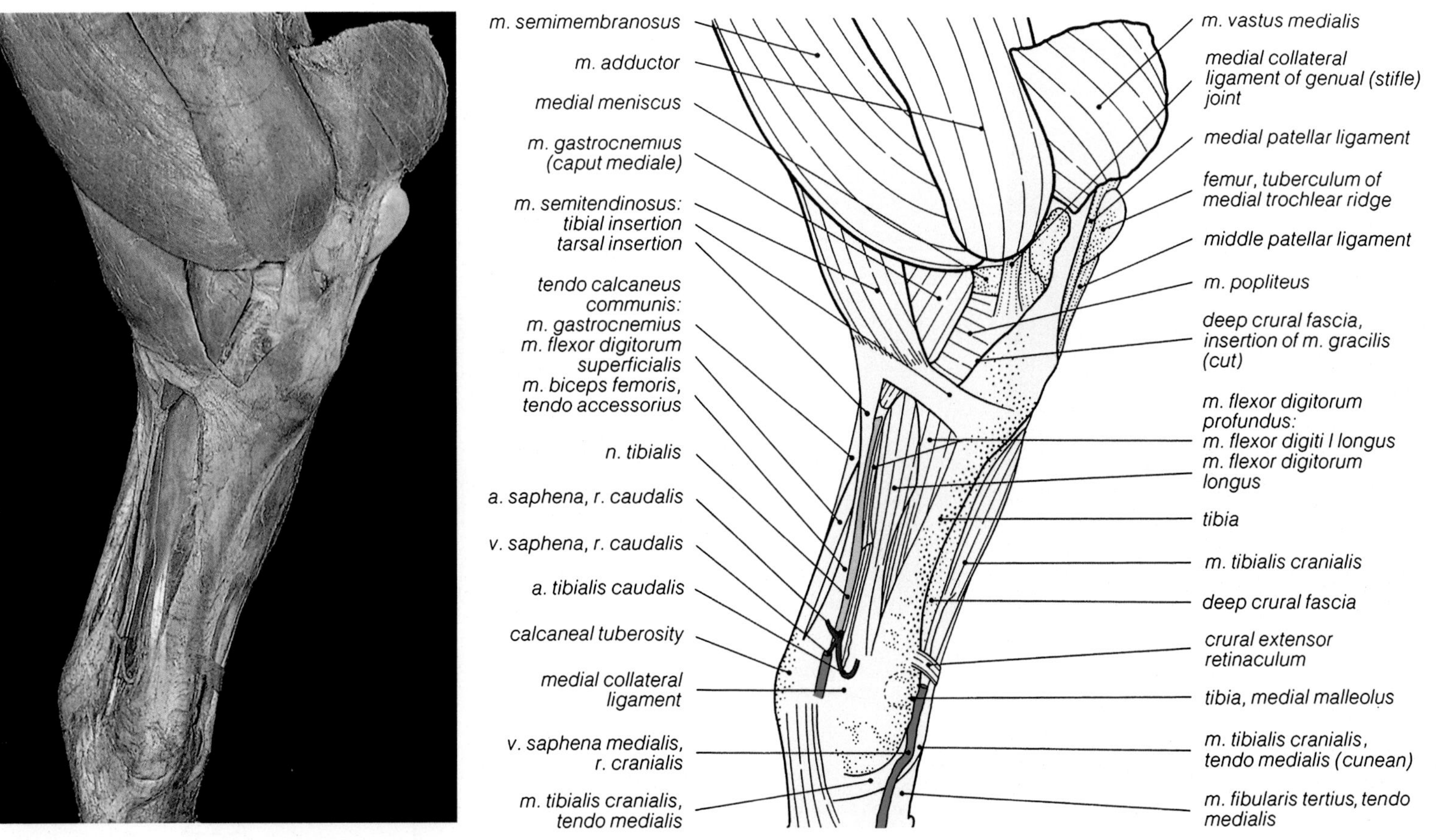
m. semimembranosus
m. adductor
medial meniscus
m. gastrocnemius (caput mediale)
m. semitendinosus: tibial insertion tarsal insertion
tendo calcaneus communis: m. gastrocnemius m. flexor digitorum superficialis m. biceps femoris, tendo accessorius
n. tibialis
a. saphena, r. caudalis
v. saphena, r. caudalis
a. tibialis caudalis
calcaneal tuberosity
medial collateral ligament
v. saphena medialis, r. cranialis
m. tibialis cranialis, tendo medialis
m. vastus medialis
medial collateral ligament of genual (stifle) joint
medial patellar ligament
femur, tuberculum of medial trochlear ridge
middle patellar ligament
m. popliteus
deep crural fascia, insertion of m. gracilis (cut)
m. flexor digitorum profundus: m. flexor digiti I longus m. flexor digitorum longus
tibia
m. tibialis cranialis
deep crural fascia
crural extensor retinaculum
tibia, medial malleolus
m. tibialis cranialis, tendo medialis (cunean)
m. fibularis tertius, tendo medialis

Fig. 6.30 Left stifle, crural and tarsal regions: medial view. The gracilis and sartorius muscles and the deep fascia have been removed. This dissection is also shown in Figs. 6.31 and 6.32.

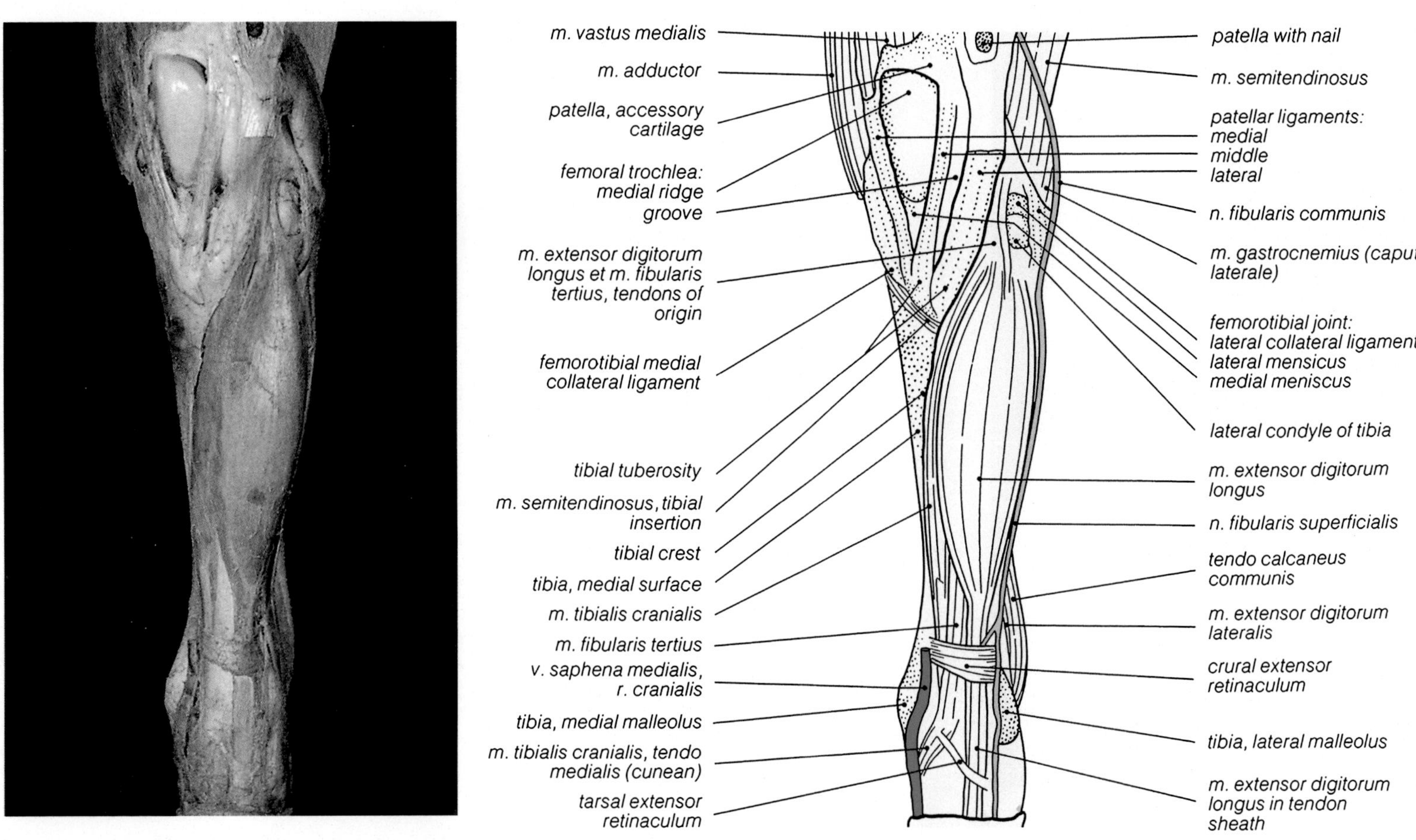
m. vastus medialis
m. adductor
patella, accessory cartilage
femoral trochlea: medial ridge groove
m. extensor digitorum longus et m. fibularis tertius, tendons of origin
femorotibial medial collateral ligament
tibial tuberosity
m. semitendinosus, tibial insertion
tibial crest
tibia, medial surface
m. tibialis cranialis
m. fibularis tertius
v. saphena medialis, r. cranialis
tibia, medial malleolus
m. tibialis cranialis, tendo medialis (cunean)
tarsal extensor retinaculum
patella with nail
m. semitendinosus
patellar ligaments: medial middle lateral
n. fibularis communis
m. gastrocnemius (caput laterale)
femorotibial joint: lateral collateral ligament lateral mensicus medial meniscus
lateral condyle of tibia
m. extensor digitorum longus
n. fibularis superficialis
tendo calcaneus communis
m. extensor digitorum lateralis
crural extensor retinaculum
tibia, lateral malleolus
m. extensor digitorum longus in tendon sheath

Fig. 6.31 Left stifle, crural and tarsal regions: cranial view. This dissection is also shown in Figs. 6.30 and 6.32.

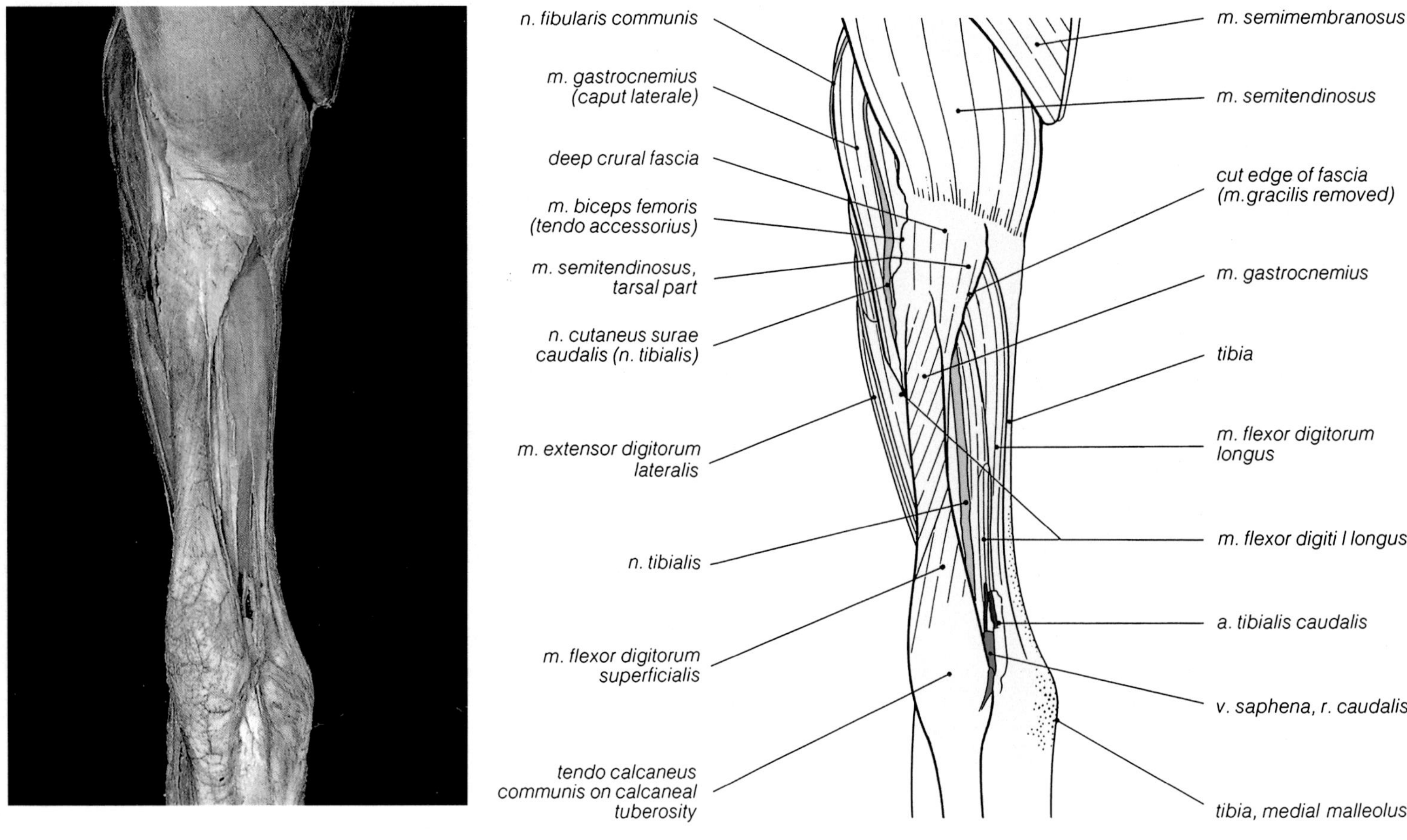
n. fibularis communis
m. gastrocnemius (caput laterale)
deep crural fascia
m. biceps femoris (tendo accessorius)
m. semitendinosus, tarsal part
n. cutaneus surae caudalis (n. tibialis)
m. extensor digitorum lateralis
n. tibialis
m. flexor digitorum superficialis
tendo calcaneus communis on calcaneal tuberosity
m. semimembranosus
m. semitendinosus
cut edge of fascia (m.gracilis removed)
m. gastrocnemius
tibia
m. flexor digitorum longus
m. flexor digiti I longus
a. tibialis caudalis
v. saphena, r. caudalis
tibia, medial malleolus

Fig. 6.32 Left stifle, crural and tarsal regions: caudal view. This dissection is also shown in Figs. 6.30 and 6.31.

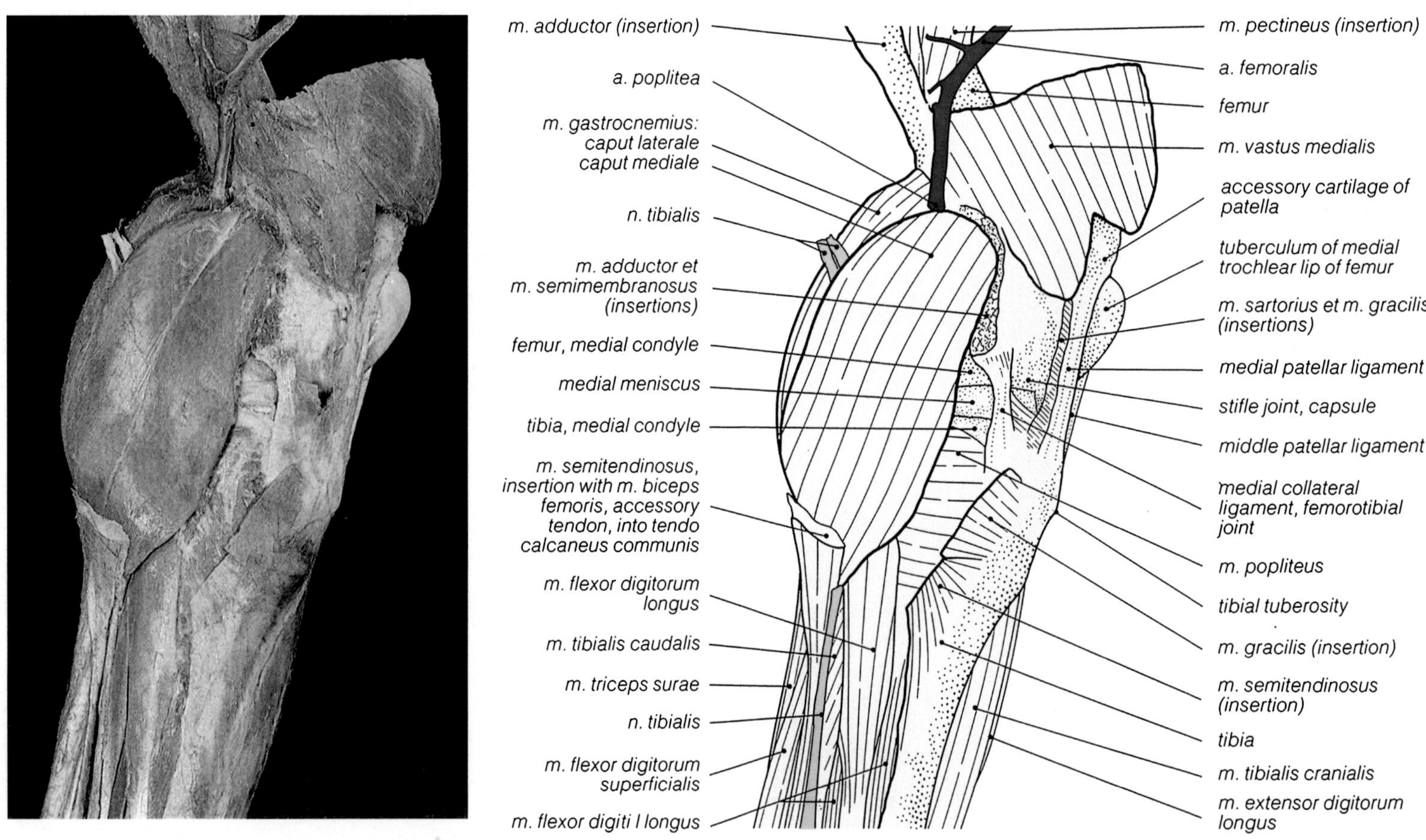
m. adductor (insertion)
a. poplitea
m. gastrocnemius:
caput laterale
caput mediale
n. tibialis
m. adductor et m. semimembranosus (insertions)
femur, medial condyle
medial meniscus
tibia, medial condyle
m. semitendinosus, insertion with m. biceps femoris, accessory tendon, into tendo calcaneus communis
m. flexor digitorum longus
m. tibialis caudalis
m. triceps surae
n. tibialis
m. flexor digitorum superficialis
m. flexor digiti I longus
m. pectineus (insertion)
a. femoralis
femur
m. vastus medialis
accessory cartilage of patella
tuberculum of medial trochlear lip of femur
m. sartorius et m. gracilis (insertions)
medial patellar ligament
stifle joint, capsule
middle patellar ligament
medial collateral ligament, femorotibial joint
m. popliteus
tibial tuberosity
m. gracilis (insertion)
m. semitendinosus (insertion)
tibia
m. tibialis cranialis
m. extensor digitorum longus

Fig. 6.33 Left stifle region: medial view. The adductor, semimembranosus and semitendinosus muscles (see Fig. 6.30) have been removed to expose the medial aspect of the stifle joint. The patella has been fixed in the 'locked' position.

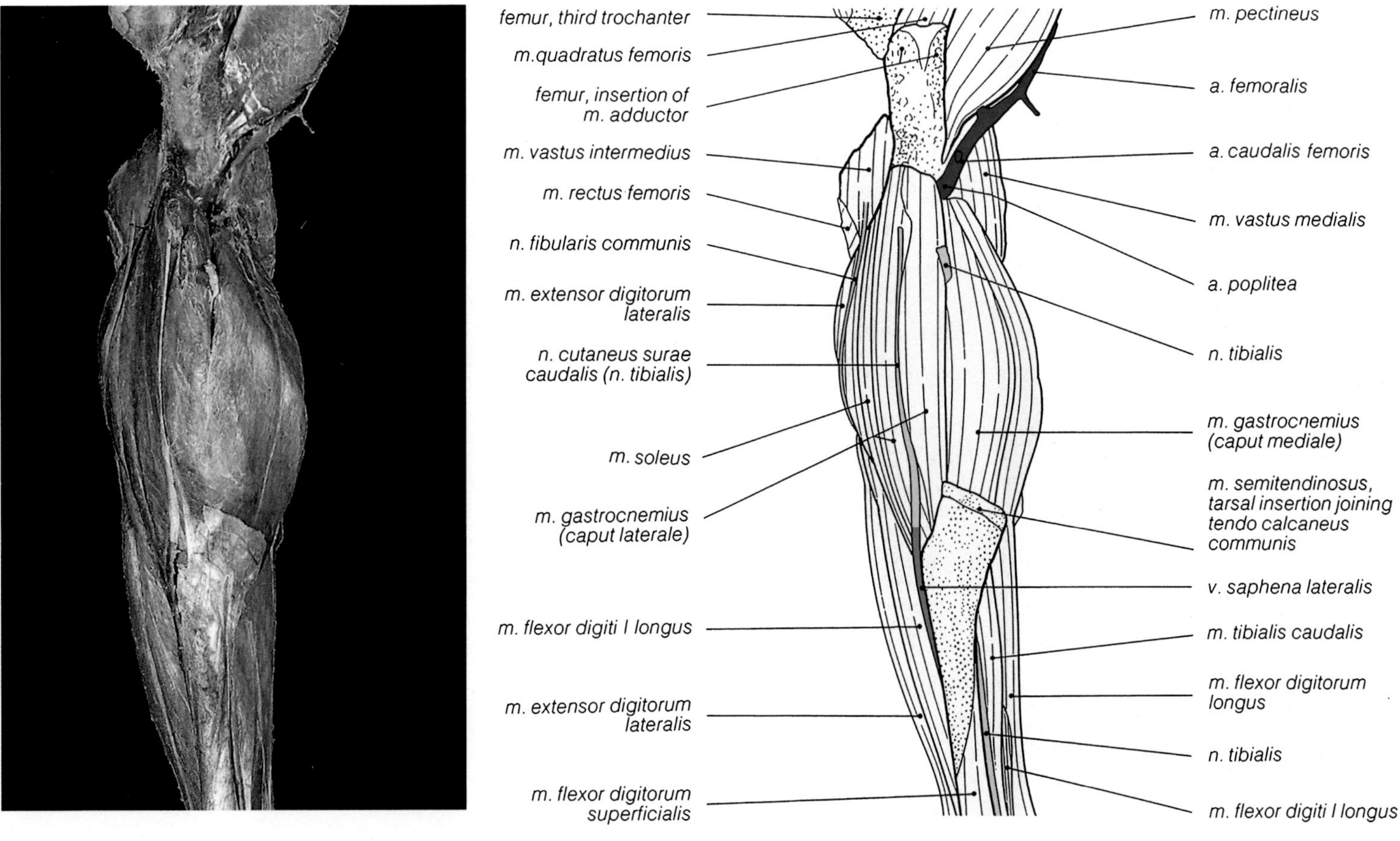
femur, third trochanter
m.quadratus femoris
femur, insertion of m. adductor
m. vastus intermedius
m. rectus femoris
n. fibularis communis
m. extensor digitorum lateralis
n. cutaneus surae caudalis (n. tibialis)
m. soleus
m. gastrocnemius (caput laterale)
m. flexor digiti I longus
m. extensor digitorum lateralis
m. flexor digitorum superficialis
m. pectineus
a. femoralis
a. caudalis femoris
m. vastus medialis
a. poplitea
n. tibialis
m. gastrocnemius (caput mediale)
m. semitendinosus, tarsal insertion joining tendo calcaneus communis
v. saphena lateralis
m. tibialis caudalis
m. flexor digitorum longus
n. tibialis
m. flexor digiti I longus

Fig. 6.34 The left crural region: caudal view. The specimen is at the same stage of dissection as that shown in Fig. 6.33.

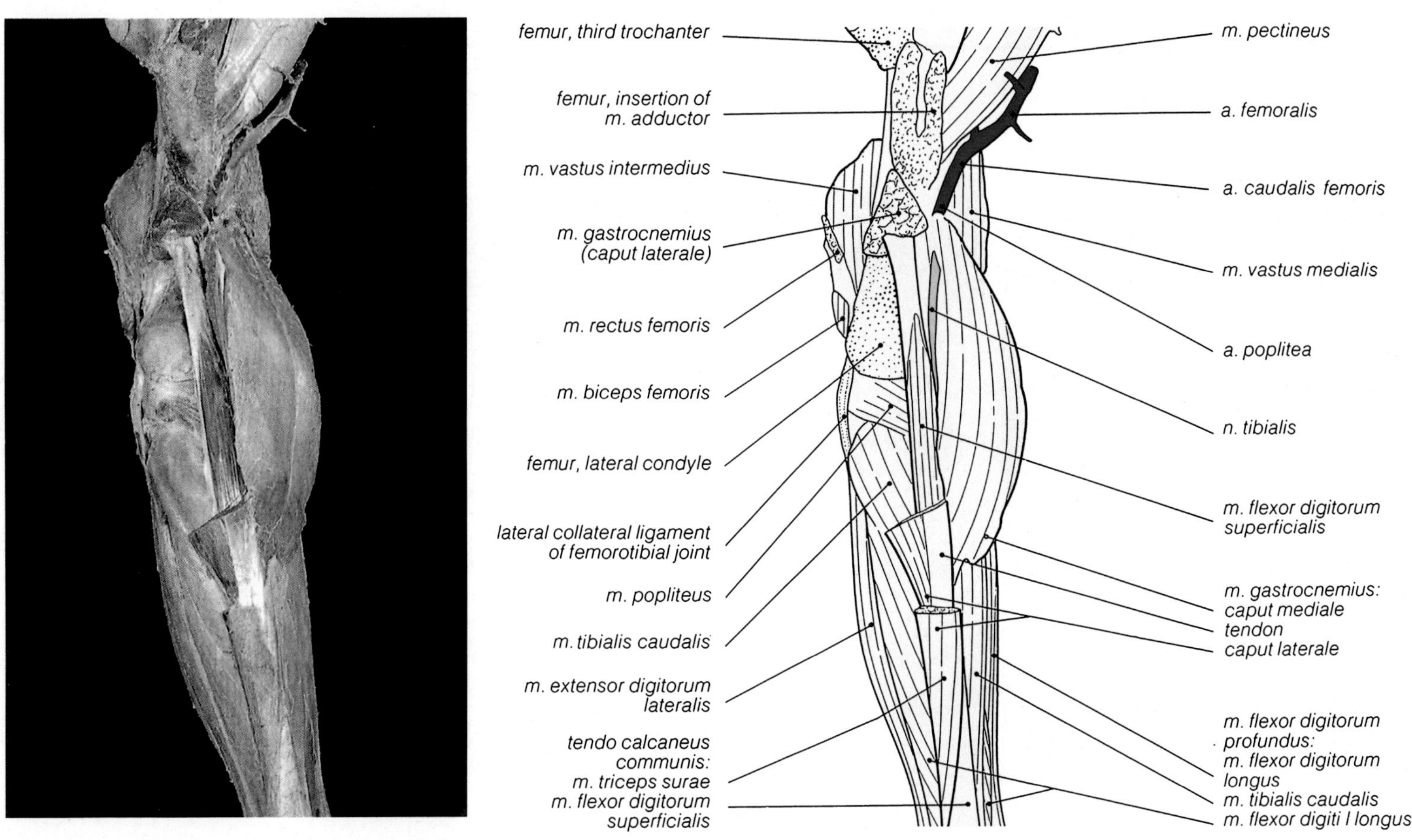
femur, third trochanter
femur, insertion of m. adductor
m. vastus intermedius
m. gastrocnemius (caput laterale)
m. rectus femoris
m. biceps femoris
femur, lateral condyle
lateral collateral ligament of femorotibial joint
m. popliteus
m. tibialis caudalis
m. extensor digitorum lateralis
tendo calcaneus communis:
m. triceps surae
m. flexor digitorum superficialis
m. pectineus
a. femoralis
a. caudalis femoris
m. vastus medialis
a. poplitea
n. tibialis
m. flexor digitorum superficialis
m. gastrocnemius:
caput mediale
tendon
caput laterale
m. flexor digitorum profundus:
m. flexor digitorum longus
m. tibialis caudalis
m. flexor digiti I longus

Fig. 6.35 The left stifle and crural regions: caudal view. The lateral head of the gastrocnemius muscle has now been removed (compare with Fig. 6.34) to show the superficial digital flexor and popliteus muscles.

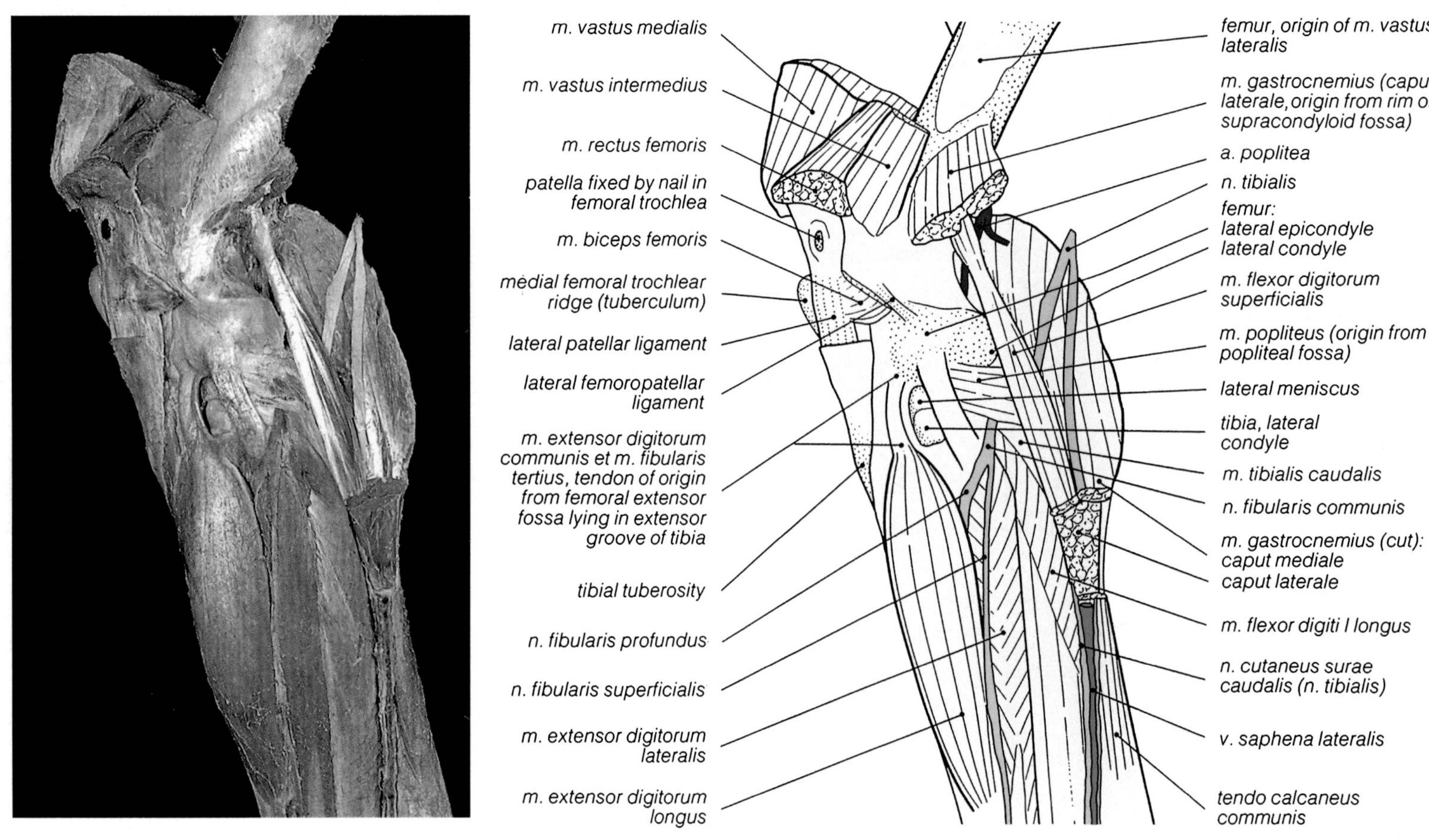
m. vastus medialis
m. vastus intermedius
m. rectus femoris
patella fixed by nail in femoral trochlea
m. biceps femoris
medial femoral trochlear ridge (tuberculum)
lateral patellar ligament
lateral femoropatellar ligament
m. extensor digitorum communis et m. fibularis tertius, tendon of origin from femoral extensor fossa lying in extensor groove of tibia
tibial tuberosity
n. fibularis profundus
n. fibularis superficialis
m. extensor digitorum lateralis
m. extensor digitorum longus
femur, origin of m. vastus lateralis
m. gastrocnemius (caput laterale, origin from rim of supracondyloid fossa)
a. poplitea
n. tibialis
femur:
lateral epicondyle
lateral condyle
m. flexor digitorum superficialis
m. popliteus (origin from popliteal fossa)
lateral meniscus
tibia, lateral condyle
m. tibialis caudalis
n. fibularis communis
m. gastrocnemius (cut):
caput mediale
caput laterale
m. flexor digiti I longus
n. cutaneus surae caudalis (n. tibialis)
v. saphena lateralis
tendo calcaneus communis

Fig. 6.36 The left stifle region and popliteal space: left lateral view. The specimen is at the same stage of dissection as that shown in Fig. 6.35.

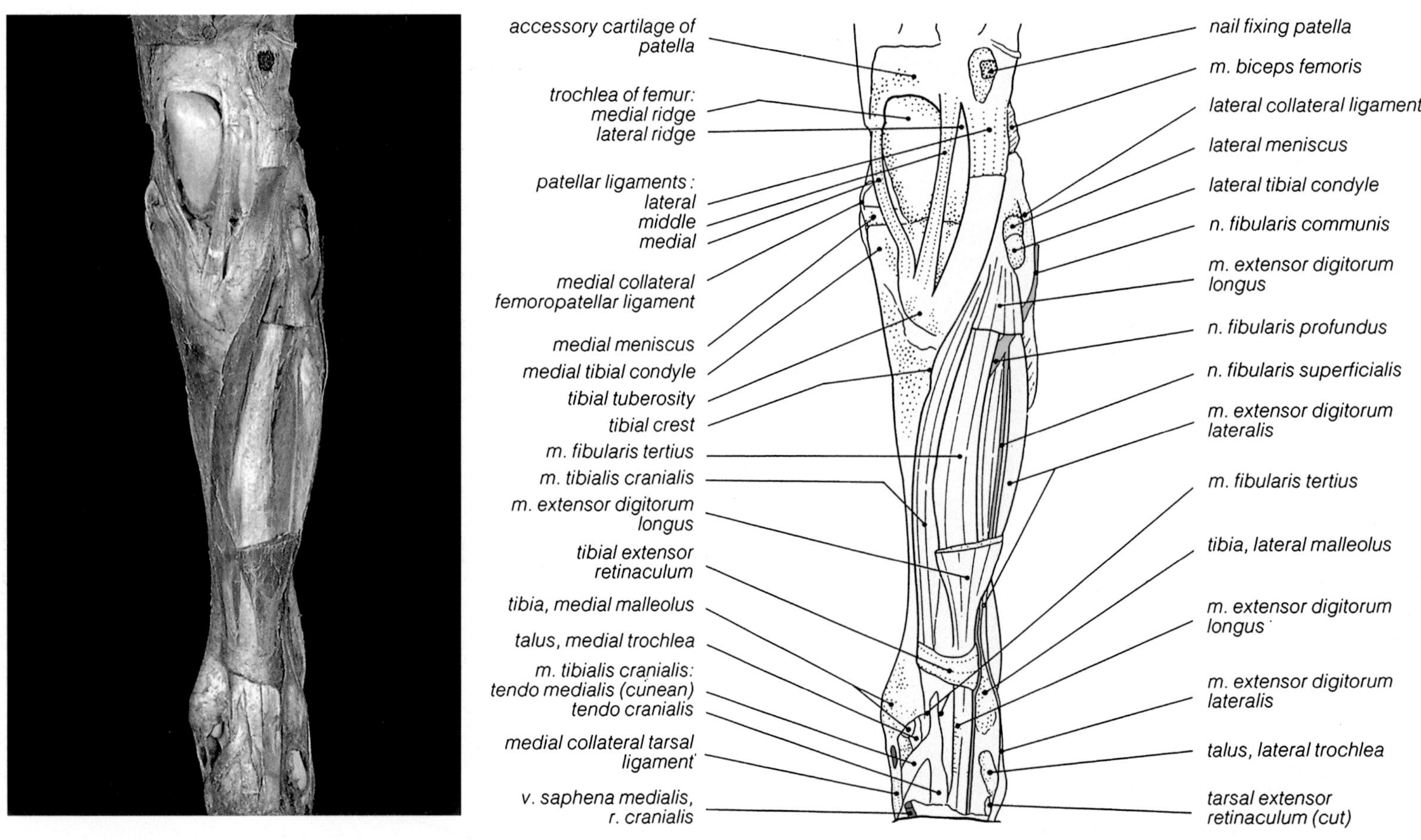
accessory cartilage of patella
trochlea of femur:
medial ridge
lateral ridge
patellar ligaments:
lateral
middle
medial
medial collateral femoropatellar ligament
medial meniscus
medial tibial condyle
tibial tuberosity
tibial crest
m. fibularis tertius
m. tibialis cranialis
m. extensor digitorum longus
tibial extensor retinaculum
tibia, medial malleolus
talus, medial trochlea
m. tibialis cranialis:
tendo medialis (cunean)
tendo cranialis
medial collateral tarsal ligament
v. saphena medialis, r. cranialis
nail fixing patella
m. biceps femoris
lateral collateral ligament
lateral meniscus
lateral tibial condyle
n. fibularis communis
m. extensor digitorum longus
n. fibularis profundus
n. fibularis superficialis
m. extensor digitorum lateralis
m. fibularis tertius
tibia, lateral malleolus
m. extensor digitorum longus
m. extensor digitorum lateralis
talus, lateral trochlea
tarsal extensor retinaculum (cut)

Fig. 6.37 The left stifle, crural and tarsal regions: cranial view. The middle part of the muscle belly of the long digital extensor muscle has been resected to show the fibrous belly of the third fibular muscle. The joint cavities of the stifle and tarsocrural joints have been opened to demonstrate their positions more definitely. This dissection is also shown in Figs. 6.38 and 6.39.

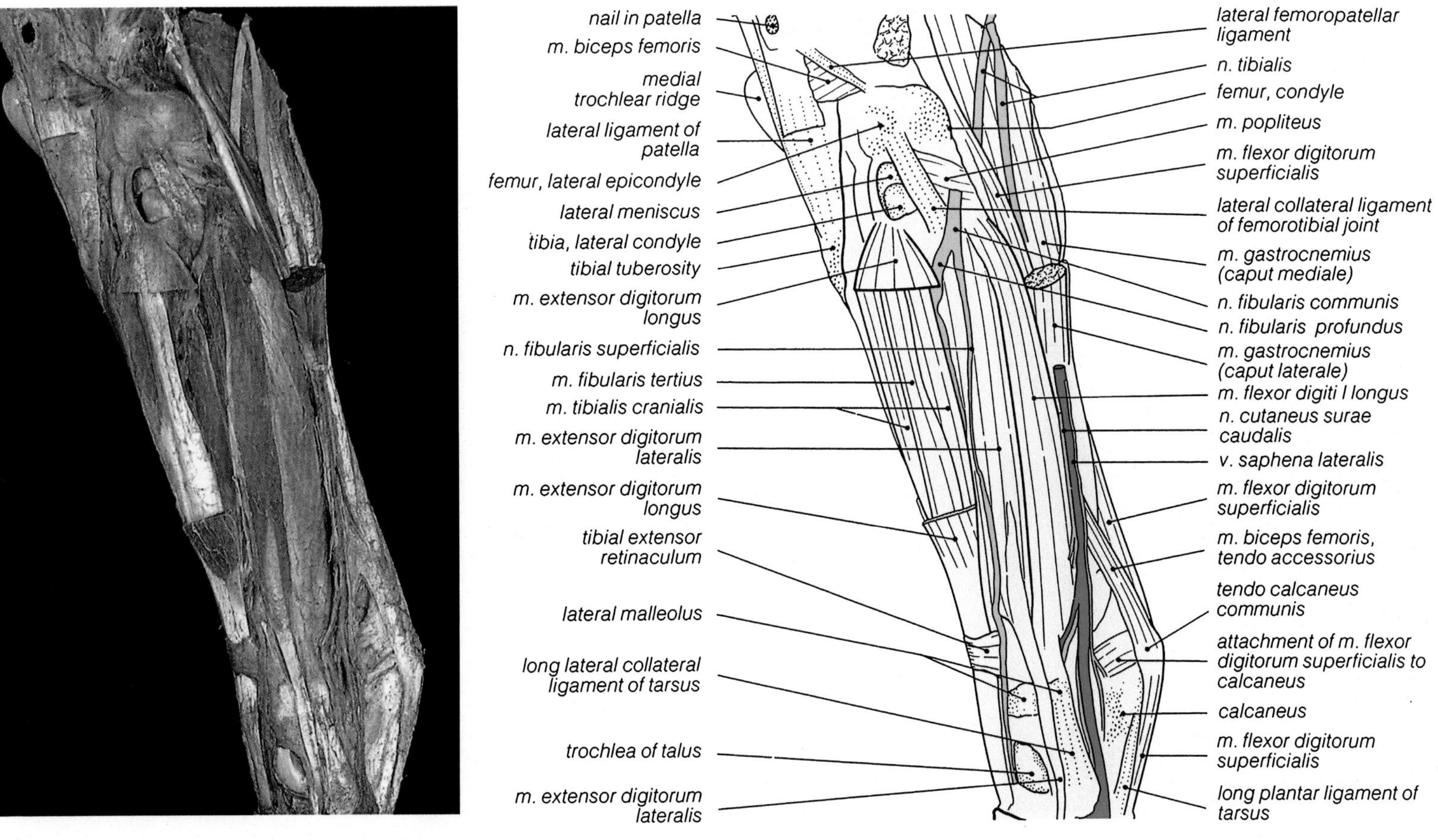

nail in patella
m. biceps femoris
medial trochlear ridge
lateral ligament of patella
femur, lateral epicondyle
lateral meniscus
tibia, lateral condyle
tibial tuberosity
m. extensor digitorum longus
n. fibularis superficialis
m. fibularis tertius
m. tibialis cranialis
m. extensor digitorum lateralis
m. extensor digitorum longus
tibial extensor retinaculum
lateral malleolus
long lateral collateral ligament of tarsus
trochlea of talus
m. extensor digitorum lateralis
lateral femoropatellar ligament
n. tibialis
femur, condyle
m. popliteus
m. flexor digitorum superficialis
lateral collateral ligament of femorotibial joint
m. gastrocnemius (caput mediale)
n. fibularis communis
n. fibularis profundus
m. gastrocnemius (caput laterale)
m. flexor digiti I longus
n. cutaneus surae caudalis
v. saphena lateralis
m. flexor digitorum superficialis
m. biceps femoris, tendo accessorius
tendo calcaneus communis
attachment of m. flexor digitorum superficialis to calcaneus
calcaneus
m. flexor digitorum superficialis
long plantar ligament of tarsus

Fig. 6.38 The left stifle, crural and tarsal regions: lateral view. The specimen is at the stage of dissection shown in Figs. 6.37 and 6.39.

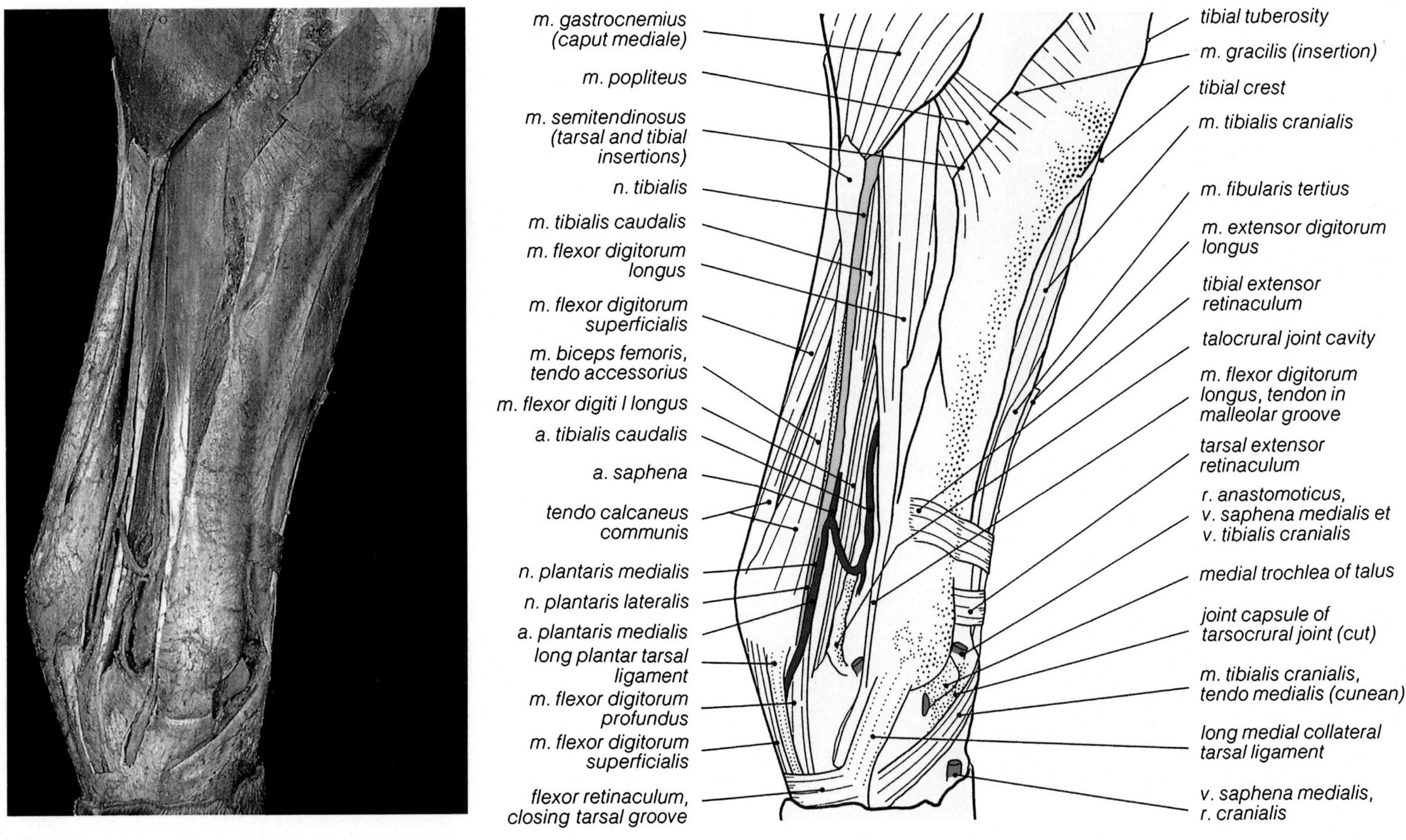

m. gastrocnemius (caput mediale)
m. popliteus
m. semitendinosus (tarsal and tibial insertions)
n. tibialis
m. tibialis caudalis
m. flexor digitorum longus
m. flexor digitorum superficialis
m. biceps femoris, tendo accessorius
m. flexor digiti I longus
a. tibialis caudalis
a. saphena
tendo calcaneus communis
n. plantaris medialis
n. plantaris lateralis
a. plantaris medialis
long plantar tarsal ligament
m. flexor digitorum profundus
m. flexor digitorum superficialis
flexor retinaculum, closing tarsal groove
tibial tuberosity
m. gracilis (insertion)
tibial crest
m. tibialis cranialis
m. fibularis tertius
m. extensor digitorum longus
tibial extensor retinaculum
talocrural joint cavity
m. flexor digitorum longus, tendon in malleolar groove
tarsal extensor retinaculum
r. anastomoticus, v. saphena medialis et v. tibialis cranialis
medial trochlea of talus
joint capsule of tarsocrural joint (cut)
m. tibialis cranialis, tendo medialis (cunean)
long medial collateral tarsal ligament
v. saphena medialis, r. cranialis

Fig. 6.39 The left crural and tarsal regions: medial view. The specimen is at the stage of dissection shown in Figs. 6.37 and 6.38.

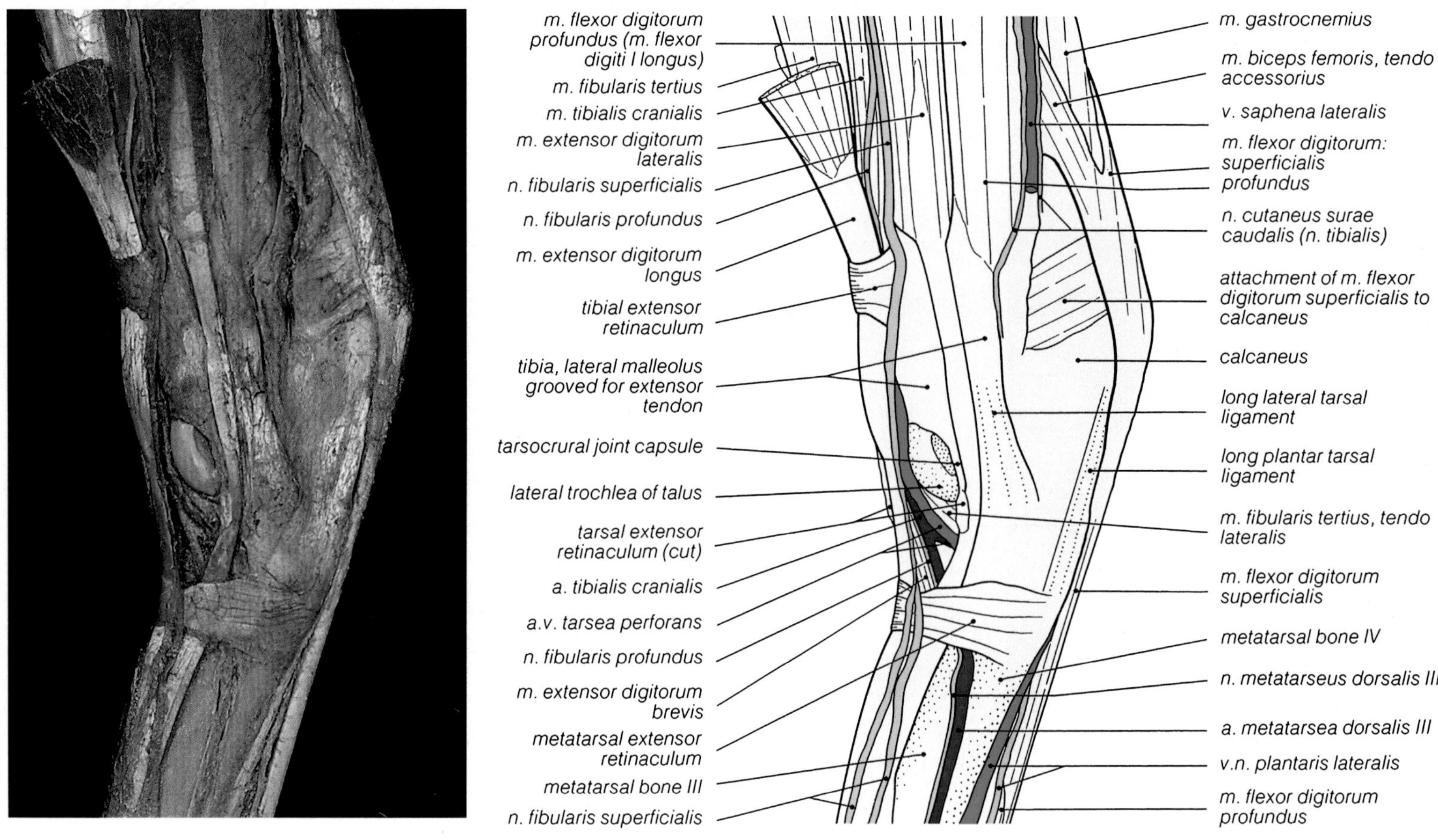
m. flexor digitorum profundus (m. flexor digiti I longus)
m. fibularis tertius
m. tibialis cranialis
m. extensor digitorum lateralis
n. fibularis superficialis
n. fibularis profundus
m. extensor digitorum longus
tibial extensor retinaculum
tibia, lateral malleolus grooved for extensor tendon
tarsocrural joint capsule
lateral trochlea of talus
tarsal extensor retinaculum (cut)
a. tibialis cranialis
a.v. tarsea perforans
n. fibularis profundus
m. extensor digitorum brevis
metatarsal extensor retinaculum
metatarsal bone III
n. fibularis superficialis
m. gastrocnemius
m. biceps femoris, tendo accessorius
v. saphena lateralis
m. flexor digitorum: superficialis profundus
n. cutaneus surae caudalis (n. tibialis)
attachment of m. flexor digitorum superficialis to calcaneus
calcaneus
long lateral tarsal ligament
long plantar tarsal ligament
m. fibularis tertius, tendo lateralis
m. flexor digitorum superficialis
metatarsal bone IV
n. metatarseus dorsalis III
a. metatarsea dorsalis III
v.n. plantaris lateralis
m. flexor digitorum profundus

Fig. 6.40 The left tarsus: lateral view. The lateral saphenous vein and the accompanying nerve have been shortened to simplify the dissection of the lateral region of the tarsus. The tarsal retinaculum has been cut to reveal the cranial tibial vessels more clearly. A medial view of the tarsus is shown in Fig. 6.44. See also Figs. 6.57 and 6.58.

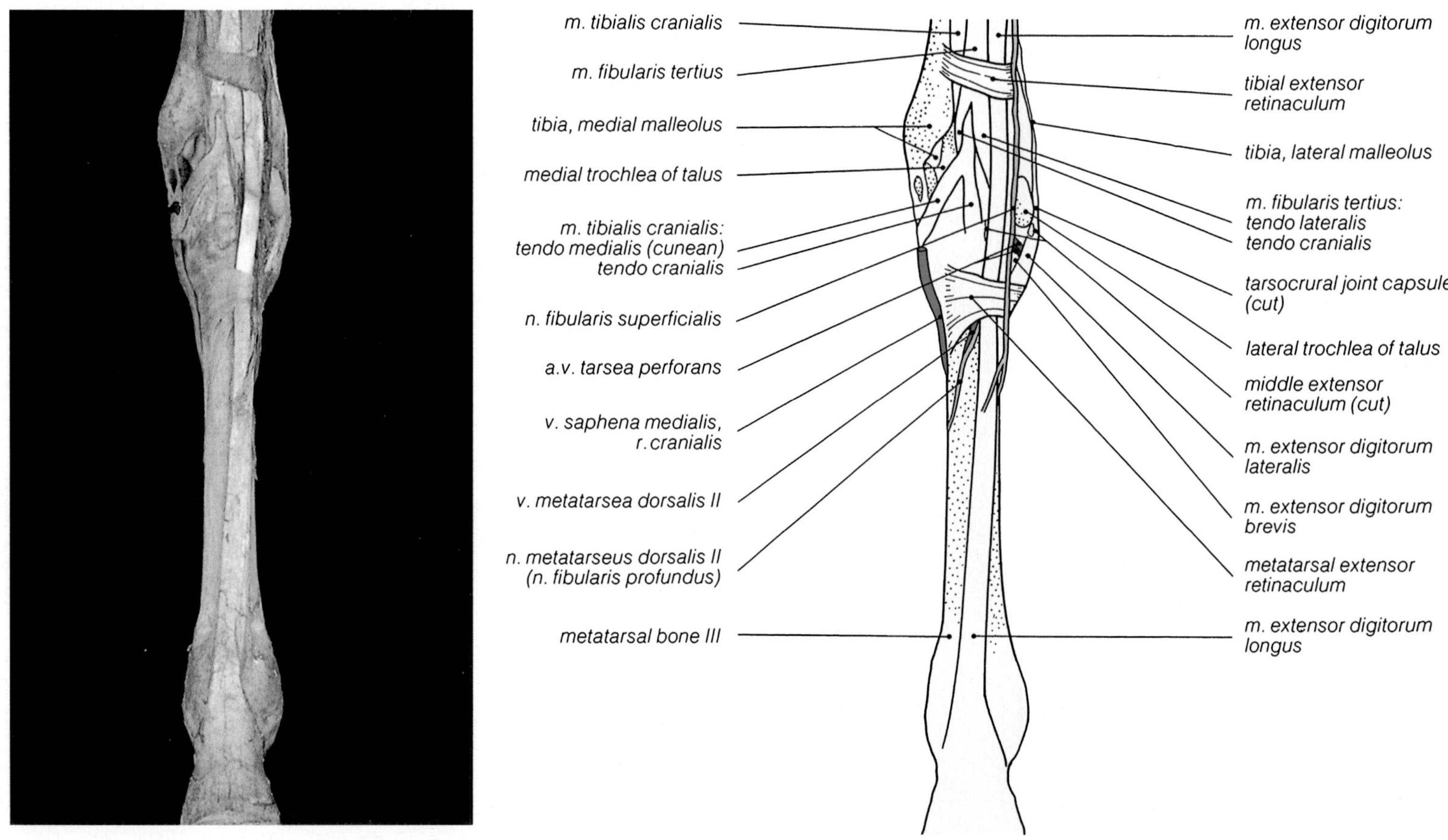
m. tibialis cranialis
m. fibularis tertius
tibia, medial malleolus
medial trochlea of talus
m. tibialis cranialis: tendo medialis (cunean) tendo cranialis
n. fibularis superficialis
a.v. tarsea perforans
v. saphena medialis, r. cranialis
v. metatarsea dorsalis II
n. metatarseus dorsalis II (n. fibularis profundus)
metatarsal bone III
m. extensor digitorum longus
tibial extensor retinaculum
tibia, lateral malleolus
m. fibularis tertius: tendo lateralis tendo cranialis
tarsocrural joint capsule (cut)
lateral trochlea of talus
middle extensor retinaculum (cut)
m. extensor digitorum lateralis
m. extensor digitorum brevis
metatarsal extensor retinaculum
m. extensor digitorum longus

Fig. 6.41 The left tarsus and metatarsus: dorsal view. The tarsal extensor retinaculum has been removed and medial and lateral parts of the tarsocrural joint cavity have been opened. This dissection is also shown in Figs. 6.42 and 6.43.

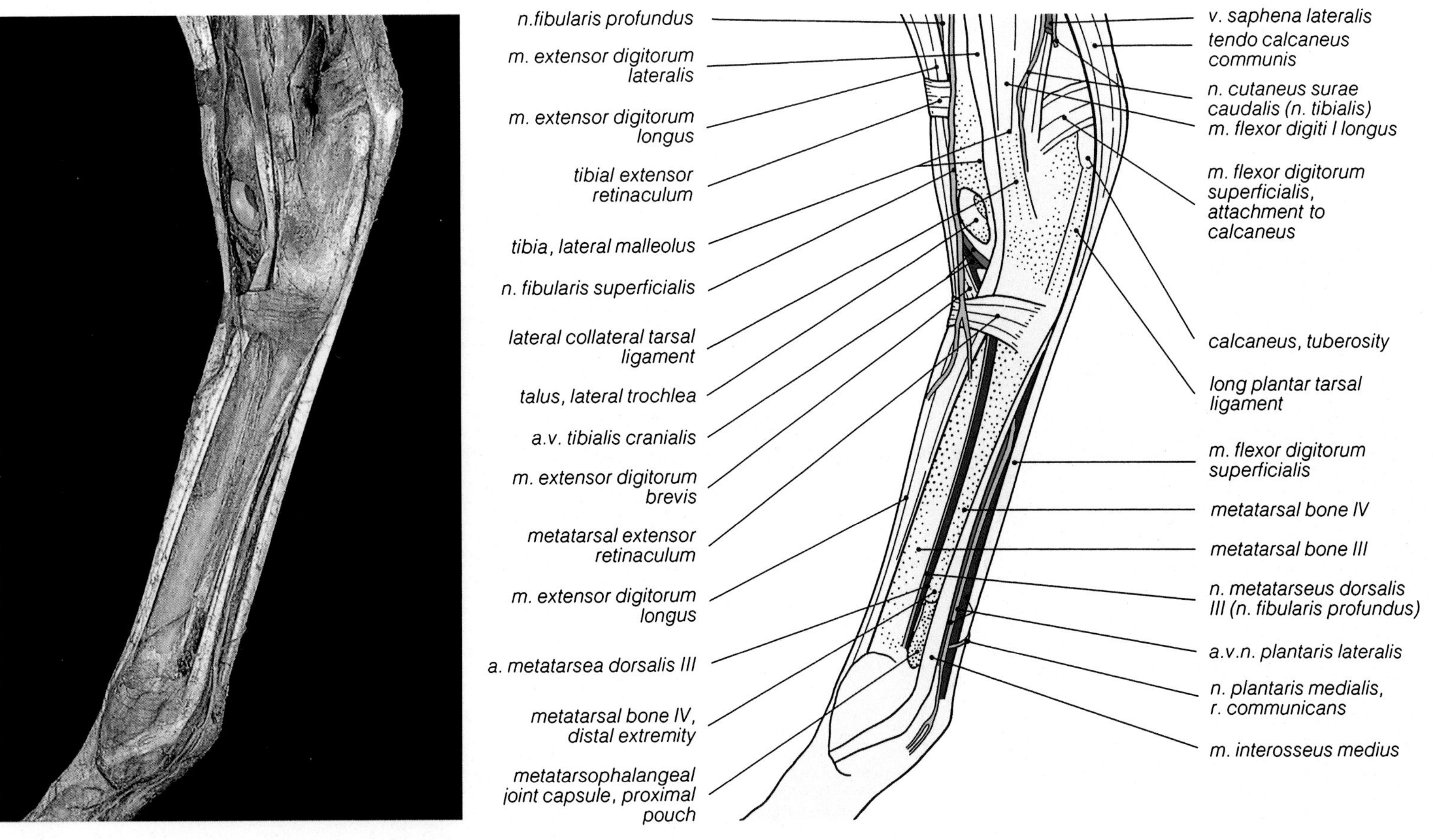
n.fibularis profundus
m. extensor digitorum lateralis
m. extensor digitorum longus
tibial extensor retinaculum
tibia, lateral malleolus
n. fibularis superficialis
lateral collateral tarsal ligament
talus, lateral trochlea
a.v. tibialis cranialis
m. extensor digitorum brevis
metatarsal extensor retinaculum
m. extensor digitorum longus
a. metatarsea dorsalis III
metatarsal bone IV, distal extremity
metatarsophalangeal joint capsule, proximal pouch
v. saphena lateralis
tendo calcaneus communis
n. cutaneus surae caudalis (n. tibialis)
m. flexor digiti I longus
m. flexor digitorum superficialis, attachment to calcaneus
calcaneus, tuberosity
long plantar tarsal ligament
m. flexor digitorum superficialis
metatarsal bone IV
metatarsal bone III
n. metatarseus dorsalis III (n. fibularis profundus)
a.v.n. plantaris lateralis
n. plantaris medialis, r. communicans
m. interosseus medius

Fig. 6.42 The left tarsus and metatarsus: lateral view. The tarsal extensor retinaculum has been removed. This dissection is also shown in Figs. 6.41 and 6.43.

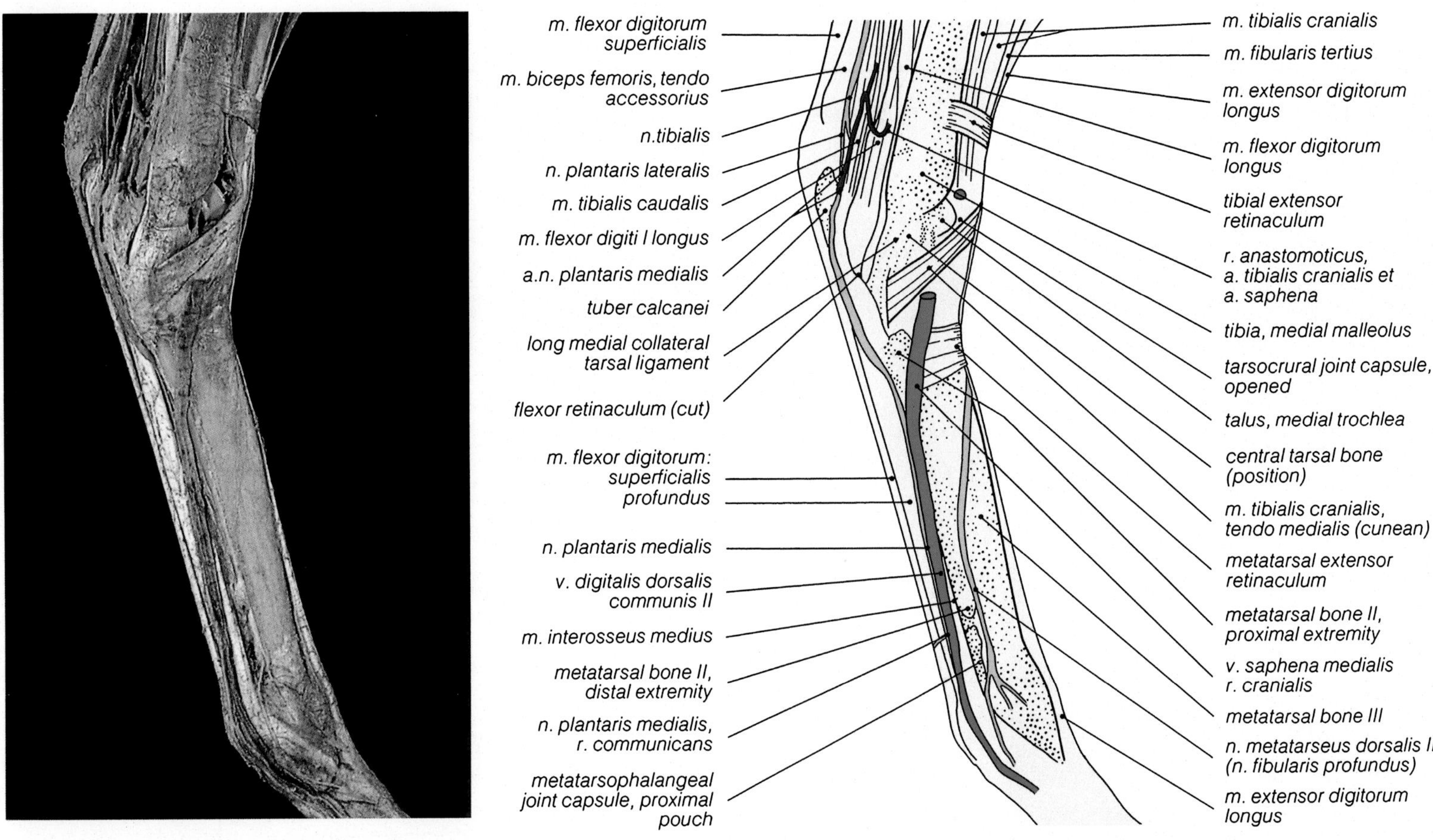
m. flexor digitorum superficialis
m. biceps femoris, tendo accessorius
n.tibialis
n. plantaris lateralis
m. tibialis caudalis
m. flexor digiti I longus
a.n. plantaris medialis
tuber calcanei
long medial collateral tarsal ligament
flexor retinaculum (cut)
m. flexor digitorum: superficialis profundus
n. plantaris medialis
v. digitalis dorsalis communis II
m. interosseus medius
metatarsal bone II, distal extremity
n. plantaris medialis, r. communicans
metatarsophalangeal joint capsule, proximal pouch
m. tibialis cranialis
m. fibularis tertius
m. extensor digitorum longus
m. flexor digitorum longus
tibial extensor retinaculum
r. anastomoticus, a. tibialis cranialis et a. saphena
tibia, medial malleolus
tarsocrural joint capsule, opened
talus, medial trochlea
central tarsal bone (position)
m. tibialis cranialis, tendo medialis (cunean)
metatarsal extensor retinaculum
metatarsal bone II, proximal extremity
v. saphena medialis r. cranialis
metatarsal bone III
n. metatarseus dorsalis II (n. fibularis profundus)
m. extensor digitorum longus

Fig. 6.43 The left tarsus and metatarsus: medial view. This dissection is also shown in Figs. 6.41 and 6.42. The flexor retinaculum which closes the medial aspect of the tarsal groove (see Fig. 6.39) has been cut to show the deep digital flexor tendon and the medial plantar vessels and nerve occupying the tarsal groove (see also Fig. 6.44).

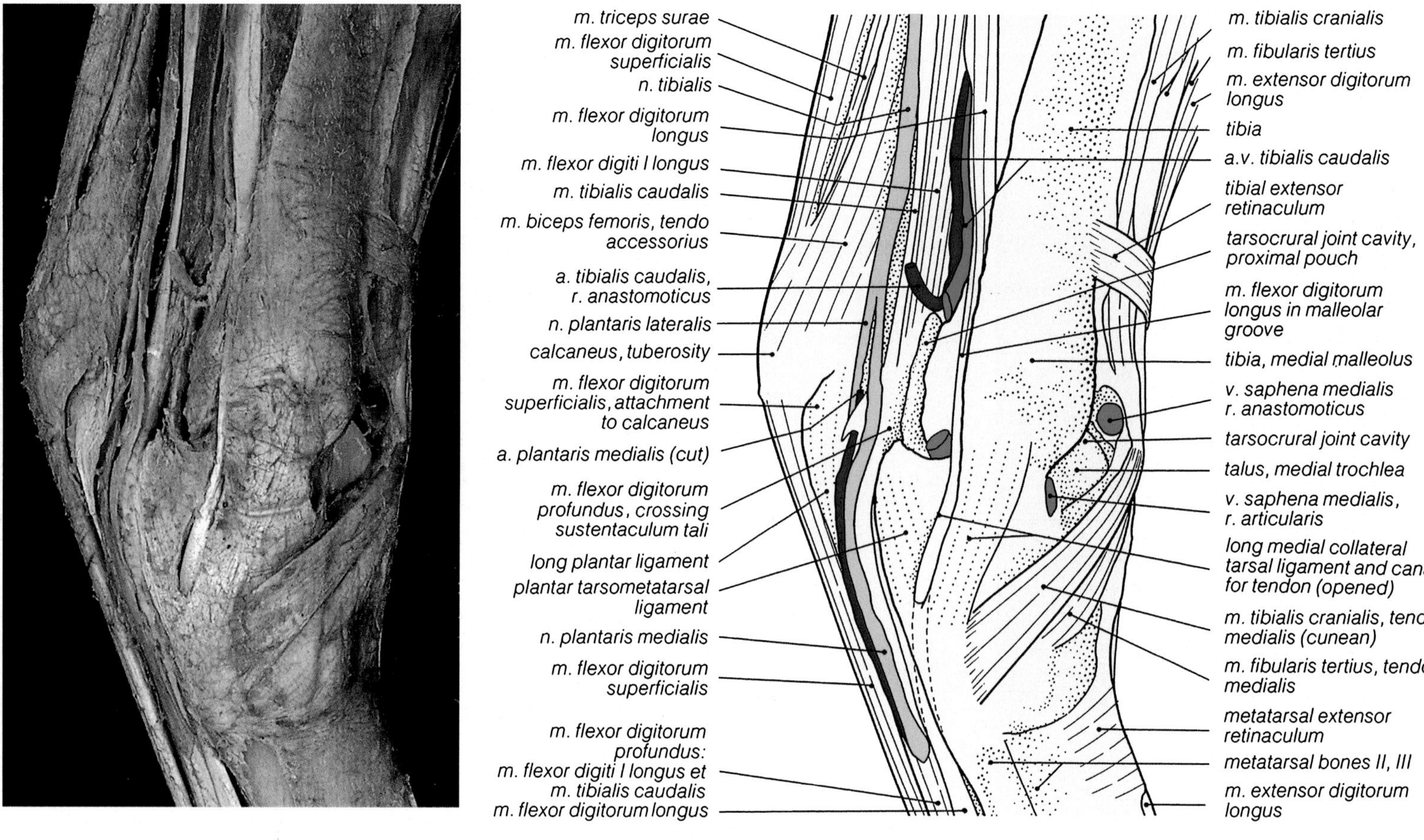
m. triceps surae
m. flexor digitorum superficialis
n. tibialis
m. flexor digitorum longus
m. flexor digiti I longus
m. tibialis caudalis
m. biceps femoris, tendo accessorius
a. tibialis caudalis, r. anastomoticus
n. plantaris lateralis
calcaneus, tuberosity
m. flexor digitorum superficialis, attachment to calcaneus
a. plantaris medialis (cut)
m. flexor digitorum profundus, crossing sustentaculum tali
long plantar ligament
plantar tarsometatarsal ligament
n. plantaris medialis
m. flexor digitorum superficialis
m. flexor digitorum profundus:
m. flexor digiti I longus et
m. tibialis caudalis
m. flexor digitorum longus
m. tibialis cranialis
m. fibularis tertius
m. extensor digitorum longus
tibia
a.v. tibialis caudalis
tibial extensor retinaculum
tarsocrural joint cavity, proximal pouch
m. flexor digitorum longus in malleolar groove
tibia, medial malleolus
v. saphena medialis r. anastomoticus
tarsocrural joint cavity
talus, medial trochlea
v. saphena medialis, r. articularis
long medial collateral tarsal ligament and canal for tendon (opened)
m. tibialis cranialis, tendo medialis (cunean)
m. fibularis tertius, tendo medialis
metatarsal extensor retinaculum
metatarsal bones II, III
m. extensor digitorum longus

Fig. 6.44 The left tarsus: medial view. The saphenous artery has been resected to show more clearly the origin of the two plantar nerves from the tibial nerve. The distal part of the canal for the tendon of the long digital flexor muscle has not been opened. It is indicated by broken blue lines. Union of this tendon with that of the rest of the muscle occurs one third of the way down the metatarsus (see Fig. 6.49). This stage of dissection is also shown in Fig. 6.45.

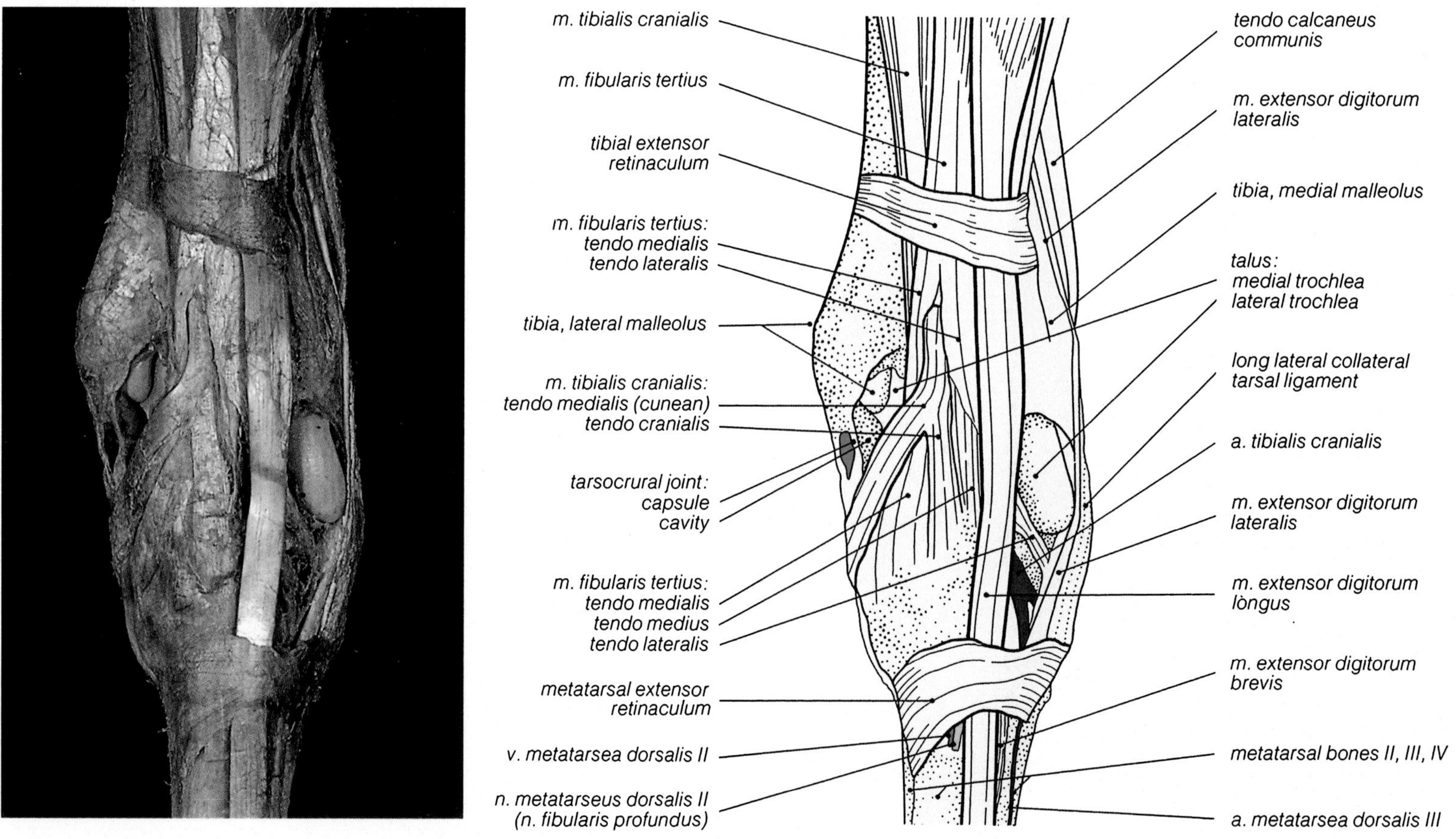
m. tibialis cranialis
m. fibularis tertius
tibial extensor retinaculum
m. fibularis tertius:
tendo medialis
tendo lateralis
tibia, lateral malleolus
m. tibialis cranialis:
tendo medialis (cunean)
tendo cranialis
tarsocrural joint:
capsule
cavity
m. fibularis tertius:
tendo medialis
tendo medius
tendo lateralis
metatarsal extensor retinaculum
v. metatarsea dorsalis II
n. metatarseus dorsalis II
(n. fibularis profundus)
tendo calcaneus communis
m. extensor digitorum lateralis
tibia, medial malleolus
talus:
medial trochlea
lateral trochlea
long lateral collateral tarsal ligament
a. tibialis cranialis
m. extensor digitorum lateralis
m. extensor digitorum longus
m. extensor digitorum brevis
metatarsal bones II, III, IV
a. metatarsea dorsalis III

Fig. 6.45 The left tarsus: dorsal view. The superficial fibular nerve has been removed and the dorsal metatarsal nerve has been resected. This stage of dissection is also shown in Fig. 6.44.

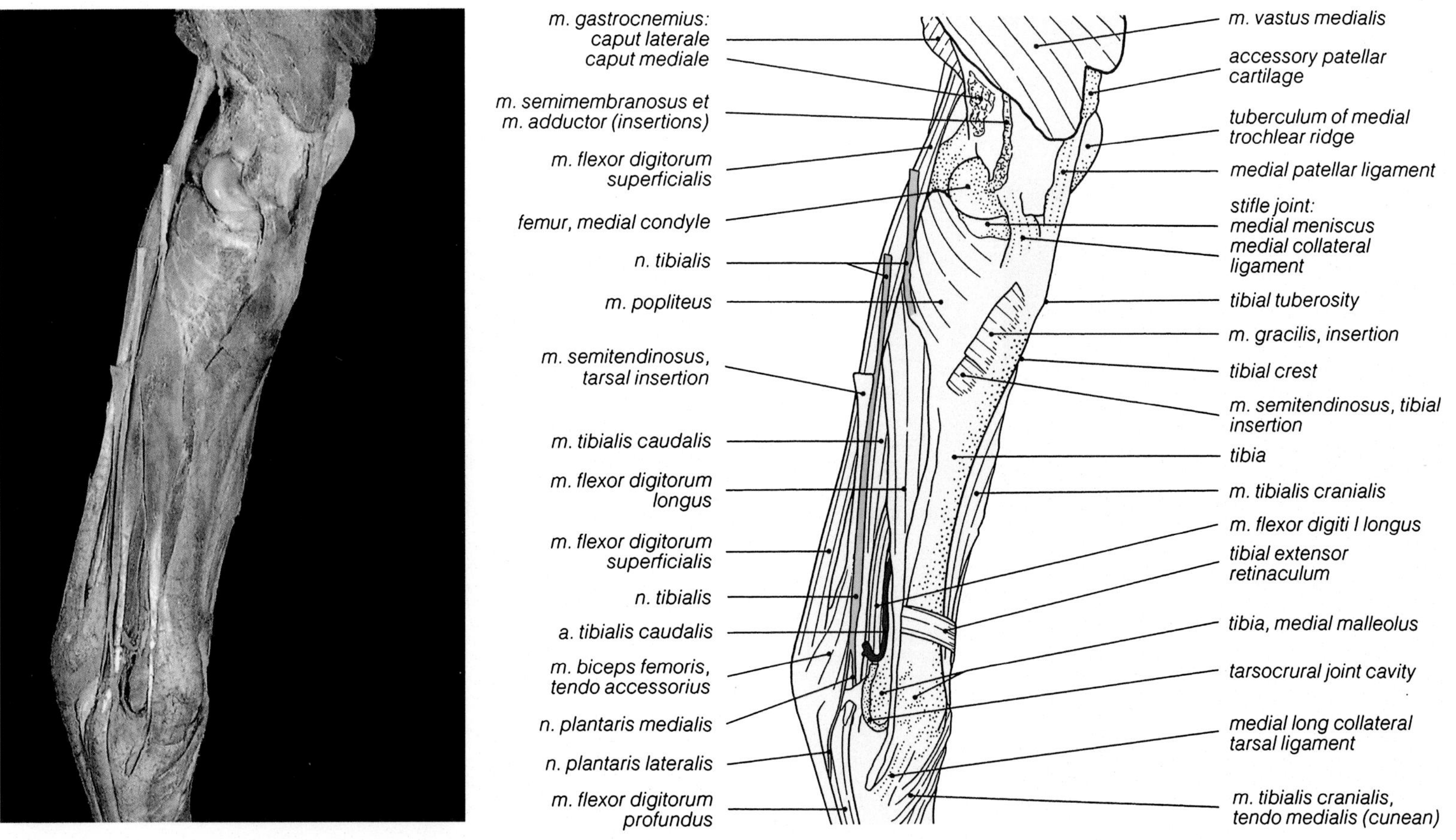
m. gastrocnemius:
caput laterale
caput mediale
m. semimembranosus et
m. adductor (insertions)
m. flexor digitorum
superficialis
femur, medial condyle
n. tibialis
m. popliteus
m. semitendinosus,
tarsal insertion
m. tibialis caudalis
m. flexor digitorum
longus
m. flexor digitorum
superficialis
n. tibialis
a. tibialis caudalis
m. biceps femoris,
tendo accessorius
n. plantaris medialis
n. plantaris lateralis
m. flexor digitorum
profundus
m. vastus medialis
accessory patellar
cartilage
tuberculum of medial
trochlear ridge
medial patellar ligament
stifle joint:
medial meniscus
medial collateral
ligament
tibial tuberosity
m. gracilis, insertion
tibial crest
m. semitendinosus, tibial
insertion
tibia
m. tibialis cranialis
m. flexor digiti I longus
tibial extensor
retinaculum
tibia, medial malleolus
tarsocrural joint cavity
medial long collateral
tarsal ligament
m. tibialis cranialis,
tendo medialis (cunean)

Fig. 6.46 Deep structures of the left crus: medial view. The gastrocnemius muscle has been resected. This stage of dissection is also shown in Fig. 6.47.

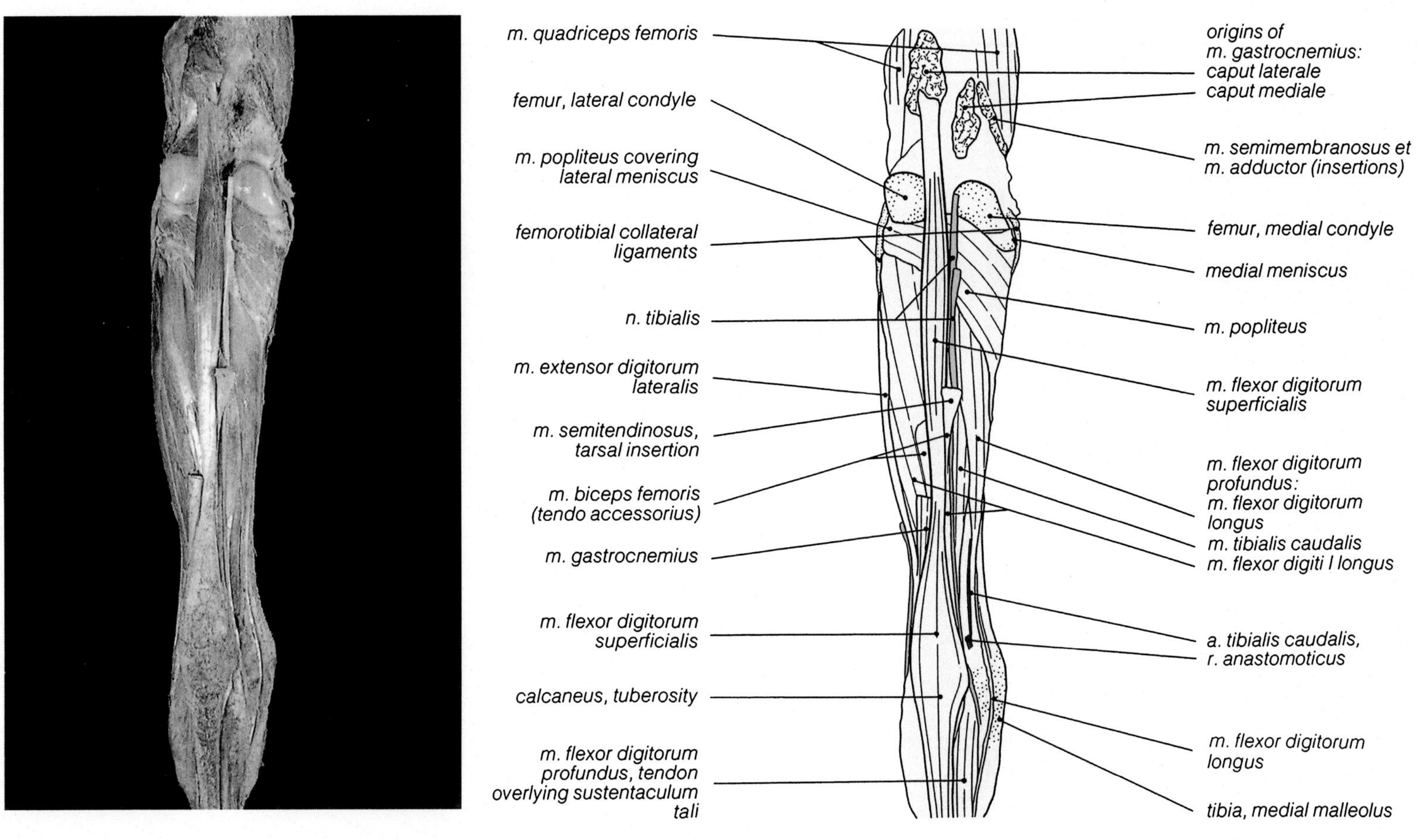
m. quadriceps femoris
femur, lateral condyle
m. popliteus covering
lateral meniscus
femorotibial collateral
ligaments
n. tibialis
m. extensor digitorum
lateralis
m. semitendinosus,
tarsal insertion
m. biceps femoris
(tendo accessorius)
m. gastrocnemius
m. flexor digitorum
superficialis
calcaneus, tuberosity
m. flexor digitorum
profundus, tendon
overlying sustentaculum
tali
origins of
m. gastrocnemius:
caput laterale
caput mediale
m. semimembranosus et
m. adductor (insertions)
femur, medial condyle
medial meniscus
m. popliteus
m. flexor digitorum
superficialis
m. flexor digitorum
profundus:
m. flexor digitorum
longus
m. tibialis caudalis
m. flexor digiti I longus
a. tibialis caudalis,
r. anastomoticus
m. flexor digitorum
longus
tibia, medial malleolus

Fig. 6.47 Deep structures of the left crus: caudal view. The gastrocnemius muscle has been resected. This stage of dissection is also shown in Fig. 6.46.

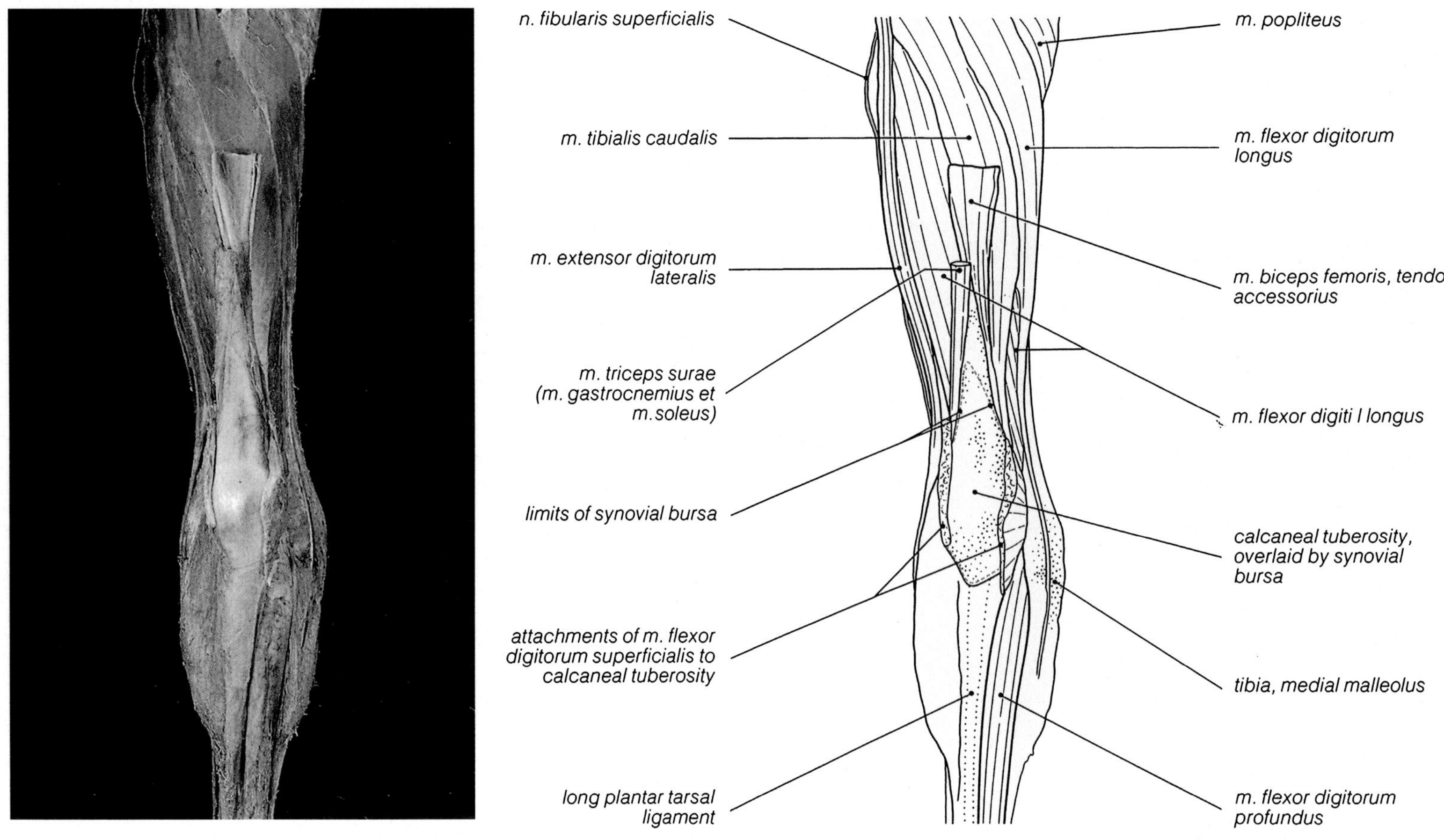
n. fibularis superficialis
m. tibialis caudalis
m. extensor digitorum lateralis
m. triceps surae (m. gastrocnemius et m.soleus)
limits of synovial bursa
attachments of m. flexor digitorum superficialis to calcaneal tuberosity
long plantar tarsal ligament
m. popliteus
m. flexor digitorum longus
m. biceps femoris, tendo accessorius
m. flexor digiti I longus
calcaneal tuberosity, overlaid by synovial bursa
tibia, medial malleolus
m. flexor digitorum profundus

Fig. 6.48 The common calcaneal tendon: caudal view. The tendon of the superficial digital flexor muscle (see Fig. 6.47) has been removed to show the synovial bursa between it and the point of the hock, and its attachments to the calcaneal tuberosity.

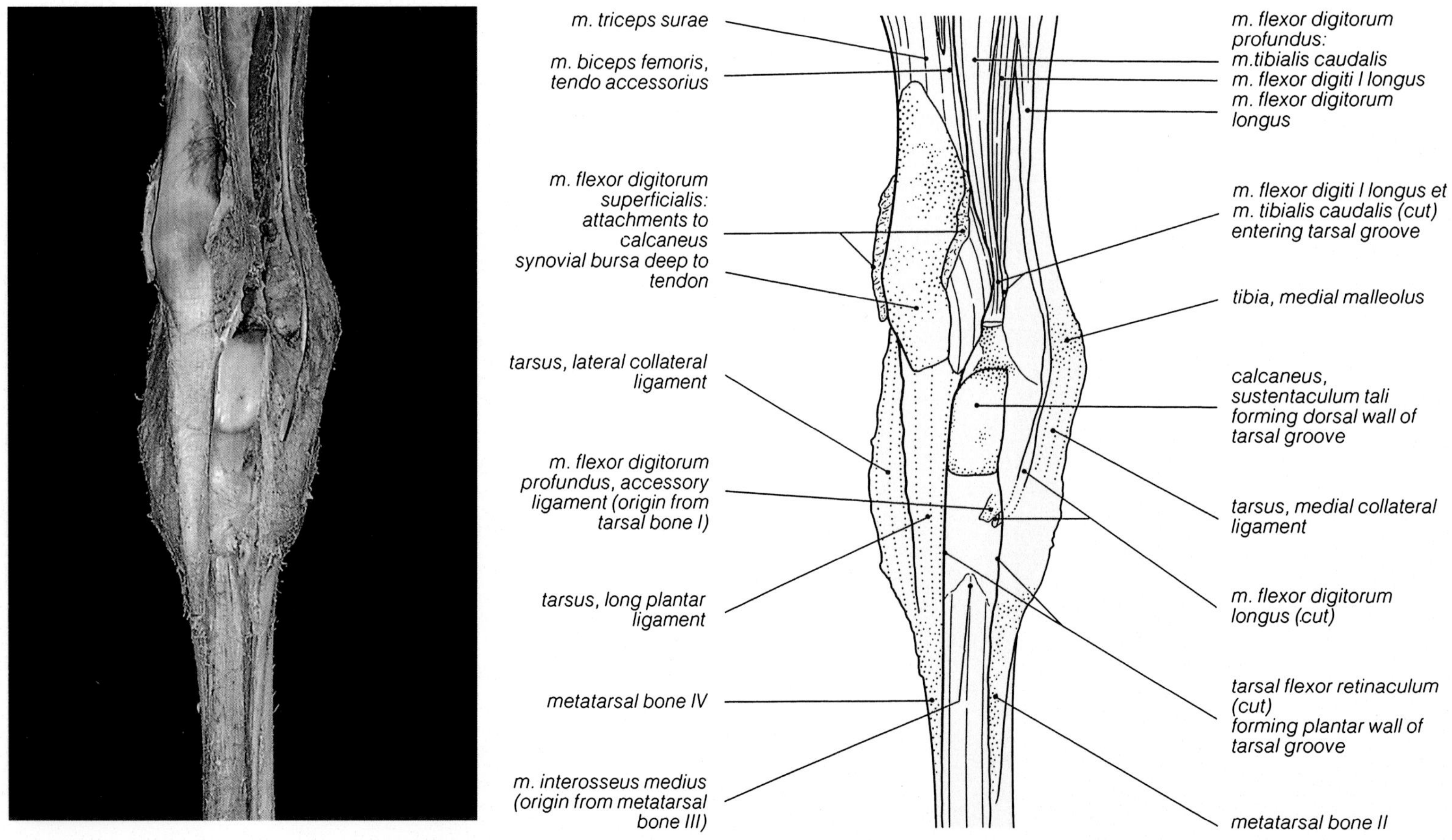
m. triceps surae
m. biceps femoris, tendo accessorius
m. flexor digitorum superficialis: attachments to calcaneus
synovial bursa deep to tendon
tarsus, lateral collateral ligament
m. flexor digitorum profundus, accessory ligament (origin from tarsal bone I)
tarsus, long plantar ligament
metatarsal bone IV
m. interosseus medius (origin from metatarsal bone III)
m. flexor digitorum profundus:
m.tibialis caudalis
m. flexor digiti I longus
m. flexor digitorum longus
m. flexor digiti I longus et m. tibialis caudalis (cut) entering tarsal groove
tibia, medial malleolus
calcaneus, sustentaculum tali forming dorsal wall of tarsal groove
tarsus, medial collateral ligament
m. flexor digitorum longus (cut)
tarsal flexor retinaculum (cut) forming plantar wall of tarsal groove
metatarsal bone II

Fig. 6.49 Tarsal groove of the left tarsus: plantar view. The tendons of the deep digital flexor muscle have been cut and removed from the tarsal groove, showing the sustentaculum tali, over which two tendons of the deep digital flexor muscle run. The origins of the accessory ligament (tarsal head of the deep digital flexor muscle) and the suspensory ligament (interosseus medius muscle) are also revealed.

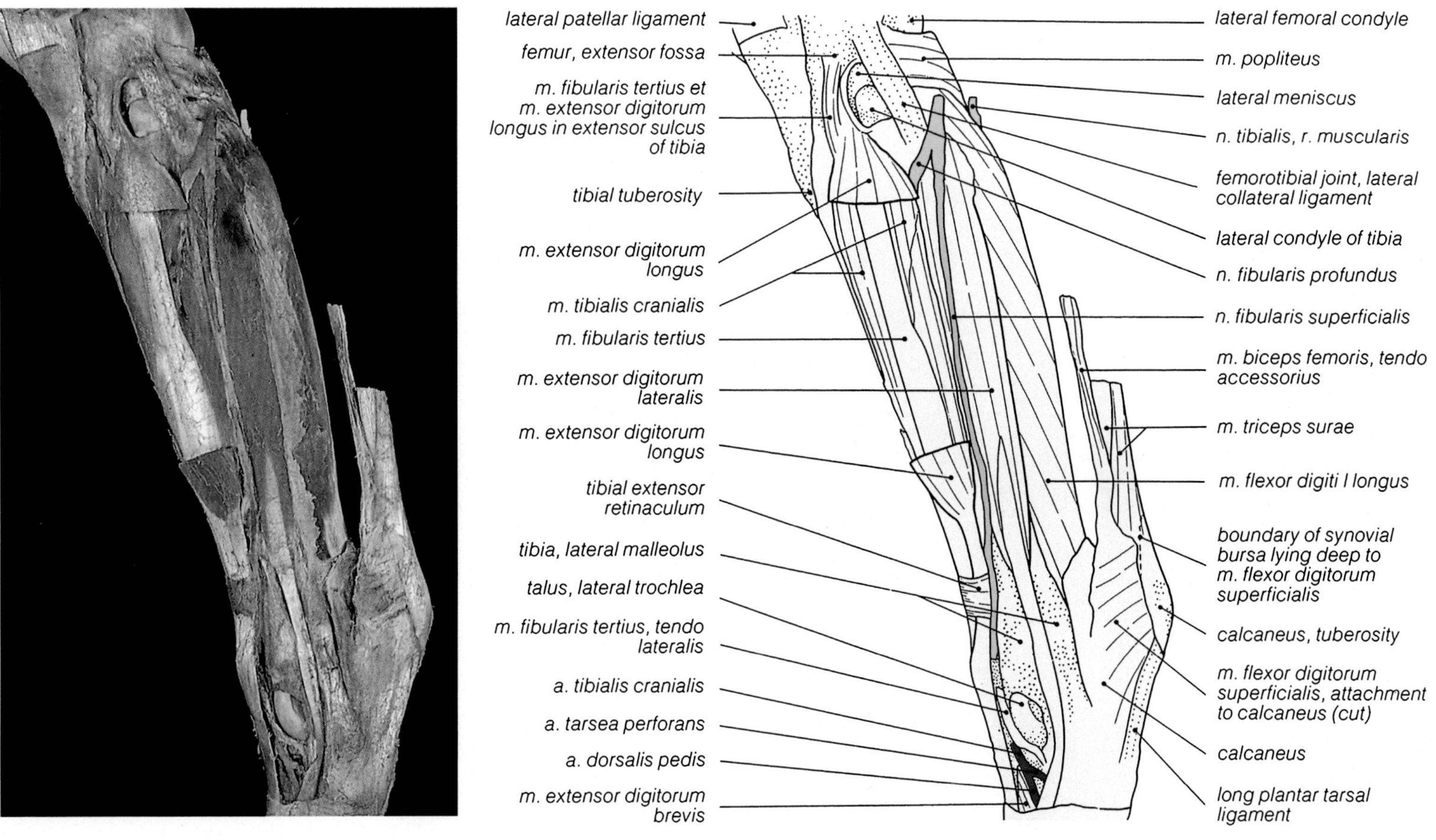
lateral patellar ligament
femur, extensor fossa
m. fibularis tertius et m. extensor digitorum longus in extensor sulcus of tibia
tibial tuberosity
m. extensor digitorum longus
m. tibialis cranialis
m. fibularis tertius
m. extensor digitorum lateralis
m. extensor digitorum longus
tibial extensor retinaculum
tibia, lateral malleolus
talus, lateral trochlea
m. fibularis tertius, tendo lateralis
a. tibialis cranialis
a. tarsea perforans
a. dorsalis pedis
m. extensor digitorum brevis
lateral femoral condyle
m. popliteus
lateral meniscus
n. tibialis, r. muscularis
femorotibial joint, lateral collateral ligament
lateral condyle of tibia
n. fibularis profundus
n. fibularis superficialis
m. biceps femoris, tendo accessorius
m. triceps surae
m. flexor digiti I longus
boundary of synovial bursa lying deep to m. flexor digitorum superficialis
calcaneus, tuberosity
m. flexor digitorum superficialis, attachment to calcaneus (cut)
calcaneus
long plantar tarsal ligament

Fig. 6.50 Deep structures of the left crus: lateral view. The specimen is at the stage of dissection shown in Figs. 6.48 and 6.51.

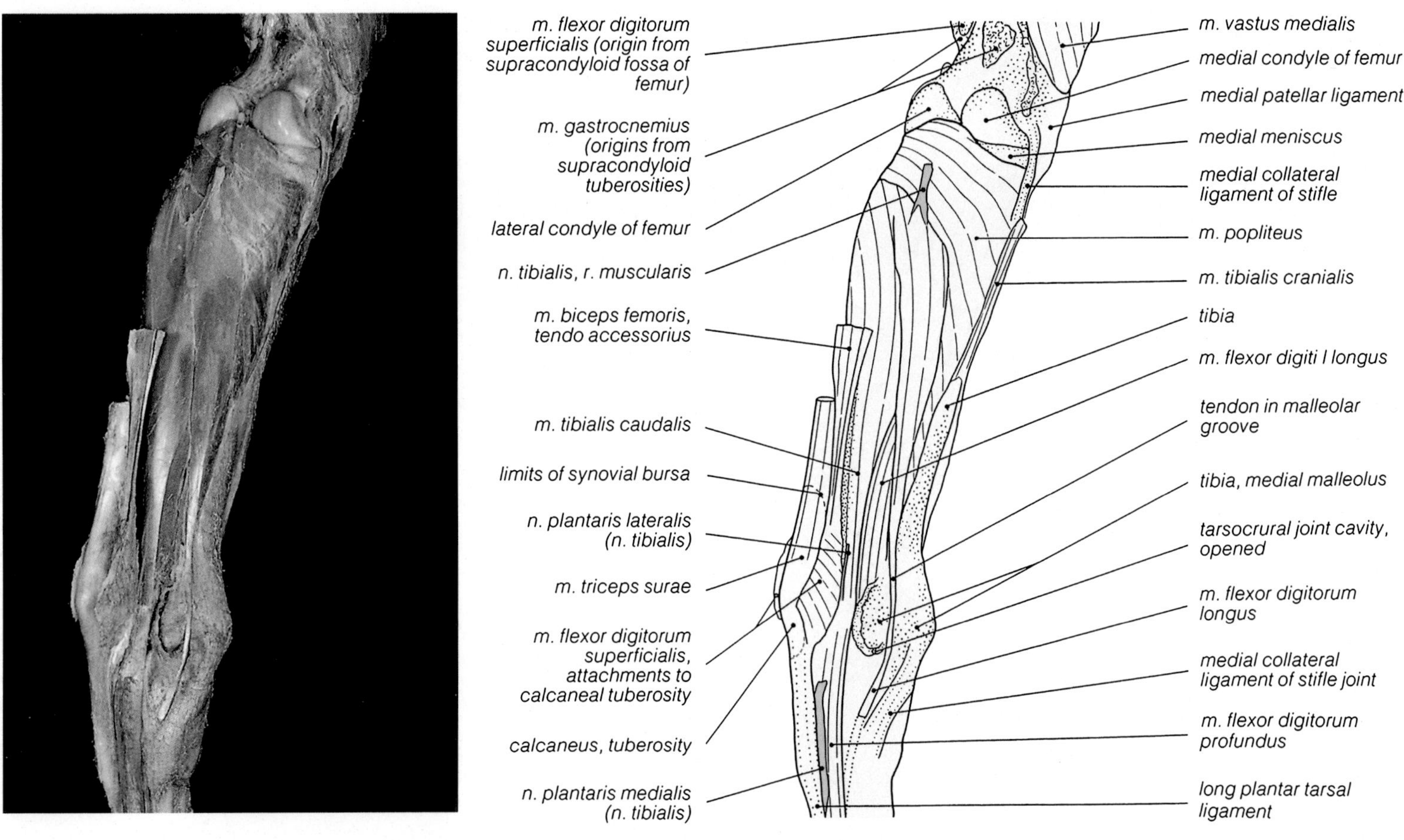
m. flexor digitorum superficialis (origin from supracondyloid fossa of femur)
m. gastrocnemius (origins from supracondyloid tuberosities)
lateral condyle of femur
n. tibialis, r. muscularis
m. biceps femoris, tendo accessorius
m. tibialis caudalis
limits of synovial bursa
n. plantaris lateralis (n. tibialis)
m. triceps surae
m. flexor digitorum superficialis, attachments to calcaneal tuberosity
calcaneus, tuberosity
n. plantaris medialis (n. tibialis)
m. vastus medialis
medial condyle of femur
medial patellar ligament
medial meniscus
medial collateral ligament of stifle
m. popliteus
m. tibialis cranialis
tibia
m. flexor digiti I longus
tendon in malleolar groove
tibia, medial malleolus
tarsocrural joint cavity, opened
m. flexor digitorum longus
medial collateral ligament of stifle joint
m. flexor digitorum profundus
long plantar tarsal ligament

Fig. 6.51 Deep structures of the left crus: caudomedial view. The specimen is at the same stage of dissection as that shown in Figs. 6.48 and 6.50.

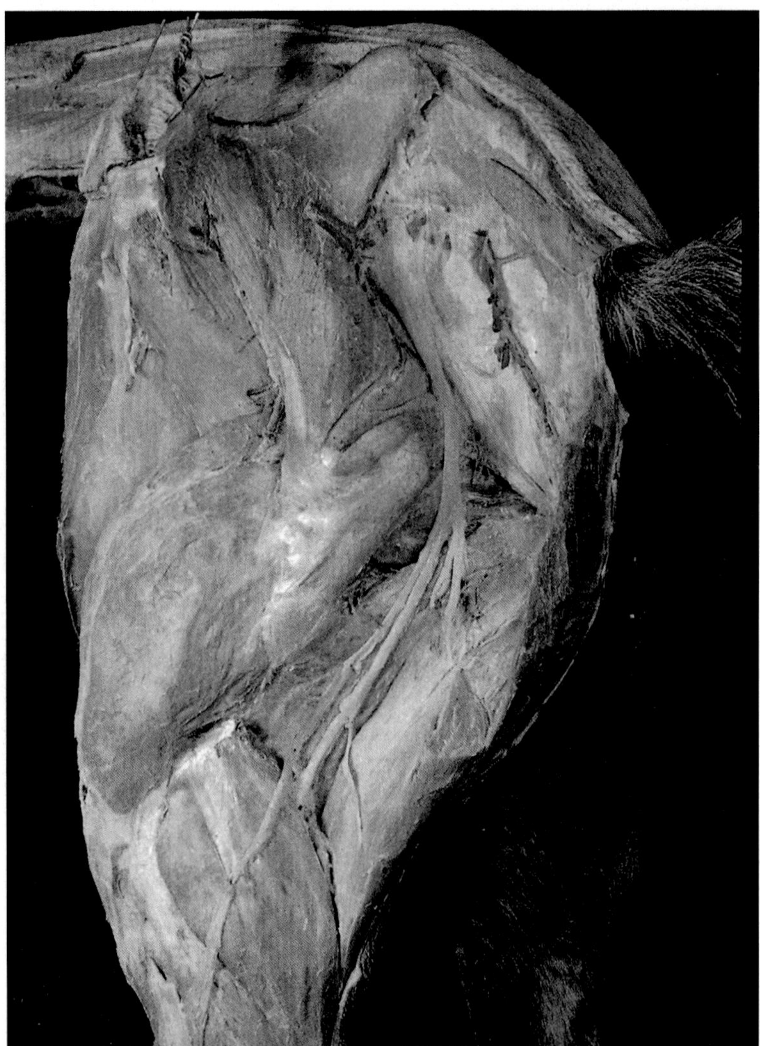

Fig. 6.52 Structures of pelvic, femoral and crural regions in the mare: left caudolateral view (1). The tensor fasciae latae, superficial gluteal and biceps femoris muscles have been removed. Parts of the middle gluteal and semitendinosus muscles have been resected. The pelvic and femoral regions of this specimen are shown in Chapter 8 (Figs. 8.62–8.64).

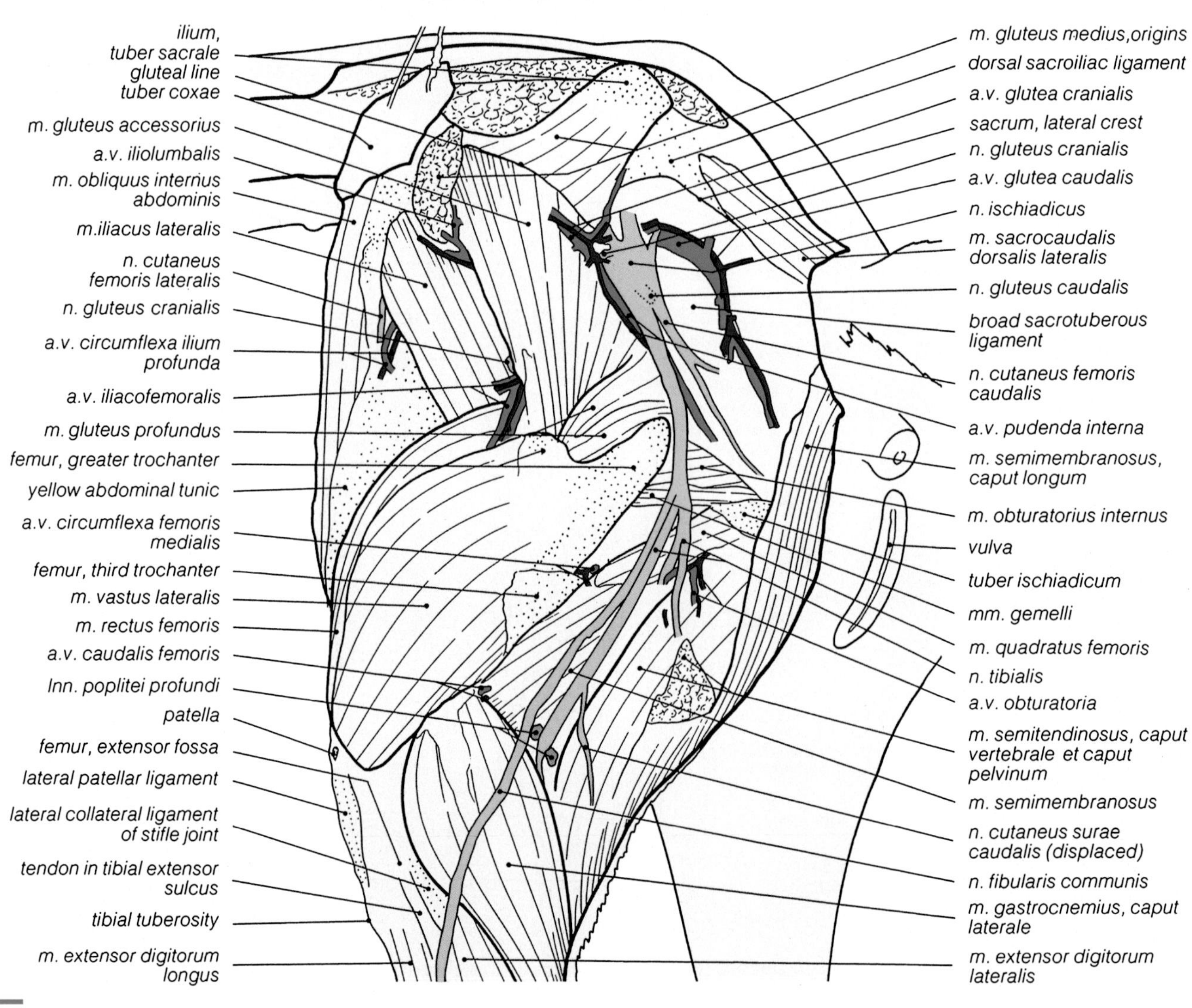

ilium,
tuber sacrale
gluteal line
tuber coxae
m. gluteus accessorius
a.v. iliolumbalis
m. obliquus internus abdominis
m.iliacus lateralis
n. cutaneus femoris lateralis
n. gluteus cranialis
a.v. circumflexa ilium profunda
a.v. iliacofemoralis
m. gluteus profundus
femur, greater trochanter
yellow abdominal tunic
a.v. circumflexa femoris medialis
femur, third trochanter
m. vastus lateralis
m. rectus femoris
a.v. caudalis femoris
lnn. poplitei profundi
patella
femur, extensor fossa
lateral patellar ligament
lateral collateral ligament of stifle joint
tendon in tibial extensor sulcus
tibial tuberosity
m. extensor digitorum longus
m. gluteus medius,origins
dorsal sacroiliac ligament
a.v. glutea cranialis
sacrum, lateral crest
n. gluteus cranialis
a.v. glutea caudalis
n. ischiadicus
m. sacrocaudalis dorsalis lateralis
n. gluteus caudalis
broad sacrotuberous ligament
n. cutaneus femoris caudalis
a.v. pudenda interna
m. semimembranosus, caput longum
m. obturatorius internus
vulva
tuber ischiadicum
mm. gemelli
m. quadratus femoris
n. tibialis
a.v. obturatoria
m. semitendinosus, caput vertebrale et caput pelvinum
m. semimembranosus
n. cutaneus surae caudalis (displaced)
n. fibularis communis
m. gastrocnemius, caput laterale
m. extensor digitorum lateralis

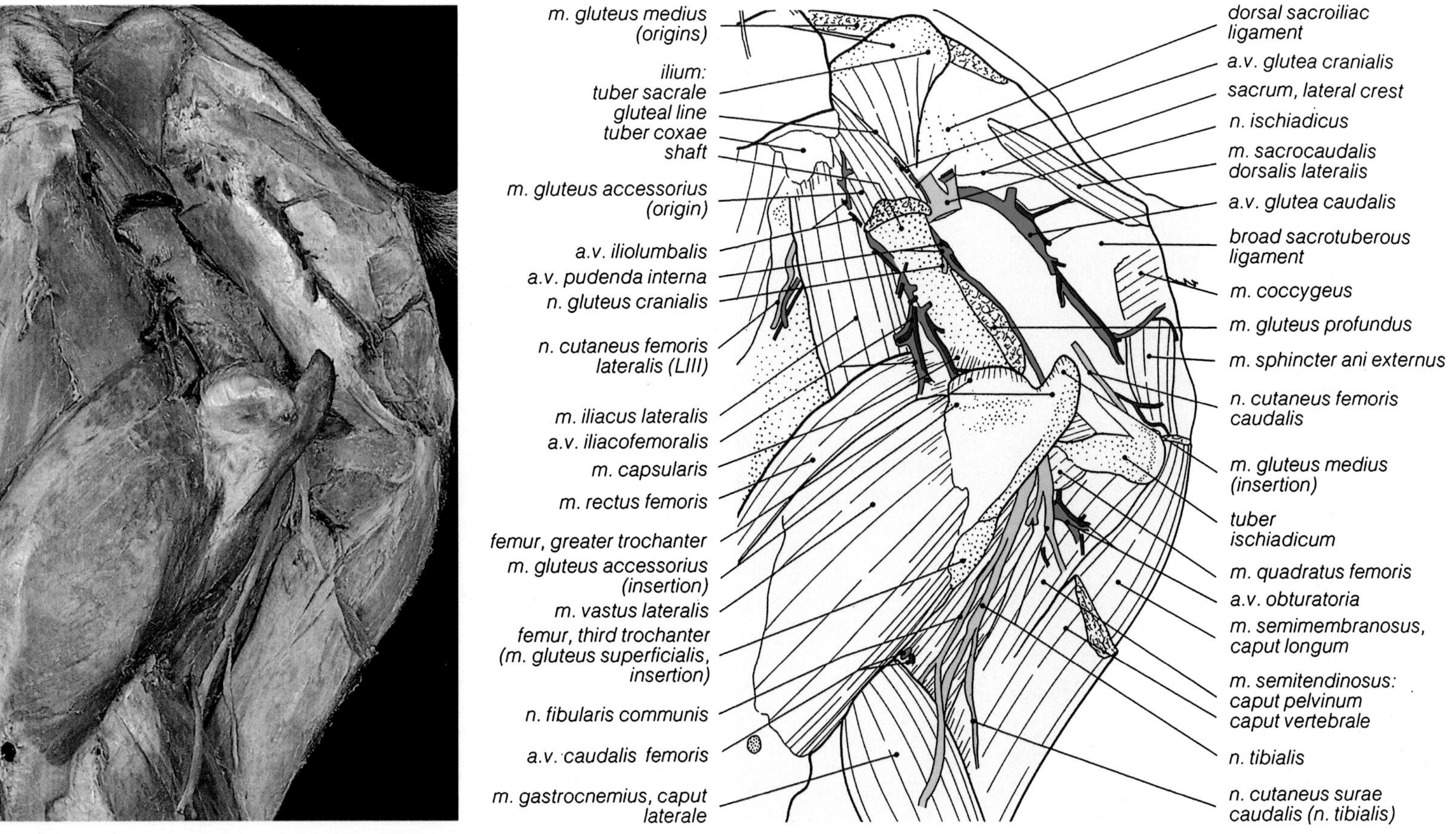
m. gluteus medius (origins)
ilium:
tuber sacrale
gluteal line
tuber coxae
shaft
m. gluteus accessorius (origin)
a.v. iliolumbalis
a.v. pudenda interna
n. gluteus cranialis
n. cutaneus femoris lateralis (LIII)
m. iliacus lateralis
a.v. iliacofemoralis
m. capsularis
m. rectus femoris
femur, greater trochanter
m. gluteus accessorius (insertion)
m. vastus lateralis
femur, third trochanter (m. gluteus superficialis, insertion)
n. fibularis communis
a.v. caudalis femoris
m. gastrocnemius, caput laterale
dorsal sacroiliac ligament
a.v. glutea cranialis
sacrum, lateral crest
n. ischiadicus
m. sacrocaudalis dorsalis lateralis
a.v. glutea caudalis
broad sacrotuberous ligament
m. coccygeus
m. gluteus profundus
m. sphincter ani externus
n. cutaneus femoris caudalis
m. gluteus medius (insertion)
tuber ischiadicum
m. quadratus femoris
a.v. obturatoria
m. semimembranosus, caput longum
m. semitendinosus: caput pelvinum caput vertebrale
n. tibialis
n. cutaneus surae caudalis (n. tibialis)

Fig. 6.53 Structures of pelvic, femoral and crural regions in the mare: left caudolateral view (2). The accessory head of the middle gluteal muscle and the deep gluteal muscles have been resected. The long head of the semimembranosus muscle has been cut away and the superficial perineal structures are displayed caudal to the caudal edge of the broad sacrotuberous ligament. The middle part of the ischiatic nerve and the caudal cutaneous femoral nerve have been removed.

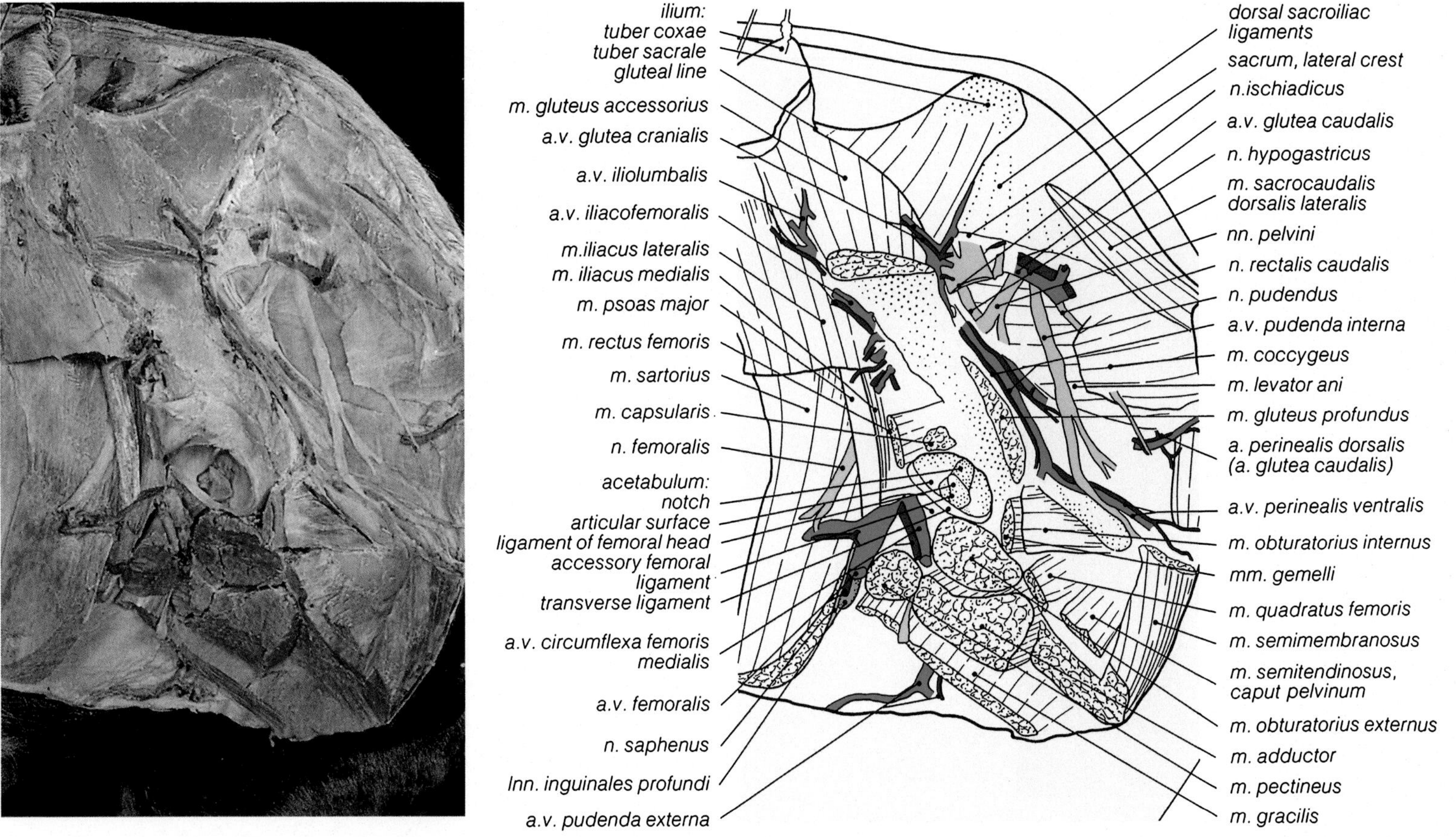
ilium:
tuber coxae
tuber sacrale
gluteal line
m. gluteus accessorius
a.v. glutea cranialis
a.v. iliolumbalis
a.v. iliacofemoralis
m.iliacus lateralis
m. iliacus medialis
m. psoas major
m. rectus femoris
m. sartorius
m. capsularis
n. femoralis
acetabulum:
notch
articular surface
ligament of femoral head
accessory femoral ligament
transverse ligament
a.v. circumflexa femoris medialis
a.v. femoralis
n. saphenus
lnn. inguinales profundi
a.v. pudenda externa
dorsal sacroiliac ligaments
sacrum, lateral crest
n.ischiadicus
a.v. glutea caudalis
n. hypogastricus
m. sacrocaudalis dorsalis lateralis
nn. pelvini
n. rectalis caudalis
n. pudendus
a.v. pudenda interna
m. coccygeus
m. levator ani
m. gluteus profundus
a. perinealis dorsalis (a. glutea caudalis)
a.v. perinealis ventralis
m. obturatorius internus
mm. gemelli
m. quadratus femoris
m. semimembranosus
m. semitendinosus, caput pelvinum
m. obturatorius externus
m. adductor
m. pectineus
m. gracilis

Fig. 6.54 The acetabulum and associated structures in the pregnant mare: left caudolateral view. The left hindlimb and broad sacrotuberous ligament have been removed. The cut ends of the muscles, vessels and nerves have been dissected to show their topographical relationships. Further dissections of this region in this specimen are shown in Chapter 8 (Figs. 8.66–8.71).

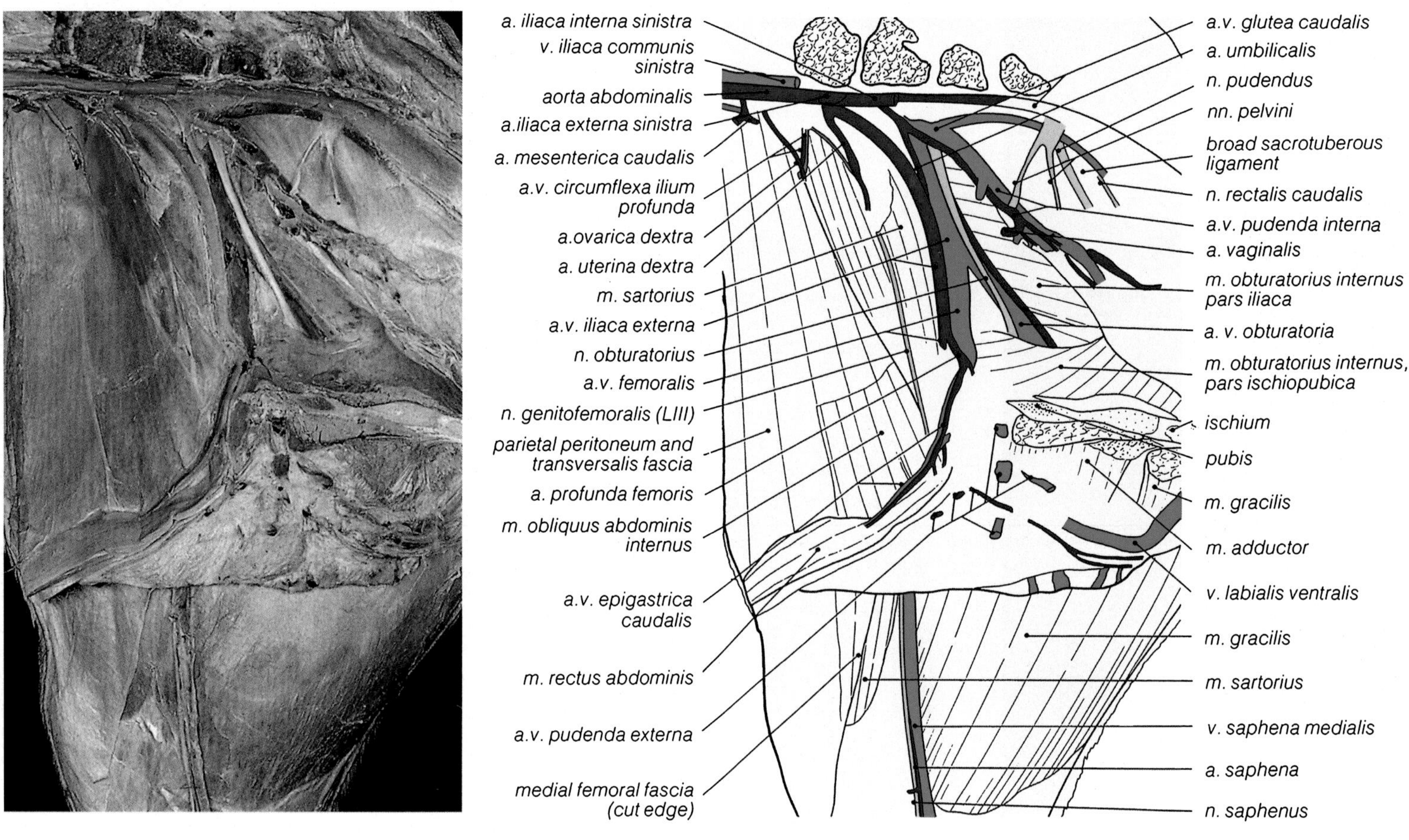
a. iliaca interna sinistra
v. iliaca communis sinistra
aorta abdominalis
a.iliaca externa sinistra
a. mesenterica caudalis
a.v. circumflexa ilium profunda
a.ovarica dextra
a. uterina dextra
m. sartorius
a.v. iliaca externa
n. obturatorius
a.v. femoralis
n. genitofemoralis (LIII)
parietal peritoneum and transversalis fascia
a. profunda femoris
m. obliquus abdominis internus
a.v. epigastrica caudalis
m. rectus abdominis
a.v. pudenda externa
medial femoral fascia (cut edge)
a.v. glutea caudalis
a. umbilicalis
n. pudendus
nn. pelvini
broad sacrotuberous ligament
n. rectalis caudalis
a.v. pudenda interna
a. vaginalis
m. obturatorius internus pars iliaca
a. v. obturatoria
m. obturatorius internus, pars ischiopubica
ischium
pubis
m. gracilis
m. adductor
v. labialis ventralis
m. gracilis
m. sartorius
v. saphena medialis
a. saphena
n. saphenus

Fig. 6.55 The right pelvic wall of a pregnant mare: medial view. The left side of the pelvis and the pelvic viscera have been removed. The dissections leading to this stage are shown in Chapter 8 (Figs. 8.62–8.92). Further stages are shown in Figs. 6.59–6.62.

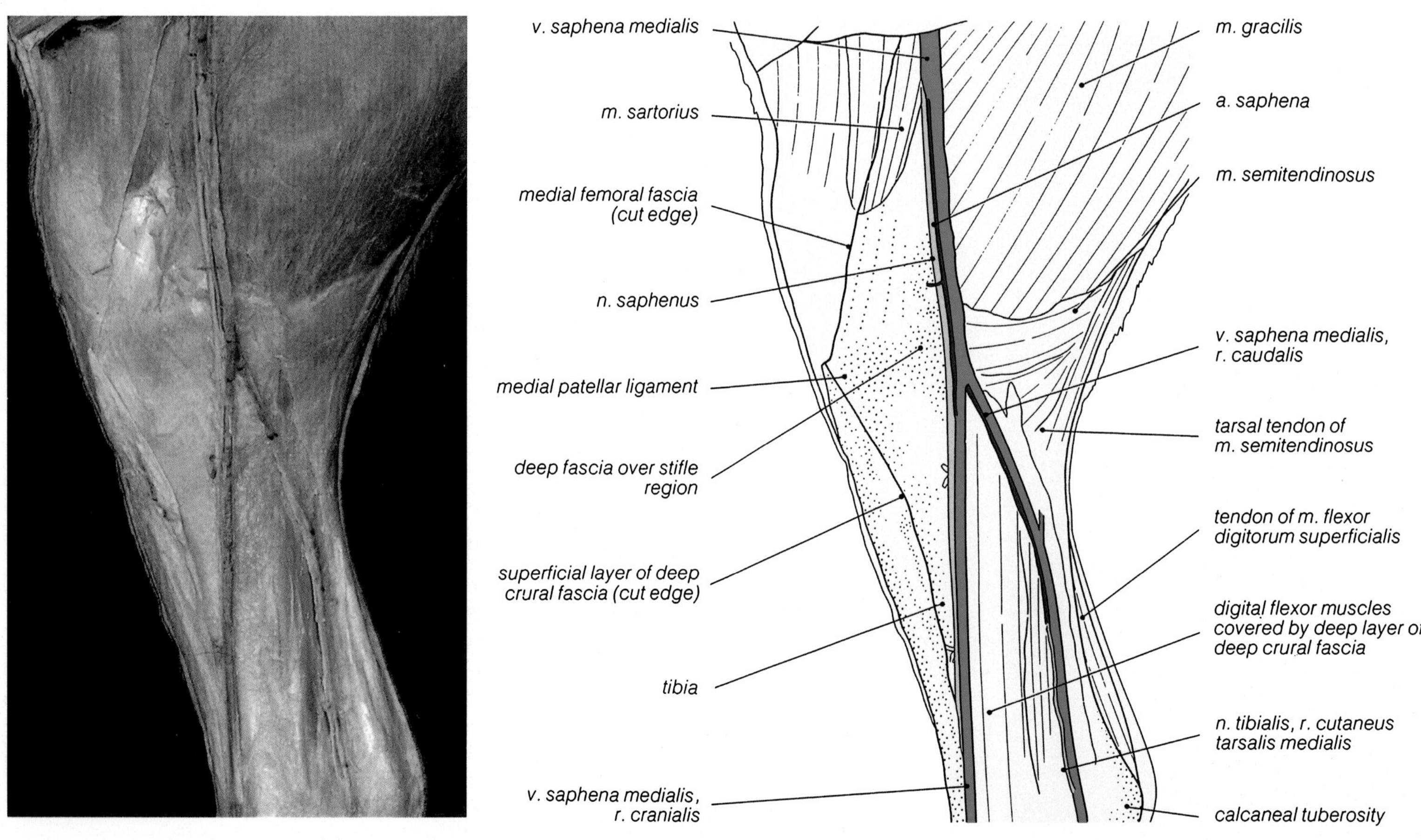
v. saphena medialis
m. sartorius
medial femoral fascia (cut edge)
n. saphenus
medial patellar ligament
deep fascia over stifle region
superficial layer of deep crural fascia (cut edge)
tibia
v. saphena medialis, r. cranialis
m. gracilis
a. saphena
m. semitendinosus
v. saphena medialis, r. caudalis
tarsal tendon of m. semitendinosus
tendon of m. flexor digitorum superficialis
digital flexor muscles covered by deep layer of deep crural fascia
n. tibialis, r. cutaneus tarsalis medialis
calcaneal tuberosity

Fig. 6.56 The right stifle and crural regions of the mare: medial view. The superficial fasciae and parts of the superficial layer of deep fascia have been removed.

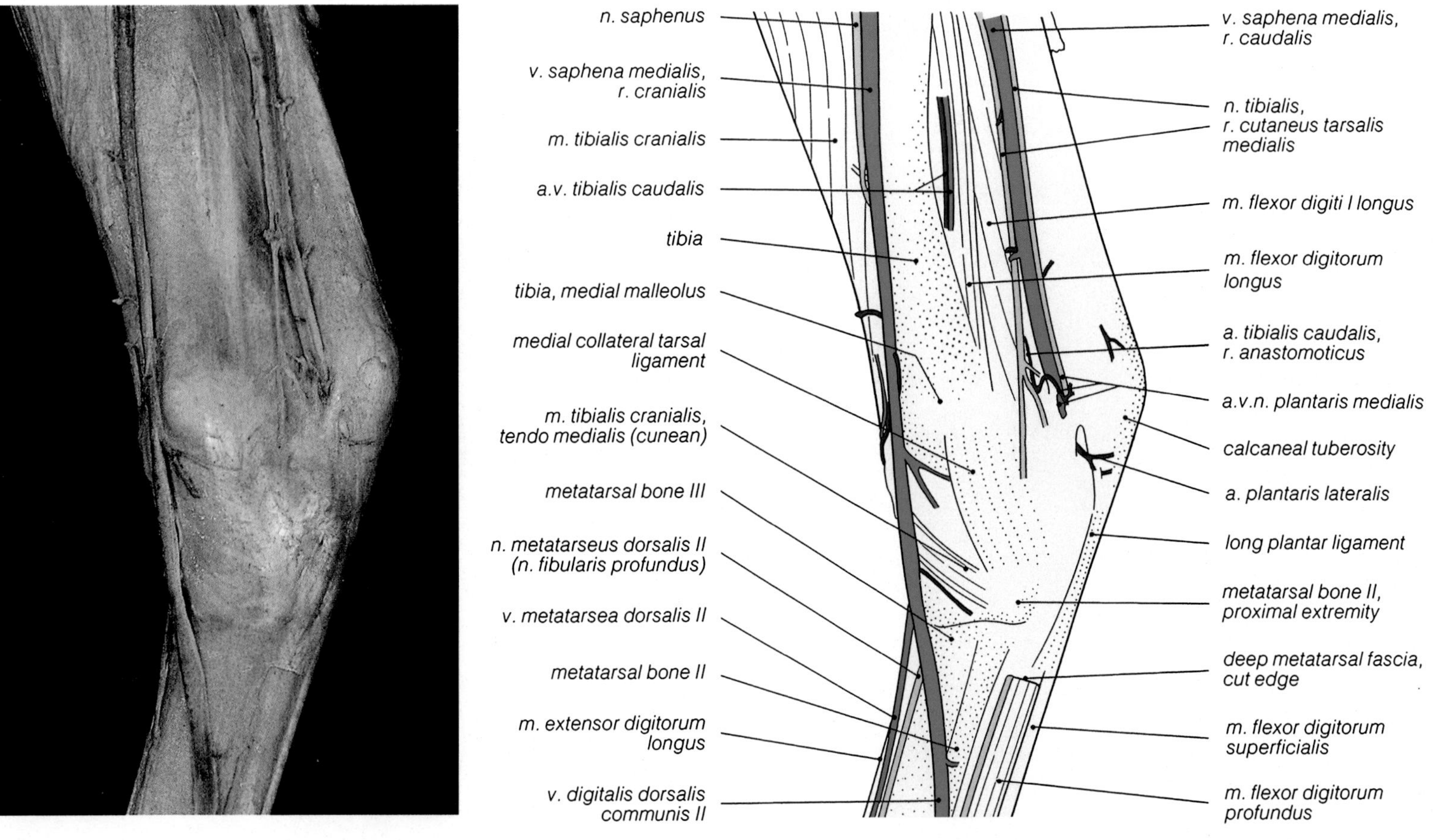
n. saphenus
v. saphena medialis, r. cranialis
m. tibialis cranialis
a.v. tibialis caudalis
tibia
tibia, medial malleolus
medial collateral tarsal ligament
m. tibialis cranialis, tendo medialis (cunean)
metatarsal bone III
n. metatarseus dorsalis II (n. fibularis profundus)
v. metatarsea dorsalis II
metatarsal bone II
m. extensor digitorum longus
v. digitalis dorsalis communis II
v. saphena medialis, r. caudalis
n. tibialis, r. cutaneus tarsalis medialis
m. flexor digiti I longus
m. flexor digitorum longus
a. tibialis caudalis, r. anastomoticus
a.v.n. plantaris medialis
calcaneal tuberosity
a. plantaris lateralis
long plantar ligament
metatarsal bone II, proximal extremity
deep metatarsal fascia, cut edge
m. flexor digitorum superficialis
m. flexor digitorum profundus

Fig. 6.57 Superficial structures of the right tarsus: medial view. More distal parts of this specimen are shown in Fig. 7.74.

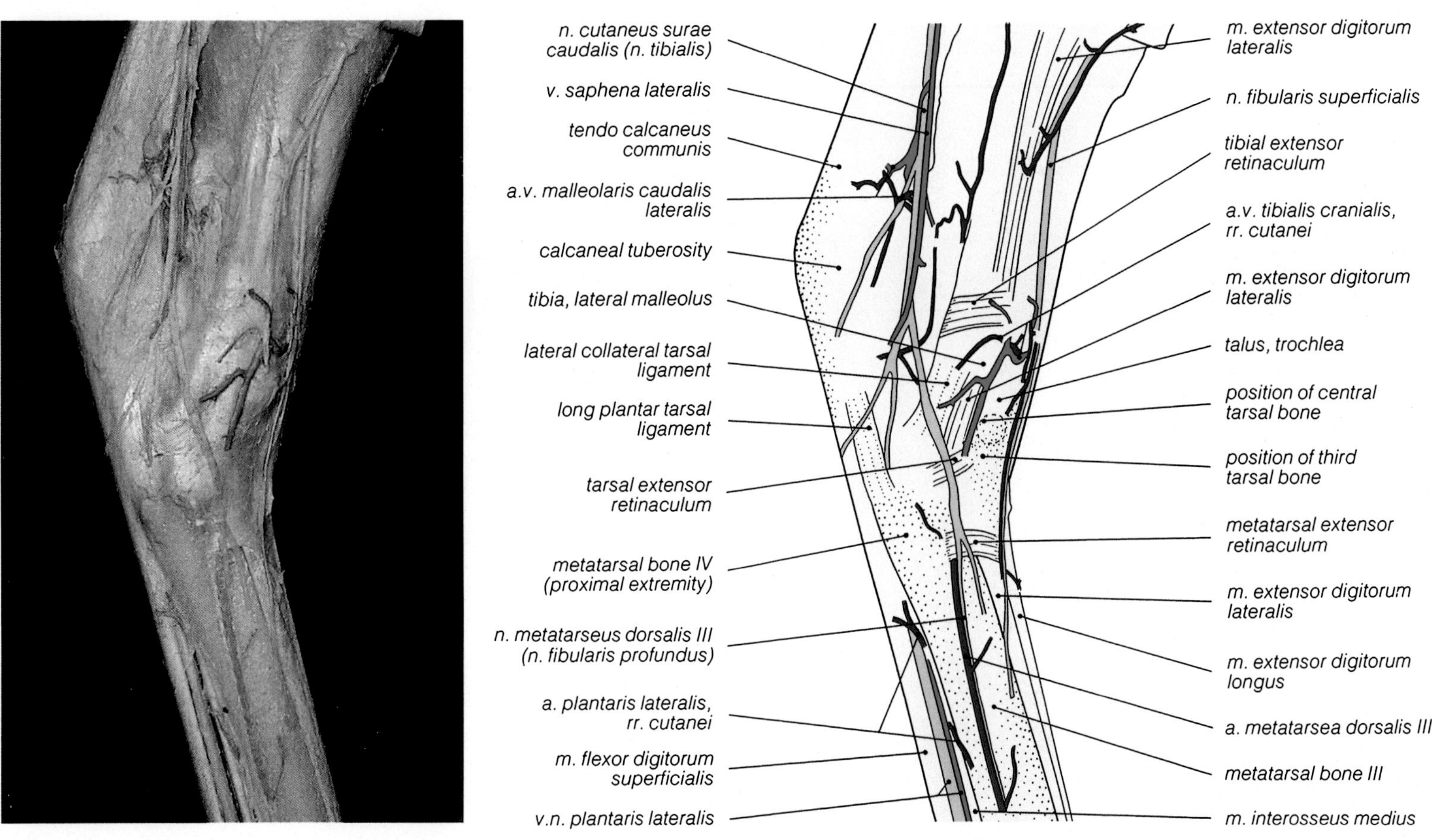
n. cutaneus surae caudalis (n. tibialis)
v. saphena lateralis
tendo calcaneus communis
a.v. malleolaris caudalis lateralis
calcaneal tuberosity
tibia, lateral malleolus
lateral collateral tarsal ligament
long plantar tarsal ligament
tarsal extensor retinaculum
metatarsal bone IV (proximal extremity)
n. metatarseus dorsalis III (n. fibularis profundus)
a. plantaris lateralis, rr. cutanei
m. flexor digitorum superficialis
v.n. plantaris lateralis
m. extensor digitorum lateralis
n. fibularis superficialis
tibial extensor retinaculum
a.v. tibialis cranialis, rr. cutanei
m. extensor digitorum lateralis
talus, trochlea
position of central tarsal bone
position of third tarsal bone
metatarsal extensor retinaculum
m. extensor digitorum lateralis
m. extensor digitorum longus
a. metatarsea dorsalis III
metatarsal bone III
m. interosseus medius

Fig. 6.58 Superficial structures of the right tarsus: lateral view. More distal parts of this specimen are shown in Fig. 7.72.

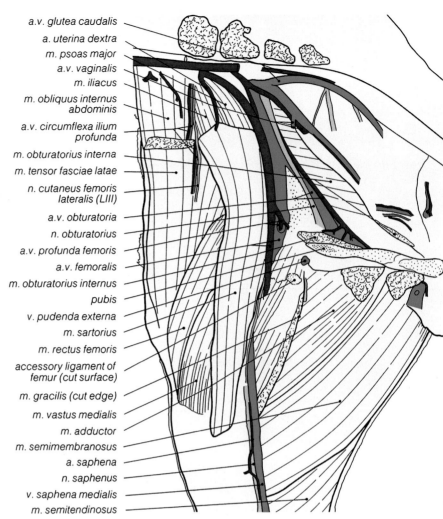

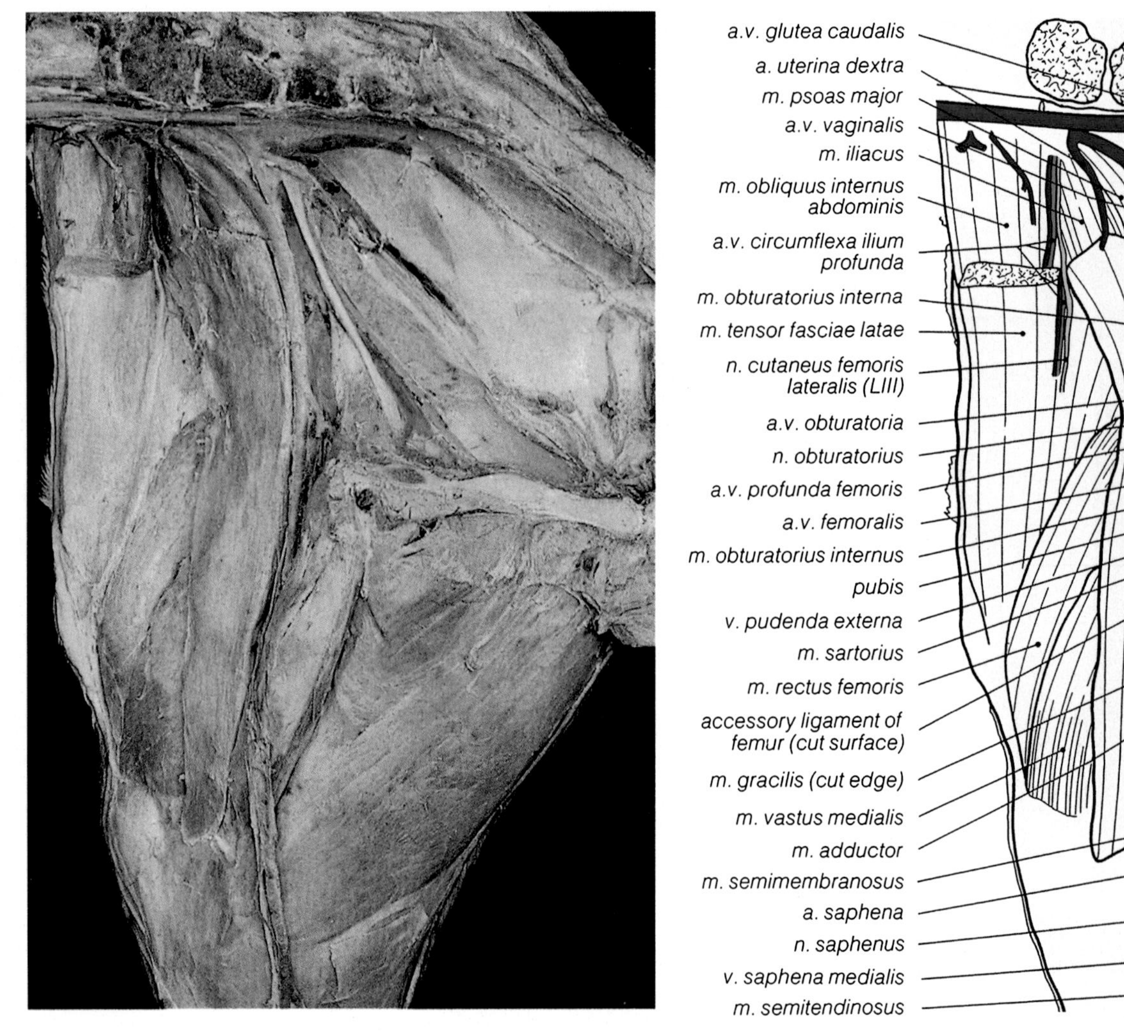
a.v. glutea caudalis
a. uterina dextra
m. psoas major
a.v. vaginalis
m. iliacus
m. obliquus internus abdominis
a.v. circumflexa ilium profunda
m. obturatorius interna
m. tensor fasciae latae
n. cutaneus femoris lateralis (LIII)
a.v. obturatoria
n. obturatorius
a.v. profunda femoris
a.v. femoralis
m. obturatorius internus
pubis
v. pudenda externa
m. sartorius
m. rectus femoris
accessory ligament of femur (cut surface)
m. gracilis (cut edge)
m. vastus medialis
m. adductor
m. semimembranosus
a. saphena
n. saphenus
v. saphena medialis
m. semitendinosus

Fig. 6.59 Vessels and nerves of the right pelvic and femoral regions in the pregnant mare: medial view. The ischiopubic part of the internal obturator muscle has been removed. The abdominal wall and most of the gracilis muscle have been resected (compare with Fig. 6.55).

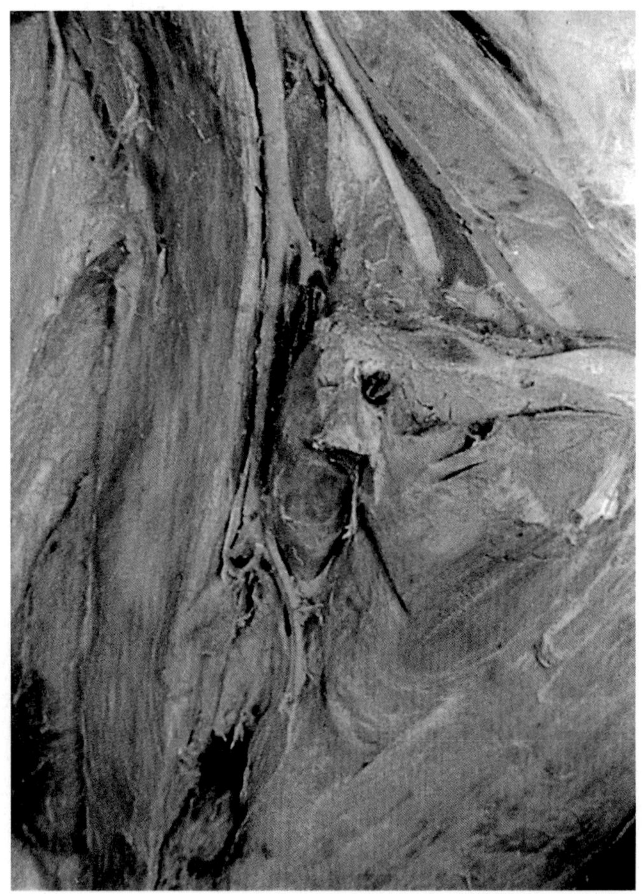

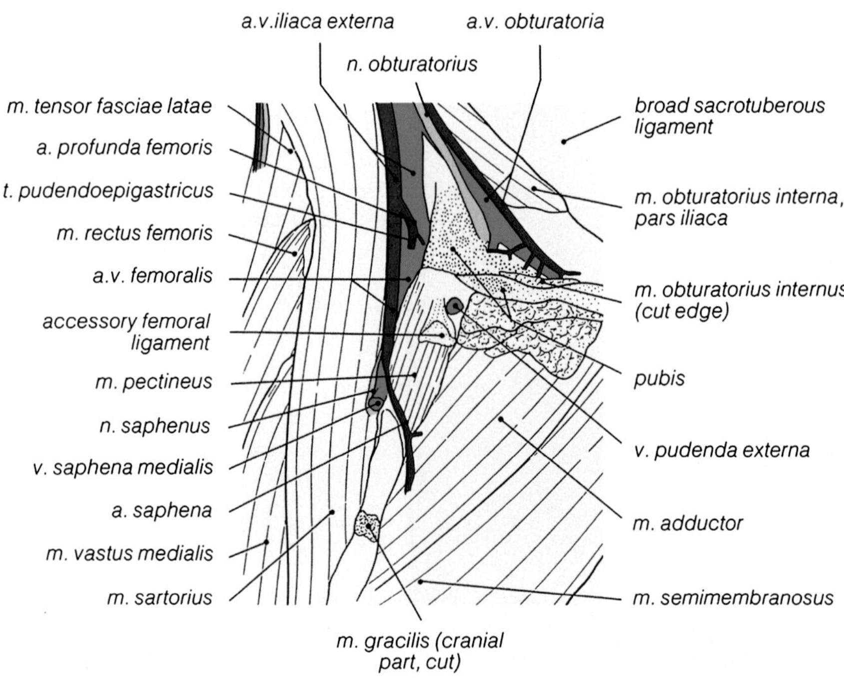
a.v.iliaca externa
a.v. obturatoria
n. obturatorius
m. tensor fasciae latae
a. profunda femoris
t. pudendoepigastricus
m. rectus femoris
a.v. femoralis
accessory femoral ligament
m. pectineus
n. saphenus
v. saphena medialis
a. saphena
m. vastus medialis
m. sartorius
broad sacrotuberous ligament
m. obturatorius interna, pars iliaca
m. obturatorius internus (cut edge)
pubis
v. pudenda externa
m. adductor
m. semimembranosus
m. gracilis (cranial part, cut)

Fig. 6.60 The right pectineus muscle: medial view. The cranial remnant of the gracilis muscle has been resected to show the pectineus muscle and the origin and termination of the saphenous vessels.

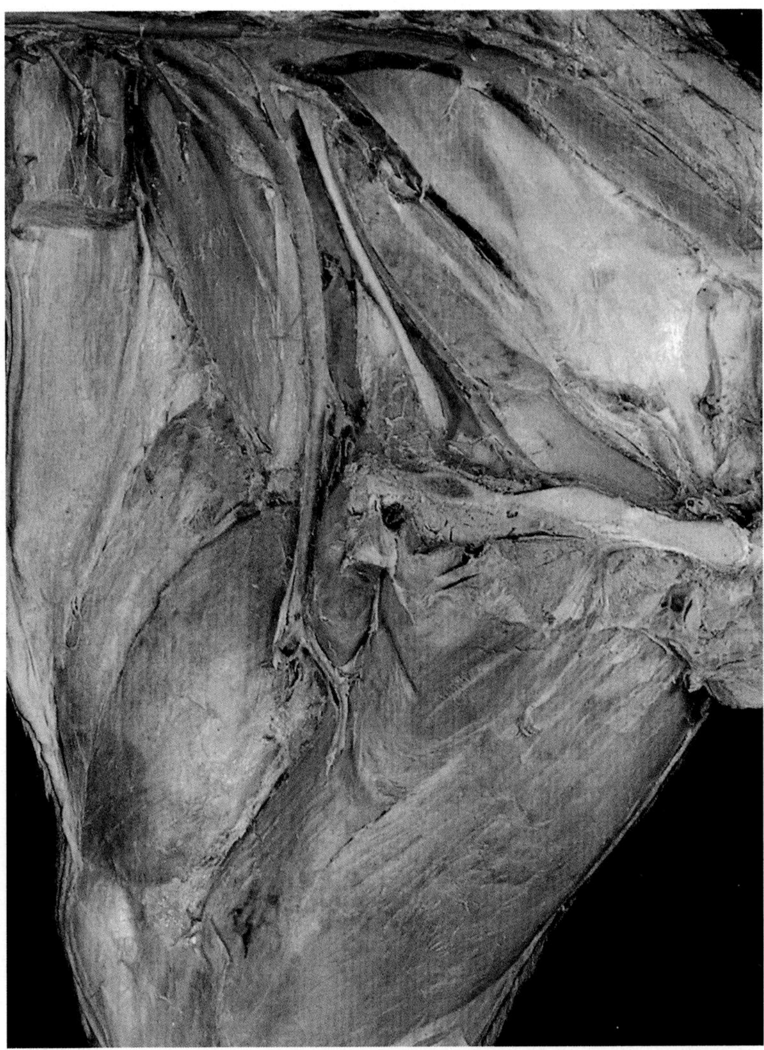

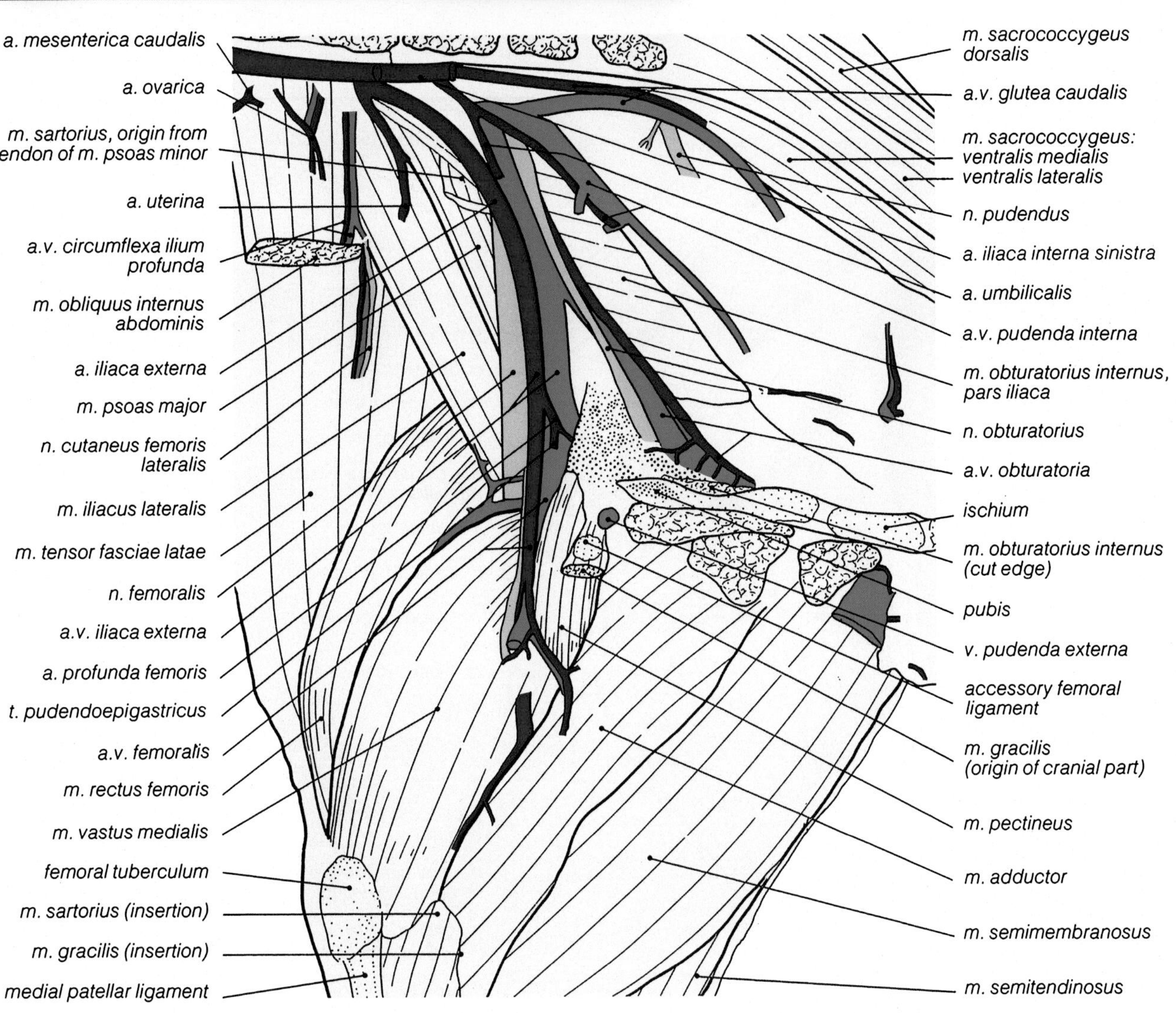
a. mesenterica caudalis
a. ovarica
m. sartorius, origin from tendon of m. psoas minor
a. uterina
a.v. circumflexa ilium profunda
m. obliquus internus abdominis
a. iliaca externa
m. psoas major
n. cutaneus femoris lateralis
m. iliacus lateralis
m. tensor fasciae latae
n. femoralis
a.v. iliaca externa
a. profunda femoris
t. pudendoepigastricus
a.v. femoralis
m. rectus femoris
m. vastus medialis
femoral tuberculum
m. sartorius (insertion)
m. gracilis (insertion)
medial patellar ligament
m. sacrococcygeus dorsalis
a.v. glutea caudalis
m. sacrococcygeus: ventralis medialis
ventralis lateralis
n. pudendus
a. iliaca interna sinistra
a. umbilicalis
a.v. pudenda interna
m. obturatorius internus, pars iliaca
n. obturatorius
a.v. obturatoria
ischium
m. obturatorius internus (cut edge)
pubis
v. pudenda externa
accessory femoral ligament
m. gracilis (origin of cranial part)
m. pectineus
m. adductor
m. semimembranosus
m. semitendinosus

Fig. 6.61 Femoral and saphenous vessels and nerves in the mare: right medial view. The sartorius muscle has been removed.

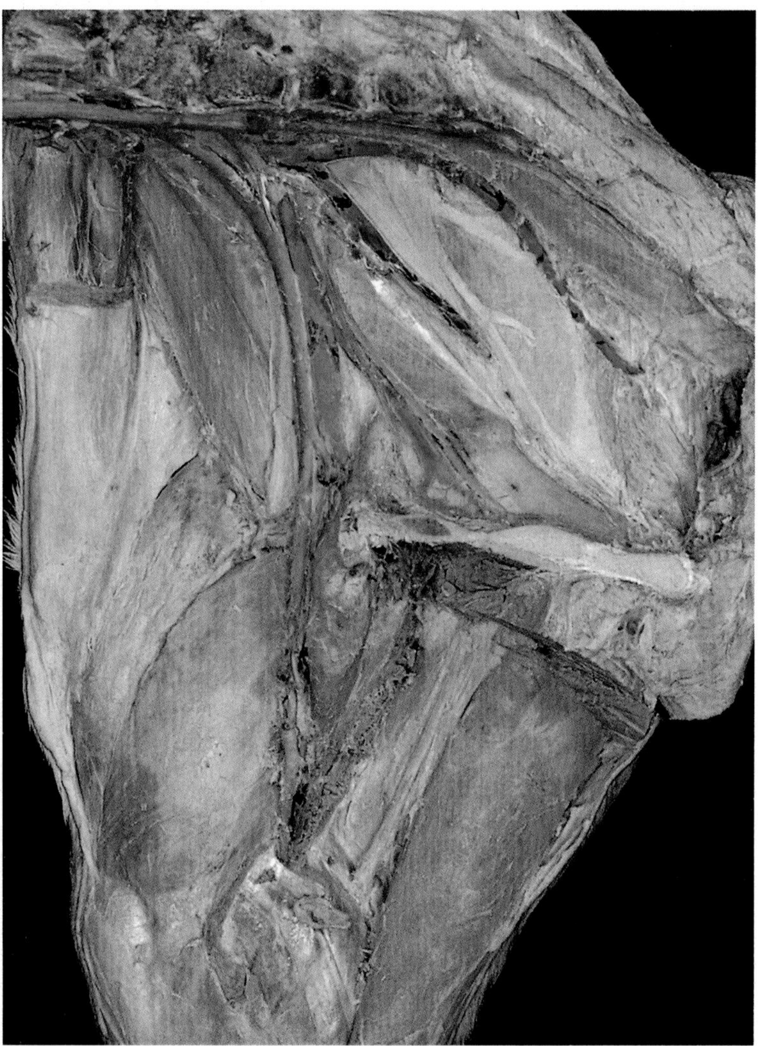

Fig. 6.62 Deep structures of the right pelvic and femoral regions in the mare: medial view. The adductor and semimembranosus muscles have been removed. The broad sacrotuberous ligament and the pudendal nerve which runs in it, have been resected to show the nerves lying lateral to the ligament.

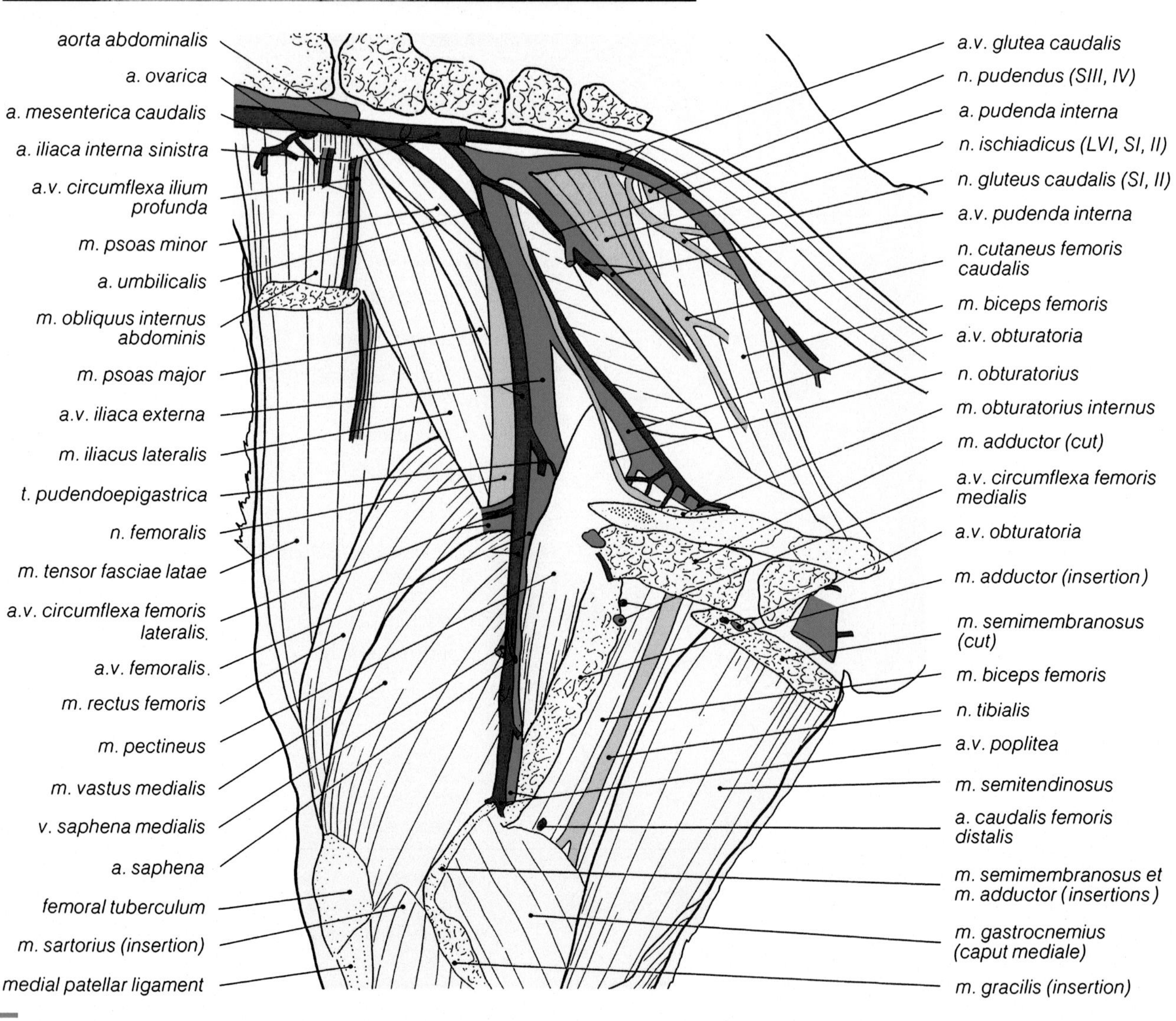
aorta abdominalis
a. ovarica
a. mesenterica caudalis
a. iliaca interna sinistra
a.v. circumflexa ilium profunda
m. psoas minor
a. umbilicalis
m. obliquus internus abdominis
m. psoas major
a.v. iliaca externa
m. iliacus lateralis
t. pudendoepigastrica
n. femoralis
m. tensor fasciae latae
a.v. circumflexa femoris lateralis
a.v. femoralis
m. rectus femoris
m. pectineus
m. vastus medialis
v. saphena medialis
a. saphena
femoral tuberculum
m. sartorius (insertion)
medial patellar ligament
a.v. glutea caudalis
n. pudendus (SIII, IV)
a. pudenda interna
n. ischiadicus (LVI, SI, II)
n. gluteus caudalis (SI, II)
a.v. pudenda interna
n. cutaneus femoris caudalis
m. biceps femoris
a.v. obturatoria
n. obturatorius
m. obturatorius internus
m. adductor (cut)
a.v. circumflexa femoris medialis
a.v. obturatoria
m. adductor (insertion)
m. semimembranosus (cut)
m. biceps femoris
n. tibialis
a.v. poplitea
m. semitendinosus
a. caudalis femoris distalis
m. semimembranosus et m. adductor (insertions)
m. gastrocnemius (caput mediale)
m. gracilis (insertion)

7. THE FOOT

Clinical importance of the foot

In vertebrate anatomy, the 'foot' includes the carpus or tarsus and the regions distal to these joints. Contact between the foot and the potentially dangerous ground underfoot (frequently mud or concrete) produces a variety of disorders which cause many clinical problems. The lower limb is subjected to tremendous stress and strain through normal locomotion, and is frequently involved in trauma. Approximately 60% of the weight of a horse is carried on the forefeet and approximately 90% of all forelimb lameness occurs in the foot.

Correct foot balance is required and is sometimes forgotten. Various imbalances of conformation can occur. The foot has to be balanced and evenly placed around its centre of weight-bearing (midpoint of the circle of the laminar suspension). In dorso-palmar imbalance, the foot has a long toe and a low heel, so the load is transferred to the heels. Latero-medial imbalance is often the result of uneven trimming which results in sheared heels; one heel (usually the medial one) strikes the ground before the other.

In young horses, fractures of the growth plates are the most common. The younger the foal when the fracture occurs the better the prognosis. If the fracture is transverse, across the bone (as is usual in the pedal bone) rather than longitudinal, along the long axis, the bone heals more quickly. Approximately 80% of the fractures of the equine foot occur in the manus. Distal limb fractures are often acute, with severe ligament damage and soft tissue swelling. The fracture may be closed or open (exposed to potential infection). Bruised or sore shins (dorsal metacarpal disease) are the result of stress or fatigue to the bone as this part of the bone receives more stress compression than the other parts of the bone. Condylar, metaphyseal and diaphyseal fractures of the third metapodial (metacarpal and metatarsal) bones may occur. Chip fractures are also quite common. In the 'proximal metapodial syndrome' there are avulsion stress fractures of the proximal palmar and plantar cortices.

'Splints' are bony exostoses of the second or fourth metapodial bones. Fractures of the second and fourth metapodial bones usually occur in the distal third of the bone. They usually result from kicks, but may also occur spontaneously. Fractures of the middle phalanx occur frequently from the sudden compression and simultaneous torsion to which the foot is often subjected. This is particularly severe with sudden stops and starts.

Fractures of the distal phalanx (pedal bone) are not uncommon. They often occur when the horse kicks out and hits something solid. The digital pulse is increased in this fracture. If the distal interphalangeal joint (DIP) is also involved, there may be considerable effusions into the joint. Fracture of the proximal sesamoid bone may result from over-extension of the suspensory apparatus, degenerative changes in the bone, direct trauma or osteoporosis. Sesamoiditis (degenerative or bony change in the proximal sesamoid bones) is an important disease of the foot in the horse. 'Ringbone' is an enlargement of one or both of the bones which form the proximal or distal interphalangeal joint. The term 'false ringbone' is often used when only the shaft of the proximal or middle phalanx is affected.

There are several types of fracture (#) of the pedal bone (distal phalanx):

Type I – non-articular fractures of the palmar/plantar process
Type II – parasagittal articular fractures from the DIP joint to the medial and lateral solar margin
Type III – mid-sagittal articular fractures
Type IV – fractures of the extensor process
Type V – comminuted fractures of the pedal bone secondary to foreign body penetration
Type VI – non-articular marginal fractures
Type VII – non-articular fractures of the palmar/plantar process.

Inflammation of the distal phalanx (pedal osteitis) is quite common. 'Sidebone' is ossification in the ungular cartilages of the pedal bone and is relatively common, whereas bone-cysts in the pedal bone are much rarer. Fracture of the distal sesamoid ('navicular bone') may be in the form of a chip fracture or a simple sagittal fracture close to the ridge of the sesamoid bone. Comminuted fractures of this bone are fortunately rare, as they are impossible to repair.

Problems of the joints of the foot involve a considerable amount of the equine practitioners time, expertise, energy and patience. In the foal, the most common cause of acute lameness is septic arthritis/osteomyelitis. Most are septicaemic infections and in at least 50% of the cases, multiple joints are involved. There are basically three types of injury. One is related to the epiphyses, the second to the epiphyseal cartilages and the third to the cuboidal bones in the carpus and tarsus. Villonodular synovitis in the form of a chronic proliferative hypertrophic response is also not uncommon.

The joints of the manus and pes of the older horse are also subjected to a wide range of abnormalities. Sub-luxations occur and must be repaired, but they have a very poor prognosis. Luxations occur in the proximal (PIP) and the distal (DIP) interphalangeal joints. Angular deformity (joint laxity) of the fetlock is also a possibility. This, and a similar interphalangeal disorder, have a poor prognosis. Flexural deformity of the fetlock is either congenital or acquired. It may be due to relative shortening of the musculo-tendinous part of the superficial digital flexor muscle, the deep digital flexor muscle, or the sesamoidean ligaments. Traumatic and degenerative arthritis of the proximal interphalangeal joint (PIP or pastern joint) and distal interphalangeal joint (DIP or coffin joint) has been described, and infectious arthritis of the joint is also known.

The joints of the foot are accessible for the collection of joint fluid samples, or the administration of anaesthesia, or treatments. The fetlock joint is accessible via its palmar/plantar synovial recess. This is located just proximal to the joint, between the palmar aspect of the distal metapodial bone III and the suspensory ligament, at a level distal to the distal end of metapodial II. With the limb in a weight-bearing position, the needle is inserted at right angles to the axis of the limb, in a slightly downward direction, to a depth of 2–3 cm. The PIP (pastern) joint is entered through a site dorsal and just lateral to the common (forelimb) or long (hindlimb) digital extensor tendon and at the level of, or just distal to, the palmar or plantar process of the proximal phalanx. With the limb in a weight-bearing position, the needle is inserted in a distal and medial direction. The DIP (coffin) joint is located by finding a depression that is approximately 2 cm dorsal to the coronary band and on the midline. The needle may be inserted just medial or lateral to the common (forelimb) or long (hindlimb) digital extensor tendon or directly through the tendon. With the limb in a weight-bearing position, the needle is inserted in a distal and palmar or plantar direction, to a depth of 2.5 cm.

Tendonitis is inflammation of the tendon sheaths. Usually the superficial (SDF) and deep (DDF) digital flexor tendons are affected. These tendons suffer severe stress in the leg of the horse. They are also damaged when the muscles are fatigued. The SDF is more likely to be damaged because it suffers much more strain in over-extension than the DDF. The damage is most likely to occur at mid metacarpal level in the SDF or, for the DDF, at the level of the fetlock joint. Both tendons are avascular and repair therefore takes time.

Tendon lacerations are quite common as a result of wire cuts, over-reaching, or striking injuries. Damage to the DDF causes lifting of the toe. Damage to the SDF causes sinking of the fetlock. If both the tendons are sectioned then the fetlock sinks to the ground.

The ligaments of the foot may also suffer damage, usually as a result of trauma. Desmitis (inflammation of a ligament) can affect the distal sesamoidean ligaments of the fetlock. Breakdown of the suspensory apparatus can also occur, usually in racehorses when going at full speed: an acute over-extension of the fetlock can disrupt any or all of the components of the suspensory apparatus – suspensory ligament, sesamoid bones, and distal sesamoidean ligaments. The most common site of any such injury is at the proximal attachment of the suspensory ligament to the proximal plantar cortex of the metacarpal/metatarsal bones.

The 'navicular syndrome' is responsible for 30% of all of forelimb lamenesses. The syndrome is chronic palmar foot lameness affecting the distal sesamoid ('navicular') bone. It involves the fibrocartilage of its flexor surface, the palmar part of the distal interphalangeal joint, the deep digital flexor tendon, the podotrochlear ('navicular') bursa, the collateral sesamoidean ('navicular' suspensory) ligaments and the distal sesamoid impar ligament. There are two theories for its cause: the vascular theory and the biomechanical theory. It is thought to be associated with abnormal pressure/vibration forces between the deep digital flexor tendon and the flexor surface of the navicular bone. Also, penetrating wounds can reach the deep digital flexor tendon and may result in necrosis in the tendon. Penetration into the podotrochlear ('navicular') bursa may also involve the impar ligament and progress into the distal interphalangeal joint (DIP) and result in infectious arthritis. The digital sheath of the deep digital flexor muscle extends to the midshaft of the middle digit. Penetration into this digital sheath may result in infectious tenosynovitis.

The hoof may be damaged by treading on something sharp or by being kicked and it is then easily infected by soil-borne pathogens. However, when the hoof is damaged, it can be supported and protected by casts and shoes.

Laminitis is a specific condition of the foot of the horse, usually affecting the forelimb. This is inflammation of the sensitive laminae of the corium (dermis) within the wall of the hoof. It is essentially a peripheral vascular disorder caused by systemic damage. Release of vasoactive substances (catecholamines) can cause ischaemic necrosis. There are many different predisposing factors, particularly grain overload and postoperative recovery after colic surgery. Laminitis can be graded as 1, 2, 3 and 4. Type 1 is developmental, type 2 foot pain and lameness, type 3 sub-clinical (recovery without mechanical failure) and type 4 chronic (this leads to displacement of the distal phalanx). The progression usually starts with excess grain overload, leading to a rise in lactic acid, then the caecal pH falls. Gram-negative bacteria rapidly multiply and extra endotoxin is released. Vasoactive agents are then released and circulate. This leads to vasoconstriction, ischaemia and necrosis. Another theory suggests that proteinases are activated in the distal lamellae and this degrades the type IV collagen which attaches the hoof to the distal phalanx. This results in loss of mechanical support.

Various other foot problems can be listed. 'Mud rash' (otherwise known as greasy-heel) is associated with bacterial infections caused by *Dermatophilus* and *Staphylococci.* Cracks in the hoof wall run vertically from the coronary band. 'Seedy toe' is separation of the hoof wall from the distal phalanx. 'Thrush' is a degenerative condition of the central and collateral sulci of the frog; it is associated with surface invasion by micro-organisms under anaerobic conditions. 'Canker' is a chronic, infectious, hypertrophic, moist, podo-dermatitis of the frog and sole. 'Keratoma' is an uncommon benign tumour of the horn between the laminar horn and dermis (corium) in the wall of the hoof. 'White line disease' is a rare, progressive crumbling of the hoof wall at the junction between the wall and sole. 'Nail bind' is a direct injury or bruising of the solar or laminar dermis caused by a shoe-nail. 'Quittor' is the necrosis of the ungular cartilages of the distal phalanx; it often results in purulent discharges and sinus formation above the coronary band.

The hoof wall is rigid except at the heels, where the laminae are attached to the ungular cartilages, which can 'expand' (move abaxially) on bearing weight. The structures within the 'rigid', box-like regions of the toe and quarters are also subjected to continuous movement on bearing weight, so there is a potential for problems of diminished blood supply to these regions. The hoof has a diminished response to injury and a slow rate of healing, yet it contains many important structures. Superficial wounds that penetrate only cornified tissue may, nevertheless, produce a sub-solar abscess. Pododermatitis is the inflammation of the solar dermis (corium) with or without secondary infection. Deep wounds that penetrate the germinal epithelium introduce infections, usually *Clostridia.* These are life-threatening emergencies with serious long-term consequences. Wounds that involve the synovial structures are particularly serious and require immediate and aggressive treatment.

Wounds greater than 1 cm in depth are dangerous as these penetrate the sole. Wounds of 1.2 cm will penetrate the hoof and wall. Wounds over 1.5 cm deep will penetrate the frog. These deep penetrating wounds can be classified into three groups: Type 1 wounds penetrate the corium and cause septic osteitis in the distal phalanx, with a distal cushion abscess. Type 2, penetrating deep puncture wounds, gain access into the caudal third of the frog and can enter many structures including the digital flexor tendons (the SDF and DDF). The hoof also contains other structures that can be penetrated, including the distal interphalangeal (DIP) joint, tendon sheaths, tendons (particularly the tendon of the DDF) and ligaments (the distal sesamoid impar ligament and the collateral ligaments of the DIP), the distal and middle phalanges and the distal sesamoid ('navicular') bone and its bursa. Type 3 wounds penetrate the coronary band, leading to septic chondritis of the cartilaginous structures such as the articular cartilages and ungular cartilages of the distal phalanx, and may subsequently extend into the distal interphalangeal (DIP) joint.

Several nerve blocks are used to localise the site of lameness in the manus or pes. Perineural analgesia of the distal digital region can be achieved by blocking the lateral and medial palmar/plantar nerves at the level of the middle phalanx. The needle is inserted subcutaneously over the palpable neurovascular bundle, just proximal to the ungular cartilage of the distal phalanx on each side. This is the Palmar/Plantar digital nerve block. These nerves can be blocked at a more proximal level by inserting the needle subcutaneously over the palpable neurovascular bundle, on the abaxial surface of the lateral and then the medial proximal sesamoid bone. This is the Abaxial sesamoid nerve block.

Perineural analgesia of the distal metacarpal and digital regions can be achieved by blocking the lateral and medial palmar, and palmar metacarpal nerves, proximal to the fetlock. The sites for subcutaneous injections are immediately distal to the distal extremities ('buttons') of the metacarpal bones II and IV, to block the palmar metacarpal nerves on both sides. At the same level, the sites for subcutaneous injections are located between the DDF and the suspensory ligament on each side, to block the palmar nerves. This is the Low 4-point nerve block for the forelimb. For the hindlimb, the same four injections are made, but there is an important anatomical difference. The dorsal metatarsal nerves exchange fibres with the plantar metatarsal nerves in the proximal phalangeal region and they innervate the hoof. It is therefore necessary to block these medial and lateral dorsal metatarsal nerves with subcutaneous circumferential ring-blocks at the dorsal aspect of the 'buttons' of the splint bones. This is the Low 6-point nerve block for the hindlimb.

Perineural analgesia of the metacarpal and digital regions can be achieved by blocking the lateral and medial palmar, and also the palmar metacarpal nerves, just distal to the carpus. The needle is inserted deeply, axial to metacarpal bone IV, until it reaches the palmar surface of metacarpal bone III. Here the lateral palmar metacarpal nerve is injected. The palmar nerve is blocked by inserting the needle subcutaneously at the same level into the space between the DDF and the suspensory ligament. This is repeated on the medial side in relation to metacarpal bone II. These constitute the High palmar nerve block. In the hindlimb, only one injection site is needed on each side to inject the nerves. The needle is inserted just distal to the tarsometatarsal joint and axial to metatarsal bone IV, until it reaches the plantar surface of metatarsal bone III. After injecting the lateral plantar metatarsal nerve at this site, the needle is partially withdrawn and a second injection is made between the DDF and the suspensory ligament, to block the lateral plantar nerve. This procedure is repeated on the medial side, in relation to metatarsal bone II and the tendon and ligament. This is the High plantar nerve block.

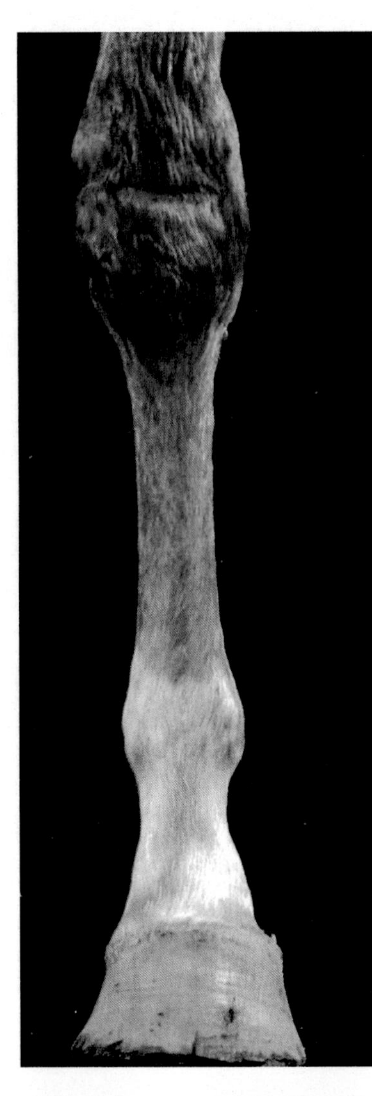

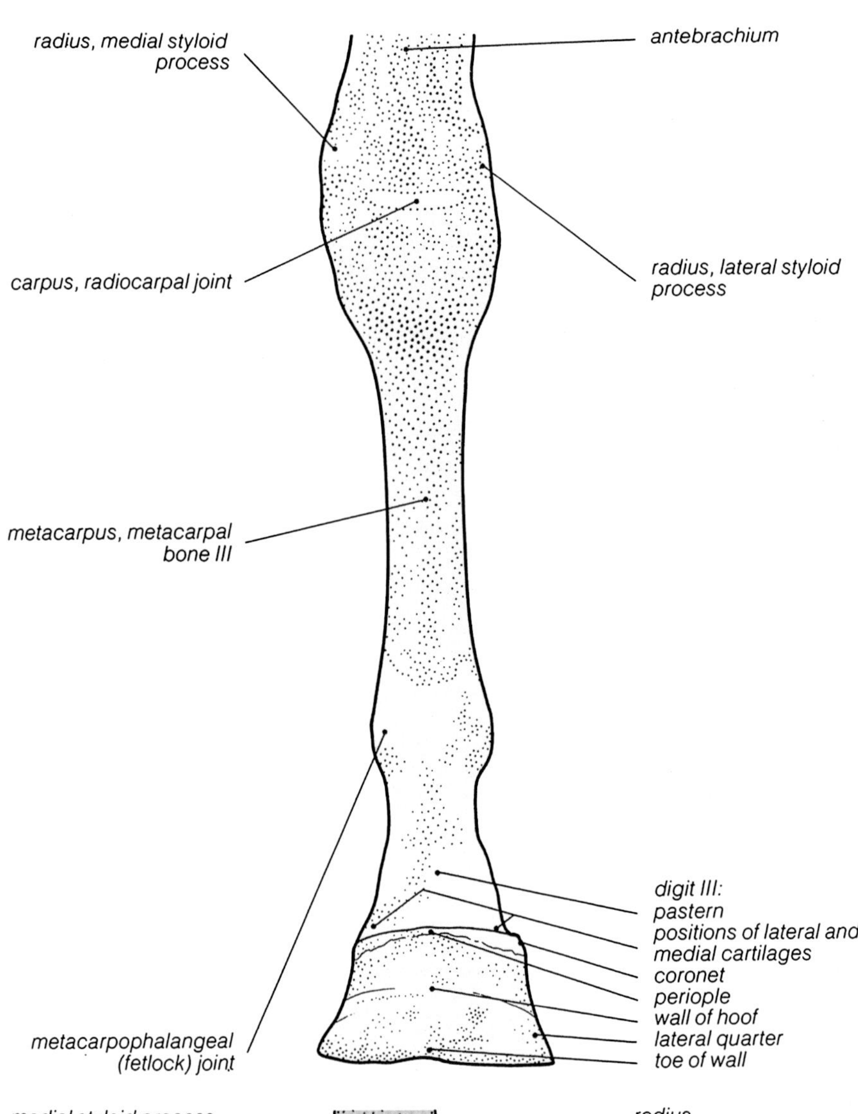
radius, medial styloid process
antebrachium
carpus, radiocarpal joint
radius, lateral styloid process
metacarpus, metacarpal bone III
digit III:
pastern
positions of lateral and medial cartilages
coronet
periople
wall of hoof
lateral quarter
toe of wall
metacarpophalangeal (fetlock) joint

Fig. 7.1 Surface features of the left manus: cranial view. Figs. 7.3, 7.5 and 7.7 show further views of this specimen. Palpable features have been shaved. Figs. 7.2, 7.4, 7.6 and 7.8 show the bones of the region. Fig. 7.9 shows the solar surfaces of the hoof.

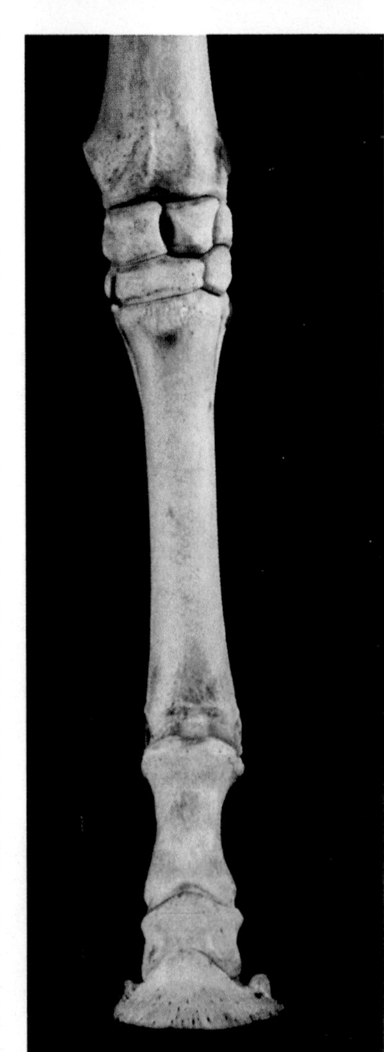

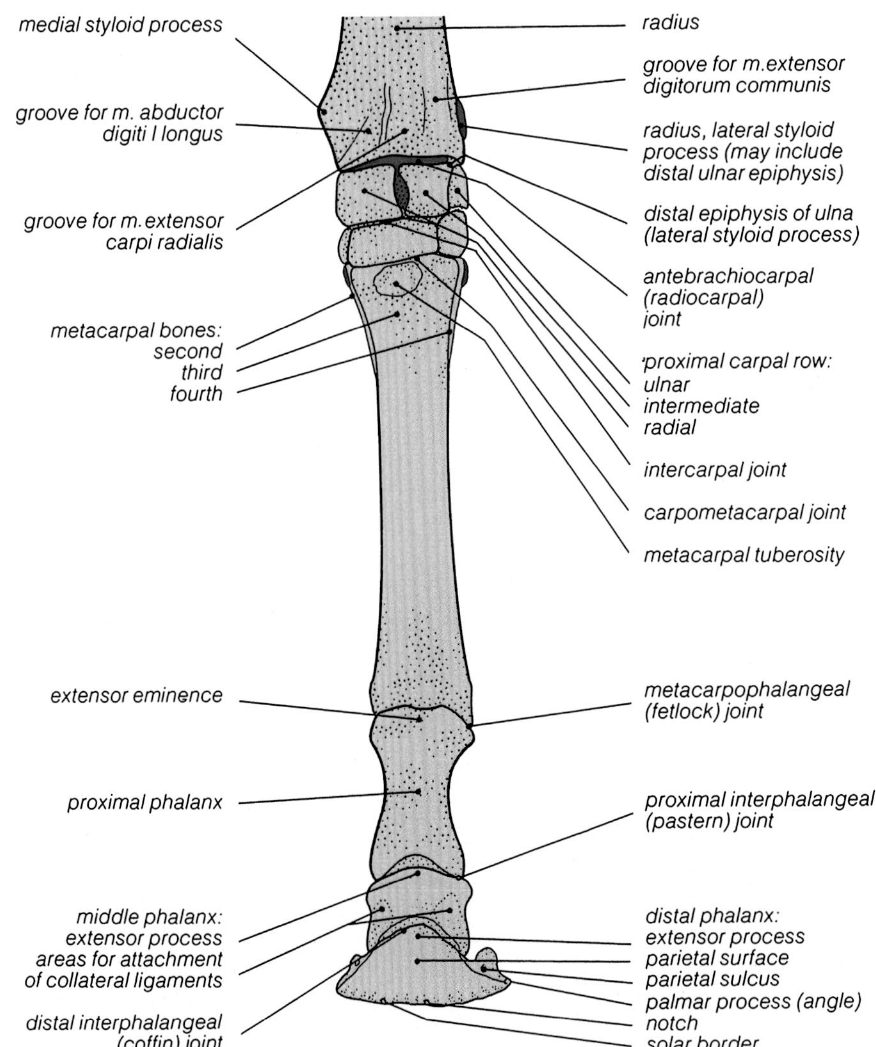
medial styloid process
radius
groove for m.extensor digitorum communis
groove for m. abductor digiti I longus
radius, lateral styloid process (may include distal ulnar epiphysis)
groove for m.extensor carpi radialis
distal epiphysis of ulna (lateral styloid process)
antebrachiocarpal (radiocarpal) joint
metacarpal bones:
second
third
fourth
proximal carpal row:
ulnar
intermediate
radial
intercarpal joint
carpometacarpal joint
metacarpal tuberosity
extensor eminence
metacarpophalangeal (fetlock) joint
proximal phalanx
proximal interphalangeal (pastern) joint
middle phalanx:
extensor process
areas for attachment of collateral ligaments
distal phalanx:
extensor process
parietal surface
parietal sulcus
palmar process (angle)
notch
solar border
distal interphalangeal (coffin) joint

Fig. 7.2 The bones of the left manus: cranial view. The prominences shaved in Fig. 7.1 have been coloured red, except for the salient medial styloid process. For a comment on the lateral styloid process, see Fig. 7.4.

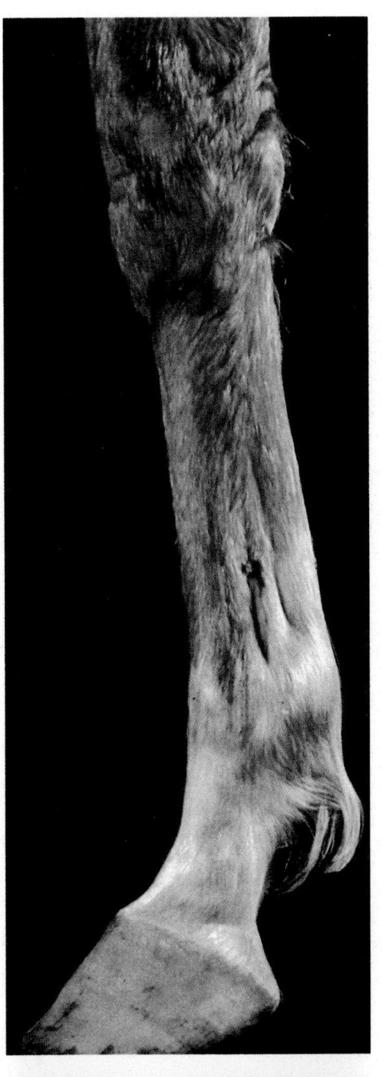

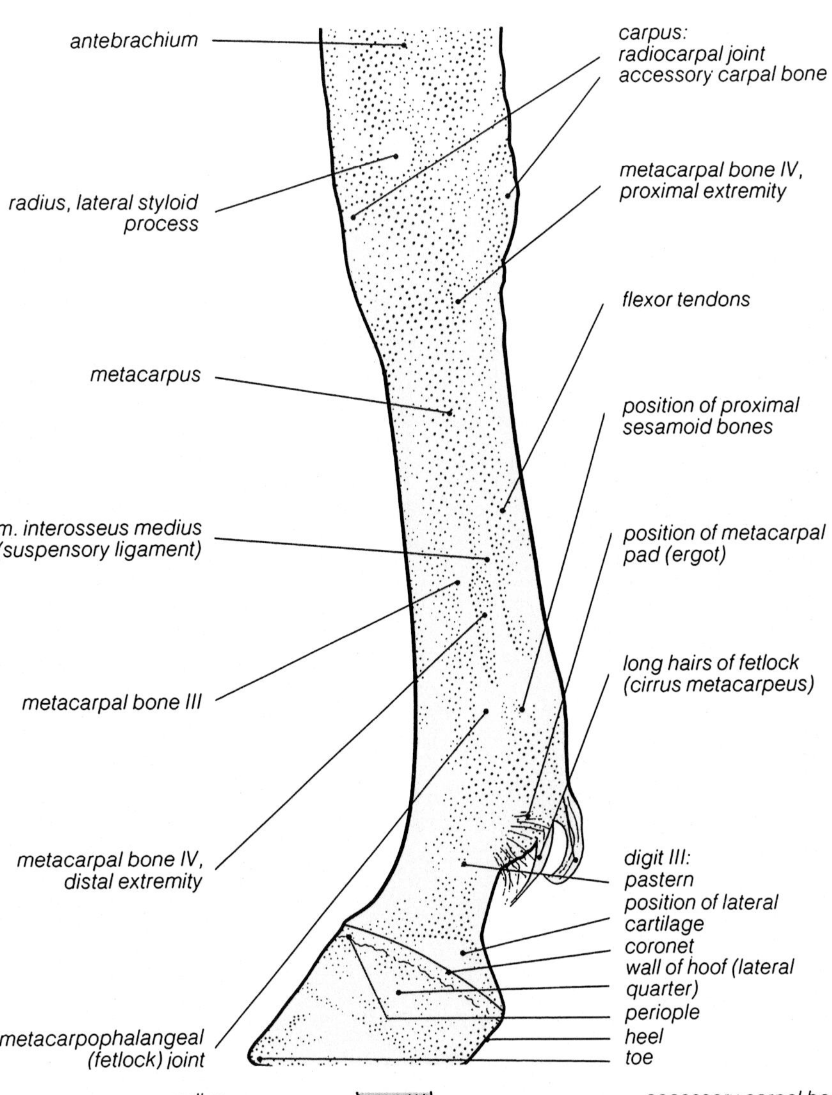
antebrachium
radius, lateral styloid process
metacarpus
m. interosseus medius (suspensory ligament)
metacarpal bone III
metacarpal bone IV, distal extremity
metacarpophalangeal (fetlock) joint
carpus:
radiocarpal joint
accessory carpal bone
metacarpal bone IV, proximal extremity
flexor tendons
position of proximal sesamoid bones
position of metacarpal pad (ergot)
long hairs of fetlock (cirrus metacarpeus)
digit III:
pastern
position of lateral cartilage
coronet
wall of hoof (lateral quarter)
periople
heel
toe

Fig. 7.3 Surface features of the left manus: lateral view. The specimen was embalmed in the standing position, with the limb arranged to imitate its position in normal level standing. Palpable features have been shaved. In some breeds of horse the long hairs of the fetlock are extremely well developed, covering the whole pastern region.

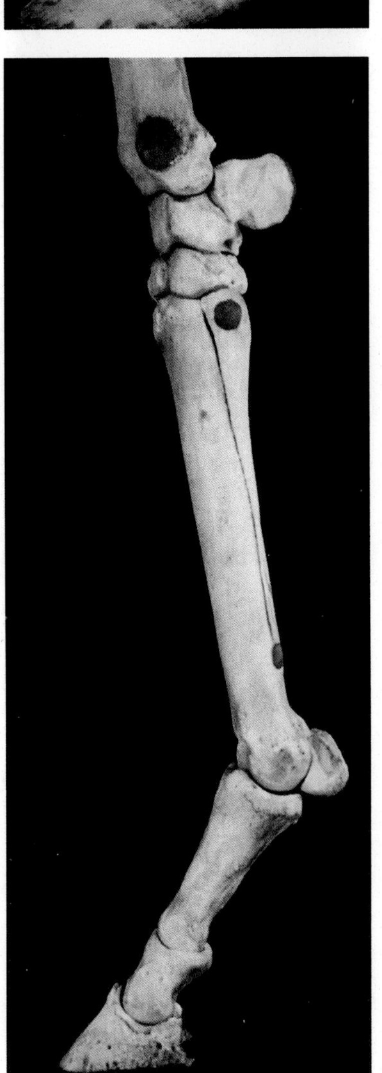

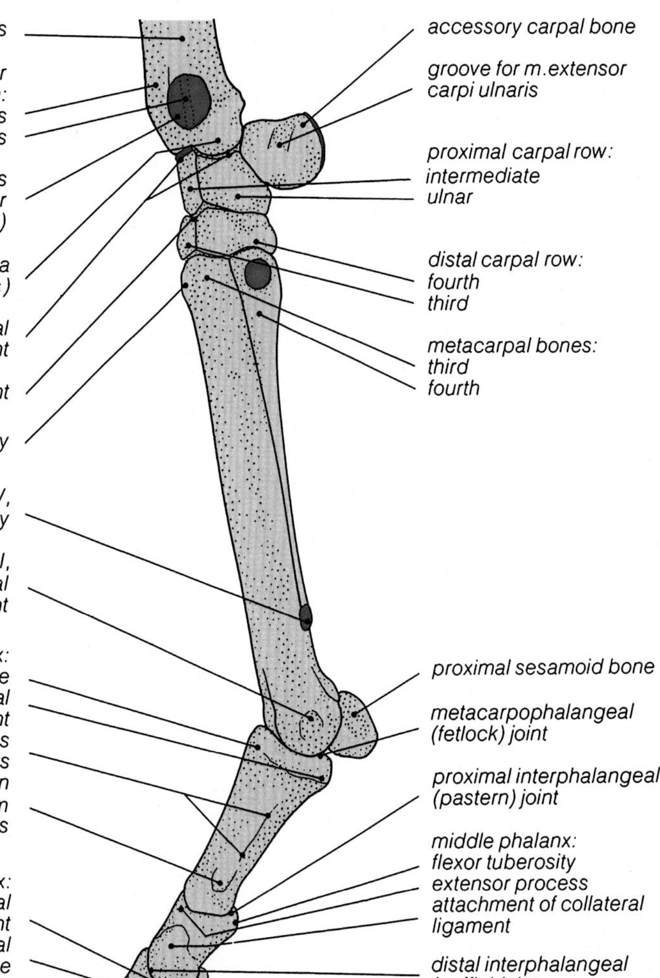
radius
groove for m. extensor digitorum:
communis
lateralis
lateral styloid process (may include distal ulnar diaphysis)
distal epiphysis of ulna (lateral styloid process)
antebrachiocarpal (radiocarpal) joint
intercarpal joint
metacarpal tuberosity
metacarpal bone IV, distal extremity
metacarpal bone III, attachment of collateral ligament
proximal phalanx:
extensor eminence
eminence for collateral ligament
ridge for ligamentous attachments
area for part of insertion of m. flexor digitorum superficialis
distal phalanx:
attachment of collateral ligament
attachment of lateral cartilage
parietal sulcus
parietal surface
palmar process (angle)
solar border
accessory carpal bone
groove for m.extensor carpi ulnaris
proximal carpal row:
intermediate
ulnar
distal carpal row:
fourth
third
metacarpal bones:
third
fourth
proximal sesamoid bone
metacarpophalangeal (fetlock) joint
proximal interphalangeal (pastern) joint
middle phalanx:
flexor tuberosity
extensor process
attachment of collateral ligament
distal interphalangeal (coffin) joint
distal sesamoid (navicular) bone

Fig. 7.4 The bones of the left manus: lateral view. The prominences shaved in Fig. 7.3 have been coloured red. The distal epiphysis of the ulna fuses with that of the radius at about 1 year, to form the lateral articular condyle. The prominence just proximal to it is probably of diaphyseal origin, but it is commonly called the lateral styloid process of the radius.

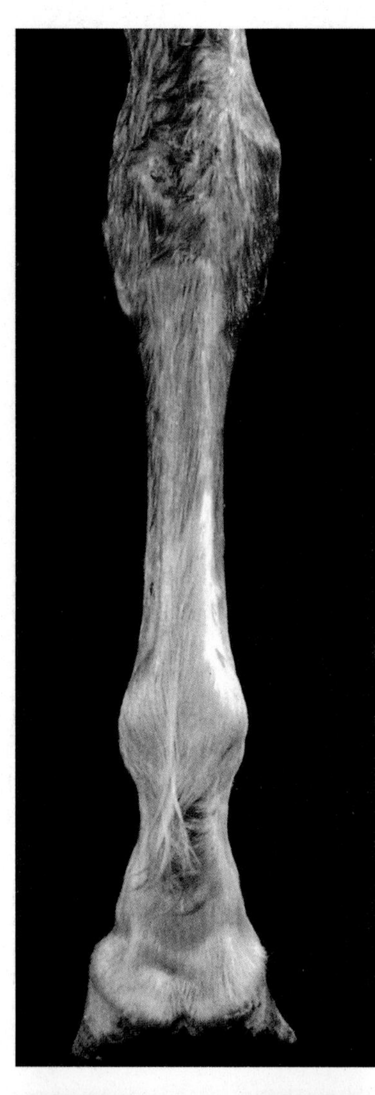

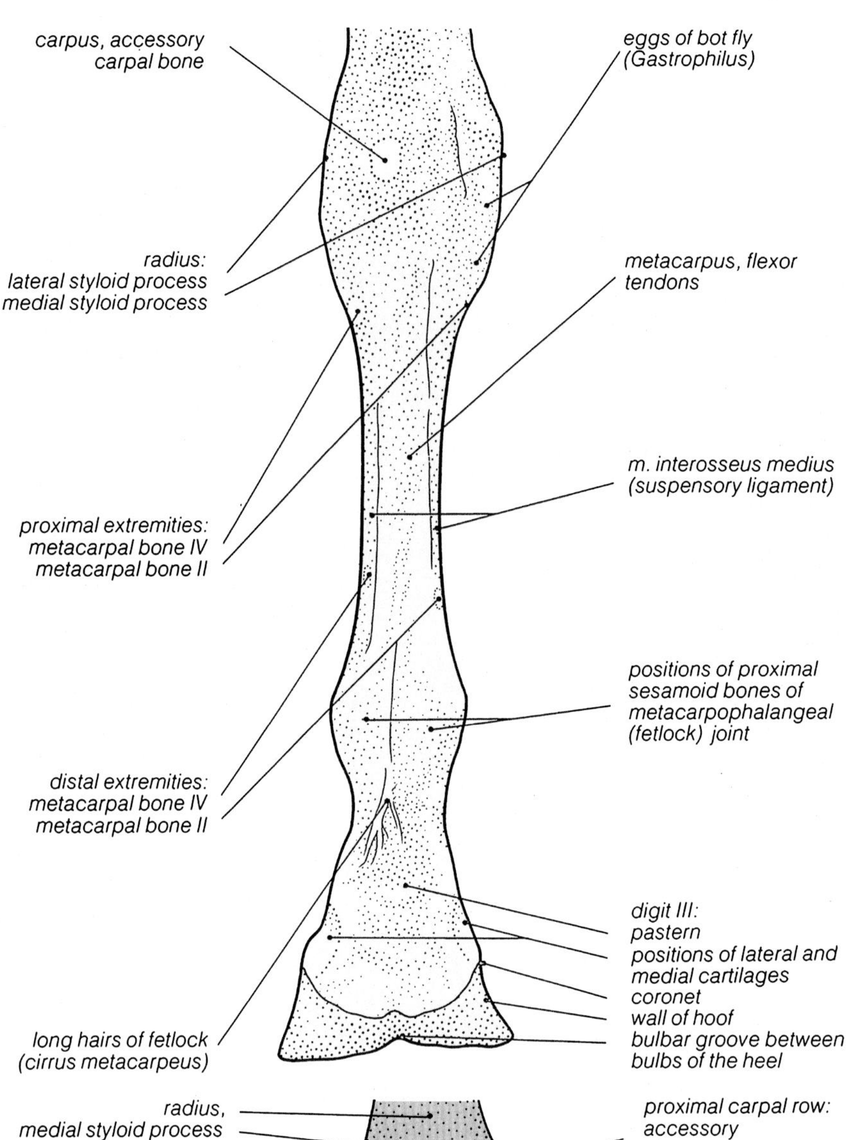
carpus, accessory carpal bone
radius:
lateral styloid process
medial styloid process
proximal extremities:
metacarpal bone IV
metacarpal bone II
distal extremities:
metacarpal bone IV
metacarpal bone II
long hairs of fetlock (cirrus metacarpeus)
eggs of bot fly (Gastrophilus)
metacarpus, flexor tendons
m. interosseus medius (suspensory ligament)
positions of proximal sesamoid bones of metacarpophalangeal (fetlock) joint
digit III:
pastern
positions of lateral and medial cartilages
coronet
wall of hoof
bulbar groove between bulbs of the heel

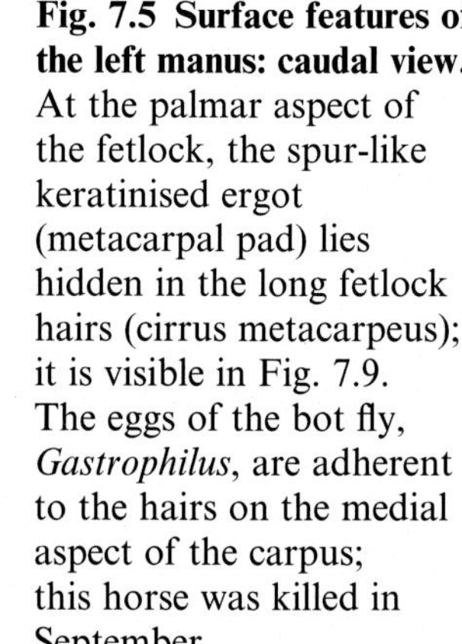

Fig. 7.5 Surface features of the left manus: caudal view. At the palmar aspect of the fetlock, the spur-like keratinised ergot (metacarpal pad) lies hidden in the long fetlock hairs (cirrus metacarpeus); it is visible in Fig. 7.9. The eggs of the bot fly, *Gastrophilus*, are adherent to the hairs on the medial aspect of the carpus; this horse was killed in September.

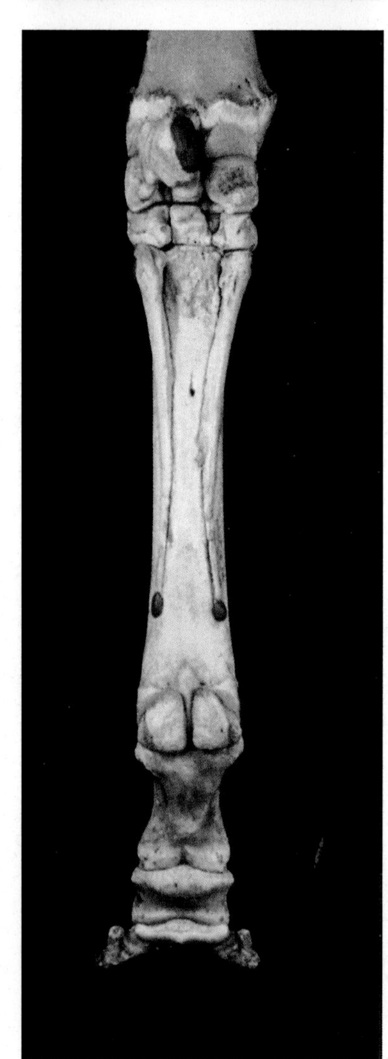

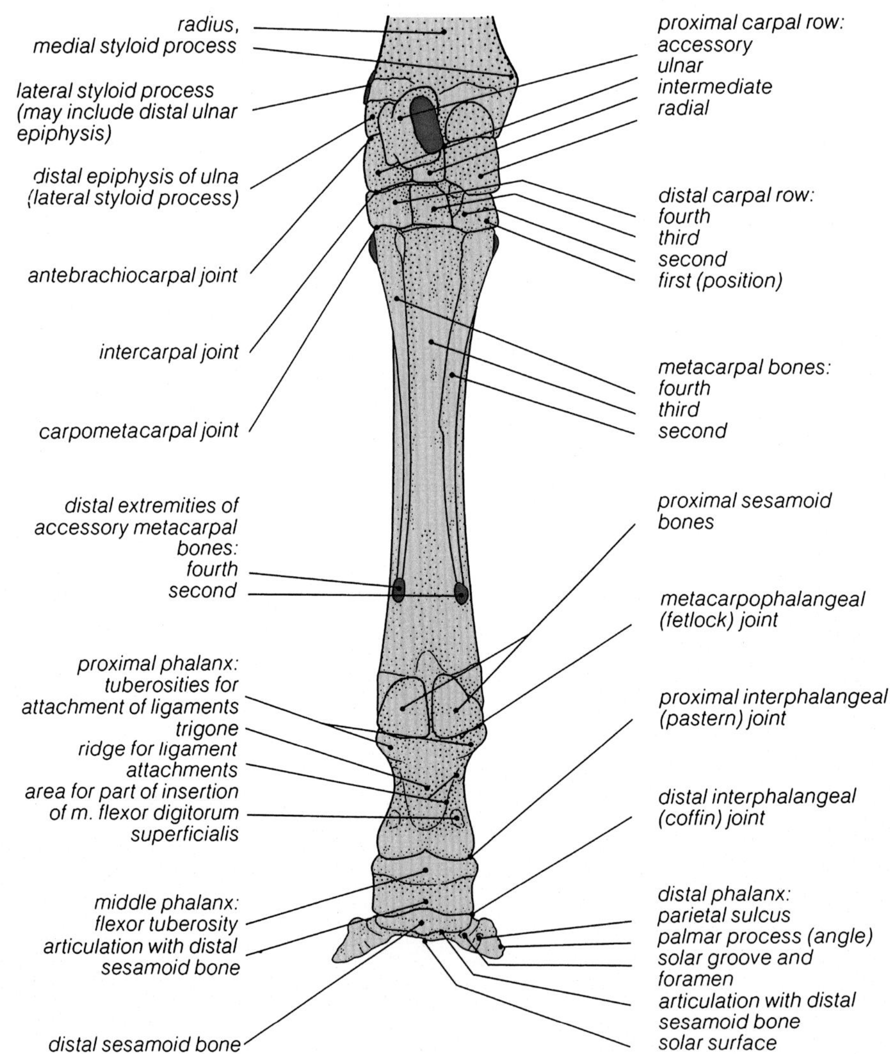
radius,
medial styloid process
lateral styloid process (may include distal ulnar epiphysis)
distal epiphysis of ulna (lateral styloid process)
antebrachiocarpal joint
intercarpal joint
carpometacarpal joint
distal extremities of accessory metacarpal bones:
fourth
second
proximal phalanx:
tuberosities for attachment of ligaments
trigone
ridge for ligament attachments
area for part of insertion of m. flexor digitorum superficialis
middle phalanx:
flexor tuberosity
articulation with distal sesamoid bone
distal sesamoid bone
proximal carpal row:
accessory
ulnar
intermediate
radial
distal carpal row:
fourth
third
second
first (position)
metacarpal bones:
fourth
third
second
proximal sesamoid bones
metacarpophalangeal (fetlock) joint
proximal interphalangeal (pastern) joint
distal interphalangeal (coffin) joint
distal phalanx:
parietal sulcus
palmar process (angle)
solar groove and foramen
articulation with distal sesamoid bone
solar surface

Fig. 7.6 The bones of the left manus: caudal view. The parts shaved in Fig. 7.5 have been coloured red, except for the salient medial styloid process. The inconstant and variable first carpal bone was not present on this skeleton, but its position is indicated in the drawing.

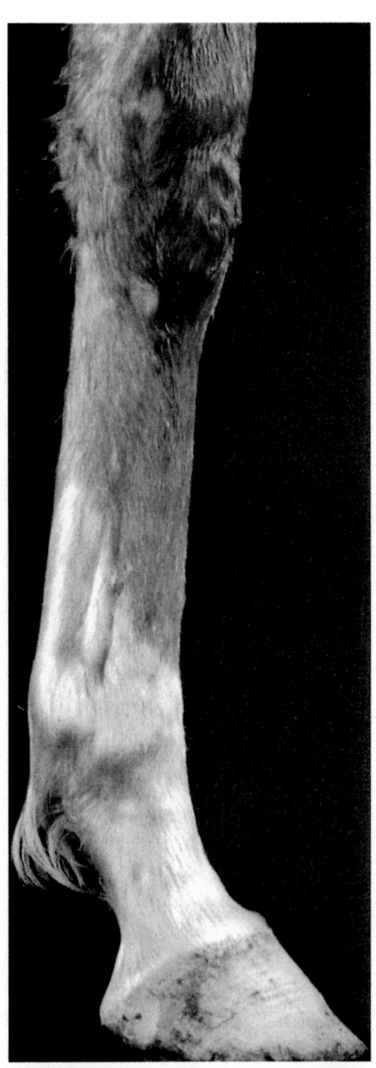

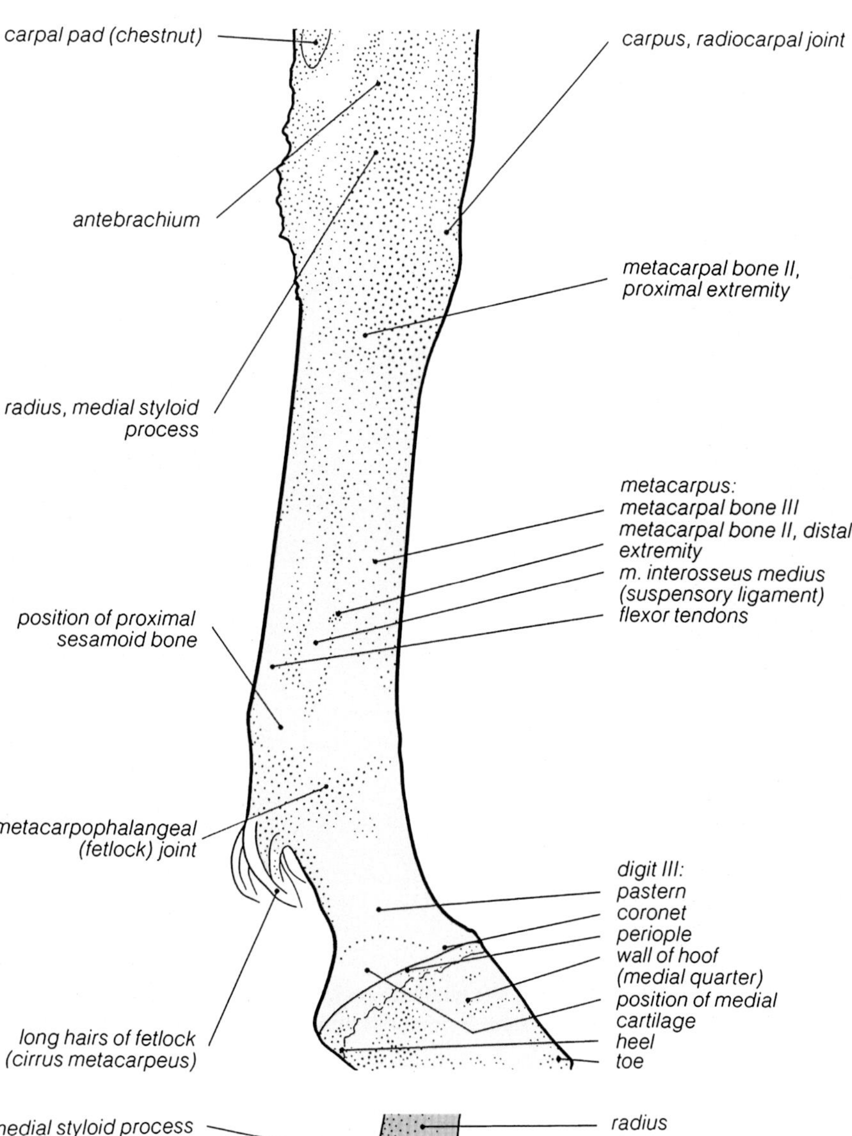
carpal pad (chestnut)
antebrachium
radius, medial styloid process
position of proximal sesamoid bone
metacarpophalangeal (fetlock) joint
long hairs of fetlock (cirrus metacarpeus)
carpus, radiocarpal joint
metacarpal bone II, proximal extremity
metacarpus:
metacarpal bone III
metacarpal bone II, distal extremity
m. interosseus medius (suspensory ligament)
flexor tendons
digit III:
pastern
coronet
periople
wall of hoof (medial quarter)
position of medial cartilage
heel
toe

Fig. 7.7 Surface features of the left manus: medial view. The position of the carpal pad or 'chestnut' in relation to the underlying structures is variable, but it is usually present in all members of the genus *Equus*, lying proximal to the carpus.

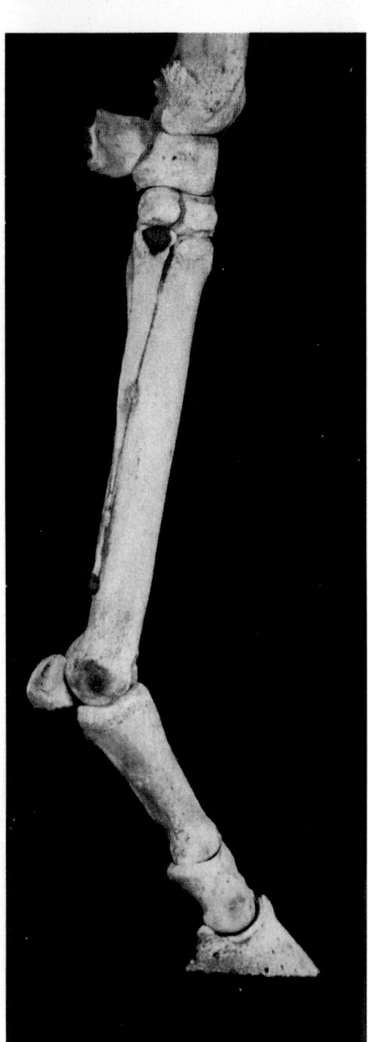

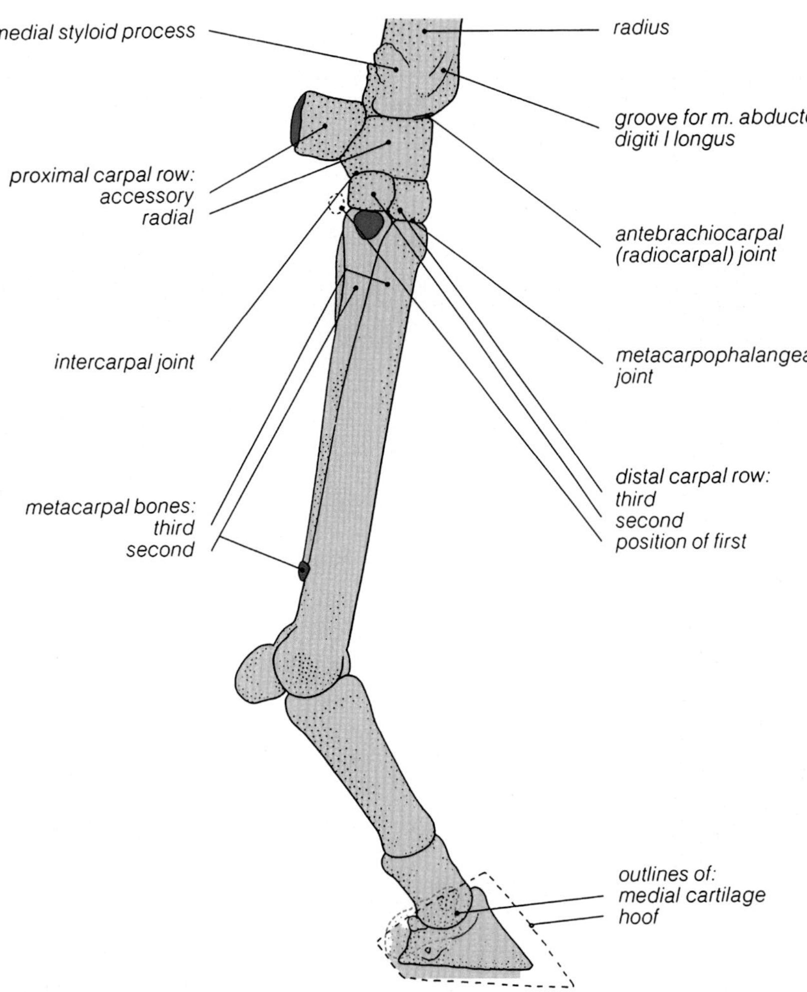
medial styloid process
proximal carpal row:
accessory
radial
intercarpal joint
metacarpal bones:
third
second
radius
groove for m. abductor digiti I longus
antebrachiocarpal (radiocarpal) joint
metacarpophalangeal joint
distal carpal row:
third
second
position of first
outlines of:
medial cartilage
hoof

Fig. 7.8 The bones of the left manus: medial view. The parts shaved in Fig. 7.7 have been coloured red, except for the medial styloid process. The inconstant first carpal bone was not present on this skeleton, but its position has been indicated. Outlines of the medial cartilage of the distal phalanx (stippled) and of the hoof have been added (see Figs. 7.61 and 7.66).

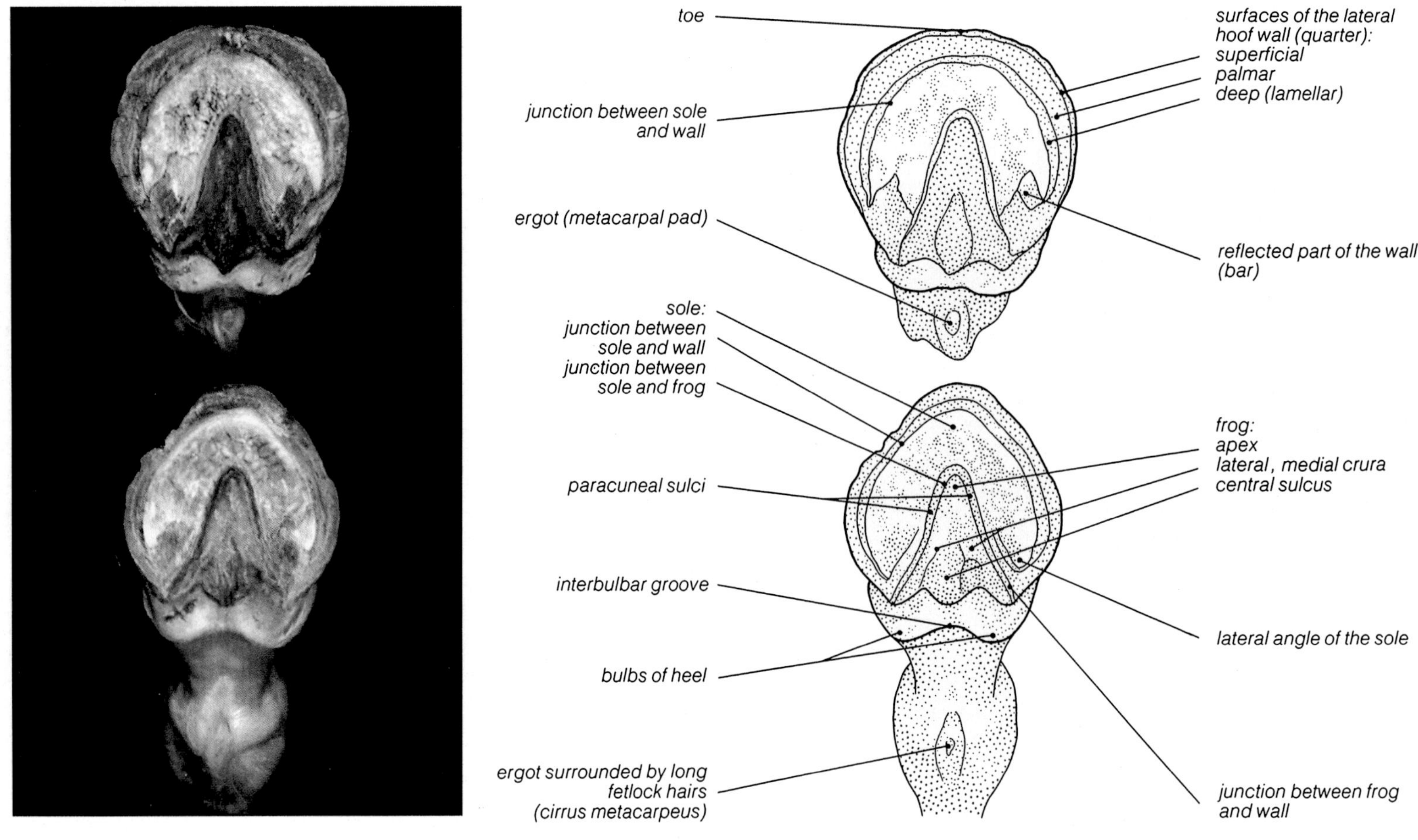
toe
junction between sole and wall
ergot (metacarpal pad)
sole:
junction between sole and wall
junction between sole and frog
paracuneal sulci
interbulbar groove
bulbs of heel
ergot surrounded by long fetlock hairs (cirrus metacarpeus)
surfaces of the lateral hoof wall (quarter):
superficial
palmar
deep (lamellar)
reflected part of the wall (bar)
frog:
apex
lateral, medial crura
central sulcus
lateral angle of the sole
junction between frog and wall

Fig. 7.9 Solar surfaces of the hooves: left forelimb (above) and left hindlimb (below). The wall is overgrown on both hooves, but no attempt has been made to trim or prepare the feet for this photograph, other than by wet brushing.

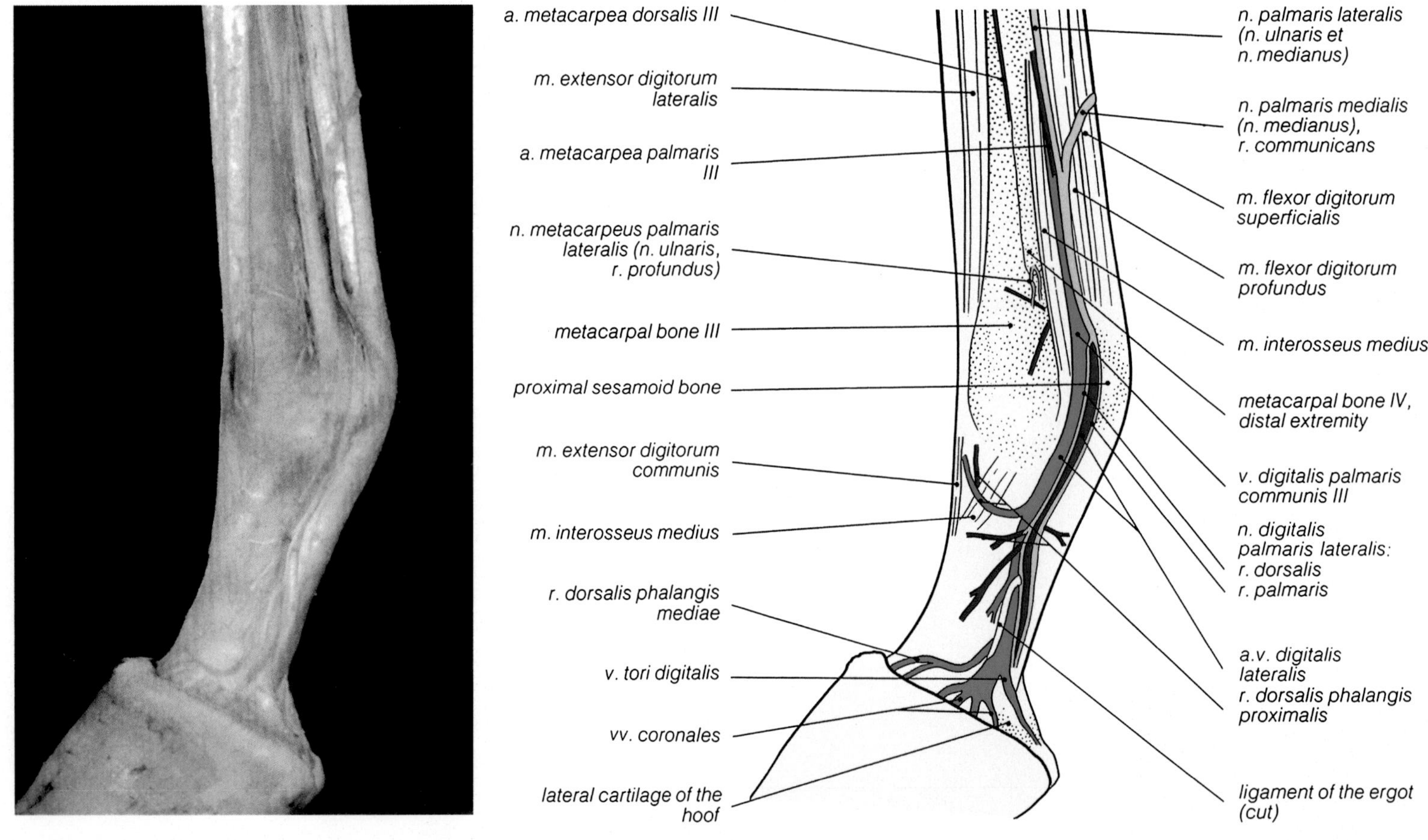
a. metacarpea dorsalis III
m. extensor digitorum lateralis
a. metacarpea palmaris III
n. metacarpeus palmaris lateralis (n. ulnaris, r. profundus)
metacarpal bone III
proximal sesamoid bone
m. extensor digitorum communis
m. interosseus medius
r. dorsalis phalangis mediae
v. tori digitalis
vv. coronales
lateral cartilage of the hoof
n. palmaris lateralis (n. ulnaris et n. medianus)
n. palmaris medialis (n. medianus), r. communicans
m. flexor digitorum superficialis
m. flexor digitorum profundus
m. interosseus medius
metacarpal bone IV, distal extremity
v. digitalis palmaris communis III
n. digitalis palmaris lateralis:
r. dorsalis
r. palmaris
a.v. digitalis lateralis
r. dorsalis phalangis proximalis
ligament of the ergot (cut)

Fig. 7.10 Superficial structures of the distal left manus (1): lateral view. The skin and superficial fascia have been removed. Other views of this dissection are shown in Figs. 7.11–7.12. The carpal and proximal metacarpal regions are shown in Figs. 3.34–3.36.

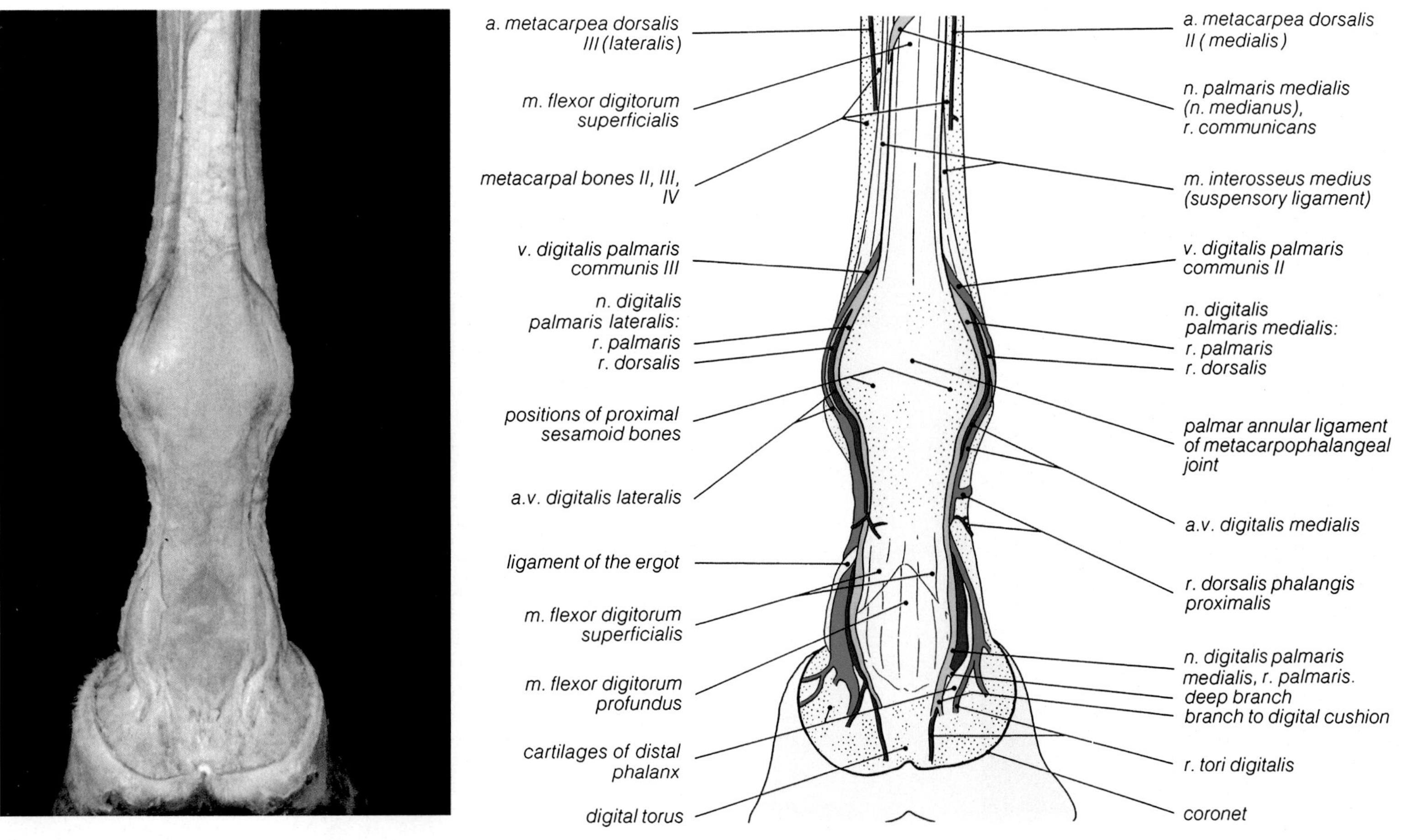
a. metacarpea dorsalis III (lateralis)
m. flexor digitorum superficialis
metacarpal bones II, III, IV
v. digitalis palmaris communis III
n. digitalis palmaris lateralis:
r. palmaris
r. dorsalis
positions of proximal sesamoid bones
a.v. digitalis lateralis
ligament of the ergot
m. flexor digitorum superficialis
m. flexor digitorum profundus
cartilages of distal phalanx
digital torus
a. metacarpea dorsalis II (medialis)
n. palmaris medialis (n. medianus), r. communicans
m. interosseus medius (suspensory ligament)
v. digitalis palmaris communis II
n. digitalis palmaris medialis:
r. palmaris
r. dorsalis
palmar annular ligament of metacarpophalangeal joint
a.v. digitalis medialis
r. dorsalis phalangis proximalis
n. digitalis palmaris medialis, r. palmaris.
deep branch
branch to digital cushion
r. tori digitalis
coronet

Fig. 7.11 Superficial structures of the distal left manus (2): palmar view. Other views of this dissection are shown in Figs. 7.10 and 7.12. The carpal and proximal metacarpal regions are shown in Figs. 3.34–3.36. The ligament of the ergot has been removed on the medial side.

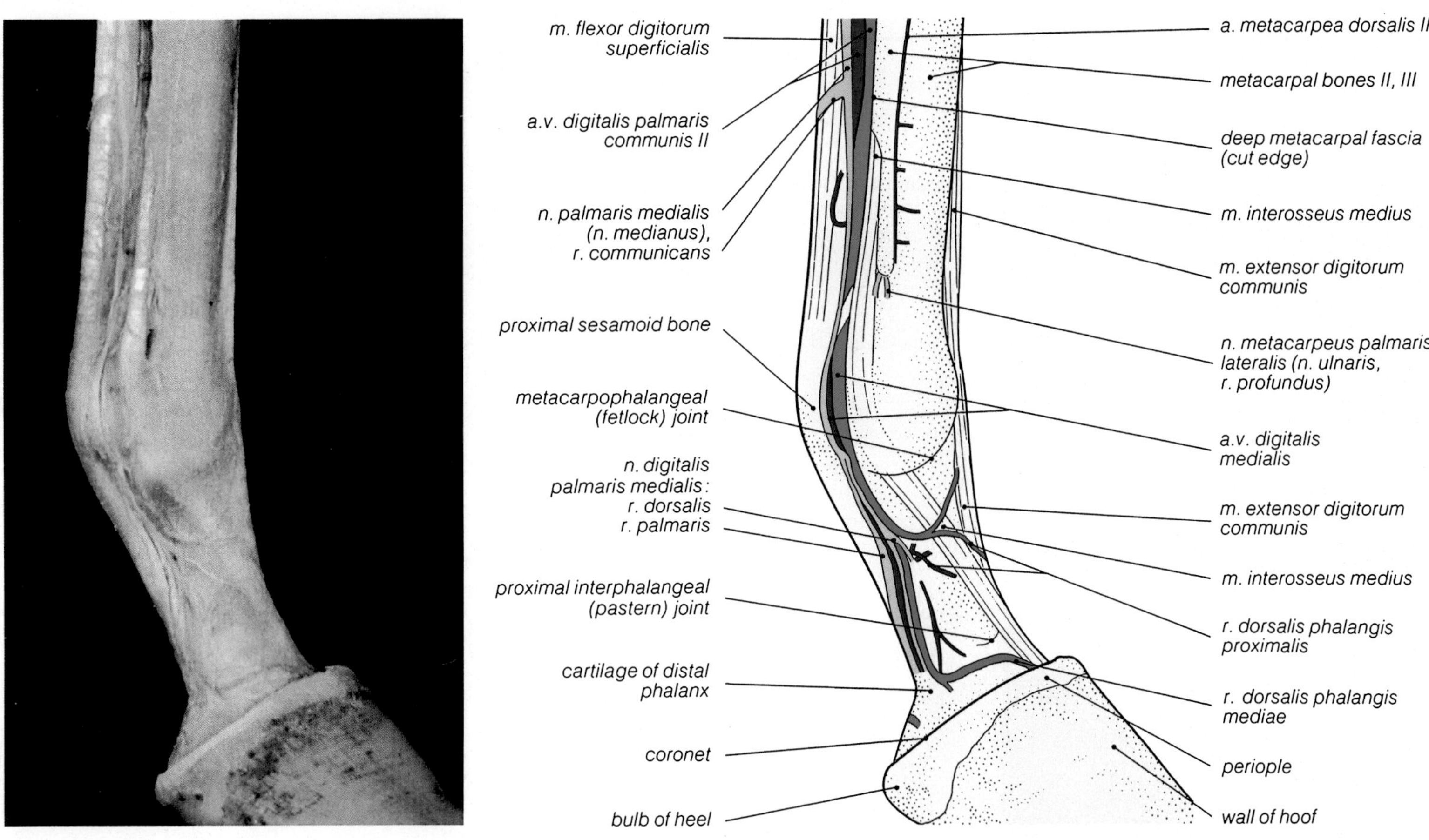
m. flexor digitorum superficialis
a.v. digitalis palmaris communis II
n. palmaris medialis (n. medianus), r. communicans
proximal sesamoid bone
metacarpophalangeal (fetlock) joint
n. digitalis palmaris medialis:
r. dorsalis
r. palmaris
proximal interphalangeal (pastern) joint
cartilage of distal phalanx
coronet
bulb of heel
a. metacarpea dorsalis II
metacarpal bones II, III
deep metacarpal fascia (cut edge)
m. interosseus medius
m. extensor digitorum communis
n. metacarpeus palmaris lateralis (n. ulnaris, r. profundus)
a.v. digitalis medialis
m. extensor digitorum communis
m. interosseus medius
r. dorsalis phalangis proximalis
r. dorsalis phalangis mediae
periople
wall of hoof

Fig. 7.12 Superficial structures of the distal manus (3): left medial view. Other views of this dissection are shown in Figs. 7.10 and 7.11. The carpal and proximal metacarpal regions are shown in Figs. 3.34–3.36. The ligament of the ergot has been removed.

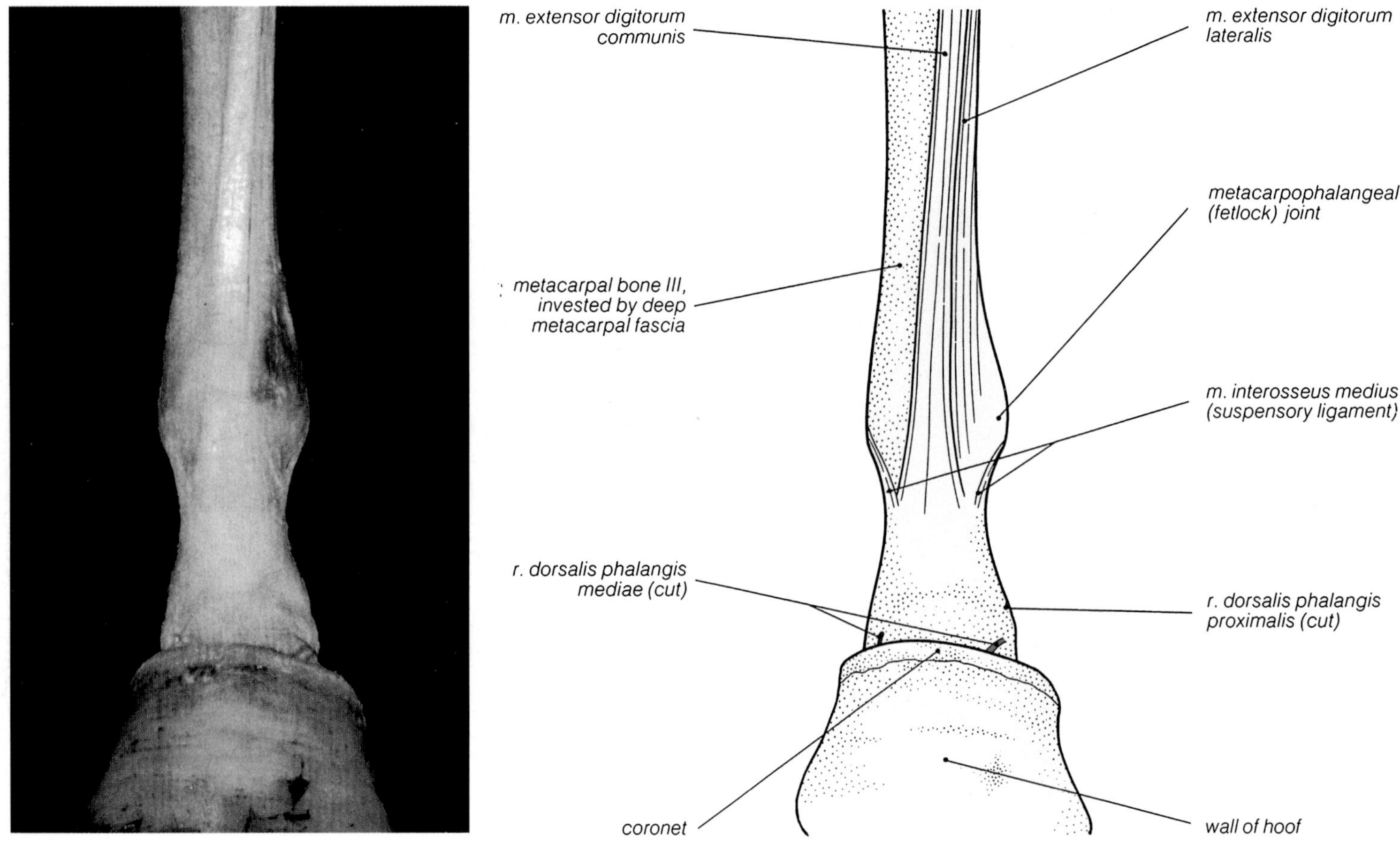
m. extensor digitorum communis
m. extensor digitorum lateralis
metacarpophalangeal (fetlock) joint
metacarpal bone III, invested by deep metacarpal fascia
m. interosseus medius (suspensory ligament)
r. dorsalis phalangis mediae (cut)
r. dorsalis phalangis proximalis (cut)
coronet
wall of hoof

Fig. 7.13 Superficial structures of the distal left manus (4): dorsal view. The nerves and veins have been removed but the arteries have been left to provide reference points for comparison with the previous dissection (Figs. 7.10–7.12). Other views of this dissection are shown in Figs. 7.14–7.16. A dorsal view of carpal and proximal metacarpal regions is shown in Fig. 3.33.

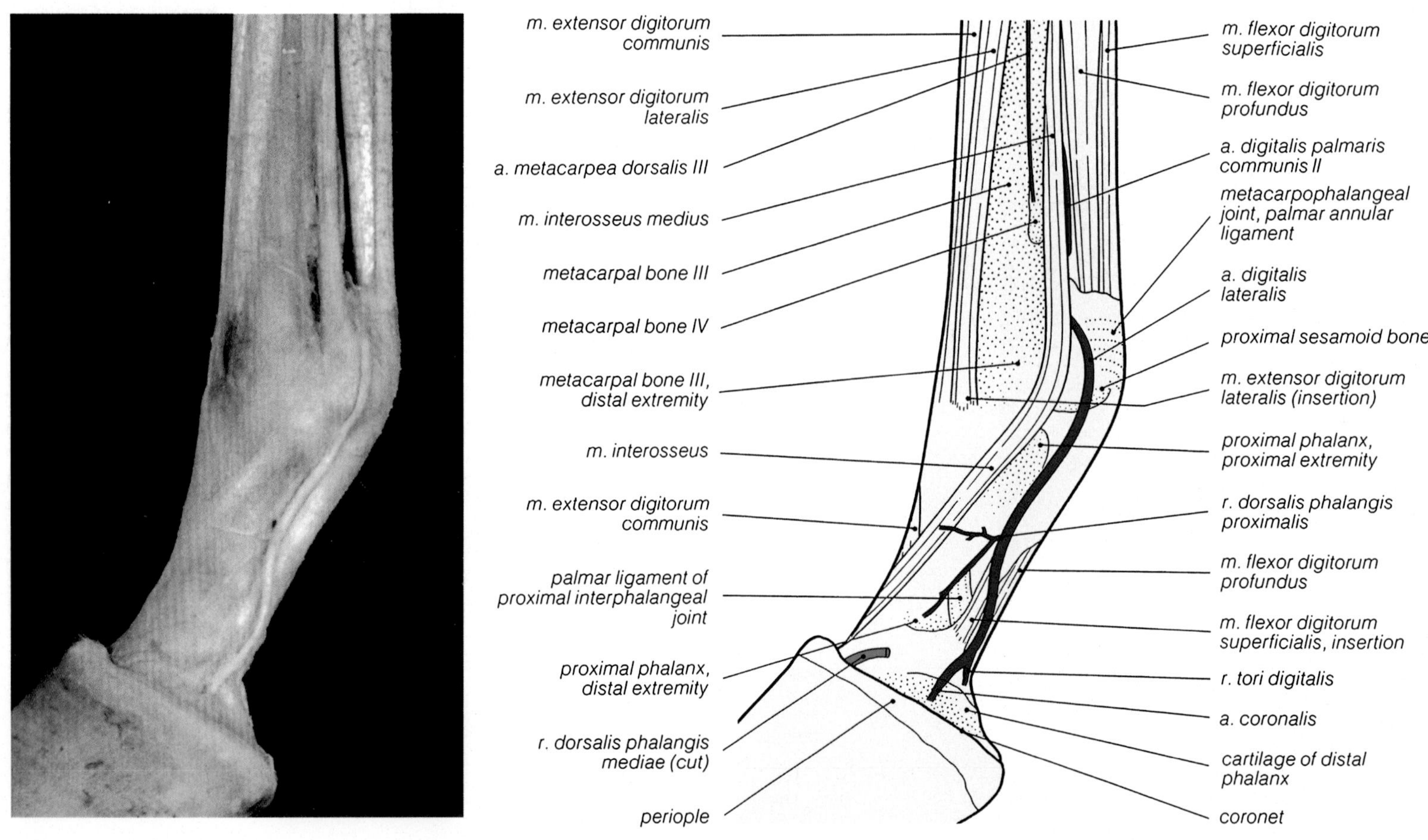
m. extensor digitorum communis
m. extensor digitorum lateralis
a. metacarpea dorsalis III
m. interosseus medius
metacarpal bone III
metacarpal bone IV
metacarpal bone III, distal extremity
m. interosseus
m. extensor digitorum communis
palmar ligament of proximal interphalangeal joint
proximal phalanx, distal extremity
r. dorsalis phalangis mediae (cut)
periople
m. flexor digitorum superficialis
m. flexor digitorum profundus
a. digitalis palmaris communis II
metacarpophalangeal joint, palmar annular ligament
a. digitalis lateralis
proximal sesamoid bone
m. extensor digitorum lateralis (insertion)
proximal phalanx, proximal extremity
r. dorsalis phalangis proximalis
m. flexor digitorum profundus
m. flexor digitorum superficialis, insertion
r. tori digitalis
a. coronalis
cartilage of distal phalanx
coronet

Fig. 7.14 Superficial structures of the distal left manus (5): lateral view. Other views of this dissection are shown in Figs. 7.13, 7.15 and 7.16.

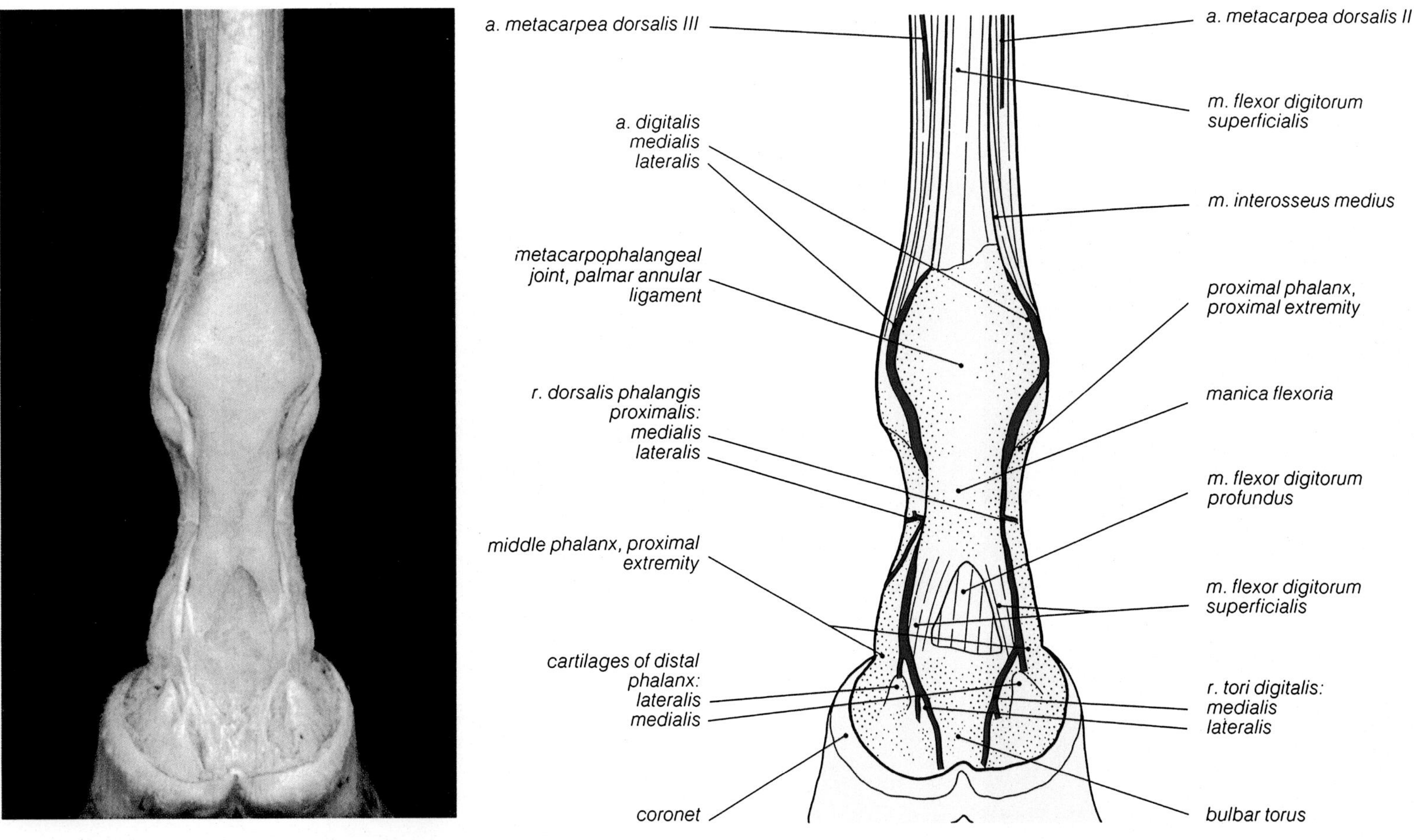
a. metacarpea dorsalis III
a. metacarpea dorsalis II
m. flexor digitorum superficialis
a. digitalis medialis lateralis
m. interosseus medius
metacarpophalangeal joint, palmar annular ligament
proximal phalanx, proximal extremity
r. dorsalis phalangis proximalis: medialis lateralis
manica flexoria
m. flexor digitorum profundus
middle phalanx, proximal extremity
m. flexor digitorum superficialis
cartilages of distal phalanx: lateralis medialis
r. tori digitalis: medialis lateralis
coronet
bulbar torus

Fig. 7.15 Superficial structures of the distal manus (6): palmar view. Other views of this dissection are shown in Figs. 7.13,7.14 and 7.16.

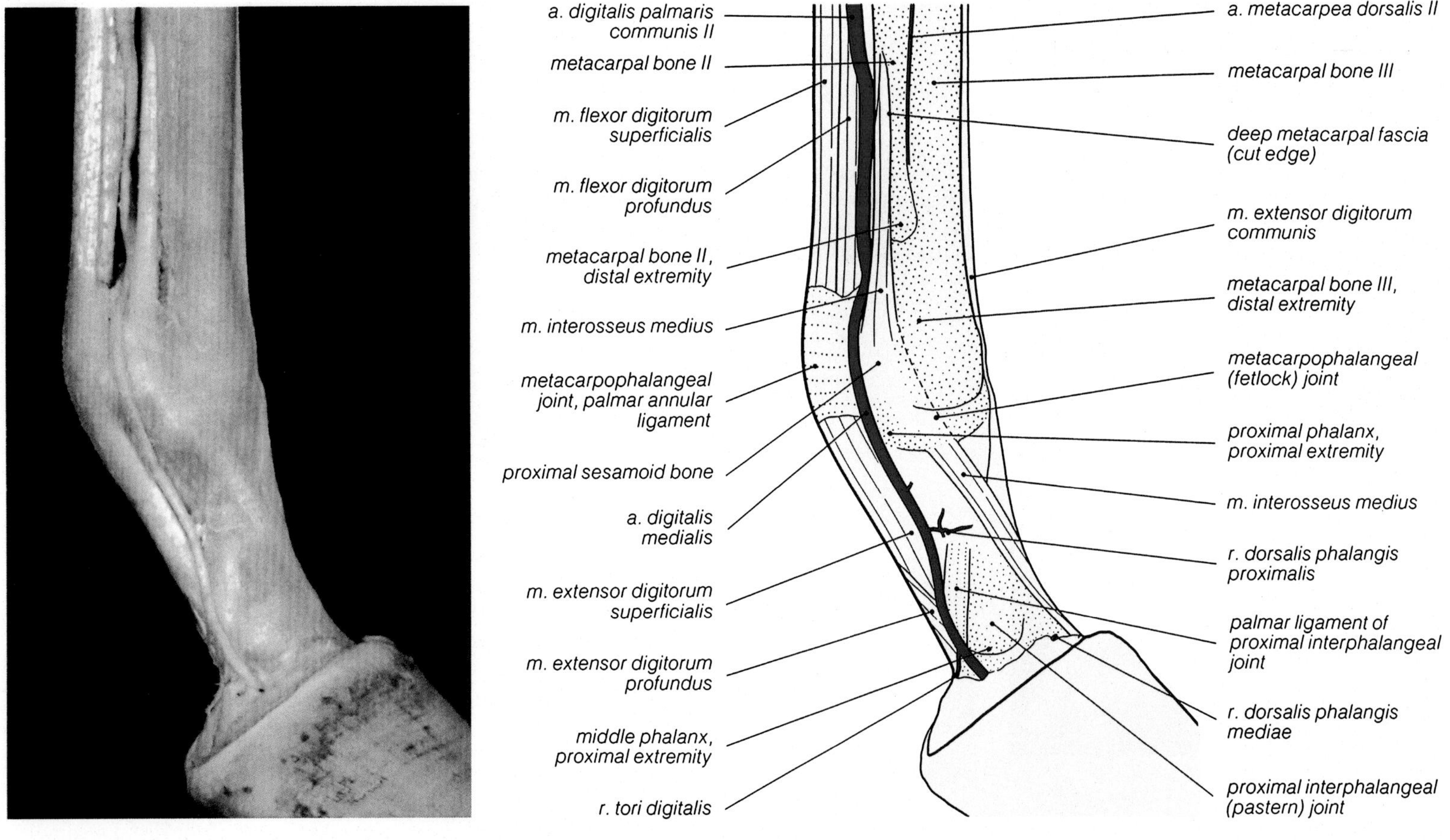
a. digitalis palmaris communis II
a. metacarpea dorsalis II
metacarpal bone II
metacarpal bone III
m. flexor digitorum superficialis
deep metacarpal fascia (cut edge)
m. flexor digitorum profundus
m. extensor digitorum communis
metacarpal bone II, distal extremity
metacarpal bone III, distal extremity
m. interosseus medius
metacarpophalangeal joint, palmar annular ligament
metacarpophalangeal (fetlock) joint
proximal phalanx, proximal extremity
proximal sesamoid bone
m. interosseus medius
a. digitalis medialis
r. dorsalis phalangis proximalis
m. extensor digitorum superficialis
palmar ligament of proximal interphalangeal joint
m. extensor digitorum profundus
r. dorsalis phalangis mediae
middle phalanx, proximal extremity
proximal interphalangeal (pastern) joint
r. tori digitalis

Fig. 7.16 Superficial structures of the distal manus (7): left medial view. Other views of this dissection are shown in Figs. 7.13, 7.14 and 7.15.

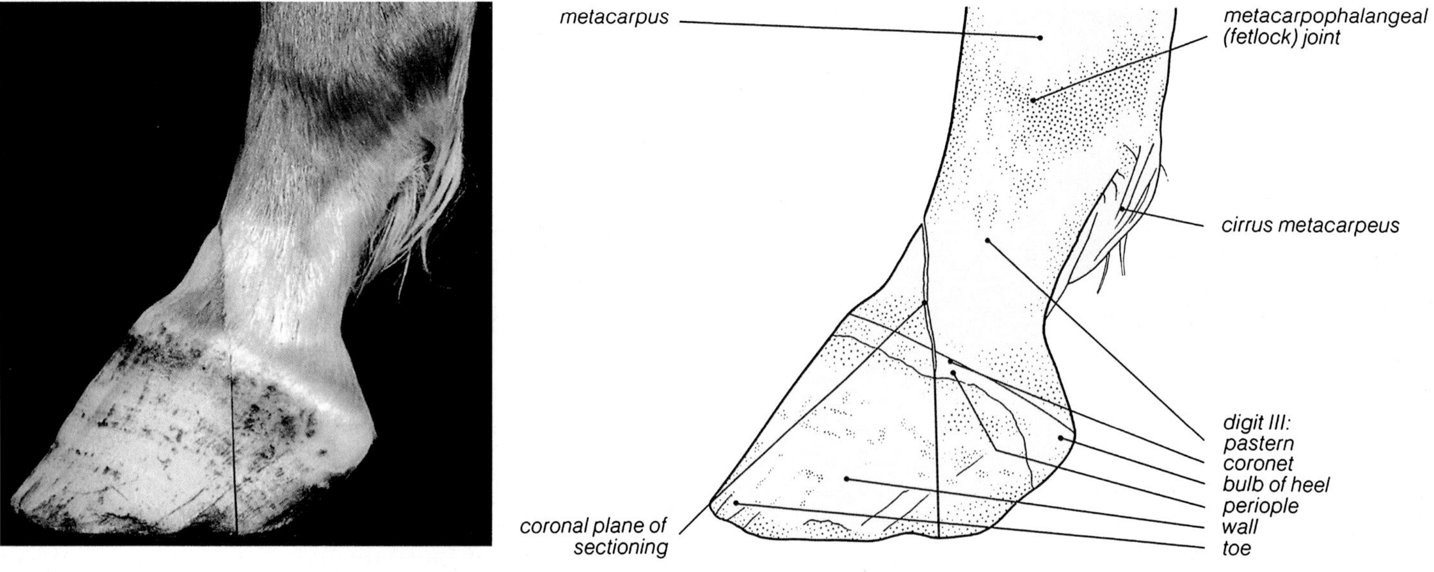
metacarpus
metacarpophalangeal (fetlock) joint
cirrus metacarpeus
digit III:
pastern
coronet
bulb of heel
periople
wall
toe
coronal plane of sectioning

Fig. 7.17 The right manus: medial view. The digit has been sawn through in a coronal plane, to produce the specimens for Figs. 7.19–7.24.

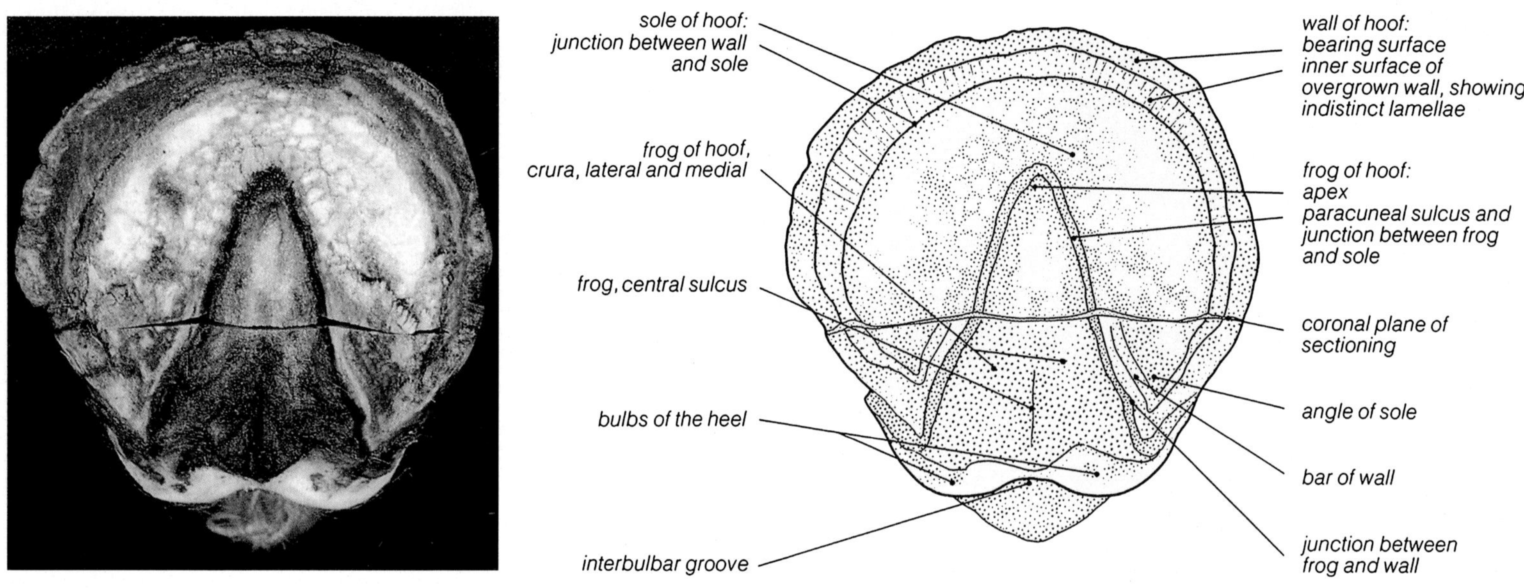
sole of hoof:
junction between wall and sole
frog of hoof, crura, lateral and medial
frog, central sulcus
bulbs of the heel
interbulbar groove
wall of hoof:
bearing surface
inner surface of overgrown wall, showing indistinct lamellae
frog of hoof:
apex
paracuneal sulcus and junction between frog and sole
coronal plane of sectioning
angle of sole
bar of wall
junction between frog and wall

Fig. 7.18 The right manus: solar surface of the hoof. The digit has been sawn through in a coronal plane, to produce the specimens for Figs. 7.19–7.24. The wall is overgrown, but the foot has not been trimmed; only wet brushing has been carried out.

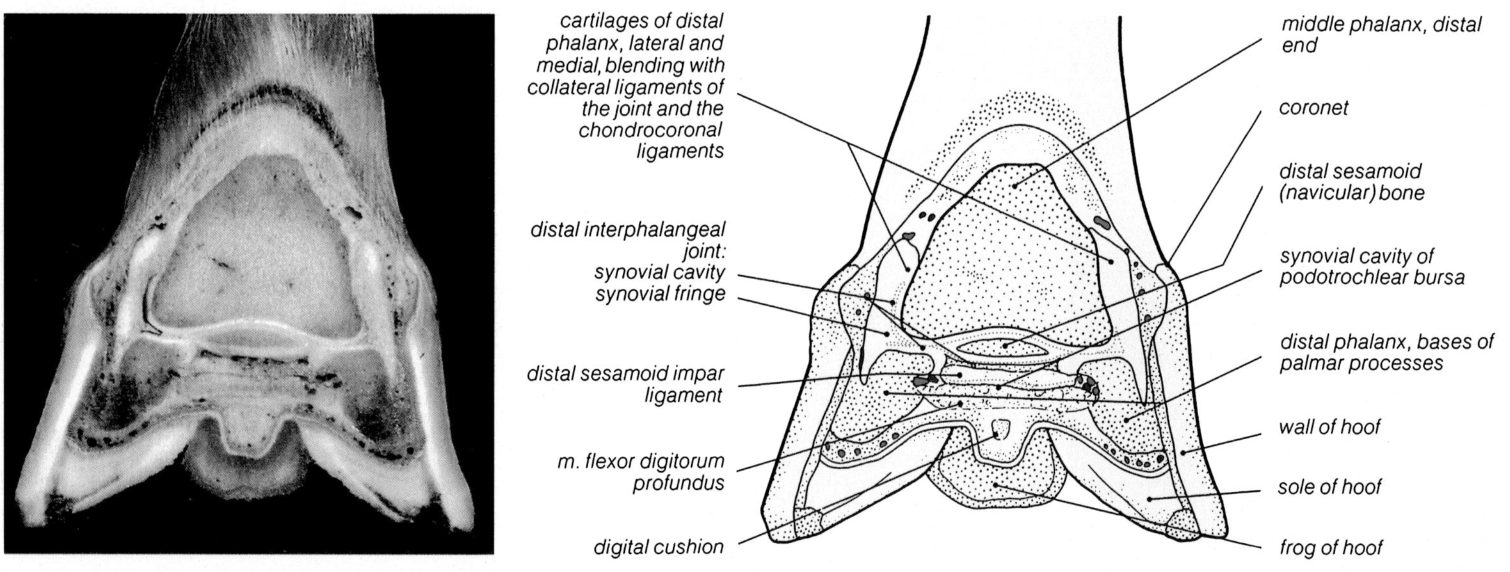
cartilages of distal phalanx, lateral and medial, blending with collateral ligaments of the joint and the chondrocoronal ligaments
distal interphalangeal joint:
synovial cavity
synovial fringe
distal sesamoid impar ligament
m. flexor digitorum profundus
digital cushion
middle phalanx, distal end
coronet
distal sesamoid (navicular) bone
synovial cavity of podotrochlear bursa
distal phalanx, bases of palmar processes
wall of hoof
sole of hoof
frog of hoof

Fig. 7.19 The right manus: coronal section through the hoof (1). The plane of sectioning passes through the extreme distal part of the distal sesamoid bone and through the ligament joining it to the distal phalanx (see Fig. 7.66). The inner surfaces of the joint cavity and synovial bursa (synovial membranes and articular cartilage) are indicated by blue dots.

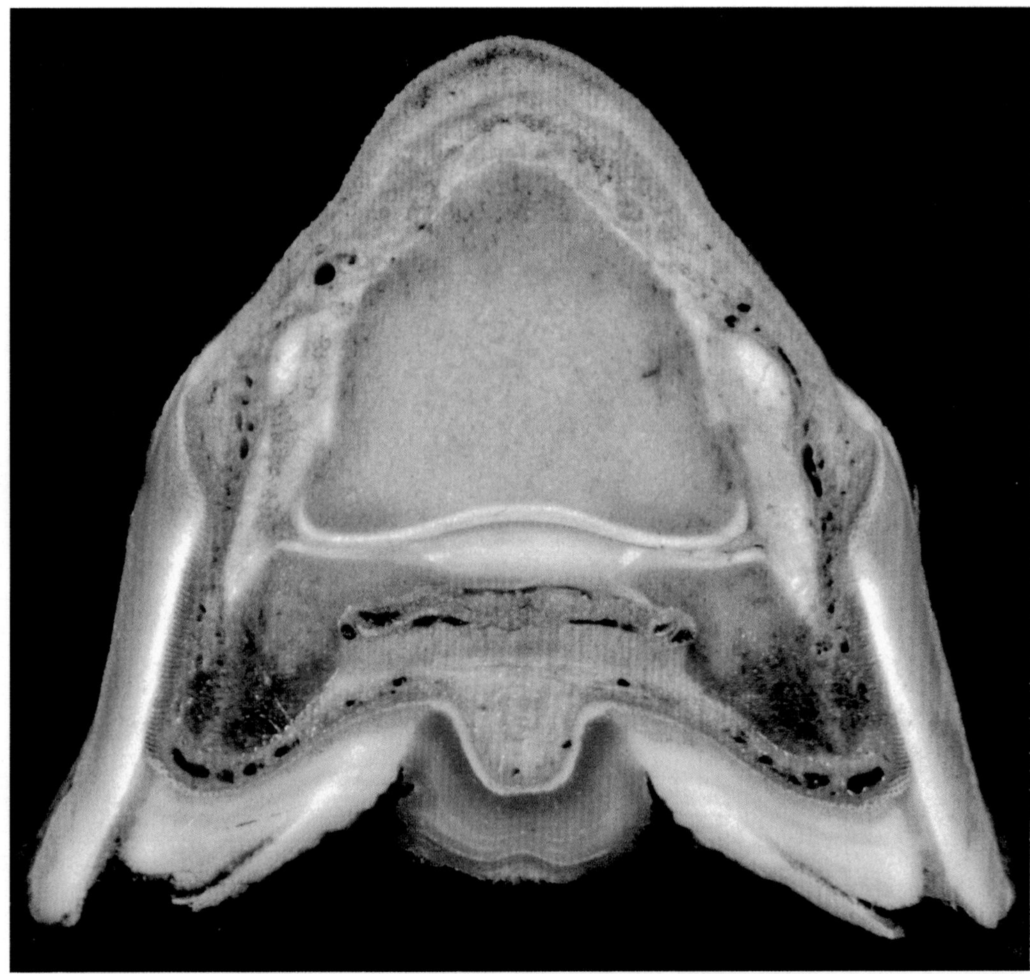

m. extensor digitorum communis

middle phalanx

cartilage of sesamoid articular surface of distal phalanx

medial cartilage of distal phalanx, blending with collateral ligament of joint and the chondrocoronal ligament

synovial membrane of distal interphalangeal joint

distal phalanx

distal sesamoid impar ligament

m. flexor digitorum profundus (tendon of insertion)

overgrown part of hoof wall, bearing lamellae on its inner surface

common integument:
epidermis
dermis (corium)
hypodermis (superficial fascia)

plexus coronarius

coronary cushion

periople

coronary corium

wall of hoof:
outer layer (glaze)
inner layer (lamellar)
middle layer (pigmented and non-pigmented layers)

plexus parietalis

plexus palmaris

sole of hoof

junction between wall and sole (white zone)

junction between frog and sole

paracuneal sulcus

digital cushion

frog of hoof

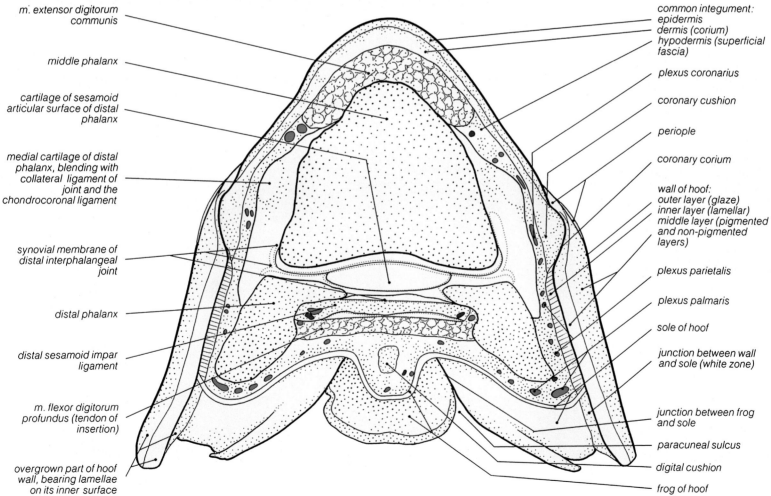

Fig. 7.20 The right manus: coronal section through the hoof (2). This is the distal part (including the toe) of the specimen shown in Fig. 7.19. A sliver of the distal sesamoid bone (see Fig. 7.66) was included on this surface of the saw cut, but it was removed from the joint cavity of the distal interphalangeal (coffin) joint to show the cartilage of the sesamoid articular surface of the distal phalanx.

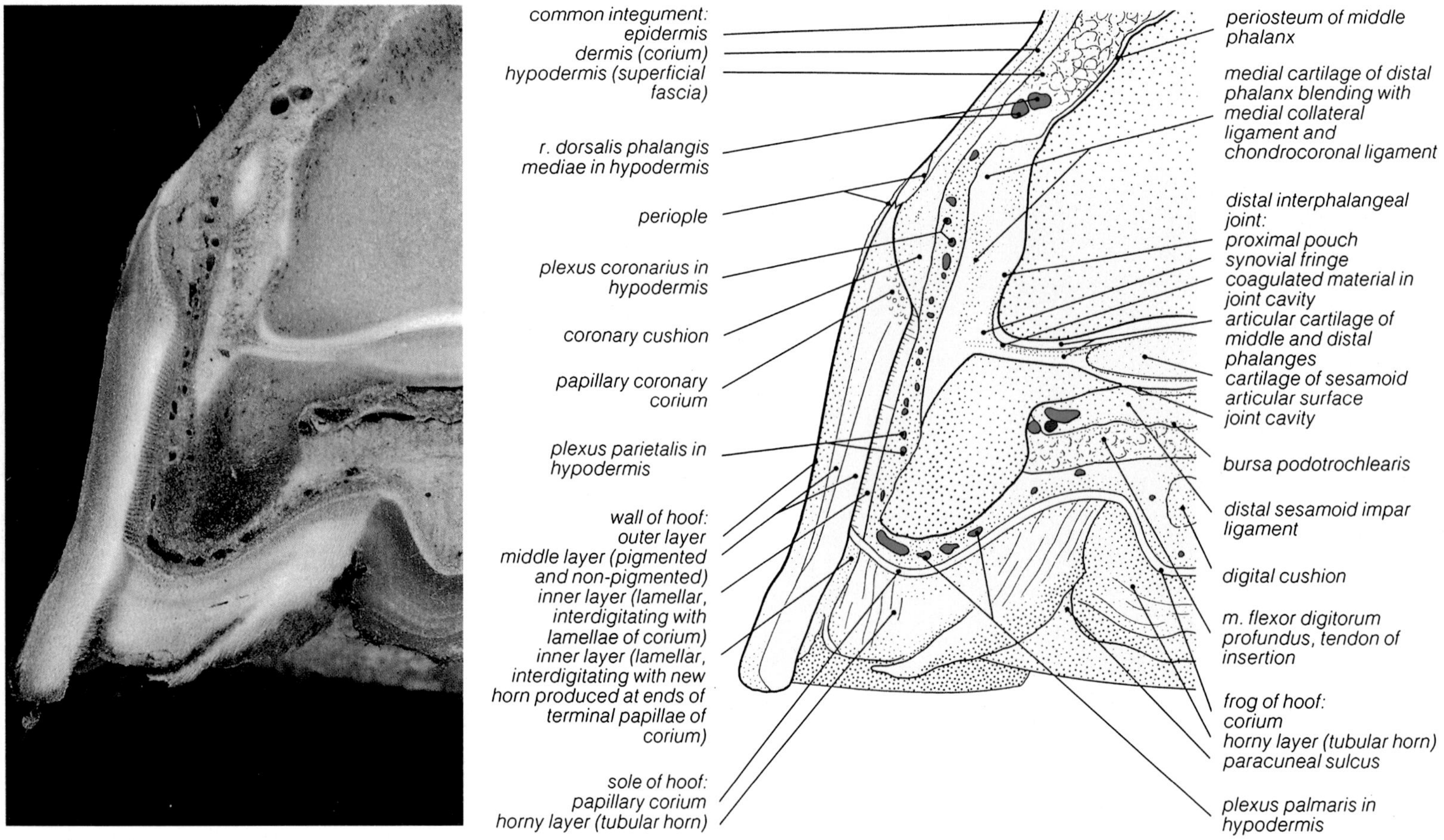

common integument:
epidermis
dermis (corium)
hypodermis (superficial fascia)
r. dorsalis phalangis mediae in hypodermis
periople
plexus coronarius in hypodermis
coronary cushion
papillary coronary corium
plexus parietalis in hypodermis
wall of hoof:
outer layer
middle layer (pigmented and non-pigmented)
inner layer (lamellar, interdigitating with lamellae of corium)
inner layer (lamellar, interdigitating with new horn produced at ends of terminal papillae of corium)
sole of hoof:
papillary corium
horny layer (tubular horn)
periosteum of middle phalanx
medial cartilage of distal phalanx blending with medial collateral ligament and chondrocoronal ligament
distal interphalangeal joint:
proximal pouch
synovial fringe
coagulated material in joint cavity
articular cartilage of middle and distal phalanges
cartilage of sesamoid articular surface
joint cavity
bursa podotrochlearis
distal sesamoid impar ligament
digital cushion
m. flexor digitorum profundus, tendon of insertion
frog of hoof:
corium
horny layer (tubular horn)
paracuneal sulcus
plexus palmaris in hypodermis

Fig. 7.21 The right manus: coronal section through the hoof (3). This is a closer view of the medial part of the specimen shown in Fig. 7.20. See also Figs. 7.75 and 7.76.

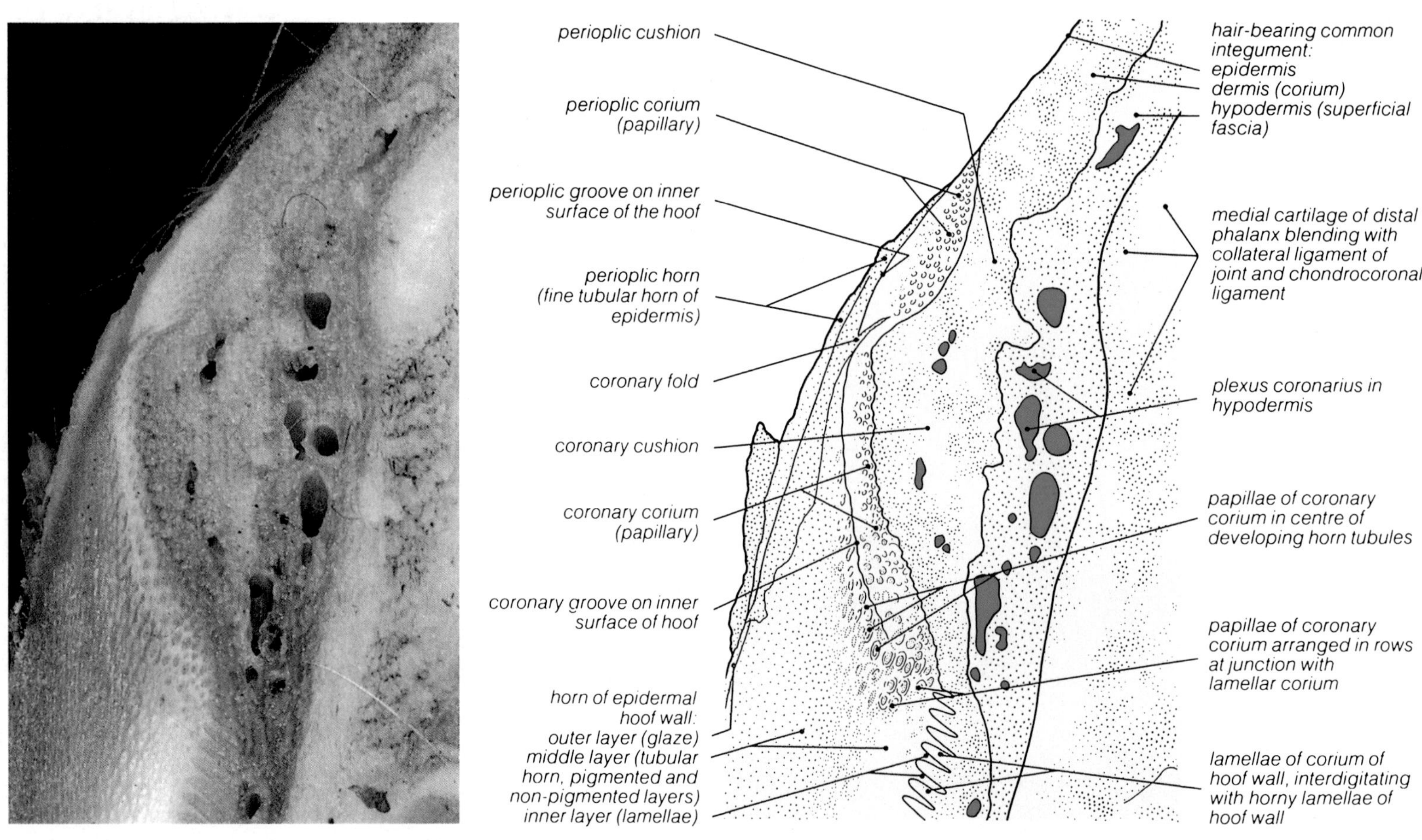
perioplic cushion
perioplic corium (papillary)
perioplic groove on inner surface of the hoof
perioplic horn (fine tubular horn of epidermis)
coronary fold
coronary cushion
coronary corium (papillary)
coronary groove on inner surface of hoof
horn of epidermal hoof wall:
outer layer (glaze)
middle layer (tubular horn, pigmented and non-pigmented layers)
inner layer (lamellae)
hair-bearing common integument:
epidermis
dermis (corium)
hypodermis (superficial fascia)
medial cartilage of distal phalanx blending with collateral ligament of joint and chondrocoronal ligament
plexus coronarius in hypodermis
papillae of coronary corium in centre of developing horn tubules
papillae of coronary corium arranged in rows at junction with lamellar corium
lamellae of corium of hoof wall, interdigitating with horny lamellae of hoof wall

Fig. 7.22 The right manus: coronal section through the hoof (4). This is part of the specimen shown in Fig. 7.21. The perioplic and coronary cushions are usually held to be derivatives of the hypodermis (superficial fascia) but appear continuous with the dermis of the common integument. The clearly visible horn tubules of the wall of the hoof are formed by the epidermal germinal layer overlying the papillae of the coronary corium. Dissections of the coronet region are shown in Figs. 7.57–7.60.

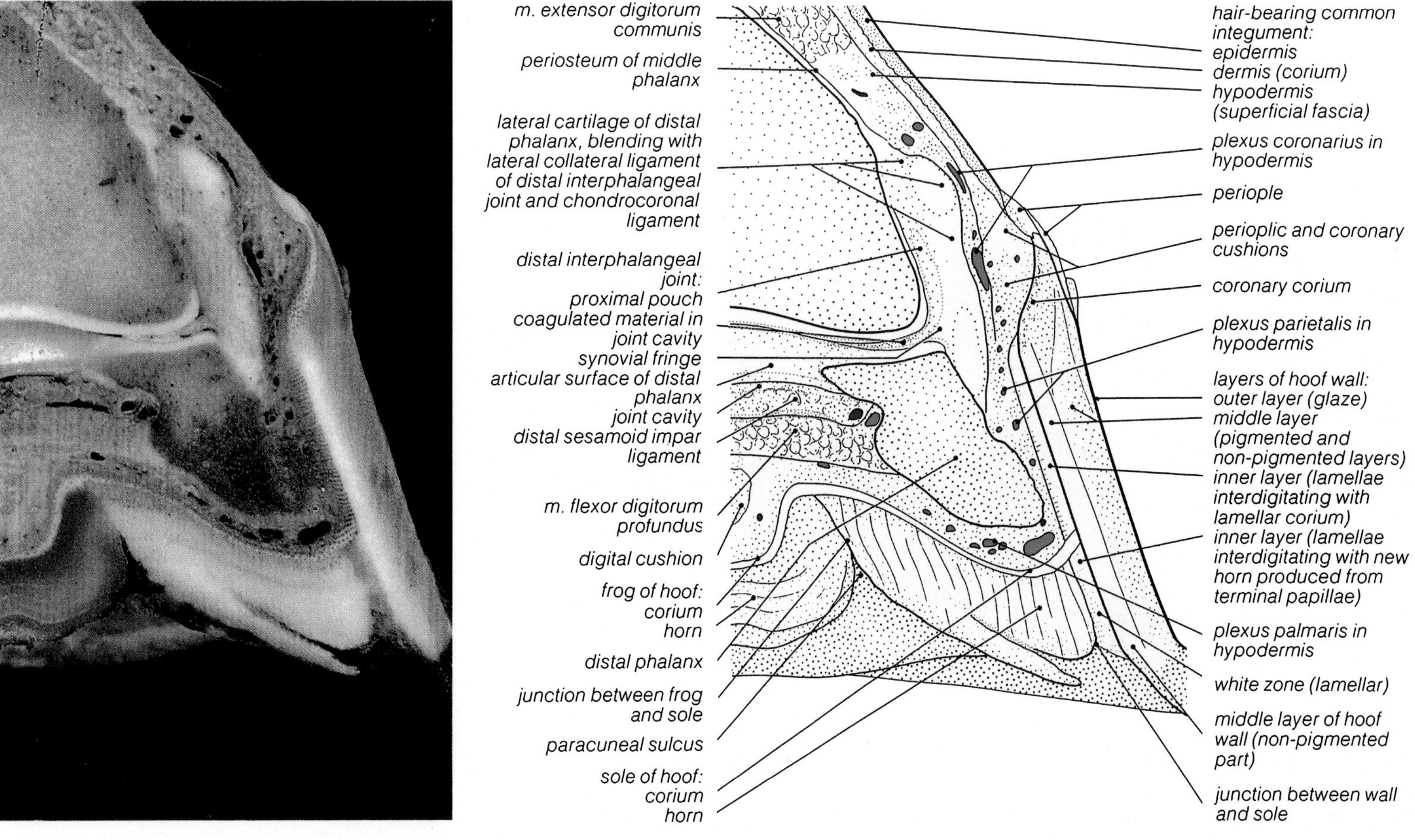
m. extensor digitorum communis
periosteum of middle phalanx
lateral cartilage of distal phalanx, blending with lateral collateral ligament of distal interphalangeal joint and chondrocoronal ligament
distal interphalangeal joint:
proximal pouch
coagulated material in joint cavity
synovial fringe
articular surface of distal phalanx
joint cavity
distal sesamoid impar ligament
m. flexor digitorum profundus
digital cushion
frog of hoof:
corium
horn
distal phalanx
junction between frog and sole
paracuneal sulcus
sole of hoof:
corium
horn
hair-bearing common integument:
epidermis
dermis (corium)
hypodermis (superficial fascia)
plexus coronarius in hypodermis
periople
perioplic and coronary cushions
coronary corium
plexus parietalis in hypodermis
layers of hoof wall:
outer layer (glaze)
middle layer (pigmented and non-pigmented layers)
inner layer (lamellae interdigitating with lamellar corium)
inner layer (lamellae interdigitating with new horn produced from terminal papillae)
plexus palmaris in hypodermis
white zone (lamellar)
middle layer of hoof wall (non-pigmented part)
junction between wall and sole

Fig. 7.23 The right manus: coronal section through the hoof (5). This is a closer view of the lateral part of the specimen shown in Fig. 7.20. A sliver of the distal sesamoid bone was removed from the surface of the slice.

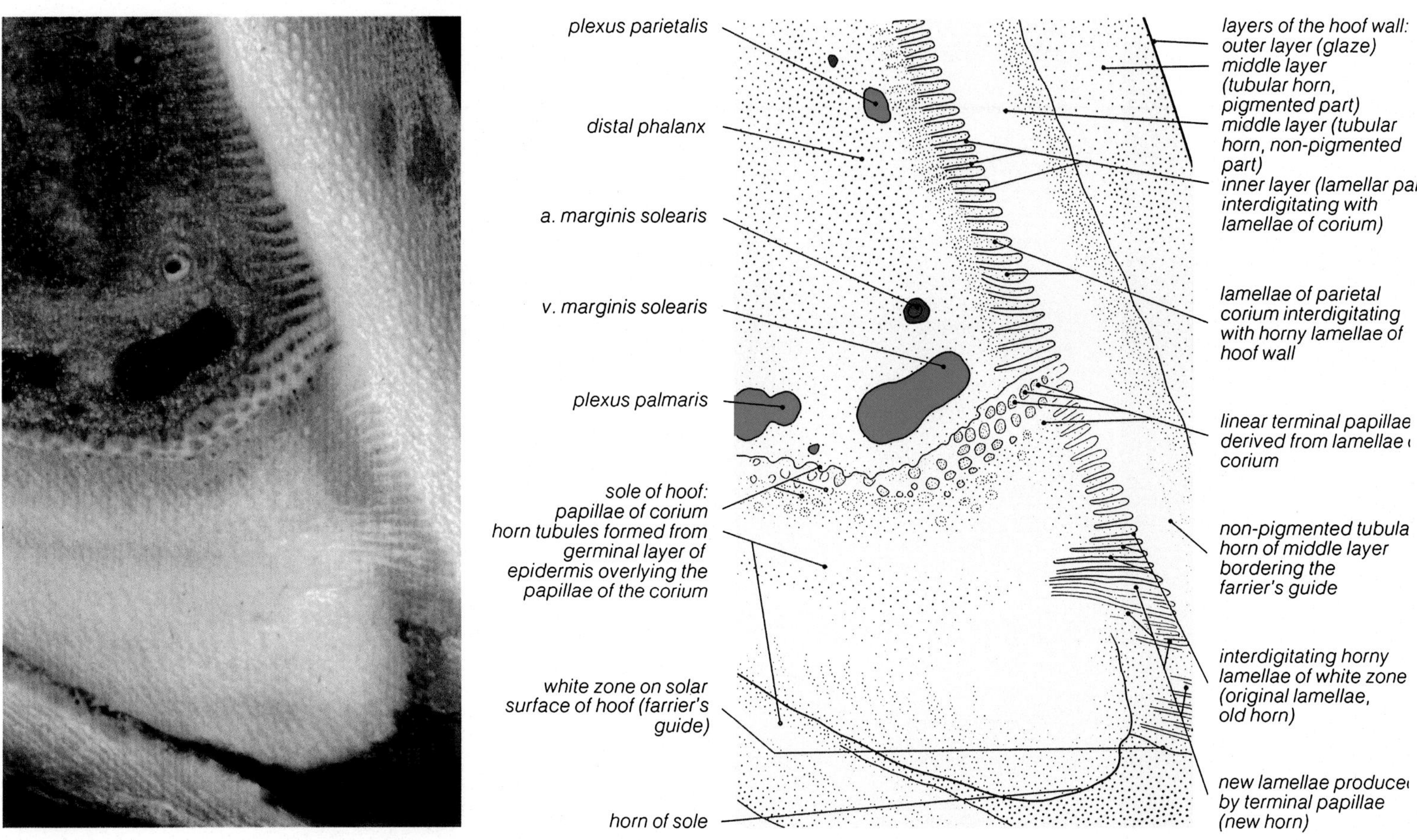
plexus parietalis
distal phalanx
a. marginis solearis
v. marginis solearis
plexus palmaris
sole of hoof:
papillae of corium
horn tubules formed from germinal layer of epidermis overlying the papillae of the corium
white zone on solar surface of hoof (farrier's guide)
horn of sole
layers of the hoof wall:
outer layer (glaze)
middle layer (tubular horn, pigmented part)
middle layer (tubular horn, non-pigmented part)
inner layer (lamellar part interdigitating with lamellae of corium)
lamellae of parietal corium interdigitating with horny lamellae of hoof wall
linear terminal papillae derived from lamellae
corium
non-pigmented tubula
horn of middle layer bordering the farrier's guide
interdigitating horny lamellae of white zone (original lamellae, old horn)
new lamellae produce
by terminal papillae (new horn)

Fig. 7.24 The right manus: coronal section through the hoof (6). This is part of the specimen shown in Fig. 7.23. At the junctional region between sole and wall the spaces left at the distal ends of the lamellae of the parietal corium are filled by new horn to produce a lamellated 'white zone' that is translucent. The white colour seen on the 'prepared' foot is that of the inner, non-pigmented horn of the wall (see Figs. 7.9, 7.18 and 7.59). Dissections of the parietal lamellae are shown in Figs. 7.57–7.60.

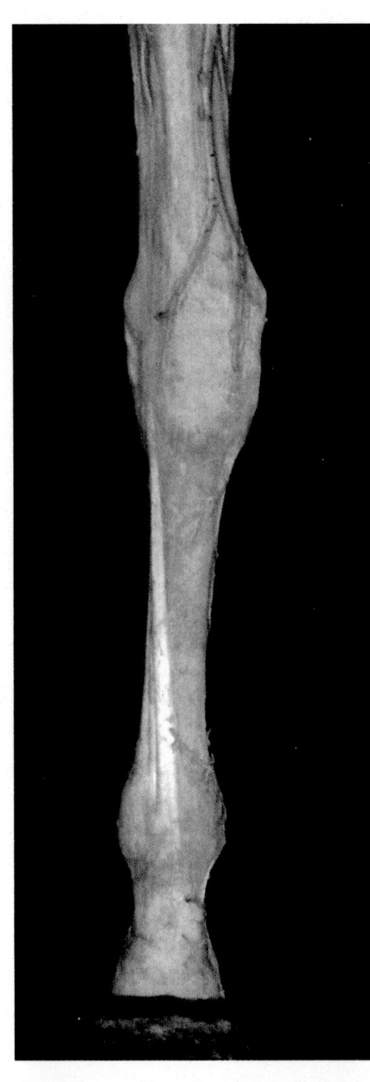

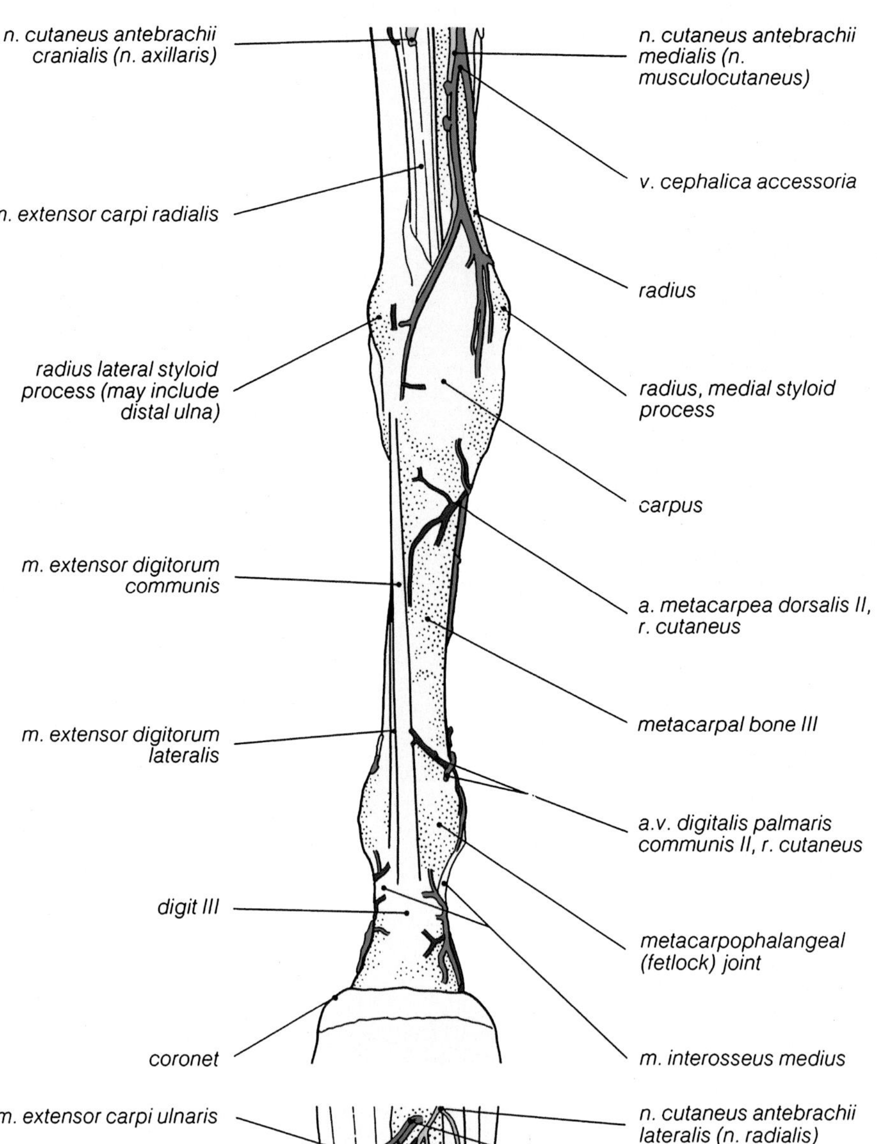
n. cutaneus antebrachii cranialis (n. axillaris)
m. extensor carpi radialis
radius lateral styloid process (may include distal ulna)
m. extensor digitorum communis
m. extensor digitorum lateralis
digit III
coronet
n. cutaneus antebrachii medialis (n. musculocutaneus)
v. cephalica accessoria
radius
radius, medial styloid process
carpus
a. metacarpea dorsalis II, r. cutaneus
metacarpal bone III
a.v. digitalis palmaris communis II, r. cutaneus
metacarpophalangeal (fetlock) joint
m. interosseus medius

Fig. 7.25 Superficial structures of the right forelimb (1): cranial view. The skin has been removed, and the vessels and nerves within the superficial fascia have been dissected. Figs 7.25–7.28 show the relationships between the superficial vessels and nerves of the digit (shown in Figs. 7.29–7.32) and those of more proximal regions of the limb.

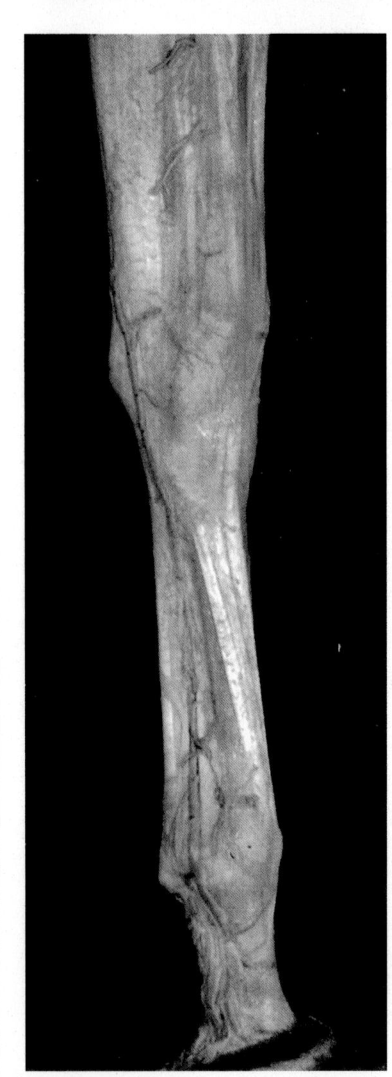

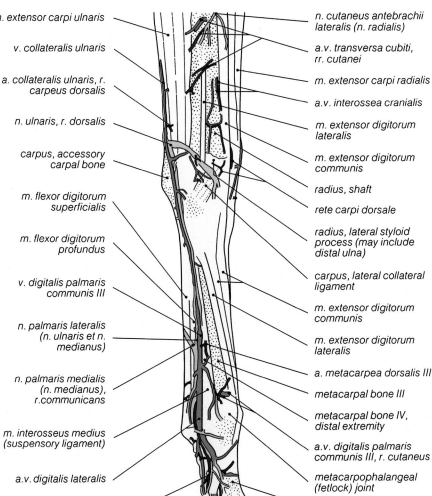

m. extensor carpi ulnaris
v. collateralis ulnaris
a. collateralis ulnaris, r. carpeus dorsalis
n. ulnaris, r. dorsalis
carpus, accessory carpal bone
m. flexor digitorum superficialis
m. flexor digitorum profundus
v. digitalis palmaris communis III
n. palmaris lateralis (n. ulnaris et n. medianus)
n. palmaris medialis (n. medianus), r.communicans
m. interosseus medius (suspensory ligament)
a.v. digitalis lateralis
ligament of the ergot (cut)
n. cutaneus antebrachii lateralis (n. radialis)
a.v. transversa cubiti, rr. cutanei
m. extensor carpi radialis
a.v. interossea cranialis
m. extensor digitorum lateralis
m. extensor digitorum communis
radius, shaft
rete carpi dorsale
radius, lateral styloid process (may include distal ulna)
carpus, lateral collateral ligament
m. extensor digitorum communis
m. extensor digitorum lateralis
a. metacarpea dorsalis III
metacarpal bone III
metacarpal bone IV, distal extremity
a.v. digitalis palmaris communis III, r. cutaneus
metacarpophalangeal (fetlock) joint
digit III
coronet

Fig. 7.26 Superficial structures of the right forelimb (2): lateral view. This dissection is also shown in Figs. 7.25, 7.27 and 7.28. For further details of the digital region see Fig. 7.30.

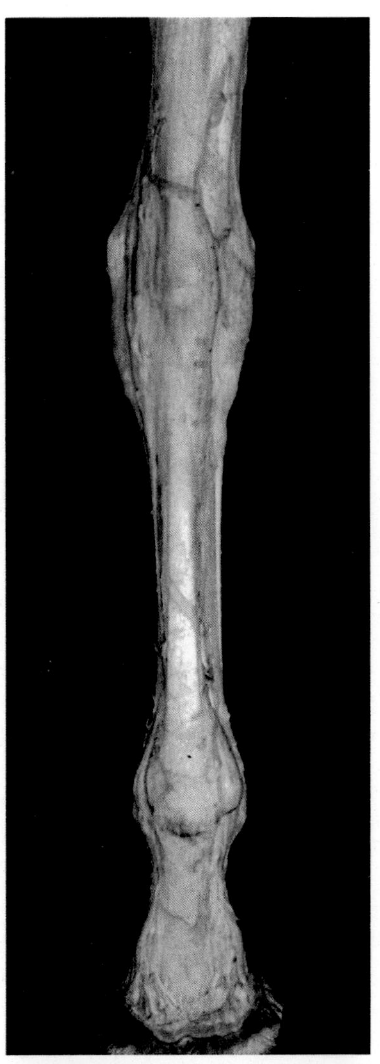

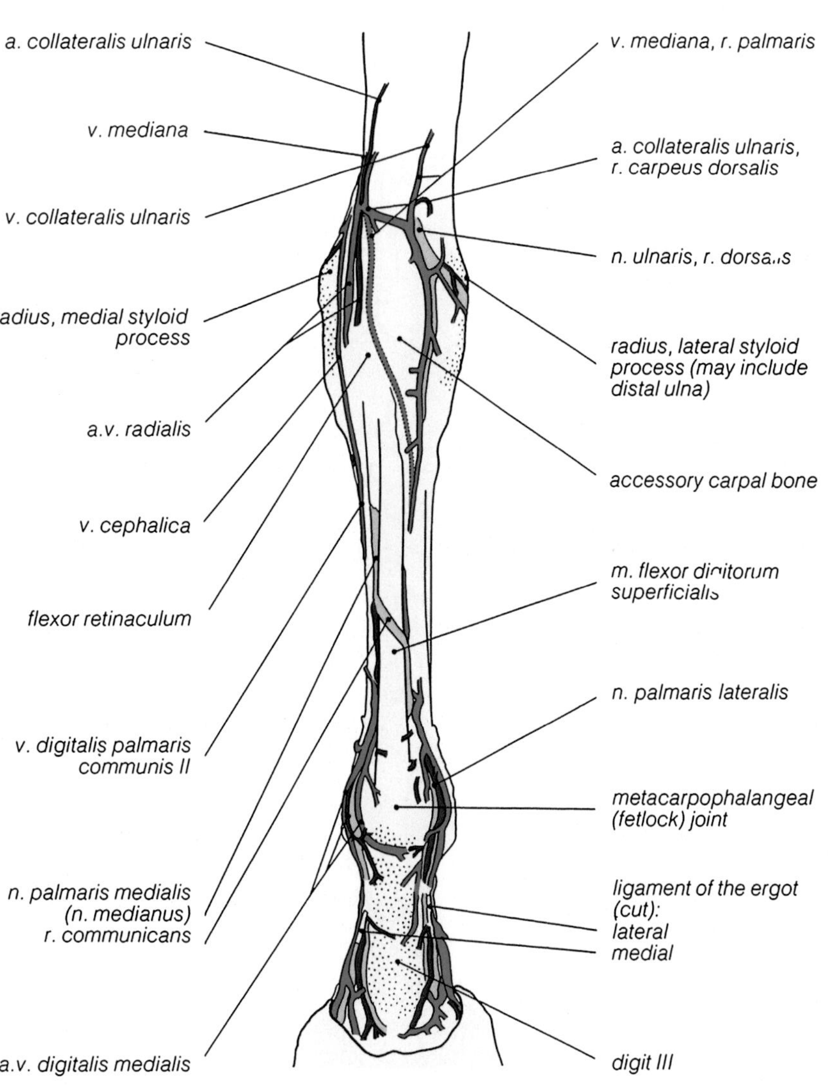

a. collateralis ulnaris
v. mediana
v. collateralis ulnaris
radius, medial styloid process
a.v. radialis
v. cephalica
flexor retinaculum
v. digitalis palmaris communis II
n. palmaris medialis (n. medianus) r. communicans
a.v. digitalis medialis
v. mediana, r. palmaris
a. collateralis ulnaris, r. carpeus dorsalis
n. ulnaris, r. dorsalis
radius, lateral styloid process (may include distal ulna)
accessory carpal bone
m. flexor digitorum superficialis
n. palmaris lateralis
metacarpophalangeal (fetlock) joint
ligament of the ergot (cut):
lateral
medial
digit III

Fig. 7.27 Superficial structures of the right forelimb (3): caudal view. This dissection is also shown in Figs. 7.25, 7.26 and 7.28. For further details of the digital region see Fig. 7.31.

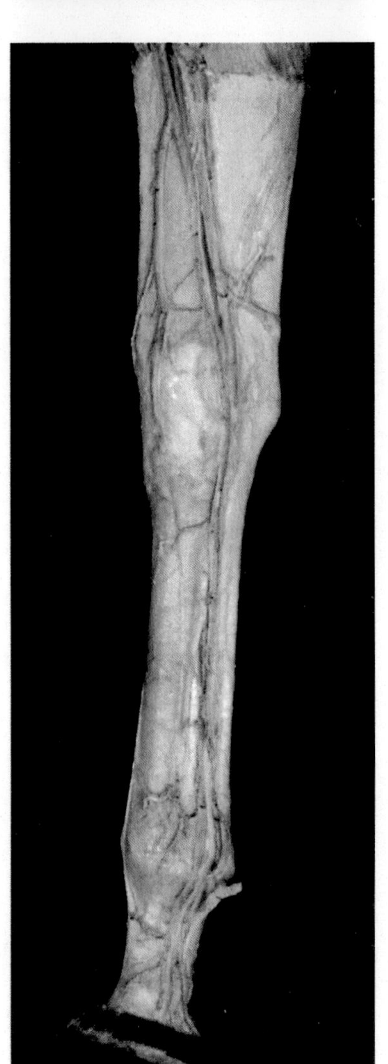

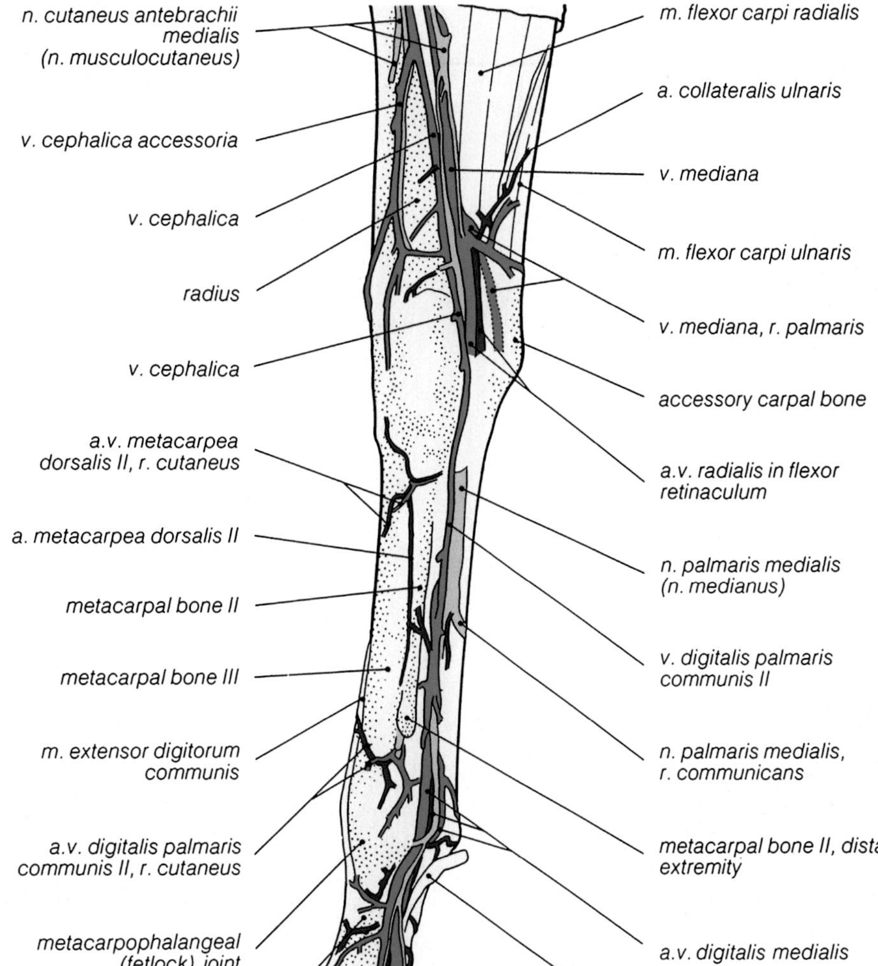

n. cutaneus antebrachii medialis (n. musculocutaneus)
v. cephalica accessoria
v. cephalica
radius
v. cephalica
a.v. metacarpea dorsalis II, r. cutaneus
a. metacarpea dorsalis II
metacarpal bone II
metacarpal bone III
m. extensor digitorum communis
a.v. digitalis palmaris communis II, r. cutaneus
metacarpophalangeal (fetlock) joint
digit III
m. flexor carpi radialis
a. collateralis ulnaris
v. mediana
m. flexor carpi ulnaris
v. mediana, r. palmaris
accessory carpal bone
a.v. radialis in flexor retinaculum
n. palmaris medialis (n. medianus)
v. digitalis palmaris communis II
n. palmaris medialis, r. communicans
metacarpal bone II, distal extremity
a.v. digitalis medialis
ligament of the ergot

Fig. 7.28 Superficial structures of the right forelimb (4): medial view. This dissection is also shown in Fig. 7.25, 7.26 and 7.27. For further details of the digital region, see Fig. 7.32. The full extent of the ligament of the ergot is shown in this figure.

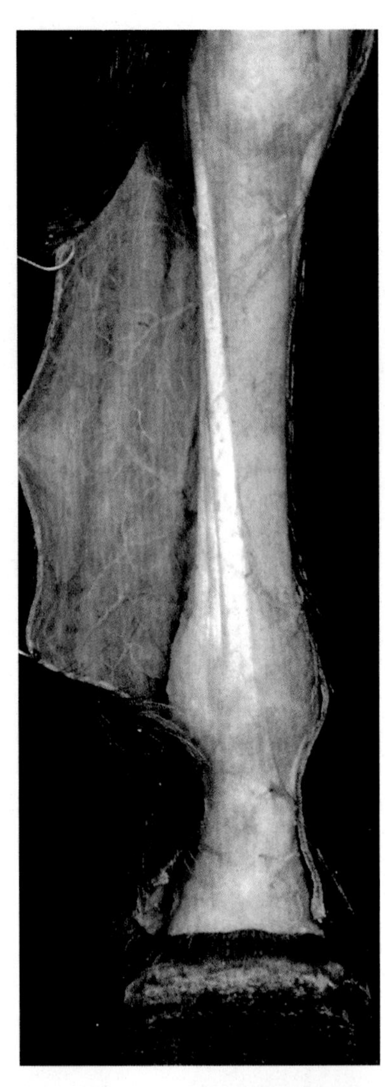

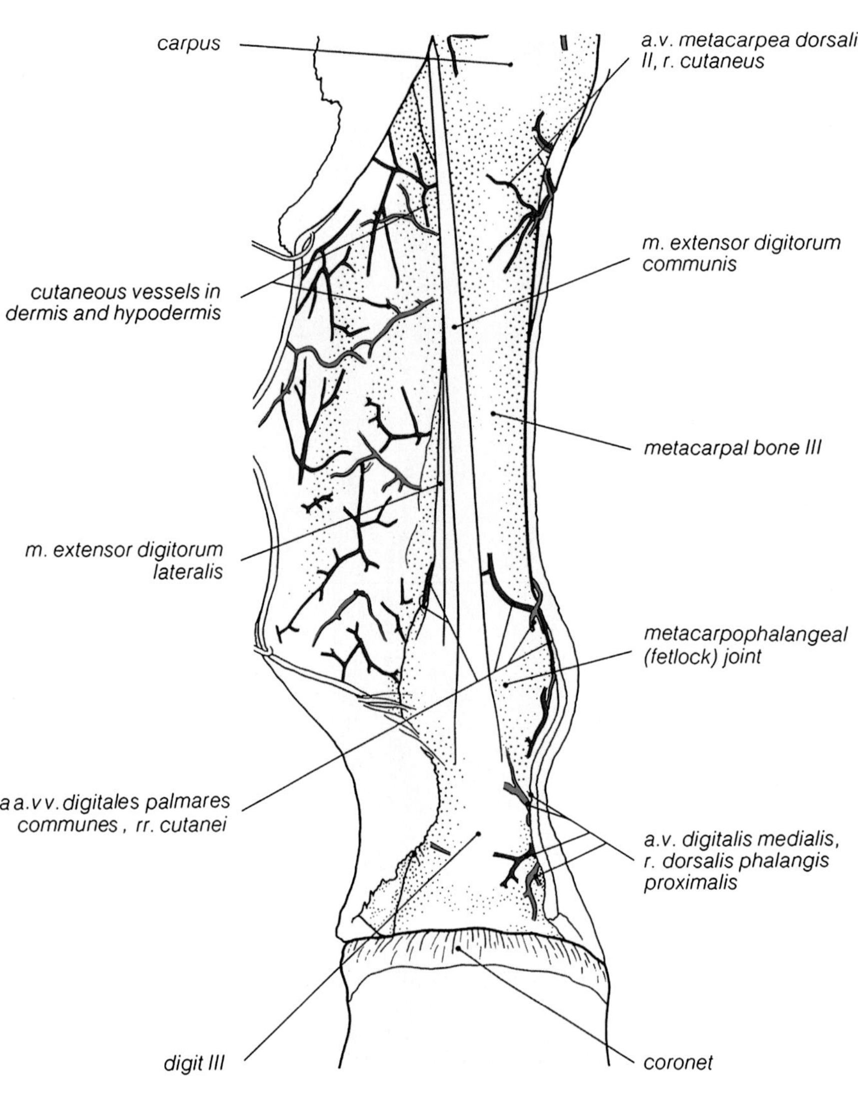
carpus
cutaneous vessels in dermis and hypodermis
m. extensor digitorum lateralis
aa.vv. digitales palmares communes, rr. cutanei
digit III
a.v. metacarpea dorsalis II, r. cutaneus
m. extensor digitorum communis
metacarpal bone III
metacarpophalangeal (fetlock) joint
a.v. digitalis medialis, r. dorsalis phalangis proximalis
coronet

Fig. 7.29 Superficial structures of the right manus (1): dorsal view. In this figure the skin has been replaced after dissection of the superficial structures in order to show the blood vessels of its deeper layers and their origins from the metacarpal and digital vessels (see also Figs. 7.30–7.32).

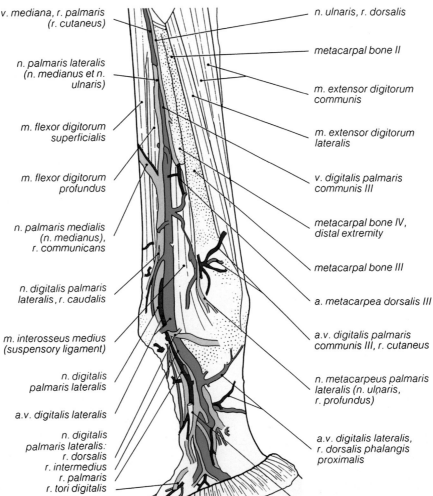

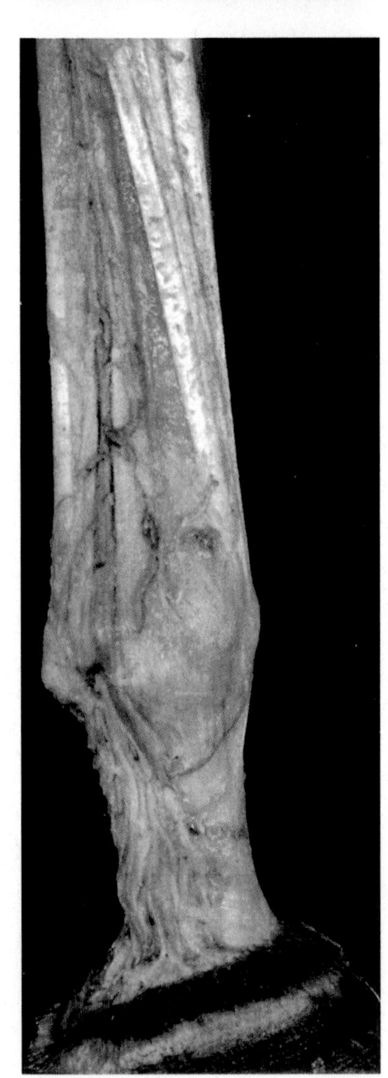
v. mediana, r. palmaris (r. cutaneus)
n. palmaris lateralis (n. medianus et n. ulnaris)
m. flexor digitorum superficialis
m. flexor digitorum profundus
n. palmaris medialis (n. medianus), r. communicans
n. digitalis palmaris lateralis, r. caudalis
m. interosseus medius (suspensory ligament)
n. digitalis palmaris lateralis
a.v. digitalis lateralis
n. digitalis palmaris lateralis:
r. dorsalis
r. intermedius
r. palmaris
r. tori digitalis
coronet
n. ulnaris, r. dorsalis
metacarpal bone II
m. extensor digitorum communis
m. extensor digitorum lateralis
v. digitalis palmaris communis III
metacarpal bone IV, distal extremity
metacarpal bone III
a. metacarpea dorsalis III
a.v. digitalis palmaris communis III, r. cutaneus
n. metacarpeus palmaris lateralis (n. ulnaris, r. profundus)
a.v. digitalis lateralis, r. dorsalis phalangis proximalis
ligament of the ergot (cut)

Fig. 7.30 Superficial structures of the right manus (2): lateral view. This is a closer view of part of the dissection shown in Fig. 7.26. Other views of this part of the specimen are shown in Figs. 7.31 and 7.32. See also Fig. 7.29.

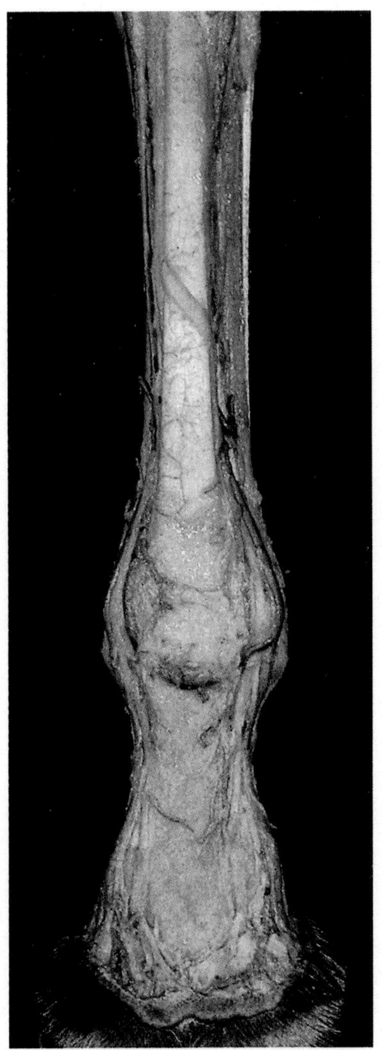

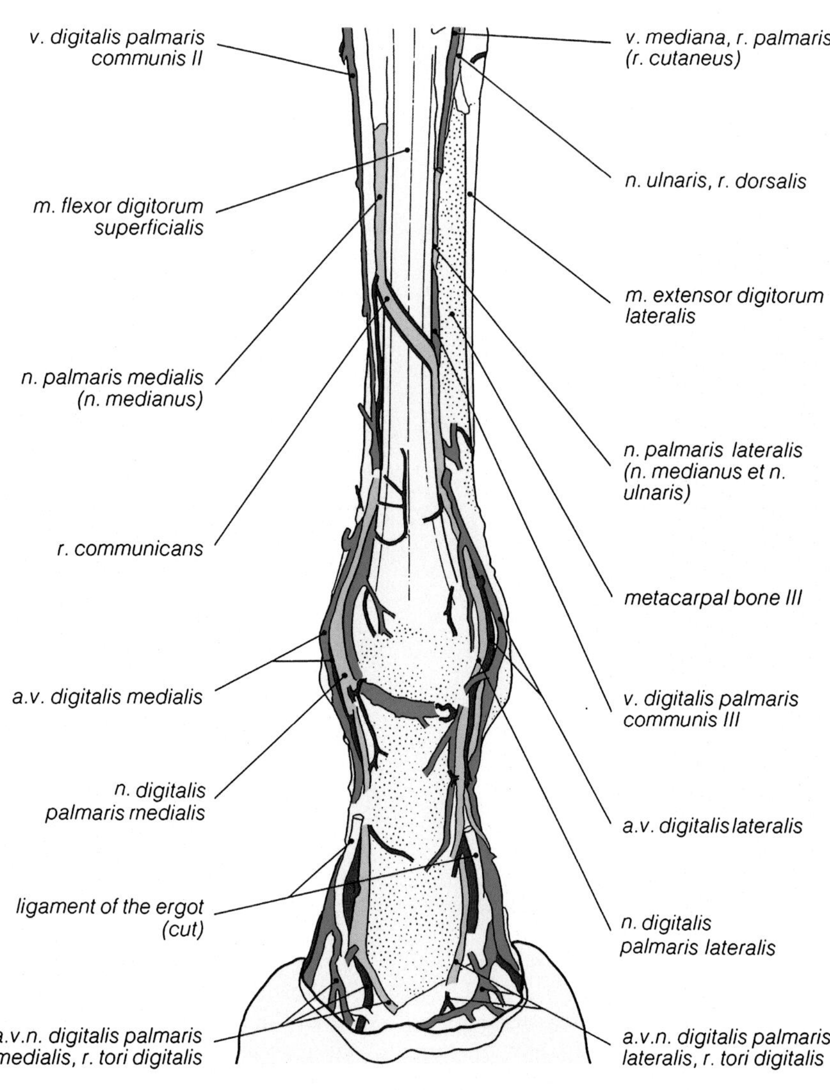
v. digitalis palmaris communis II
m. flexor digitorum superficialis
n. palmaris medialis (n. medianus)
r. communicans
a.v. digitalis medialis
n. digitalis palmaris medialis
ligament of the ergot (cut)
a.v.n. digitalis palmaris medialis, r. tori digitalis
v. mediana, r. palmaris (r. cutaneus)
n. ulnaris, r. dorsalis
m. extensor digitorum lateralis
n. palmaris lateralis (n. medianus et n. ulnaris)
metacarpal bone III
v. digitalis palmaris communis III
a.v. digitalis lateralis
n. digitalis palmaris lateralis
a.v.n. digitalis palmaris lateralis, r. tori digitalis

Fig. 7.31 Superficial structures of the right manus (3): palmar view. This is a closer view of a part of the dissection shown in Fig. 7.27. Other views of this part of the specimen are shown in Figs. 7.30 and 7.32 (see also Fig. 7.29).

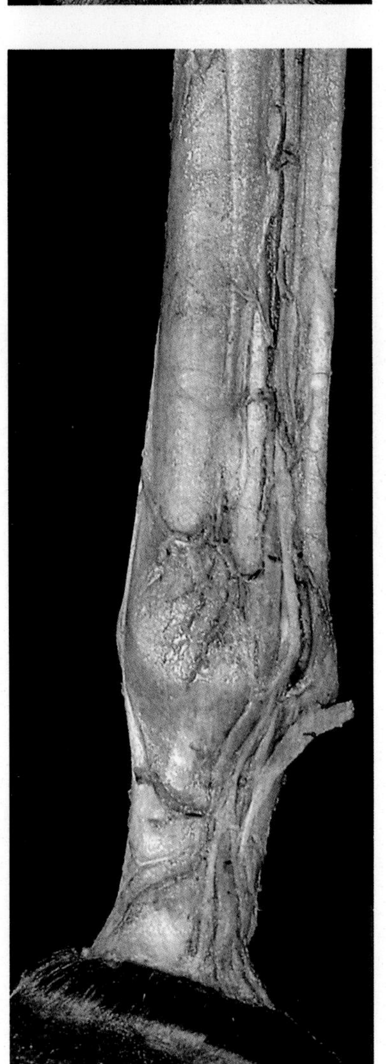

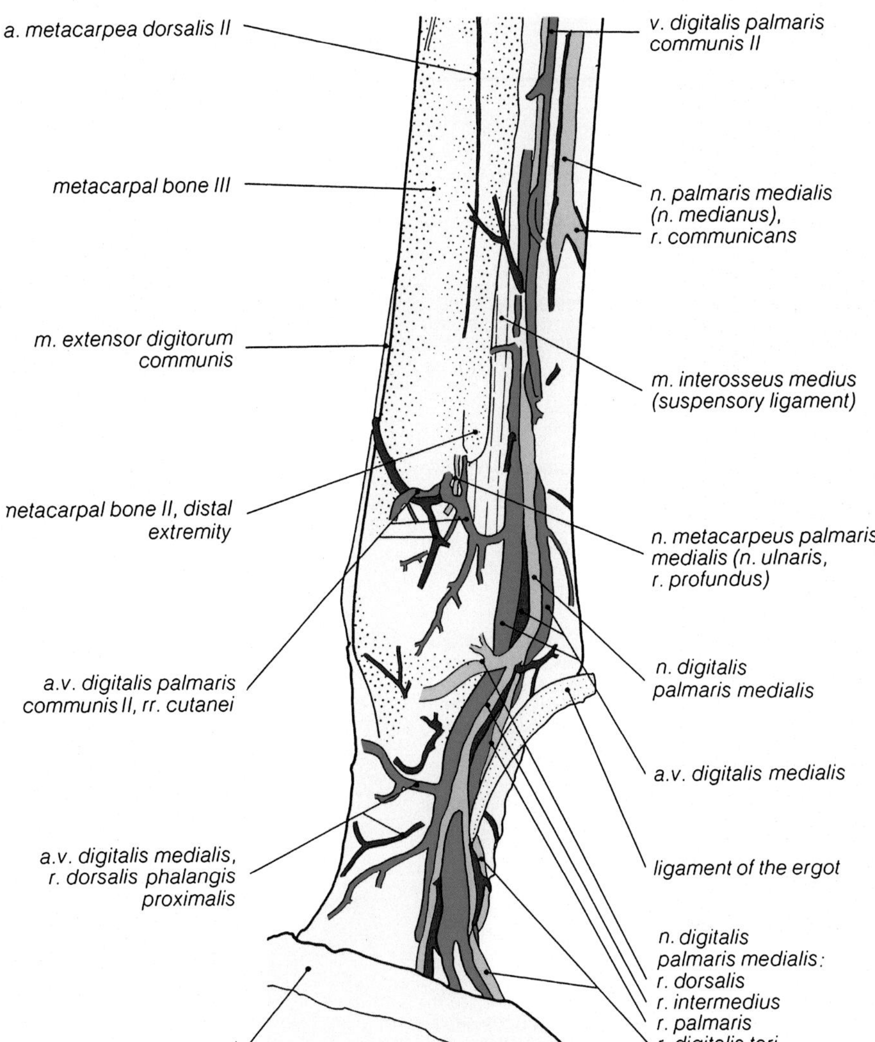
a. metacarpea dorsalis II
metacarpal bone III
m. extensor digitorum communis
netacarpal bone II, distal extremity
a.v. digitalis palmaris communis II, rr. cutanei
a.v. digitalis medialis, r. dorsalis phalangis proximalis
coronet
v. digitalis palmaris communis II
n. palmaris medialis (n. medianus), r. communicans
m. interosseus medius (suspensory ligament)
n. metacarpeus palmaris medialis (n. ulnaris, r. profundus)
n. digitalis palmaris medialis
a.v. digitalis medialis
ligament of the ergot
n. digitalis palmaris medialis:
r. dorsalis
r. intermedius
r. palmaris
r. digitalis tori

Fig. 7.32 Superficial structures of the right manus (4): medial view. This is a closer view of a part of the dissection shown in Fig. 7.28. Other views of this part of this specimen are shown in Figs. 7.30 and 7.31 but note that in this figure the medial ligament of the ergot has not yet been cut short. See also Fig. 7.29.

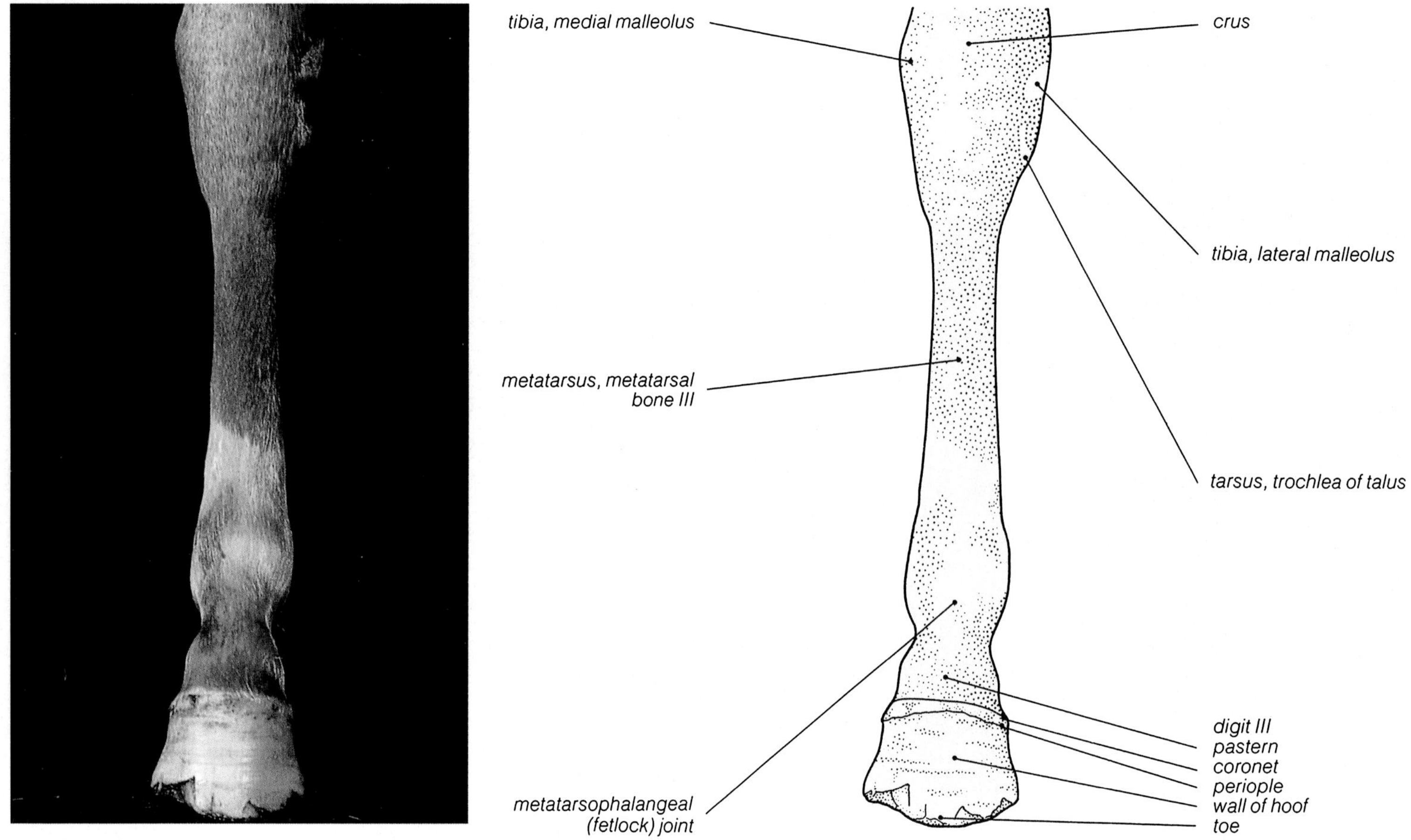
tibia, medial malleolus
crus
tibia, lateral malleolus
metatarsus, metatarsal bone III
tarsus, trochlea of talus
metatarsophalangeal (fetlock) joint
digit III
pastern
coronet
periople
wall of hoof
toe

Fig. 7.33 Surface features of the left pes: cranial view. Figs. 7.35, 7.37 and 7.39 show further views of this specimen. Palpable features have been shaved. Note that in this specimen the palpable structures on the medial aspect of the hock were demonstrated on the right leg (see Fig. 7.39) and are not seen in this figure. Figs. 7.34, 7.36, 7.38 and 7.40 show the bones of this region and Fig. 7.9 shows the solar surface of the hoof. A note on the terminology applied to the lateral prominence of the tibia is given in Fig. 7.36.

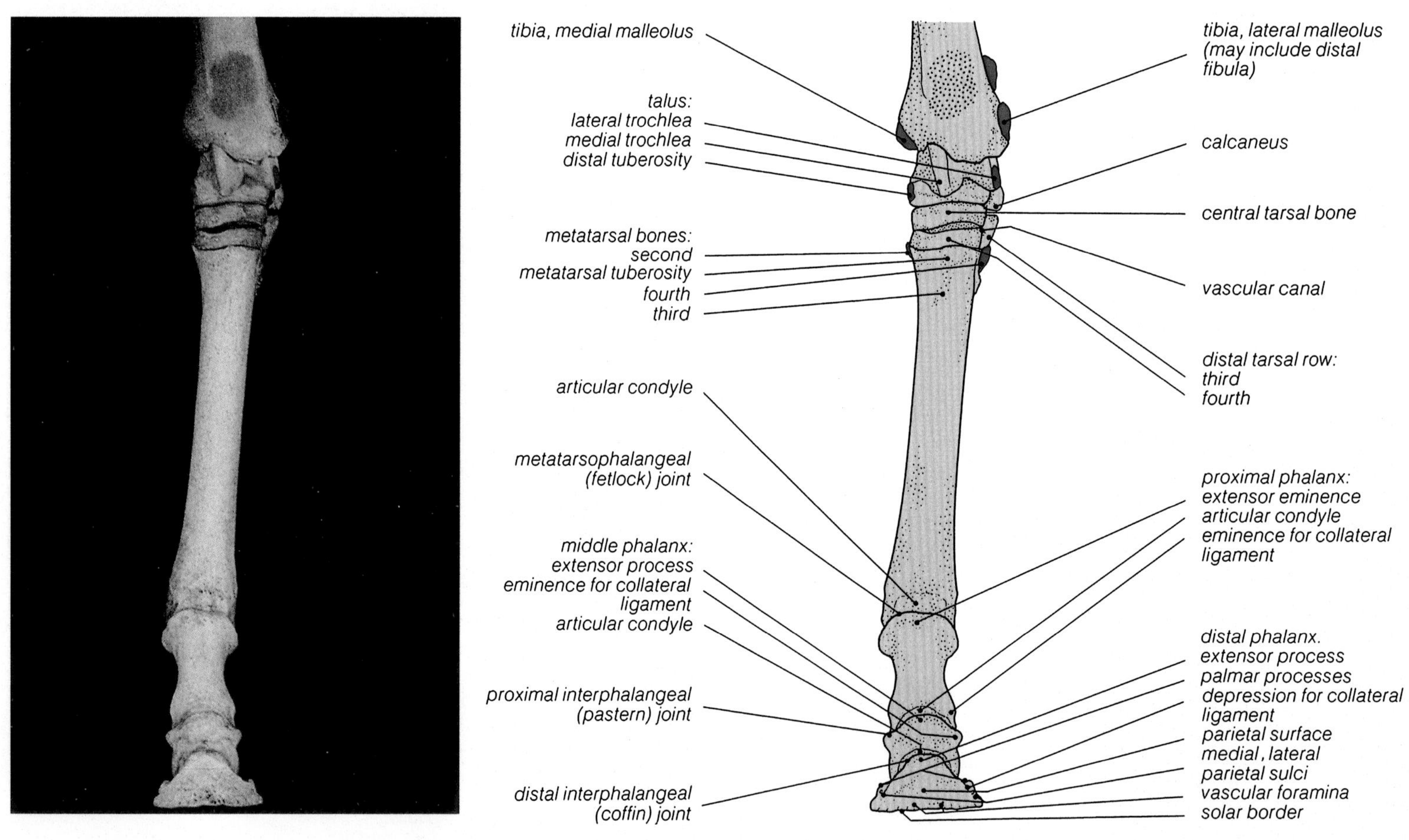
tibia, medial malleolus
talus:
lateral trochlea
medial trochlea
distal tuberosity
metatarsal bones:
second
metatarsal tuberosity
fourth
third
articular condyle
metatarsophalangeal (fetlock) joint
middle phalanx:
extensor process
eminence for collateral ligament
articular condyle
proximal interphalangeal (pastern) joint
distal interphalangeal (coffin) joint
tibia, lateral malleolus (may include distal fibula)
calcaneus
central tarsal bone
vascular canal
distal tarsal row:
third
fourth
proximal phalanx:
extensor eminence
articular condyle
eminence for collateral ligament
distal phalanx.
extensor process
palmar processes
depression for collateral ligament
parietal surface
medial, lateral
parietal sulci
vascular foramina
solar border

Fig. 7.34 The bones of the left pes: cranial view. The prominences shaved in Fig. 7.33 have been coloured red.

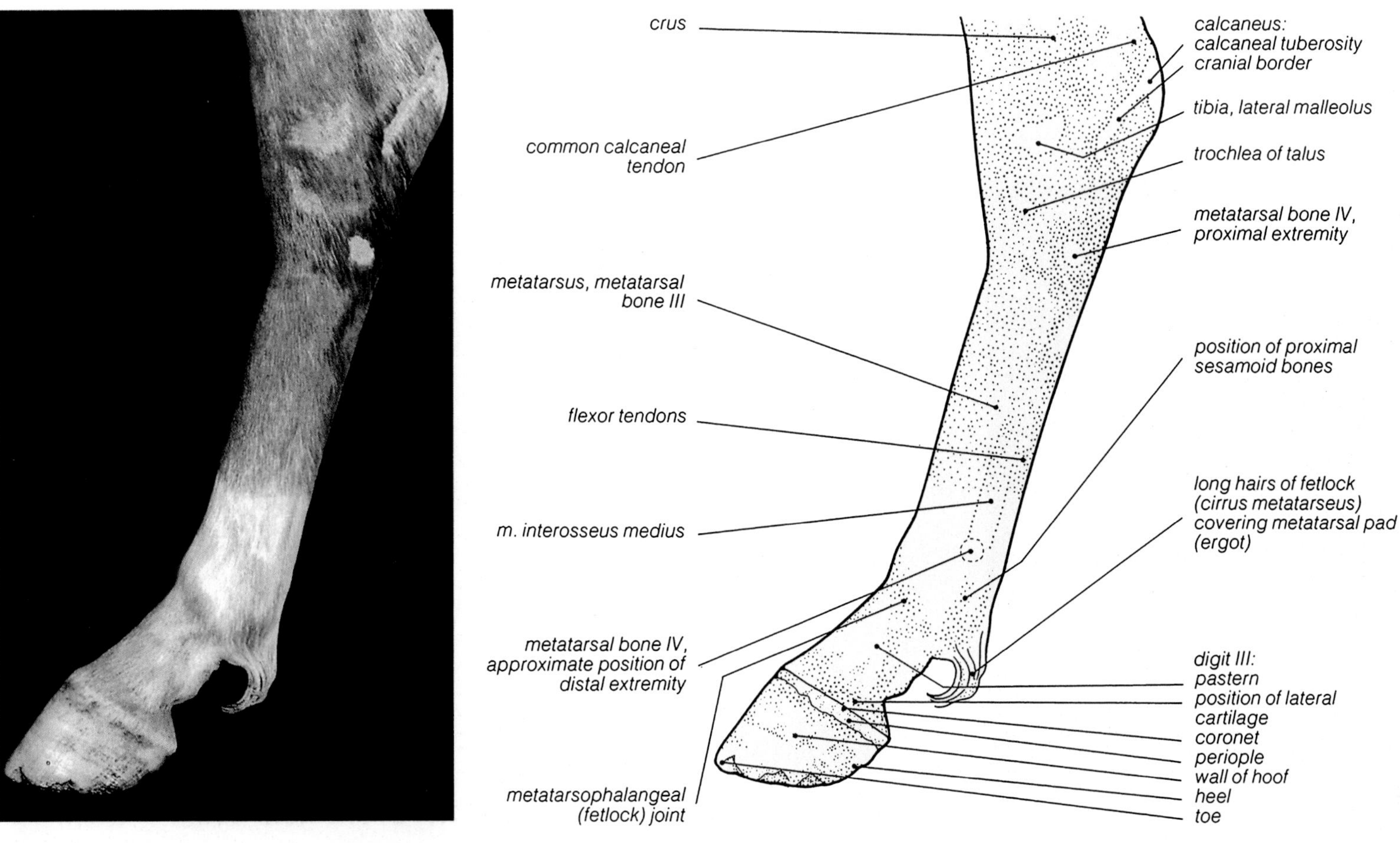
crus
common calcaneal tendon
metatarsus, metatarsal bone III
flexor tendons
m. interosseus medius
metatarsal bone IV, approximate position of distal extremity
metatarsophalangeal (fetlock) joint
calcaneus:
calcaneal tuberosity
cranial border
tibia, lateral malleolus
trochlea of talus
metatarsal bone IV, proximal extremity
position of proximal sesamoid bones
long hairs of fetlock (cirrus metatarseus) covering metatarsal pad (ergot)
digit III:
pastern
position of lateral cartilage
coronet
periople
wall of hoof
heel
toe

Fig. 7.35 Surface features of the left pes: lateral view. The specimen was embalmed in the standing position, with the limb arranged to imitate its position in normal level standing, but the metatarsus should be more vertical. The position of the distal end of the fourth metatarsal bone has not been shaved; it can be seen in Fig. 7.42.

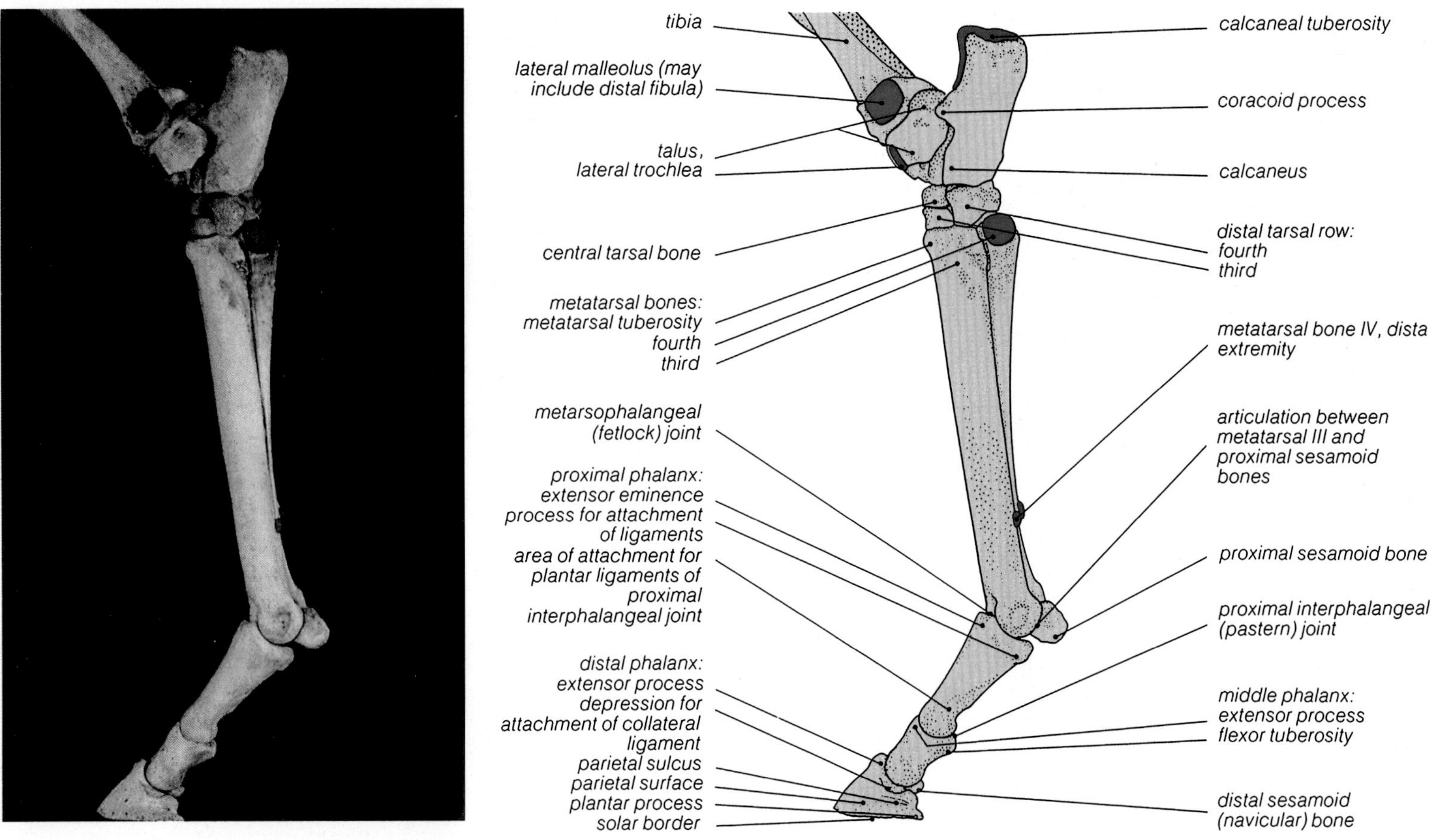
tibia
lateral malleolus (may include distal fibula)
talus,
lateral trochlea
central tarsal bone
metatarsal bones:
metatarsal tuberosity
fourth
third
metarsophalangeal (fetlock) joint
proximal phalanx:
extensor eminence
process for attachment of ligaments
area of attachment for plantar ligaments of proximal interphalangeal joint
distal phalanx:
extensor process
depression for attachment of collateral ligament
parietal sulcus
parietal surface
plantar process
solar border
calcaneal tuberosity
coracoid process
calcaneus
distal tarsal row:
fourth
third
metatarsal bone IV, dista extremity
articulation between metatarsal III and proximal sesamoid bones
proximal sesamoid bone
proximal interphalangeal (pastern) joint
middle phalanx:
extensor process
flexor tuberosity
distal sesamoid (navicular) bone

Fig. 7.36 The bones of the left pes: lateral view. The prominences shaved in Fig. 7.35 have been coloured red. The distal epiphysis of the fibula fuses with that of the tibia during the first year of life. It forms part of the lateral articular surface and may contribute to the palpable lateral malleolus.

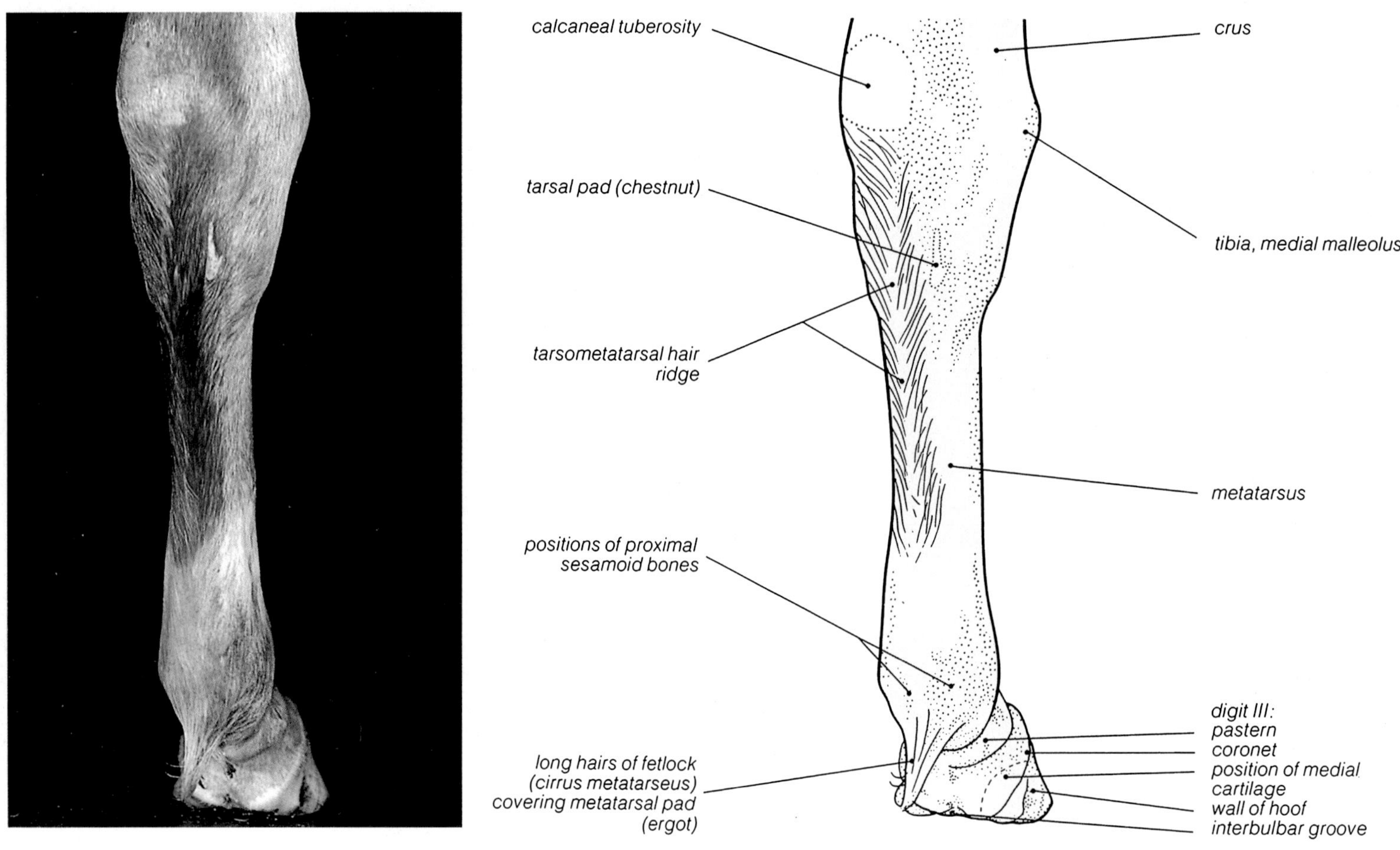
calcaneal tuberosity
crus
tarsal pad (chestnut)
tibia, medial malleolus
tarsometatarsal hair ridge
metatarsus
positions of proximal sesamoid bones
digit III:
pastern
coronet
position of medial cartilage
wall of hoof
interbulbar groove
long hairs of fetlock (cirrus metatarseus) covering metatarsal pad (ergot)

Fig. 7.37 Surface features of the left pes: caudomedial view. The specimen is viewed from a slightly medial angle to show the tarsal pad or 'chestnut' more clearly. This structure is usually superficial to the fused 1st and 2nd tarsal bones; it may be absent in the horse, and it is not found in other species of the genus *Equus*.

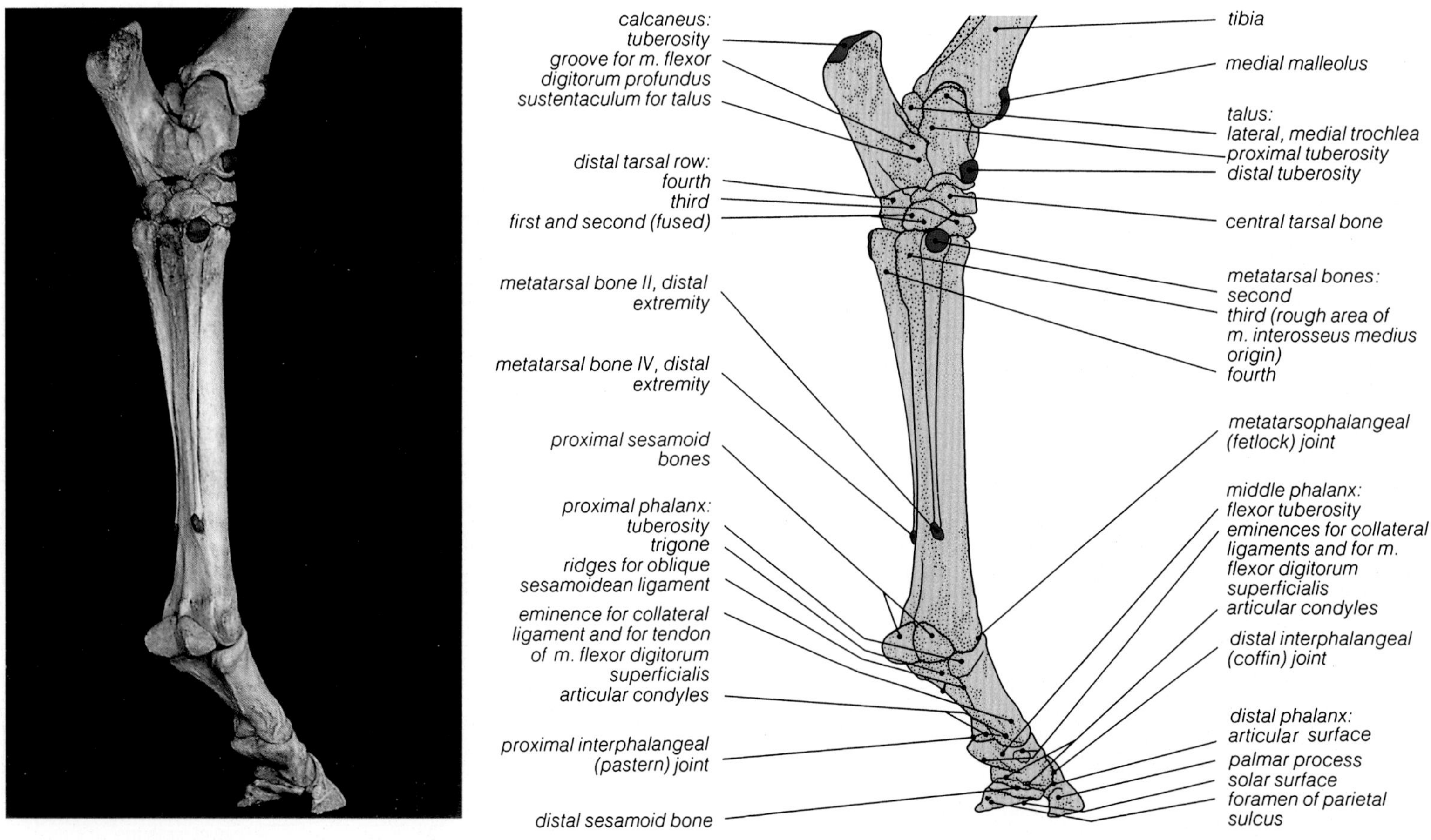
calcaneus:
tuberosity
groove for m. flexor digitorum profundus
sustentaculum for talus
distal tarsal row:
fourth
third
first and second (fused)
metatarsal bone II, distal extremity
metatarsal bone IV, distal extremity
proximal sesamoid bones
proximal phalanx:
tuberosity
trigone
ridges for oblique sesamoidean ligament
eminence for collateral ligament and for tendon of m. flexor digitorum superficialis
articular condyles
proximal interphalangeal (pastern) joint
distal sesamoid bone
tibia
medial malleolus
talus:
lateral, medial trochlea
proximal tuberosity
distal tuberosity
central tarsal bone
metatarsal bones:
second
third (rough area of m. interosseus medius origin)
fourth
metatarsophalangeal (fetlock) joint
middle phalanx:
flexor tuberosity
eminences for collateral ligaments and for m. flexor digitorum superficialis
articular condyles
distal interphalangeal (coffin) joint
distal phalanx:
articular surface
palmar process
solar surface
foramen of parietal sulcus

Fig. 7.38 The bones of the left pes: caudomedial view. The prominences, shaved in Fig. 7.37 and 7.39 have been coloured red.

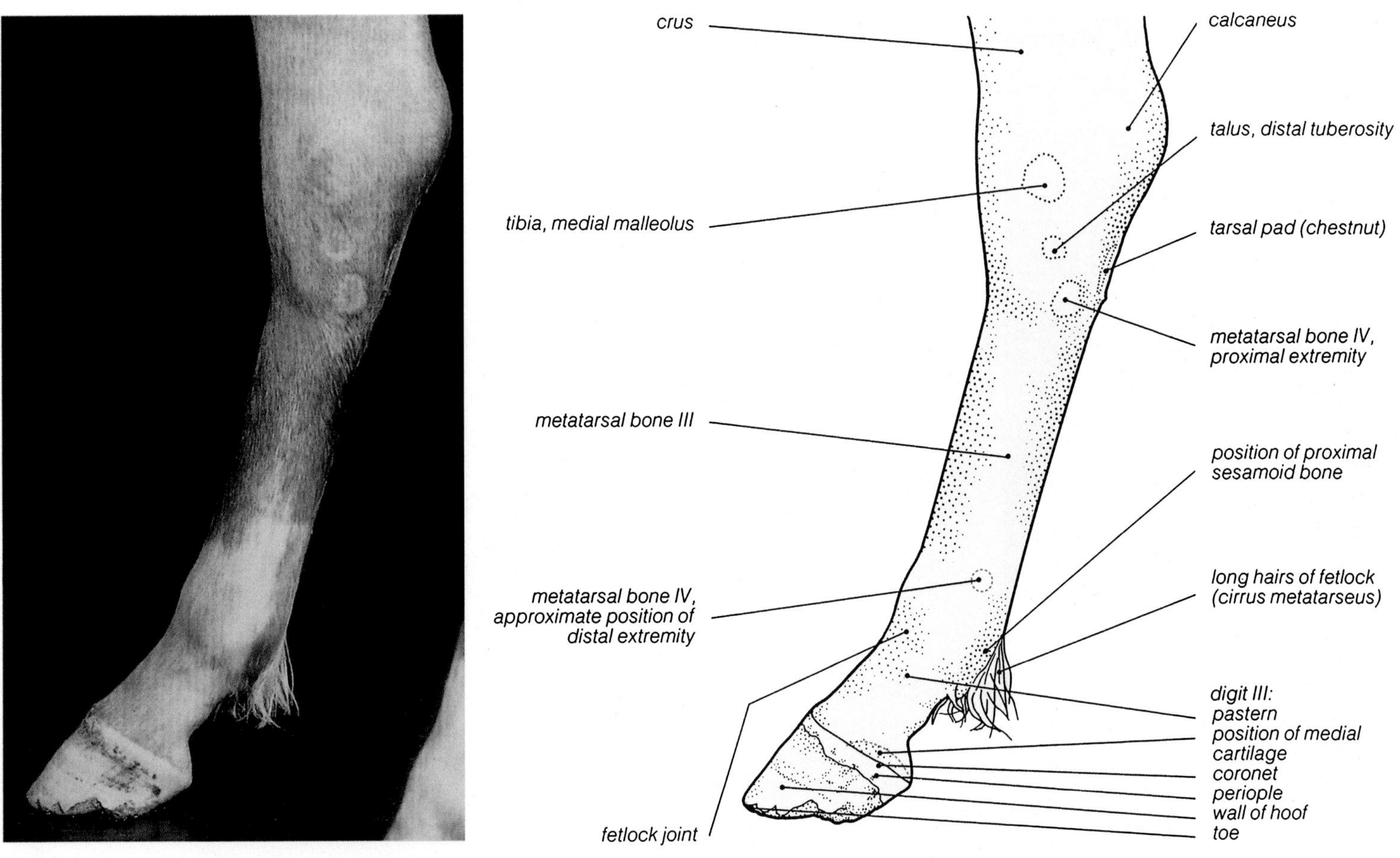
crus
calcaneus
talus, distal tuberosity
tibia, medial malleolus
tarsal pad (chestnut)
metatarsal bone IV, proximal extremity
metatarsal bone III
position of proximal sesamoid bone
long hairs of fetlock (cirrus metatarseus)
metatarsal bone IV, approximate position of distal extremity
digit III:
pastern
position of medial cartilage
coronet
periople
wall of hoof
toe
fetlock joint

Fig. 7.39 Surface features of the right pes: medial view. The position of the distal extremity of the fourth metatarsal bone has not been shaved; it can be seen in Fig. 7.44. The medial hoof wall is severely damaged along its solar surface (see Fig. 7.9).

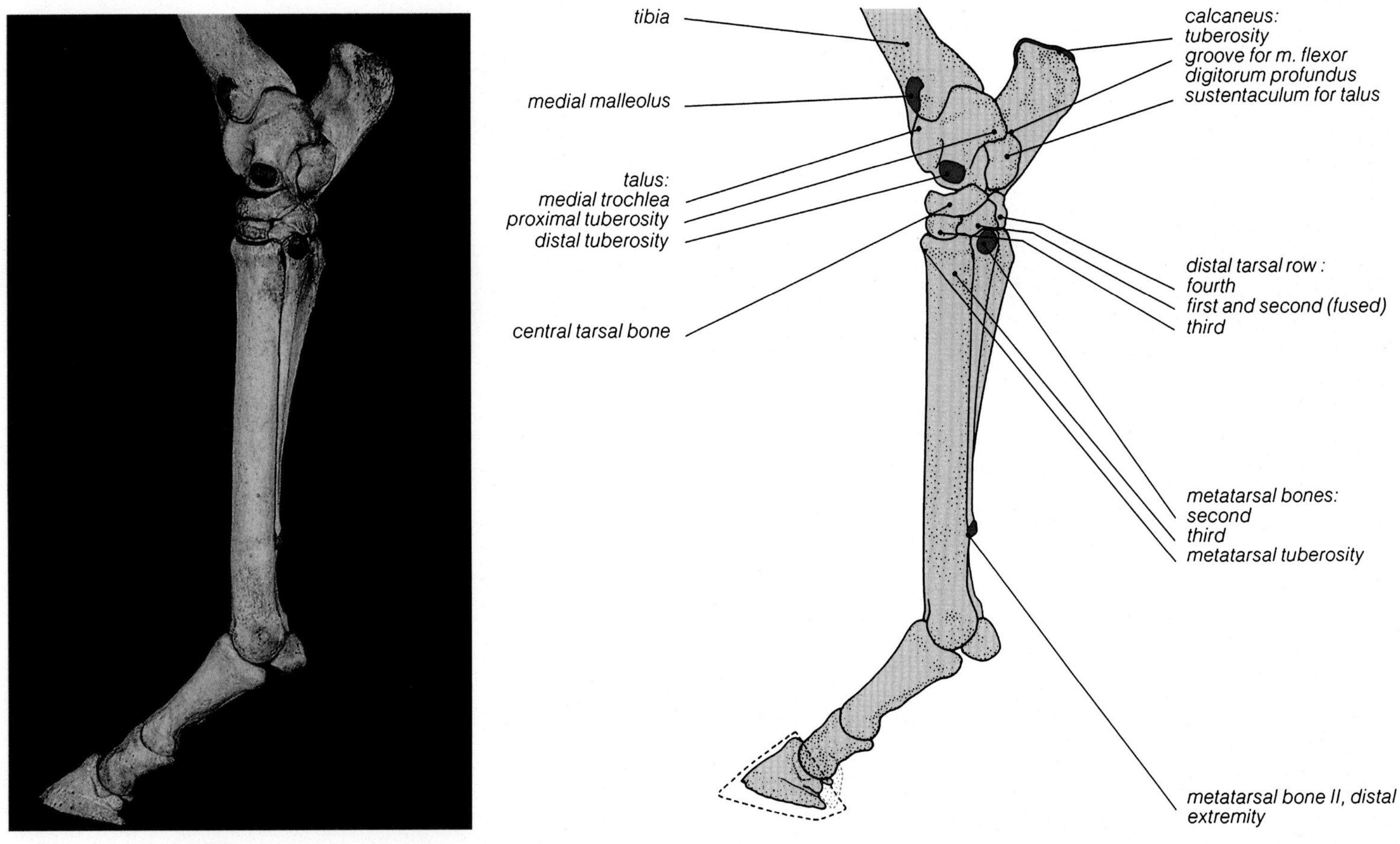
tibia
calcaneus:
tuberosity
groove for m. flexor digitorum profundus
sustentaculum for talus
medial malleolus
talus:
medial trochlea
proximal tuberosity
distal tuberosity
central tarsal bone
distal tarsal row :
fourth
first and second (fused)
third
metatarsal bones:
second
third
metatarsal tuberosity
metatarsal bone II, distal extremity

Fig. 7.40 The bones of the right pes: medial view. The prominences shaved in Fig. 7.37 and 7.39 have been coloured red. Outlines of the medial cartilage of the distal phalanx (stippled), and of the hoof, have been added (see Figs. 7.61 and 7.66).

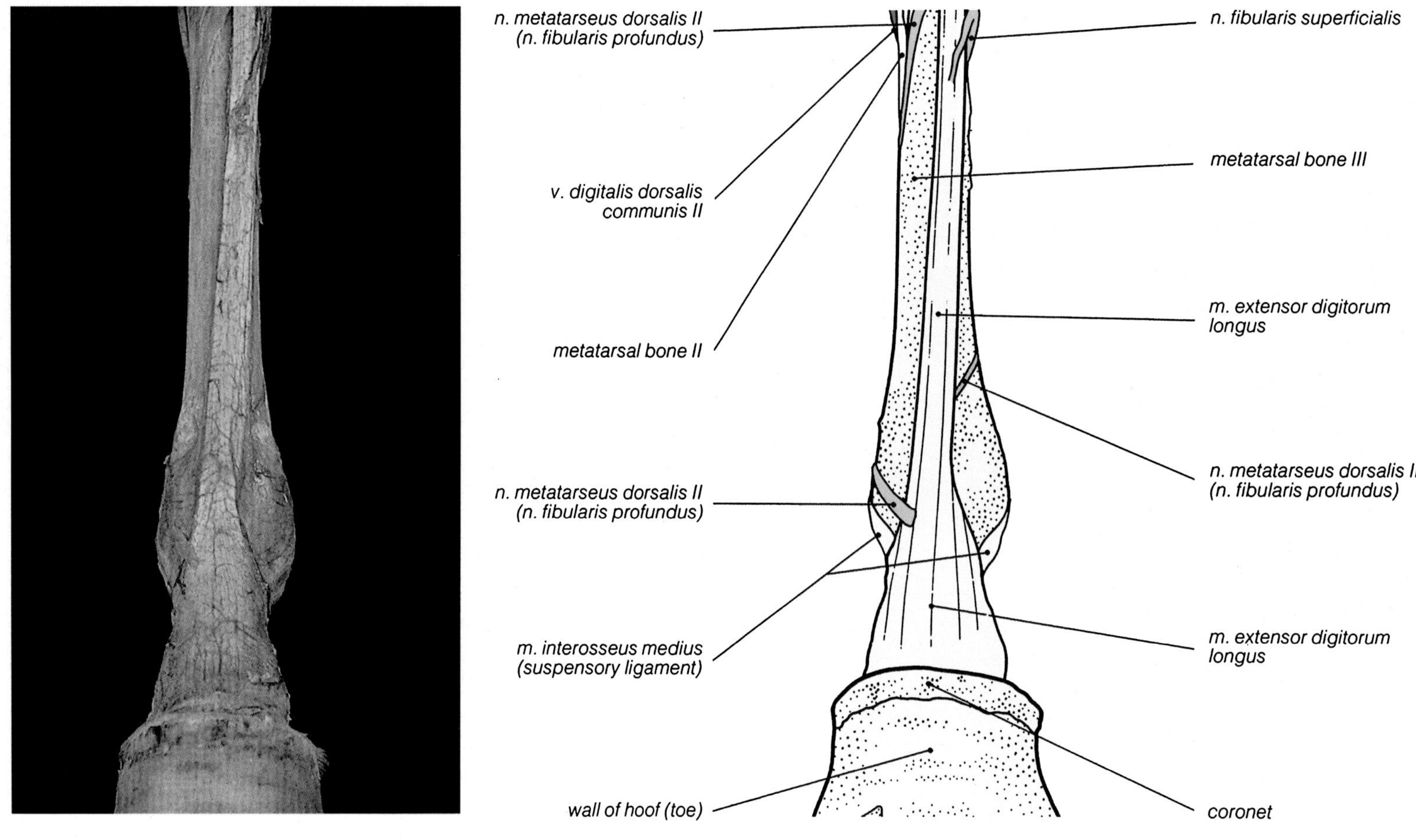
n. metatarseus dorsalis II
(n. fibularis profundus)
v. digitalis dorsalis
communis II
metatarsal bone II
n. metatarseus dorsalis II
(n. fibularis profundus)
m. interosseus medius
(suspensory ligament)
wall of hoof (toe)
n. fibularis superficialis
metatarsal bone III
m. extensor digitorum
longus
n. metatarseus dorsalis III
(n. fibularis profundus)
m. extensor digitorum
longus
coronet

Fig. 7.41 Superficial structures of the distal left pes (1): dorsal view. The more proximal parts of this specimen are shown in Fig. 6.41. This dissection is also shown in Figs. 7.42–7.44.

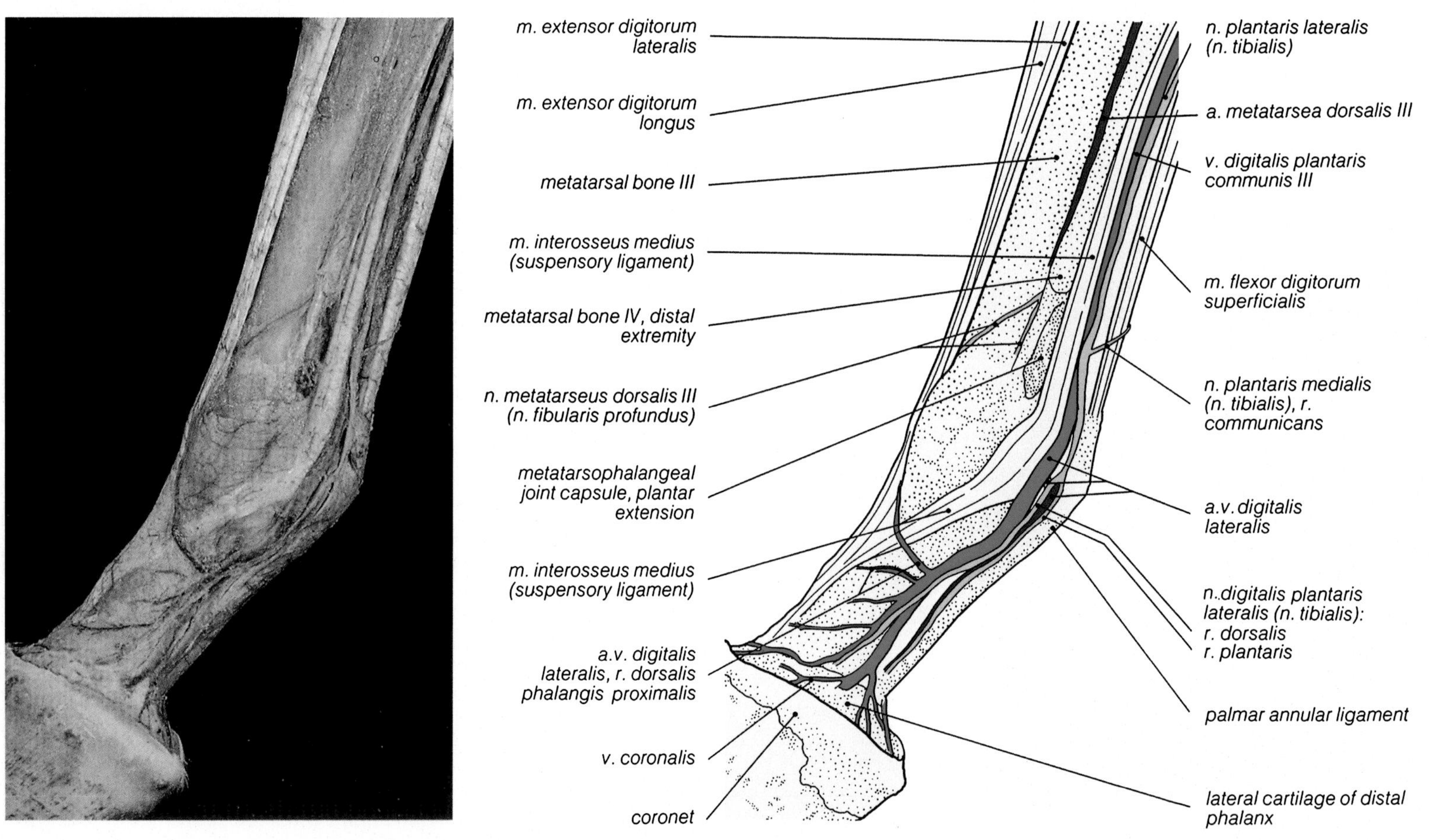
m. extensor digitorum
lateralis
m. extensor digitorum
longus
metatarsal bone III
m. interosseus medius
(suspensory ligament)
metatarsal bone IV, distal
extremity
n. metatarseus dorsalis III
(n. fibularis profundus)
metatarsophalangeal
joint capsule, plantar
extension
m. interosseus medius
(suspensory ligament)
a.v. digitalis
lateralis, r. dorsalis
phalangis proximalis
v. coronalis
coronet
n. plantaris lateralis
(n. tibialis)
a. metatarsea dorsalis III
v. digitalis plantaris
communis III
m. flexor digitorum
superficialis
n. plantaris medialis
(n. tibialis), r.
communicans
a.v. digitalis
lateralis
n..digitalis plantaris
lateralis (n. tibialis):
r. dorsalis
r. plantaris
palmar annular ligament
lateral cartilage of distal
phalanx

Fig. 7.42 Superficial structures of the distal left pes (2): lateral view. The more proximal parts of this dissection are shown in Fig.6.42. This dissection is also shown in Figs. 7.41, 7.43 and 7.44.

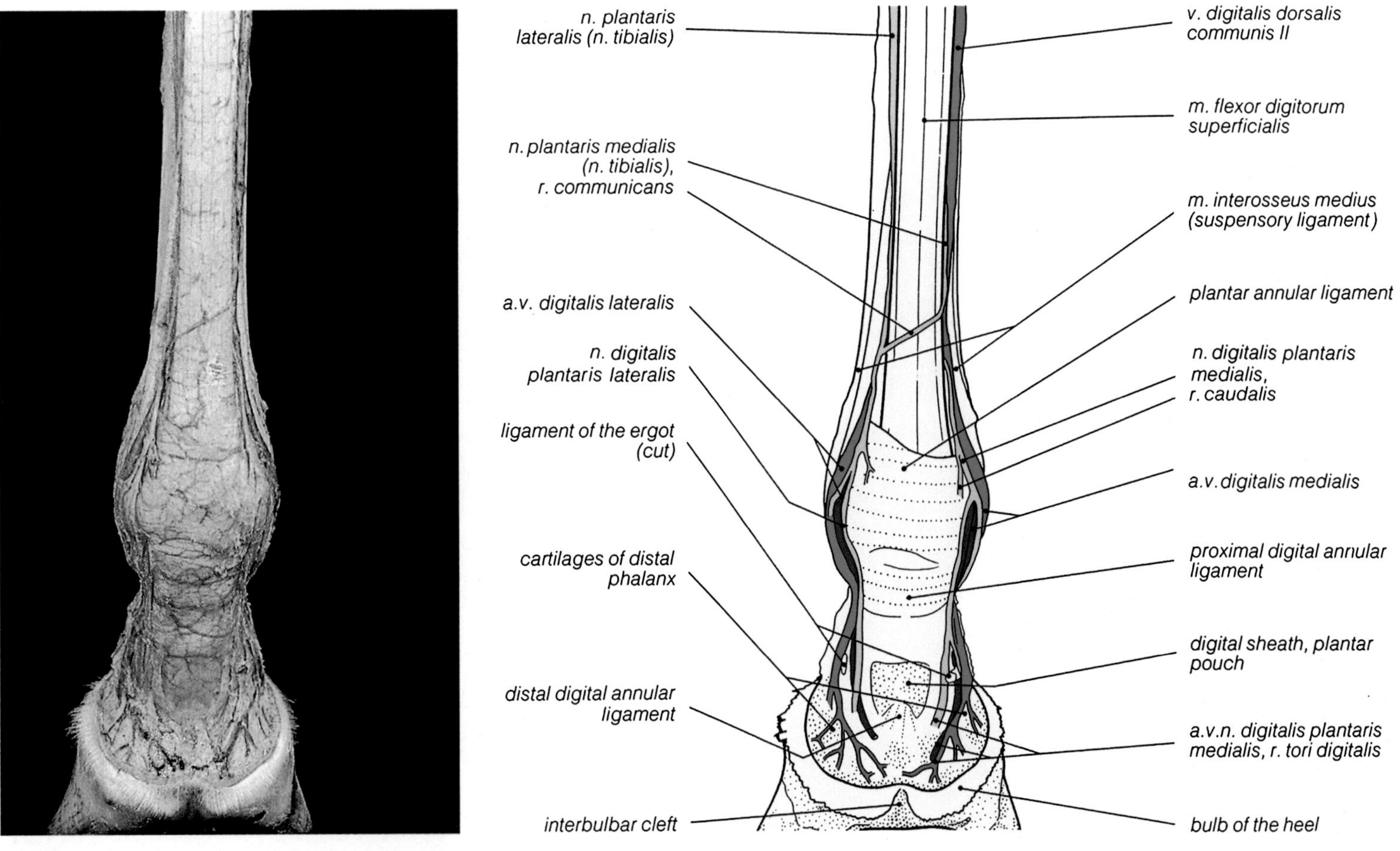
n. plantaris lateralis (n. tibialis)
n. plantaris medialis (n. tibialis), r. communicans
a.v. digitalis lateralis
n. digitalis plantaris lateralis
ligament of the ergot (cut)
cartilages of distal phalanx
distal digital annular ligament
interbulbar cleft
v. digitalis dorsalis communis II
m. flexor digitorum superficialis
m. interosseus medius (suspensory ligament)
plantar annular ligament
n. digitalis plantaris medialis, r. caudalis
a.v. digitalis medialis
proximal digital annular ligament
digital sheath, plantar pouch
a.v.n. digitalis plantaris medialis, r. tori digitalis
bulb of the heel

Fig. 7.43 Superficial structures of the distal left pes (3): plantar view. This dissection is also shown in Figs. 7.41, 7.42 and 7.44.

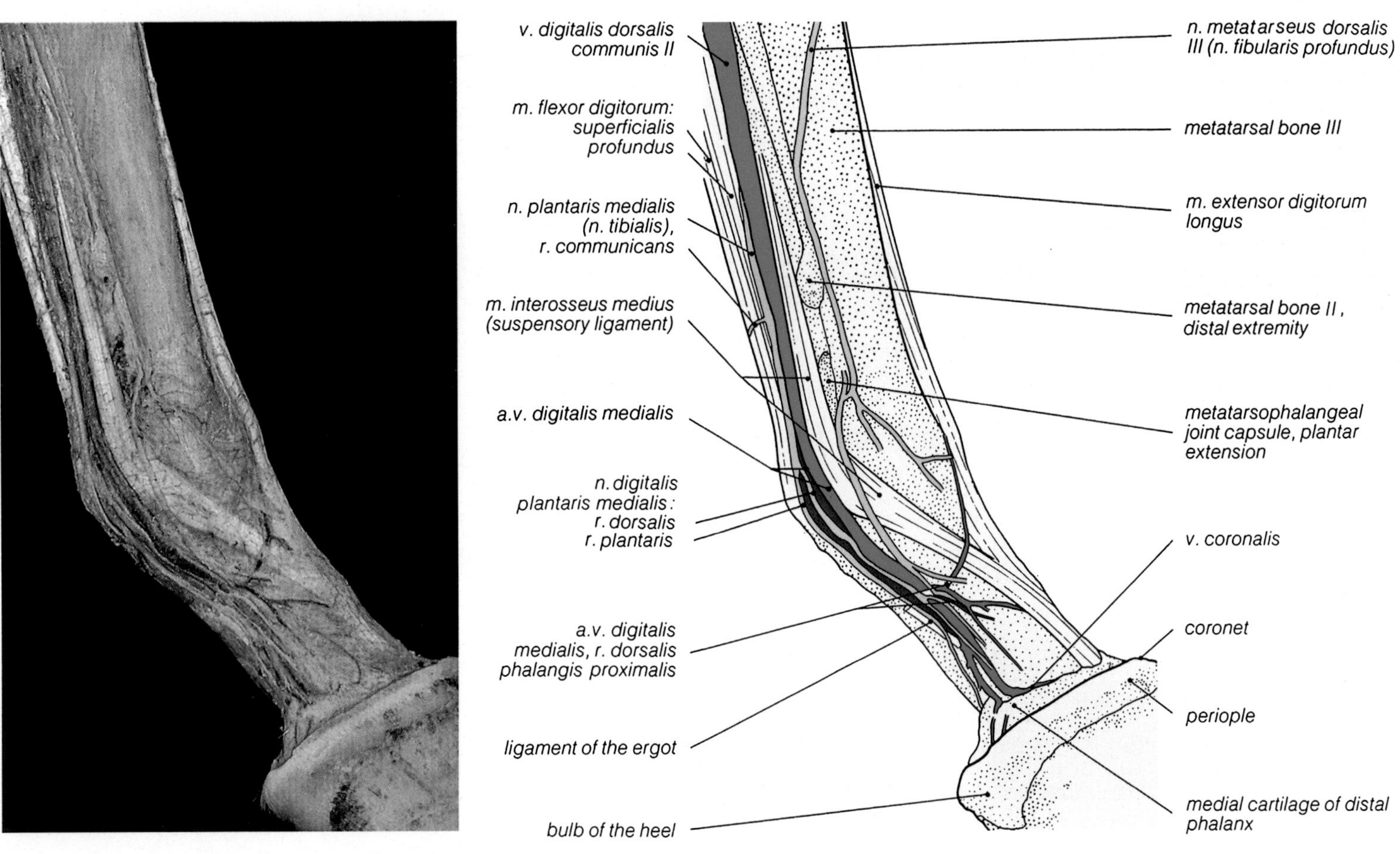
v. digitalis dorsalis communis II
m. flexor digitorum: superficialis profundus
n. plantaris medialis (n. tibialis), r. communicans
m. interosseus medius (suspensory ligament)
a.v. digitalis medialis
n. digitalis plantaris medialis: r. dorsalis r. plantaris
a.v. digitalis medialis, r. dorsalis phalangis proximalis
ligament of the ergot
bulb of the heel
n. metatarseus dorsalis III (n. fibularis profundus)
metatarsal bone III
m. extensor digitorum longus
metatarsal bone II, distal extremity
metatarsophalangeal joint capsule, plantar extension
v. coronalis
coronet
periople
medial cartilage of distal phalanx

Fig. 7.44 Superficial structures of the distal left pes (4): medial view. The more proximal parts of this dissection are shown in Fig. 6.43. This dissection is also seen in Figs. 7.41–7.43.

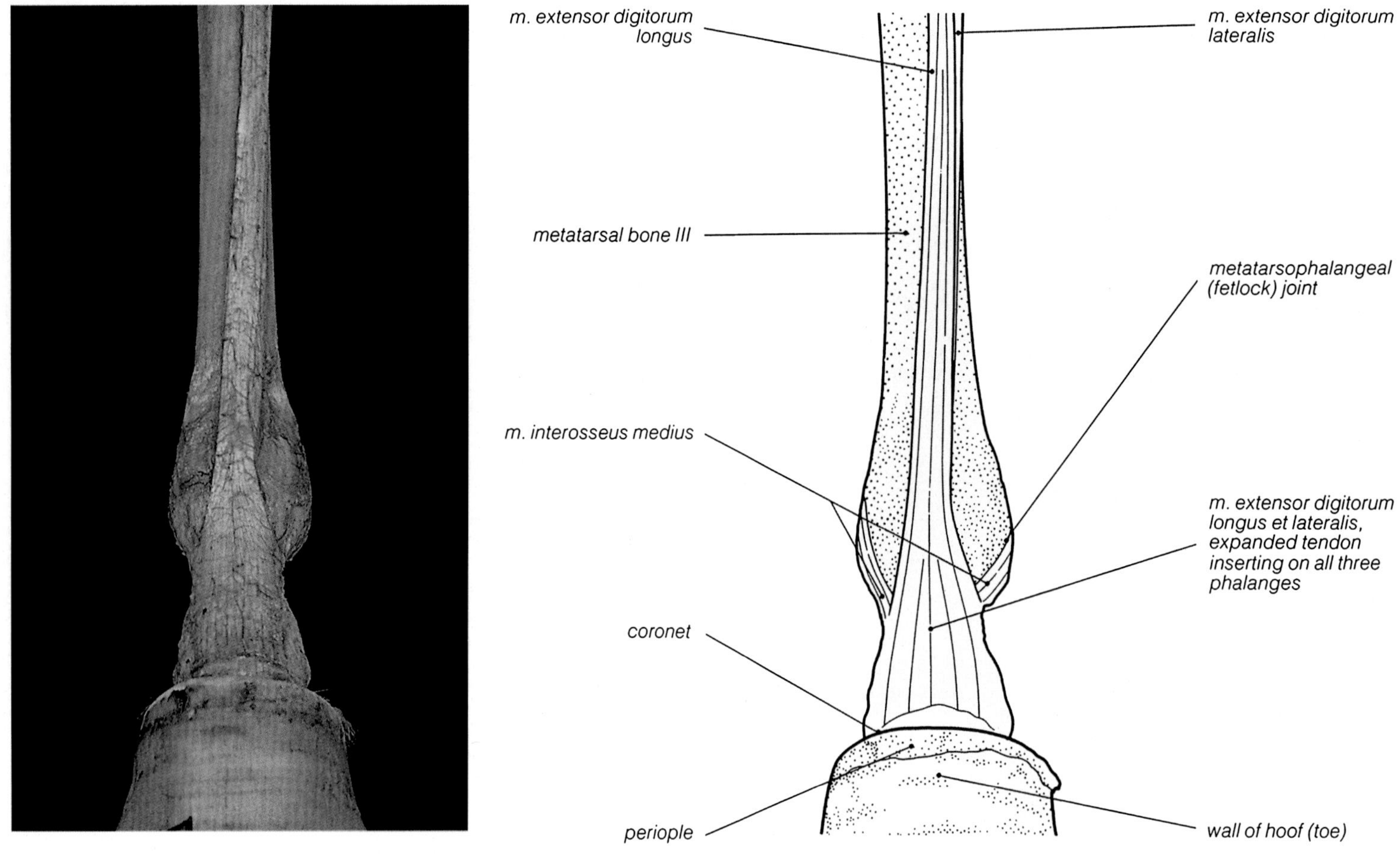
m. extensor digitorum longus
m. extensor digitorum lateralis
metatarsal bone III
metatarsophalangeal (fetlock) joint
m. interosseus medius
m. extensor digitorum longus et lateralis, expanded tendon inserting on all three phalanges
coronet
periople
wall of hoof (toe)

Fig. 7.45 Superficial structures of the distal left pes (5): dorsal view. The vessels and nerves have been removed to show the tendons and superficial ligaments more clearly. Figs. 7.46–7.48 show further views of this dissection.

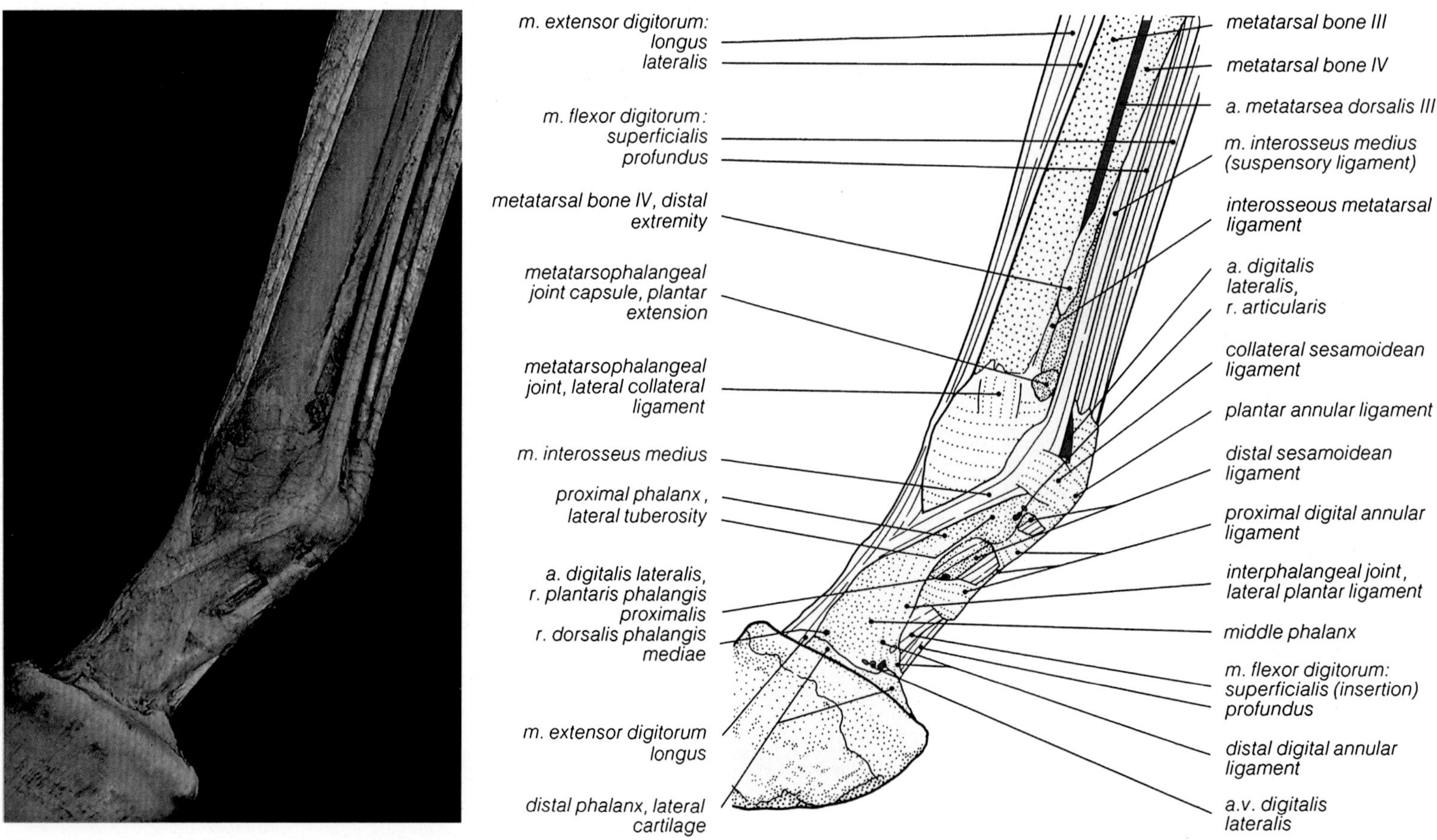
m. extensor digitorum: longus lateralis
m. flexor digitorum: superficialis profundus
metatarsal bone IV, distal extremity
metatarsophalangeal joint capsule, plantar extension
metatarsophalangeal joint, lateral collateral ligament
m. interosseus medius
proximal phalanx, lateral tuberosity
a. digitalis lateralis, r. plantaris phalangis proximalis r. dorsalis phalangis mediae
m. extensor digitorum longus
distal phalanx, lateral cartilage
metatarsal bone III
metatarsal bone IV
a. metatarsea dorsalis III
m. interosseus medius (suspensory ligament)
interosseous metatarsal ligament
a. digitalis lateralis, r. articularis
collateral sesamoidean ligament
plantar annular ligament
distal sesamoidean ligament
proximal digital annular ligament
interphalangeal joint, lateral plantar ligament
middle phalanx
m. flexor digitorum: superficialis (insertion) profundus
distal digital annular ligament
a.v. digitalis lateralis

Fig. 7.46 Superficial structures of the distal left pes (6): lateral view. The major artery of the foot (third dorsal metatarsal) has been retained, together with the cut ends of other vessels (compare with earlier dissection, Fig. 7.42). Other views of this dissection are shown in Figs. 7.45, 7.47 and 7.48.

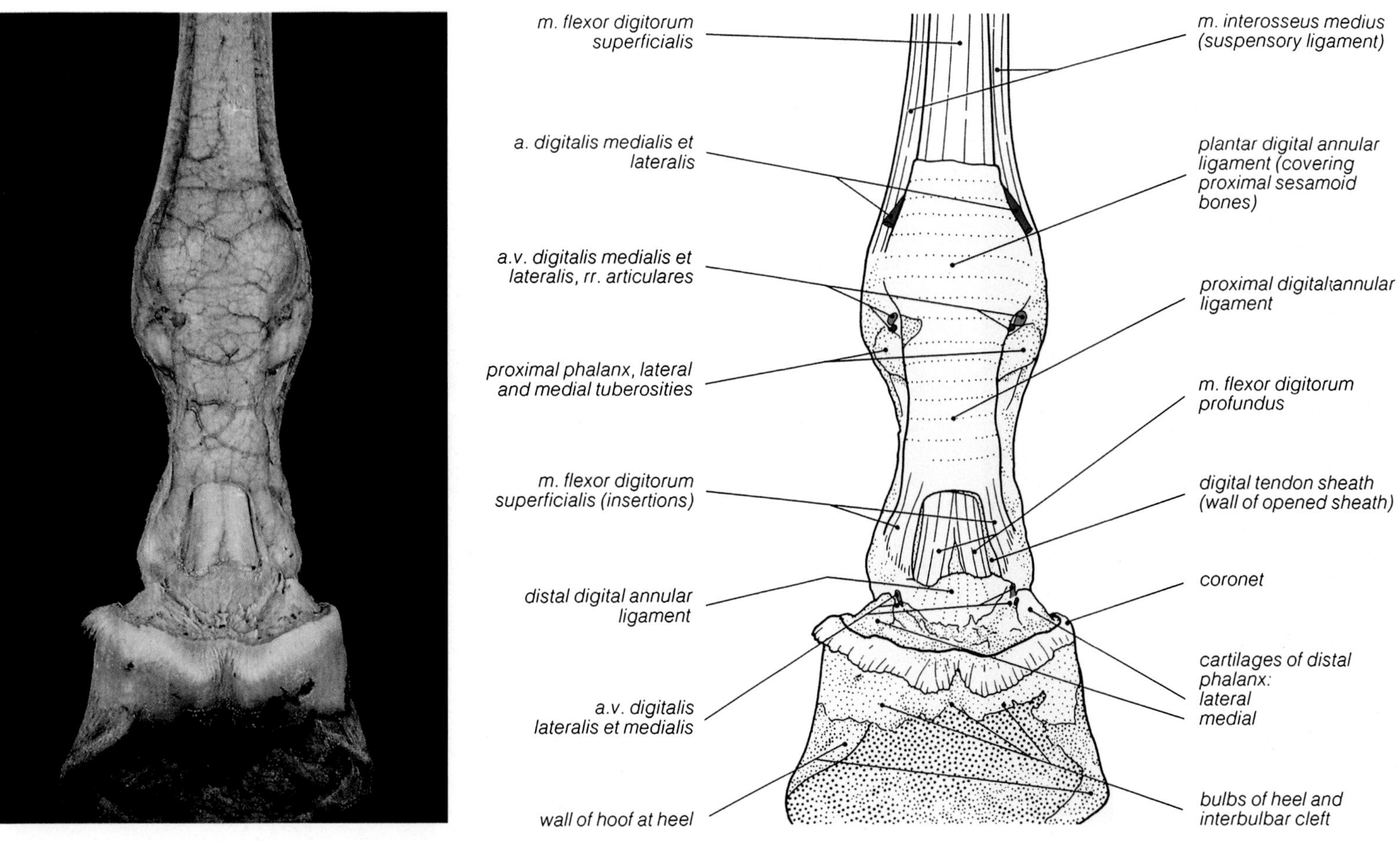
m. flexor digitorum superficialis
a. digitalis medialis et lateralis
a.v. digitalis medialis et lateralis, rr. articulares
proximal phalanx, lateral and medial tuberosities
m. flexor digitorum superficialis (insertions)
distal digital annular ligament
a.v. digitalis lateralis et medialis
wall of hoof at heel
m. interosseus medius (suspensory ligament)
plantar digital annular ligament (covering proximal sesamoid bones)
proximal digital annular ligament
m. flexor digitorum profundus
digital tendon sheath (wall of opened sheath)
coronet
cartilages of distal phalanx: lateral medial
bulbs of heel and interbulbar cleft

Fig. 7.47 Superficial structures of the distal left pes (7): plantar view. The heel of the hoof has been lifted slightly, to obtain a better view of the plantar surface of the digit. Other views of this dissection are shown in Figs. 7.45, 7.46 and 7.48.

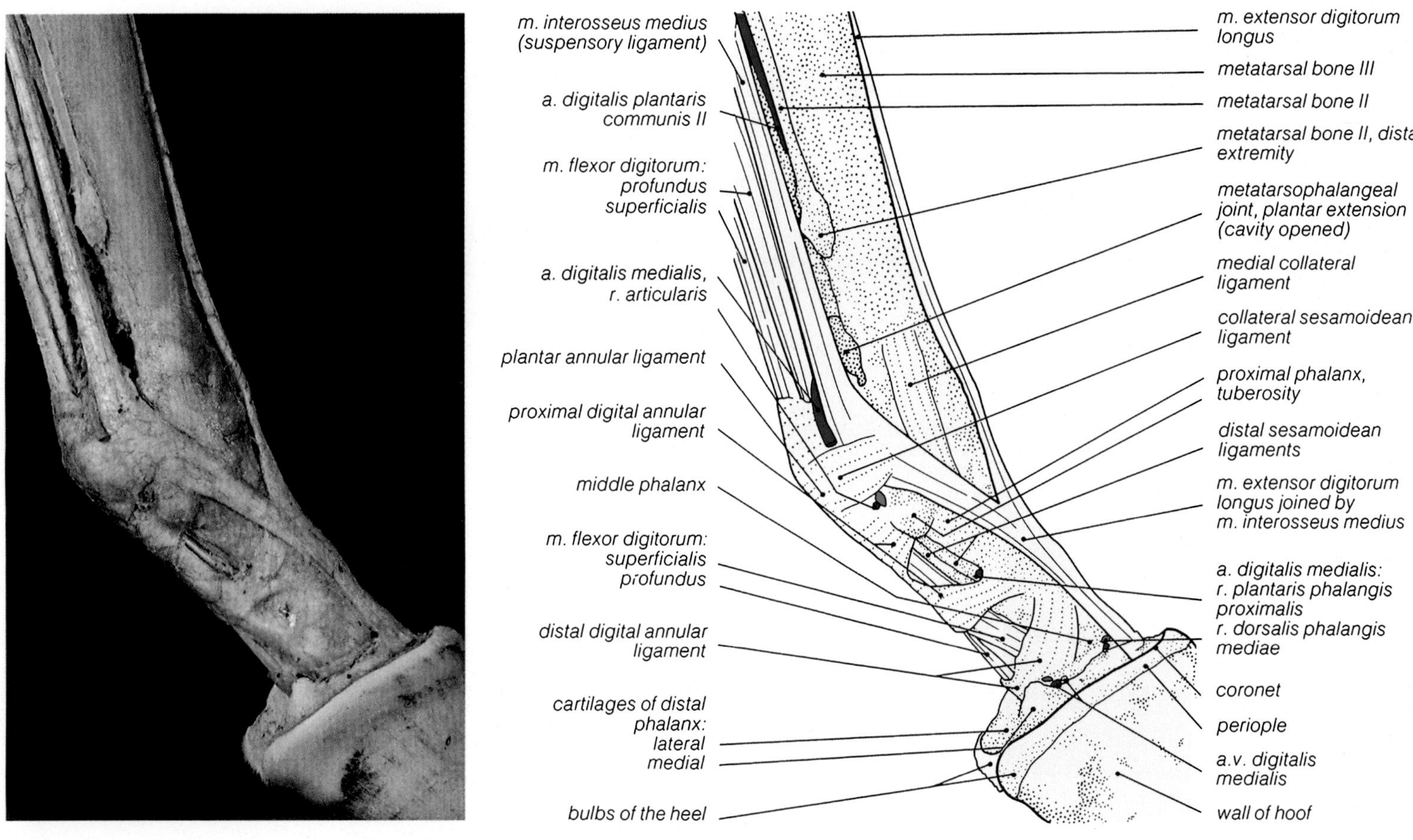
m. interosseus medius (suspensory ligament)
a. digitalis plantaris communis II
m. flexor digitorum: profundus superficialis
a. digitalis medialis, r. articularis
plantar annular ligament
proximal digital annular ligament
middle phalanx
m. flexor digitorum: superficialis profundus
distal digital annular ligament
cartilages of distal phalanx: lateral medial
bulbs of the heel
m. extensor digitorum longus
metatarsal bone III
metatarsal bone II
metatarsal bone II, distal extremity
metatarsophalangeal joint, plantar extension (cavity opened)
medial collateral ligament
collateral sesamoidean ligament
proximal phalanx, tuberosity
distal sesamoidean ligaments
m. extensor digitorum longus joined by m. interosseus medius
a. digitalis medialis: r. plantaris phalangis proximalis r. dorsalis phalangis mediae
coronet
periople
a.v. digitalis medialis
wall of hoof

Fig. 7.48 Superficial structures of the distal left pes (8): medial view. No dorsal metatarsal artery occupies the intermetatarsal groove on the medial side (compare with Fig. 7.46). Other views of this dissection are shown in Figs. 7.45–7.47.

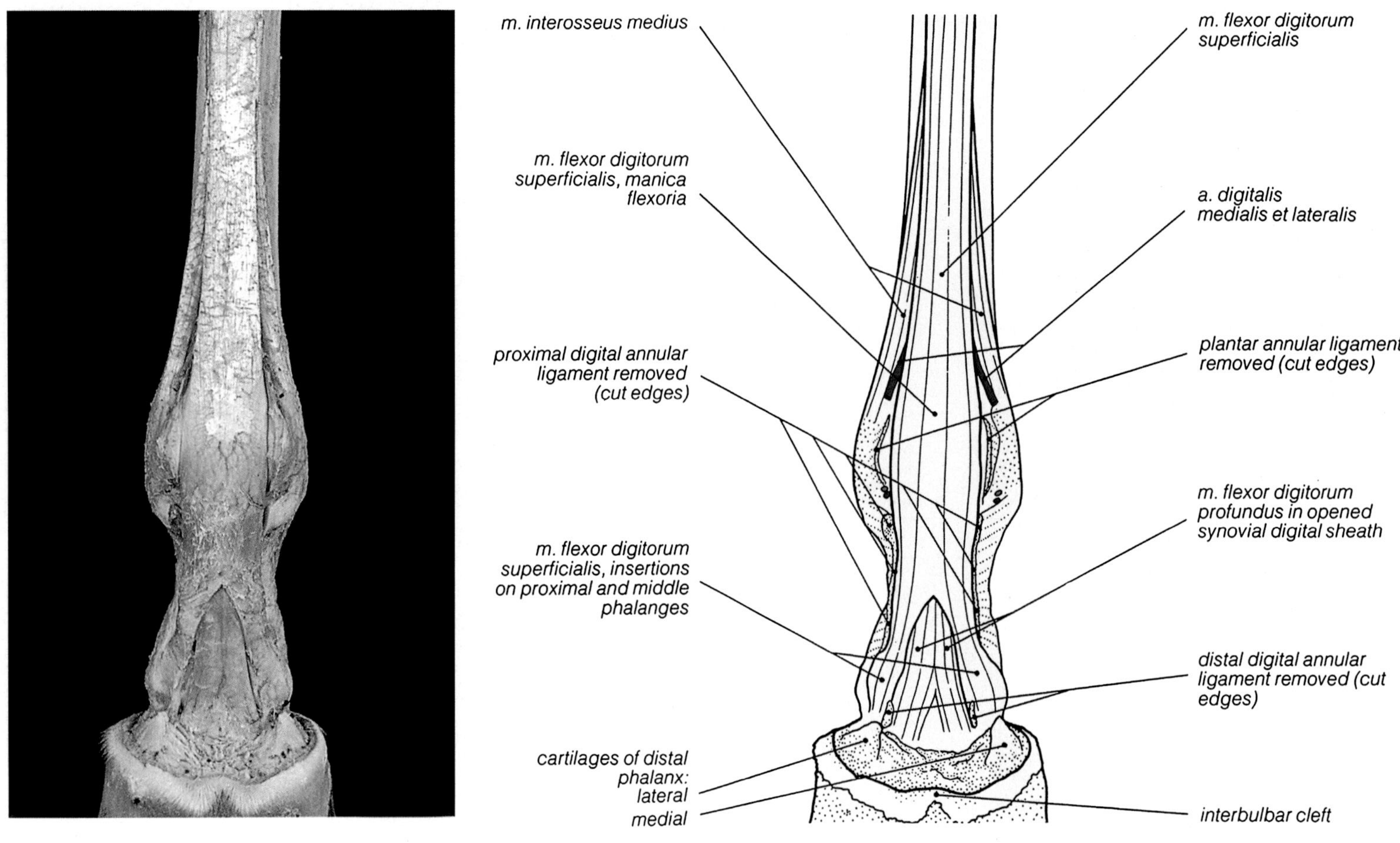
m. interosseus medius
m. flexor digitorum superficialis, manica flexoria
proximal digital annular ligament removed (cut edges)
m. flexor digitorum superficialis, insertions on proximal and middle phalanges
cartilages of distal phalanx: lateral medial
m. flexor digitorum superficialis
a. digitalis medialis et lateralis
plantar annular ligament removed (cut edges)
m. flexor digitorum profundus in opened synovial digital sheath
distal digital annular ligament removed (cut edges)
interbulbar cleft

Fig. 7.49 The flexor tendons of the left digit: plantar view (1). The annular ligaments have been removed from the fetlock and the digit.

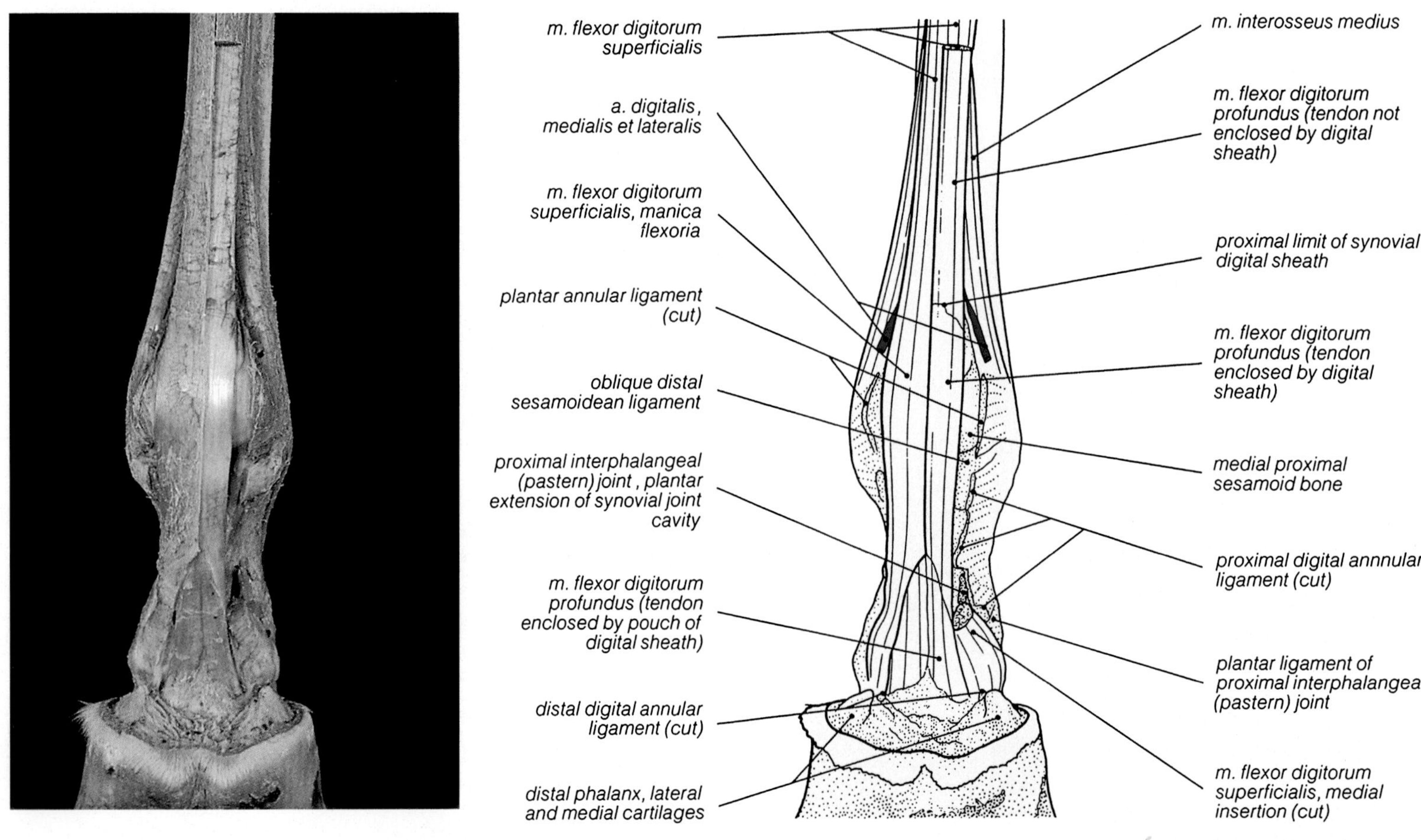
m. flexor digitorum superficialis
a. digitalis, medialis et lateralis
m. flexor digitorum superficialis, manica flexoria
plantar annular ligament (cut)
oblique distal sesamoidean ligament
proximal interphalangeal (pastern) joint, plantar extension of synovial joint cavity
m. flexor digitorum profundus (tendon enclosed by pouch of digital sheath)
distal digital annular ligament (cut)
distal phalanx, lateral and medial cartilages
m. interosseus medius
m. flexor digitorum profundus (tendon not enclosed by digital sheath)
proximal limit of synovial digital sheath
m. flexor digitorum profundus (tendon enclosed by digital sheath)
medial proximal sesamoid bone
proximal digital annnular ligament (cut)
plantar ligament of proximal interphalangeal (pastern) joint
m. flexor digitorum superficialis, medial insertion (cut)

Fig. 7.50 The flexor tendons of the left digit: plantar view (2). The medial half of the superficial digital flexor muscle has been excised to reveal the deep digital flexor muscle lying beneath it. The proximal limit of the synovial digital tendon sheath is visible, but its distal limit lies within the hoof (see Fig. 7.66).

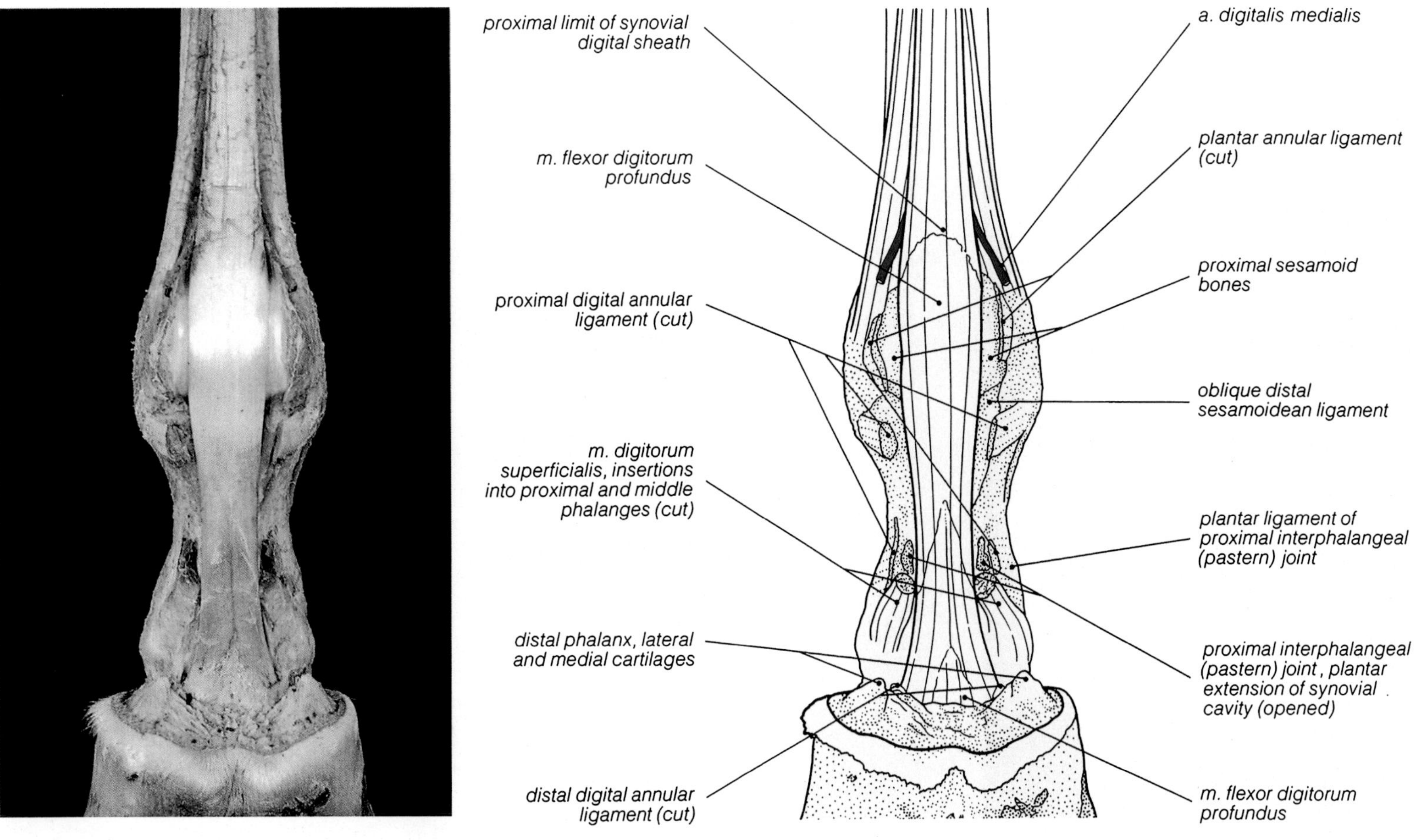
proximal limit of synovial digital sheath
m. flexor digitorum profundus
proximal digital annular ligament (cut)
m. digitorum superficialis, insertions into proximal and middle phalanges (cut)
distal phalanx, lateral and medial cartilages
distal digital annular ligament (cut)
a. digitalis medialis
plantar annular ligament (cut)
proximal sesamoid bones
oblique distal sesamoidean ligament
plantar ligament of proximal interphalangeal (pastern) joint
proximal interphalangeal (pastern) joint, plantar extension of synovial cavity (opened)
m. flexor digitorum profundus

Fig. 7.51 The deep digital flexor tendon of the left pes: plantar view. The lateral and medial halves of the superficial digital flexor tendon have been removed. This dissection is also seen in Fig. 7.52. The insertion of the deep digital flexor tendon into the distal phalanx within the hoof is shown in Fig. 7.54.

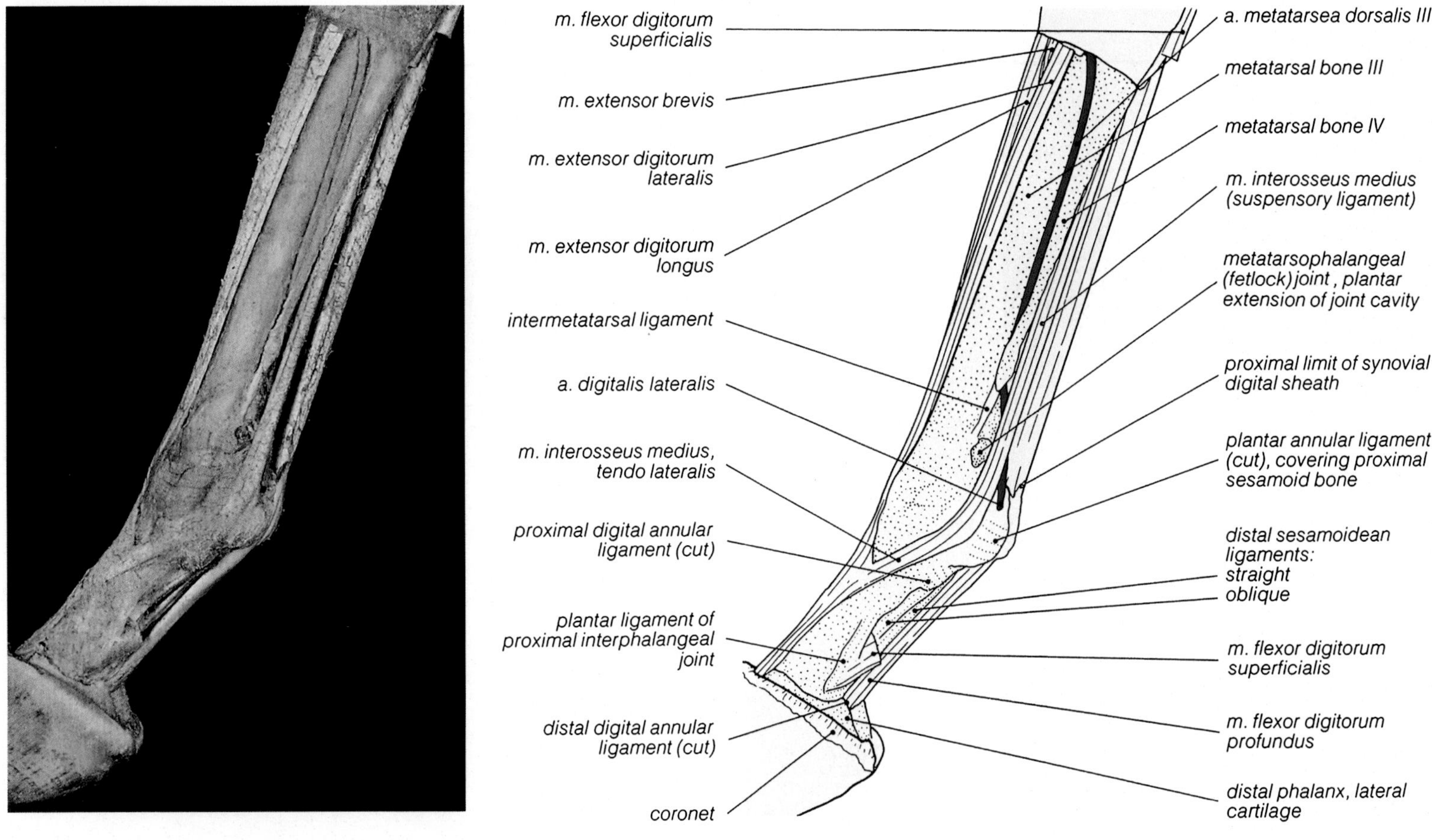
m. flexor digitorum superficialis
m. extensor brevis
m. extensor digitorum lateralis
m. extensor digitorum longus
intermetatarsal ligament
a. digitalis lateralis
m. interosseus medius, tendo lateralis
proximal digital annular ligament (cut)
plantar ligament of proximal interphalangeal joint
distal digital annular ligament (cut)
coronet
a. metatarsea dorsalis III
metatarsal bone III
metatarsal bone IV
m. interosseus medius (suspensory ligament)
metatarsophalangeal (fetlock) joint, plantar extension of joint cavity
proximal limit of synovial digital sheath
plantar annular ligament (cut), covering proximal sesamoid bone
distal sesamoidean ligaments:
straight
oblique
m. flexor digitorum superficialis
m. flexor digitorum profundus
distal phalanx, lateral cartilage

Fig. 7.52 The deep digital flexor tendon of the left pes: lateral view. The specimen is at the same stage of dissection as that shown in Fig. 7.51.

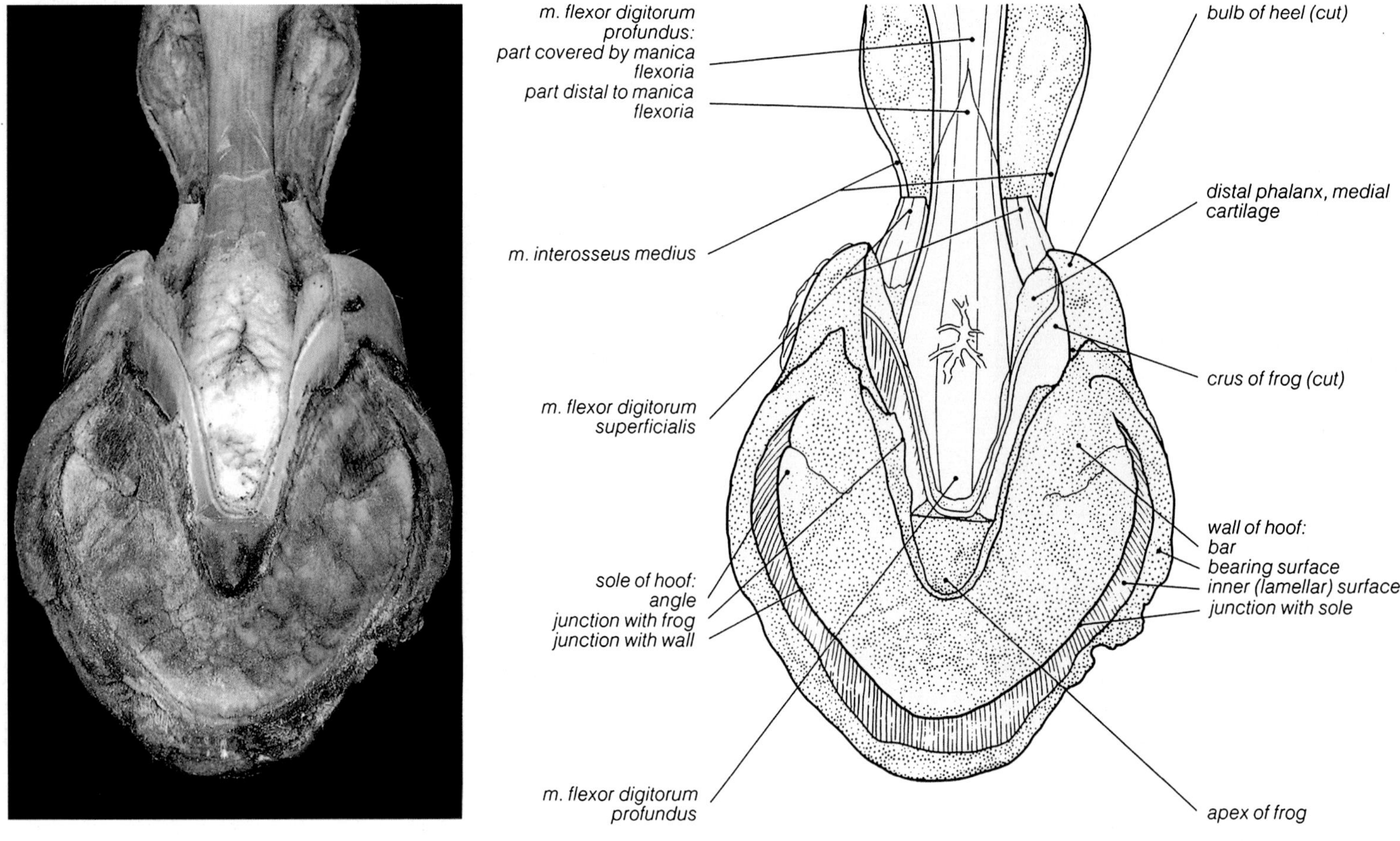
m. flexor digitorum profundus:
part covered by manica flexoria
part distal to manica flexoria
m. interosseus medius
m. flexor digitorum superficialis
sole of hoof:
angle
junction with frog
junction with wall
m. flexor digitorum profundus
bulb of heel (cut)
distal phalanx, medial cartilage
crus of frog (cut)
wall of hoof:
bar
bearing surface
inner (lamellar) surface
junction with sole
apex of frog

Fig. 7.53 The left deep digital flexor tendon: plantar and solar view. A wedge of tissue has been resected from the plantar aspect of the hoof to show the tendon in relationship to the bulbs of the heel, the frog and the sole of the hoof.

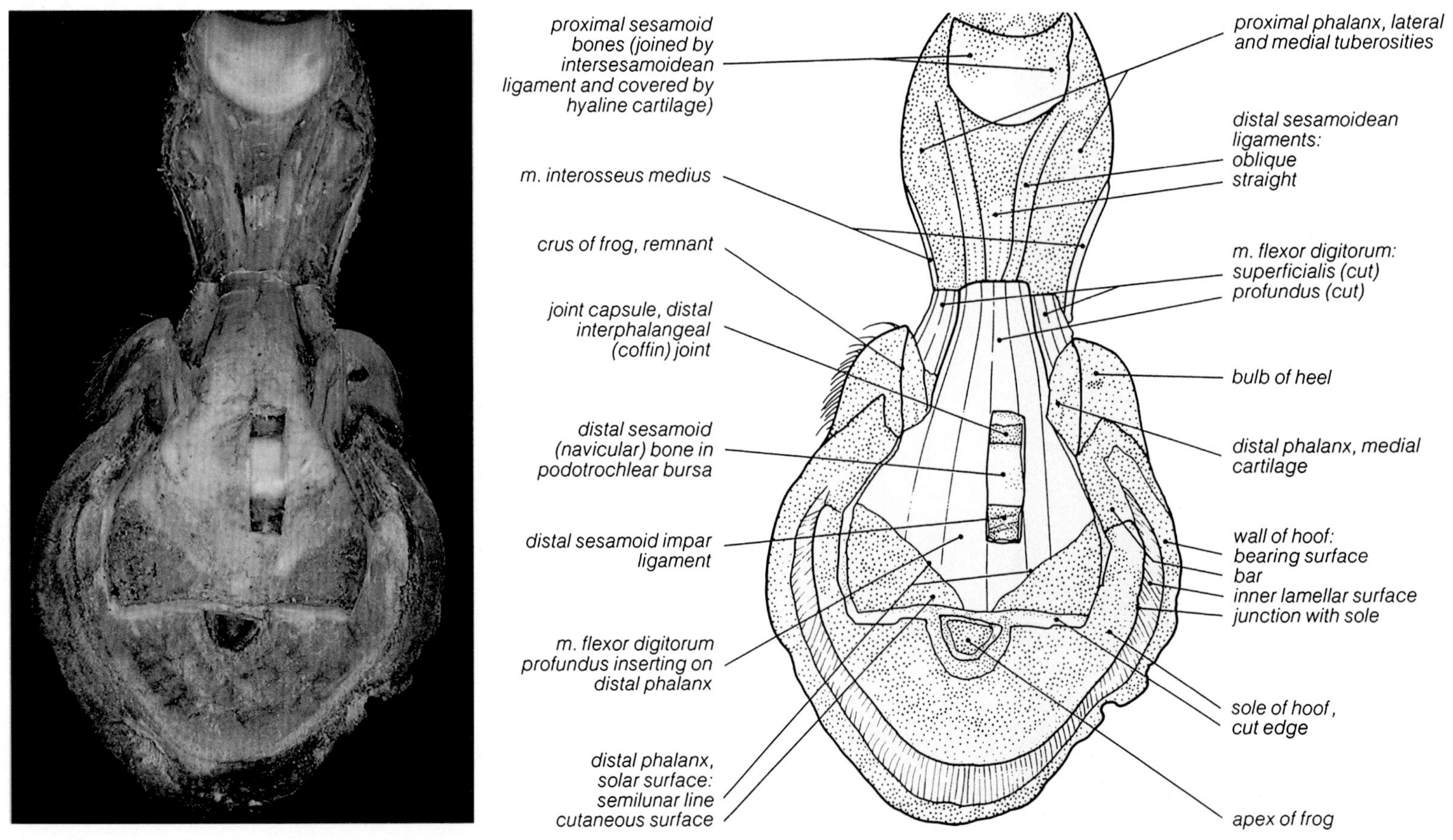
proximal sesamoid bones (joined by intersesamoidean ligament and covered by hyaline cartilage)
m. interosseus medius
crus of frog, remnant
joint capsule, distal interphalangeal (coffin) joint
distal sesamoid (navicular) bone in podotrochlear bursa
distal sesamoid impar ligament
m. flexor digitorum profundus inserting on distal phalanx
distal phalanx, solar surface:
semilunar line
cutaneous surface
proximal phalanx, lateral and medial tuberosities
distal sesamoidean ligaments:
oblique
straight
m. flexor digitorum:
superficialis (cut)
profundus (cut)
bulb of heel
distal phalanx, medial cartilage
wall of hoof:
bearing surface
bar
inner lamellar surface
junction with sole
sole of hoof, cut edge
apex of frog

Fig. 7.54 The left distal sesamoid (navicular) bone: plantar and solar view. Removal of further parts of the sole shows the insertion of the flexor tendon. A window has been cut in this tendon to show the distal sesamoid bone and its podotrochlear bursa. Removal of part of the deep flexor tendon reveals the intersesamoidean and sesamoidean ligaments. See also Fig. 7.80.

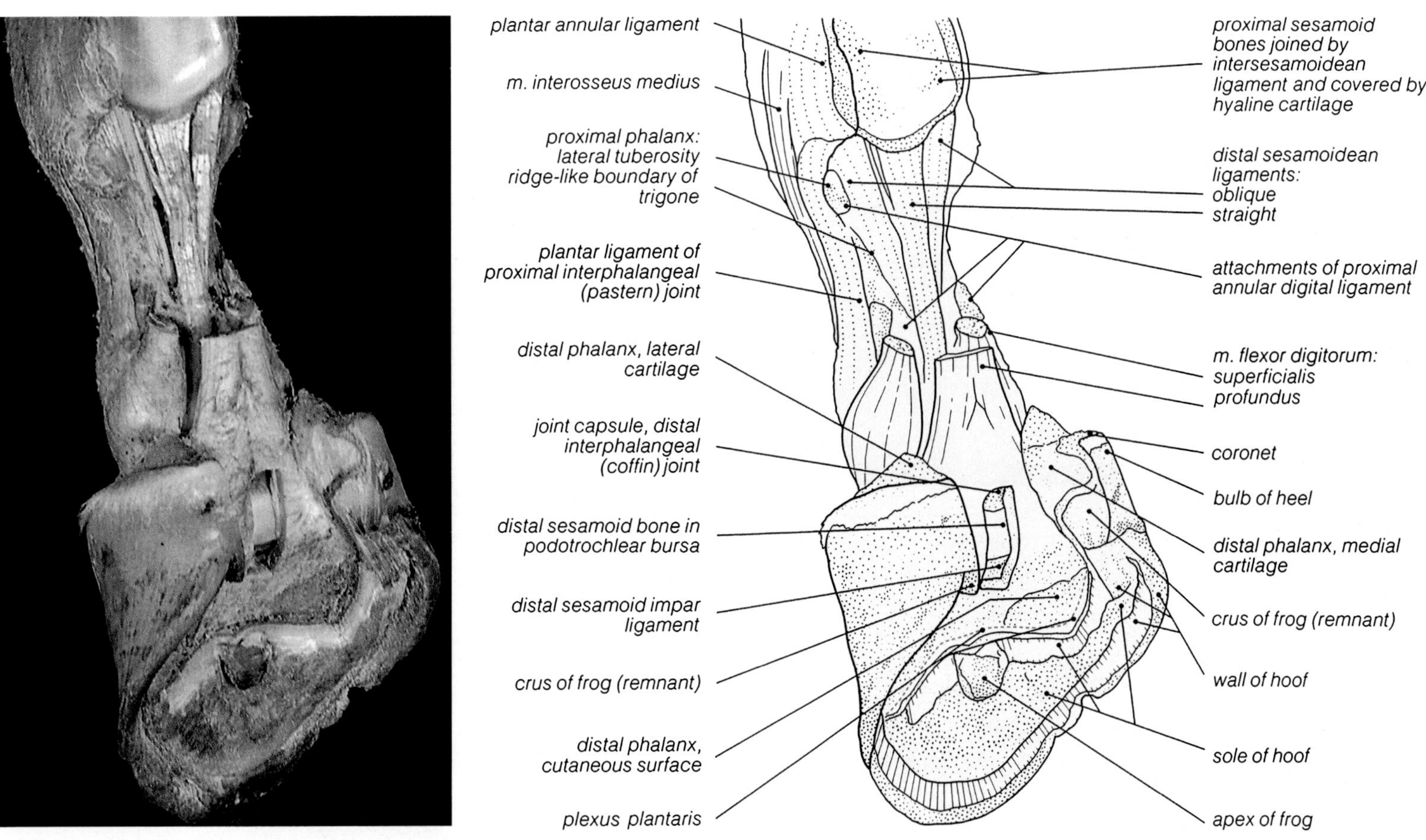
plantar annular ligament
m. interosseus medius
proximal phalanx: lateral tuberosity
ridge-like boundary of trigone
plantar ligament of proximal interphalangeal (pastern) joint
distal phalanx, lateral cartilage
joint capsule, distal interphalangeal (coffin) joint
distal sesamoid bone in podotrochlear bursa
distal sesamoid impar ligament
crus of frog (remnant)
distal phalanx, cutaneous surface
plexus plantaris
proximal sesamoid bones joined by intersesamoidean ligament and covered by hyaline cartilage
distal sesamoidean ligaments:
oblique
straight
attachments of proximal annular digital ligament
m. flexor digitorum:
superficialis
profundus
coronet
bulb of heel
distal phalanx, medial cartilage
crus of frog (remnant)
wall of hoof
sole of hoof
apex of frog

Fig. 7.55 The sesamoidean ligaments and the left distal sesamoid (navicular) bone: lateroplantar view. The dissection is at the same stage as that shown in Fig. 7.54. The cruciate and short sesamoidean ligaments are shown in Figs. 7.78 and 7.79. See also Fig. 7.77.

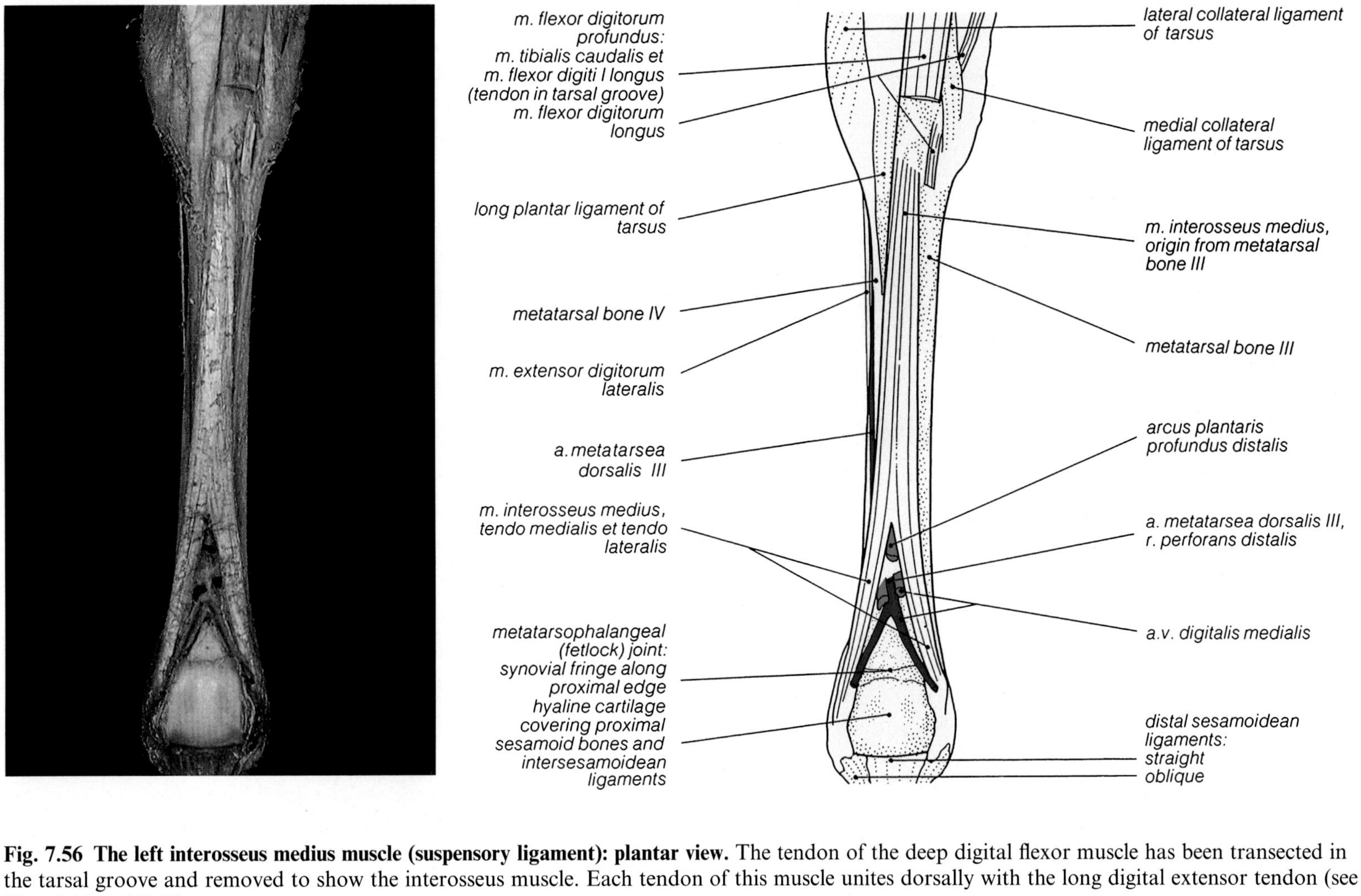

m. flexor digitorum profundus:
m. tibialis caudalis et m. flexor digiti I longus (tendon in tarsal groove)
m. flexor digitorum longus
long plantar ligament of tarsus
metatarsal bone IV
m. extensor digitorum lateralis
a. metatarsea dorsalis III
m. interosseus medius, tendo medialis et tendo lateralis
metatarsophalangeal (fetlock) joint: synovial fringe along proximal edge
hyaline cartilage covering proximal sesamoid bones and intersesamoidean ligaments
lateral collateral ligament of tarsus
medial collateral ligament of tarsus
m. interosseus medius, origin from metatarsal bone III
metatarsal bone III
arcus plantaris profundus distalis
a. metatarsea dorsalis III, r. perforans distalis
a.v. digitalis medialis
distal sesamoidean ligaments:
straight
oblique

Fig. 7.56 The left interosseus medius muscle (suspensory ligament): plantar view. The tendon of the deep digital flexor muscle has been transected in the tarsal groove and removed to show the interosseus muscle. Each tendon of this muscle unites dorsally with the long digital extensor tendon (see Figs. 7.45 and 7.52).

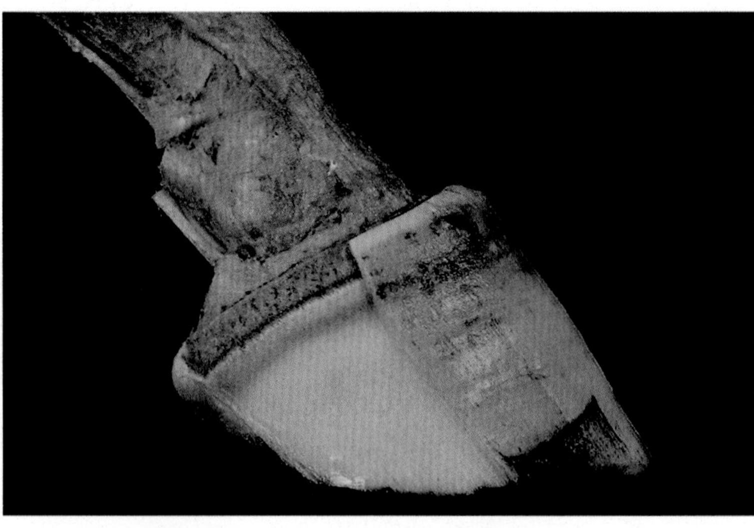

Fig. 7.57 The structure of the hoof wall: medial view (1). The superficial part of the middle layer has been removed from the plantar part of the medial quarter of the hoof wall. Further dissections are shown in Figs. 7.58–7.62. See also Figs. 7.75 and 7.76.

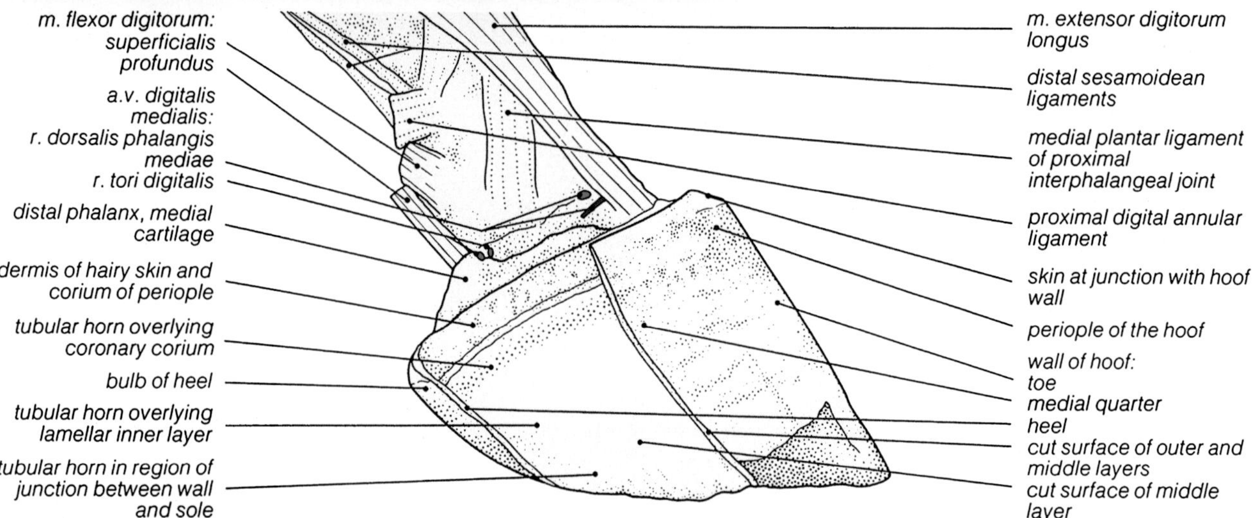
m. flexor digitorum:
superficialis
profundus
a.v. digitalis medialis:
r. dorsalis phalangis mediae
r. tori digitalis
distal phalanx, medial cartilage
dermis of hairy skin and corium of periople
tubular horn overlying coronary corium
bulb of heel
tubular horn overlying lamellar inner layer
tubular horn in region of junction between wall and sole
m. extensor digitorum longus
distal sesamoidean ligaments
medial plantar ligament of proximal interphalangeal joint
proximal digital annular ligament
skin at junction with hoof wall
periople of the hoof
wall of hoof:
toe
medial quarter
heel
cut surface of outer and middle layers
cut surface of middle layer

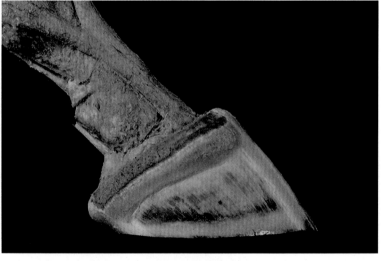

Fig. 7.58 The structure of the hoof wall: medial view (2). The outer and middle layers of the wall have been removed from the medial quarter of the hoof. The depth of wall removed from the bearing surface is shown in Fig. 7.59.

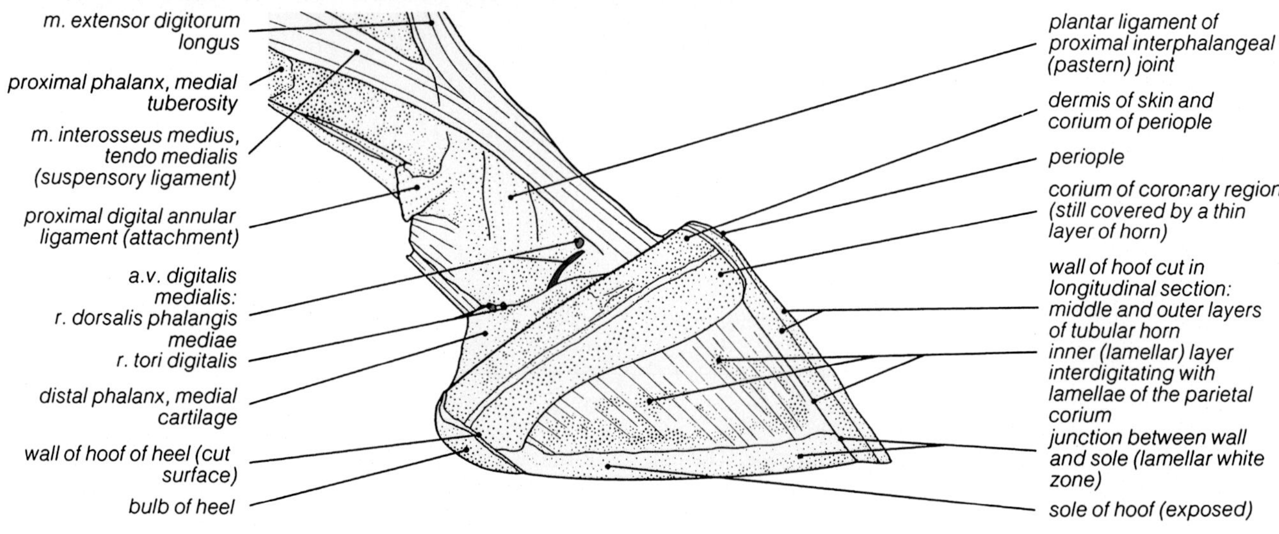
m. extensor digitorum longus
proximal phalanx, medial tuberosity
m. interosseus medius, tendo medialis (suspensory ligament)
proximal digital annular ligament (attachment)
a.v. digitalis medialis:
r. dorsalis phalangis mediae
r. tori digitalis
distal phalanx, medial cartilage
wall of hoof of heel (cut surface)
bulb of heel
plantar ligament of proximal interphalangeal (pastern) joint
dermis of skin and corium of periople
periople
corium of coronary region (still covered by a thin layer of horn)
wall of hoof cut in longitudinal section:
middle and outer layers of tubular horn
inner (lamellar) layer interdigitating with lamellae of the parietal corium
junction between wall and sole (lamellar white zone)
sole of hoof (exposed)

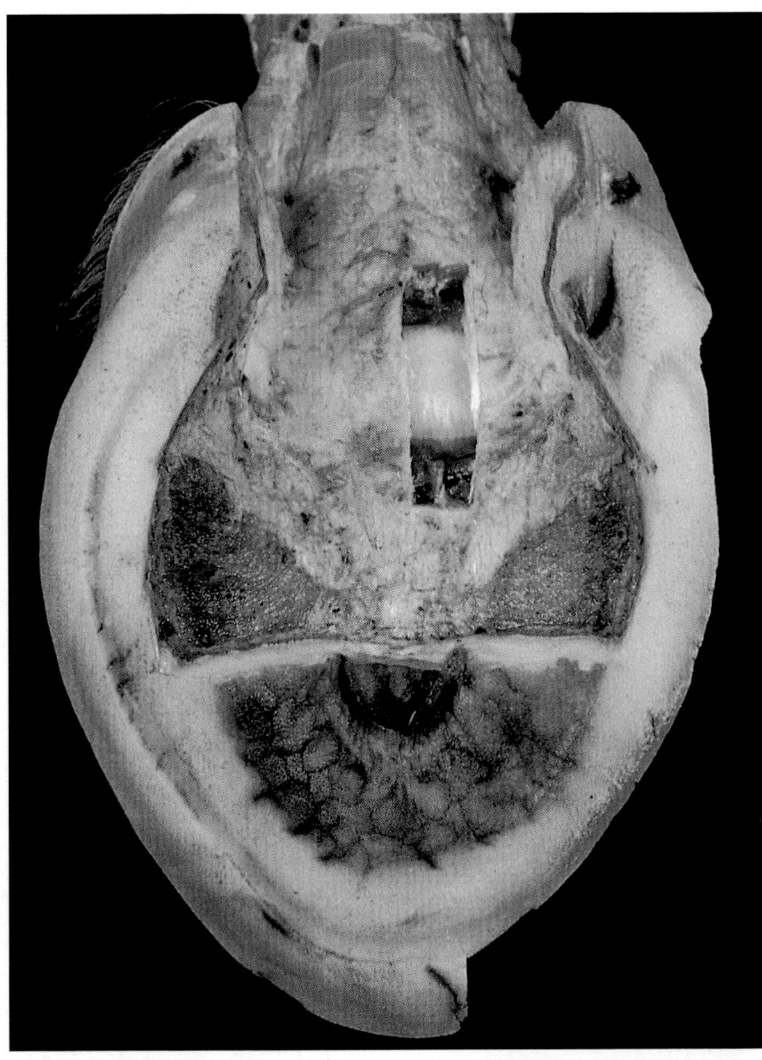

Fig. 7.59 The structure of the hoof wall: plantar and solar view. The bearing surface of sole and wall has been trimmed to show more clearly the so-called 'white' zone of the wall which forms the junction between wall and sole (see Fig. 7.24). In the untrimmed hoof this lamellar zone is less clearly seen (see Fig. 7.54). The removed parts of the medial wall, (see Fig. 7.58), are indicated by broken lines.

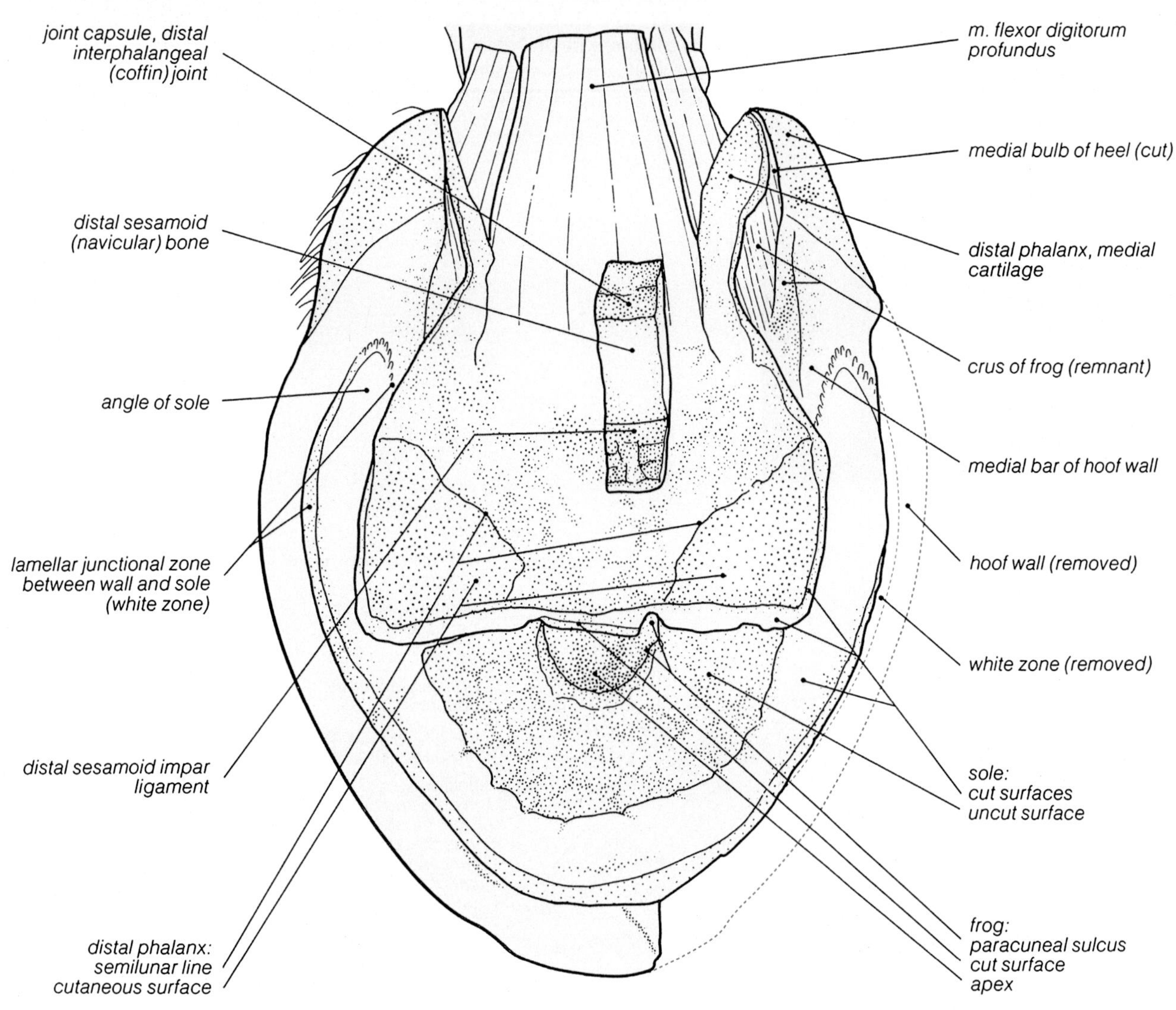
joint capsule, distal interphalangeal (coffin) joint
distal sesamoid (navicular) bone
angle of sole
lamellar junctional zone between wall and sole (white zone)
distal sesamoid impar ligament
distal phalanx:
semilunar line
cutaneous surface
m. flexor digitorum profundus
medial bulb of heel (cut)
distal phalanx, medial cartilage
crus of frog (remnant)
medial bar of hoof wall
hoof wall (removed)
white zone (removed)
sole:
cut surfaces
uncut surface
frog:
paracuneal sulcus
cut surface
apex

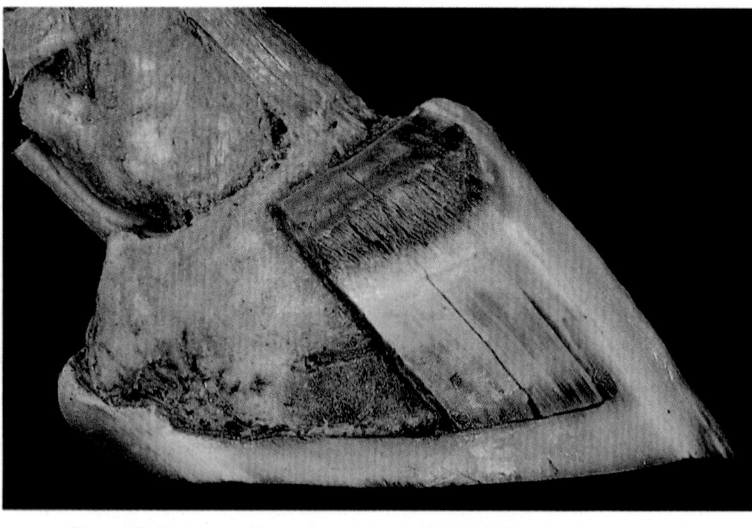

Fig. 7.60 The structure of the hoof wall: medial view (3). The middle layer of hoof wall has been removed from the more dorsal half of the medial wall, exposing the long coronary papillae. The entire hoof wall has been removed from the more plantar half of the wall, together with the parietal venous plexus, to expose the medial cartilage of the distal phalanx.

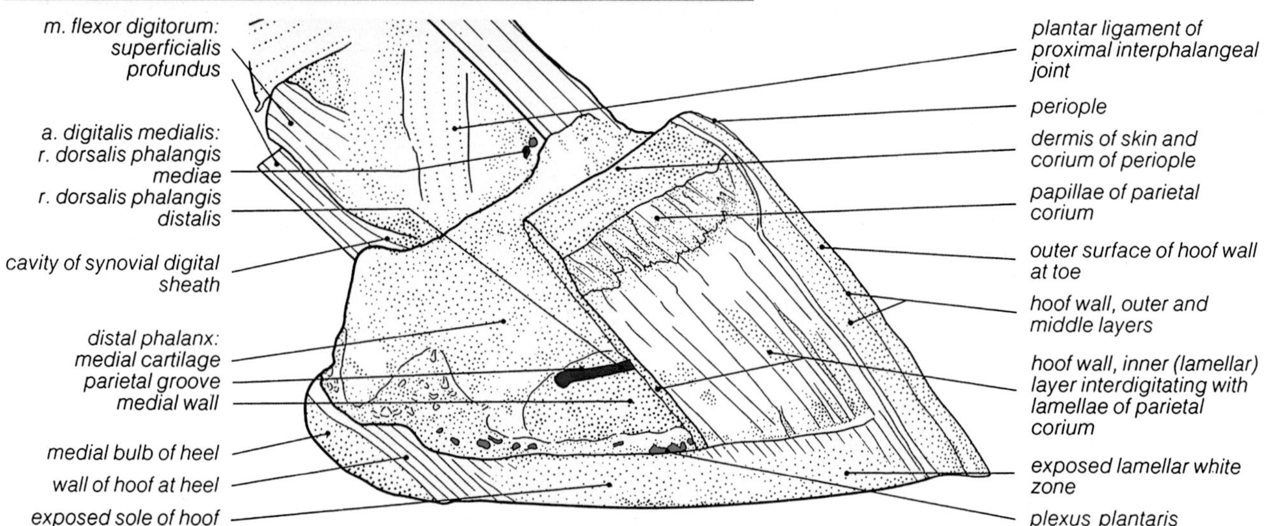
m. flexor digitorum:
superficialis
profundus
a. digitalis medialis:
r. dorsalis phalangis mediae
r. dorsalis phalangis distalis
cavity of synovial digital sheath
distal phalanx:
medial cartilage
parietal groove
medial wall
medial bulb of heel
wall of hoof at heel
exposed sole of hoof
plantar ligament of proximal interphalangeal joint
periople
dermis of skin and corium of periople
papillae of parietal corium
outer surface of hoof wall at toe
hoof wall, outer and middle layers
hoof wall, inner (lamellar) layer interdigitating with lamellae of parietal corium
exposed lamellar white zone
plexus plantaris

Fig. 7.61 The structure of the hoof wall and the medial cartilage of the distal phalanx: medial view. Removal of most of the remaining inner layer of the wall exposes the whole abaxial surface of the medial cartilage. The lamellae are also seen within the remaining part of the hoof wall.

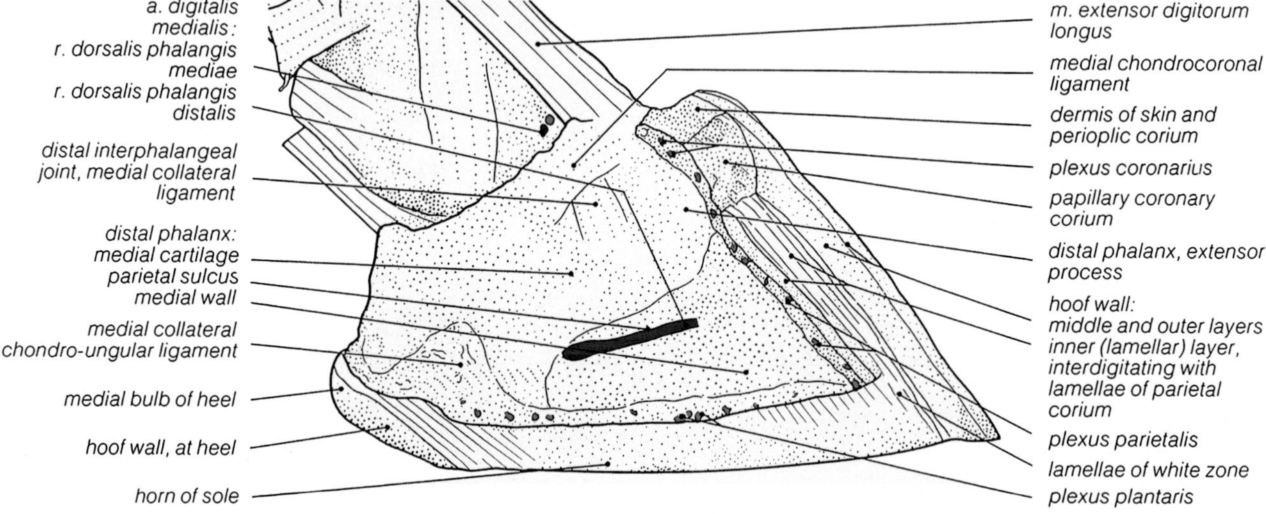
a. digitalis medialis:
r. dorsalis phalangis mediae
r. dorsalis phalangis distalis
distal interphalangeal joint, medial collateral ligament
distal phalanx:
medial cartilage
parietal sulcus
medial wall
medial collateral chondro-ungular ligament
medial bulb of heel
hoof wall, at heel
horn of sole
m. extensor digitorum longus
medial chondrocoronal ligament
dermis of skin and perioplic corium
plexus coronarius
papillary coronary corium
distal phalanx, extensor process
hoof wall:
middle and outer layers
inner (lamellar) layer, interdigitating with lamellae of parietal corium
plexus parietalis
lamellae of white zone
plexus plantaris

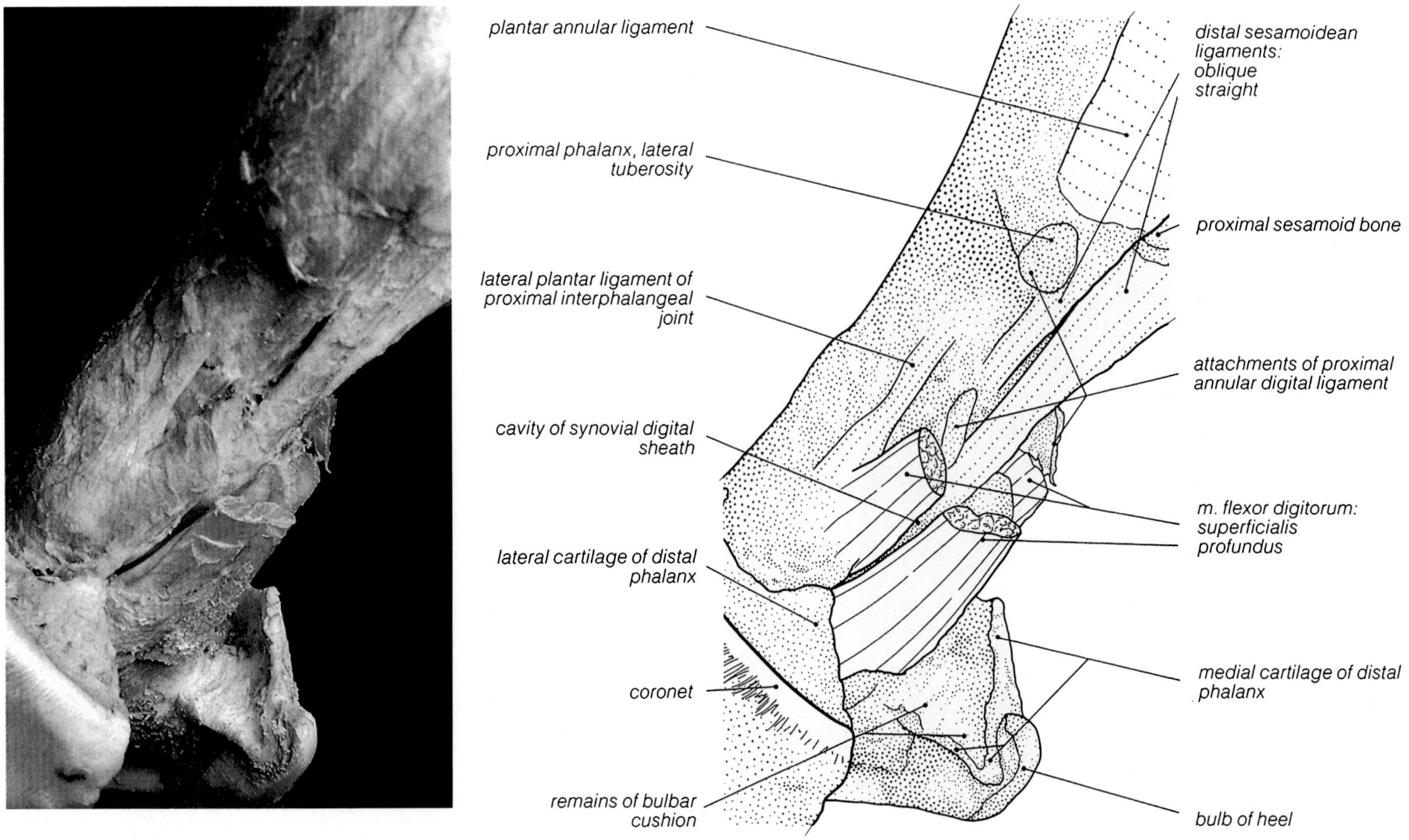

plantar annular ligament
proximal phalanx, lateral tuberosity
lateral plantar ligament of proximal interphalangeal joint
cavity of synovial digital sheath
lateral cartilage of distal phalanx
coronet
remains of bulbar cushion
distal sesamoidean ligaments:
oblique
straight
proximal sesamoid bone
attachments of proximal annular digital ligament
m. flexor digitorum:
superficialis
profundus
medial cartilage of distal phalanx
bulb of heel

Fig. 7.62 The medial cartilage of the distal phalanx: lateroplantar view. The dissection is at the same stage as that shown in Fig. 7.61. The medial cartilage curls behind and beneath the bulbar cushion, which has been removed.

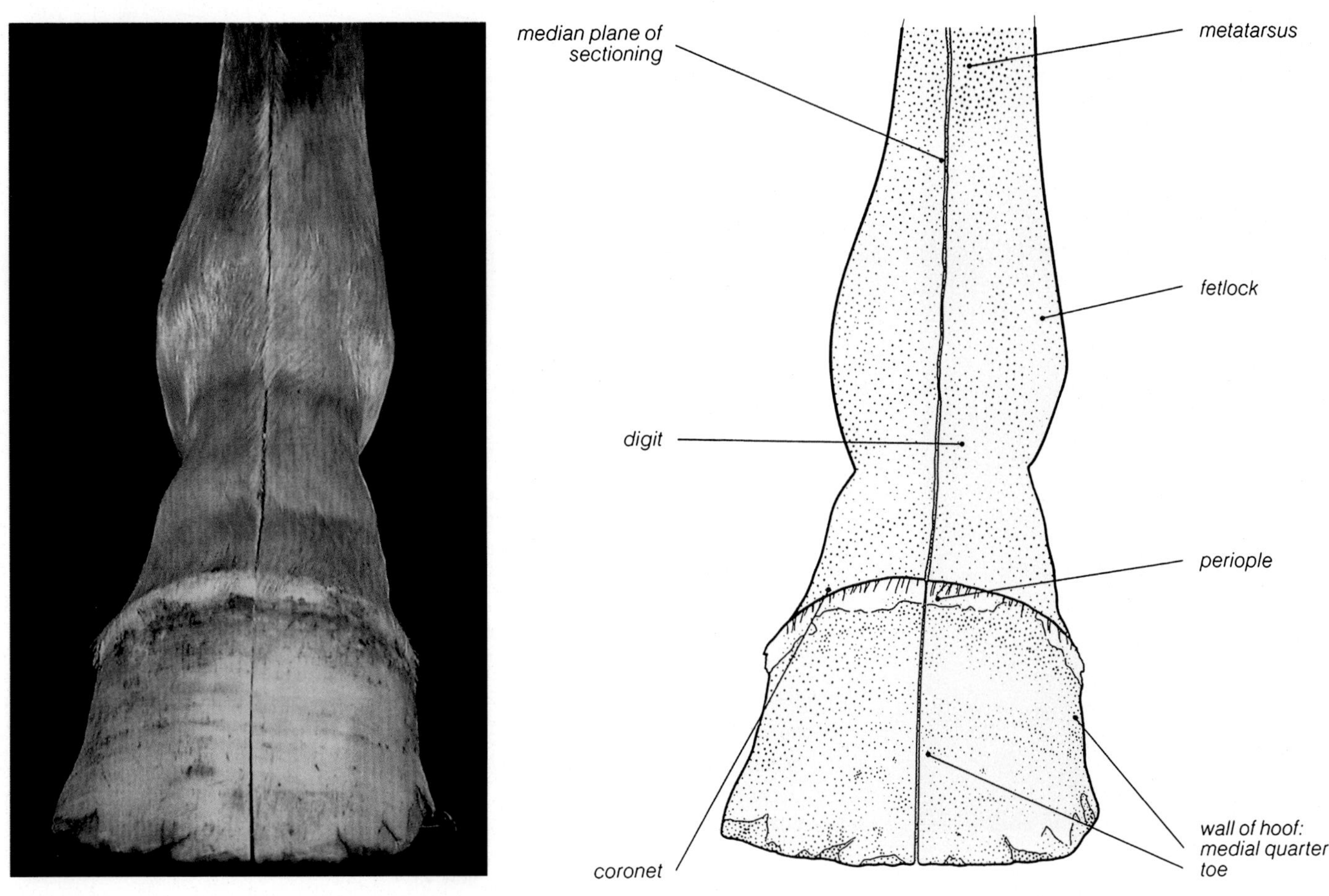
median plane of sectioning
digit
coronet
metatarsus
fetlock
periople
wall of hoof:
medial quarter
toe

Fig. 7.63 The right pes: dorsal view. The specimen has been sawn through the median plane, to produce the specimen for Figs. 7.65 and 7.66.

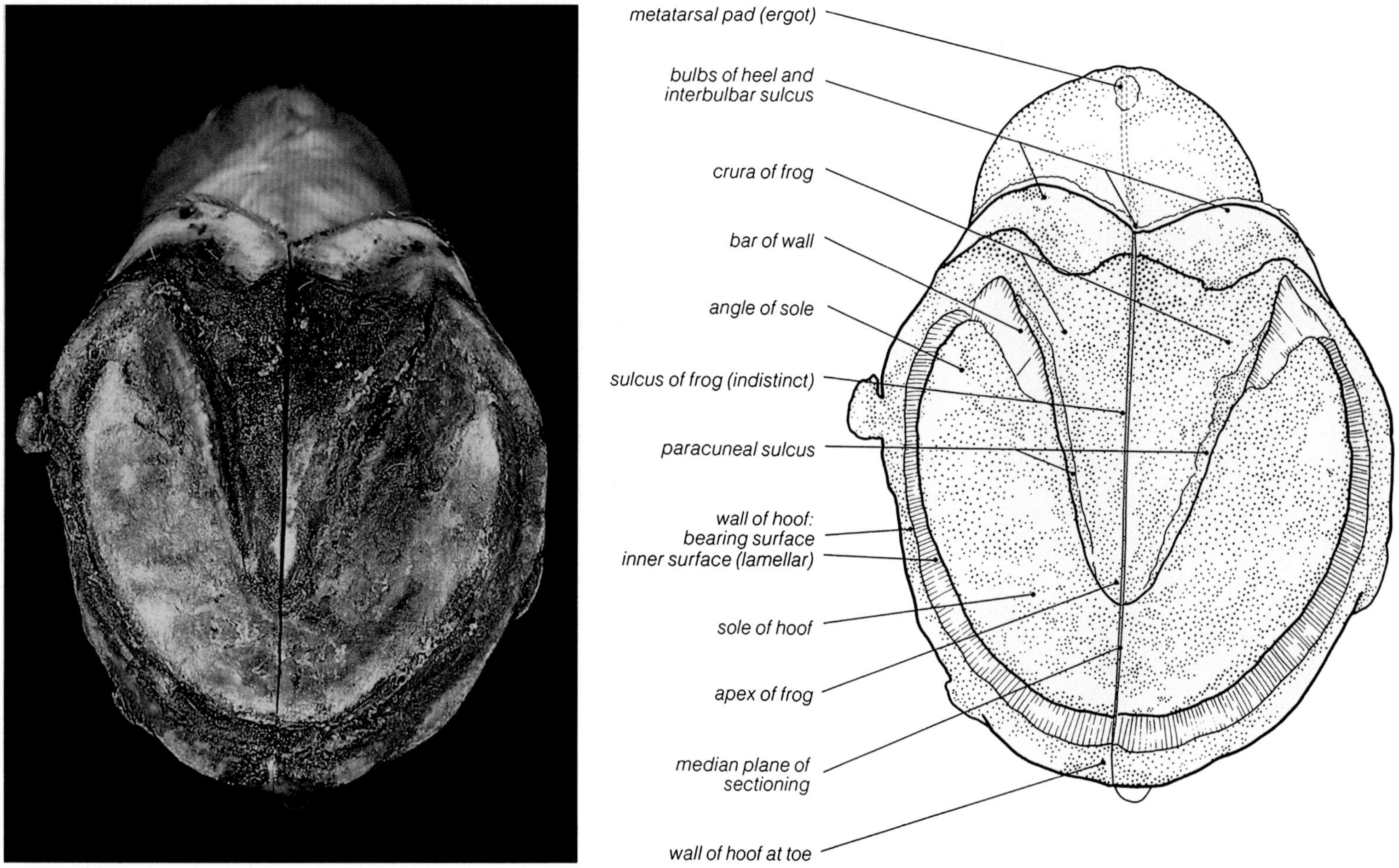

metatarsal pad (ergot)
bulbs of heel and interbulbar sulcus
crura of frog
bar of wall
angle of sole
sulcus of frog (indistinct)
paracuneal sulcus
wall of hoof:
bearing surface
inner surface (lamellar)
sole of hoof
apex of frog
median plane of sectioning
wall of hoof at toe

Fig. 7.64 The right pes: solar view. The specimen has been sawn through in the median plane to produce the specimen for Figs. 7.65 and 7.66.

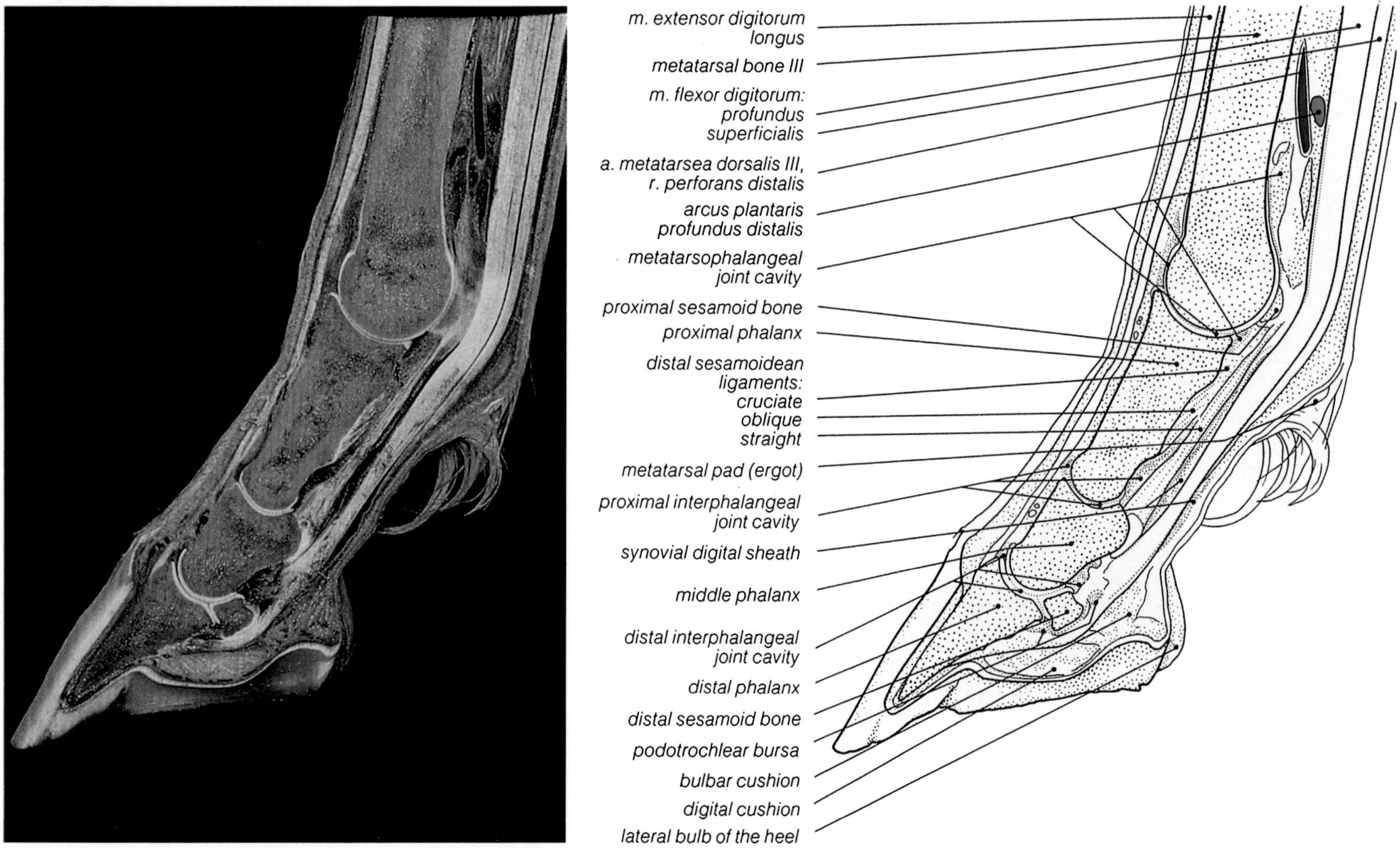

m. extensor digitorum longus
metatarsal bone III
m. flexor digitorum:
profundus
superficialis
a. metatarsea dorsalis III, r. perforans distalis
arcus plantaris profundus distalis
metatarsophalangeal joint cavity
proximal sesamoid bone
proximal phalanx
distal sesamoidean ligaments:
cruciate
oblique
straight
metatarsal pad (ergot)
proximal interphalangeal joint cavity
synovial digital sheath
middle phalanx
distal interphalangeal joint cavity
distal phalanx
distal sesamoid bone
podotrochlear bursa
bulbar cushion
digital cushion
lateral bulb of the heel

Fig. 7.65 The right pes in median section: medial view. This is the lateral half of the specimen. The limits of the synovial cavities are indicated by blue dotted lines. Epiphyseal fusion is completed in metatarsal bones and phalanges; this occurs at about 12 months of age (range 6–15 months) in each bone.

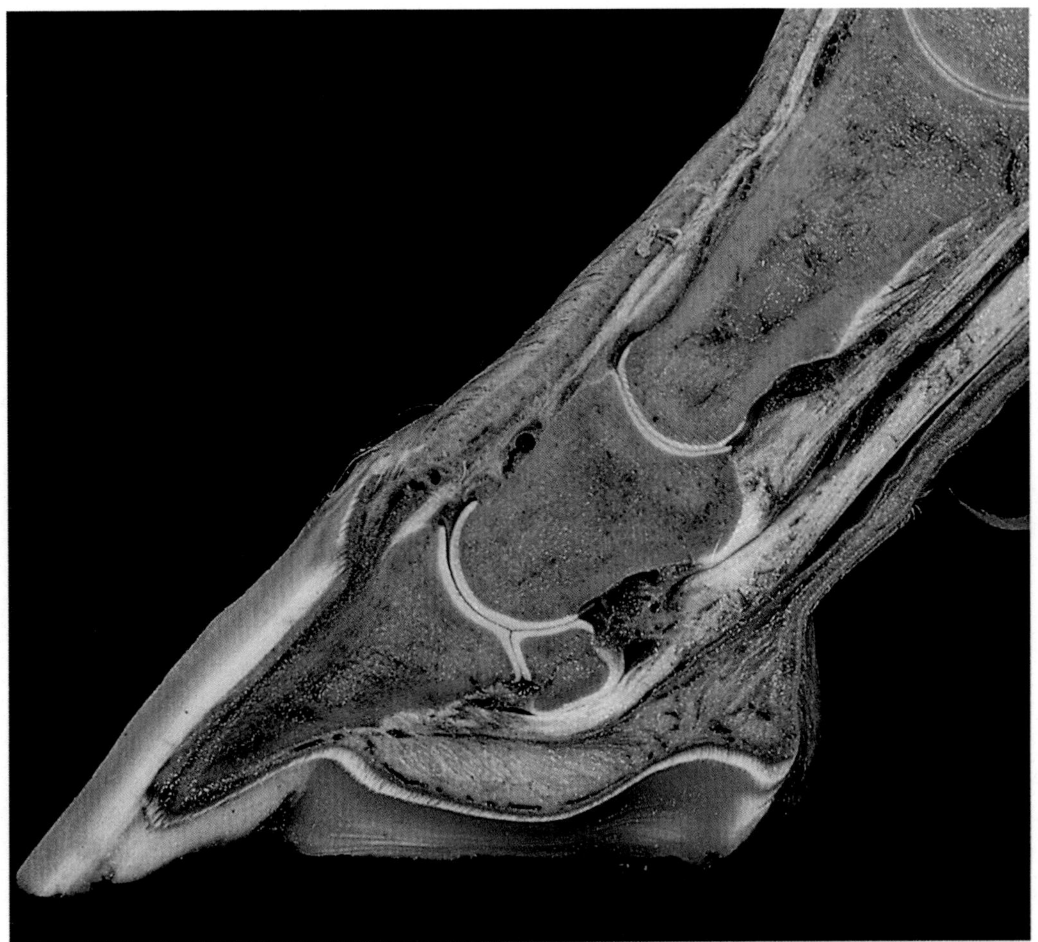

Fig. 7.66 The right digit in median section: medial view. This is a closer view of a part of the specimen shown in Fig. 7.65. The limits of the synovial cavities are indicated by blue dotted lines. The line marked by arrows indicates the plane of sectioning shown in Figs. 7.19 and 7.20.

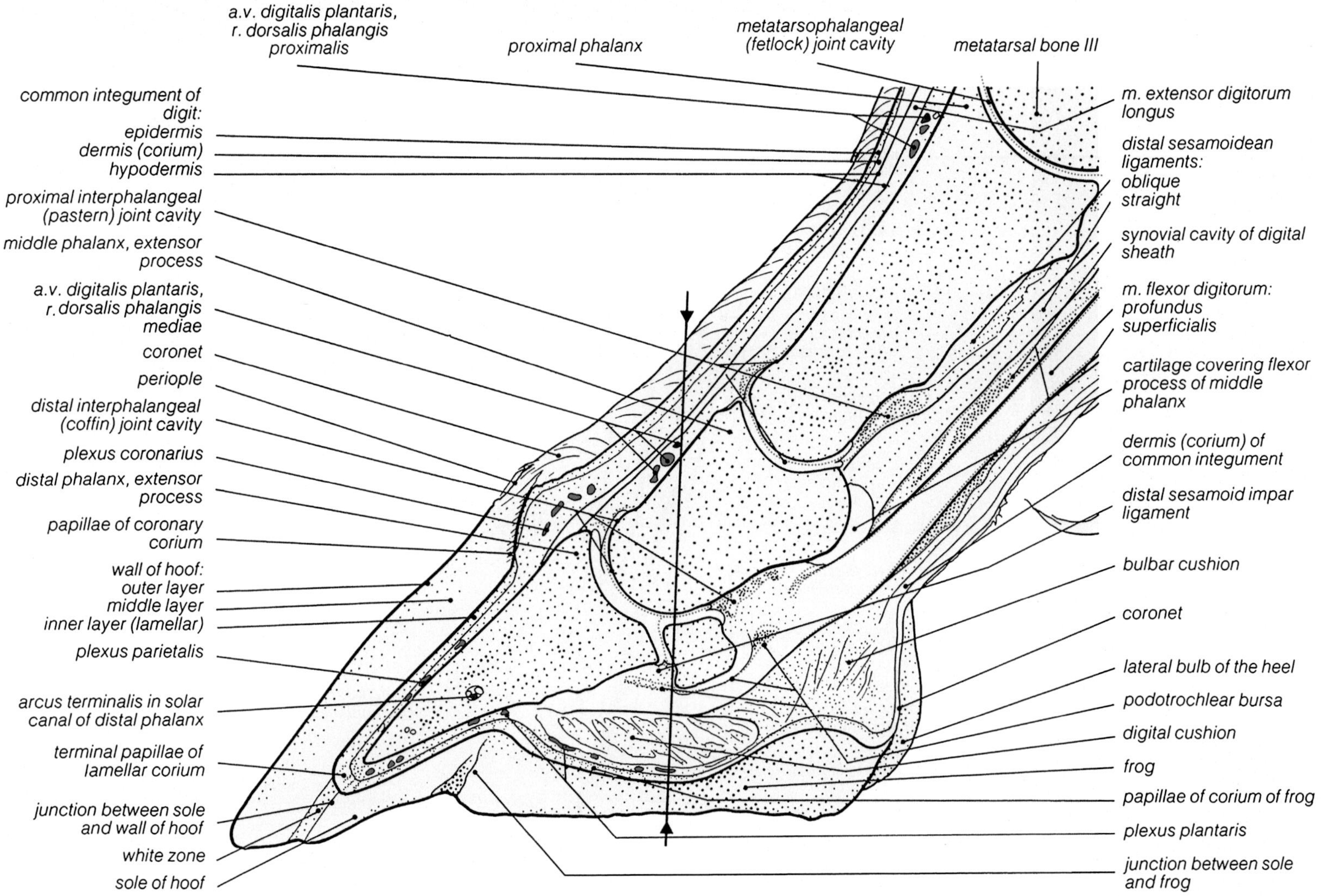

a.v. digitalis plantaris, r. dorsalis phalangis proximalis
proximal phalanx
metatarsophalangeal (fetlock) joint cavity
metatarsal bone III
common integument of digit:
epidermis
dermis (corium)
hypodermis
proximal interphalangeal (pastern) joint cavity
middle phalanx, extensor process
a.v. digitalis plantaris, r. dorsalis phalangis mediae
coronet
periople
distal interphalangeal (coffin) joint cavity
plexus coronarius
distal phalanx, extensor process
papillae of coronary corium
wall of hoof:
outer layer
middle layer
inner layer (lamellar)
plexus parietalis
arcus terminalis in solar canal of distal phalanx
terminal papillae of lamellar corium
junction between sole and wall of hoof
white zone
sole of hoof
m. extensor digitorum longus
distal sesamoidean ligaments:
oblique
straight
synovial cavity of digital sheath
m. flexor digitorum:
profundus
superficialis
cartilage covering flexor process of middle phalanx
dermis (corium) of common integument
distal sesamoid impar ligament
bulbar cushion
coronet
lateral bulb of the heel
podotrochlear bursa
digital cushion
frog
papillae of corium of frog
plexus plantaris
junction between sole and frog

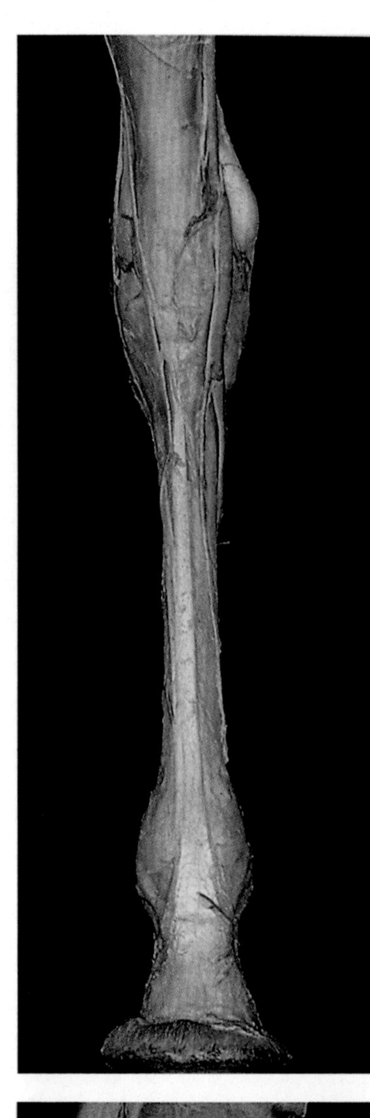

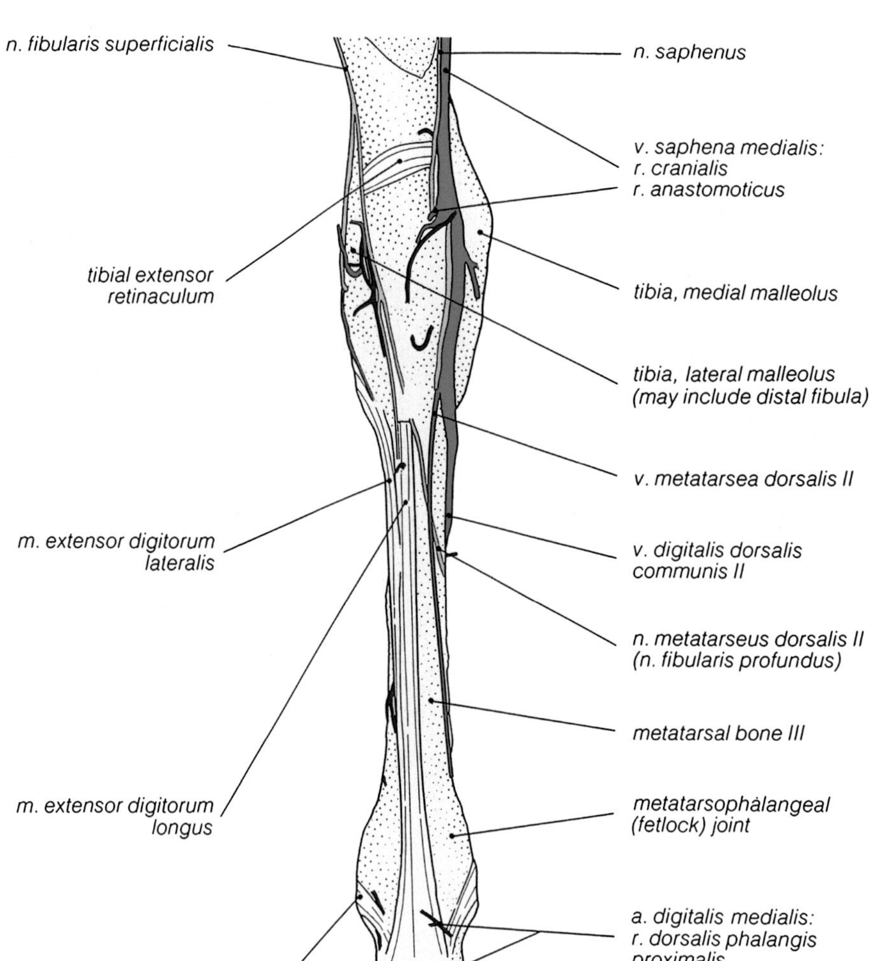
n. fibularis superficialis
tibial extensor retinaculum
m. extensor digitorum lateralis
m. extensor digitorum longus
m. interosseus medius, tendo lateralis
n. saphenus
v. saphena medialis: r. cranialis
r. anastomoticus
tibia, medial malleolus
tibia, lateral malleolus (may include distal fibula)
v. metatarsea dorsalis II
v. digitalis dorsalis communis II
n. metatarseus dorsalis II (n. fibularis profundus)
metatarsal bone III
metatarsophalangeal (fetlock) joint
a. digitalis medialis: r. dorsalis phalangis proximalis
r. dorsalis phalangis mediae
coronet

Fig. 7.67 Superficial structures of the right hindlimb (1): cranial view. The skin has been removed and the vessels and nerves within the superficial fascia have been dissected. Figs. 7.68–7.70 also show this specimen. The dissection shows the relationship between the superficial vessels and nerves of the digit (Figs. 7.71–7.74) and those of the more proximal regions of the limb.

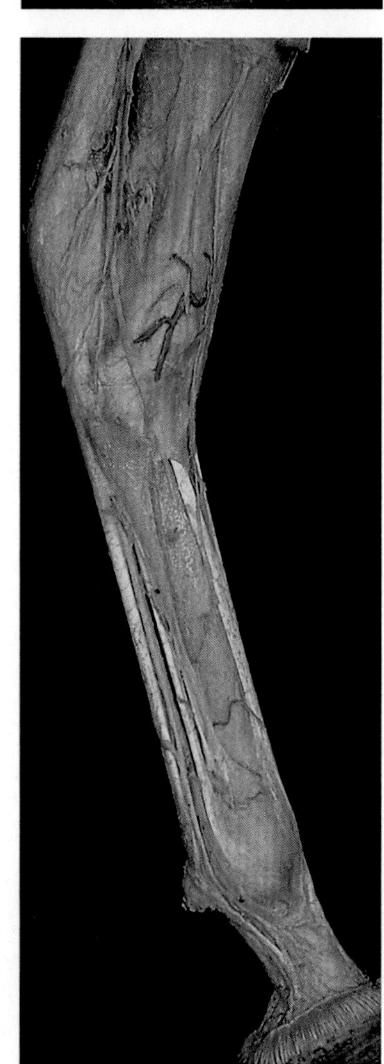

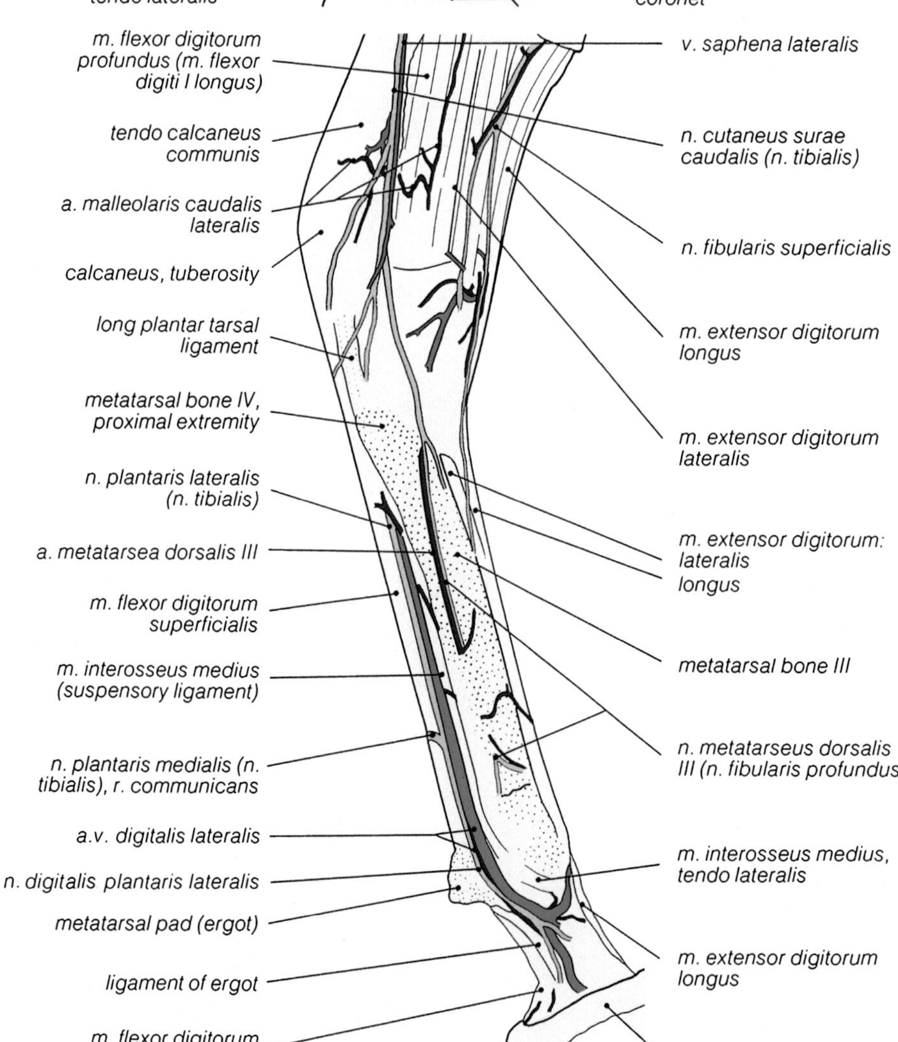
m. flexor digitorum profundus (m. flexor digiti I longus)
tendo calcaneus communis
a. malleolaris caudalis lateralis
calcaneus, tuberosity
long plantar tarsal ligament
metatarsal bone IV, proximal extremity
n. plantaris lateralis (n. tibialis)
a. metatarsea dorsalis III
m. flexor digitorum superficialis
m. interosseus medius (suspensory ligament)
n. plantaris medialis (n. tibialis), r. communicans
a.v. digitalis lateralis
n. digitalis plantaris lateralis
metatarsal pad (ergot)
ligament of ergot
m. flexor digitorum profundus
v. saphena lateralis
n. cutaneus surae caudalis (n. tibialis)
n. fibularis superficialis
m. extensor digitorum longus
m. extensor digitorum lateralis
m. extensor digitorum: lateralis longus
metatarsal bone III
n. metatarseus dorsalis III (n. fibularis profundus)
m. interosseus medius, tendo lateralis
m. extensor digitorum longus
coronet

Fig. 7.68 Superficial structures of the right hindlimb (2): lateral view. Figs. 7.67, 7.69 and 7.70 also show this specimen.

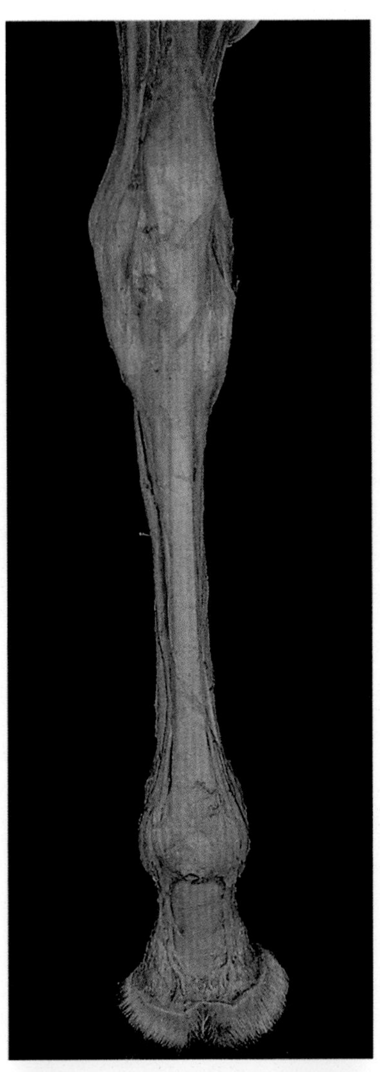

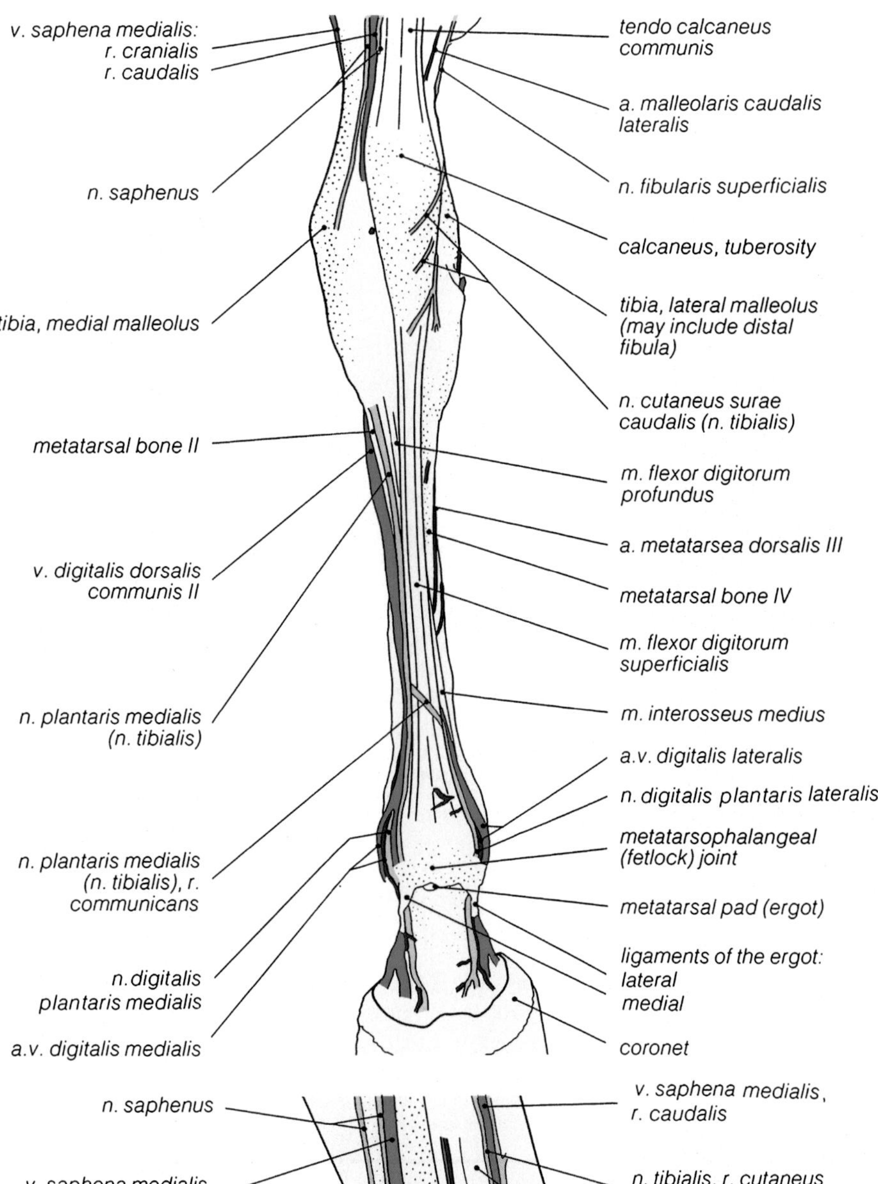
v. saphena medialis:
r. cranialis
r. caudalis
n. saphenus
tibia, medial malleolus
metatarsal bone II
v. digitalis dorsalis communis II
n. plantaris medialis (n. tibialis)
n. plantaris medialis (n. tibialis), r. communicans
n. digitalis plantaris medialis
a.v. digitalis medialis
tendo calcaneus communis
a. malleolaris caudalis lateralis
n. fibularis superficialis
calcaneus, tuberosity
tibia, lateral malleolus (may include distal fibula)
n. cutaneus surae caudalis (n. tibialis)
m. flexor digitorum profundus
a. metatarsea dorsalis III
metatarsal bone IV
m. flexor digitorum superficialis
m. interosseus medius
a.v. digitalis lateralis
n. digitalis plantaris lateralis
metatarsophalangeal (fetlock) joint
metatarsal pad (ergot)
ligaments of the ergot:
lateral
medial
coronet

Fig. 7.69 Superficial structures of the right hindlimb (3): caudal view. Figs. 7.67, 7.68 and 7.70 also show this specimen.

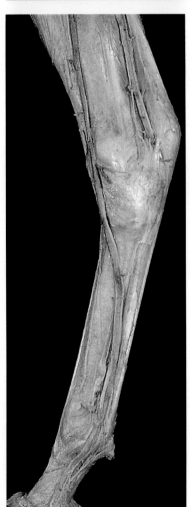

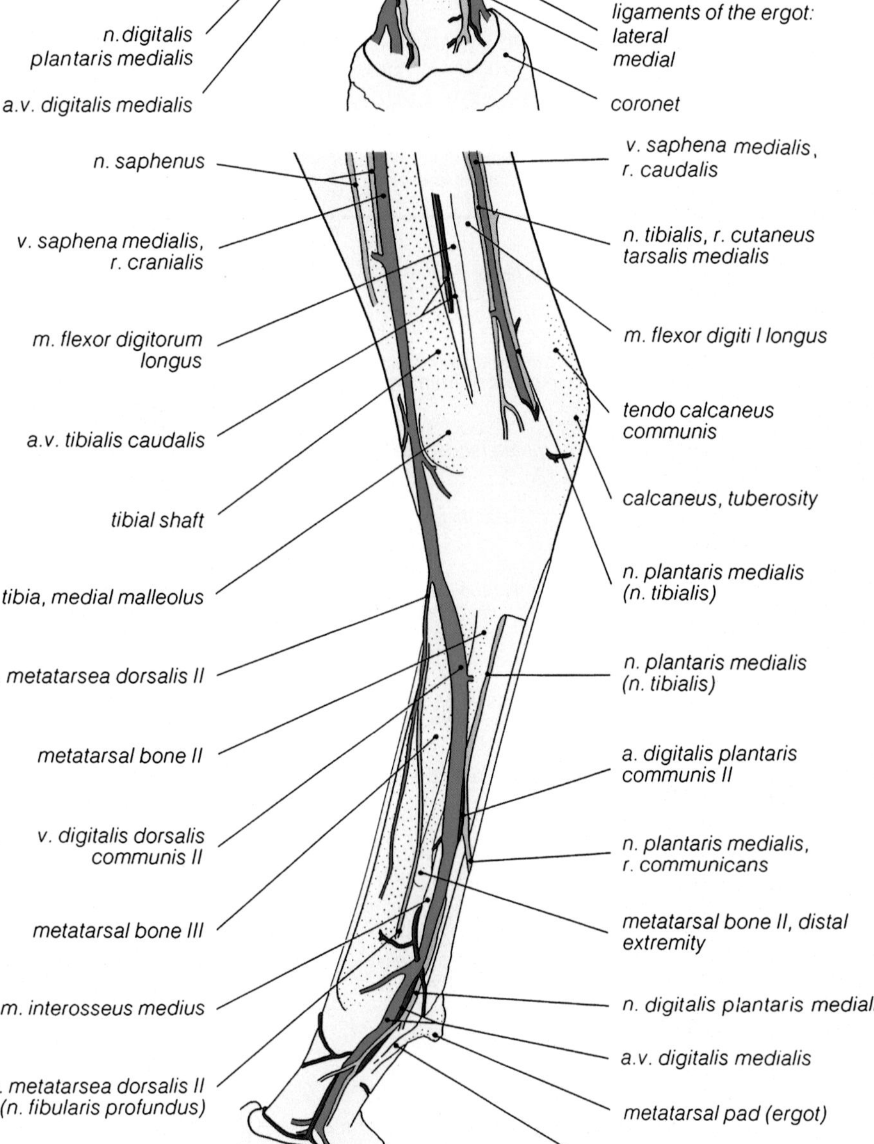
n. saphenus
v. saphena medialis, r. cranialis
m. flexor digitorum longus
a.v. tibialis caudalis
tibial shaft
tibia, medial malleolus
v. metatarsea dorsalis II
metatarsal bone II
v. digitalis dorsalis communis II
metatarsal bone III
m. interosseus medius
n. metatarsea dorsalis II (n. fibularis profundus)
coronet
v. saphena medialis, r. caudalis
n. tibialis, r. cutaneus tarsalis medialis
m. flexor digiti I longus
tendo calcaneus communis
calcaneus, tuberosity
n. plantaris medialis (n. tibialis)
n. plantaris medialis (n. tibialis)
a. digitalis plantaris communis II
n. plantaris medialis, r. communicans
metatarsal bone II, distal extremity
n. digitalis plantaris medialis
a.v. digitalis medialis
metatarsal pad (ergot)
ligament of the ergot

Fig. 7.70 Superficial structures of the right hindlimb (4): medial view. Figs. 7.67–7.69 also show this specimen. The more proximal parts of this dissection are shown in Fig. 6.56.

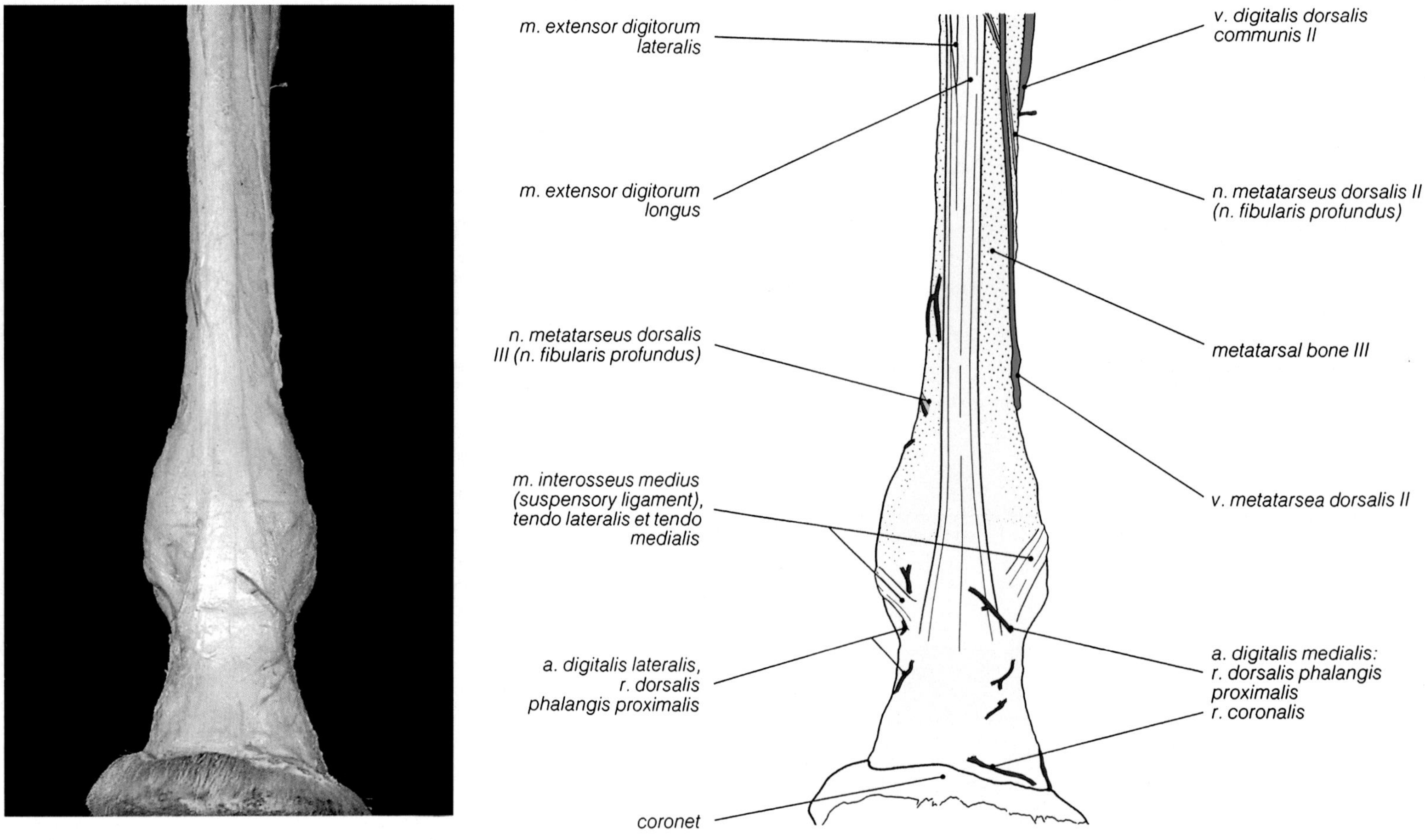

m. extensor digitorum lateralis
v. digitalis dorsalis communis II
m. extensor digitorum longus
n. metatarseus dorsalis II (n. fibularis profundus)
n. metatarseus dorsalis III (n. fibularis profundus)
metatarsal bone III
m. interosseus medius (suspensory ligament), tendo lateralis et tendo medialis
v. metatarsea dorsalis II
a. digitalis lateralis, r. dorsalis phalangis proximalis
a. digitalis medialis: r. dorsalis phalangis proximalis r. coronalis
coronet

Fig. 7.71 Superficial structures of the distal right pes (1): dorsal view. This is a closer view of a part of the specimen shown in Fig. 7.67.

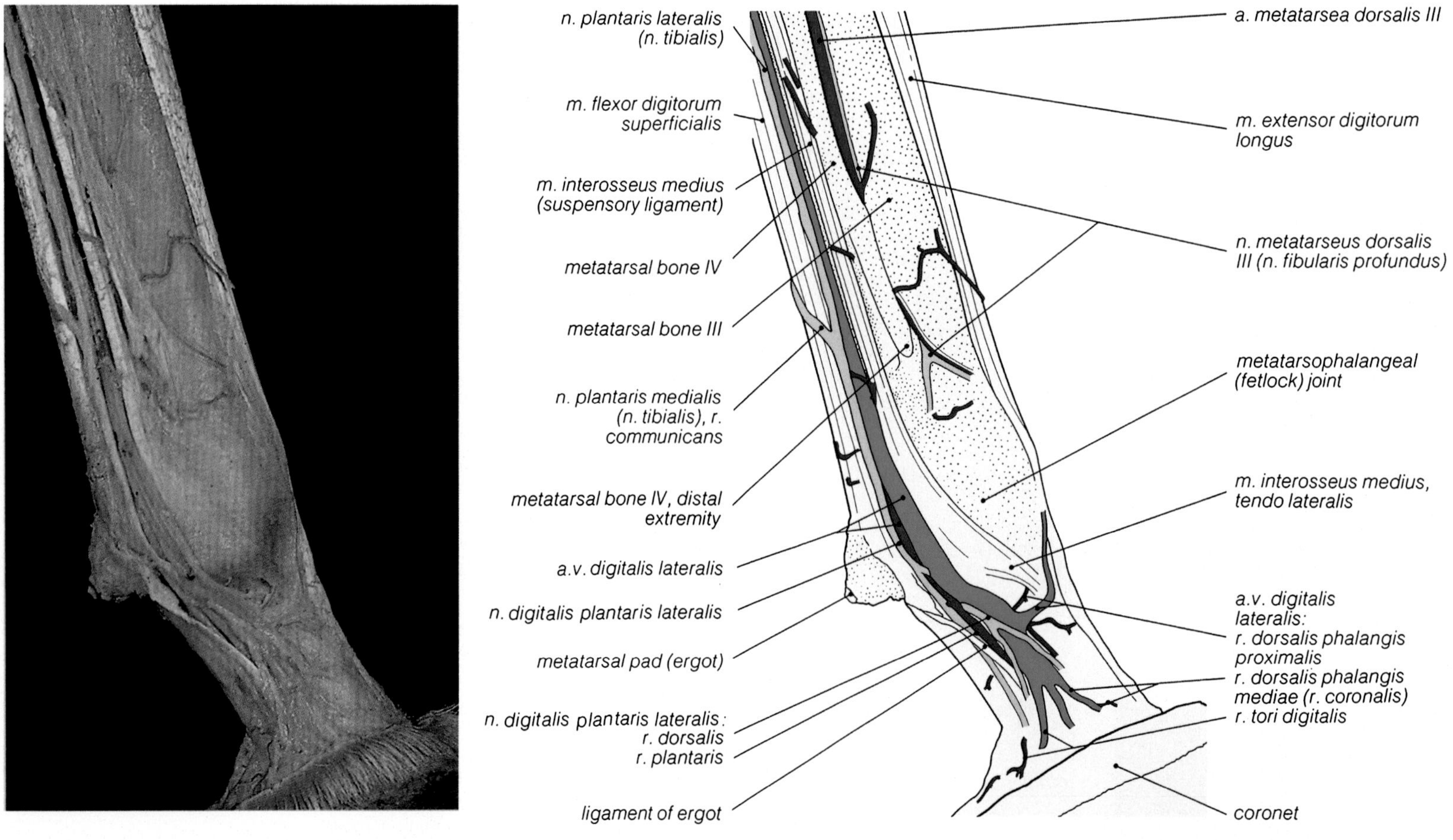

n. plantaris lateralis (n. tibialis)
a. metatarsea dorsalis III
m. flexor digitorum superficialis
m. extensor digitorum longus
m. interosseus medius (suspensory ligament)
metatarsal bone IV
n. metatarseus dorsalis III (n. fibularis profundus)
metatarsal bone III
metatarsophalangeal (fetlock) joint
n. plantaris medialis (n. tibialis), r. communicans
metatarsal bone IV, distal extremity
m. interosseus medius, tendo lateralis
a.v. digitalis lateralis
n. digitalis plantaris lateralis
a.v. digitalis lateralis: r. dorsalis phalangis proximalis r. dorsalis phalangis mediae (r. coronalis) r. tori digitalis
metatarsal pad (ergot)
n. digitalis plantaris lateralis: r. dorsalis r. plantaris
ligament of ergot
coronet

Fig. 7.72 Superficial structures of the distal right pes (2): lateral view. This is a closer view of a part of the specimen seen in Fig. 7.68.

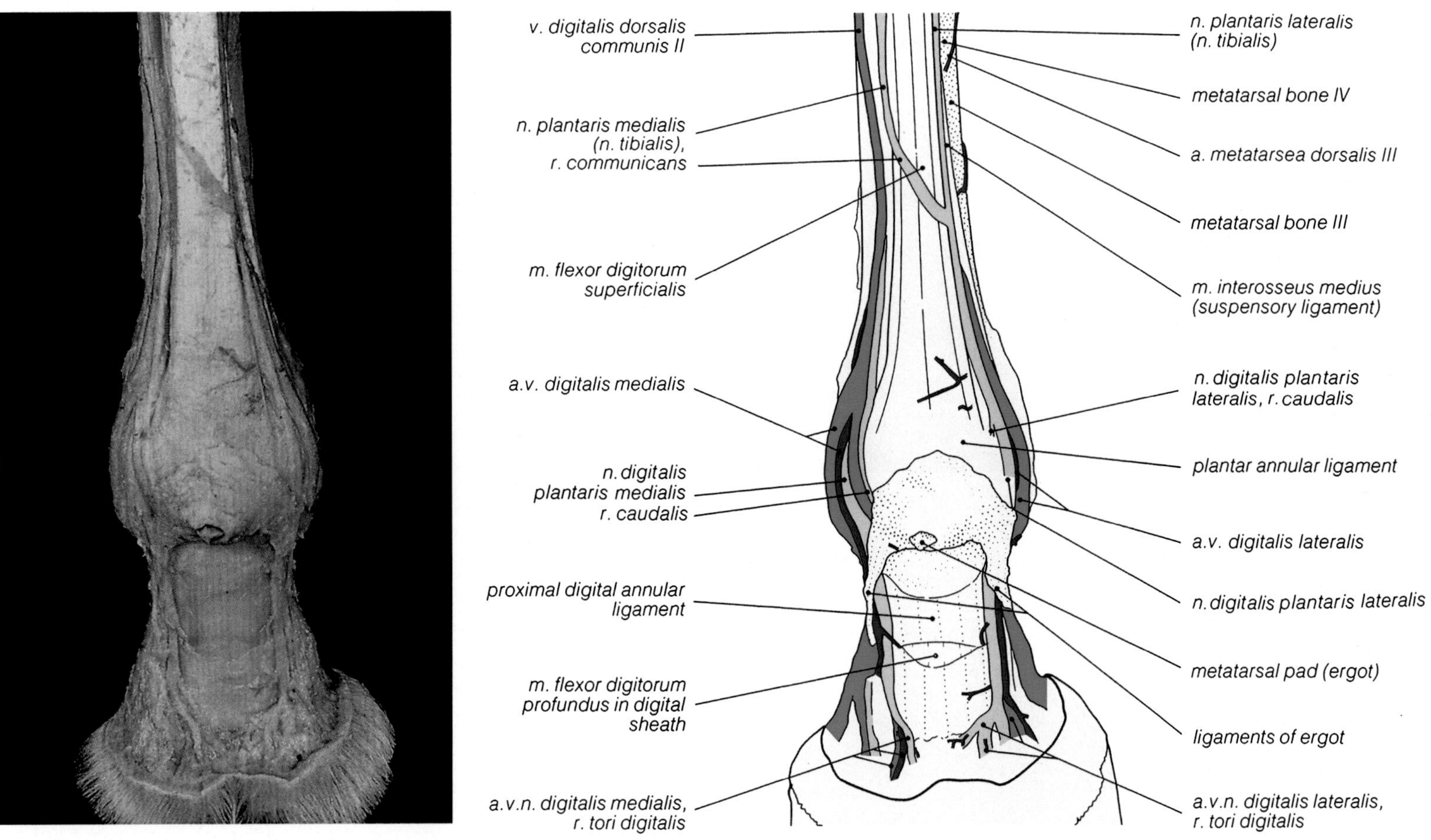
v. digitalis dorsalis communis II
n. plantaris medialis (n. tibialis), r. communicans
m. flexor digitorum superficialis
a.v. digitalis medialis
n. digitalis plantaris medialis r. caudalis
proximal digital annular ligament
m. flexor digitorum profundus in digital sheath
a.v.n. digitalis medialis, r. tori digitalis
n. plantaris lateralis (n. tibialis)
metatarsal bone IV
a. metatarsea dorsalis III
metatarsal bone III
m. interosseus medius (suspensory ligament)
n. digitalis plantaris lateralis, r. caudalis
plantar annular ligament
a.v. digitalis lateralis
n. digitalis plantaris lateralis
metatarsal pad (ergot)
ligaments of ergot
a.v.n. digitalis lateralis, r. tori digitalis

Fig. 7.73 Superficial structures of the distal right pes (3): plantar view. This is a closer view of a part of the specimen seen in Fig. 7.69.

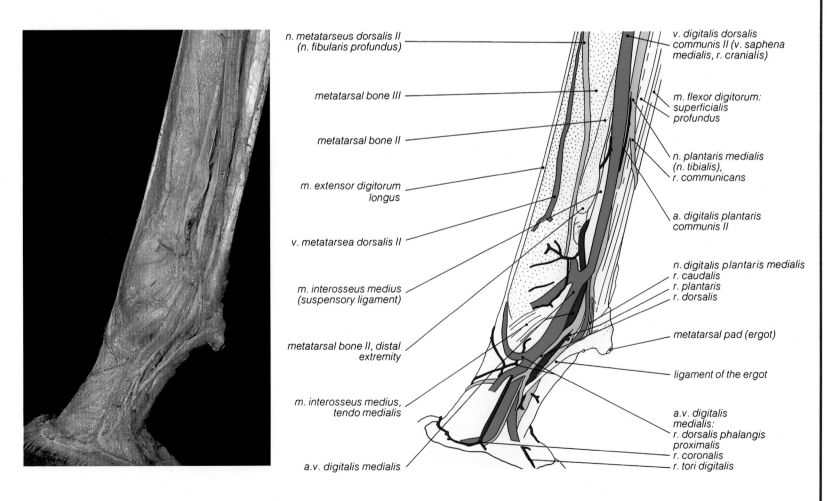

n. metatarseus dorsalis II (n. fibularis profundus)
metatarsal bone III
metatarsal bone II
m. extensor digitorum longus
v. metatarsea dorsalis II
m. interosseus medius (suspensory ligament)
metatarsal bone II, distal extremity
m. interosseus medius, tendo medialis
a.v. digitalis medialis
v. digitalis dorsalis communis II (v. saphena medialis, r. cranialis)
m. flexor digitorum: superficialis profundus
n. plantaris medialis (n. tibialis), r. communicans
a. digitalis plantaris communis II
n. digitalis plantaris medialis r. caudalis r. plantaris r. dorsalis
metatarsal pad (ergot)
ligament of the ergot
a.v. digitalis medialis: r. dorsalis phalangis proximalis r. coronalis r. tori digitalis

Fig. 7.74 Superficial structures of the distal right pes (4): medial view. This is a closer view of a part of the specimen shown in Fig. 7.70. Note the origin of the coronal ramus from the dorsal artery of the proximal phalanx. It usually arises from the dorsal artery of the middle phalanx.

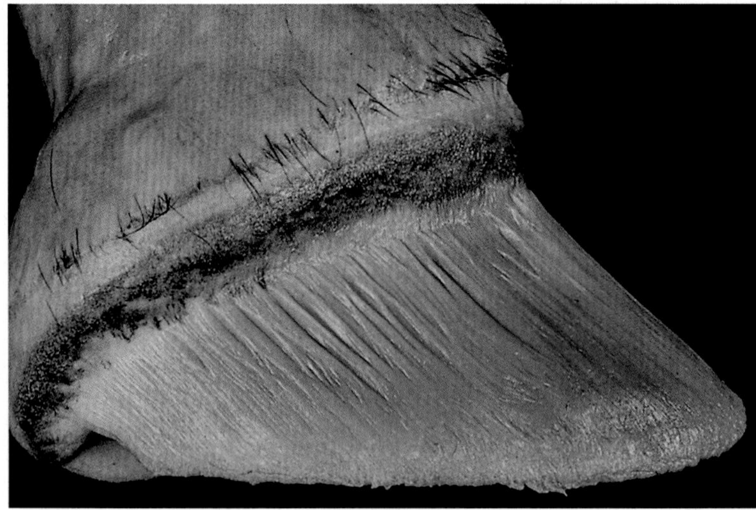

Fig. 7.75 The corium of the hoof: right lateral view. The keratinised hoof (epidermis) has been removed after cold water maceration, exposing the corium (dermis). Most of the hair has been lost in this method of preparation but the papillary and lamellar structure of the corium has been preserved.

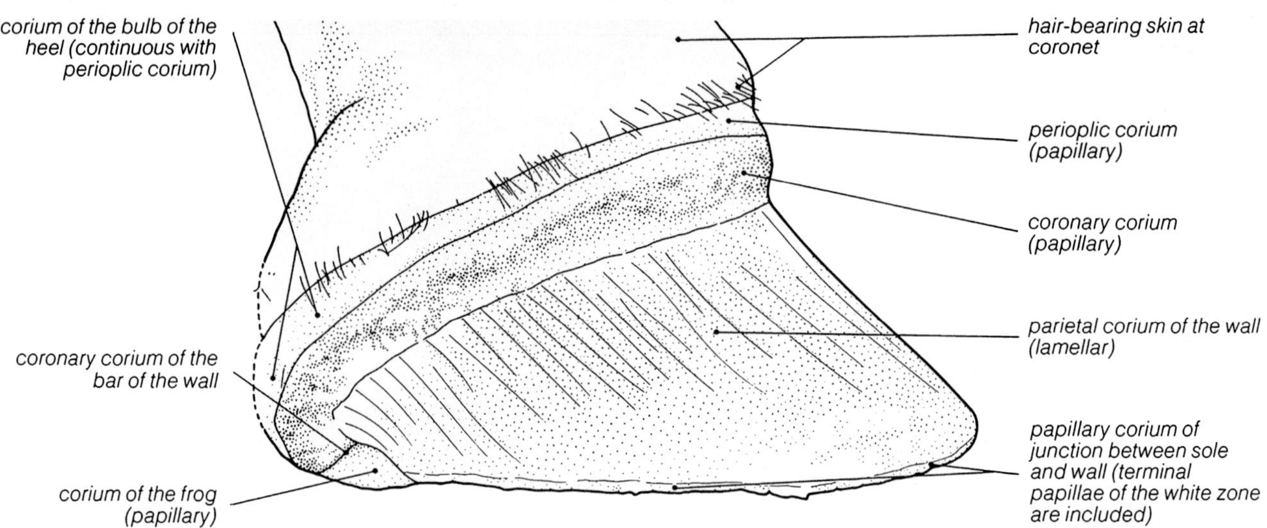

corium of the bulb of the heel (continuous with perioplic corium)
coronary corium of the bar of the wall
corium of the frog (papillary)
hair-bearing skin at coronet
perioplic corium (papillary)
coronary corium (papillary)
parietal corium of the wall (lamellar)
papillary corium of junction between sole and wall (terminal papillae of the white zone are included)

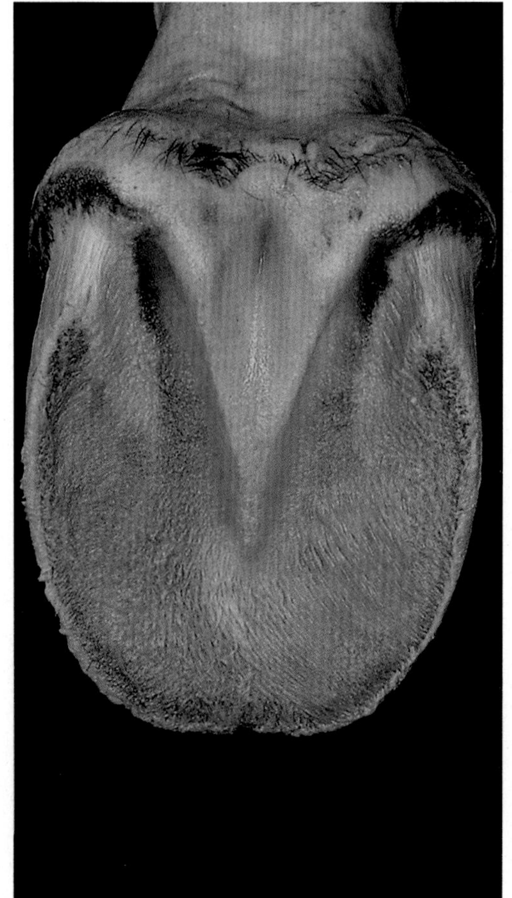

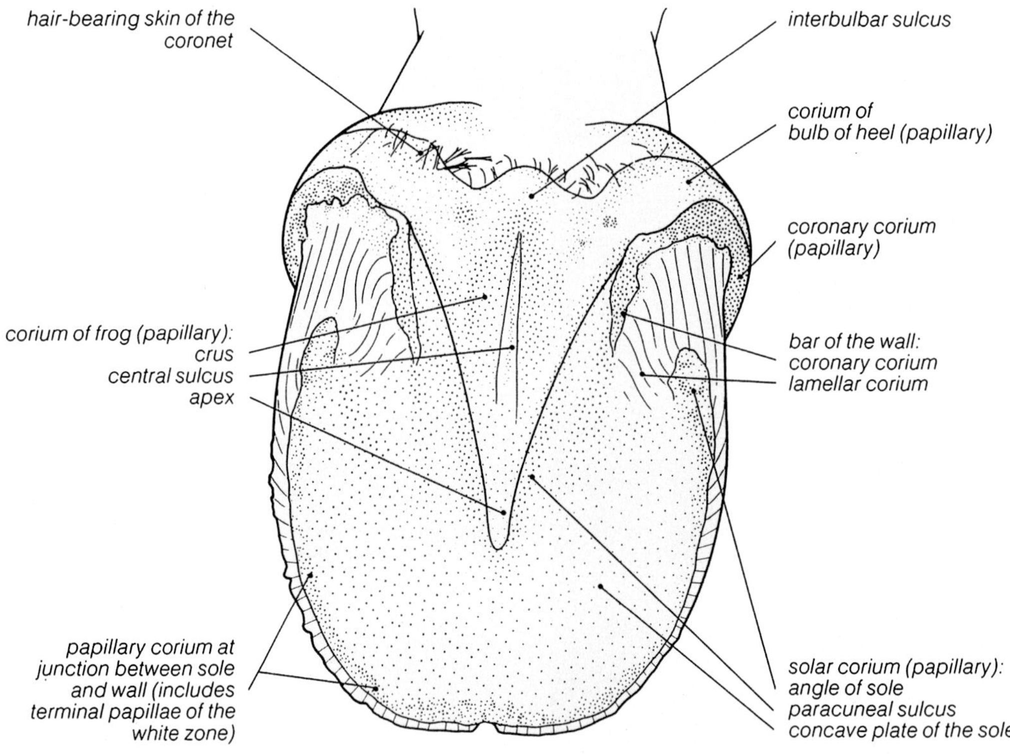

hair-bearing skin of the coronet
interbulbar sulcus
corium of bulb of heel (papillary)
coronary corium (papillary)
corium of frog (papillary): crus
central sulcus
apex
bar of the wall: coronary corium
lamellar corium
papillary corium at junction between sole and wall (includes terminal papillae of the white zone)
solar corium (papillary): angle of sole
paracuneal sulcus
concave plate of the sole

Fig. 7.76 The corium of the hoof: solar view. The periople (Fig. 7.75), bulbs and frog form a proximal collar ('frog' and 'frogband') around the wall and sole. Modern anatomical terminology however, fails to recognise the unity of these three parts of the hoof.

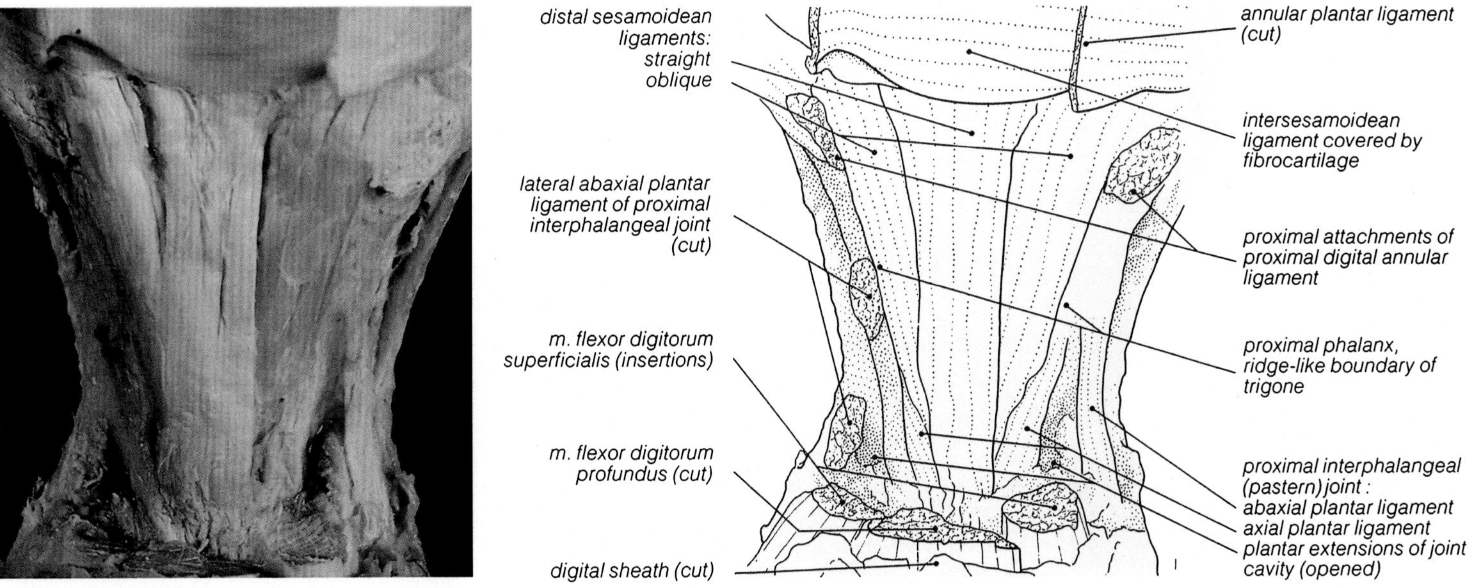
distal sesamoidean ligaments: straight oblique
lateral abaxial plantar ligament of proximal interphalangeal joint (cut)
m. flexor digitorum superficialis (insertions)
m. flexor digitorum profundus (cut)
digital sheath (cut)
annular plantar ligament (cut)
intersesamoidean ligament covered by fibrocartilage
proximal attachments of proximal digital annular ligament
proximal phalanx, ridge-like boundary of trigone
proximal interphalangeal (pastern) joint:
abaxial plantar ligament
axial plantar ligament
plantar extensions of joint cavity (opened)

Fig. 7.77 The sesamoidean and plantar ligaments of the digit: plantar view (1). The superficial and deep flexor tendons have been resected, and the lateral abaxial plantar ligament has been removed.

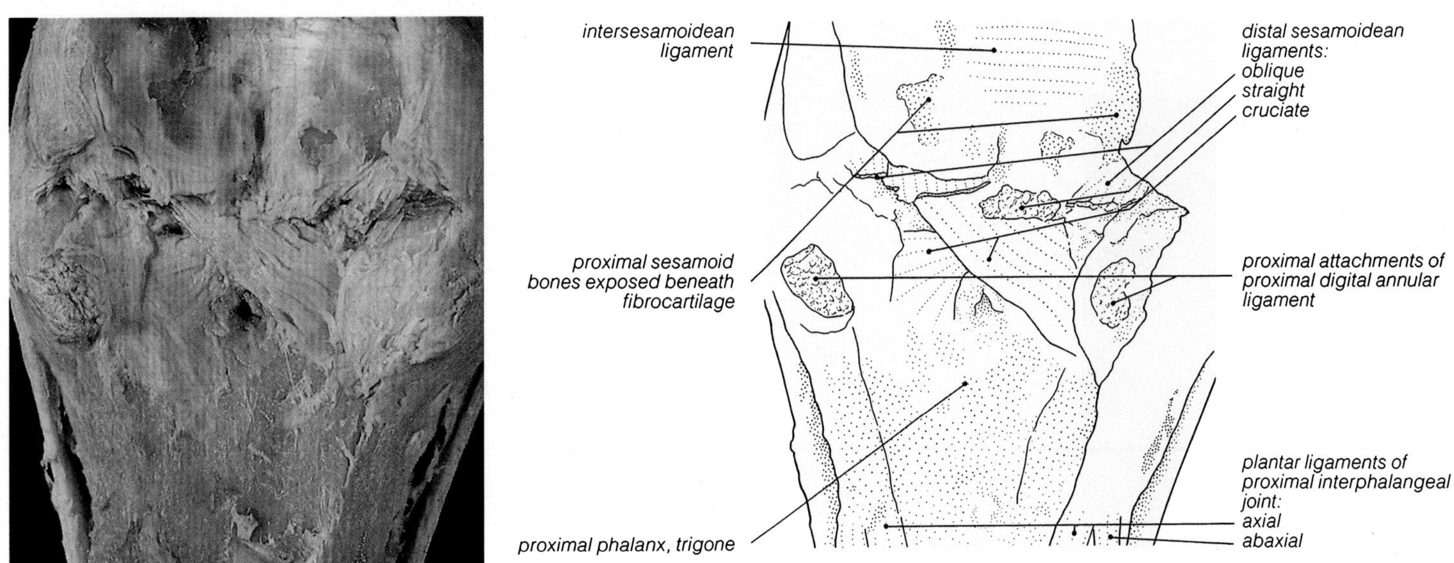
intersesamoidean ligament
proximal sesamoid bones exposed beneath fibrocartilage
proximal phalanx, trigone
distal sesamoidean ligaments:
oblique
straight
cruciate
proximal attachments of proximal digital annular ligament
plantar ligaments of proximal interphalangeal joint:
axial
abaxial

Fig. 7.78 The sesamoidean and plantar ligaments of the digit: plantar view (2). The straight and oblique ligaments have been removed to expose the cruciate ligaments which lie close to the capsule of the metatarsophalangeal (fetlock) joint.

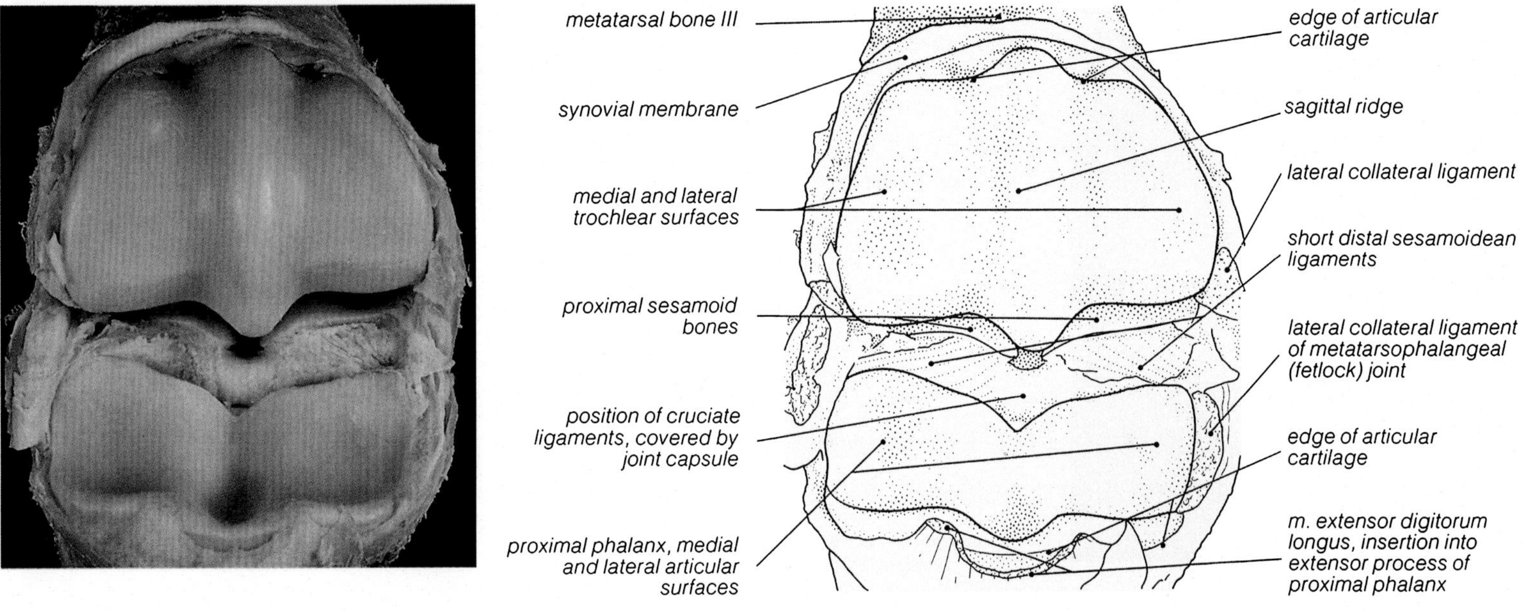
metatarsal bone III
synovial membrane
medial and lateral trochlear surfaces
proximal sesamoid bones
position of cruciate ligaments, covered by joint capsule
proximal phalanx, medial and lateral articular surfaces
edge of articular cartilage
sagittal ridge
lateral collateral ligament
short distal sesamoidean ligaments
lateral collateral ligament of metatarsophalangeal (fetlock) joint
edge of articular cartilage
m. extensor digitorum longus, insertion into extensor process of proximal phalanx

Fig. 7.79 The metatarsophalangeal joint cavity: dorsal view. The joint has been opened from its dorsal aspect, and flexed to show the joint surfaces. The plantar part of the joint capsule has been dissected to show the short sesamoidean ligaments within it.

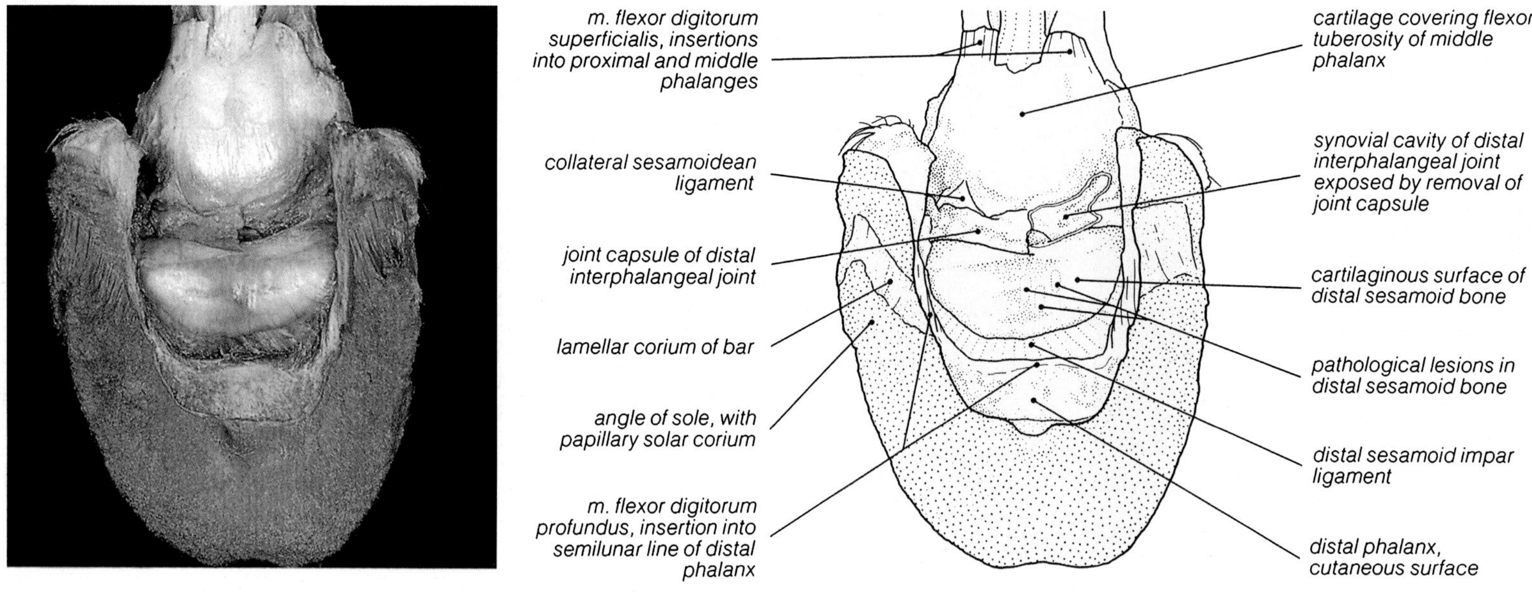
m. flexor digitorum superficialis, insertions into proximal and middle phalanges
collateral sesamoidean ligament
joint capsule of distal interphalangeal joint
lamellar corium of bar
angle of sole, with papillary solar corium
m. flexor digitorum profundus, insertion into semilunar line of distal phalanx
cartilage covering flexor tuberosity of middle phalanx
synovial cavity of distal interphalangeal joint exposed by removal of joint capsule
cartilaginous surface of distal sesamoid bone
pathological lesions in distal sesamoid bone
distal sesamoid impar ligament
distal phalanx, cutaneous surface

Fig. 7.80 The distal sesamoid bone: plantar and solar view. Removal of the tendon of the deep digital flexor muscle has opened up the podotrochlear bursa to reveal the distal sesamoid bone. Partial excision of the roof of the podotrochlear bursa reveals the synovial cavity of the distal interphalangeal joint. The cartilage covering the podotrochlear surface of the distal sesamoid bone shows evidence of pathological change ('navicular' disease).

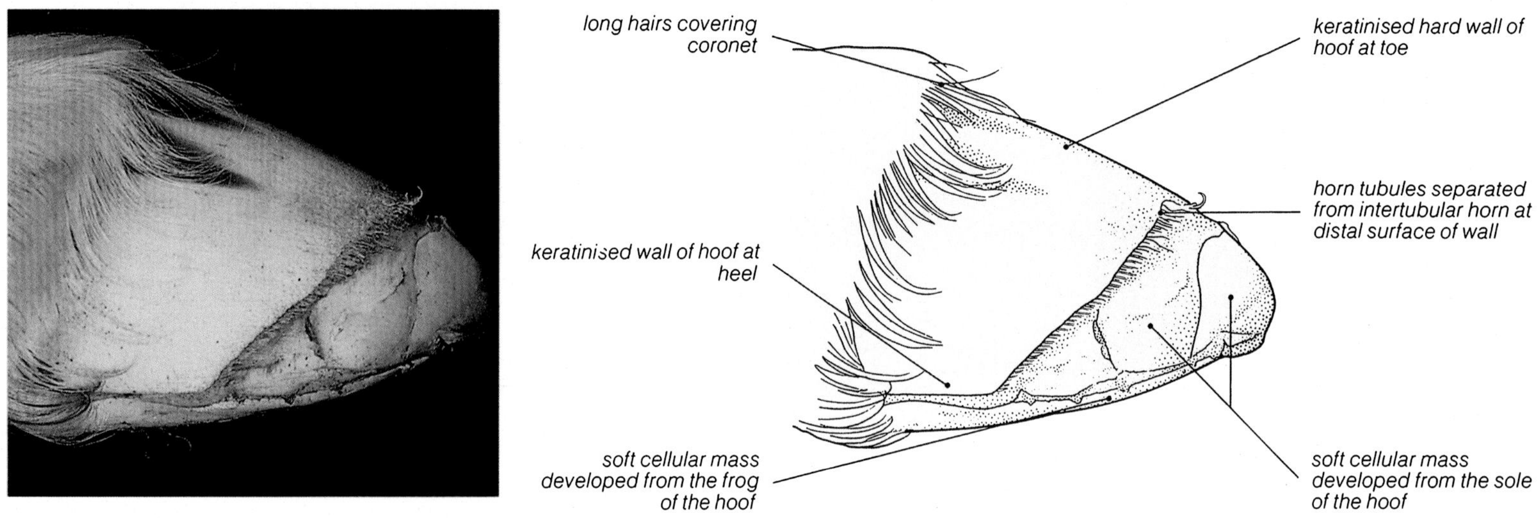
long hairs covering coronet
keratinised wall of hoof at heel
soft cellular mass developed from the frog of the hoof
keratinised hard wall of hoof at toe
horn tubules separated from intertubular horn at distal surface of wall
soft cellular mass developed from the sole of the hoof

Fig. 7.81 The hoof of an unborn foal: lateral view. The soft cellular masses developed from the sole and the frog rapidly dry out after birth, and when weight is taken on the foot they are quickly worn away to expose the hard keratinised structures beneath (compare with Fig. 7.39).

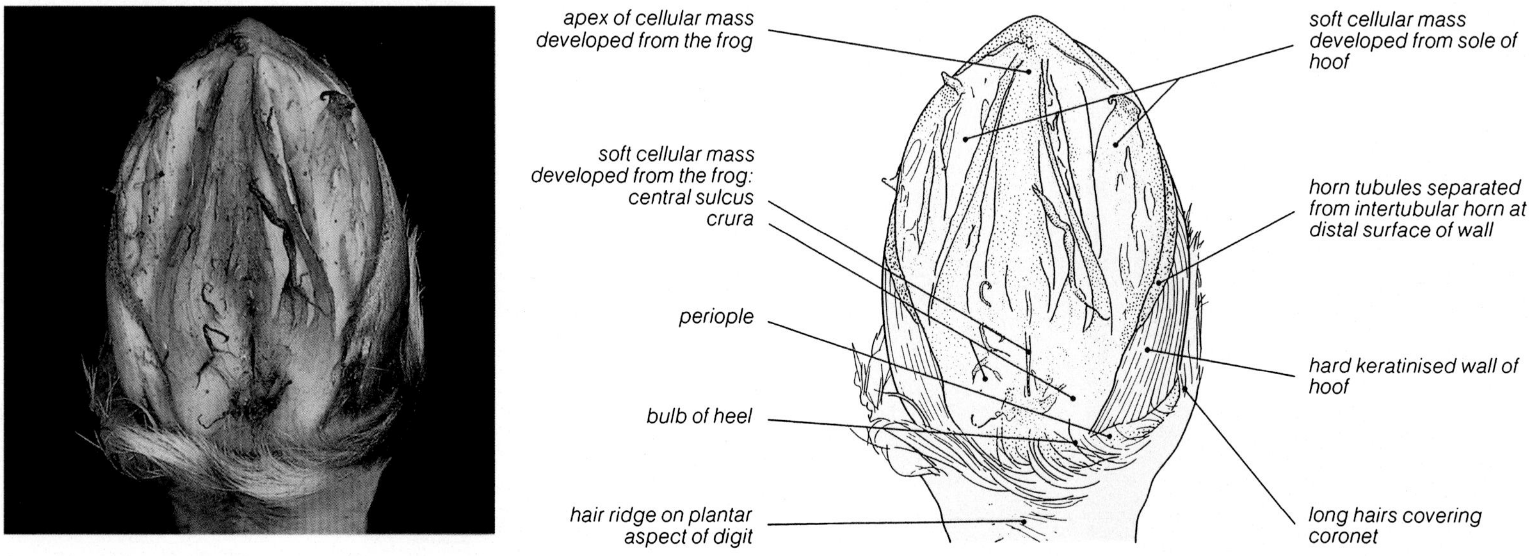
apex of cellular mass developed from the frog
soft cellular mass developed from the frog: central sulcus crura
periople
bulb of heel
hair ridge on plantar aspect of digit
soft cellular mass developed from sole of hoof
horn tubules separated from intertubular horn at distal surface of wall
hard keratinised wall of hoof
long hairs covering coronet

Fig. 7.82 The hoof of the unborn foal: solar and plantar view. The overgrowth of the cellular masses derived from the angle of the sole and from the frog hide the inflected parts of the wall (the bars). When the foal begins to walk, however, the soft tissues dry and are worn away. The solar surface of the hoof quickly becomes like that of the adult horse (see Fig. 7.9).

8. THE PELVIS (INCLUDING THE SPINE)

Clinical importance of the pelvis

Lameness associated with the pelvis can be investigated by clinical examination, ultrasonography, scintigraphy, radiology in the young horse, local anaesthesia and nerve blocks. The pelvis has a very important function in providing the link between the spine (for support) and the hindlimb (for propulsion). At times the pelvis may be carrying the whole weight of the horse. It transfers the propulsive effort but, because of the strong ligamentous and musculature attachments, has very limited movement itself. It is continuously subjected to non-compressive forces. It could be said that the sacro-iliac ligaments and joint are subjected to the most disruptive forces in the locomotory system. The pelvis gives passage, through the greater sciatic foramen, to the cranial gluteal artery and vein and the gluteal nerves; also to the largest single nerve in the equine body, the sciatic nerve. In addition, the obturator foramen gives passage to the obturator nerves and vessels.

Fractures of the pelvis are relatively rare, as the pelvis is protected by such strong muscle groups. They do, however, occur in traumatic accidents or may present as stress fractures. Often the horse with a pelvic injury may be in shock and may be very reluctant to bear weight or move. There may be fractures of the wing or the shaft of the ilium, acetabulum, pubic bone or ischium. The most common fracture is probably that of the *tuber coxae*. Pelvic fractures present as a sudden onset of very acute unilateral or bilateral lameness, often following exercise and trauma. The sacral or ischiatic tuberosities often appear uneven in height when viewed from behind.

The sacro-iliac joint is clinically the most important locomotory structure in the pelvis. It is a diarthrodial joint; it has a joint capsule, is thin and tight, with a total capacity of only 1–2 ml. There is hyaline cartilage on the sacral joint surface and fibro-cartilage on the ilial surface. The shape of the articulation varies with age and between individuals so there is considerable variation. The joint is stabilized by three pairs of sacro-iliac ligaments. The dorsal sacro-iliac ligament is divided into dorsal and lateral parts. There is an interosseus ligament and also a ventral ligament. Hunters and jumpers are particularly affected by damage to these ligaments. Which results in a sore back or persistent hindlimb lameness. The injuries fall into two groups. Firstly, there are acute injuries, desmitis, and luxation/subluxation of the joint. Secondly, there is chronic injury in the form of sacro-iliac osteoarthritis or desmitis or both. Both are seen as hindlimb lameness and/or poor performance. The acute injuries result from a fall, from slipping, or from overwork. Which often causes overstretching of the dorsal and ventral ligaments. Sometimes, if the sacro-iliac joint is particularly unstable, it is possible to see movement of the *tuber sacrale* when the affected horse moves forward at a walk. Chronic sacro-iliac injury results from over-use, trauma, and the saddle. It has a high incidence of 8–15% in racehorses. There is usually a history of poor performance, resisting jumping, lack of hindlimb impulsion, behavioural changes and back soreness. Examination of the joint by ultrasonography often reveals degenerative changes in the joint. Anaesthesia of the joint will confirm the seat of lameness. For the right sacro-iliac joint, a site 2 cm cranial to the left *tuber sacrale*, at a 45–60 degree angle to the joint and slightly caudal towards the right greater trochanter of the femur, along the medial aspect of the right ilial wing, will reach the joint and *vice versa* for the left joint. Nerve damage within the pelvic cavity may affect the obturator nerve, which is sometimes damaged in foaling. This nerve innervates the adductor, gracilis, and pectineus muscles. Loss of adduction of the hindlimb results in a wide stance, with inability to keep the limb under the body.Trauma to the cranial and caudal gluteal nerves occurs sometimes, with a resultant atrophy of the gluteo-biceps (biceps femoris) muscle.

'Ruptures' occur when a part of the body is displaced through a break in bodily structure. ('Hernias' are displacements through natural bodily openings.) Ruptures are often associated with kicks, being stuck half over fences, and road traffic accidents. Damage to the prepubic tendon, followed by rupture, is occasionally described in association with the presence of twin foals, hydro-allantois or giant fetal oversize. Rupture of the abdominal muscles may occur following trauma. Inguinal or scrotal hernias may occur in colts (usually congenital), stallions, or (rarely) mares or geldings. A segment of small intestine, or part of the great omentum, or both, enter the vaginal process through the vaginal ring. These parts may remain close to the superficial inguinal ring (inguinal hernia) or may enter the scrotum (scrotal hernia). In scrotal hernia, the hernial sac comprises the scrotal skin, tunica dartos, and the tunica vaginalis of the vaginal process, and also contains the testis, and epididymis. If the blood supply to the contents of the hernial sac is affected (strangulated hernia), surgery is urgently needed. Surgical treatment usually involves replacing the abdominal contents by twisting the vaginal process. The twisted neck of the process is then sutured to the edges of the superficial inguinal ring (abdominal and pelvic tendons of the external abdominal oblique muscle). The vaginal tunic is incised and the testis and epidymis are removed. Femoral hernia (or ?rupture) occurs through the femoral ring, alongside the femoral artery, and is rare, but (as in the human cases) may be more common in females than in males.

Examination of the pelvis by rectal examination is not so easy in the horse as in the ox because the rectum is friable and easily torn. It can be used to evaluate inguinal hernias and cryptorchidism (undescended testis). If a stallion has colic, it can be used to investigate whether there is an incarceration of the intestine in the inguinal canal. The superficial inguinal ring is located 6–8 cm cranial to the iliopectineal eminence of the pubis and 10–12 cm lateral to the midline. The perineal region is a favoured area for the occurrence of melanoma in grey horses.

The male and female reproductive tracts are associated with the pelvic region and will be discussed here. The intra-abdominal features of both female and male systems can be viewed by laparoscopy. The horse is a long-day breeder and is seasonally polyoestrus. Examination of the external and internal genital tract of the mare is an important aspect of stud practice. Vaginal examination using a speculum, and digital examination, are possible. Vulval bleeding occurs occasionally. One of the more unusual conditions is pneumo-vagina (wind-sucking) which constitutes a risk for subsequent bacterial infection. There may be fibroids and sacculations of the uterus. Trans-rectal ultrasonography is very useful in pregnancy, to assess the ovarian follicles and corpora lutea, the presence of small or hypoplastic ovaries, the presence and size of follicles, and the state of the uterus. It is particularly important to detect endometritis or chronic endometriosis. The most important diagnosis is Contagious Equine 'Metritis' caused by *Tayloriella equigenitalis* which is the most important infectious genital disease of the mare and stallion. Endometrial cysts, peri-glandular fibrosis, and cystic glandular distension, may also be revealed. Mucometra (mucus accumulations in the uterus) also occurs occasionally. Enlarged ovaries may indicate tumours such as granulosa-cell tumours. Endoscopy can be used to collect microbiological samples and samples for endometrial biopsy or cytology.

Uterine torsion is not uncommon as a cause of colic in the late term mare (usually at around 8 months). It may be 180–540 degrees torsion, cranial to the cervix and vagina, and rupture of the uterus may result from the torsion.

Placentitis is an unusual occurrence. It may be necessary to carry out ovariectomy because of abnormal behaviour, to curtail reproductive activity, or for pathological conditions such as granulosa-cell tumours or haematomas in the ovary. The operation can be carried out through the flank or by ventral midline, oblique paramedian or vaginal approaches. Inflammation of the Fallopian tubes (oophritis) may also require their removal.

Pregnancy failure in the mare is not uncommon as a result of embryonic death or abortion. Pregnancy diagnosis in the mare is possible *per rectum* and is accurate after about 28 days and optimal around day 42. Trans-rectal ultra-sonography will give results from day 10 to term. Usually the first scan is 14–15 days. To detect twins before implantation, scan at 16 days. The heart beat should be visible at 26–28 days. Transabdominal ultra-sonography can be used from day 80 to term. It is possible during pregnancy to have umbilical cord abnormalities, placental insufficiencies, pregnancy in the uterine body, insufficiency of hormones from the corpora lutea and, the worst possibility of all, uterine torsion. Prolonged gestation is rare, with only 1% exceeding 370 days. Premature udder development occurs occasionally. There are several causes of abortion including bacterial, fungal, and viral agents. In the latter group, equine infectious anaemia, equine herpes virus 1 and equine viral arteritis, are the most important.

Parturition is a time when intervention may be necessary. Caesarean section is essential if second stage labour is delayed, but it is rare to get a live foal delivered by this operation. From the mare's point of view it is preferable to perform an embryotomy. Parturition occurs in 3 stages. The first stage, which lasts about one hour, is rupture of the fetal membranes; the second stage lasts about 30 minutes and the foal is born. Stage three relates to expulsion of the foetal membranes and lasts about 1 hour. Uterine involution takes about 6–10 days and the foaling heat occurs 7–9 days after foaling. *Post-partum* complications include retained placenta, haemorrhage, recto-vaginal fistula, perineal lacerations, uterine rupture, endometrial haemorrhage, uterine prolapse, and endometritis. Dystocia (difficult parturition) is a rare event with only about 4% of foalings having difficulty. It may be followed by acute septic metritis or necrotic vaginitis; rupture of the internal iliac artery rupture has been known after a long period of dystocia. Interventions which may prove necessary include retropulsion, forced extraction, amputation of fetal parts (foetotomy), or Caesarean section. The latter operation requires mid-line laparotomy with an incision along the greater curvature of the uterus.

Examination of the stallion for soundness requires examination of the musculo-skeletal, respiratory, and cardiovascular systems, as well as the reproductive tract and semen evaluation. The semen should have a high progressive motility, a pH of 7.2–7.6, a volume of around 70 ml (quite variable but not too important), a concentration of 8×10^6 and, in terms of morphology, at least 60% should be normal and 10% still motile after 6 hours. If a second sample is taken on the same day, the values should be at least 50% of the first sample. There are ejaculatory dysfunctions, some of which may have an anatomical basis, or an abnormality of the locomotory system may make it difficult to mount. The external genitalia have to be examined. Penile trauma is quite common and includes abrasions, lacerations and rupture of the *corpus cavernosum penis*. The penis can be affected by a variety of conditions including inability to retract the organ (due to inanition or debility after breeding), haematomas, coital exanthema, inflammation (balanitis) and, rarely, squamous cell carcinoma and papilloma. Removal of these tumours may require surgery. Contraction of the preputial ring can also occur following injury and may prevent extrusion of the penis (acquired phimosis). The prepuce can be an important source of bacterial pathogens, particularly for the mare at mating. Examination of the scrotum may reveal acquired swellings, acute trauma, scrotal lacerations, testicular torsions or even hydrocoele (fluid within the vaginal process).

The scrotum is an area that is often involved in trauma, so may show signs of scars on its surface. Torsion of the spermatic cords is an extremely rare event. Congenital abnormalities of the scrotum may be a result of male pseudo-hermaphroditism or the testicular feminization syndrome. The testes should be palpated and their size and consistency are related to the use of the stallion and his daily sperm output. The left testis is often larger and more pendulous than the right. Abnormalities may include hypoplasia (revealed in the young horse), degeneration of the testes following trauma, inflammation (orchitis) which may follow trauma or bacterial infection or both, and neoplasia in the form of a seminoma. It may also be possible to palpate the epididymis (which is on the dorso-lateral border of the testis) for abnormalities. The tail of the epididymis is at the caudal pole of the testis. The internal genitalia may be palpated *per rectum.*

Castration of the stallion (also known as gelding) is one of the most common operations carried out in equine practice and is usually carried out to prevent male behaviour, rather than for medical or surgical reasons. The exception to this is for the horse that has an undescended testis (cryptorchid). There are open and closed techniques for castration. The operation can be carried out in the field, in the standing position, or in lateral recumbency. The operation can be followed by a variety of complications (infection, haemorrhage, swellings, septicaemia, tetanus, schirrhous cord, hydrocoele, penile prolapse, evisceration, and furunculosis) so care must be taken with hygiene. In the cryptorchid horse ('rig') the testis and epididymis fail to descend into the scrotum. In half of these cases, the testis is retained in the abdomen (usually near the deep inguinal ring) and the vaginal process is absent, or short (containing only the tail of the epididymis). In the other cases the testis lies in the inguinal region or canal. It may lie superficial to the superficial inguinal ring of the external abdominal oblique muscle, but it may not be palpable externally. In this position it will be lying between the origin of the lateral scrotal lamina from the dorsolateral edge of the ring (abdominal tendon of the external abdominal oblique muscle) and the origin of the medial scrotal lamina from the yellow elastic lamina medial to the ring. The cryptorchid testis in the inguinal position is usually much smaller than the descended testis, and the scrotum may be poorly developed. In most cases it can be removed by surgery in the inguinal region but some cases require a paramedian abdominal incision.

Clinical importance of the spine

Clinical considerations of the spine involve the regions of the head, neck, thorax, abdomen, and pelvis. Changes in the conformation, musculature and general well-being may affect the spinal column. Clinical examination, lameness tests, regional anaesthesia, diagnostic and contrast radiography and scintigraphy, are widely used in diagnosis. Clinical examination at exercise, either in hand or by lunging, are used in diagnosis. Also, marks may be seen and swellings detected on palpation.

There are only 36 bones in the equine vertebral column (excluding the tail), but there are many ligaments. Some are extremely powerful, such as the nuchal and supra-spinous ligaments, and there are many smaller ligaments such as the interspinous, sacroiliac, sacrotuberous, iliolumbar, intertransverse and dorsal and ventral longitudinal ligaments. Clinical signs that suggest spinal problems include acute or chronic 'back' pain, reduced flexibility of the spine, lateral curvature of the spine, asymmetry of the hindquarters, neurological deficits and atrophy of the dorsal muscles and hindquarters.

The diseases and disorders of the spinal column, dorsal musculature, and central nervous system are sometimes extremely difficult to differentiate. Many conditions of the back are diagnosed by elimination of the other possibilities, rather than by the finding of probable diagnostic indicators. 'Back problems' often have very indeterminate clinical signs such as poor performance, behavioural or temperamental changes, and difficulty of control when being mounted or ridden. Reluctance to go faster or to jump is also a very common feature. Vertebral trauma occurs quite often when horses fall at speed, when taking jumps, or in serious collisions. Fracture of the spinous processes, vertebral body and neural arches is most likely in the first three thoracic, first three lumbar and T12 vetebrae. If the horse falls over backwards it is more likely to suffer from fractures of the dorsal spinous processes. In many of these cases the horse will remain on the ground or be 'winded'. Fractures or other injuries of the cervical, thoracic, and lumbar vertebrae are not uncommon in these types of trauma, and may be accompanied by fractures of the long bones and/or accessory carpal bone, making diagnosis even more difficult. A horse pulling up lame is more likely to have problems with the superficial digital flexor tendons, or fracture of the accessory carpal bone or a lateral condyle.

The spine may be subjected to a variety of conditions. Abnormalities of conformation are seen in foals; congenital scoliosis (lateral curvature) is not uncommon; much less common are lordosis (ventral curvature), kyphosis (dorsal curvature) and synostosis (fusion of the vertebrae). Muscular damage affecting the spine includes strains, myopathies, myositis, white muscle disease (vitamin E and selenium deficiency) and external rhabdomyolysis. Ligamentous strains are also very common. Misalignment of the vertebrae leading to pinched nerves is also not uncommon. One of the most common conditions is over-riding or fracture of the spinal processes of the thoracic vertebrae. Spondylitis is inflammation of a vertebra; ossifying spondylitis and discospondylolisthesis are associated with traumatic incidents and are not uncommon.

One of the most common causes of back pain in the horse is the condition known as 'kissing spines', in which there is crowding or over-riding of the spinous processes of the vertebrae under the saddle area. It has a high incidence and a very low mortality and is caused by conformational abnormalities. It causes pressure points between the adjacent spines with over-riding. Adventitious bursae develop between the spines in response to the persistent rubbing, and where there is persistent over-riding new bone develops in response. Affected horses buck when ridden, have a very poor hindlimb action, and a poor jumping performance. The rider's weight is usually carried by T12–T18 and the most likely sites of lesions are in T15–T17.

In older horses there are also conditions associated with loss of strength in the ligaments around the small joints of the vertebrae, causing lesions in the transverse processes and the articular processes of the vertebrae.

In considering the spine as a whole it is important to realise that most of the conditions likely to be a common cause of abnormalities are found in the pelvic region. The sacral vertebrae are an important part of the spinal column and the sacroiliac ligaments can be easily damaged (see Pelvic section). One of the conditions not mentioned in the pelvic section is fracture of the sacrum. In this injury, the peripheral nerves of the hindleg (sciatic, fibular, tibial and obturator) are often involved. The femoral nerve is extremely well protected and less likely to be damaged. Fracture of the sacrum may also cause neuritis of the *cauda equina*, which affects sacral and coccygeal nerve roots.

The neurological problems of the equine spine can be investigated by radiography, ultrasonography, myelography, and by collection and analysis of cerebrospinal fluid. The fluid is best collected with the horse under a general anaesthetic, in lateral recumbency, with the head flexed to ninety degrees and with a straight spinal column. The needle is inserted in the midline between the cranial borders of the wings of the atlas, to a depth of 5–8 cm. Fluid can also be collected from the lumbo-sacral space. For this the horse, needs to be sedated, restrained and standing level on all four feet. The needle is inserted on a line that joins the cranial borders of the left and right *tuber coxae*, at the intersection with the midline. One to two cm behind this intersection is a depression; the caudal aspect of the 6th lumbar vertebra lies cranially and the cranial border of the 2nd sacral spinous process lies caudally; the rim of the tuber sacrale lies laterally. It is important to remember that L5 is less prominent than L6 and sometimes difficult to palpate, as is S1 which is heads promiuent than S2. The sub-arachnoid space can then be located at a depth of 12–13 cm.

Infectious disease of the equine spine is not an uncommon phenomenon. In many parts of the world viral encephalitides are common, including Eastern, Western and Venezuelan equine encephalomyelitis. Equine herpes virus 1 and West Nile virus infections may also occur. Various other disorders also affect the central nervous system including equine degenerating myelo-encephalopathy (EDM), verminous encephalitis (associated with aberrant parasites), equine protozoal myelitis, 'ryegrass staggers', skeletal mycotoxicoses, bacterial meningitis, botulism, tetanic hypocalcaemia, hyperkalaemic periodic paralysis and fungal meningitis.

Neural disorders of uncertain aetiology include post-endurance-race cerebral syndrome, pareses associated with upper and lower motor neuron diseases, trembling, and ataxia. This latter may be induced by plant poisons and may be seen as a lack of proprioception, and a syndrome involving both the vestibular system and the cerebellum. Neuroses include crib-biting, head-shaking, nodding (may be associated with allergy to inhaled antigens), self-mutilation syndrome and wind-sucking.

Tail damage is usually seen as a tail with 'kinks' or with a tendency to be flaccid. However, these signs can be caused by sacral fractures which result in nerve damage and neurogenic atrophy of sacral and coccygeal muscles.

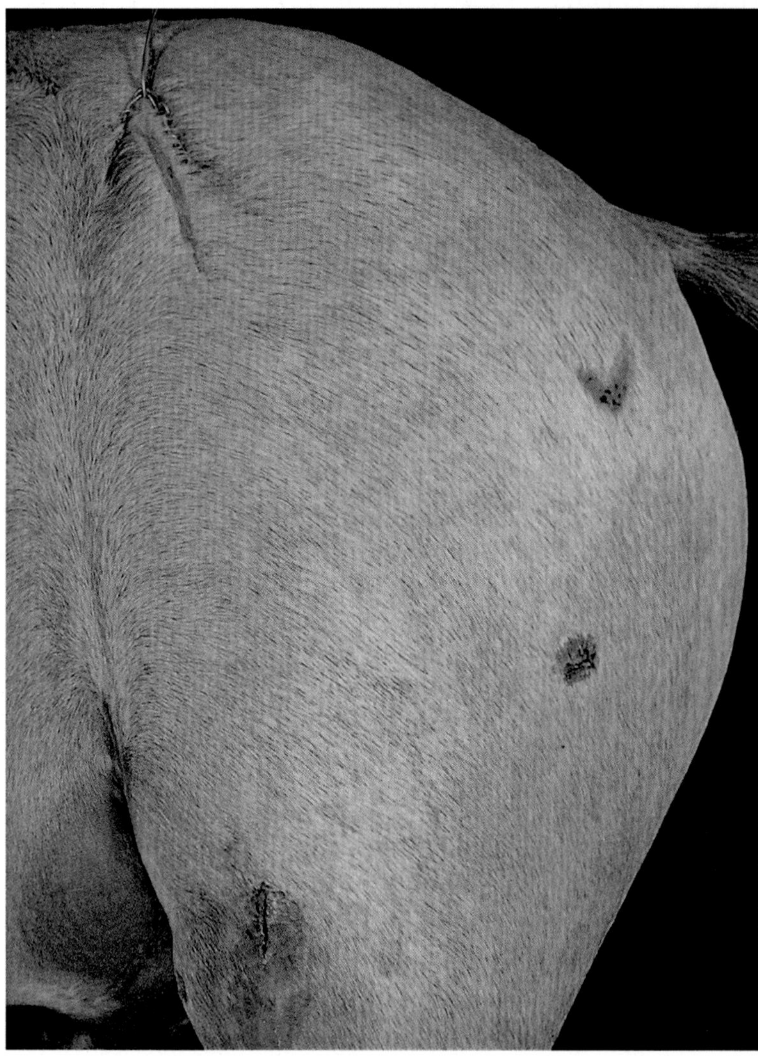
convexity of m. gluteus medius
ilium, tuber coxae (divergent hair vortex has been obscured)
tail head
femur, greater trochanter:
caudal part
notch
cranial part
intermuscular groove between m. biceps femoris and m. semitendinosus
convexity of m. semitendinosus
converging hair ridge
femur, third trochanter
hair vortex of stifle fold
incision (through which patella was nailed to femoral trochlea)
femoral trochlea, lateral and medial ridges
lateral patellar ligament
tibia, extensor sulcus

Fig. 8.1 Surface features of the pelvic and femoral regions of the gelding: left lateral view. The palpable bony features have been shaved. The rounded conformation of the gluteal musculature obscures the sacral tuberosity of the ilium in this horizontal lateral view, and the ischiatic tuberosity is similarly obscured by the semitendinosus muscle (see Fig. 8.3). The deep intermuscular groove between the biceps femoris and semitendinosus muscles (so-called 'poverty line') is much less conspicuous after embalming; in emaciated horses it is very prominent.

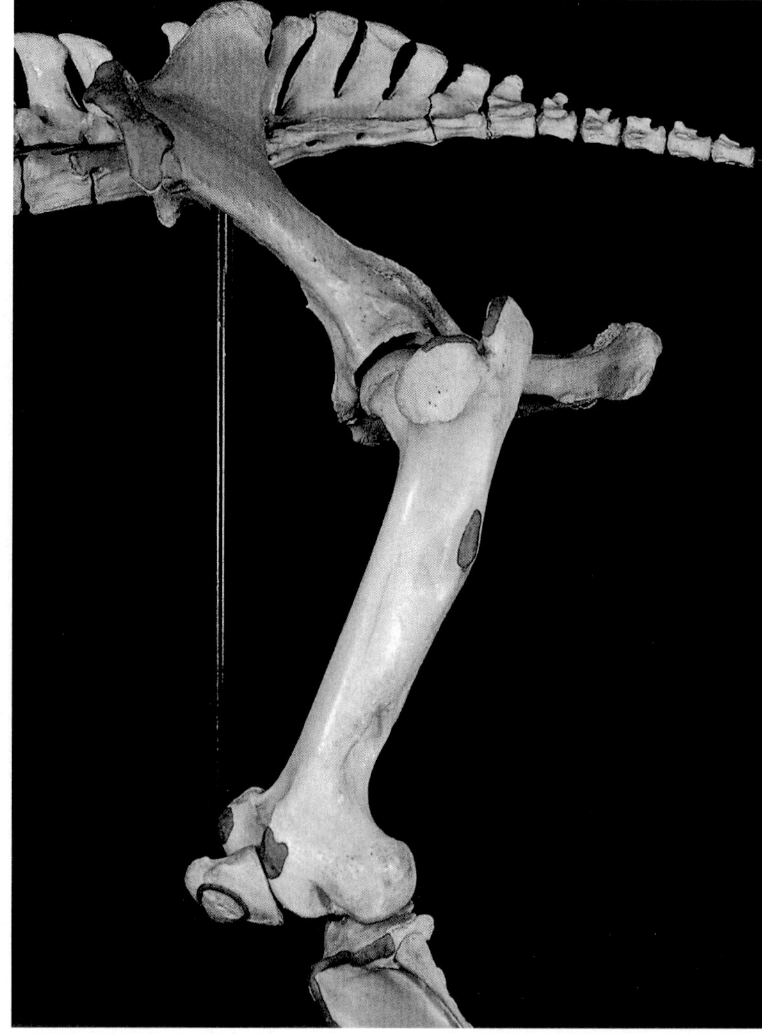

Fig. 8.2 Bones of the pelvic, femoral and stifle regions: left lateral view. The bony features shown in Fig. 8.1 are coloured red.

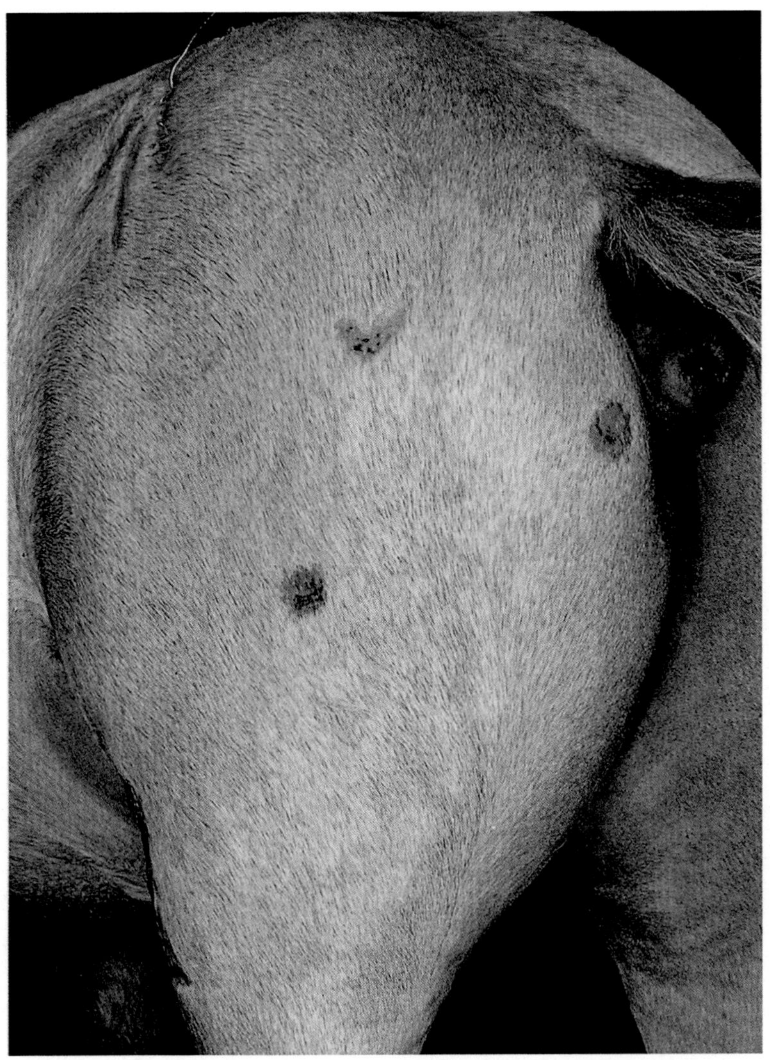

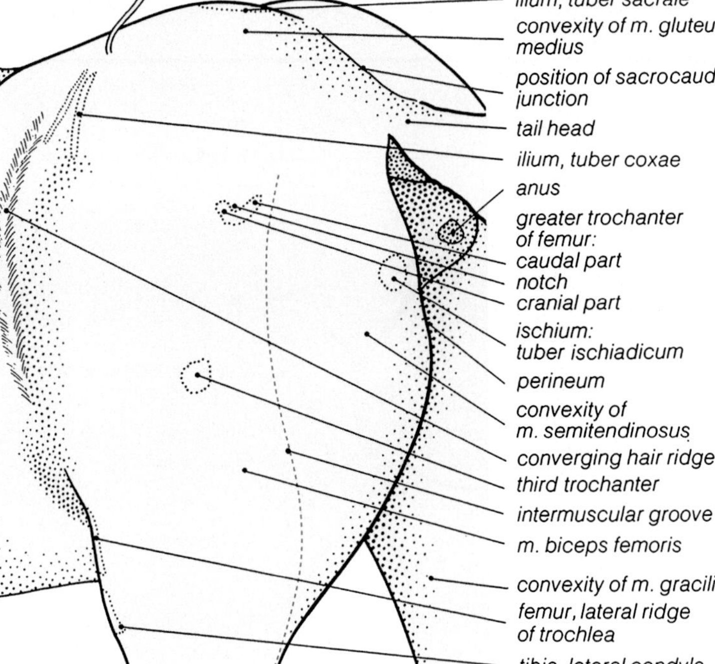
ilium, tuber sacrale
convexity of m. gluteus medius
position of sacrocaudal junction
tail head
ilium, tuber coxae
anus
greater trochanter of femur:
caudal part
notch
cranial part
ischium:
tuber ischiadicum
perineum
convexity of m. semitendinosus
converging hair ridge
third trochanter
intermuscular groove
m. biceps femoris
convexity of m. gracilis
femur, lateral ridge of trochlea
tibia, lateral condyle

Fig. 8.3 Surface features of the pelvic and femoral regions of the gelding: left caudolateral view. The positions of the sacral and caudal vertebrae are shown in Figs. 8.93 and 8.95.

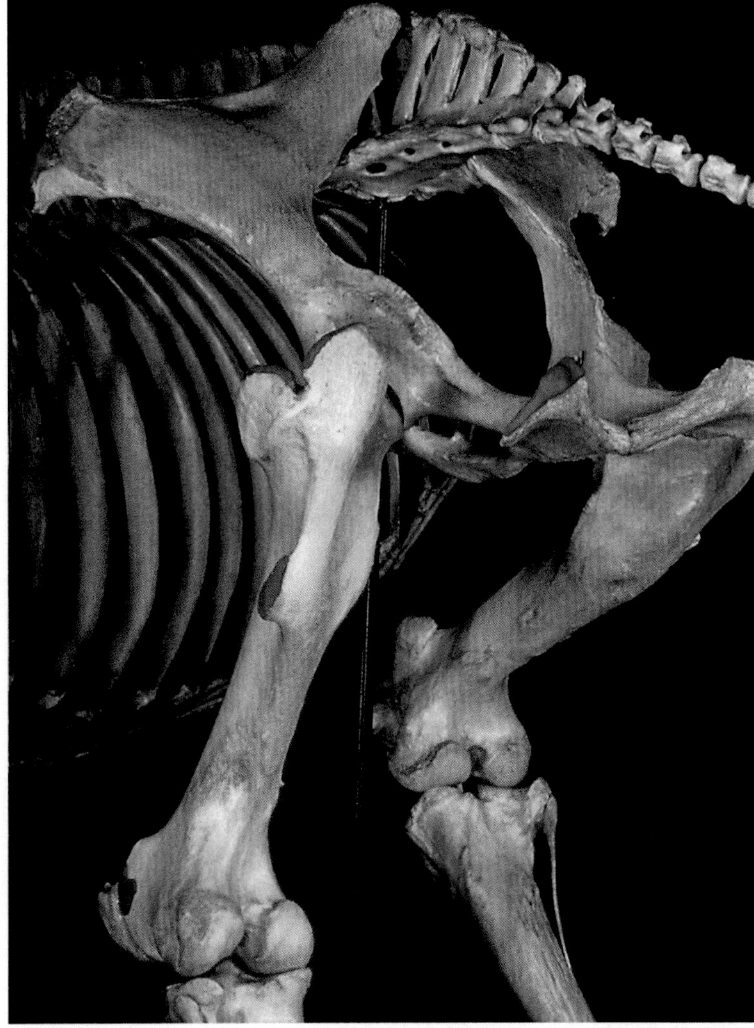

Fig. 8.4 Bones of the pelvic, femoral and stifle regions: left caudolateral view. The bony features shown in Fig. 8.3 are coloured red, except for the tuber sacrale.

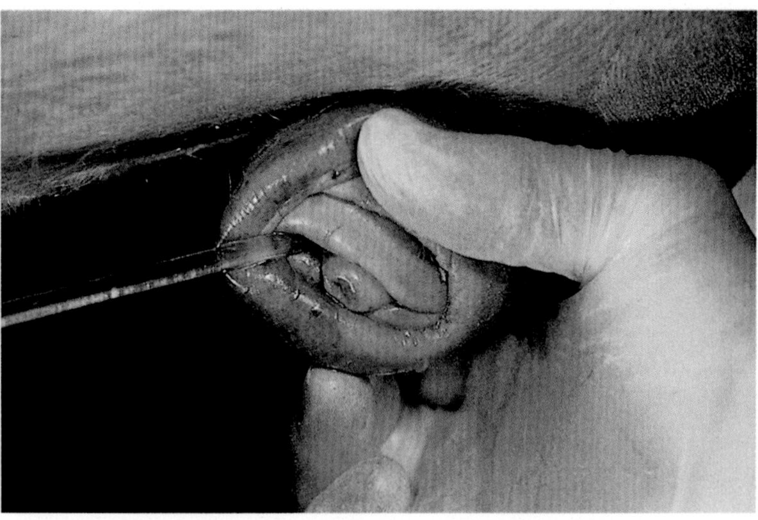

Fig. 8.5 Surface features of the penis and prepuce of the gelding: left lateral view. At birth, the free part of the penis is adherent to the internal lamina of the prepuce (see Fig. 8.47) but this adherence rapidly breaks down (Figs. 8.48 to 8.53) and in geldings and stallions the free part of the penis is separated from the prepuce by the preputial cavity. The urethral process is enclosed by a narrow cavity, the fossa glandis; the sinus urethralis is a dorsal enlargement of this fossa, and its position is indicated by the probe.

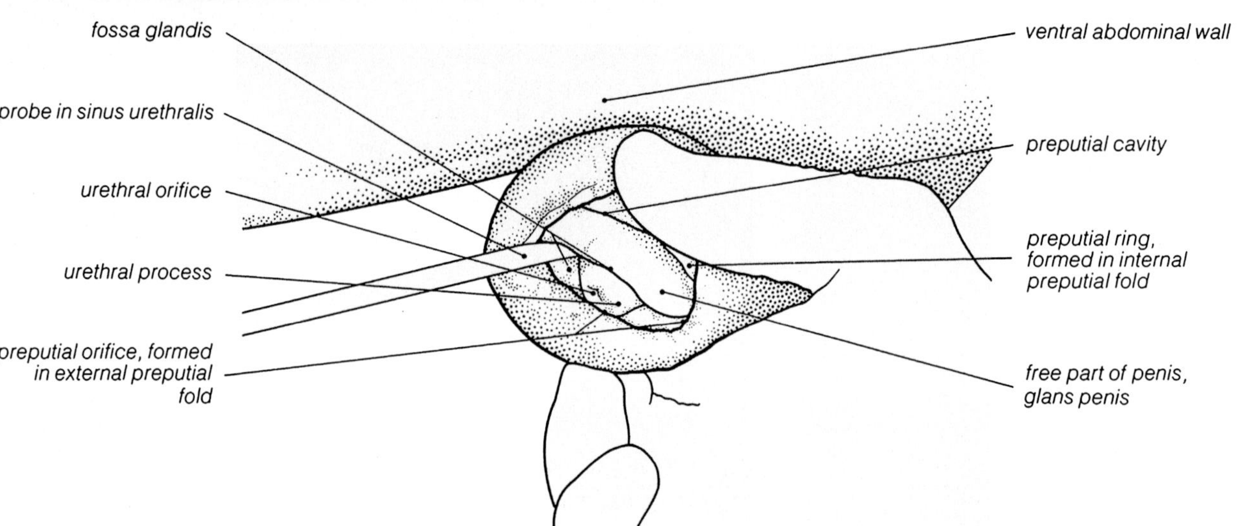
fossa glandis
probe in sinus urethralis
urethral orifice
urethral process
preputial orifice, formed in external preputial fold
ventral abdominal wall
preputial cavity
preputial ring, formed in internal preputial fold
free part of penis, glans penis

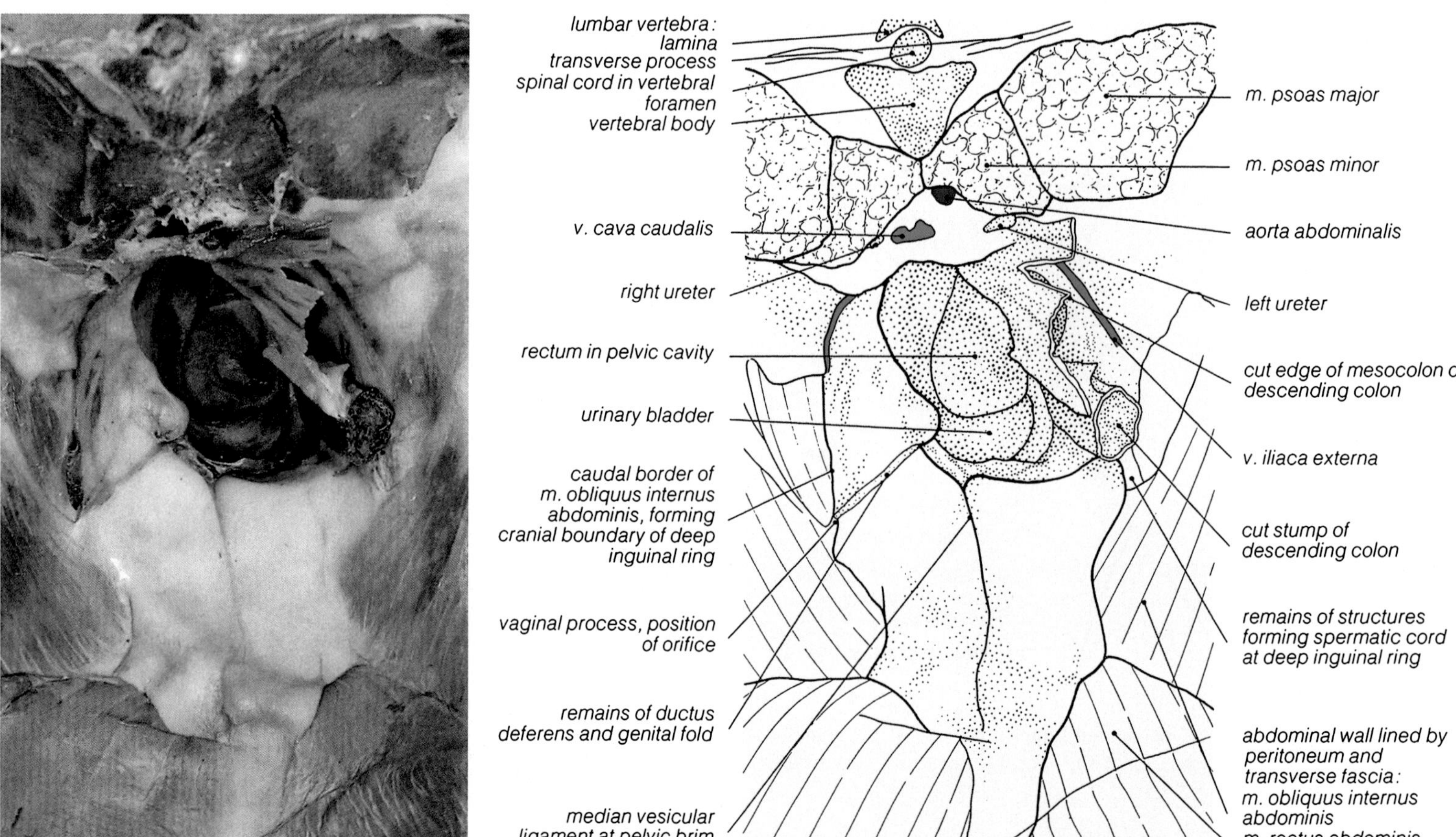
lumbar vertebra:
lamina
transverse process
spinal cord in vertebral foramen
vertebral body
v. cava caudalis
right ureter
rectum in pelvic cavity
urinary bladder
caudal border of m. obliquus internus abdominis, forming cranial boundary of deep inguinal ring
vaginal process, position of orifice
remains of ductus deferens and genital fold
median vesicular ligament at pelvic brim
m. psoas major
m. psoas minor
aorta abdominalis
left ureter
cut edge of mesocolon of descending colon
v. iliaca externa
cut stump of descending colon
remains of structures forming spermatic cord at deep inguinal ring
abdominal wall lined by peritoneum and transverse fascia:
m. obliquus internus abdominis
m. rectus abdominis

Fig. 8.6 The pelvic inlet of the gelding: cranial view. The trunk has been cut through at the level of the third lumbar vertebra after removal of the abdominal viscera. The urinary bladder is empty and entirely pelvic in position. The peritoneum of the inguinal regions remains intact. The corresponding region of the mare is shown in Fig. 5.45 (non-pregnant) and Fig. 8.57.

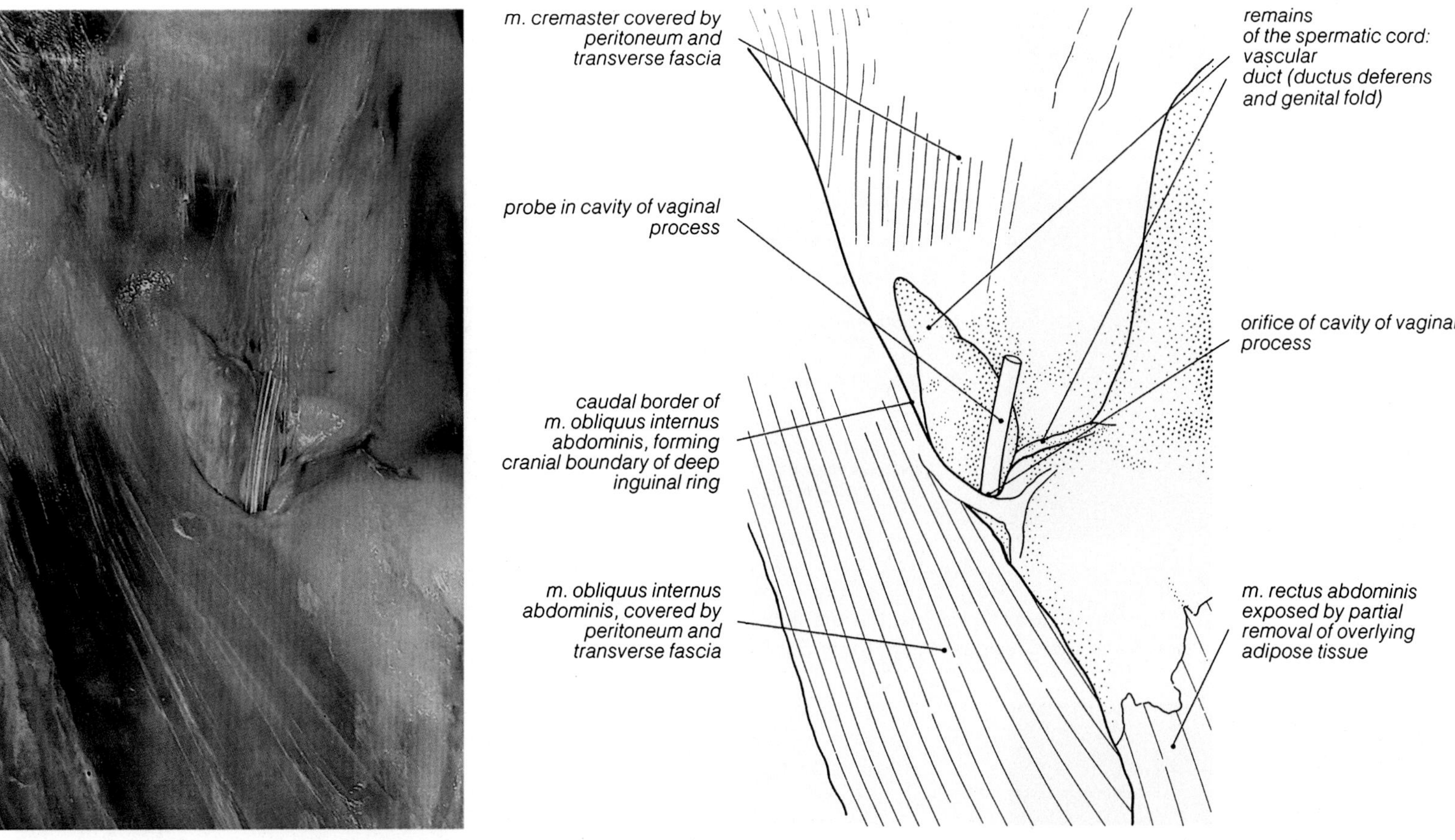
m. cremaster covered by peritoneum and transverse fascia
remains of the spermatic cord: vascular duct (ductus deferens and genital fold)
probe in cavity of vaginal process
orifice of cavity of vaginal process
caudal border of m. obliquus internus abdominis, forming cranial boundary of deep inguinal ring
m. obliquus internus abdominis, covered by peritoneum and transverse fascia
m. rectus abdominis exposed by partial removal of overlying adipose tissue

Fig. 8.7 The right inguinal canal of the gelding: cranial view. This is a closer view of a part of the specimen shown in Fig. 8.6, at a slightly later stage in the dissection. After castration, the components of the spermatic cord atrophy. A probe has been inserted into the persistent and still patent orifice leading to the cavity of the remaining stump of the vaginal process.

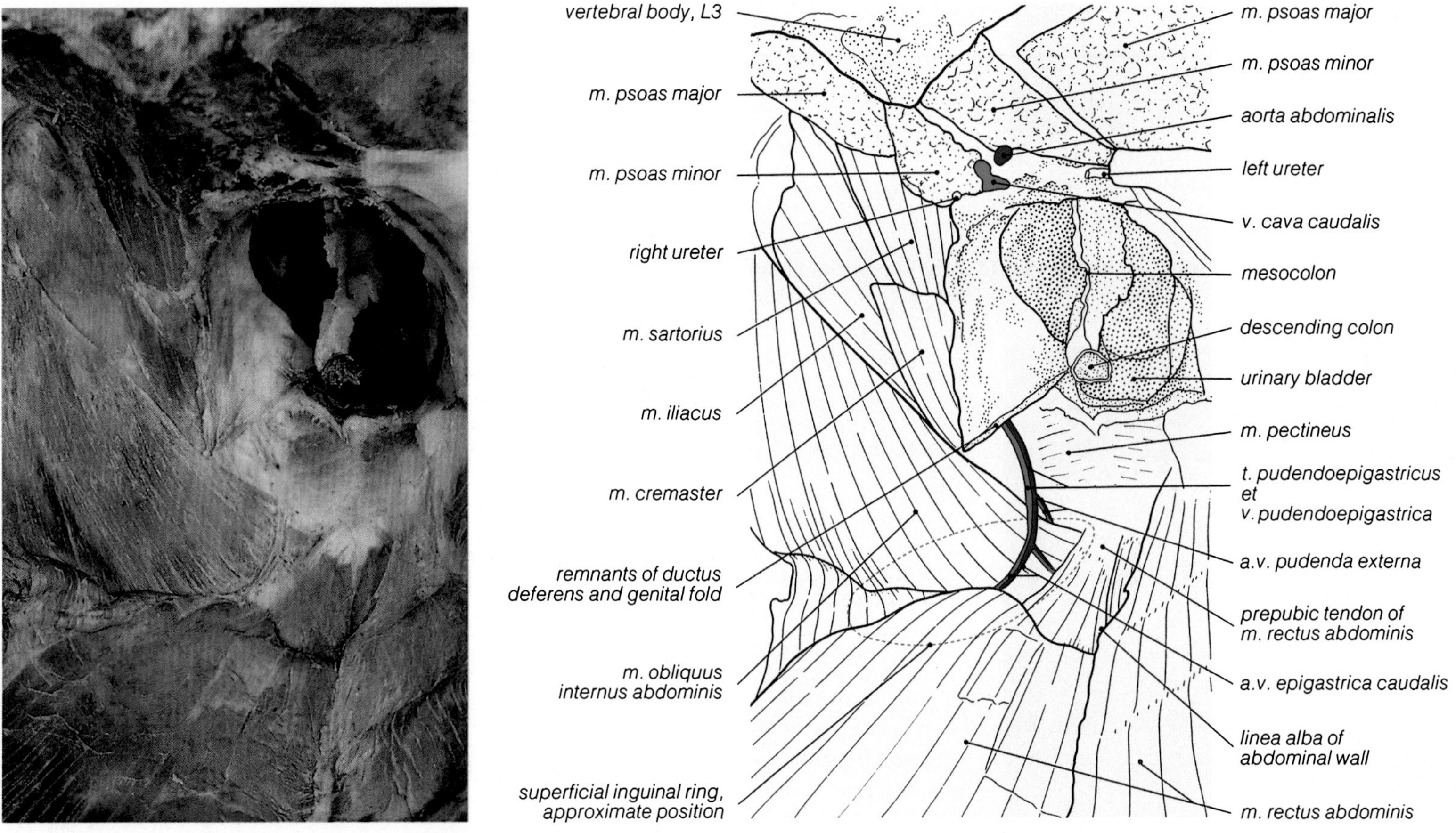
vertebral body, L3
m. psoas major
m. psoas minor
right ureter
m. sartorius
m. iliacus
m. cremaster
remnants of ductus deferens and genital fold
m. obliquus internus abdominis
superficial inguinal ring, approximate position
m. psoas major
m. psoas minor
aorta abdominalis
left ureter
v. cava caudalis
mesocolon
descending colon
urinary bladder
m. pectineus
t. pudendoepigastricus et v. pudendoepigastrica
a.v. pudenda externa
prepubic tendon of m. rectus abdominis
a.v. epigastrica caudalis
linea alba of abdominal wall
m. rectus abdominis

Fig. 8.8 The right inguinal region of the gelding: cranial view. Removal of the peritoneum and transverse fascia reveals the musculature bordering the deep inguinal ring. The iliac fascia has also been removed to reveal the muscles arising from the ilium which lie lateral to the inguinal region. The position of the superficial inguinal ring, formed within the tendon of the external oblique abdominal muscle, is indicated by a broken blue line.

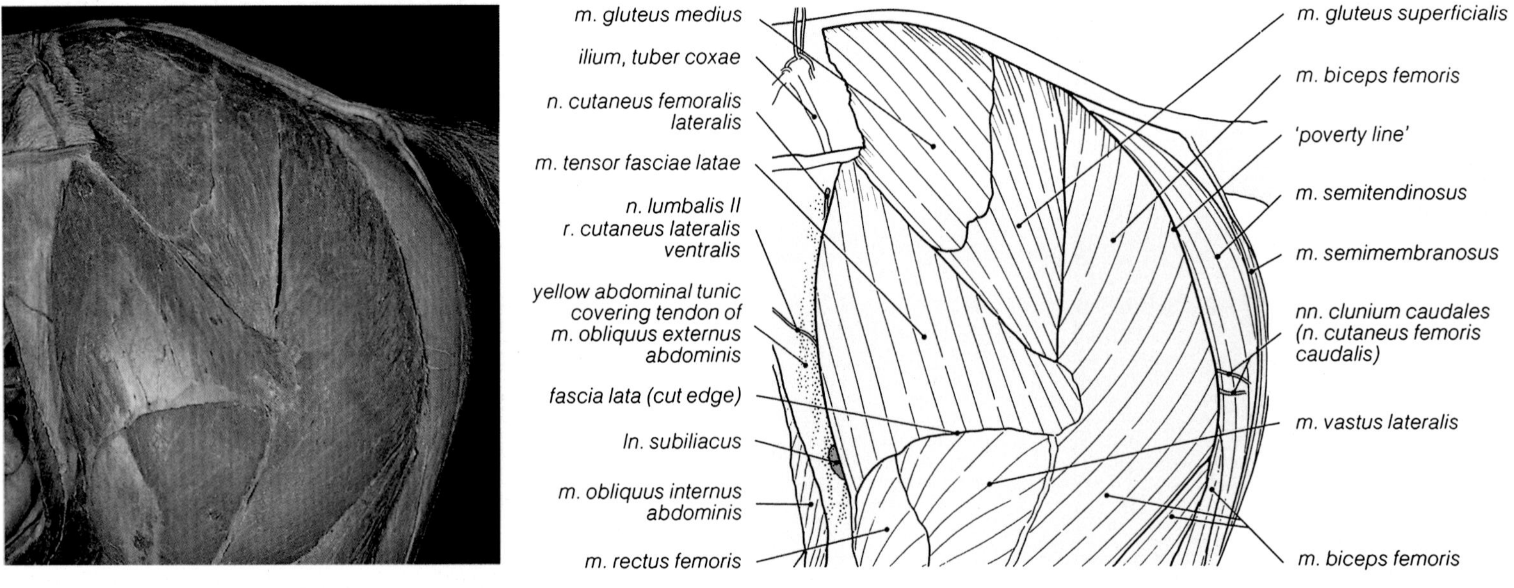
m. gluteus medius
ilium, tuber coxae
n. cutaneus femoralis lateralis
m. tensor fasciae latae
n. lumbalis II r. cutaneus lateralis ventralis
yellow abdominal tunic covering tendon of m. obliquus externus abdominis
fascia lata (cut edge)
ln. subiliacus
m. obliquus internus abdominis
m. rectus femoris
m. gluteus superficialis
m. biceps femoris
'poverty line'
m. semitendinosus
m. semimembranosus
nn. clunium caudales (n. cutaneus femoris caudalis)
m. vastus lateralis
m. biceps femoris

Fig. 8.9 The lateral pelvic wall: left lateral view (1). Removal of the skin and superficial fascia exposes the muscles of the hindlimb that lie lateral to the bony pelvis. The surface features of these regions are shown in Figs. 8.1 and 8.3.

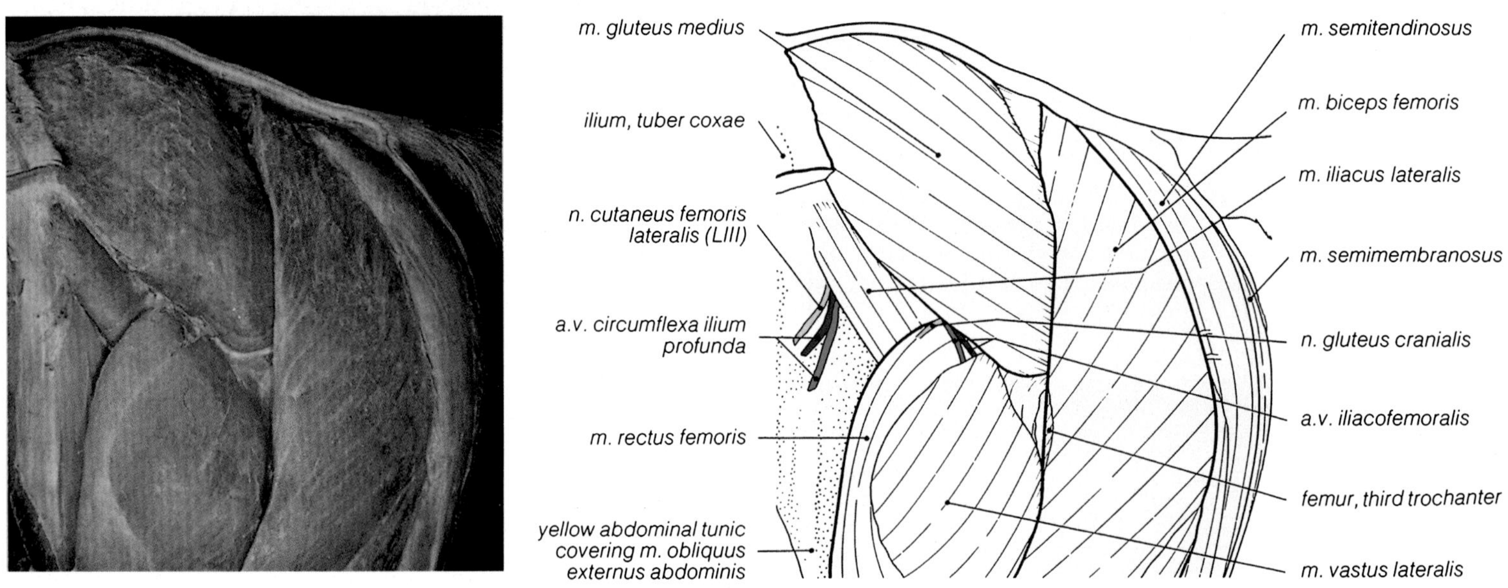
m. gluteus medius
ilium, tuber coxae
n. cutaneus femoris lateralis (LIII)
a.v. circumflexa ilium profunda
m. rectus femoris
yellow abdominal tunic covering m. obliquus externus abdominis
m. semitendinosus
m. biceps femoris
m. iliacus lateralis
m. semimembranosus
n. gluteus cranialis
a.v. iliacofemoralis
femur, third trochanter
m. vastus lateralis

Fig. 8.10 The lateral pelvic wall: left lateral view (2). The superficial gluteal muscle and the tensor muscle of the lateral fascia have been removed.

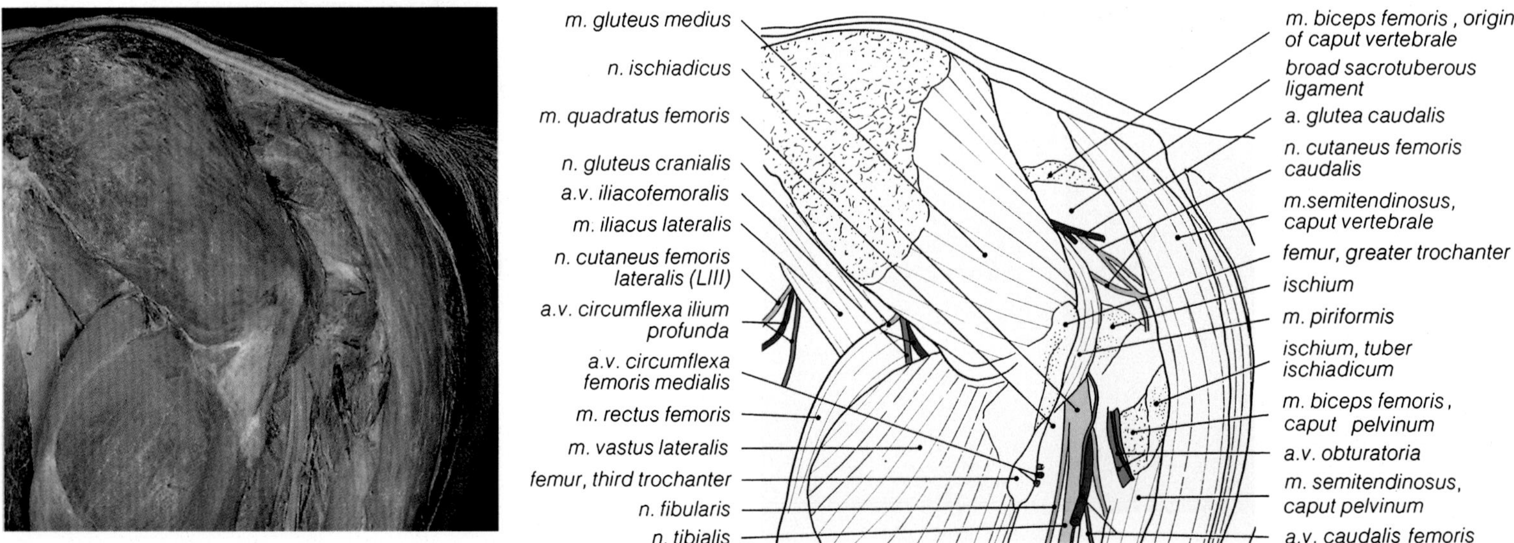
m. gluteus medius
n. ischiadicus
m. quadratus femoris
n. gluteus cranialis
a.v. iliacofemoralis
m. iliacus lateralis
n. cutaneus femoris lateralis (LIII)
a.v. circumflexa ilium profunda
a.v. circumflexa femoris medialis
m. rectus femoris
m. vastus lateralis
femur, third trochanter
n. fibularis
n. tibialis
m. biceps femoris, origin of caput vertebrale
broad sacrotuberous ligament
a. glutea caudalis
n. cutaneus femoris caudalis
m.semitendinosus, caput vertebrale
femur, greater trochanter
ischium
m. piriformis
ischium, tuber ischiadicum
m. biceps femoris, caput pelvinum
a.v. obturatoria
m. semitendinosus, caput pelvinum
a.v. caudalis femoris

Fig. 8.11 The lateral pelvic wall: left lateral view (3). The biceps femoris muscle has been removed, exposing part of the broad sacrotuberous ligament which stretches from the vertebrae to the ischium. The vertebral head of the biceps femoris muscle is thought to be of gluteal origin.

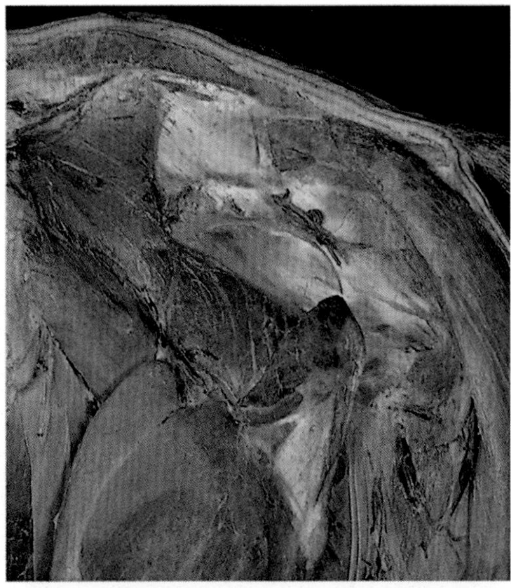

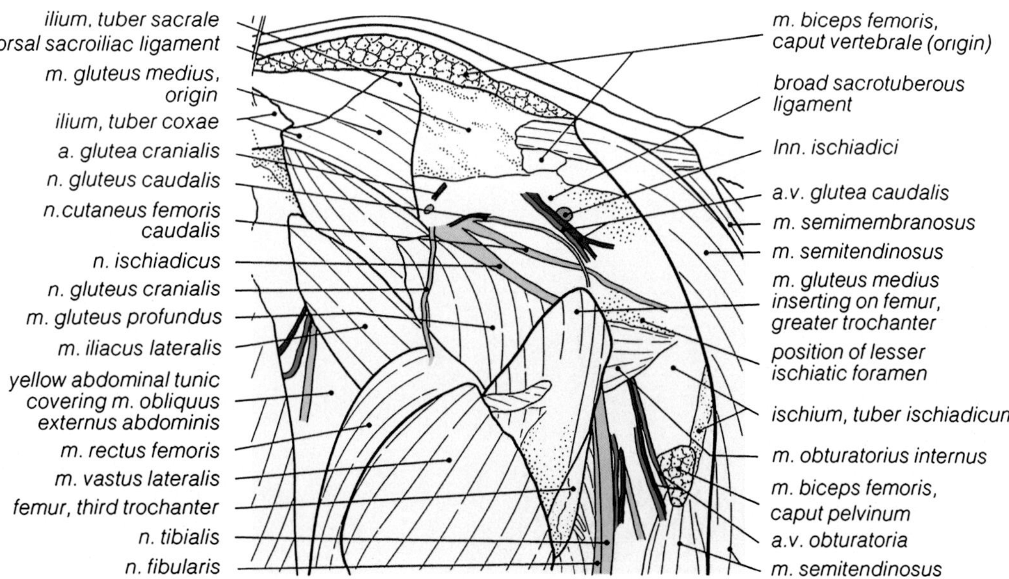

ilium, tuber sacrale
dorsal sacroiliac ligament
m. gluteus medius, origin
ilium, tuber coxae
a. glutea cranialis
n. gluteus caudalis
n. cutaneus femoris caudalis
n. ischiadicus
n. gluteus cranialis
m. gluteus profundus
m. iliacus lateralis
yellow abdominal tunic covering m. obliquus externus abdominis
m. rectus femoris
m. vastus lateralis
femur, third trochanter
n. tibialis
n. fibularis
m. biceps femoris, caput vertebrale (origin)
broad sacrotuberous ligament
lnn. ischiadici
a.v. glutea caudalis
m. semimembranosus
m. semitendinosus
m. gluteus medius inserting on femur, greater trochanter
position of lesser ischiatic foramen
ischium, tuber ischiadicum
m. obturatorius internus
m. biceps femoris, caput pelvinum
a.v. obturatoria
m. semitendinosus

Fig. 8.12 The lateral pelvic wall: left lateral view (4). The removal of the middle gluteal muscle exposes the broad sacrotuberous ligament, its greater ischiatic foramen and the structures that run lateral to it.

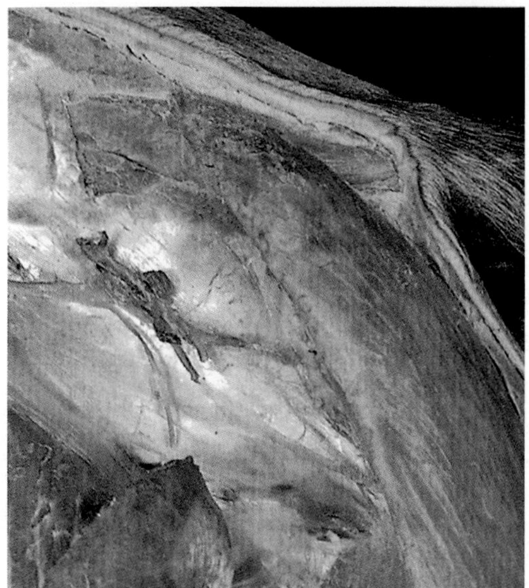

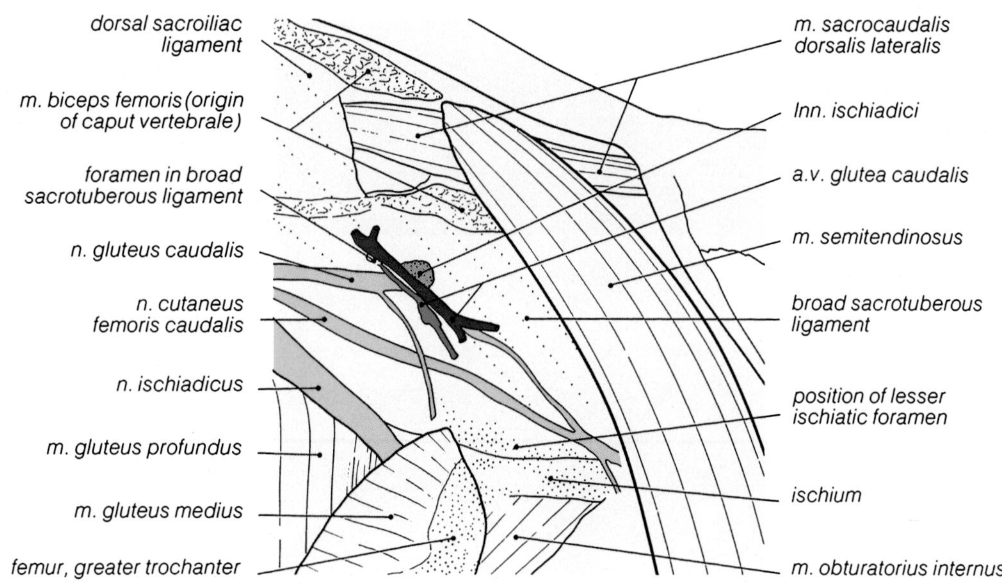

dorsal sacroiliac ligament
m. biceps femoris (origin of caput vertebrale)
foramen in broad sacrotuberous ligament
n. gluteus caudalis
n. cutaneus femoris caudalis
n. ischiadicus
m. gluteus profundus
m. gluteus medius
femur, greater trochanter
m. sacrocaudalis dorsalis lateralis
lnn. ischiadici
a.v. glutea caudalis
m. semitendinosus
broad sacrotuberous ligament
position of lesser ischiatic foramen
ischium
m. obturatorius internus

Fig. 8.13 The broad sacrotuberous ligament: left lateral view (1). This is a closer view of a part of the dissection shown in Fig. 8.12. In the horse, no major vessels or nerves traverse the lesser ischiatic foramen; the caudal gluteal vessels traverse a more dorsal and cranial foramen in the broad sacrotuberous ligament (see Fig. 8.14).

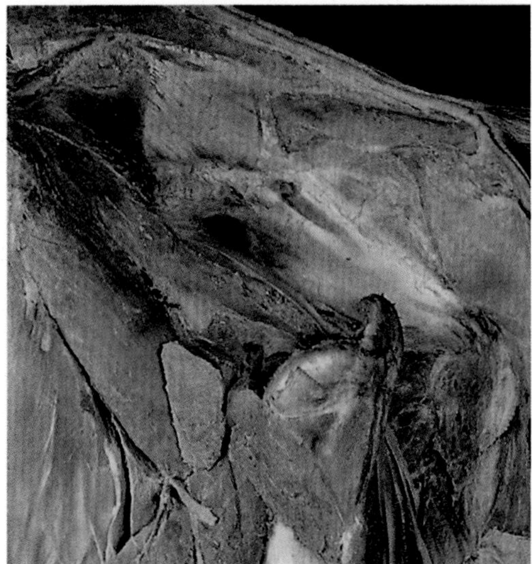

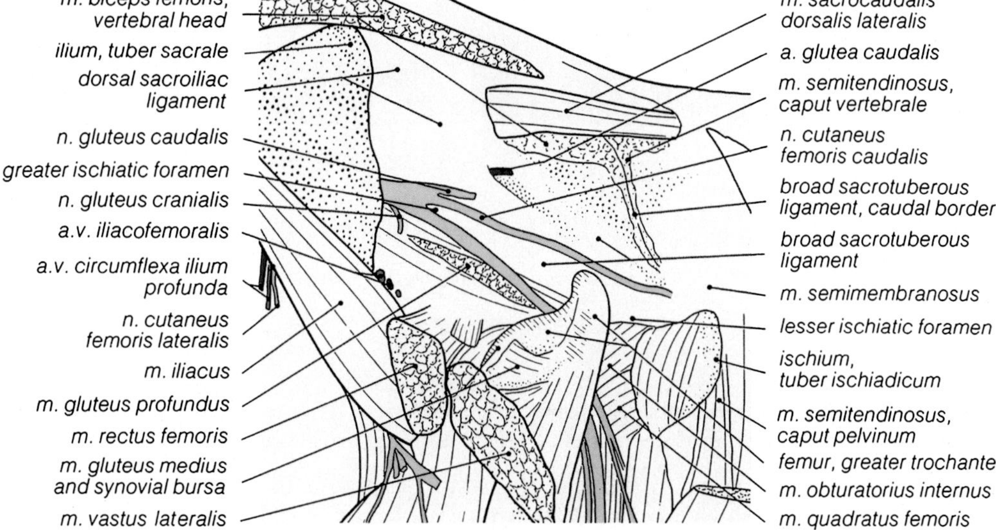

m. biceps femoris, vertebral head
ilium, tuber sacrale
dorsal sacroiliac ligament
n. gluteus caudalis
greater ischiatic foramen
n. gluteus cranialis
a.v. iliacofemoralis
a.v. circumflexa ilium profunda
n. cutaneus femoris lateralis
m. iliacus
m. gluteus profundus
m. rectus femoris
m. gluteus medius and synovial bursa
m. vastus lateralis
m. sacrocaudalis dorsalis lateralis
a. glutea caudalis
m. semitendinosus, caput vertebrale
n. cutaneus femoris caudalis
broad sacrotuberous ligament, caudal border
broad sacrotuberous ligament
m. semimembranosus
lesser ischiatic foramen
ischium, tuber ischiadicum
m. semitendinosus, caput pelvinum
femur, greater trochanter
m. obturatorius internus
m. quadratus femoris

Fig. 8.14 The broad sacrotuberous ligament: left lateral view (2). Removal of the vertebral head of the semitendinosus muscle exposes the caudal border of the ligament, from which all three 'hamstring' muscles arise. The three large foramina in the broad sacrotuberous ligament have been demonstrated more clearly in this dissection.

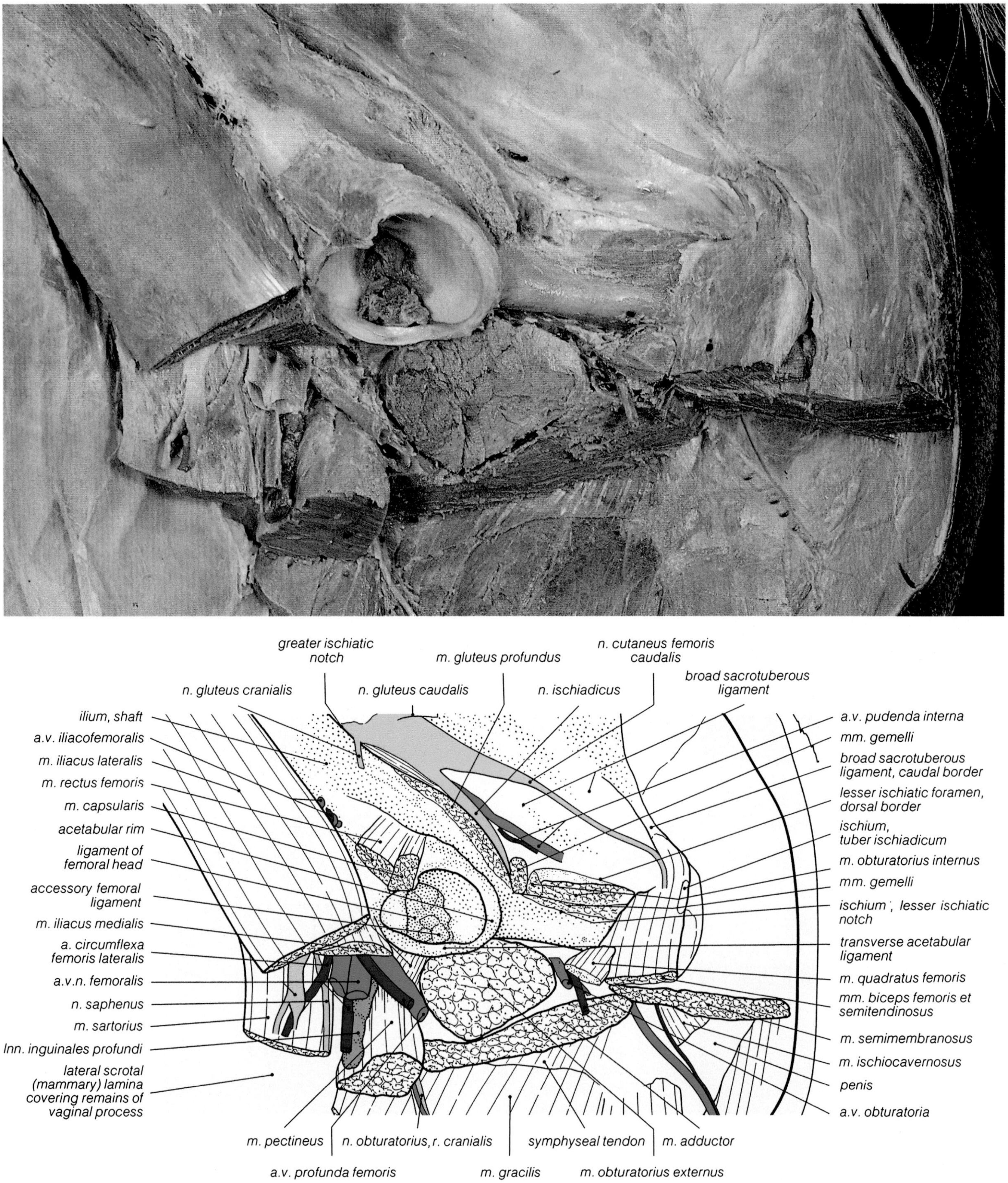

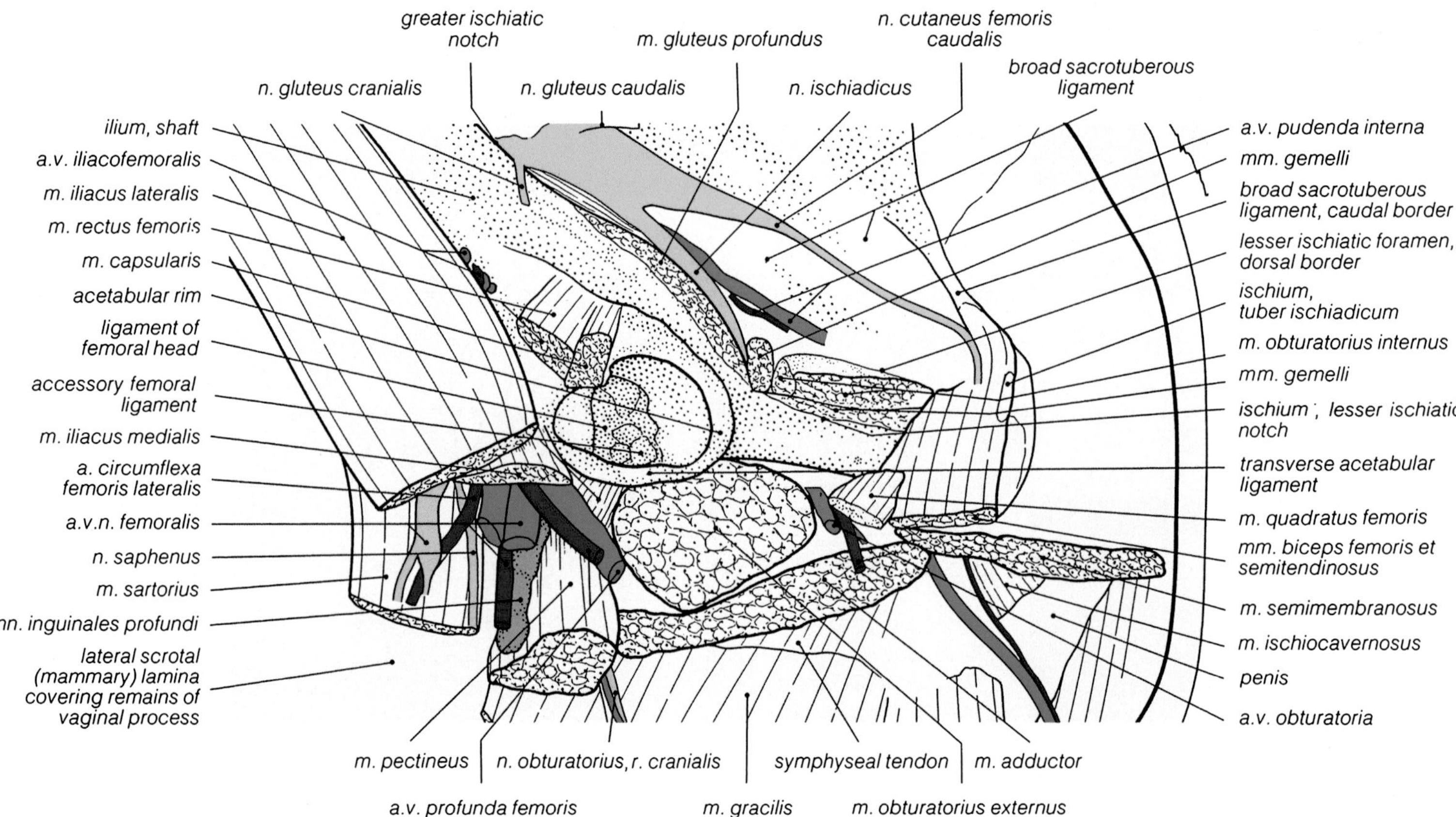
greater ischiatic notch
m. gluteus profundus
n. cutaneus femoris caudalis
n. gluteus cranialis
n. gluteus caudalis
n. ischiadicus
broad sacrotuberous ligament
ilium, shaft
a.v. iliacofemoralis
m. iliacus lateralis
m. rectus femoris
m. capsularis
acetabular rim
ligament of femoral head
accessory femoral ligament
m. iliacus medialis
a. circumflexa femoris lateralis
a.v.n. femoralis
n. saphenus
m. sartorius
lnn. inguinales profundi
lateral scrotal (mammary) lamina covering remains of vaginal process
a.v. pudenda interna
mm. gemelli
broad sacrotuberous ligament, caudal border
lesser ischiatic foramen, dorsal border
ischium, tuber ischiadicum
m. obturatorius internus
mm. gemelli
ischium ; lesser ischiatic notch
transverse acetabular ligament
m. quadratus femoris
mm. biceps femoris et semitendinosus
m. semimembranosus
m. ischiocavernosus
penis
a.v. obturatoria
m. pectineus
n. obturatorius, r. cranialis
symphyseal tendon
m. adductor
a.v. profunda femoris
m. gracilis
m. obturatorius externus

Fig. 8.15 The hip joint after removal of the femur: left lateral view. After removal of the hindlimb, the muscles that attached the limb to the body have been cut back to show the related vessels and nerves of the hindlimb.

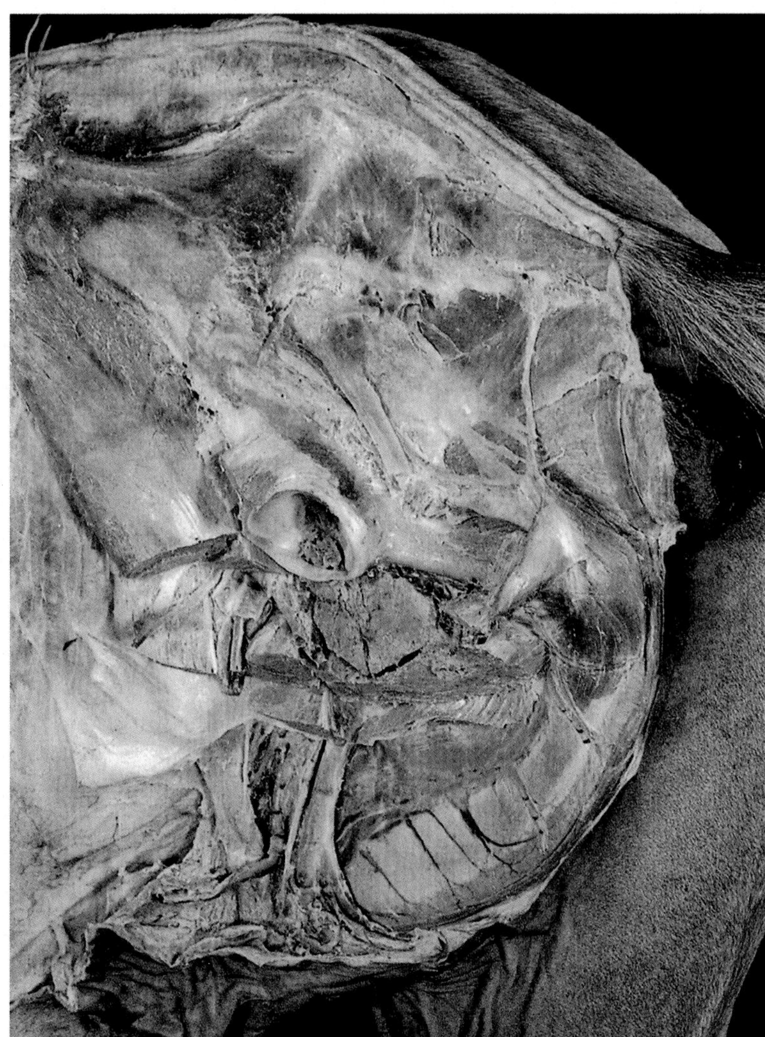

Fig. 8.16 The pelvic cavity and the inguinal region: left lateral view (1). The broad sacrotuberous ligament has been removed, exposing the muscles and nerves of the pelvis. Removal of parts of the gracilis muscle reveals a superficial view of the inguinal and penile regions. The next stage of the dissection is shown in Fig. 8.20.

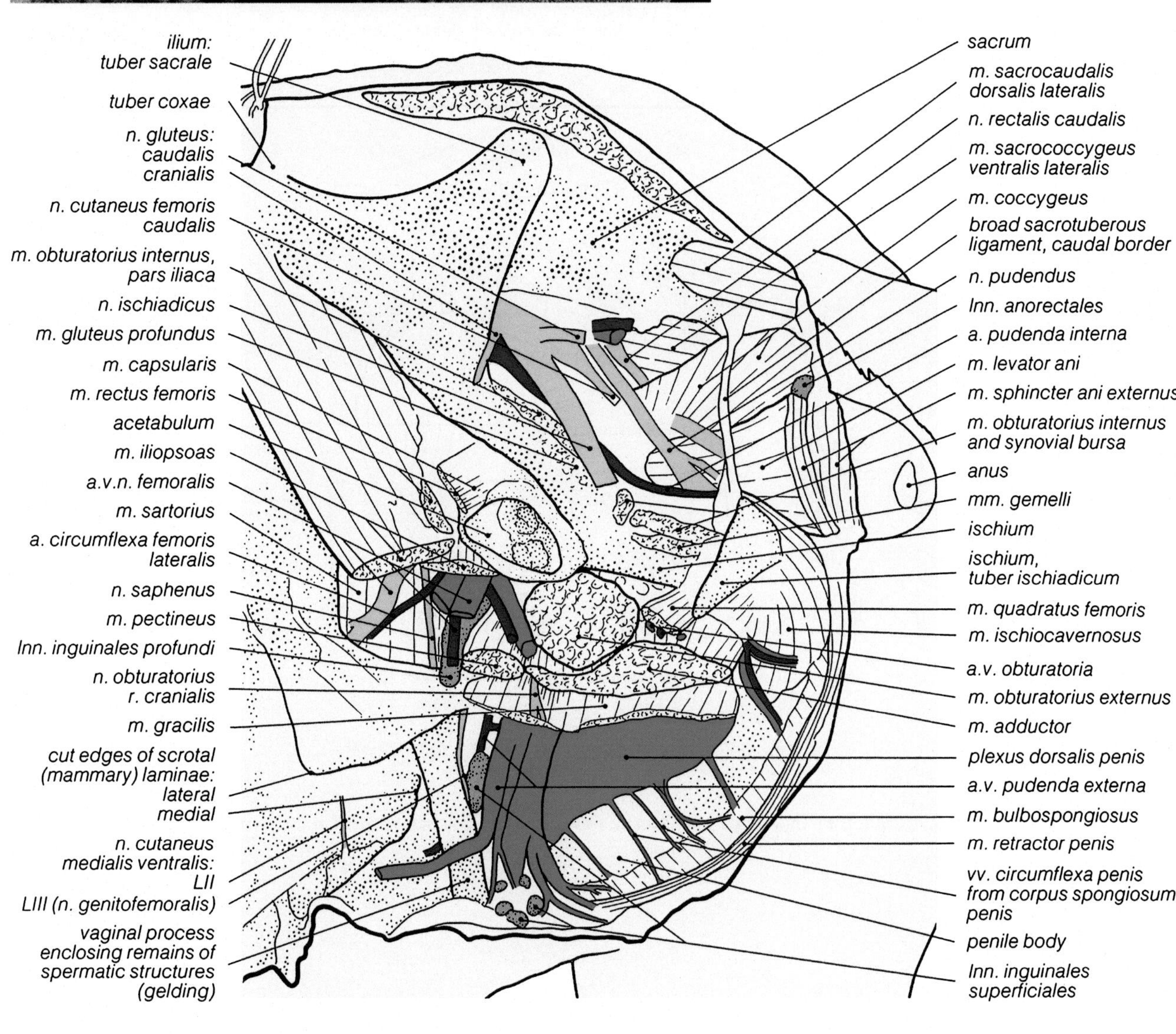
ilium:
tuber sacrale
tuber coxae
n. gluteus:
caudalis
cranialis
n. cutaneus femoris
caudalis
m. obturatorius internus,
pars iliaca
n. ischiadicus
m. gluteus profundus
m. capsularis
m. rectus femoris
acetabulum
m. iliopsoas
a.v.n. femoralis
m. sartorius
a. circumflexa femoris
lateralis
n. saphenus
m. pectineus
lnn. inguinales profundi
n. obturatorius
r. cranialis
m. gracilis
cut edges of scrotal
(mammary) laminae:
lateral
medial
n. cutaneus
medialis ventralis:
LII
LIII (n. genitofemoralis)
vaginal process
enclosing remains of
spermatic structures
(gelding)
sacrum
m. sacrocaudalis
dorsalis lateralis
n. rectalis caudalis
m. sacrococcygeus
ventralis lateralis
m. coccygeus
broad sacrotuberous
ligament, caudal border
n. pudendus
lnn. anorectales
a. pudenda interna
m. levator ani
m. sphincter ani externus
m. obturatorius internus
and synovial bursa
anus
mm. gemelli
ischium
ischium,
tuber ischiadicum
m. quadratus femoris
m. ischiocavernosus
a.v. obturatoria
m. obturatorius externus
m. adductor
plexus dorsalis penis
a.v. pudenda externa
m. bulbospongiosus
m. retractor penis
vv. circumflexa penis
from corpus spongiosum
penis
penile body
lnn. inguinales
superficiales

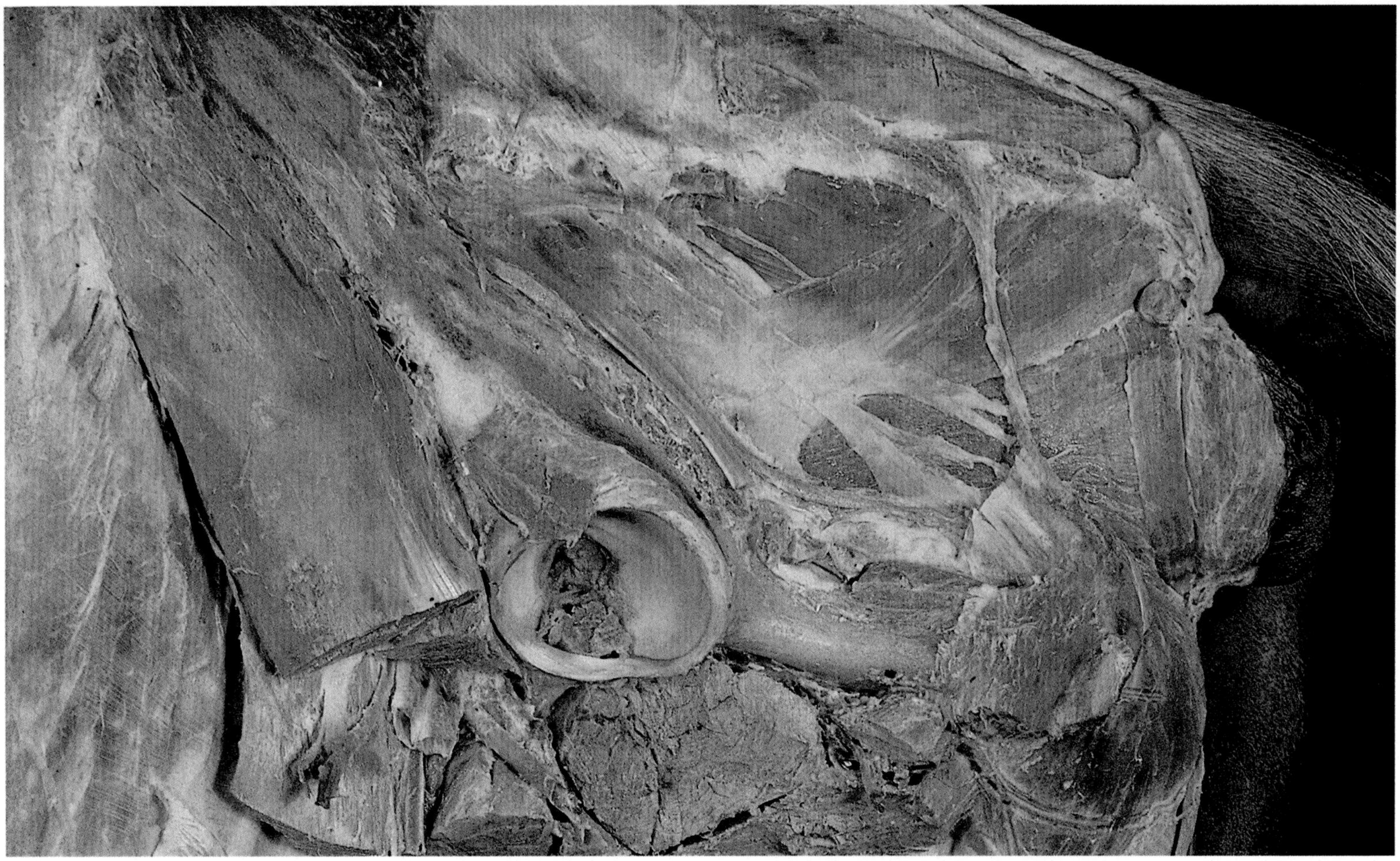

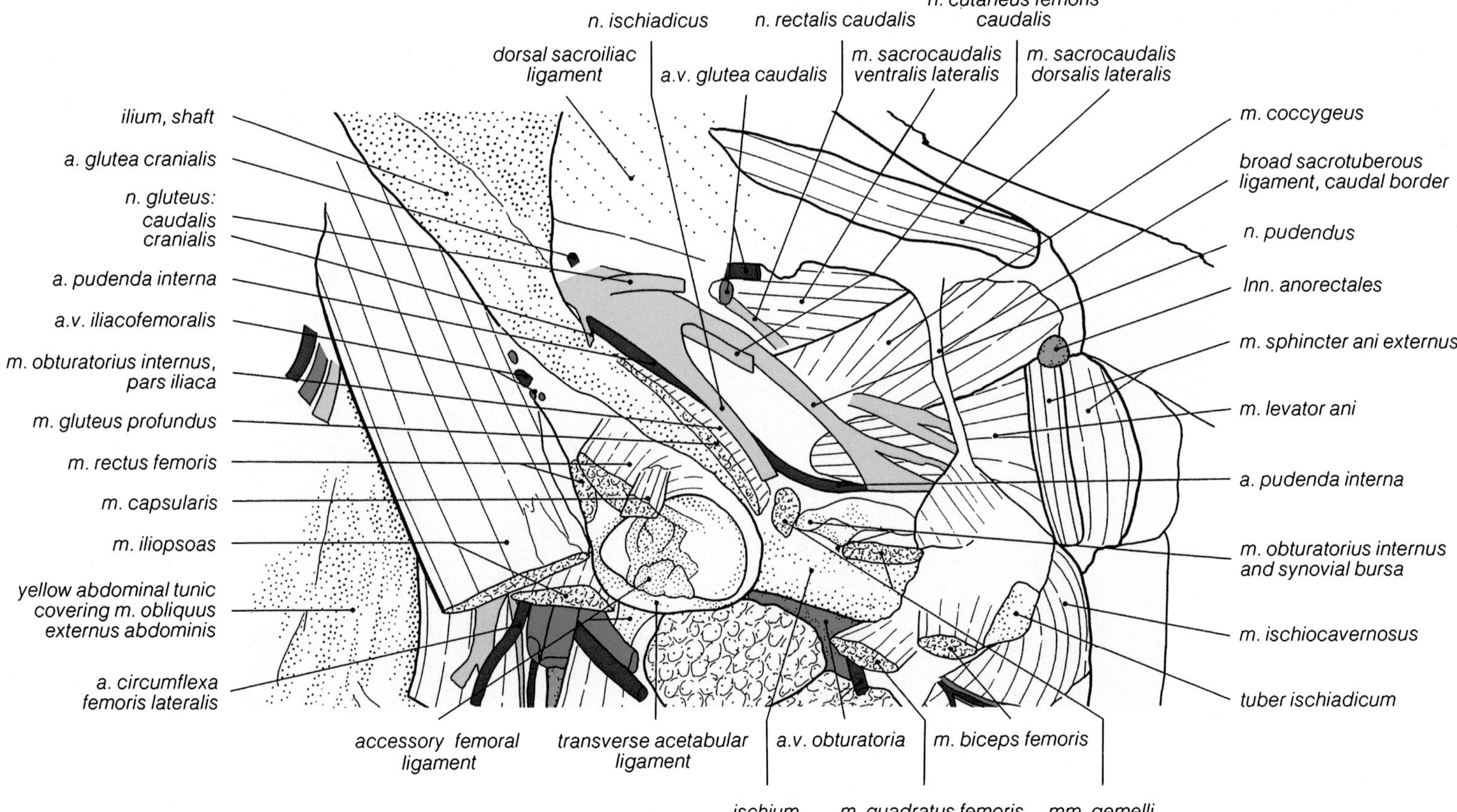
n. ischiadicus
n. rectalis caudalis
n. cutaneus femoris caudalis
dorsal sacroiliac ligament
a.v. glutea caudalis
m. sacrocaudalis ventralis lateralis
m. sacrocaudalis dorsalis lateralis
ilium, shaft
a. glutea cranialis
n. gluteus: caudalis cranialis
a. pudenda interna
a.v. iliacofemoralis
m. obturatorius internus, pars iliaca
m. gluteus profundus
m. rectus femoris
m. capsularis
m. iliopsoas
yellow abdominal tunic covering m. obliquus externus abdominis
a. circumflexa femoris lateralis
m. coccygeus
broad sacrotuberous ligament, caudal border
n. pudendus
lnn. anorectales
m. sphincter ani externus
m. levator ani
a. pudenda interna
m. obturatorius internus and synovial bursa
m. ischiocavernosus
tuber ischiadicum
accessory femoral ligament
transverse acetabular ligament
a.v. obturatoria
m. biceps femoris
ischium
m. quadratus femoris
mm. gemelli

Fig. 8.17 The pelvic cavity after removal of the broad sacrotuberous ligament: left lateral view. This is a closer view of a part of the dissection shown in Fig. 8.16.

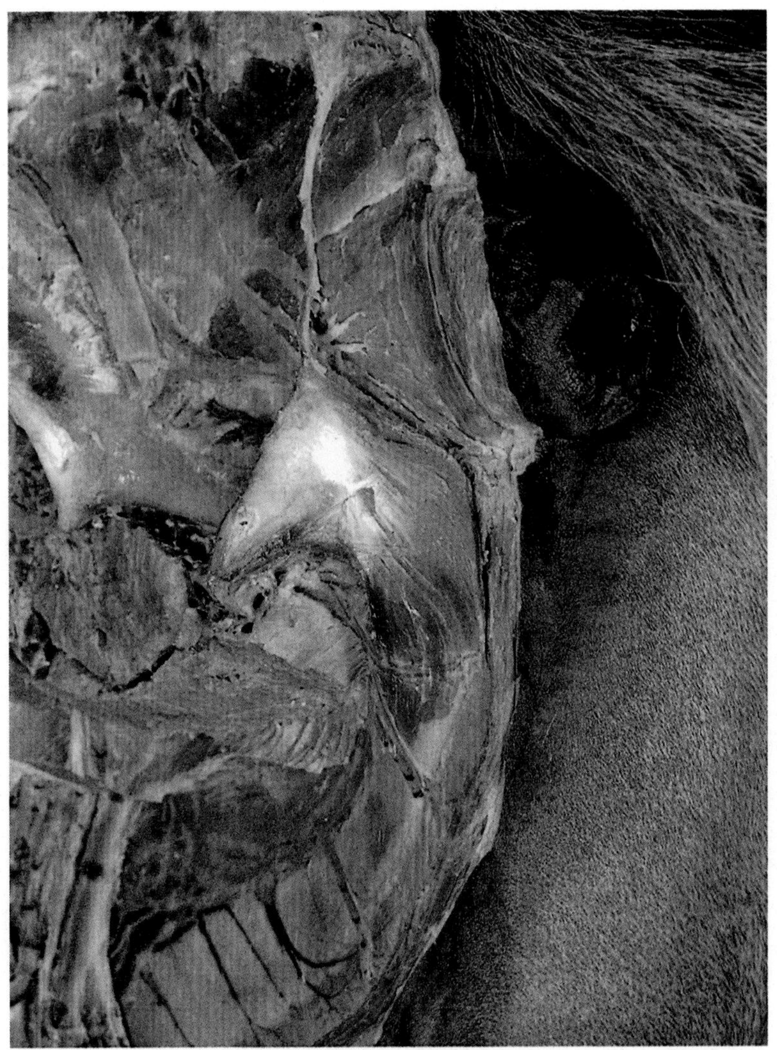

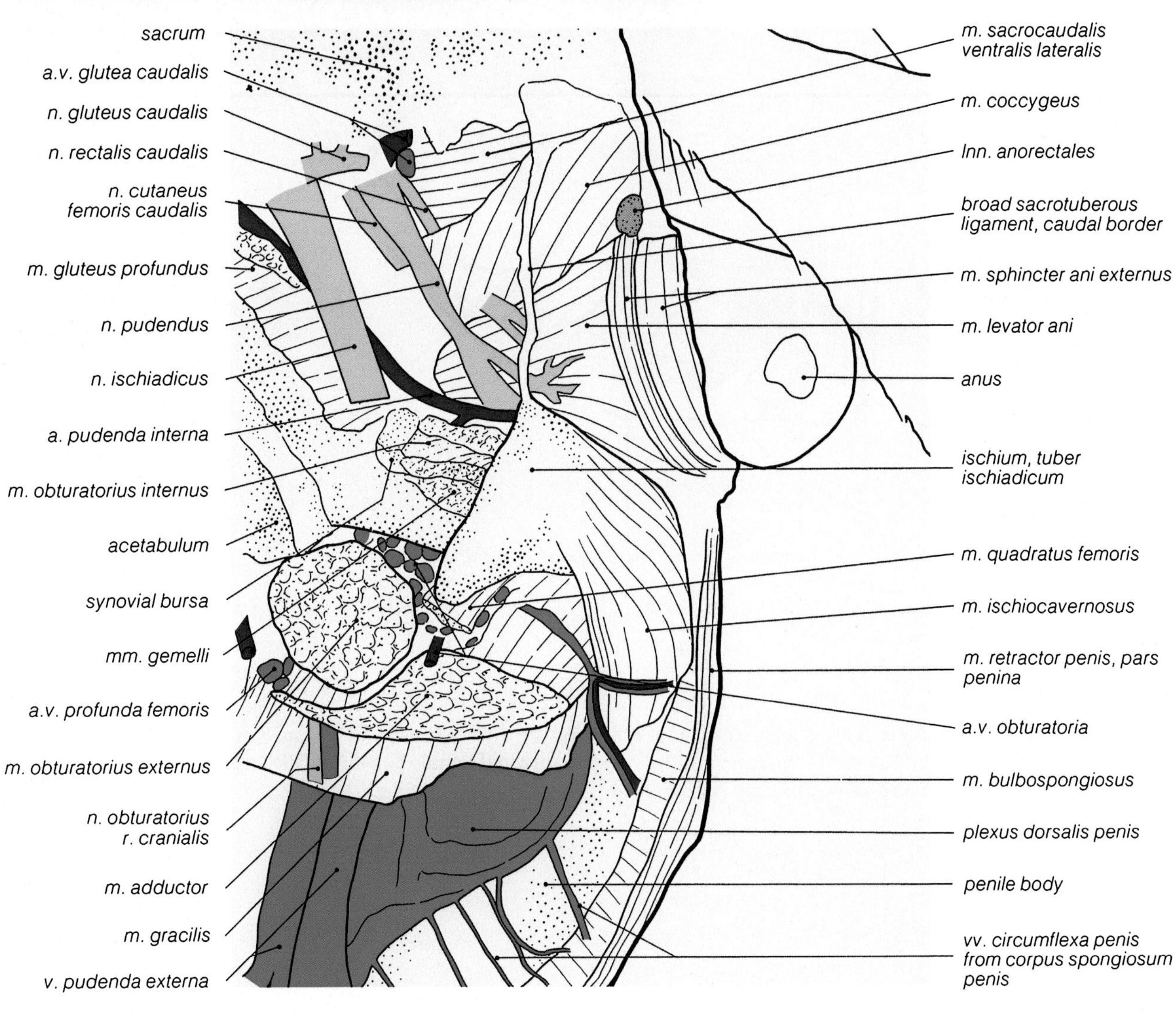
sacrum
a.v. glutea caudalis
n. gluteus caudalis
n. rectalis caudalis
n. cutaneus femoris caudalis
m. gluteus profundus
n. pudendus
n. ischiadicus
a. pudenda interna
m. obturatorius internus
acetabulum
synovial bursa
mm. gemelli
a.v. profunda femoris
m. obturatorius externus
n. obturatorius r. cranialis
m. adductor
m. gracilis
v. pudenda externa
m. sacrocaudalis ventralis lateralis
m. coccygeus
lnn. anorectales
broad sacrotuberous ligament, caudal border
m. sphincter ani externus
m. levator ani
anus
ischium, tuber ischiadicum
m. quadratus femoris
m. ischiocavernosus
m. retractor penis, pars penina
a.v. obturatoria
m. bulbospongiosus
plexus dorsalis penis
penile body
vv. circumflexa penis from corpus spongiosum penis

Fig. 8.18 The pelvic outlet and the penile root: left caudolateral view. This is a closer view of a part of the dissection shown in Fig. 8.16. The more caudal view shows the relationship of the structures in the perianal region.

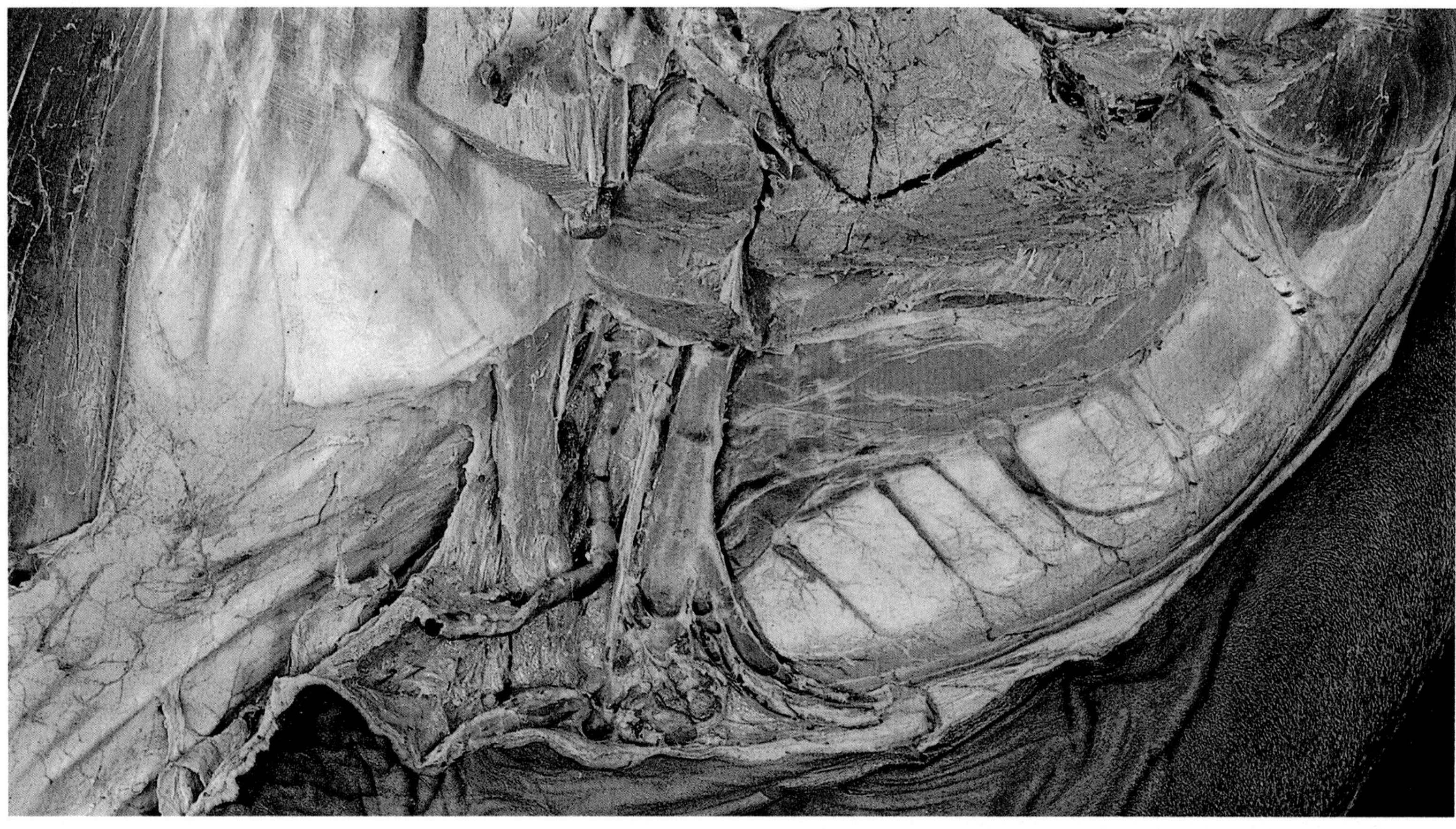

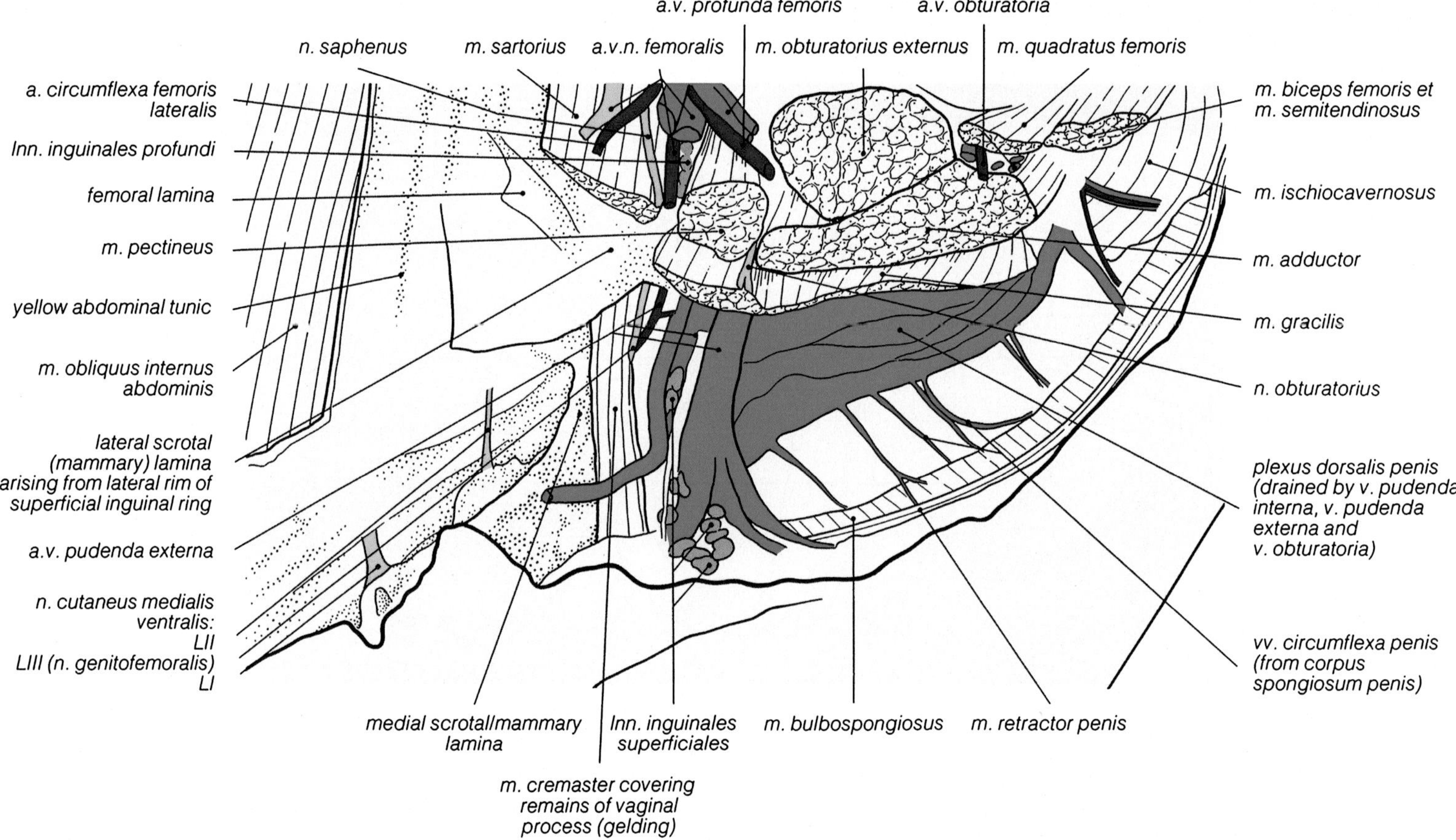
a.v. profunda femoris
a.v. obturatoria
n. saphenus
m. sartorius
a.v.n. femoralis
m. obturatorius externus
m. quadratus femoris
a. circumflexa femoris lateralis
lnn. inguinales profundi
femoral lamina
m. pectineus
yellow abdominal tunic
m. obliquus internus abdominis
lateral scrotal (mammary) lamina arising from lateral rim of superficial inguinal ring
a.v. pudenda externa
n. cutaneus medialis ventralis:
LII
LIII (n. genitofemoralis)
LI
m. biceps femoris et m. semitendinosus
m. ischiocavernosus
m. adductor
m. gracilis
n. obturatorius
plexus dorsalis penis (drained by v. pudenda interna, v. pudenda externa and v. obturatoria)
vv. circumflexa penis (from corpus spongiosum penis)
medial scrotal/mammary lamina
lnn. inguinales superficiales
m. bulbospongiosus
m. retractor penis
m. cremaster covering remains of vaginal process (gelding)

Fig. 8.19 The inguinal region and the penis: left lateral view. This is a closer view of a part of the dissection shown in Fig. 8.16. The lateral scrotal/ mammary lamina has been partly removed to reveal the structures entering and leaving the inguinal canal, but the superficial inguinal ring is not yet distinct. The scrotal structures and penis of the stallion are shown in Figs. 8.36 to 8.44

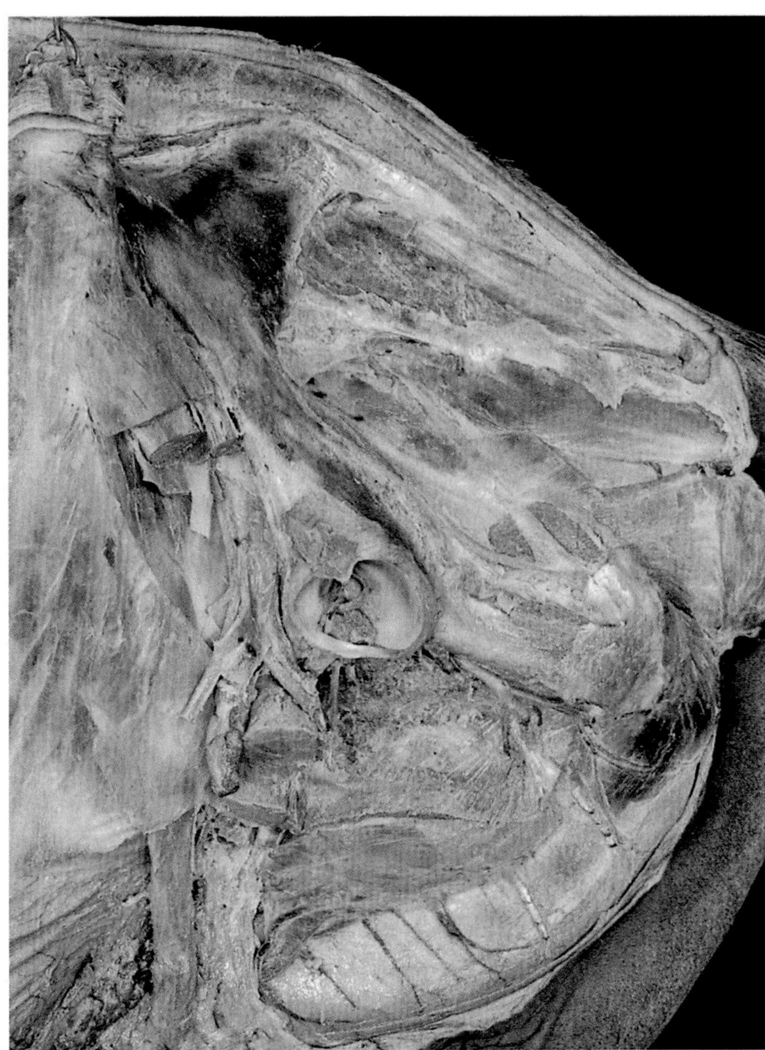

Fig. 8.20 The pelvic cavity and the inguinal region: left lateral view (2). The adductor and external obturator muscles have been removed. The ischiatic nerve and the coccygeus muscle have been shortened. The iliopsoas and sartorius muscles have been shortened and the large external pudendal veins have been partially excised.

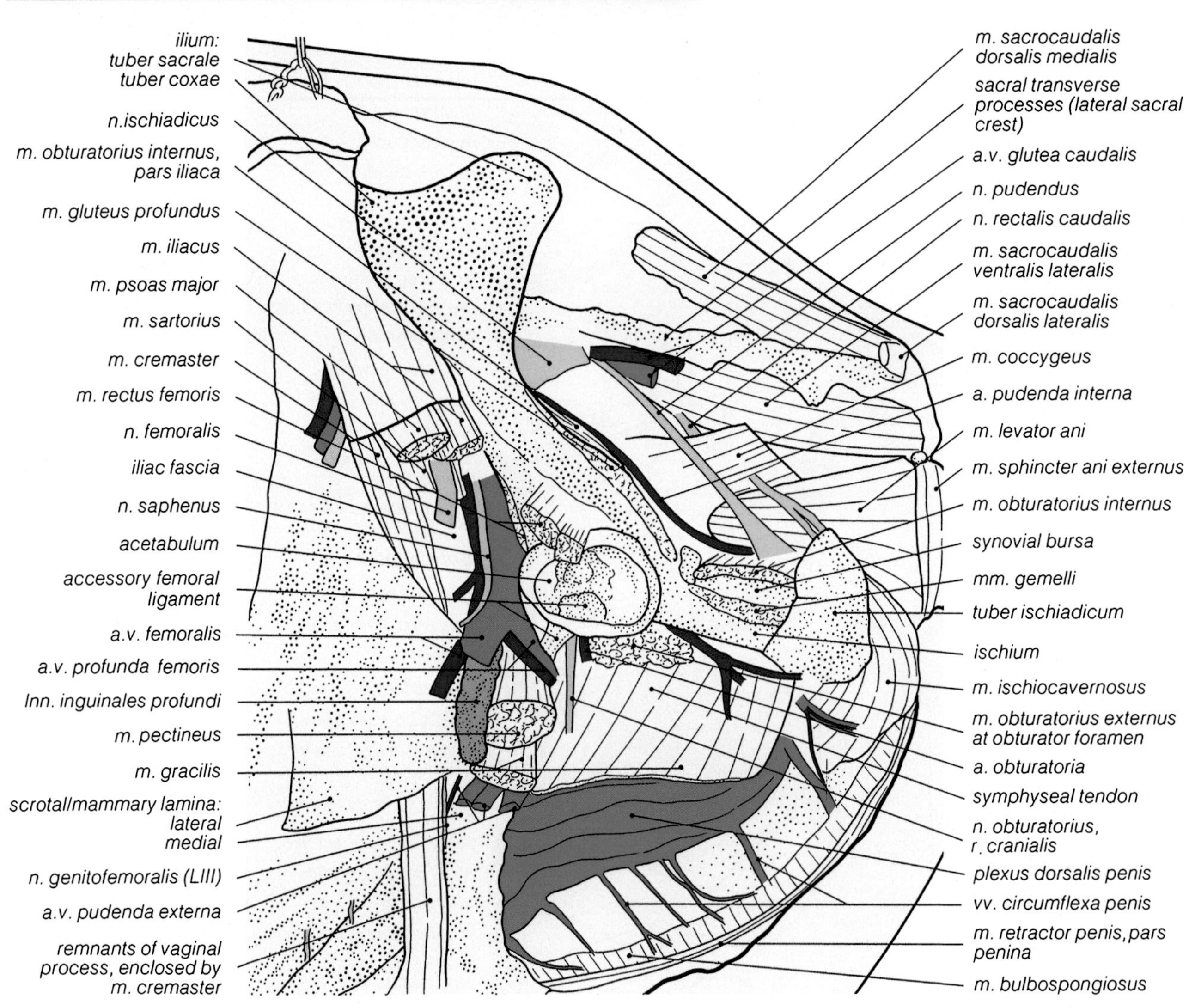
ilium:
tuber sacrale
tuber coxae
n.ischiadicus
m. obturatorius internus, pars iliaca
m. gluteus profundus
m. iliacus
m. psoas major
m. sartorius
m. cremaster
m. rectus femoris
n. femoralis
iliac fascia
n. saphenus
acetabulum
accessory femoral ligament
a.v. femoralis
a.v. profunda femoris
lnn. inguinales profundi
m. pectineus
m. gracilis
scrotal/mammary lamina:
lateral
medial
n. genitofemoralis (LIII)
a.v. pudenda externa
remnants of vaginal process, enclosed by m. cremaster
m. sacrocaudalis dorsalis medialis
sacral transverse processes (lateral sacral crest)
a.v. glutea caudalis
n. pudendus
n. rectalis caudalis
m. sacrocaudalis ventralis lateralis
m. sacrocaudalis dorsalis lateralis
m. coccygeus
a. pudenda interna
m. levator ani
m. sphincter ani externus
m. obturatorius internus
synovial bursa
mm. gemelli
tuber ischiadicum
ischium
m. ischiocavernosus
m. obturatorius externus at obturator foramen
a. obturatoria
symphyseal tendon
n. obturatorius, r. cranialis
plexus dorsalis penis
vv. circumflexa penis
m. retractor penis, pars penina
m. bulbospongiosus

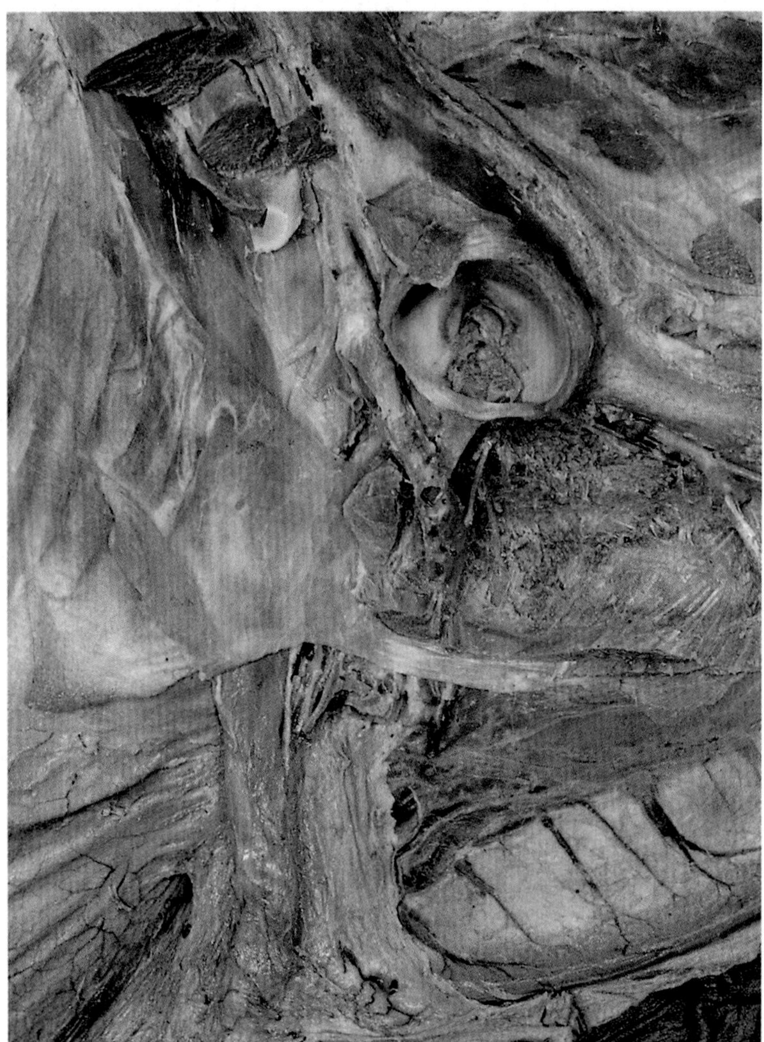

Fig. 8.21 Inguinal structures of the gelding: left lateral view (1). The origin of the lateral scrotal/mammary lamina from the deep abdominal fascia (yellow abdominal tunic) has been cut at the base of the superficial inguinal ring to reveal more clearly the structures that traverse the inguinal canal. A blue rod indicates one of the several components of the external pudendal vein that traverse the thigh muscles, and do not traverse the inguinal canal.

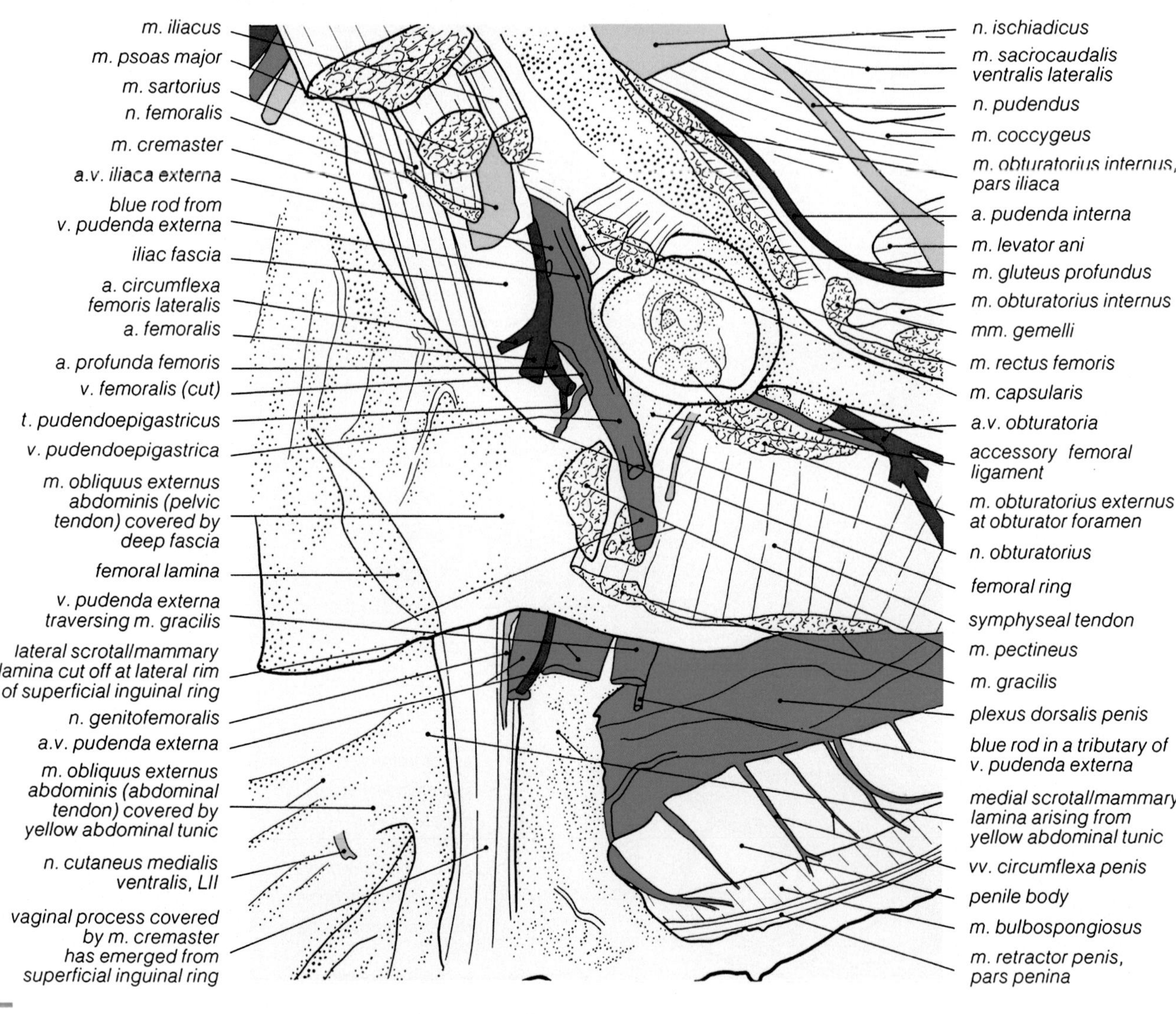
m. iliacus
m. psoas major
m. sartorius
n. femoralis
m. cremaster
a.v. iliaca externa
blue rod from v. pudenda externa
iliac fascia
a. circumflexa femoris lateralis
a. femoralis
a. profunda femoris
v. femoralis (cut)
t. pudendoepigastricus
v. pudendoepigastrica
m. obliquus externus abdominis (pelvic tendon) covered by deep fascia
femoral lamina
v. pudenda externa traversing m. gracilis
lateral scrotal/mammary lamina cut off at lateral rim of superficial inguinal ring
n. genitofemoralis
a.v. pudenda externa
m. obliquus externus abdominis (abdominal tendon) covered by yellow abdominal tunic
n. cutaneus medialis ventralis, LII
vaginal process covered by m. cremaster has emerged from superficial inguinal ring
n. ischiadicus
m. sacrocaudalis ventralis lateralis
n. pudendus
m. coccygeus
m. obturatorius internus, pars iliaca
a. pudenda interna
m. levator ani
m. gluteus profundus
m. obturatorius internus
mm. gemelli
m. rectus femoris
m. capsularis
a.v. obturatoria
accessory femoral ligament
m. obturatorius externus at obturator foramen
n. obturatorius
femoral ring
symphyseal tendon
m. pectineus
m. gracilis
plexus dorsalis penis
blue rod in a tributary of v. pudenda externa
medial scrotal/mammary lamina arising from yellow abdominal tunic
vv. circumflexa penis
penile body
m. bulbospongiosus
m. retractor penis, pars penina

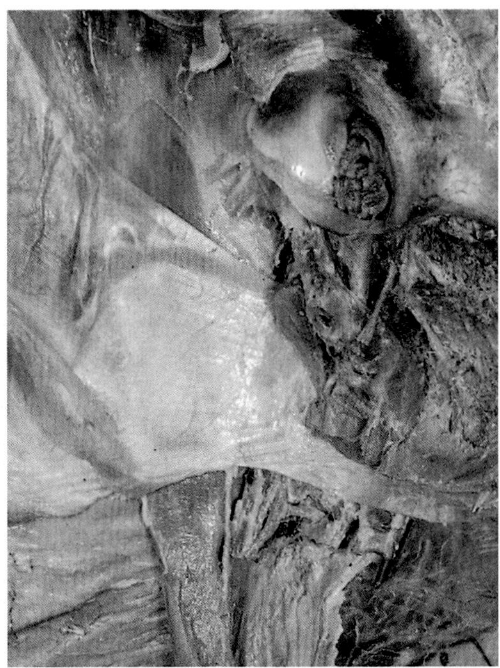
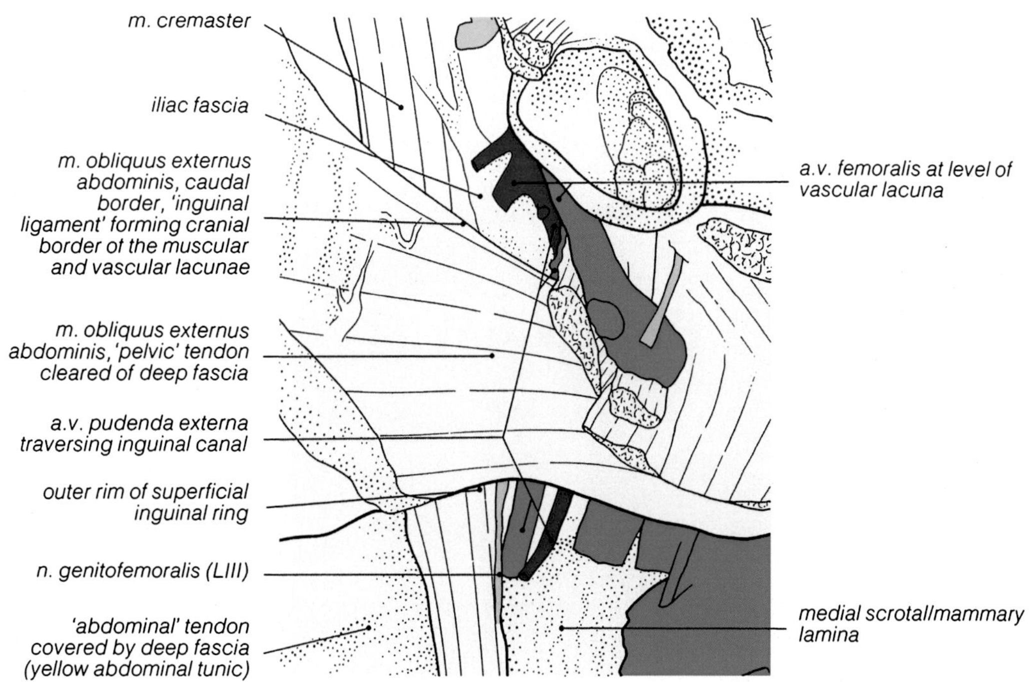
m. cremaster
iliac fascia
m. obliquus externus abdominis, caudal border, 'inguinal ligament' forming cranial border of the muscular and vascular lacunae
m. obliquus externus abdominis, 'pelvic' tendon cleared of deep fascia
a.v. pudenda externa traversing inguinal canal
outer rim of superficial inguinal ring
n. genitofemoralis (LIII)
'abdominal' tendon covered by deep fascia (yellow abdominal tunic)
a.v. femoralis at level of vascular lacuna
medial scrotal/mammary lamina

Fig. 8.22 Inguinal structures of the gelding: left lateral view (2). The specimen is at the same stage of dissection shown in Fig. 8.21 except that the deep fascia (from which the lateral scrotal/mammary lamina arises) has been removed from the pelvic tendon of the external oblique abdominal muscle. The deep fascia covering the abdominal tendon of the external oblique muscle gives rise to the medial scrotal/mammary lamina and has not been removed.

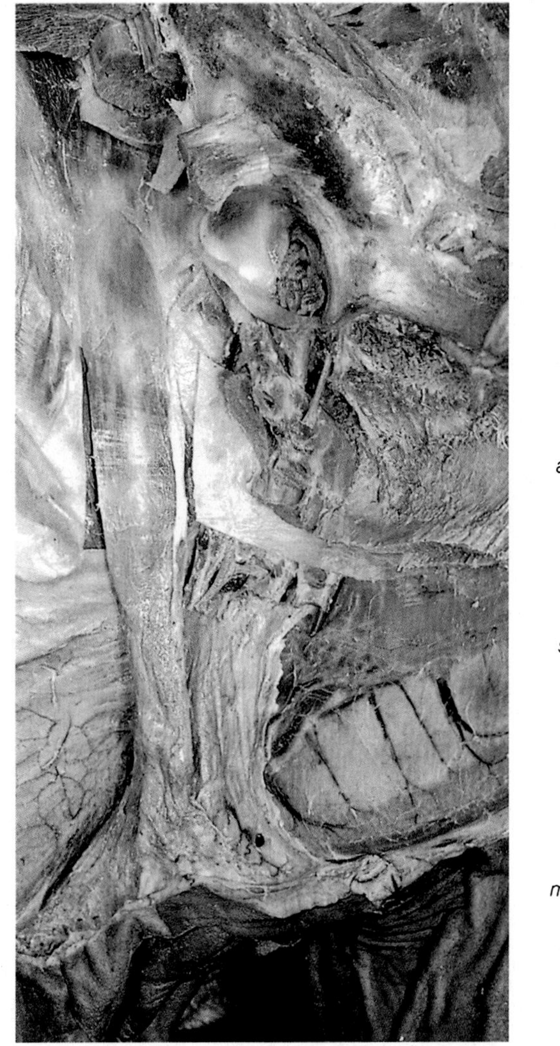
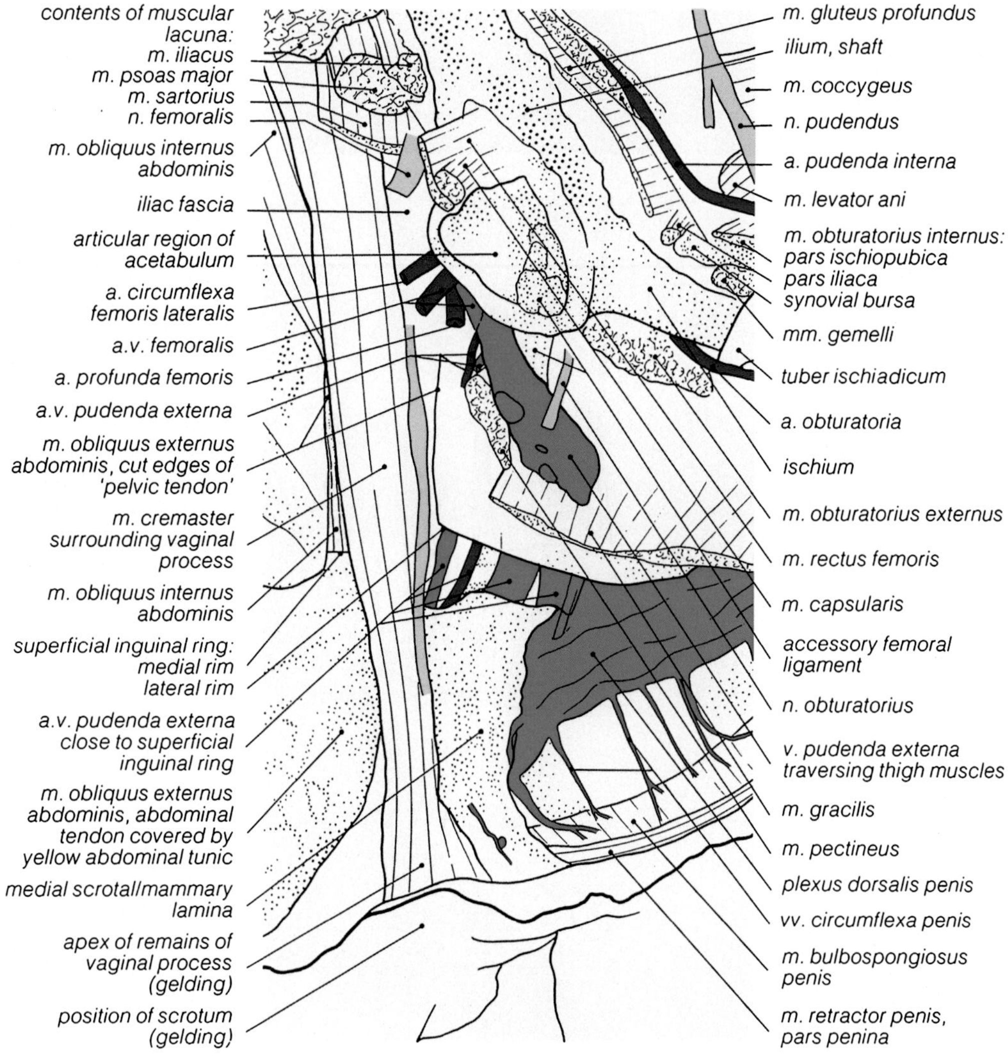
contents of muscular lacuna:
m. iliacus
m. psoas major
m. sartorius
n. femoralis
m. obliquus internus abdominis
iliac fascia
articular region of acetabulum
a. circumflexa femoris lateralis
a.v. femoralis
a. profunda femoris
a.v. pudenda externa
m. obliquus externus abdominis, cut edges of 'pelvic tendon'
m. cremaster surrounding vaginal process
m. obliquus internus abdominis
superficial inguinal ring:
medial rim
lateral rim
a.v. pudenda externa close to superficial inguinal ring
m. obliquus externus abdominis, abdominal tendon covered by yellow abdominal tunic
medial scrotal/mammary lamina
apex of remains of vaginal process (gelding)
position of scrotum (gelding)
m. gluteus profundus
ilium, shaft
m. coccygeus
n. pudendus
a. pudenda interna
m. levator ani
m. obturatorius internus:
pars ischiopubica
pars iliaca
synovial bursa
mm. gemelli
tuber ischiadicum
a. obturatoria
ischium
m. obturatorius externus
m. rectus femoris
m. capsularis
accessory femoral ligament
n. obturatorius
v. pudenda externa traversing thigh muscles
m. gracilis
m. pectineus
plexus dorsalis penis
vv. circumflexa penis
m. bulbospongiosus penis
m. retractor penis, pars penina

Fig. 8.23 Inguinal structures of the gelding: left lateral view (3). The pelvic tendon of the external oblique abdominal muscle has been sectioned to expose the contents of the inguinal canal. The dorsal (lateral) edge of the abdominal tendon of this muscle can just be seen – it forms the medial rim of the superficial inguinal ring. The internal abdominal oblique muscle, around whose caudal border the vaginal process passes at the deep inguinal ring (see Fig. 8.25) can also be glimpsed. The scrotal viscera and penis of the adult stallion are shown in Figs. 8.36–8.44.

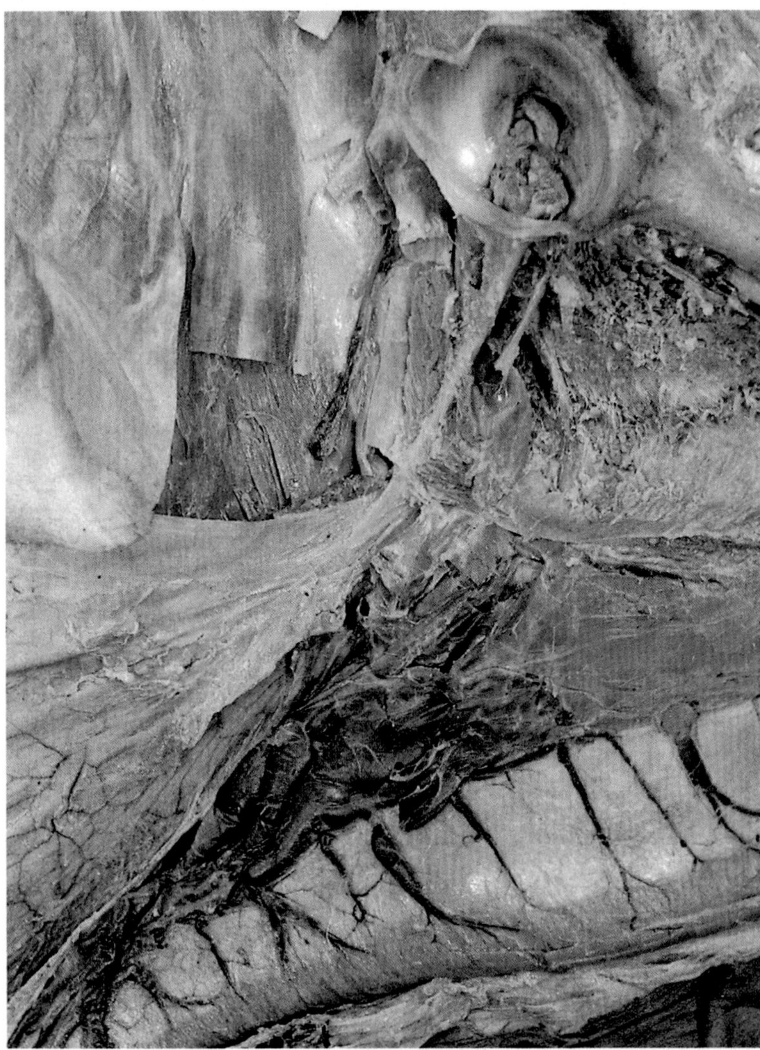

Fig. 8.24 Inguinal structures of the gelding: left lateral view (4). Removal of the apex of the vaginal process and cremaster muscle exposes the medial rim of the superficial inguinal ring and the origin of the accessory ligament of the femur from the deep fascia of the abdominal wall. The origin of the medial scrotal/mammary lamina from this fascia is also clearly seen. The deep inguinal ring lies caudal to the internal oblique abdominal muscle.

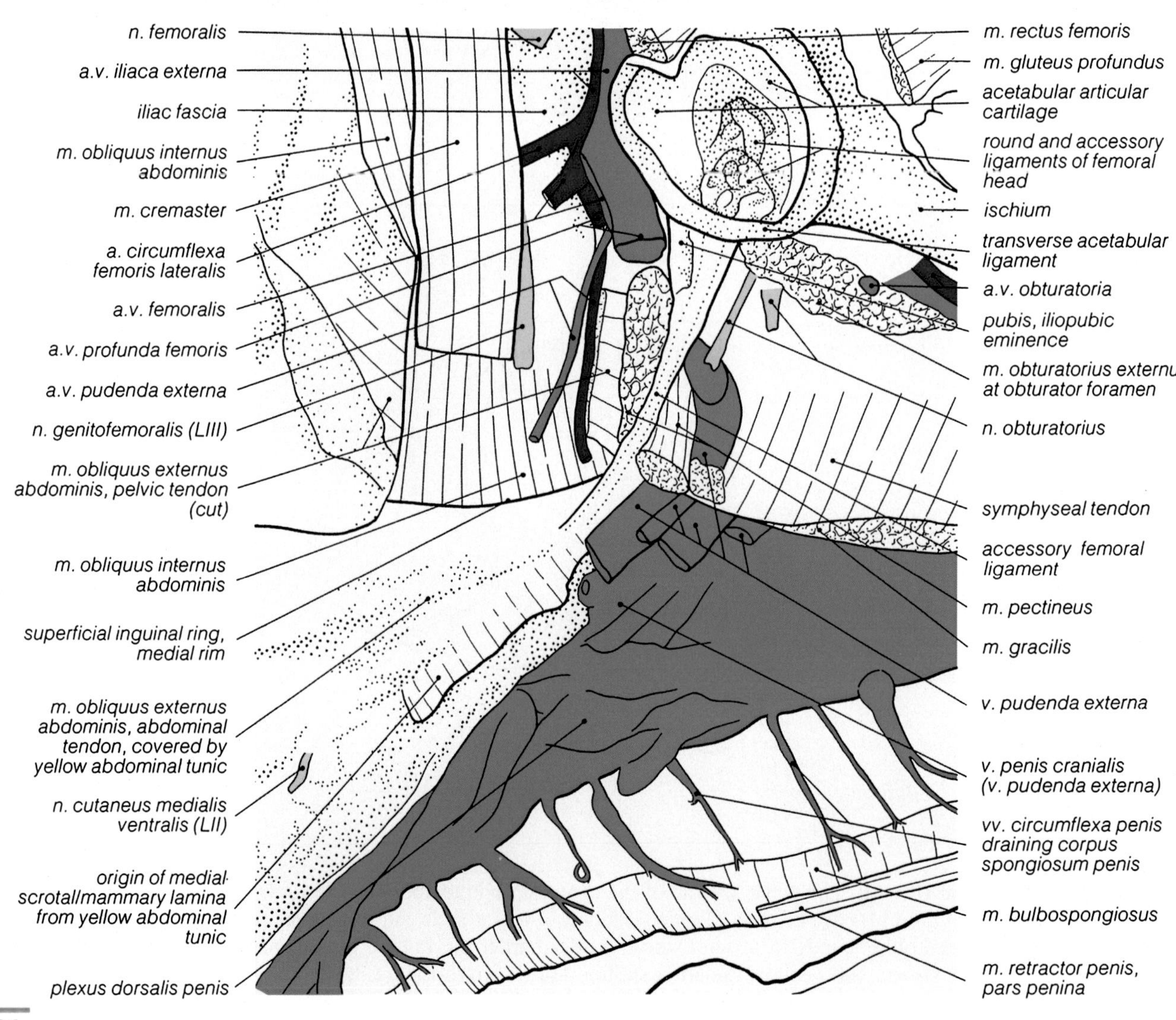
n. femoralis
a.v. iliaca externa
iliac fascia
m. obliquus internus abdominis
m. cremaster
a. circumflexa femoris lateralis
a.v. femoralis
a.v. profunda femoris
a.v. pudenda externa
n. genitofemoralis (LIII)
m. obliquus externus abdominis, pelvic tendon (cut)
m. obliquus internus abdominis
superficial inguinal ring, medial rim
m. obliquus externus abdominis, abdominal tendon, covered by yellow abdominal tunic
n. cutaneus medialis ventralis (LII)
origin of medial scrotal/mammary lamina from yellow abdominal tunic
plexus dorsalis penis
m. rectus femoris
m. gluteus profundus
acetabular articular cartilage
round and accessory ligaments of femoral head
ischium
transverse acetabular ligament
a.v. obturatoria
pubis, iliopubic eminence
m. obturatorius externus at obturator foramen
n. obturatorius
symphyseal tendon
accessory femoral ligament
m. pectineus
m. gracilis
v. pudenda externa
v. penis cranialis (v. pudenda externa)
vv. circumflexa penis draining corpus spongiosum penis
m. bulbospongiosus
m. retractor penis, pars penina

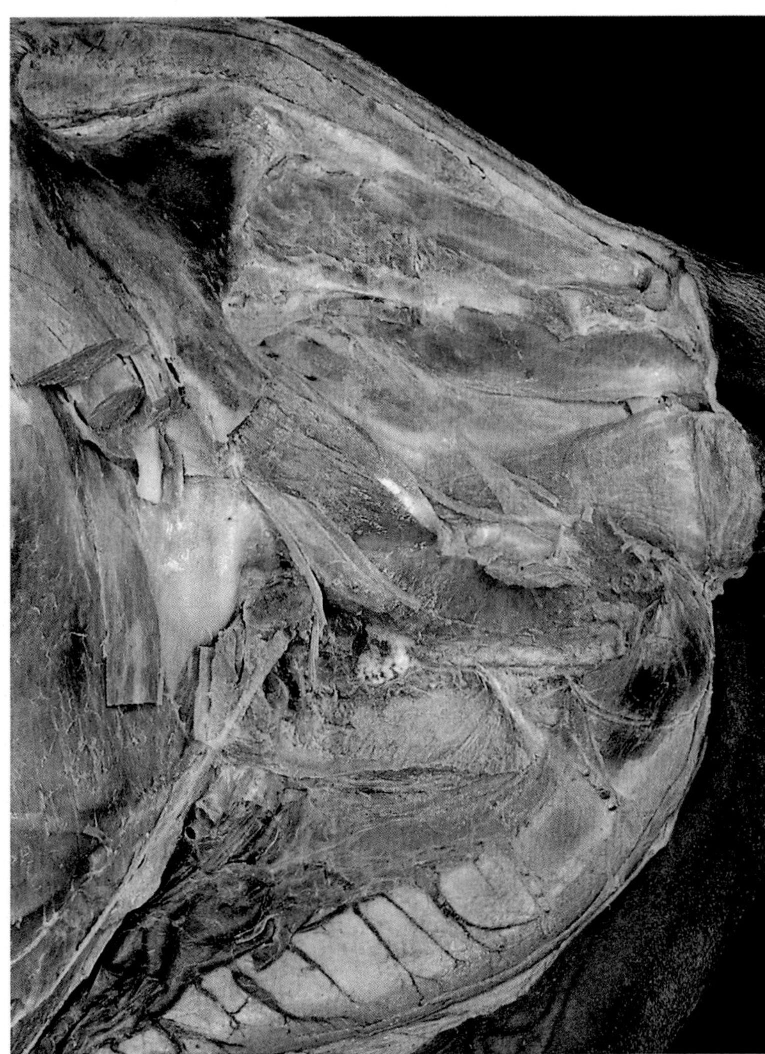

Fig. 8.25 The pelvic cavity of the gelding: left lateral view. The pubis and ischium have been cut just lateral to the pelvic symphysis. The shaft of the ilium has been transected and the left coxal bone removed, taking care to preserve the muscles attached to its internal surface (ischiocavernosus and internal obturator) and to its ischiatic spine (levator ani). Most of the coccygeus muscle has been removed to display the levator ani muscle more completely.

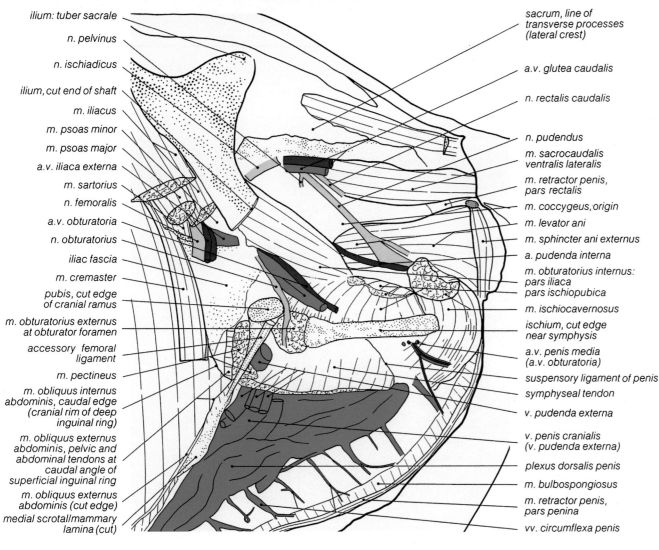

ilium: tuber sacrale
n. pelvinus
n. ischiadicus
ilium, cut end of shaft
m. iliacus
m. psoas minor
m. psoas major
a.v. iliaca externa
m. sartorius
n. femoralis
a.v. obturatoria
n. obturatorius
iliac fascia
m. cremaster
pubis, cut edge of cranial ramus
m. obturatorius externus at obturator foramen
accessory femoral ligament
m. pectineus
m. obliquus internus abdominis, caudal edge (cranial rim of deep inguinal ring)
m. obliquus externus abdominis, pelvic and abdominal tendons at caudal angle of superficial inguinal ring
m. obliquus externus abdominis (cut edge)
medial scrotal/mammary lamina (cut)

sacrum, line of transverse processes (lateral crest)
a.v. glutea caudalis
n. rectalis caudalis
n. pudendus
m. sacrocaudalis ventralis lateralis
m. retractor penis, pars rectalis
m. coccygeus, origin
m. levator ani
m. sphincter ani externus
a. pudenda interna
m. obturatorius internus: pars iliaca pars ischiopubica
m. ischiocavernosus
ischium, cut edge near symphysis
a.v. penis media (a.v. obturatoria)
suspensory ligament of penis
symphyseal tendon
v. pudenda externa
v. penis cranialis (v. pudenda externa)
plexus dorsalis penis
m. bulbospongiosus
m. retractor penis, pars penina
vv. circumflexa penis

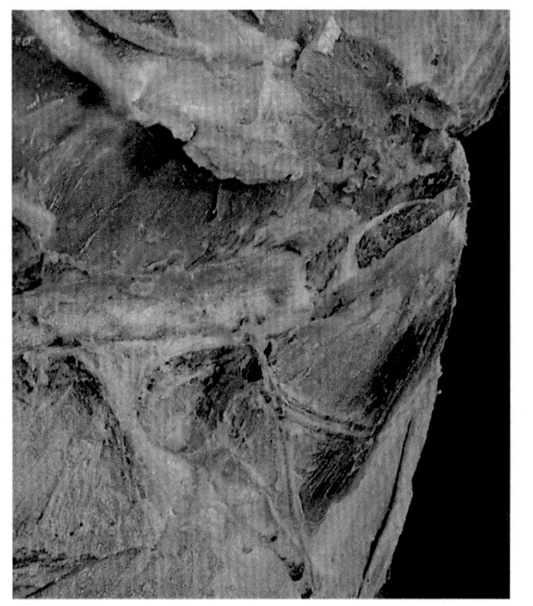

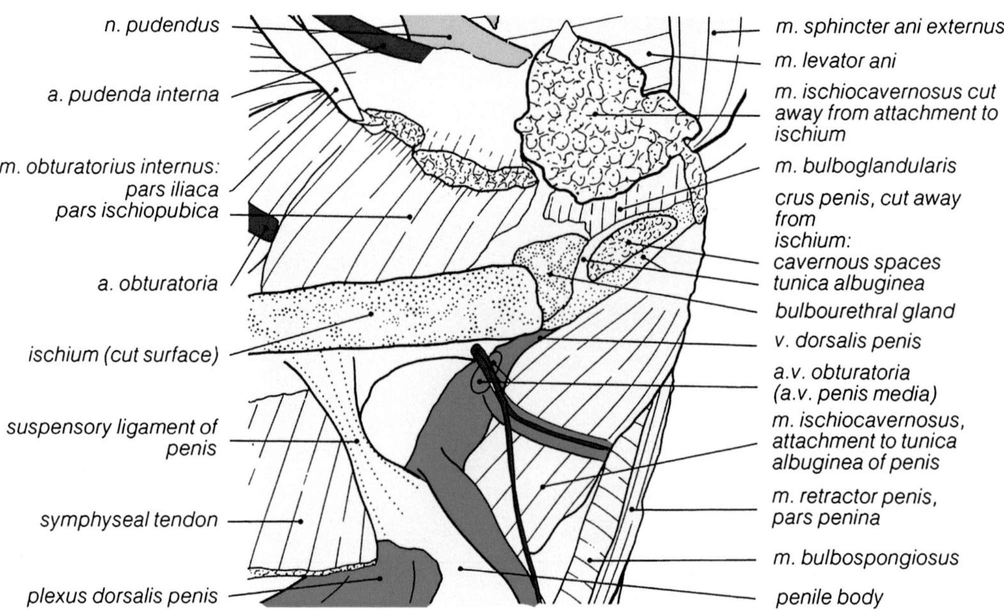
n. pudendus
a. pudenda interna
m. obturatorius internus:
pars iliaca
pars ischiopubica
a. obturatoria
ischium (cut surface)
suspensory ligament of penis
symphyseal tendon
plexus dorsalis penis
m. sphincter ani externus
m. levator ani
m. ischiocavernosus cut away from attachment to ischium
m. bulboglandularis
crus penis, cut away from ischium:
cavernous spaces
tunica albuginea
bulbourethral gland
v. dorsalis penis
a.v. obturatoria (a.v. penis media)
m. ischiocavernosus, attachment to tunica albuginea of penis
m. retractor penis, pars penina
m. bulbospongiosus
penile body

Fig. 8.26 The penile root: left lateral view. This is a closer view of a part of the specimen shown in Fig. 8.25.

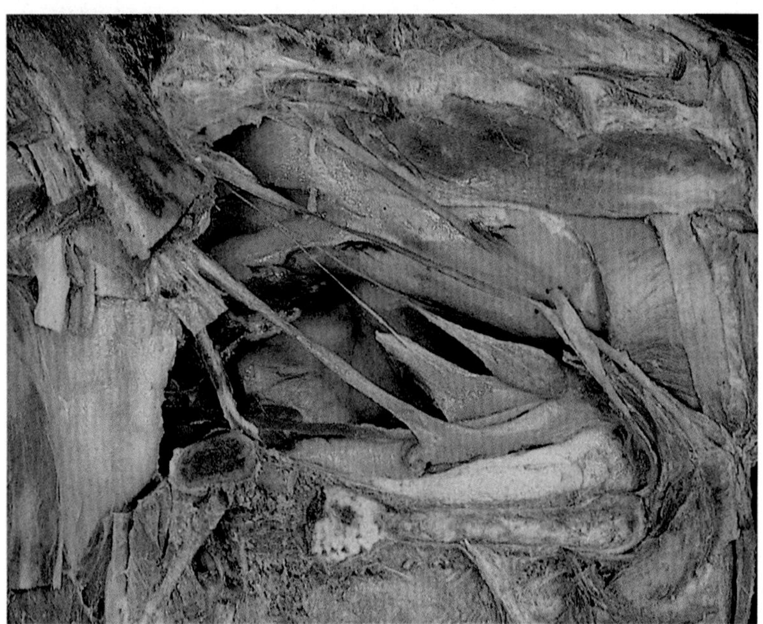

Fig. 8.27 The pelvic viscera of the gelding: left lateral view. The internal obturator muscle has been removed and the ischiocavernosus muscle dissected off from the penile crus. The internal pudendal artery and the pudendal nerve have been displaced dorsally. The rectum in this specimen was kinked close to its line of peritoneal reflection and the urinary bladder was empty and contracted. The bulbourethral gland has been removed; it is shown in Fig. 8.26. The hypogastric nerves, which leave the caudal mesenteric ganglion and enter the pelvis, are shown in Fig. 8.70.

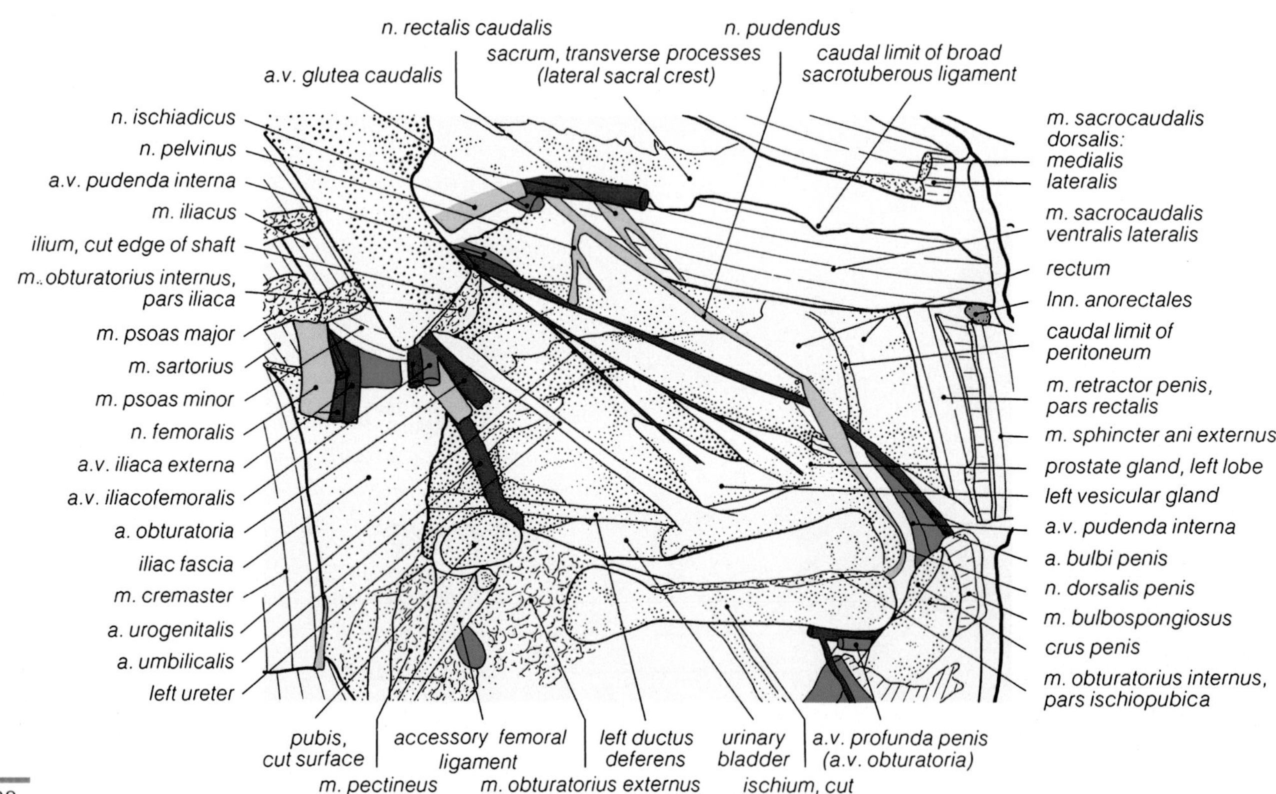
n. rectalis caudalis
n. pudendus
a.v. glutea caudalis
sacrum, transverse processes (lateral sacral crest)
caudal limit of broad sacrotuberous ligament
n. ischiadicus
n. pelvinus
a.v. pudenda interna
m. iliacus
ilium, cut edge of shaft
m. obturatorius internus, pars iliaca
m. psoas major
m. sartorius
m. psoas minor
n. femoralis
a.v. iliaca externa
a.v. iliacofemoralis
a. obturatoria
iliac fascia
m. cremaster
a. urogenitalis
a. umbilicalis
left ureter
m. sacrocaudalis dorsalis:
medialis
lateralis
m. sacrocaudalis ventralis lateralis
rectum
lnn. anorectales
caudal limit of peritoneum
m. retractor penis, pars rectalis
m. sphincter ani externus
prostate gland, left lobe
left vesicular gland
a.v. pudenda interna
a. bulbi penis
n. dorsalis penis
m. bulbospongiosus
crus penis
m. obturatorius internus, pars ischiopubica
pubis, cut surface
accessory femoral ligament
left ductus deferens
urinary bladder
a.v. profunda penis (a.v. obturatoria)
m. pectineus
m. obturatorius externus origin at obturator foramen
ischium, cut surface

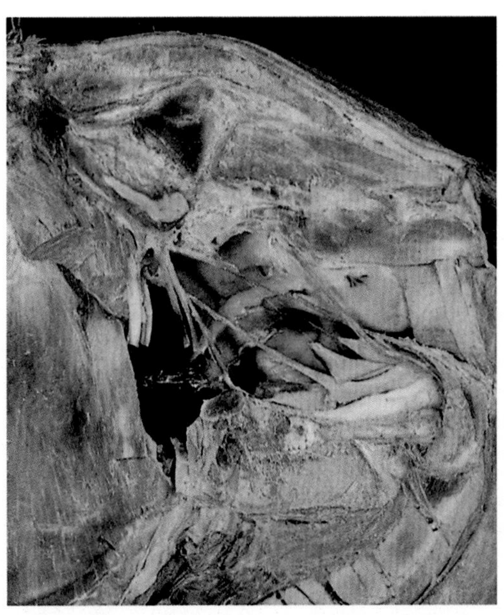

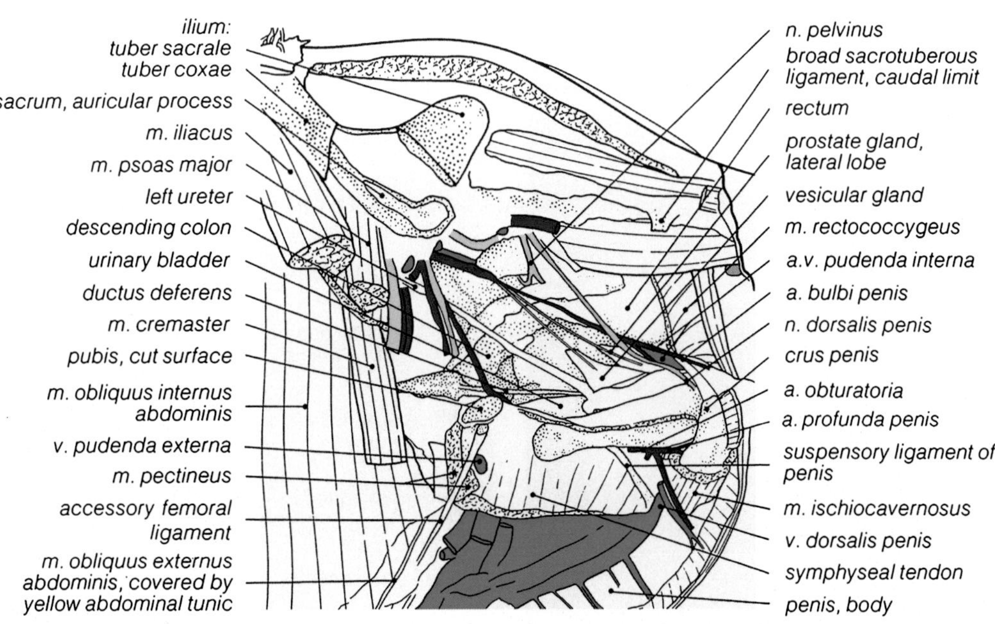
ilium:
tuber sacrale
tuber coxae
sacrum, auricular process
m. iliacus
m. psoas major
left ureter
descending colon
urinary bladder
ductus deferens
m. cremaster
pubis, cut surface
m. obliquus internus abdominis
v. pudenda externa
m. pectineus
accessory femoral ligament
m. obliquus externus abdominis, covered by yellow abdominal tunic
n. pelvinus
broad sacrotuberous ligament, caudal limit
rectum
prostate gland, lateral lobe
vesicular gland
m. rectococcygeus
a.v. pudenda interna
a. bulbi penis
n. dorsalis penis
crus penis
a. obturatoria
a. profunda penis
suspensory ligament of penis
m. ischiocavernosus
v. dorsalis penis
symphyseal tendon
penis, body

Fig. 8.28 The pelvis after removal of the left pelvic bone. Further details of parts of this dissection are shown in Figs. 8.29 and 8.30.

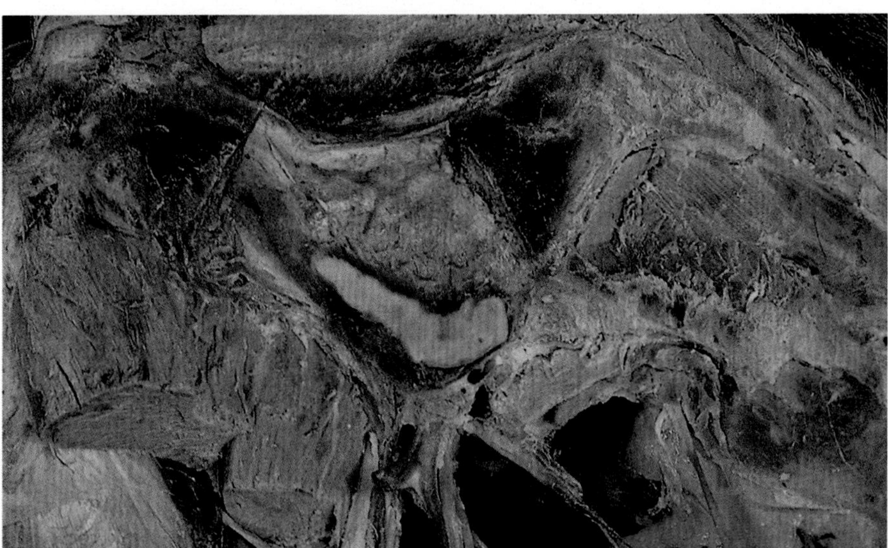

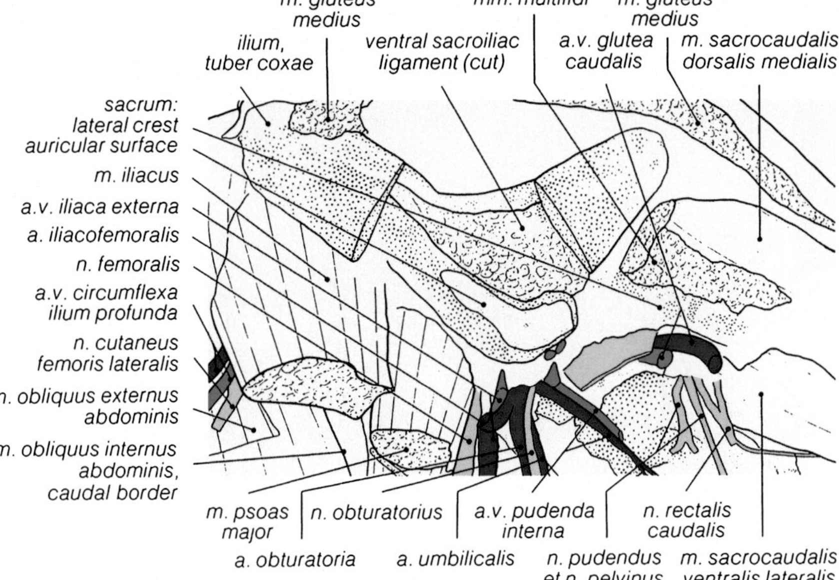
m. gluteus medius
mm. multifidi
m. gluteus medius
ilium, tuber coxae
ventral sacroiliac ligament (cut)
a.v. glutea caudalis
m. sacrocaudalis dorsalis medialis
sacrum:
lateral crest
auricular surface
m. iliacus
a.v. iliaca externa
a. iliacofemoralis
n. femoralis
a.v. circumflexa ilium profunda
n. cutaneus femoris lateralis
m. obliquus externus abdominis
m. obliquus internus abdominis, caudal border
m. psoas major
n. obturatorius
a.v. pudenda interna
n. rectalis caudalis
a. obturatoria
a. umbilicalis
n. pudendus et n. pelvinus
m. sacrocaudalis ventralis lateralis

Fig. 8.29 The sacroiliac joint and adjacent structures: left lateral view. The middle part of the blade of the ilium has been removed to reveal the articulating auricular surface of the sacrum.

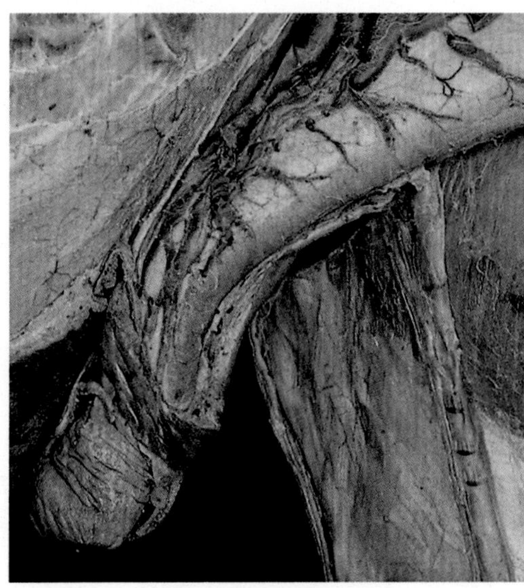
m. obliquus externus abdominis
m. rectus abdominis covered by aponeurosis of m. obliquus internus abdominis
v. pudenda externa
medial scrotal/mammary lamina
m. retractor penis, pars penina
vv. circumflexa penis
plexus dorsalis penis
m. bulbospongiosus
m. gracilis
prepuce:
prepenile part
preputial fold
preputial ring
n. saphenus
v. saphena medialis
free part of penis
glans penis
medial femoral fascia

Fig. 8.30 The distal parts of the penis and the prepuce: left lateral view. This is a slightly more cranial view of a part of the specimen shown in Fig. 8.28. Most of the prepenile part of the prepuce has been removed to show the preputial fold. The preputial fold has been partly resected to show the free part of the penis which it encloses. The free part of the penis is shown in Fig. 8.5. The penis of the adult stallion is shown in Figs. 8.42–8.44. Developmental aspects are shown in Figs. 8.46–8.53.

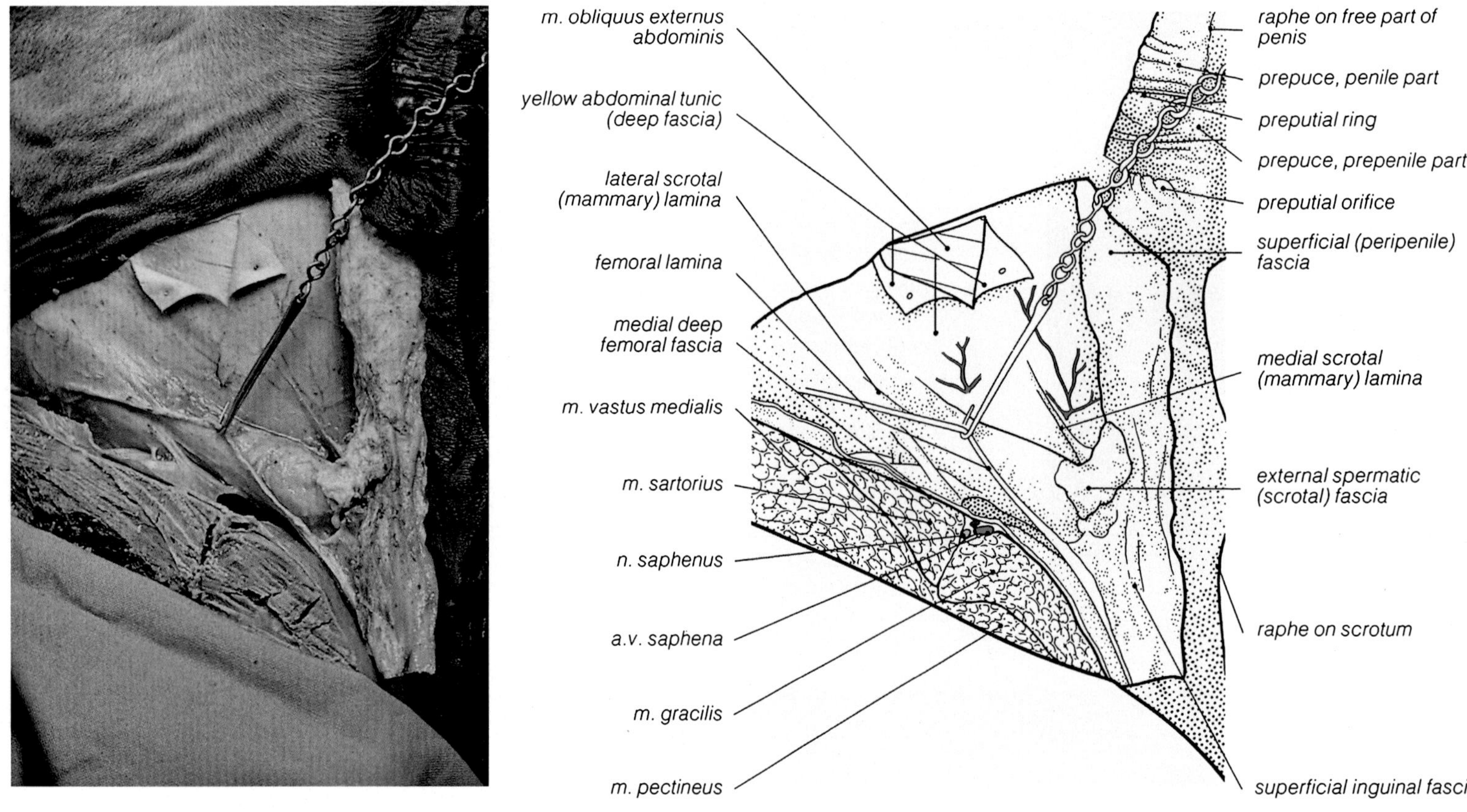
m. obliquus externus abdominis
yellow abdominal tunic (deep fascia)
lateral scrotal (mammary) lamina
femoral lamina
medial deep femoral fascia
m. vastus medialis
m. sartorius
n. saphenus
a.v. saphena
m. gracilis
m. pectineus
raphe on free part of penis
prepuce, penile part
preputial ring
prepuce, prepenile part
preputial orifice
superficial (peripenile) fascia
medial scrotal (mammary) lamina
external spermatic (scrotal) fascia
raphe on scrotum
superficial inguinal fascia

Fig. 8.31 Superficial structures of the right inguinal region in a young stallion: right ventral view. The right hindlimb has been cut away and the stump is draped with a green cloth. The yellow abdominal tunic has been incised to reveal the tendon of the oblique external abdominal mucles to which it adheres closely. Figs. 8.31–8.35 show ventral views of inguinal structures for comparison with the lateral dissections of the gelding shown in Figs. 8.21–8.24. See also Figs. 8.73–8.75.

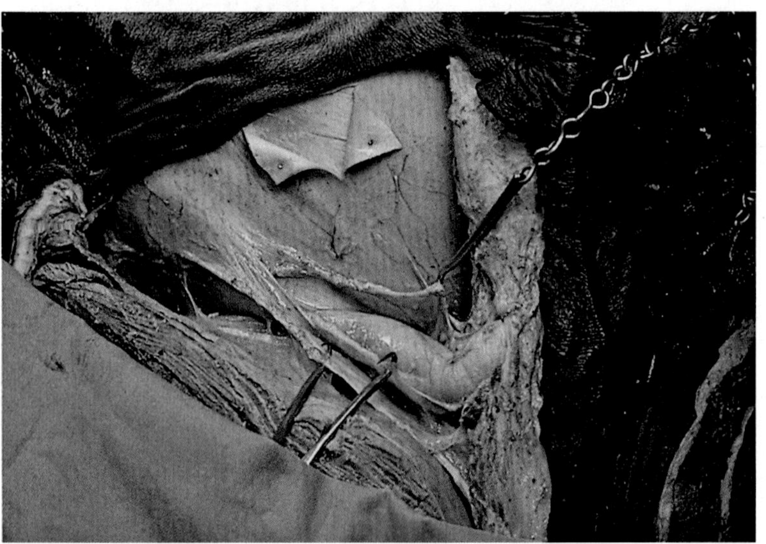

Fig. 8.32 The external spermatic fascia and the right vaginal process of the yearling stallion: ventral view. The external spermatic (scrotal) fascia has been incised and held open with hooks to show the vaginal process. The lateral part of the fascia is, in fact, the lateral scrotal (mammary) lamina. The medial part of the fascia is not adherent to the medial edge of the superficial inguinal ring; the abdominal tendon of the oblique external abdominal muscle is therefore not covered by deep fascia at this location.

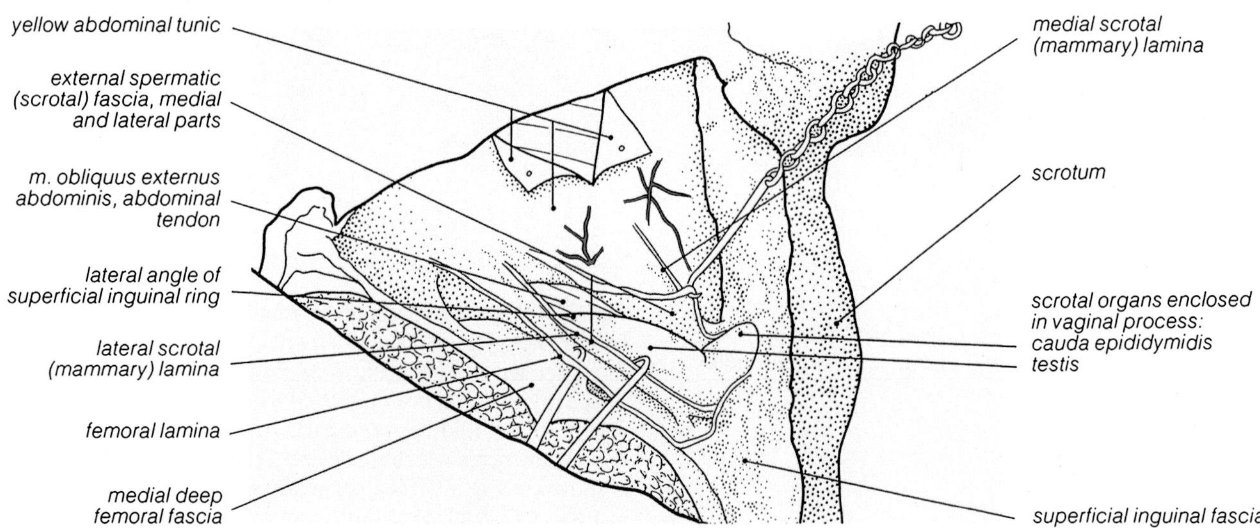
yellow abdominal tunic
external spermatic (scrotal) fascia, medial and lateral parts
m. obliquus externus abdominis, abdominal tendon
lateral angle of superficial inguinal ring
lateral scrotal (mammary) lamina
femoral lamina
medial deep femoral fascia
medial scrotal (mammary) lamina
scrotum
scrotal organs enclosed in vaginal process:
cauda epididymidis
testis
superficial inguinal fascia

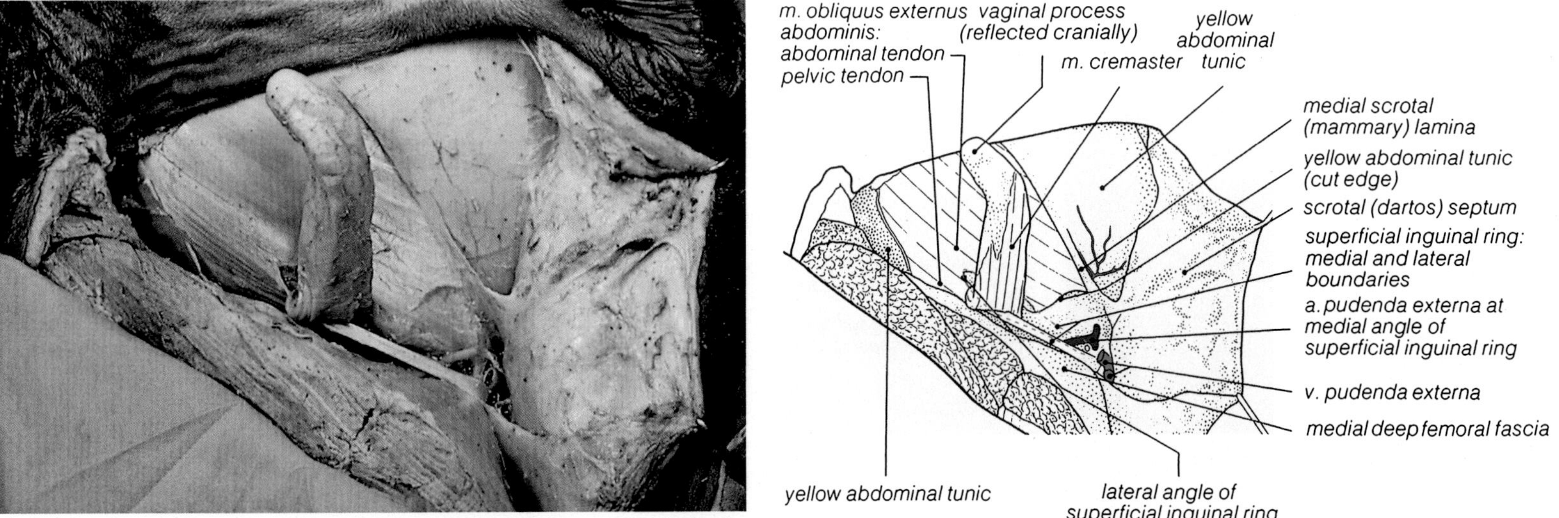

m. obliquus externus abdominis: abdominal tendon
pelvic tendon
vaginal process (reflected cranially)
m. cremaster
yellow abdominal tunic
medial scrotal (mammary) lamina
yellow abdominal tunic (cut edge)
scrotal (dartos) septum
superficial inguinal ring: medial and lateral boundaries
a. pudenda externa at medial angle of superficial inguinal ring
v. pudenda externa
medial deep femoral fascia
yellow abdominal tunic
lateral angle of superficial inguinal ring

Fig. 8.33 The right superficial inguinal ring of the yearling stallion: ventral view. The deep fascia (yellow abdominal tunic) overlying the superficial inguinal ring has been removed together with the external spermatic (scrotal) fascia. The superficial inguinal ring (indicated by the broken blue line) is revealed, dividing the tendon of the oblique external abdominal muscle into parts with pelvic and abdominal insertions. The vaginal process has been reflected cranially to show the medial aspect of the superficial ring.

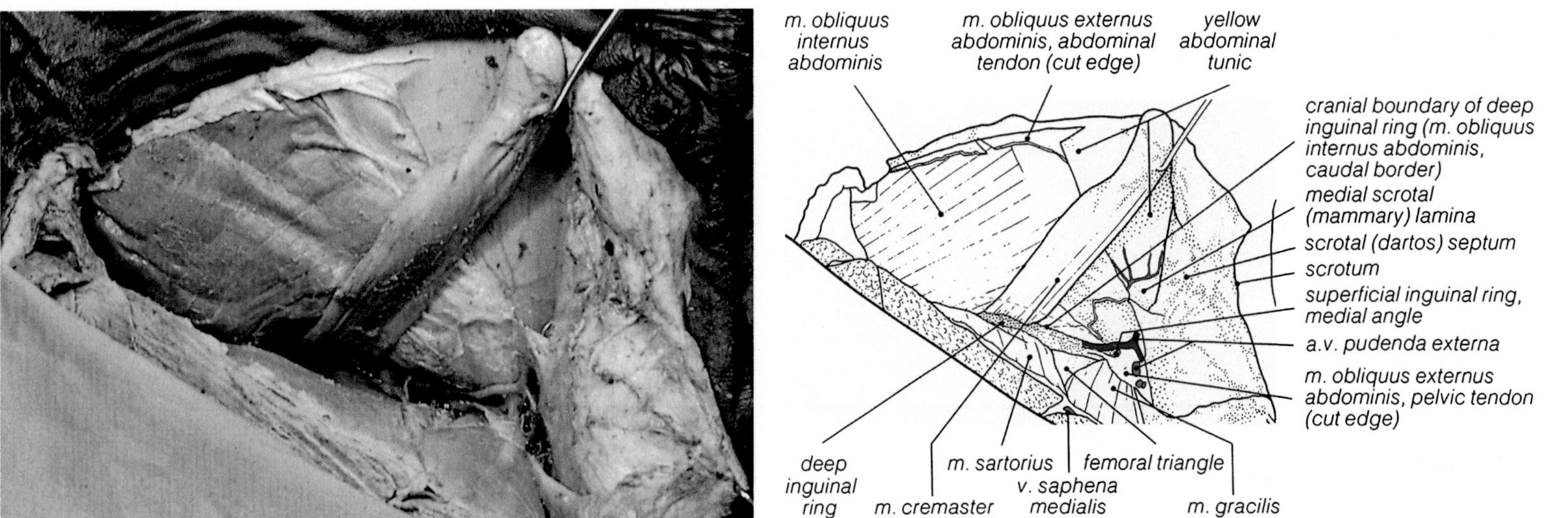

m. obliquus internus abdominis
m. obliquus externus abdominis, abdominal tendon (cut edge)
yellow abdominal tunic
cranial boundary of deep inguinal ring (m. obliquus internus abdominis, caudal border)
medial scrotal (mammary) lamina
scrotal (dartos) septum
scrotum
superficial inguinal ring, medial angle
a.v. pudenda externa
m. obliquus externus abdominis, pelvic tendon (cut edge)
deep inguinal ring
m. cremaster
m. sartorius
v. saphena medialis
femoral triangle
m. gracilis

Fig. 8.34 The right deep inguinal ring of the yearling stallion: ventral view. A part of the oblique external abdominal muscle, including the superficial inguinal ring, has been removed to display the oblique internal abdominal muscle. The vaginal process has been displaced cranially and the deep inguinal ring is just visible lying caudal to the oblique internal muscle. The position of the superficial inguinal ring is shown by a broken blue line.

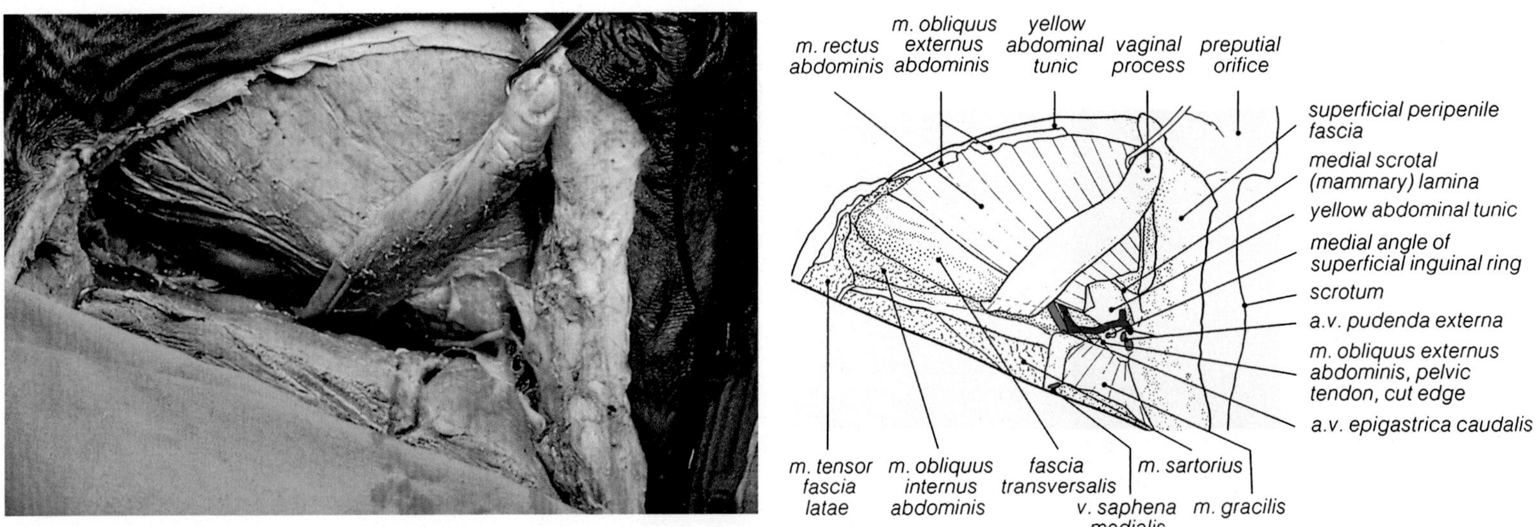

m. rectus abdominis
m. obliquus externus abdominis
yellow abdominal tunic
vaginal process
preputial orifice
superficial peripenile fascia
medial scrotal (mammary) lamina
yellow abdominal tunic
medial angle of superficial inguinal ring
scrotum
a.v. pudenda externa
m. obliquus externus abdominis, pelvic tendon, cut edge
a.v. epigastrica caudalis
m. tensor fascia latae
m. obliquus internus abdominis
fascia transversalis
v. saphena medialis
m. sartorius
m. gracilis

Fig. 8.35 Deep structures of the right inguinal region, yearling stallion: ventral view. The internal and external oblique abdominal muscles have been removed from the inguinal region to display the rectus abdominis muscle and the transverse fascia. The vaginal process has been displaced cranially. The position of the superficial inguinal ring is shown by a broken blue line.

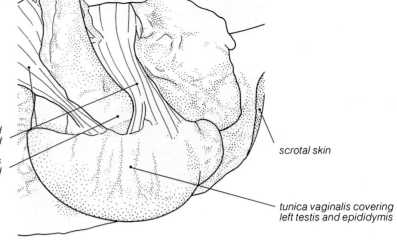

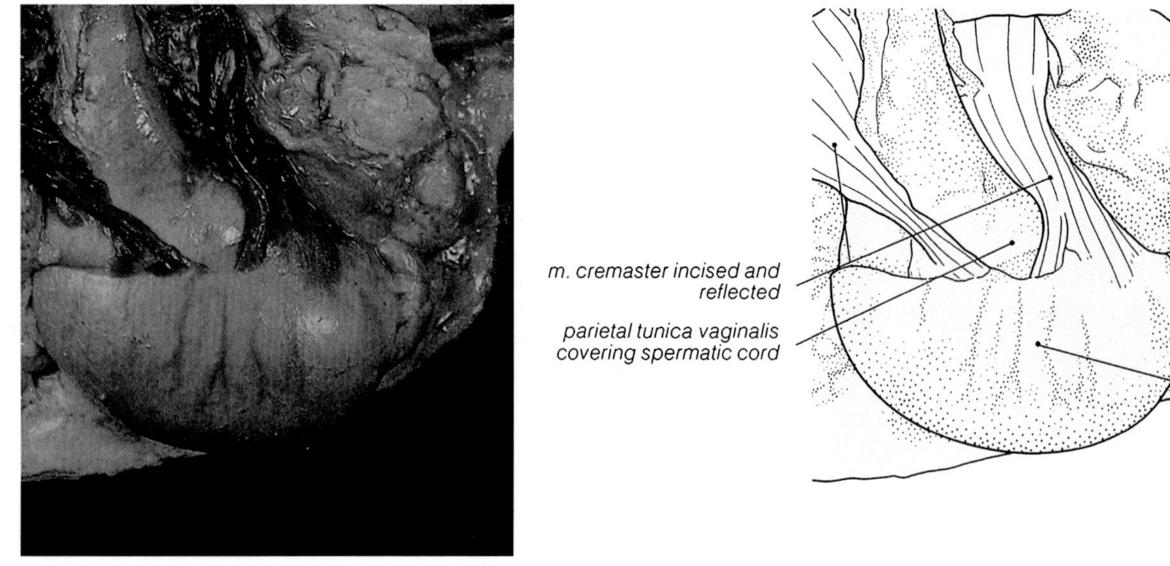
m. cremaster incised and reflected
parietal tunica vaginalis covering spermatic cord
scrotal skin
tunica vaginalis covering left testis and epididymis

Fig. 8.36 The vaginal process of the adult stallion: left lateral view. The left scrotal wall has been removed. The cremaster muscle has been incised and reflected from its insertion on the tunica vaginalis to reveal the tubular part of the vaginal process which encloses the spermatic cord. Figs. 8.37–8.41 show further dissections of fresh organs from this stallion to complement the dissections of the gelding shown in Figs. 8.21–8.30.

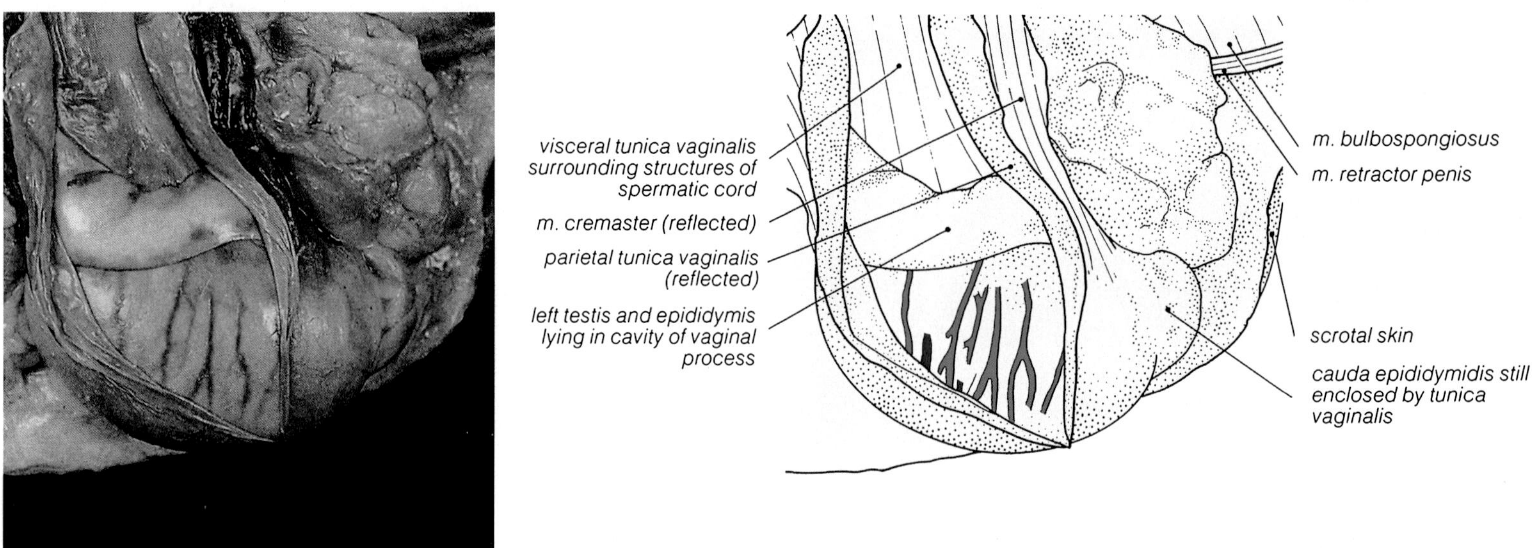
visceral tunica vaginalis surrounding structures of spermatic cord
m. cremaster (reflected)
parietal tunica vaginalis (reflected)
left testis and epididymis lying in cavity of vaginal process
m. bulbospongiosus
m. retractor penis
scrotal skin
cauda epididymidis still enclosed by tunica vaginalis

Fig. 8.37 The contents of the vaginal process of the adult stallion: left lateral view. A longitudinal incision through the wall of the vaginal process (parietal tunica vaginalis) reveals the viscera lying in the cavity of the process. The smooth muscle investing the spermatic cord is often called the 'internal cremaster muscle' – it extends distally onto the tunica albuginea of the testis.

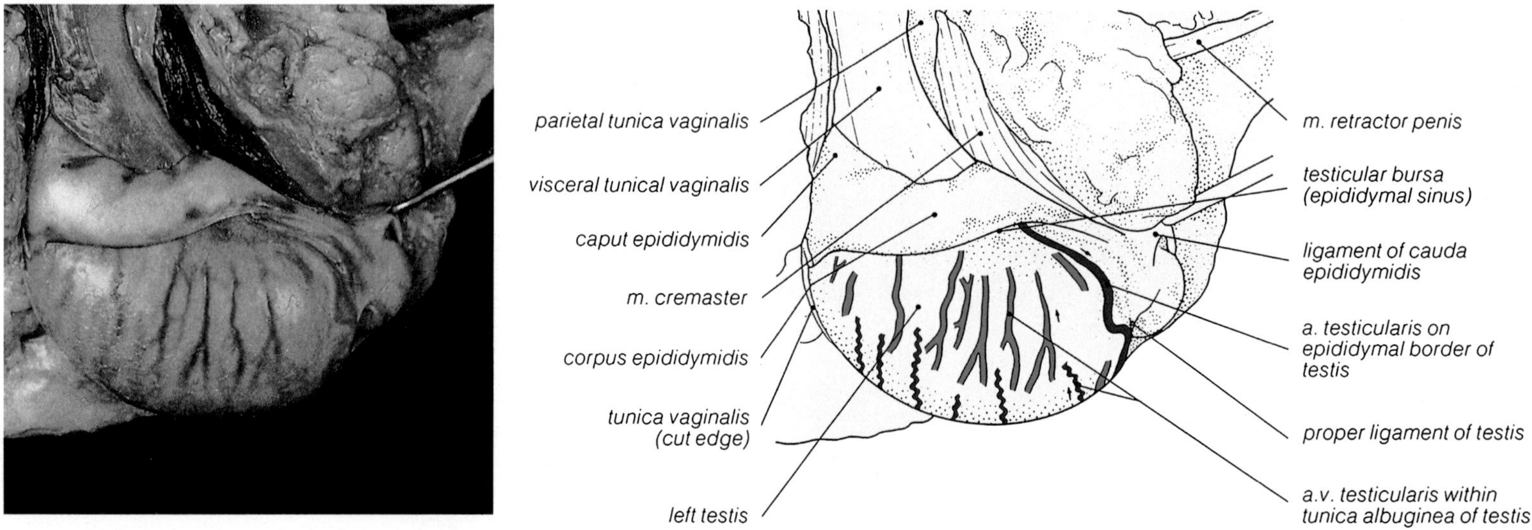
parietal tunica vaginalis
visceral tunical vaginalis
caput epididymidis
m. cremaster
corpus epididymidis
tunica vaginalis (cut edge)
left testis
m. retractor penis
testicular bursa (epididymal sinus)
ligament of cauda epididymidis
a. testicularis on epididymal border of testis
proper ligament of testis
a.v. testicularis within tunica albuginea of testis

Fig. 8.38 The left testis and epididymis of the adult stallion: lateral view. The lateral wall of the vaginal process has been removed. Arrows show the direction of flow of blood within the testicular vessels.

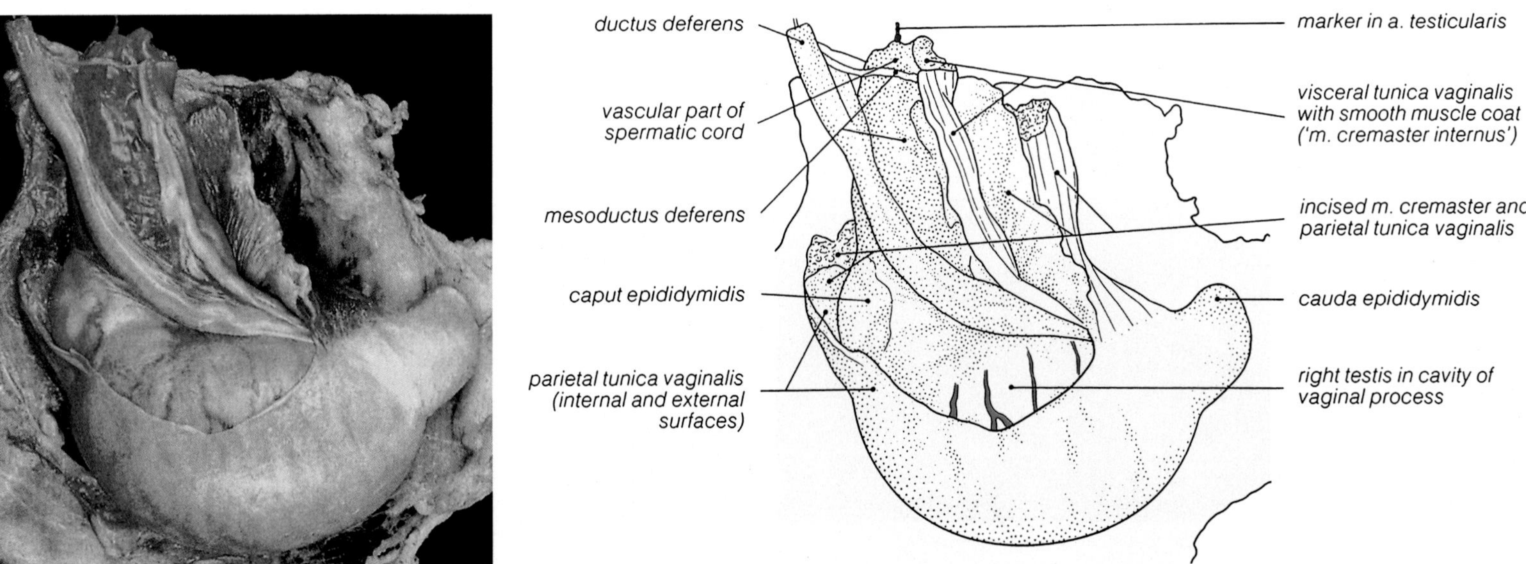
ductus deferens
vascular part of spermatic cord
mesoductus deferens
caput epididymidis
parietal tunica vaginalis (internal and external surfaces)
marker in a. testicularis
visceral tunica vaginalis with smooth muscle coat ('m. cremaster internus')
incised m. cremaster and parietal tunica vaginalis
cauda epididymidis
right testis in cavity of vaginal process

Fig. 8.39 The contents of the right vaginal process of the adult stallion: medial view (1). The excised viscera have been arranged to show the disposition within the body. The medial wall of the vaginal process (parietal tunica vaginalis) has been opened to show the contents.

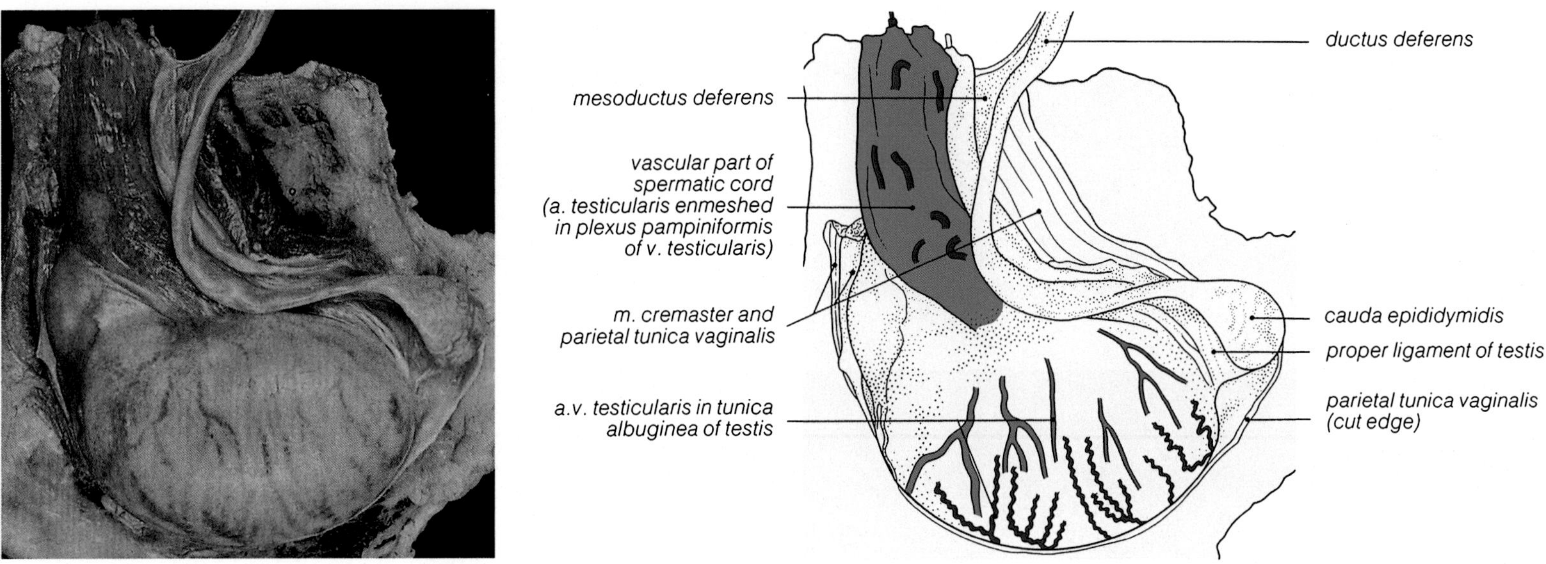
mesoductus deferens
vascular part of spermatic cord (a. testicularis enmeshed in plexus pampiniformis of v. testicularis)
m. cremaster and parietal tunica vaginalis
a.v. testicularis in tunica albuginea of testis
ductus deferens
cauda epididymidis
proper ligament of testis
parietal tunica vaginalis (cut edge)

Fig. 8.40 The contents of the right vaginal process of the adult stallion: medial view (2). The ductus deferens has been displaced caudally to show the vascular part of the spermatic cord which is still enclosed by the visceral tunica vaginalis and its muscular layers ('internal cremaster muscle').

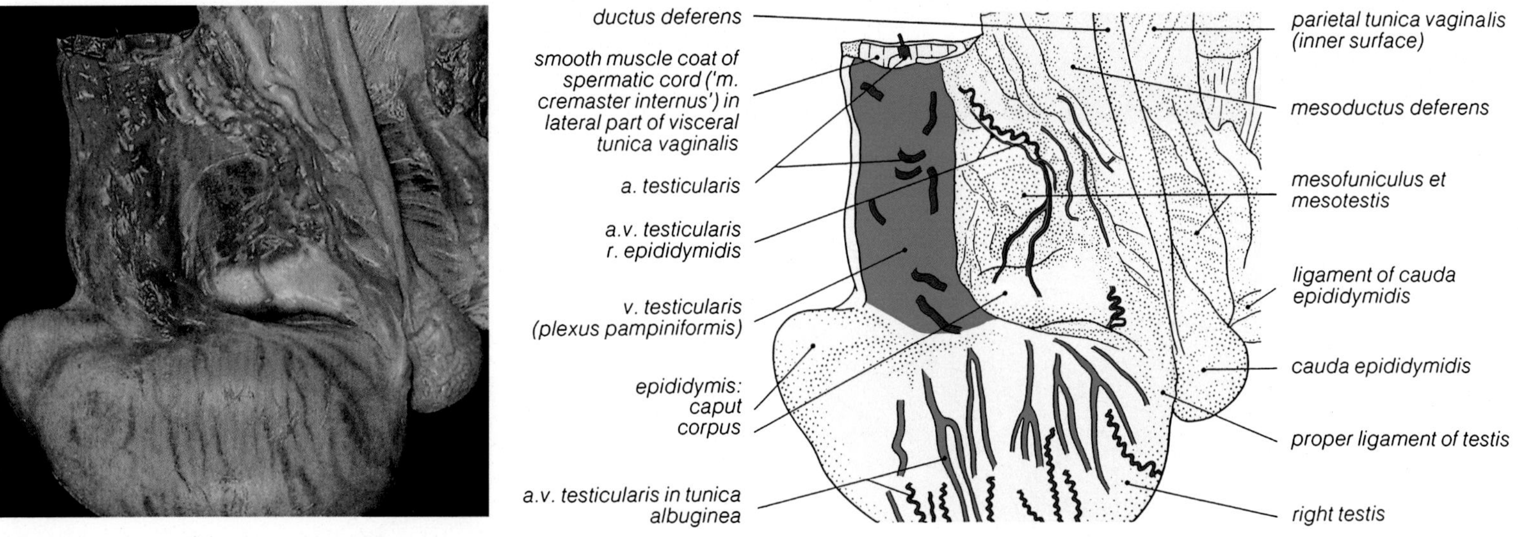
ductus deferens
smooth muscle coat of spermatic cord ('m. cremaster internus') in lateral part of visceral tunica vaginalis
a. testicularis
a.v. testicularis r. epididymidis
v. testicularis (plexus pampiniformis)
epididymis: caput corpus
a.v. testicularis in tunica albuginea
parietal tunica vaginalis (inner surface)
mesoductus deferens
mesofuniculus et mesotestis
ligament of cauda epididymidis
cauda epididymidis
proper ligament of testis
right testis

Fig. 8.41 The contents of the right vaginal process of the adult stallion: medial view (3). The excised organs have been arranged to display the peritoneal suspension of the testis, epididymis and spermatic cord within the opened vaginal process.

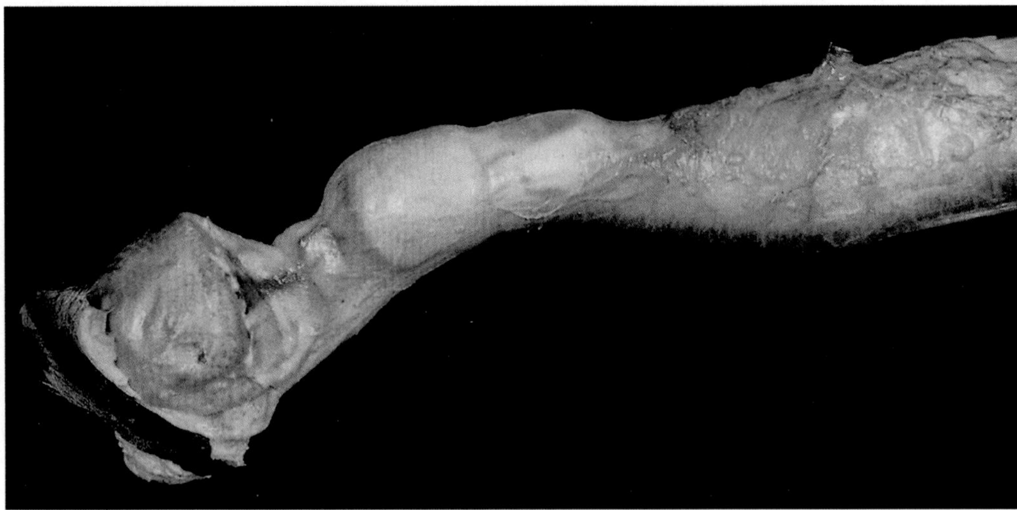

Fig. 8.42 Penis and prepuce of the adult stallion: left lateral view (1). The excised organs have been arranged to represent their disposition in the body. Coloured markers have been inserted in the cranial penile artery and in one main stem of the cranial penile vein that drains the dorsal penile plexus into the external pudendal vein.

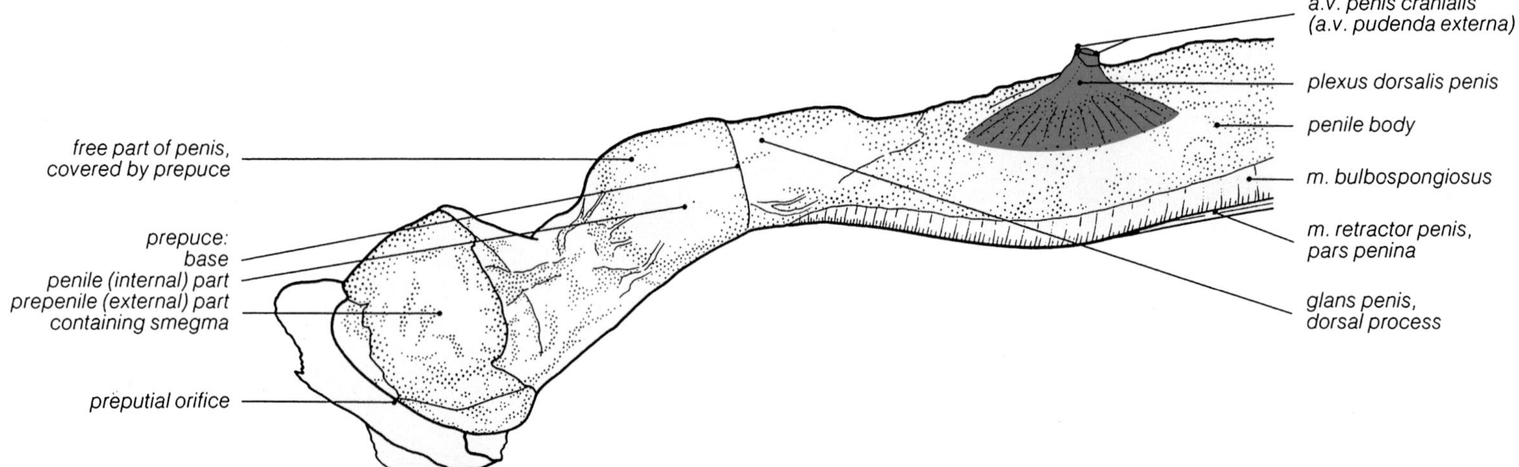
a.v. penis cranialis
(a.v. pudenda externa)
plexus dorsalis penis
penile body
m. bulbospongiosus
m. retractor penis,
pars penina
glans penis,
dorsal process
free part of penis,
covered by prepuce
prepuce:
base
penile (internal) part
prepenile (external) part
containing smegma
preputial orifice

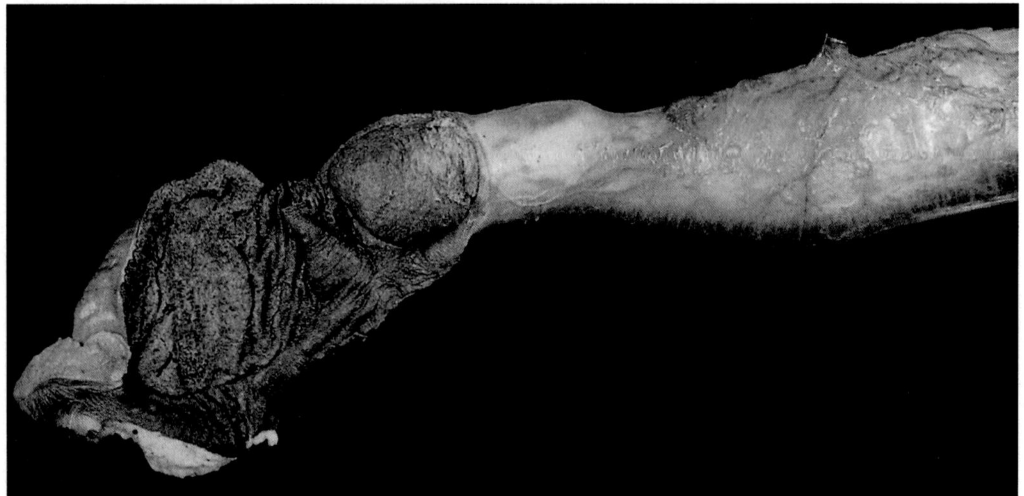

Fig. 8.43 Penis and prepuce of the adult stallion: left lateral view (2). The left side of the prepuce has been removed to display the 'double' inner structure of the prepuce and the free part of the penis. The extensive deposits of smegma normally found within the prepuce have been removed.

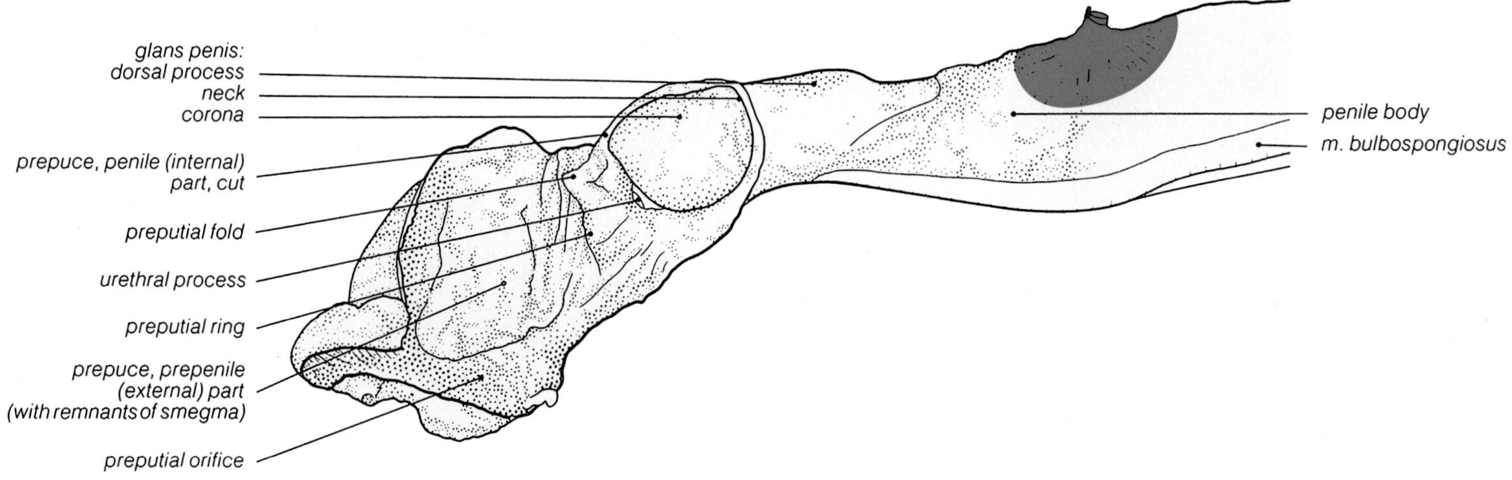
glans penis:
dorsal process
neck
corona
prepuce, penile (internal)
part, cut
preputial fold
urethral process
preputial ring
prepuce, prepenile
(external) part
(with remnants of smegma)
preputial orifice
penile body
m. bulbospongiosus

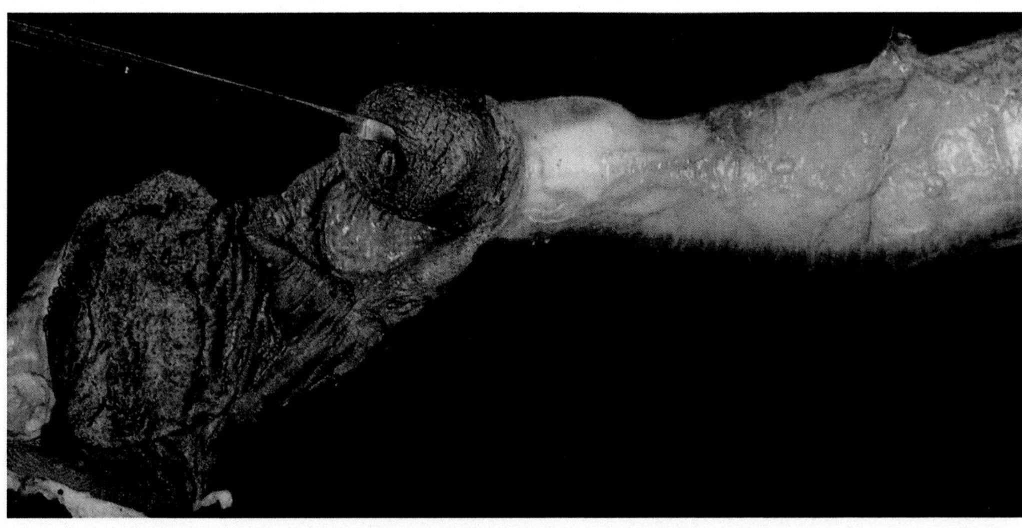

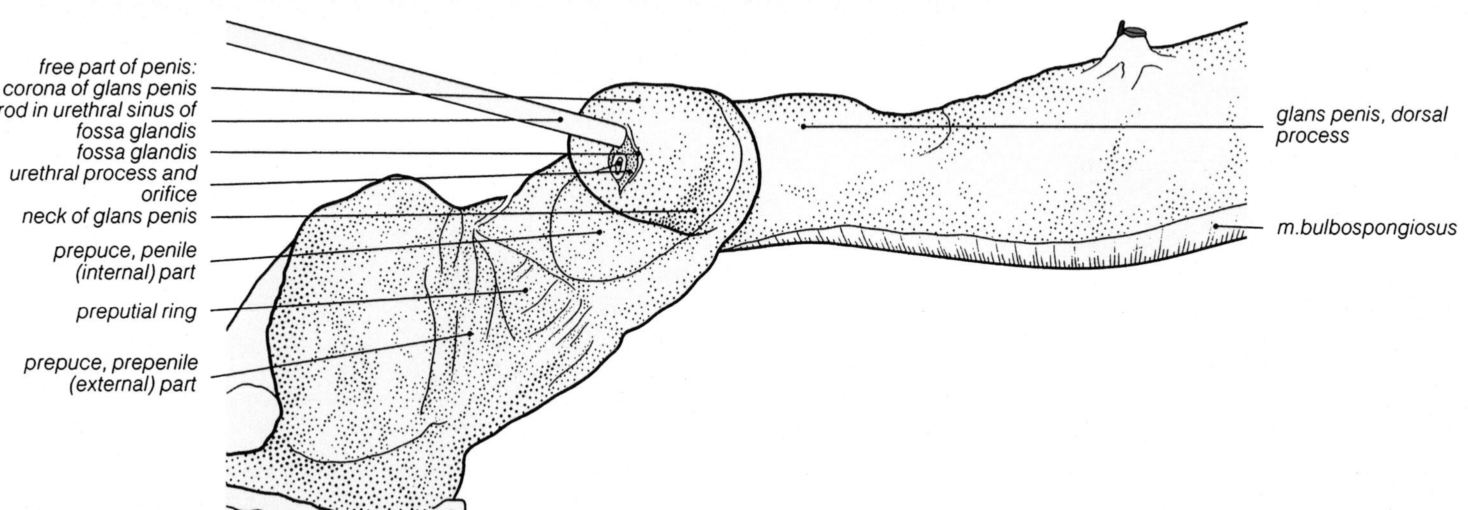
free part of penis:
corona of glans penis
rod in urethral sinus of
fossa glandis
fossa glandis
urethral process and
orifice
neck of glans penis
prepuce, penile
(internal) part
preputial ring
prepuce, prepenile
(external) part
glans penis, dorsal
process
m.bulbospongiosus

Fig. 8.44 Penis and prepuce of the adult stallion: left lateral view (3). A perspex rod has been inserted into the dorsal diverticulum of the fossa glandis (urethral sinus).

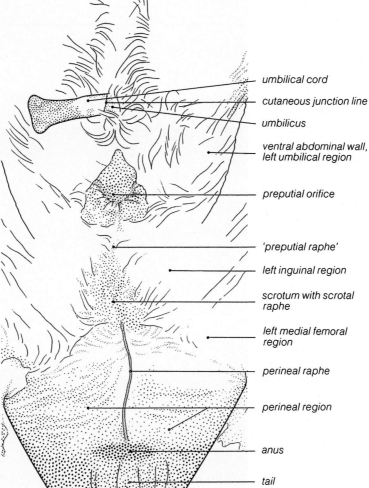

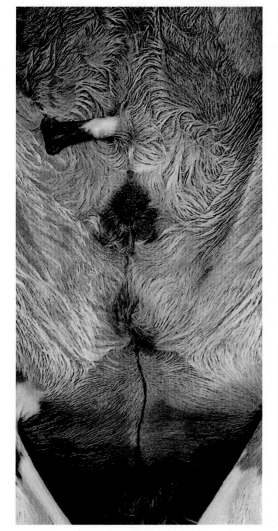

umbilical cord
cutaneous junction line
umbilicus
ventral abdominal wall,
left umbilical region
preputial orifice
'preputial raphe'
left inguinal region
scrotum with scrotal
raphe
left medial femoral
region
perineal raphe
perineal region
anus
tail

Fig. 8.45 Umbilical, inguinal and perineal regions of the new-born colt: ventral view. The perineal region extends from the anus to the scrotum, and is marked by a distinct mid-line raphe. The skin overlying the prepuce is marked by a raphe and the left and right sides of the scrotum are divided by a scrotal raphe. The umbilical cord dries to a shrivelled thread in the normal, live foal soon after birth (see Fig. 8.48). Further details of this specimen are shown in Figs. 8.46 and 8.47.

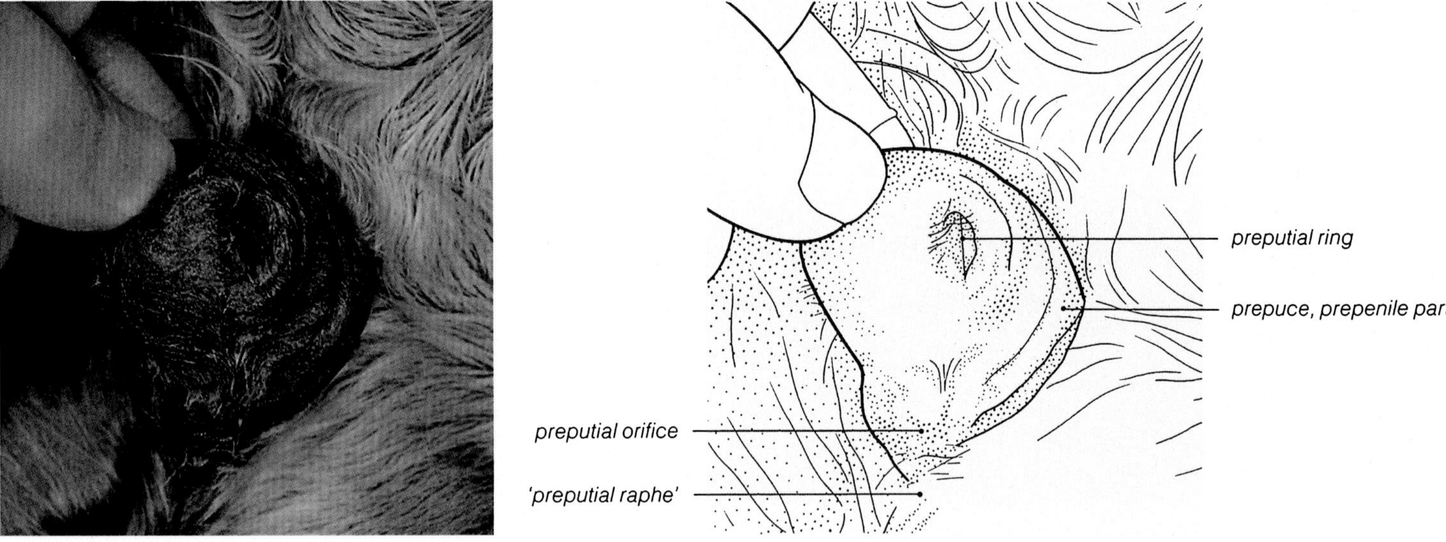
preputial ring
prepuce, prepenile part
preputial orifice
'preputial raphe'

Fig. 8.46 The preputial orifice of the new-born colt: ventral view. The prepenile part of the prepuce has been everted to show the preputial ring, but no attempt has been made to protrude the free part of the penis from the penile part of the prepuce.

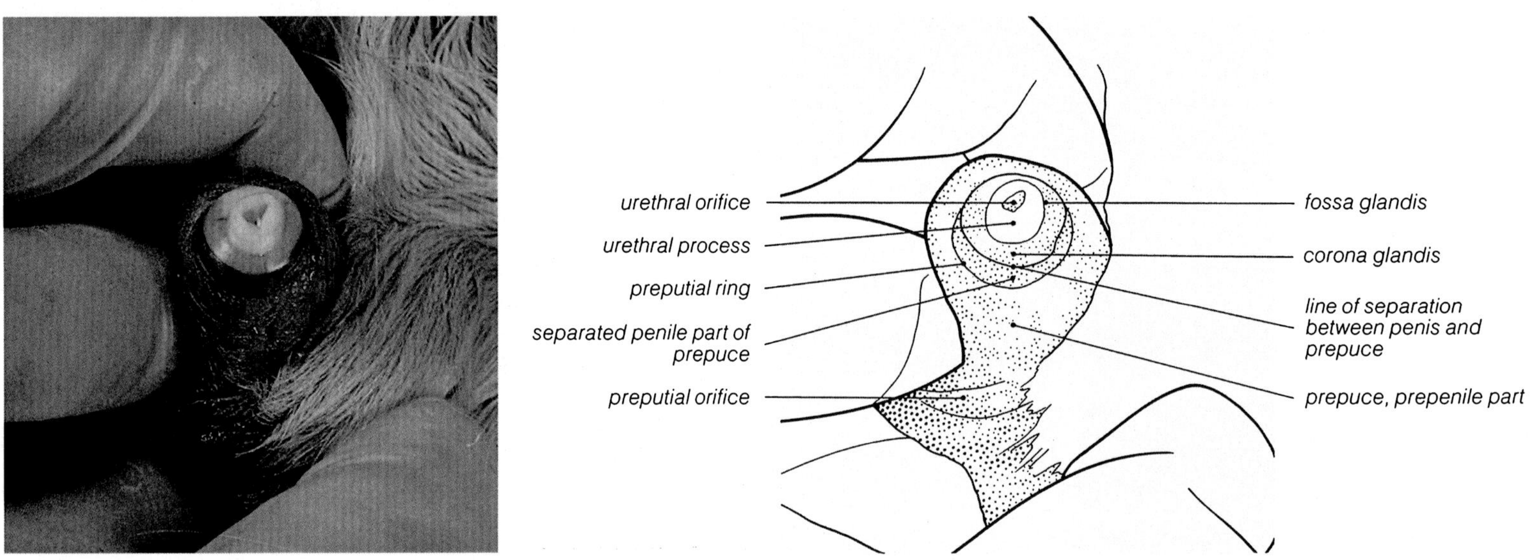
urethral orifice
urethral process
preputial ring
separated penile part of prepuce
preputial orifice
fossa glandis
corona glandis
line of separation between penis and prepuce
prepuce, prepenile part

Fig. 8.47 The non-protrusive penis of the new-born colt: ventral view. At birth, the epithelium of the free part of the penis is fused with that of the penile part of the prepuce. Only the urethral orifice and a small part of the glans penis can be protruded through the preputial ring. Separation of the free part of the penis from the penile part of the prepuce takes place in the first month after birth. (Figs. 8.48–8.53).

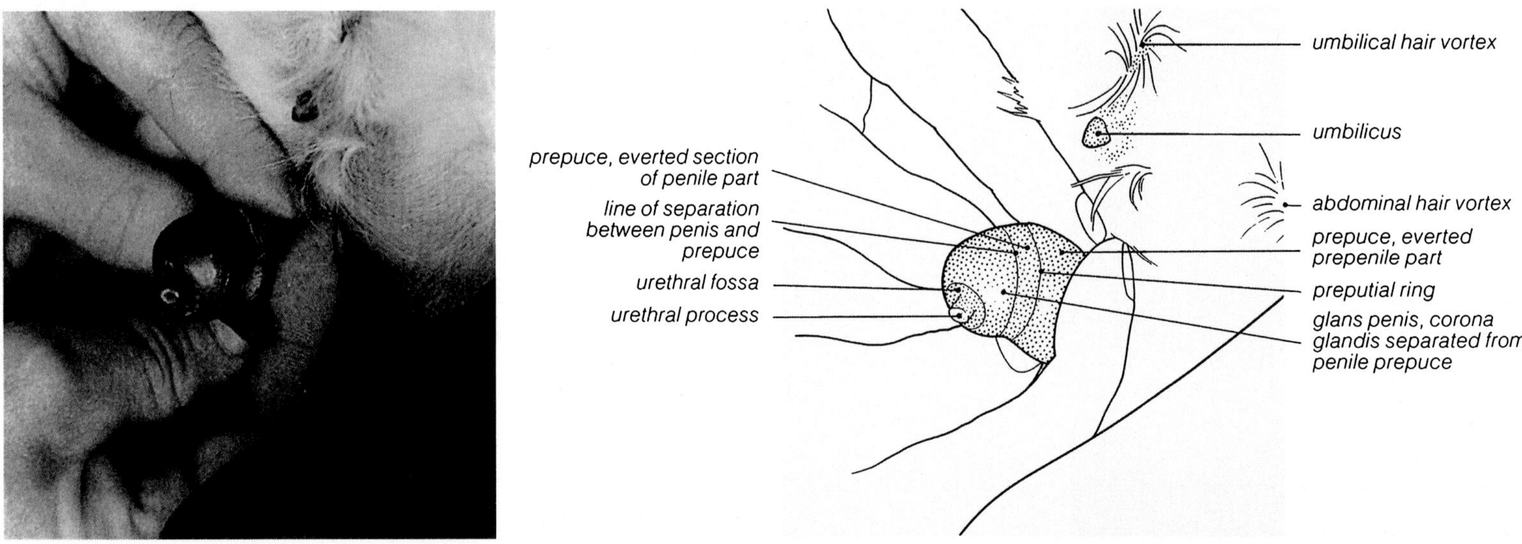
prepuce, everted section of penile part
line of separation between penis and prepuce
urethral fossa
urethral process
umbilical hair vortex
umbilicus
abdominal hair vortex
prepuce, everted prepenile part
preputial ring
glans penis, corona glandis separated from penile prepuce

Fig. 8.48 Penile development in a grey colt: 2 days, left ventrolateral view. Separation between penile integument and the penile part of the prepuce extends only very slowly over the corona glandis during the first 2 to 3 weeks after birth; the rest of the penile integument remains firmly adherent to the prepuce. The adherent epithelia of the penile integument and the penile prepuce are separated by keratinisation of the middle layer of ectodermal cells.

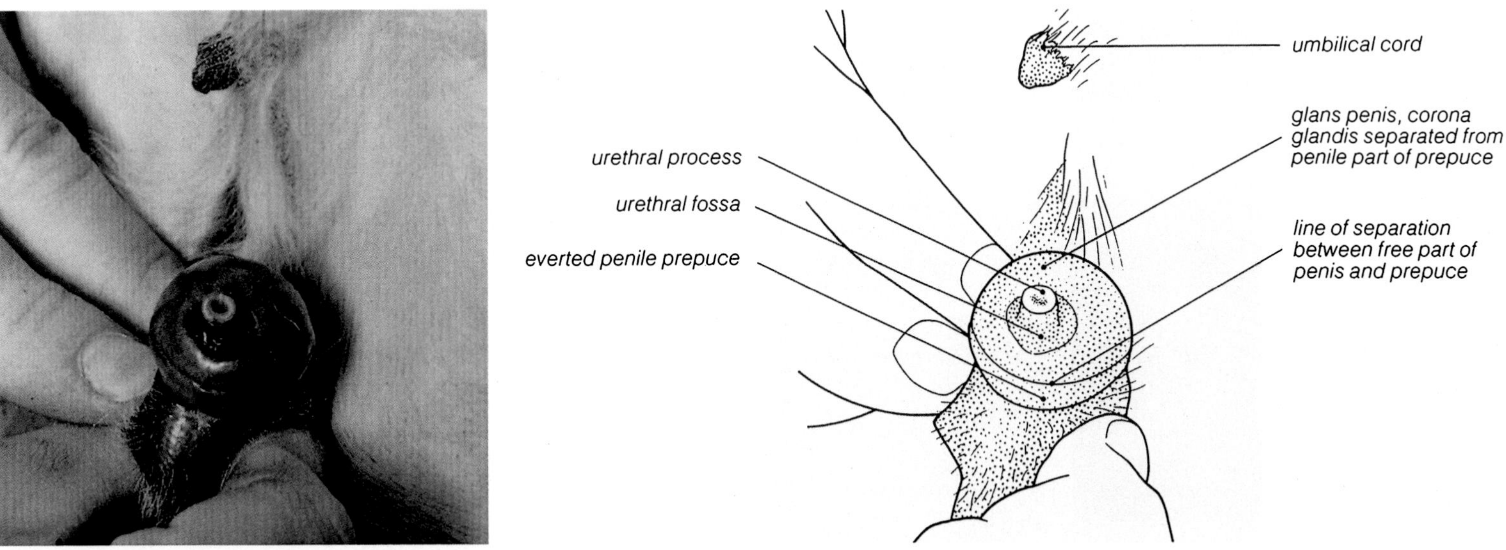
umbilical cord
glans penis, corona glandis separated from penile part of prepuce
urethral process
urethral fossa
everted penile prepuce
line of separation between free part of penis and prepuce

Fig. 8.49 Penile development in a grey colt: 9 days, left ventrolateral view. The line of separation between penile integument and penile prepuce is clearly shown.

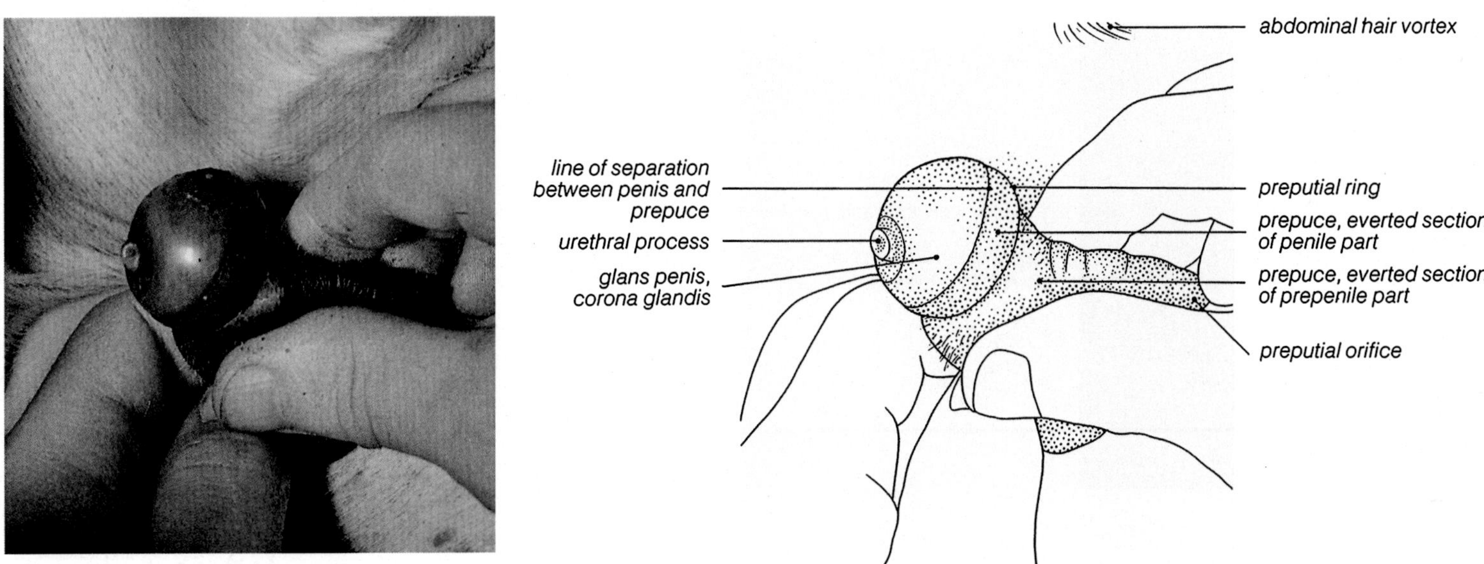
abdominal hair vortex
line of separation between penis and prepuce
preputial ring
prepuce, everted section of penile part
urethral process
glans penis, corona glandis
prepuce, everted section of prepenile part
preputial orifice

Fig. 8.50 Penile development in a grey colt: 15 days, left lateral view. The line of separation between penis and penile prepuce moves back gradually over the corona glandis during the first two weeks of life.

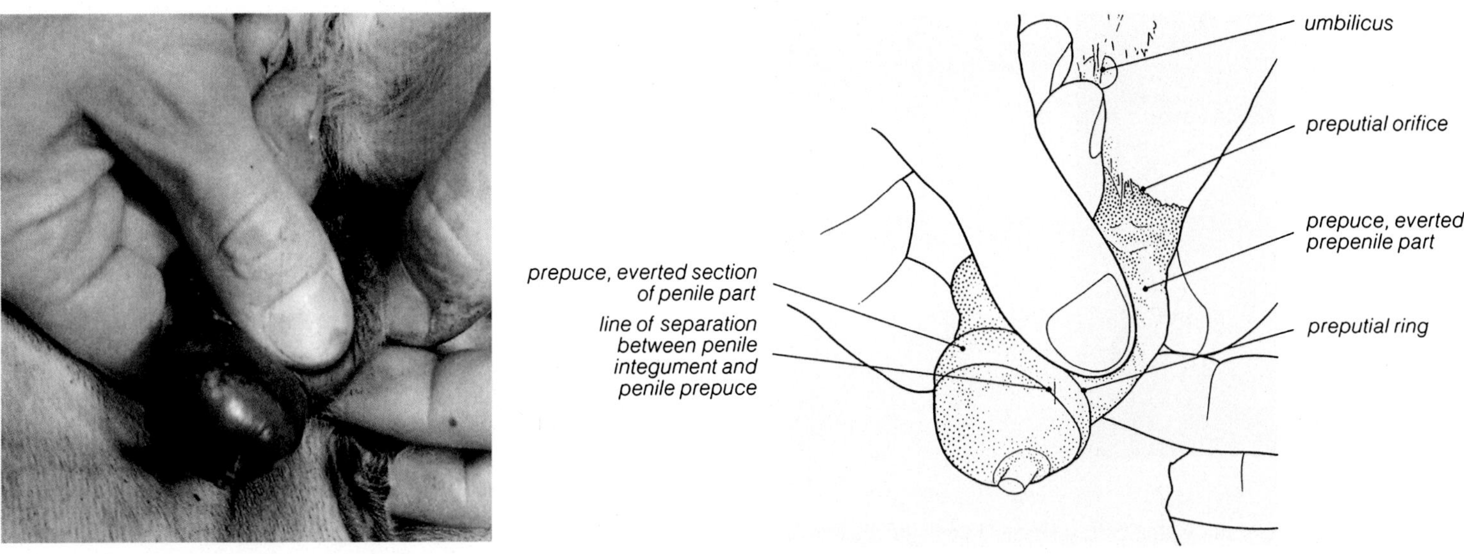
umbilicus
preputial orifice
prepuce, everted prepenile part
prepuce, everted section of penile part
line of separation between penile integument and penile prepuce
preputial ring

Fig. 8.51 Penile development in a grey colt: 22 days, left lateral view. The organ has been bent caudally during manipulation.

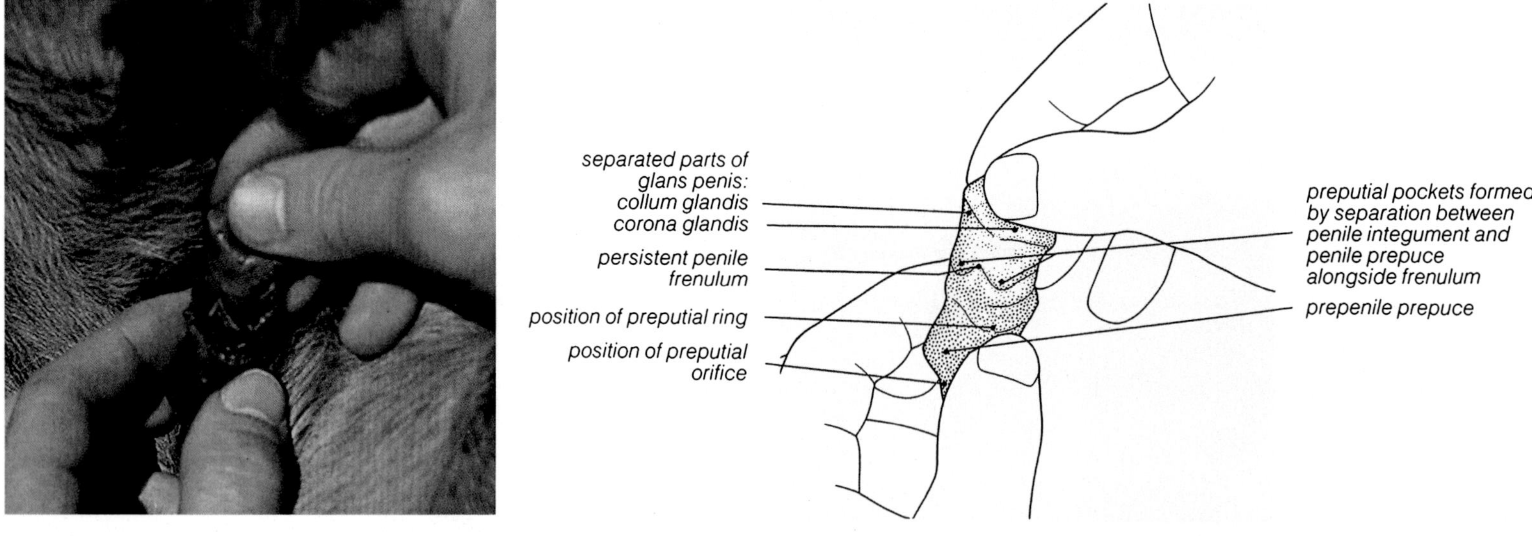
separated parts of glans penis:
collum glandis
corona glandis
persistent penile frenulum
position of preputial ring
position of preputial orifice
preputial pockets formed by separation between penile integument and penile prepuce alongside frenulum
prepenile prepuce

Fig. 8.52 Penile development in a dun colt: 24 days, ventral view. This figure and Fig. 8.53 show the final stages leading to completion of the process of separation at the end of the first month after birth. At 24 days, separation between penile integument and penile prepuce has extended past the corona glandis, and is rapidly proceeding down the shaft of the free part of the penis. However, the frenulum is still intact.

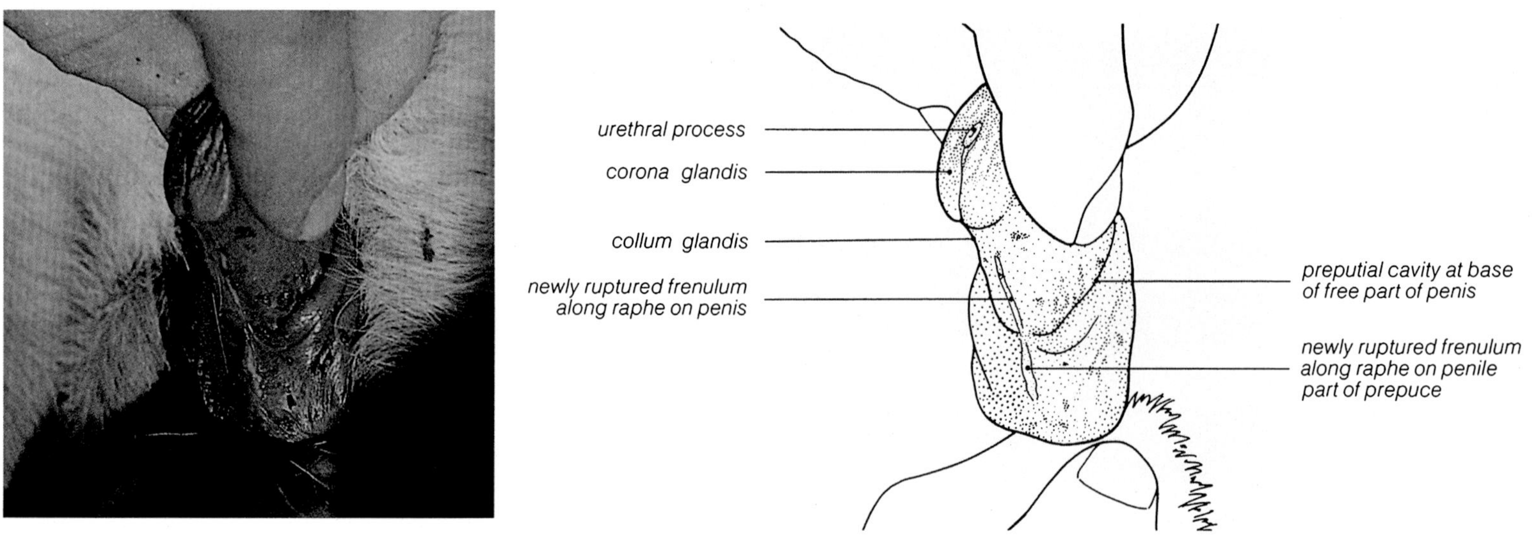
urethral process
corona glandis
collum glandis
newly ruptured frenulum along raphe on penis
preputial cavity at base of free part of penis
newly ruptured frenulum along raphe on penile part of prepuce

Fig. 8.53 Penile development in a dun colt: 32 days, ventral view. Separation between the free part of the penis and its penile prepuce is now complete. The frenulum, a direct connective tissue union, often resists rupture after keratinisation of the ectodermal lamella (controlled by male hormone) has separated the rest of the penis from its prepuce. In this colt, the persistent frenulum seen at 24 days (Fig. 8.52) has ruptured by 32 days leaving a linear sore along the ventral surfaces of penis and penile prepuce.

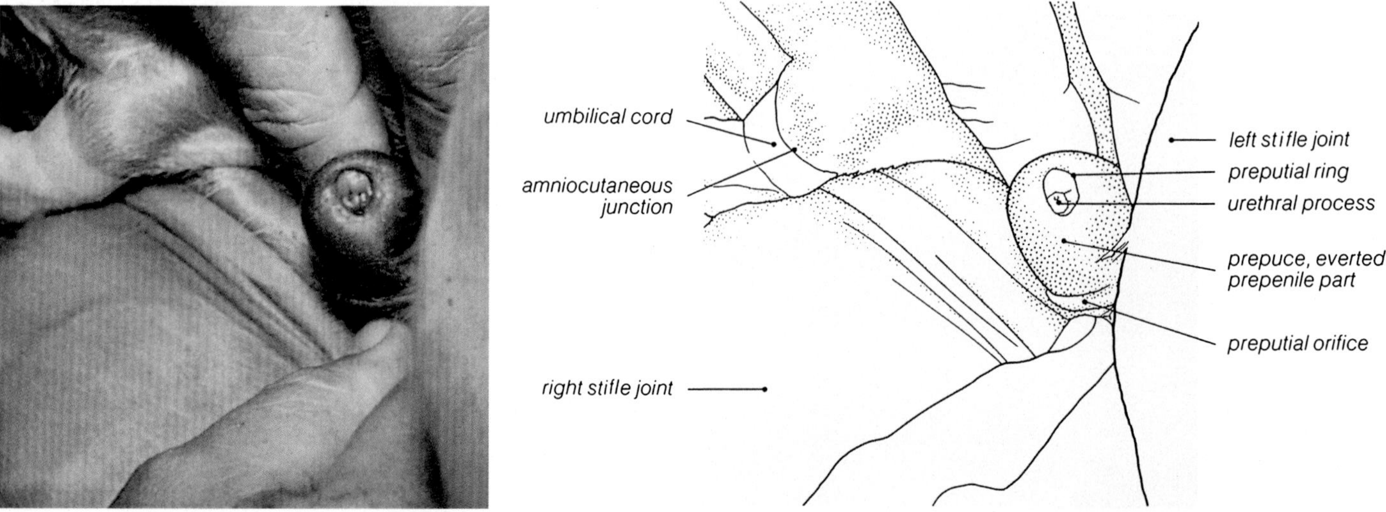
umbilical cord
amniocutaneous junction
right stifle joint
left stifle joint
preputial ring
urethral process
prepuce, everted prepenile part
preputial orifice

Fig. 8.54 Penile development in the young colt; protruded penis of the foetus: ventral view. In this 9-month foetus, the penis is still adherent to its penile prepuce and could not be protruded through the preputial ring, even though the prepenile part of the prepuce has been everted. The urethral orifice is not occluded and urination is possible during foetal life. Figs. 8.49–8.53 show the process by which the corona of the glans penis slowly separates from the penile part of the prepuce during the first month after birth.

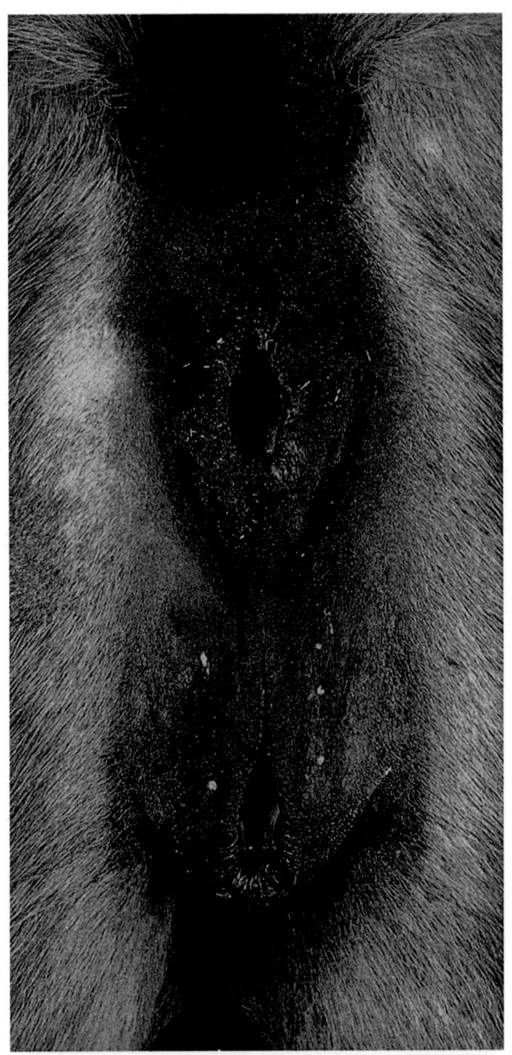

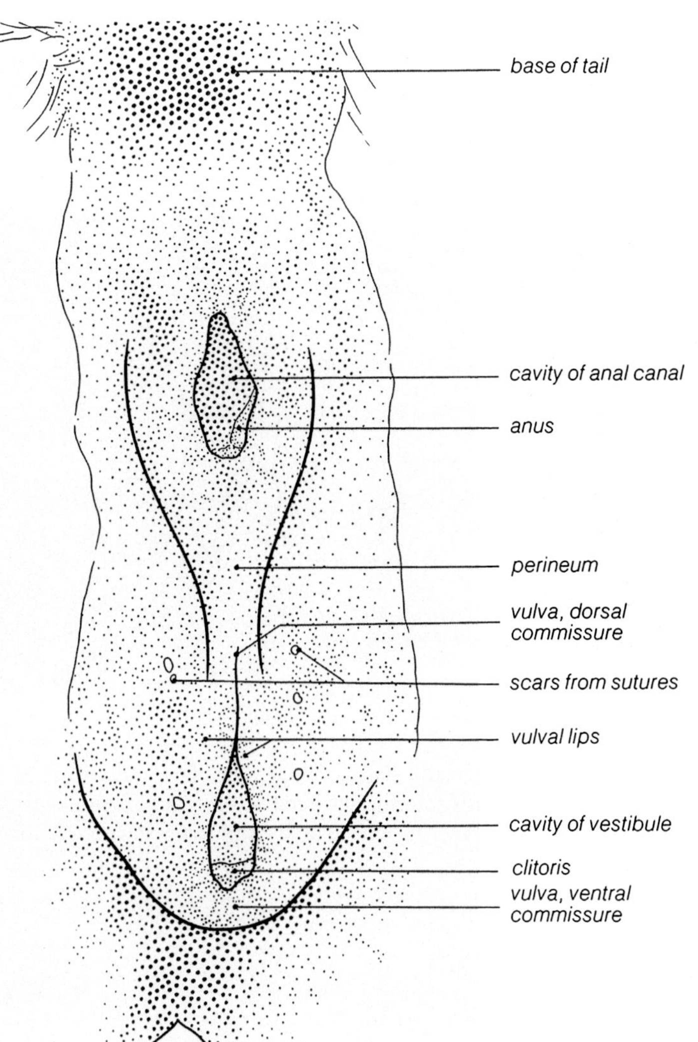
base of tail
cavity of anal canal
anus
perineum
vulva, dorsal commissure
scars from sutures
vulval lips
cavity of vestibule
clitoris
vulva, ventral commissure

Fig. 8.55 The perineal region of a pregnant mare: caudal view. This mare was 100 days pregnant. The dorsal parts of the vulval lips have been sutured together ('Caslick's operation') and scars remain. This mare was photographed immediately before embalming was commenced. Fig. 8.56 shows further details of this specimen.

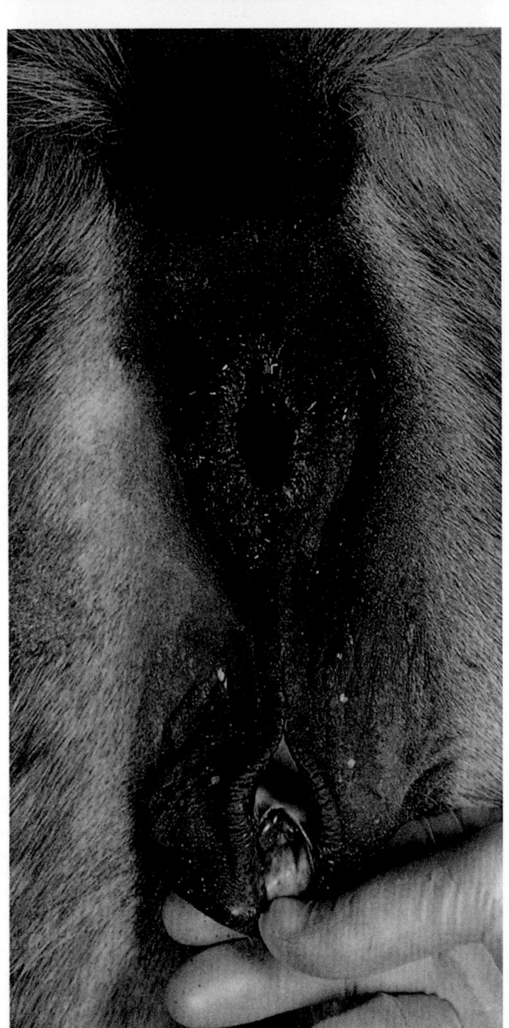

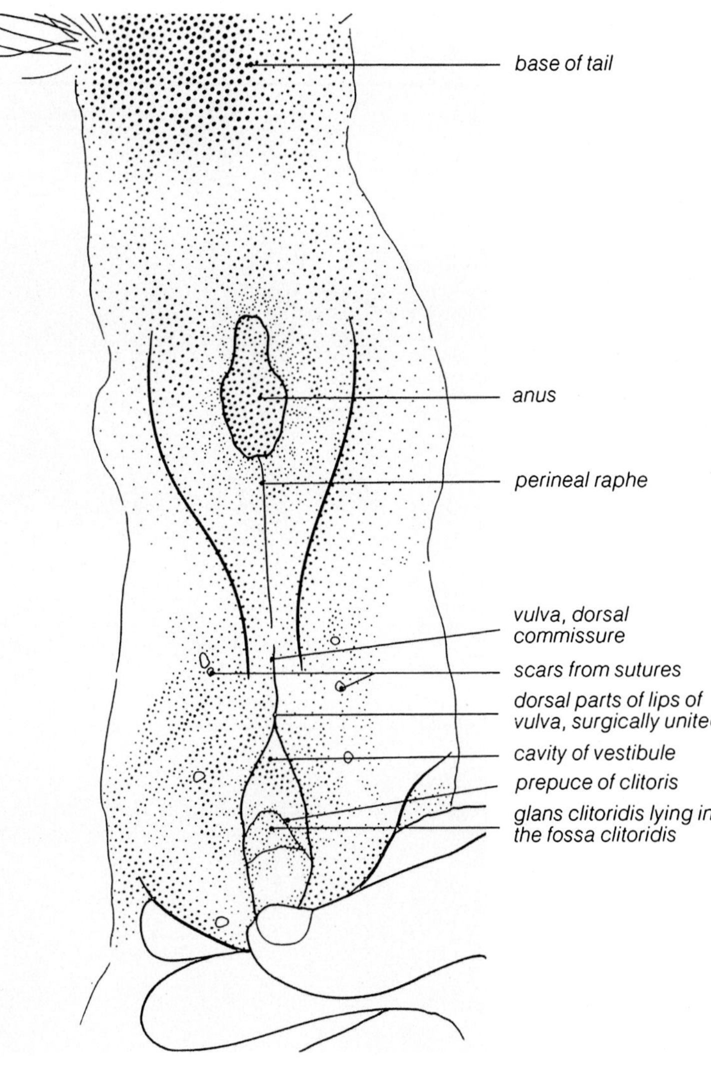
base of tail
anus
perineal raphe
vulva, dorsal commissure
scars from sutures
dorsal parts of lips of vulva, surgically united
cavity of vestibule
prepuce of clitoris
glans clitoridis lying in the fossa clitoridis

Fig. 8.56 The clitoris of a pregnant mare: caudal view. The thumb has been placed in the ventral vulval commissure in order to expose the glans, lying in the fossa of the clitoris.

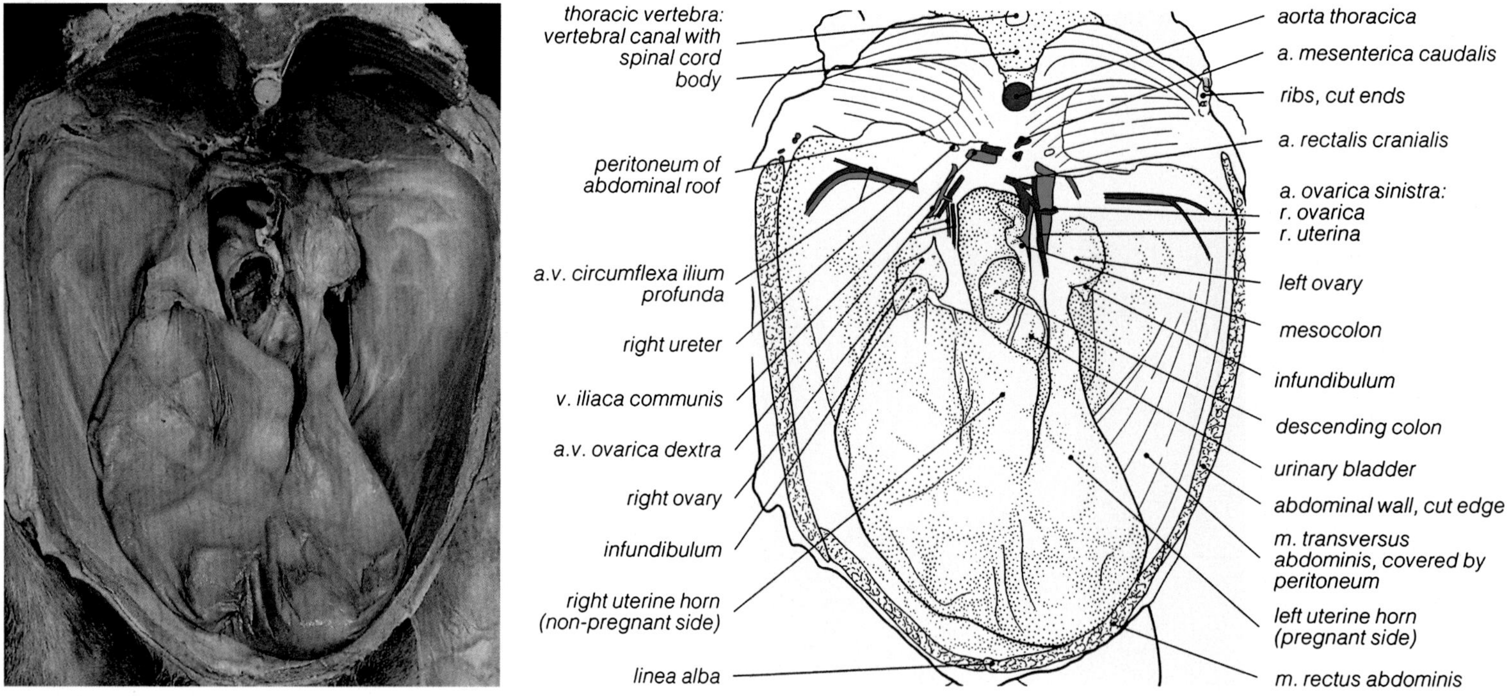

thoracic vertebra:
vertebral canal with
spinal cord
body
peritoneum of
abdominal roof
a.v. circumflexa ilium
profunda
right ureter
v. iliaca communis
a.v. ovarica dextra
right ovary
infundibulum
right uterine horn
(non-pregnant side)
linea alba
aorta thoracica
a. mesenterica caudalis
ribs, cut ends
a. rectalis cranialis
a. ovarica sinistra:
r. ovarica
r. uterina
left ovary
mesocolon
infundibulum
descending colon
urinary bladder
abdominal wall, cut edge
m. transversus
abdominis, covered by
peritoneum
left uterine horn
(pregnant side)
m. rectus abdominis

Fig. 8.57 Reproductive organs and pelvic inlet of a pregnant mare: cranial view. The abdominal organs have been removed, and the abdominal wall sectioned just cranial to the tuber coxae. The vertebral column has been sectioned at caudal thoracic level. The mare was 100 days pregnant, the foetus being located in the body and left horn of the uterus. The arteries and veins have been filled with red and blue neoprene latex.

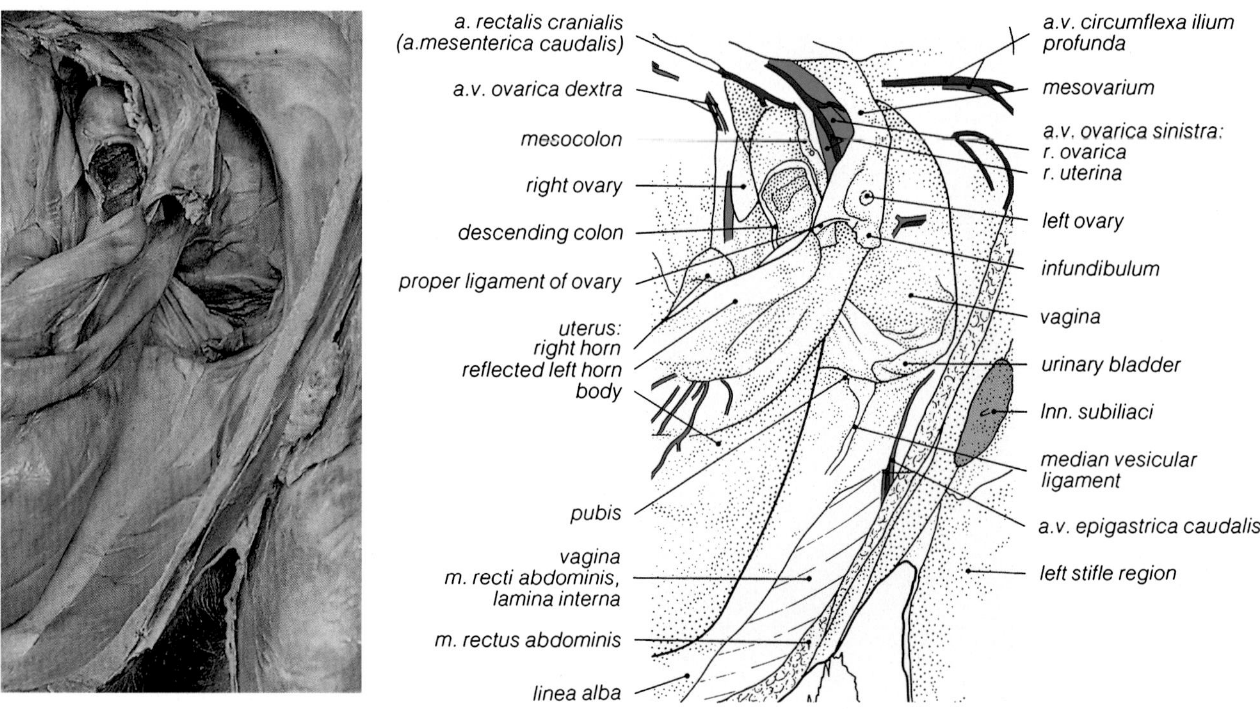

a. rectalis cranialis
(a.mesenterica caudalis)
a.v. ovarica dextra
mesocolon
right ovary
descending colon
proper ligament of ovary
uterus:
right horn
reflected left horn
body
pubis
vagina
m. recti abdominis,
lamina interna
m. rectus abdominis
linea alba
a.v. circumflexa ilium
profunda
mesovarium
a.v. ovarica sinistra:
r. ovarica
r. uterina
left ovary
infundibulum
vagina
urinary bladder
lnn. subiliaci
median vesicular
ligament
a.v. epigastrica caudalis
left stifle region

Fig. 8.58 Reproductive organs and pelvic inlet of a pregnant mare: left cranio-lateral view. The pregnant body and left horn of the uterus have been displaced to the right to show the pelvic inlet.

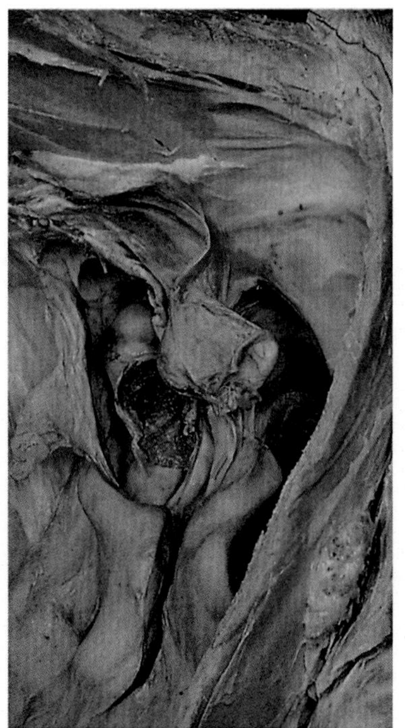

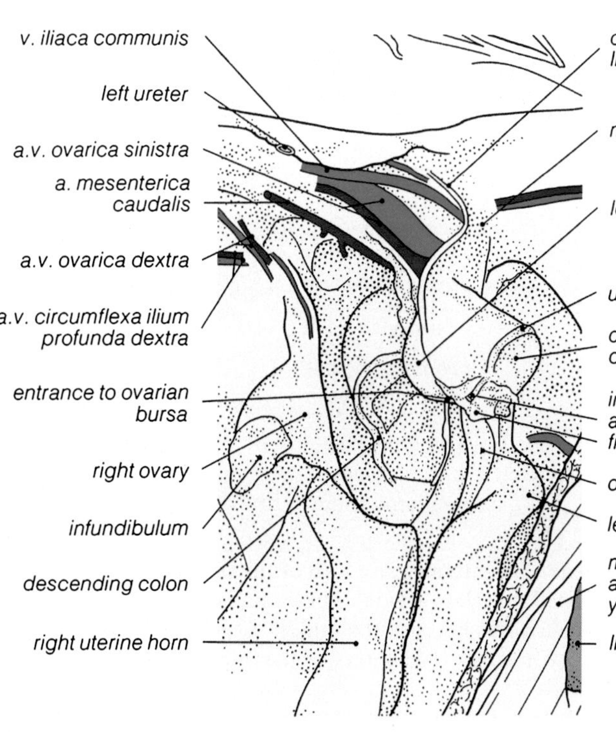

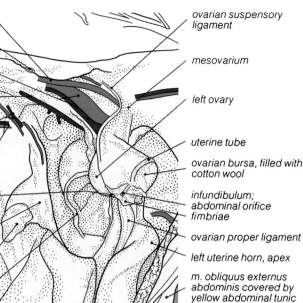

v. iliaca communis
left ureter
a.v. ovarica sinistra
a. mesenterica caudalis
a.v. ovarica dextra
a.v. circumflexa ilium profunda dextra
entrance to ovarian bursa
right ovary
infundibulum
descending colon
right uterine horn
ovarian suspensory ligament
mesovarium
left ovary
uterine tube
ovarian bursa, filled with cotton wool
infundibulum; abdominal orifice fimbriae
ovarian proper ligament
left uterine horn, apex
m. obliquus externus abdominis covered by yellow abdominal tunic
lnn. subiliaci

Fig. 8.59 The left ovary of a pregnant mare: left lateral view. The left ovary contained a single corpus luteum (pregnant 100 days) and was larger than the right ovary. The ovarian bursa of the left ovary has been filled with cotton wool; it bulges out laterally and the uterine tube traversing its wall is clearly recognisable. The fimbriae of the infundibulum have been spread out to show the orifice leading into the lumen of the left uterine tube. See also Figs. 8.76 and 8.77.

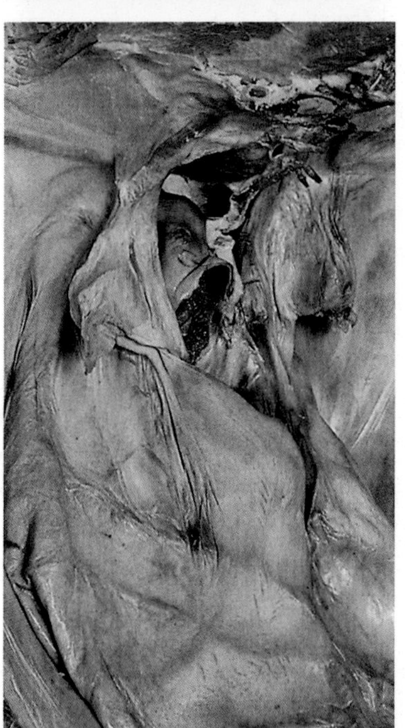

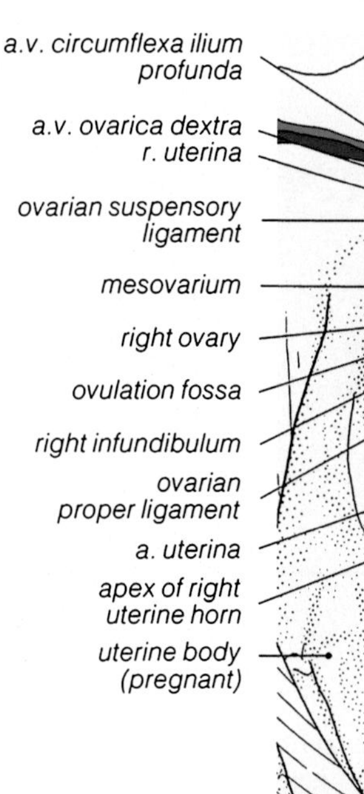

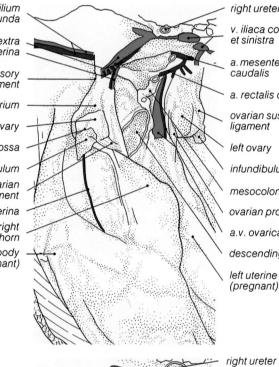

a.v. circumflexa ilium profunda
a.v. ovarica dextra r. uterina
ovarian suspensory ligament
mesovarium
right ovary
ovulation fossa
right infundibulum
ovarian proper ligament
a. uterina
apex of right uterine horn
uterine body (pregnant)
right ureter
v. iliaca communis dextra et sinistra
a. mesenterica caudalis
a. rectalis cranialis
ovarian suspensory ligament
left ovary
infundibulum
mesocolon
ovarian proper ligament
a.v. ovarica sinistra
descending colon
left uterine horn (pregnant)

Fig. 8.60 The right ovary of a pregnant mare: right cranio-lateral view. The right ovary has been positioned to show its medial surface. It contains no corpus luteum, and is considerably smaller than the left ovary. The ovarian bursa and uterine tube are shown in Fig. 8.61.

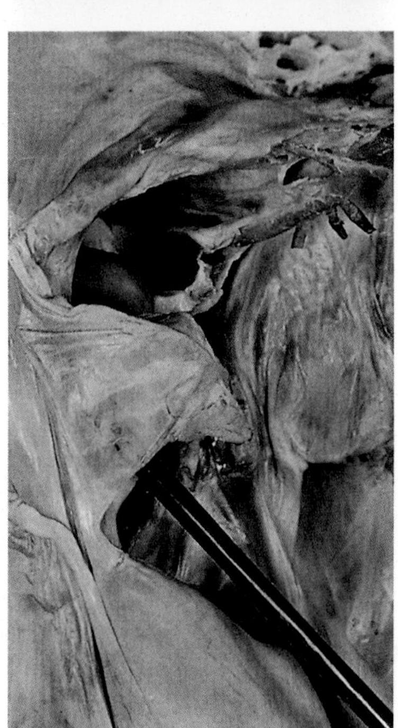

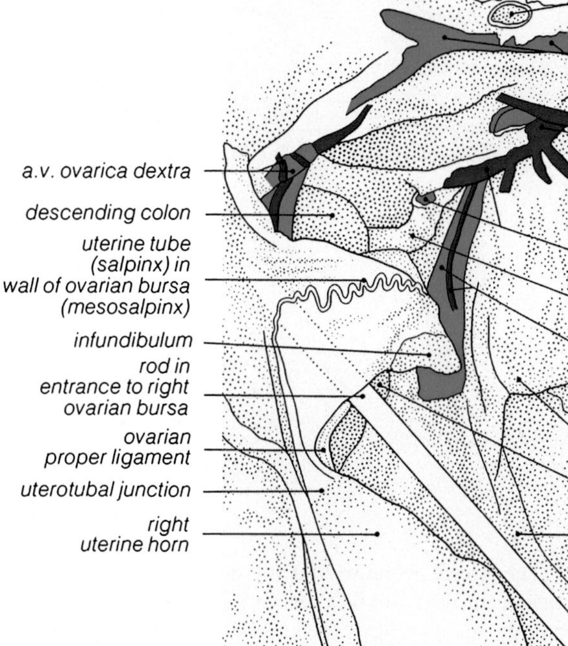

a.v. ovarica dextra
descending colon
uterine tube (salpinx) in wall of ovarian bursa (mesosalpinx)
infundibulum
rod in entrance to right ovarian bursa
ovarian proper ligament
uterotubal junction
right uterine horn
right ureter
v. iliaca communis dextra et sinistra
a. mesenterica caudalis
ovarian suspensory ligament
a.v. rectalis cranialis
mesocolon
a.v. ovarica sinistra r. uterina
infundibulum
left ovary
descending colon
left uterine horn

Fig. 8.61 The ovarian bursa and the uterine tube: right craniolateral view. The right ovary has been pushed medially, and a rod has been inserted into the ovarian bursa. The uterine tube, or salpinx, runs in the mesosalpinx, which forms the lateral wall of the ovarian bursa.

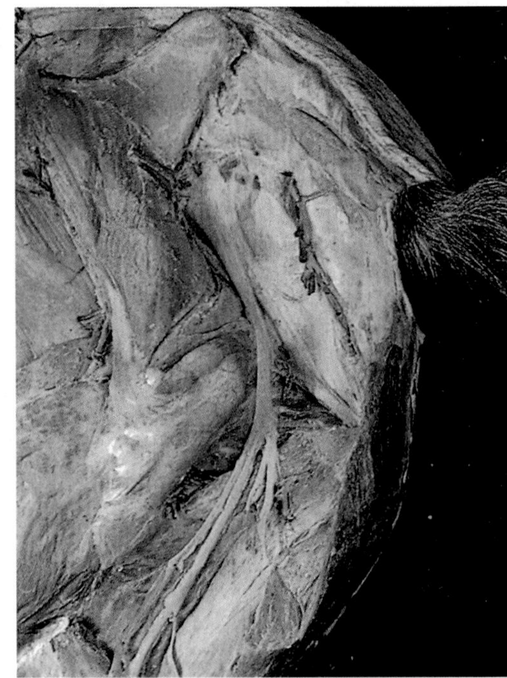

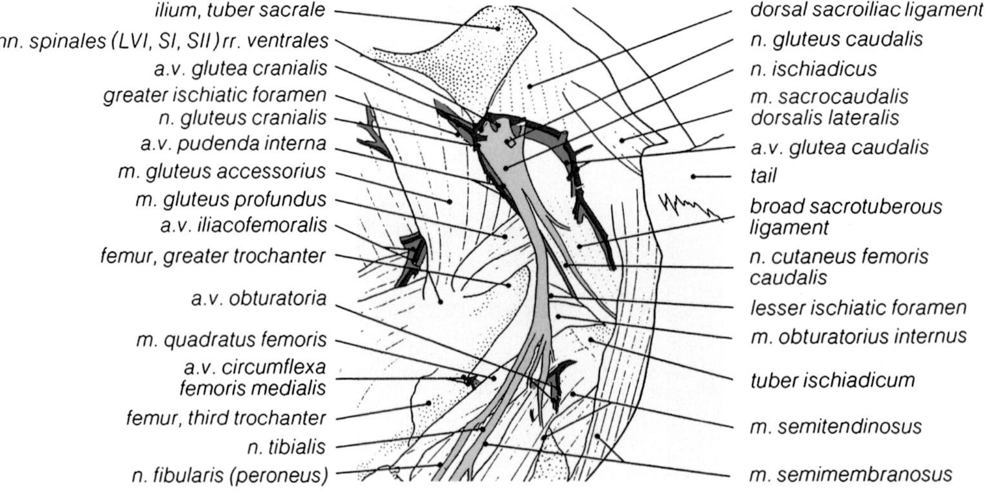
ilium, tuber sacrale
nn. spinales (LVI, SI, SII) rr. ventrales
a.v. glutea cranialis
greater ischiatic foramen
n. gluteus cranialis
a.v. pudenda interna
m. gluteus accessorius
m. gluteus profundus
a.v. iliacofemoralis
femur, greater trochanter
a.v. obturatoria
m. quadratus femoris
a.v. circumflexa femoris medialis
femur, third trochanter
n. tibialis
n. fibularis (peroneus)
dorsal sacroiliac ligament
n. gluteus caudalis
n. ischiadicus
m. sacrocaudalis dorsalis lateralis
a.v. glutea caudalis
tail
broad sacrotuberous ligament
n. cutaneus femoris caudalis
lesser ischiatic foramen
m. obturatorius internus
tuber ischiadicum
m. semitendinosus
m. semimembranosus

Fig. 8.62 The lateral pelvic wall of the mare: the sacrotuberous ligament, left caudolateral view. The superficial muscles (tensor fasciae latae, superficial gluteal, biceps femoris, the vertebral head of the semitendinosus, and the middle gluteal) have been removed to expose the sacrotuberous ligament. Further dissections of the lateral pelvic wall in this pregnant mare are shown in Figs, 8.63 to 8.70.

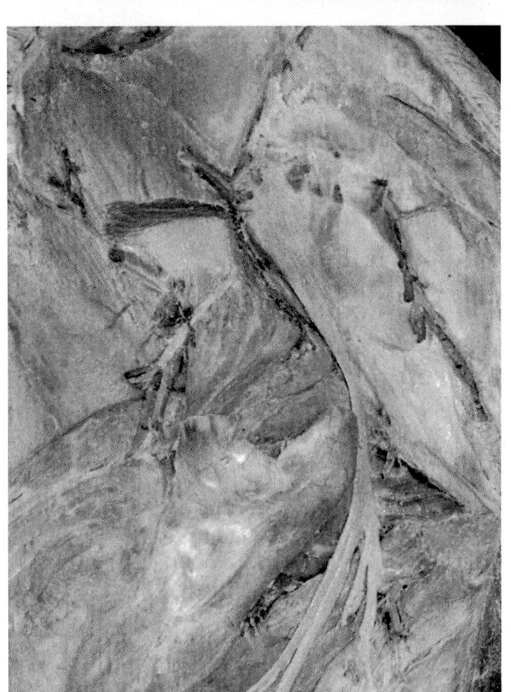

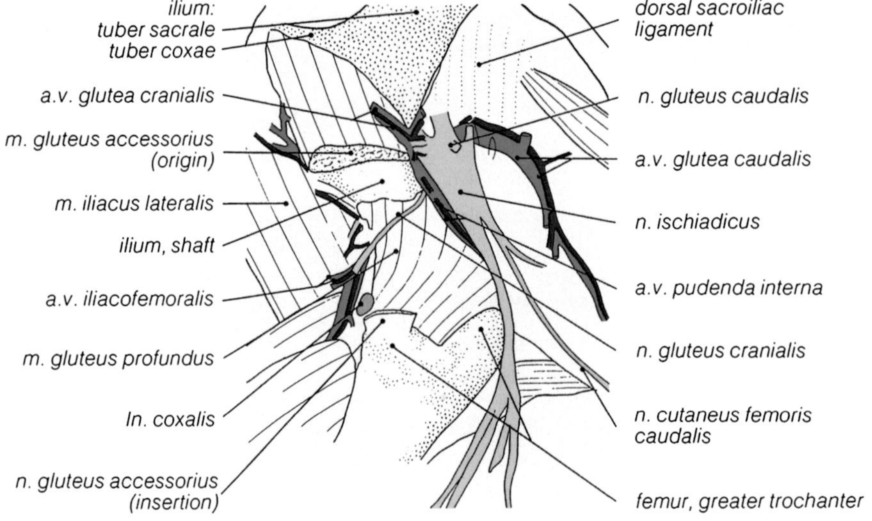
ilium:
tuber sacrale
tuber coxae
a.v. glutea cranialis
m. gluteus accessorius (origin)
m. iliacus lateralis
ilium, shaft
a.v. iliacofemoralis
m. gluteus profundus
ln. coxalis
n. gluteus accessorius (insertion)
dorsal sacroiliac ligament
n. gluteus caudalis
a.v. glutea caudalis
n. ischiadicus
a.v. pudenda interna
n. gluteus cranialis
n. cutaneus femoris caudalis
femur, greater trochanter

Fig. 8.63 The cranial gluteal nerve and the coxal lymph node of the mare: left caudolateral view. The middle part of the accessory gluteal muscle has been removed to show the cranial gluteal nerve passing between it and the deep gluteal muscle. This nerve supplies the tensor fasciae latae muscle. The coxal lymph node is not always present in the horse.

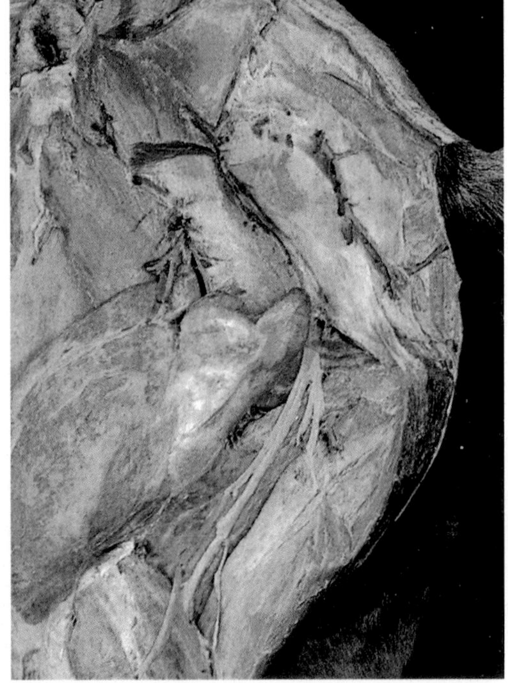

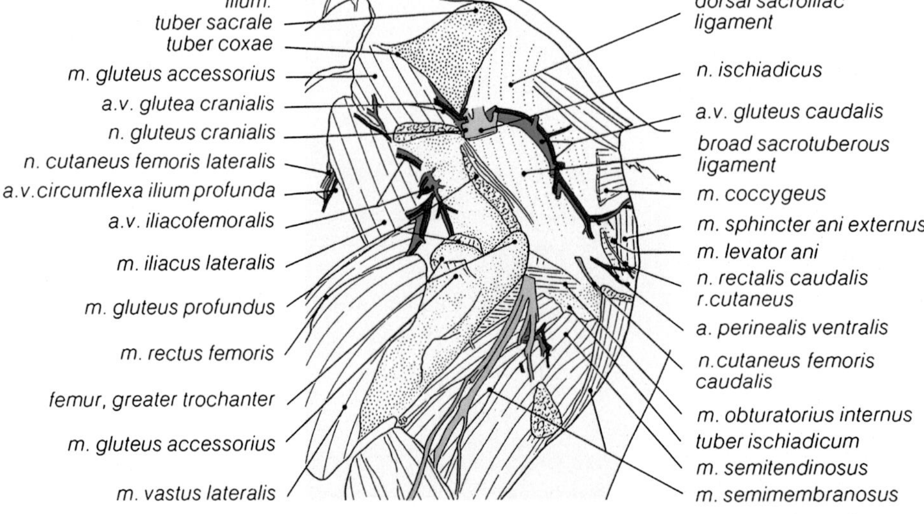
ilium:
tuber sacrale
tuber coxae
m. gluteus accessorius
a.v. glutea cranialis
n. gluteus cranialis
n. cutaneus femoris lateralis
a.v.circumflexa ilium profunda
a.v. iliacofemoralis
m. iliacus lateralis
m. gluteus profundus
m. rectus femoris
femur, greater trochanter
m. gluteus accessorius
m. vastus lateralis
dorsal sacroiliac ligament
n. ischiadicus
a.v. gluteus caudalis
broad sacrotuberous ligament
m. coccygeus
m. sphincter ani externus
m. levator ani
n. rectalis caudalis r.cutaneus
a. perinealis ventralis
n.cutaneus femoris caudalis
m. obturatorius internus
tuber ischiadicum
m. semitendinosus
m. semimembranosus

Fig. 8.64 The lateral pelvic wall of the mare: the sacrotuberous ligament, left lateral view. The deep gluteal muscle and the ischiatic nerve have been partly resected. The attachments of the semimembranosus muscle to the caudal edge of the sacrotuberous ligament have been removed, and the perineal structures displayed.

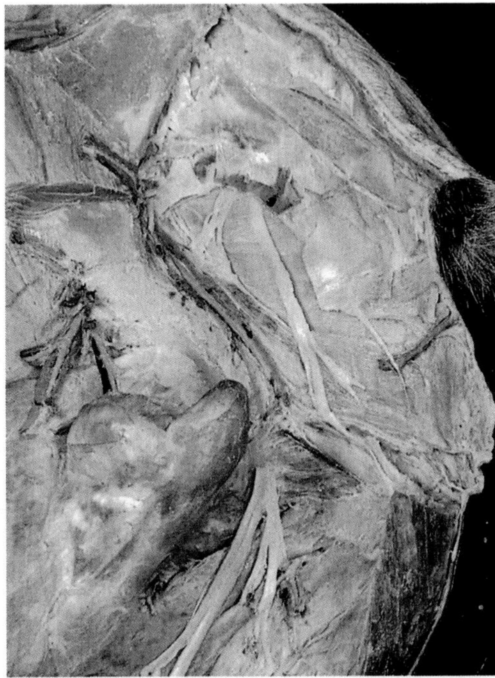

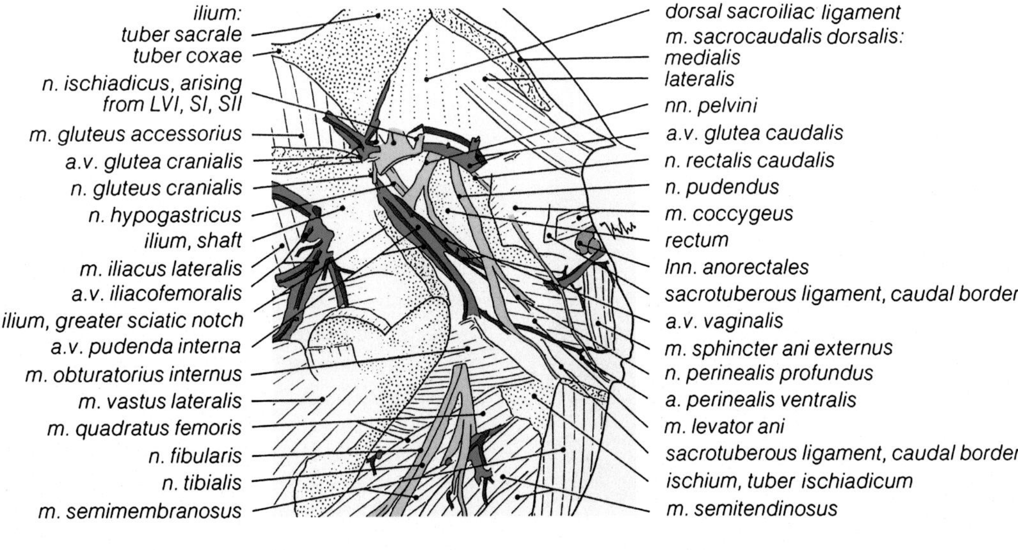
ilium:
tuber sacrale
tuber coxae
n. ischiadicus, arising from LVI, SI, SII
m. gluteus accessorius
a.v. glutea cranialis
n. gluteus cranialis
n. hypogastricus
ilium, shaft
m. iliacus lateralis
a.v. iliacofemoralis
ilium, greater sciatic notch
a.v. pudenda interna
m. obturatorius internus
m. vastus lateralis
m. quadratus femoris
n. fibularis
n. tibialis
m. semimembranosus
dorsal sacroiliac ligament
m. sacrocaudalis dorsalis:
medialis
lateralis
nn. pelvini
a.v. glutea caudalis
n. rectalis caudalis
n. pudendus
m. coccygeus
rectum
lnn. anorectales
sacrotuberous ligament, caudal border
a.v. vaginalis
m. sphincter ani externus
n. perinealis profundus
a. perinealis ventralis
m. levator ani
sacrotuberous ligament, caudal border
ischium, tuber ischiadicum
m. semitendinosus

Fig. 8.65 The lateral pelvic wall of the mare: blood vessels and nerves in left lateral view. The broad sacrotuberous ligament has been removed to expose the blood vessels and nerves that lie deep to it.

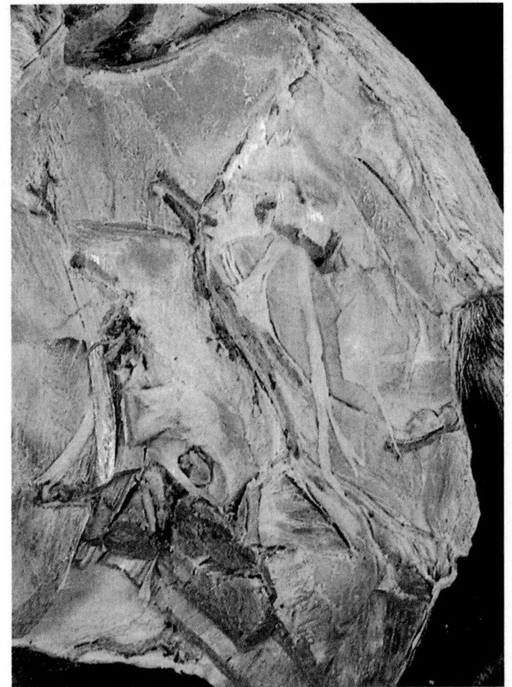

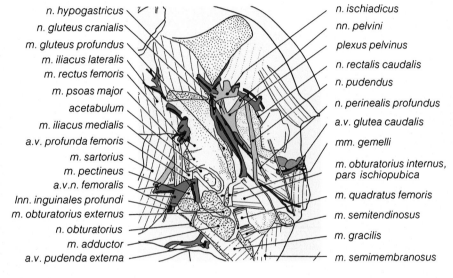

n. hypogastricus
n. gluteus cranialis
m. gluteus profundus
m. iliacus lateralis
m. rectus femoris
m. psoas major
acetabulum
m. iliacus medialis
a.v. profunda femoris
m. sartorius
m. pectineus
a.v.n. femoralis
lnn. inguinales profundi
m. obturatorius externus
n. obturatorius
m. adductor
a.v. pudenda externa
n. ischiadicus
nn. pelvini
plexus pelvinus
n. rectalis caudalis
n. pudendus
n. perinealis profundus
a.v. glutea caudalis
mm. gemelli
m. obturatorius internus, pars ischiopubica
m. quadratus femoris
m. semitendinosus
m. gracilis
m. semimembranosus

Fig. 8.66 The pelvis of the mare after removal of the hind leg: left lateral view. The muscles joining the leg to the pelvis have been cut short.

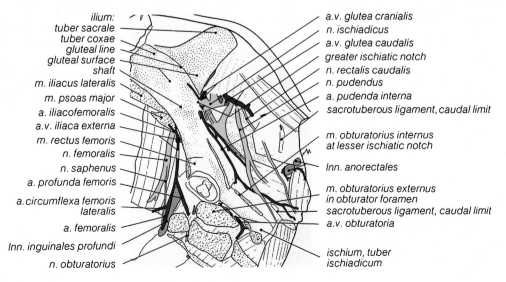

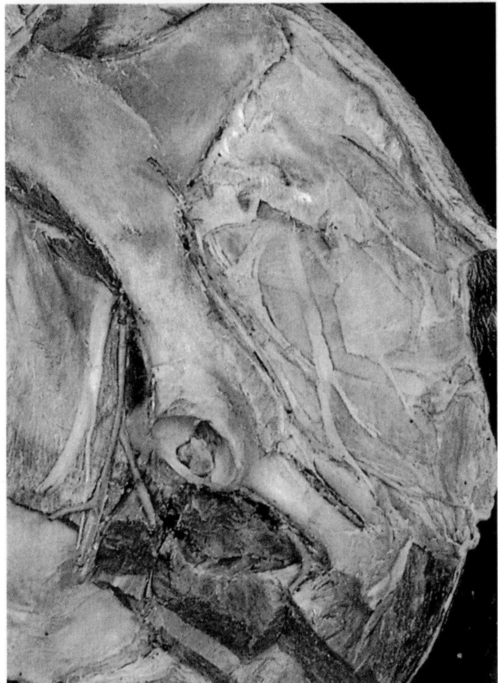

ilium:
tuber sacrale
tuber coxae
gluteal line
gluteal surface
shaft
m. iliacus lateralis
m. psoas major
a. iliacofemoralis
a.v. iliaca externa
m. rectus femoris
n. femoralis
n. saphenus
a. profunda femoris
a. circumflexa femoris lateralis
a. femoralis
lnn. inguinales profundi
n. obturatorius
a.v. glutea cranialis
n. ischiadicus
a.v. glutea caudalis
greater ischiatic notch
n. rectalis caudalis
n. pudendus
a. pudenda interna
sacrotuberous ligament, caudal limit
m. obturatorius internus at lesser ischiatic notch
lnn. anorectales
m. obturatorius externus in obturator foramen
sacrotuberous ligament, caudal limit
a.v. obturatoria
ischium, tuber ischiadicum

Fig. 8.67 The bony pelvis of the mare *in situ*: left lateral view. Structures overlying the bony pelvis have been removed to show the position of the bones in relationship to the arteries, nerves and lymph nodes. The veins have been removed to show the arteries and nerves more clearly.

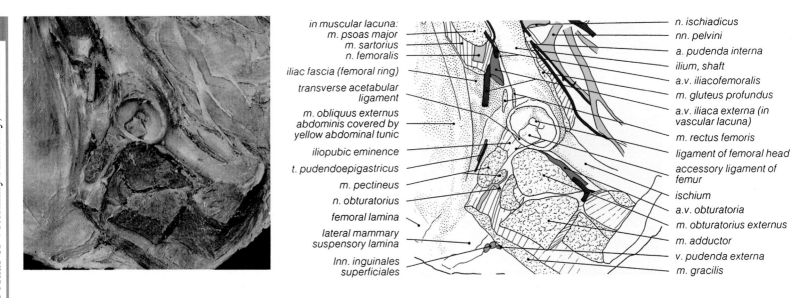

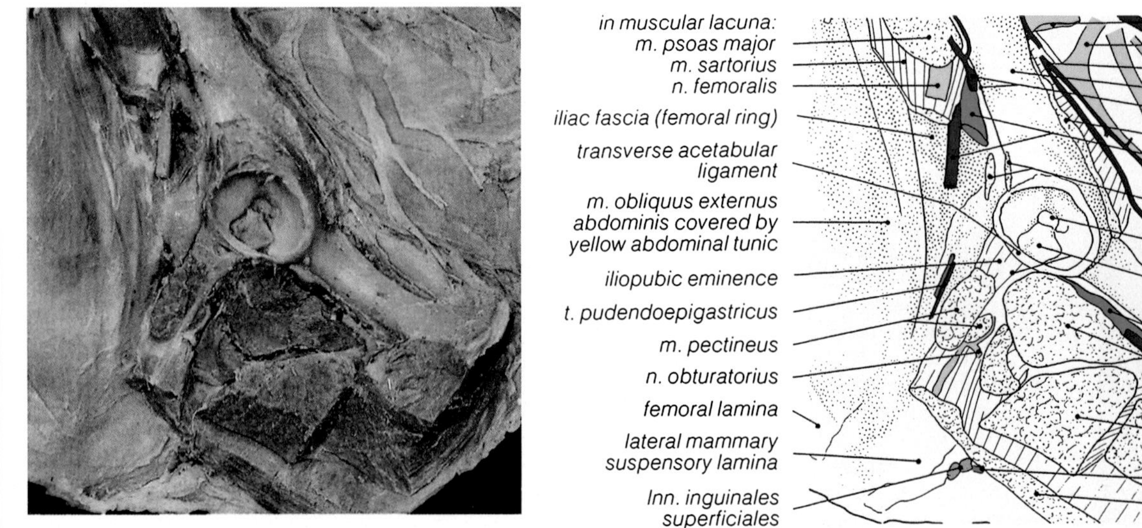
in muscular lacuna:
m. psoas major
m. sartorius
n. femoralis
iliac fascia (femoral ring)
transverse acetabular ligament
m. obliquus externus abdominis covered by yellow abdominal tunic
iliopubic eminence
t. pudendoepigastricus
m. pectineus
n. obturatorius
femoral lamina
lateral mammary suspensory lamina
lnn. inguinales superficiales
n. ischiadicus
nn. pelvini
a. pudenda interna
ilium, shaft
a.v. iliacofemoralis
m. gluteus profundus
a.v. iliaca externa (in vascular lacuna)
m. rectus femoris
ligament of femoral head
accessory ligament of femur
ischium
a.v. obturatoria
m. obturatorius externus
m. adductor
v. pudenda externa
m. gracilis

Fig. 8.68 The iliac fascia of the mare: left lateral view. The superficial inguinal ring is covered by the lateral mammary lamina. The pudendoepigastric vessels are seen passing towards the inguinal canal. The contents of the muscular and vascular lacunae of the iliac fascia are also seen.

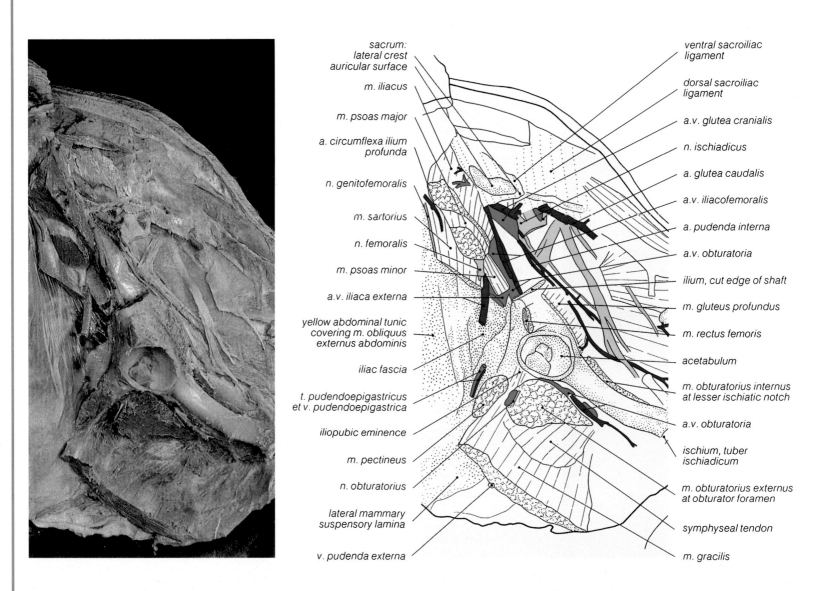

sacrum:
lateral crest
auricular surface
m. iliacus
m. psoas major
a. circumflexa ilium profunda
n. genitofemoralis
m. sartorius
n. femoralis
m. psoas minor
a.v. iliaca externa
yellow abdominal tunic covering m. obliquus externus abdominis
iliac fascia
t. pudendoepigastricus et v. pudendoepigastrica
iliopubic eminence
m. pectineus
n. obturatorius
lateral mammary suspensory lamina
v. pudenda externa
ventral sacroiliac ligament
dorsal sacroiliac ligament
a.v. glutea cranialis
n. ischiadicus
a. glutea caudalis
a.v. iliacofemoralis
a. pudenda interna
a.v. obturatoria
ilium, cut edge of shaft
m. gluteus profundus
m. rectus femoris
acetabulum
m. obturatorius internus at lesser ischiatic notch
a.v. obturatoria
ischium, tuber ischiadicum
m. obturatorius externus at obturator foramen
symphyseal tendon
m. gracilis

Fig. 8.69 The vessels and nerves of the pelvis of the pregnant mare: left lateral view. The shaft of the ilium has been sawn through, and the wing of the ilium carefully removed to expose the auricular surface of the sacrum, which forms the sacroiliac articulation. The muscles of the hindlimb arising from the tuber ischiadicum and the ventral surface of the ischium have been removed to show more clearly the symphyseal tendon of the gracilis muscle.

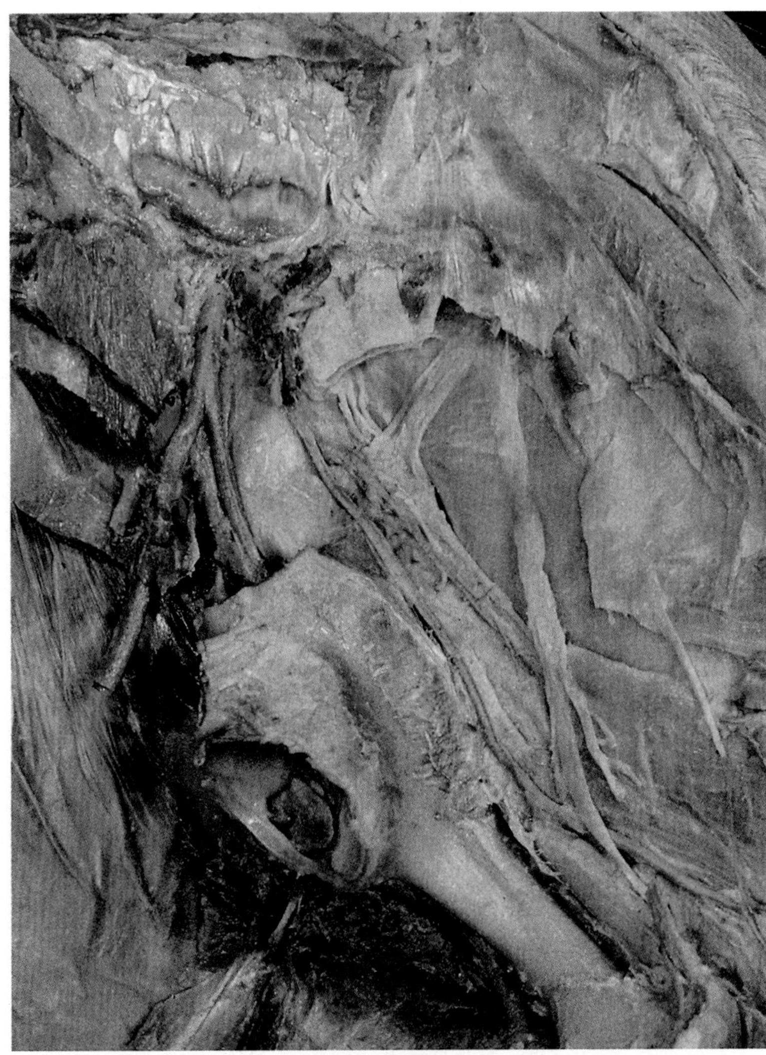

Fig. 8.70 The sacroiliac region of the pregnant mare: left lateral view. This is a closer view of a part of the dissection shown in Fig. 8.69.

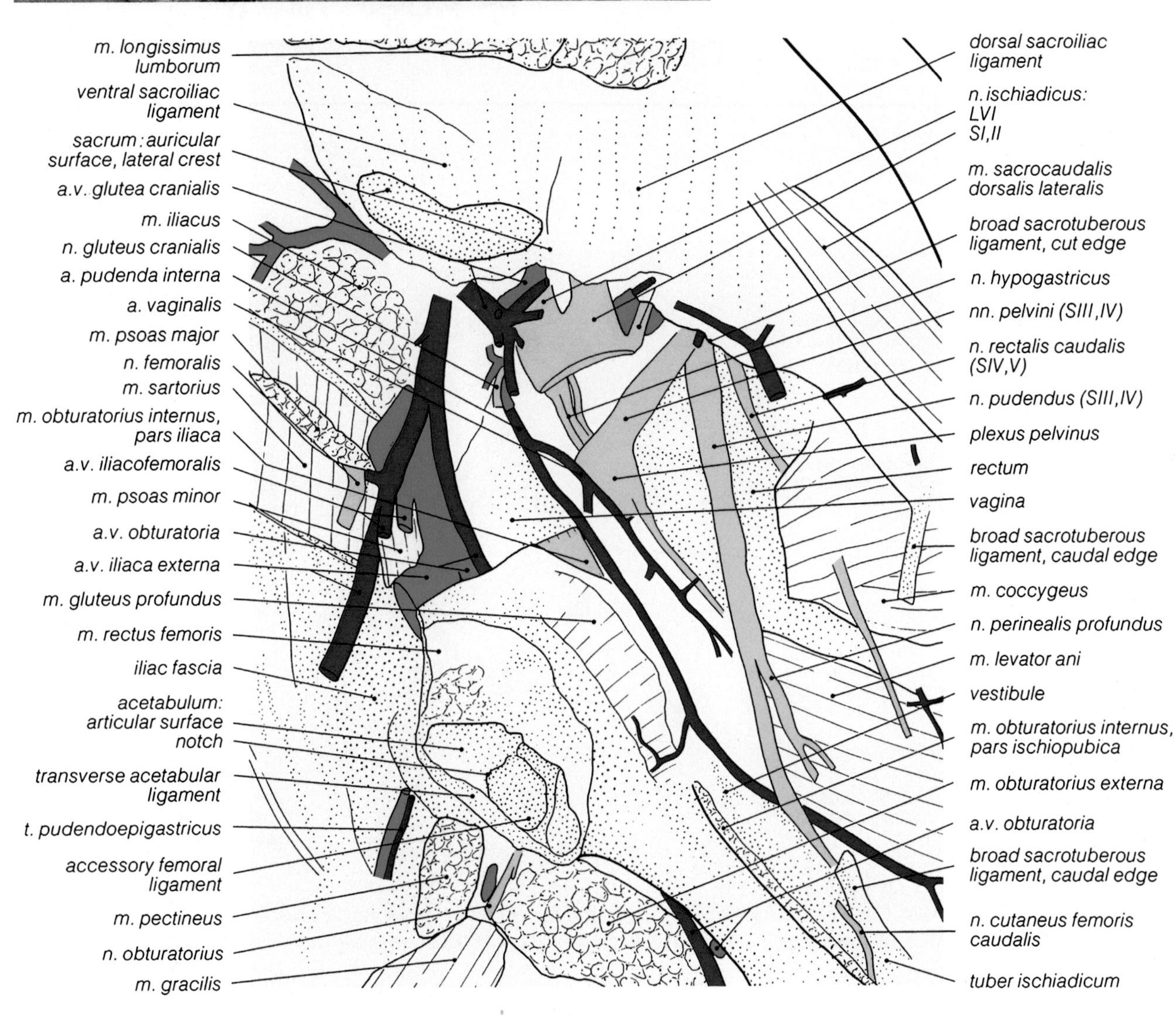
m. longissimus lumborum
ventral sacroiliac ligament
sacrum: auricular surface, lateral crest
a.v. glutea cranialis
m. iliacus
n. gluteus cranialis
a. pudenda interna
a. vaginalis
m. psoas major
n. femoralis
m. sartorius
m. obturatorius internus, pars iliaca
a.v. iliacofemoralis
m. psoas minor
a.v. obturatoria
a.v. iliaca externa
m. gluteus profundus
m. rectus femoris
iliac fascia
acetabulum: articular surface notch
transverse acetabular ligament
t. pudendoepigastricus
accessory femoral ligament
m. pectineus
n. obturatorius
m. gracilis
dorsal sacroiliac ligament
n. ischiadicus: LVI SI,II
m. sacrocaudalis dorsalis lateralis
broad sacrotuberous ligament, cut edge
n. hypogastricus
nn. pelvini (SIII,IV)
n. rectalis caudalis (SIV,V)
n. pudendus (SIII,IV)
plexus pelvinus
rectum
vagina
broad sacrotuberous ligament, caudal edge
m. coccygeus
n. perinealis profundus
m. levator ani
vestibule
m. obturatorius internus, pars ischiopubica
m. obturatorius externa
a.v. obturatoria
broad sacrotuberous ligament, caudal edge
n. cutaneus femoris caudalis
tuber ischiadicum

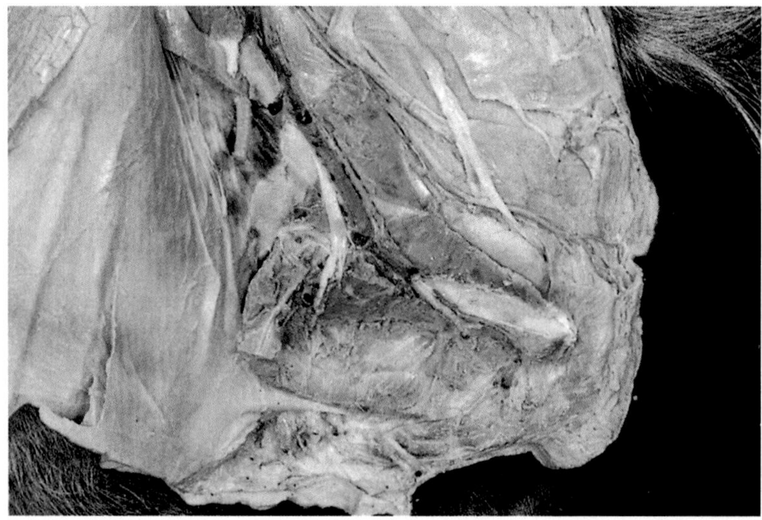

Fig. 8.71 **The pelvis of the pregnant mare: left lateral view (1).** The bony pelvis has been sawn through close to the iliopubic eminence and the pelvic symphysis, and the left side has been removed to expose the internal obturator muscle.

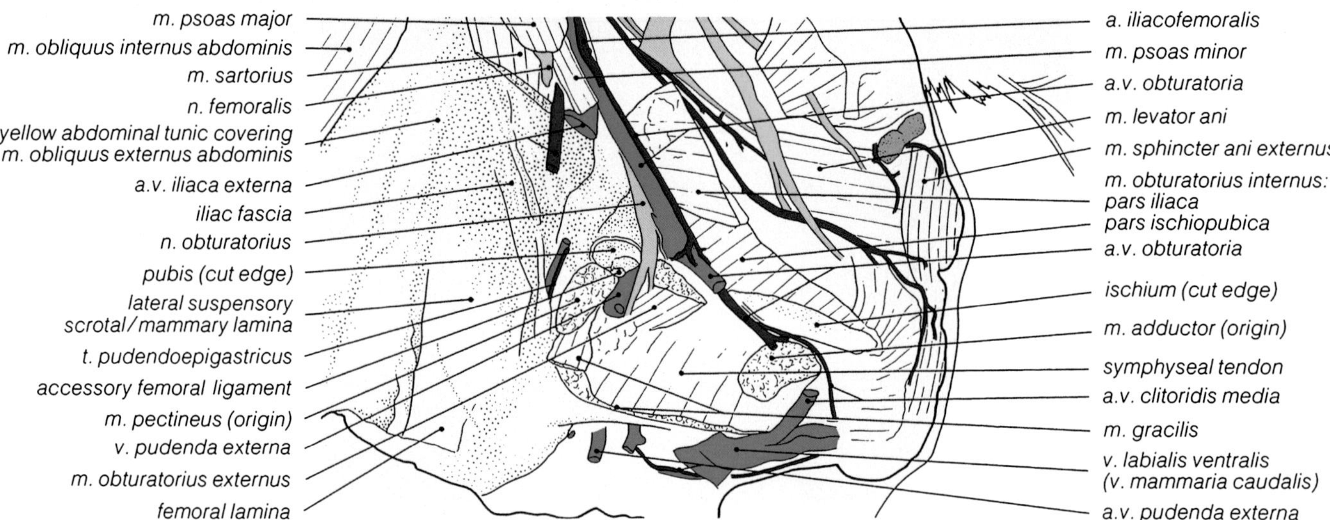
m. psoas major
m. obliquus internus abdominis
m. sartorius
n. femoralis
yellow abdominal tunic covering m. obliquus externus abdominis
a.v. iliaca externa
iliac fascia
n. obturatorius
pubis (cut edge)
lateral suspensory scrotal/mammary lamina
t. pudendoepigastricus
accessory femoral ligament
m. pectineus (origin)
v. pudenda externa
m. obturatorius externus
femoral lamina
a. iliacofemoralis
m. psoas minor
a.v. obturatoria
m. levator ani
m. sphincter ani externus
m. obturatorius internus:
pars iliaca
pars ischiopubica
a.v. obturatoria
ischium (cut edge)
m. adductor (origin)
symphyseal tendon
a.v. clitoridis media
m. gracilis
v. labialis ventralis (v. mammaria caudalis)
a.v. pudenda externa

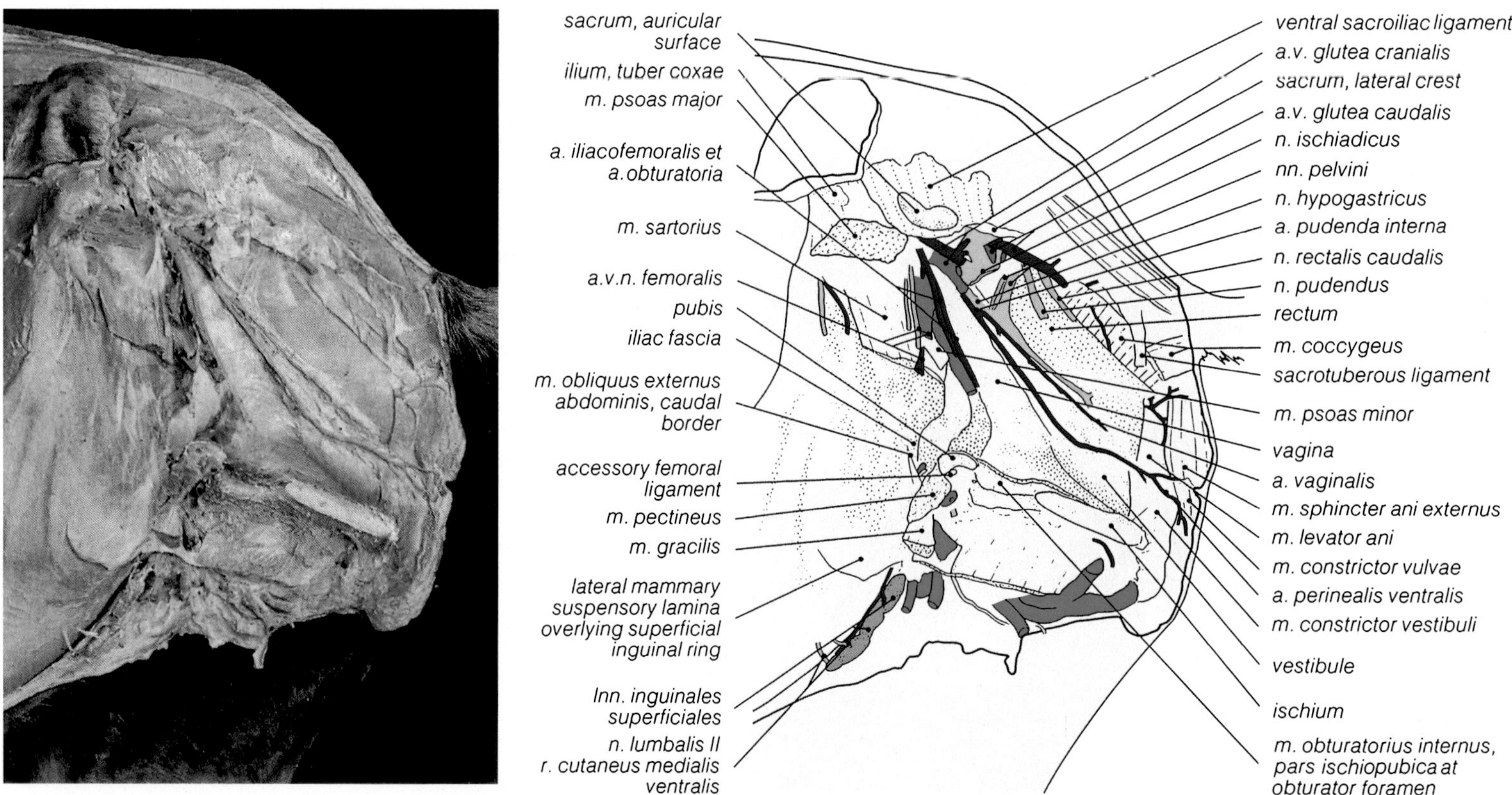
sacrum, auricular surface
ilium, tuber coxae
m. psoas major
a. iliacofemoralis et a. obturatoria
m. sartorius
a.v.n. femoralis
pubis
iliac fascia
m. obliquus externus abdominis, caudal border
accessory femoral ligament
m. pectineus
m. gracilis
lateral mammary suspensory lamina overlying superficial inguinal ring
lnn. inguinales superficiales
n. lumbalis II
r. cutaneus medialis ventralis
ventral sacroiliac ligament
a.v. glutea cranialis
sacrum, lateral crest
a.v. glutea caudalis
n. ischiadicus
nn. pelvini
n. hypogastricus
a. pudenda interna
n. rectalis caudalis
n. pudendus
rectum
m. coccygeus
sacrotuberous ligament
m. psoas minor
vagina
a. vaginalis
m. sphincter ani externus
m. levator ani
m. constrictor vulvae
a. perinealis ventralis
m. constrictor vestibuli
vestibule
ischium
m. obturatorius internus, pars ischiopubica at obturator foramen

Fig. 8.72 The pelvis of the pregnant mare: left lateral view (2). The muscles of the pelvic diaphragm (coccygeus and levator ani muscles) have been cut short to reveal the pelvic viscera. The remaining part of the left pelvic bone has been cleared of muscle to show the position of the obturator foramen.

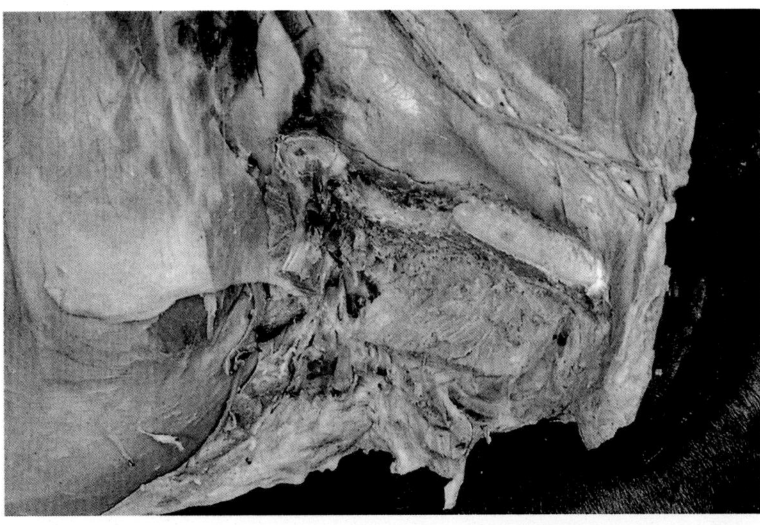

Fig. 8.73 The inguinal canal of the pregnant mare: the superficial inguinal ring in left lateral view. The lateral mammary suspensory ligament has been cut away along the medial edge of the pelvic tendon of the external oblique abdominal muscle; this line is the lateral rim of the superficial inguinal ring. The sharply defined medial rim of the ring (also the lateral edge of the abdominal tendon) is exposed.

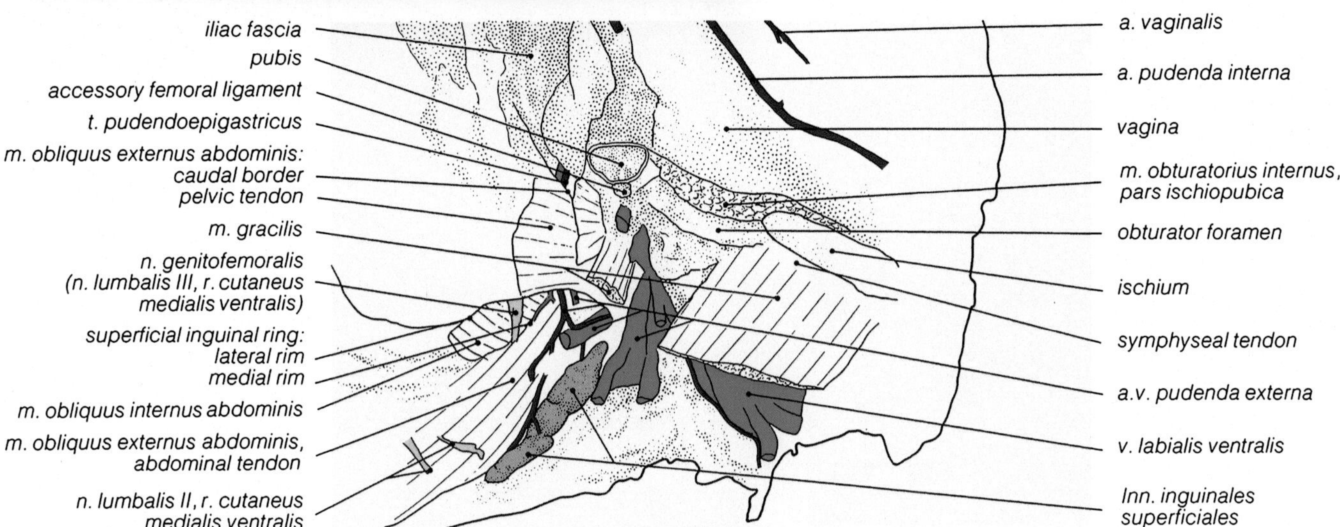

iliac fascia
pubis
accessory femoral ligament
t. pudendoepigastricus
m. obliquus externus abdominis: caudal border
pelvic tendon
m. gracilis
n. genitofemoralis (n. lumbalis III, r. cutaneus medialis ventralis)
superficial inguinal ring: lateral rim
medial rim
m. obliquus internus abdominis
m. obliquus externus abdominis, abdominal tendon
n. lumbalis II, r. cutaneus medialis ventralis
a. vaginalis
a. pudenda interna
vagina
m. obturatorius internus, pars ischiopubica
obturator foramen
ischium
symphyseal tendon
a.v. pudenda externa
v. labialis ventralis
lnn. inguinales superficiales

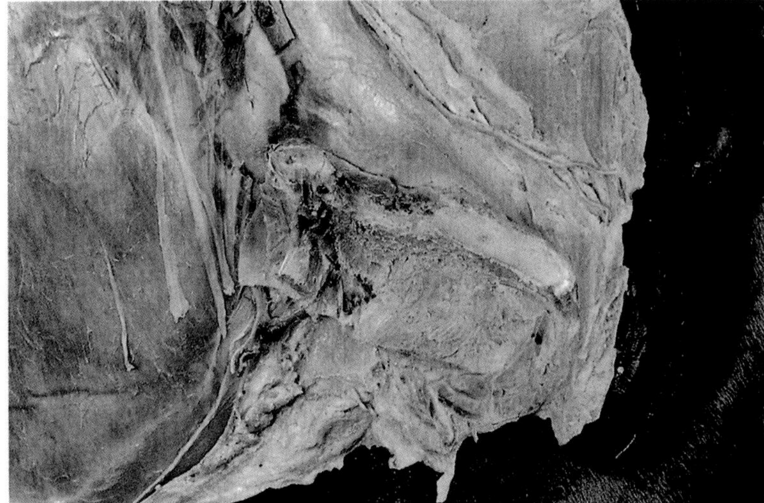

Fig. 8.74 The inguinal canal of the pregnant mare: the deep inguinal ring in left lateral view. The external oblique abdominal muscle has been removed, but parts of the pelvic and abdominal tendons of insertion have been left in order to indicate the position of the superficial inguinal ring, which lies between them. The caudal edge of the internal oblique muscle is the cranial boundary of the deep ring, while the lateral edge of the rectus abdominis muscle forms its medial boundary.

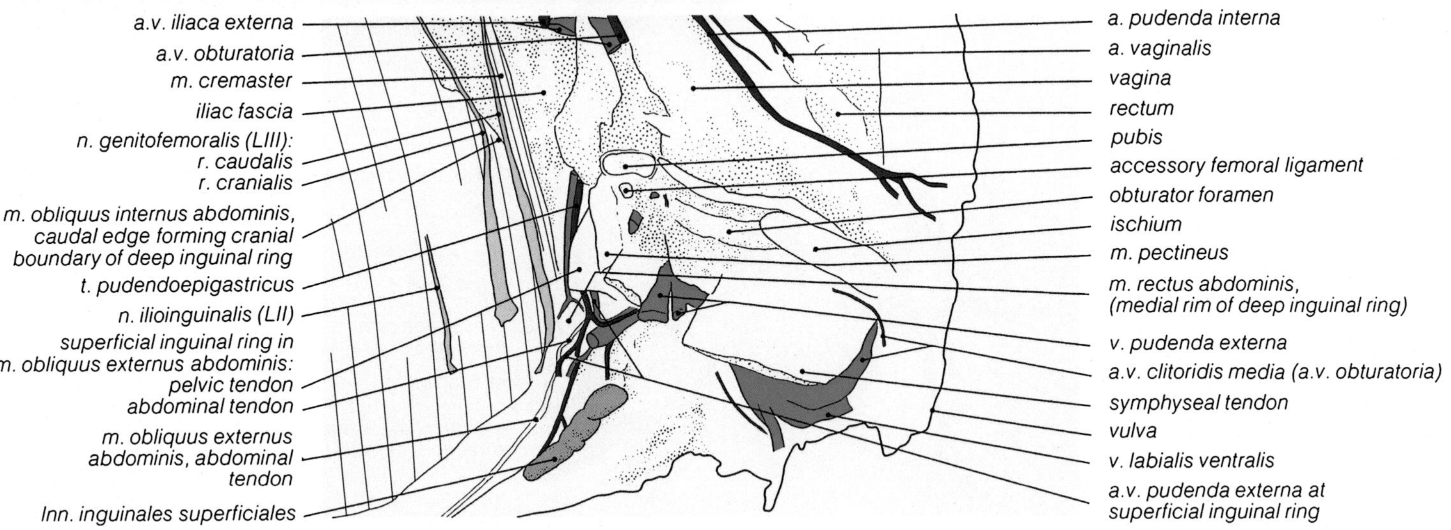

a.v. iliaca externa
a.v. obturatoria
m. cremaster
iliac fascia
n. genitofemoralis (LIII): r. caudalis
r. cranialis
m. obliquus internus abdominis, caudal edge forming cranial boundary of deep inguinal ring
t. pudendoepigastricus
n. ilioinguinalis (LII)
superficial inguinal ring in m. obliquus externus abdominis: pelvic tendon
abdominal tendon
m. obliquus externus abdominis, abdominal tendon
lnn. inguinales superficiales
a. pudenda interna
a. vaginalis
vagina
rectum
pubis
accessory femoral ligament
obturator foramen
ischium
m. pectineus
m. rectus abdominis, (medial rim of deep inguinal ring)
v. pudenda externa
a.v. clitoridis media (a.v. obturatoria)
symphyseal tendon
vulva
v. labialis ventralis
a.v. pudenda externa at superficial inguinal ring

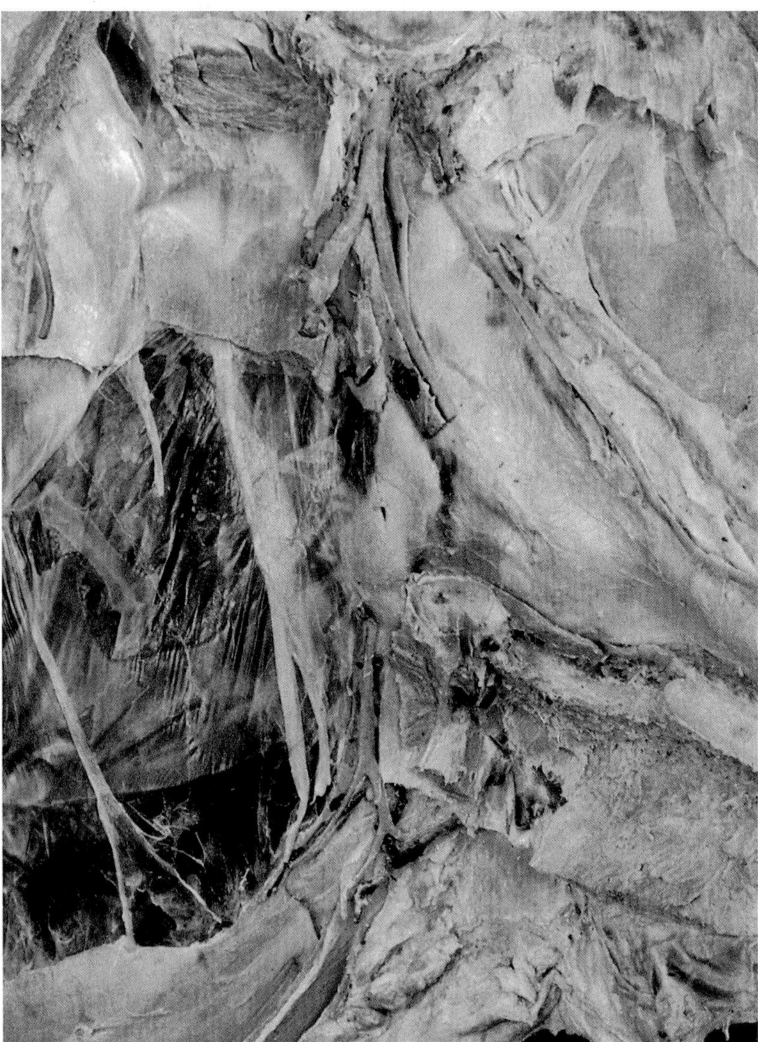

Fig. 8.75 The inguinal canal of the pregnant mare: the transverse fascia in left lateral view. The internal oblique abdominal muscle has been removed, but the pelvic and abdominal tendons of the external oblique muscle have been retained to show the position of the superficial inguinal ring. The rectus abdominis muscle is clearly visible. The origin of the caudal epigastric vessels can be seen situated within the inguinal canal. The transverse abdominal muscle does not extend caudally into the inguinal region of the horse.

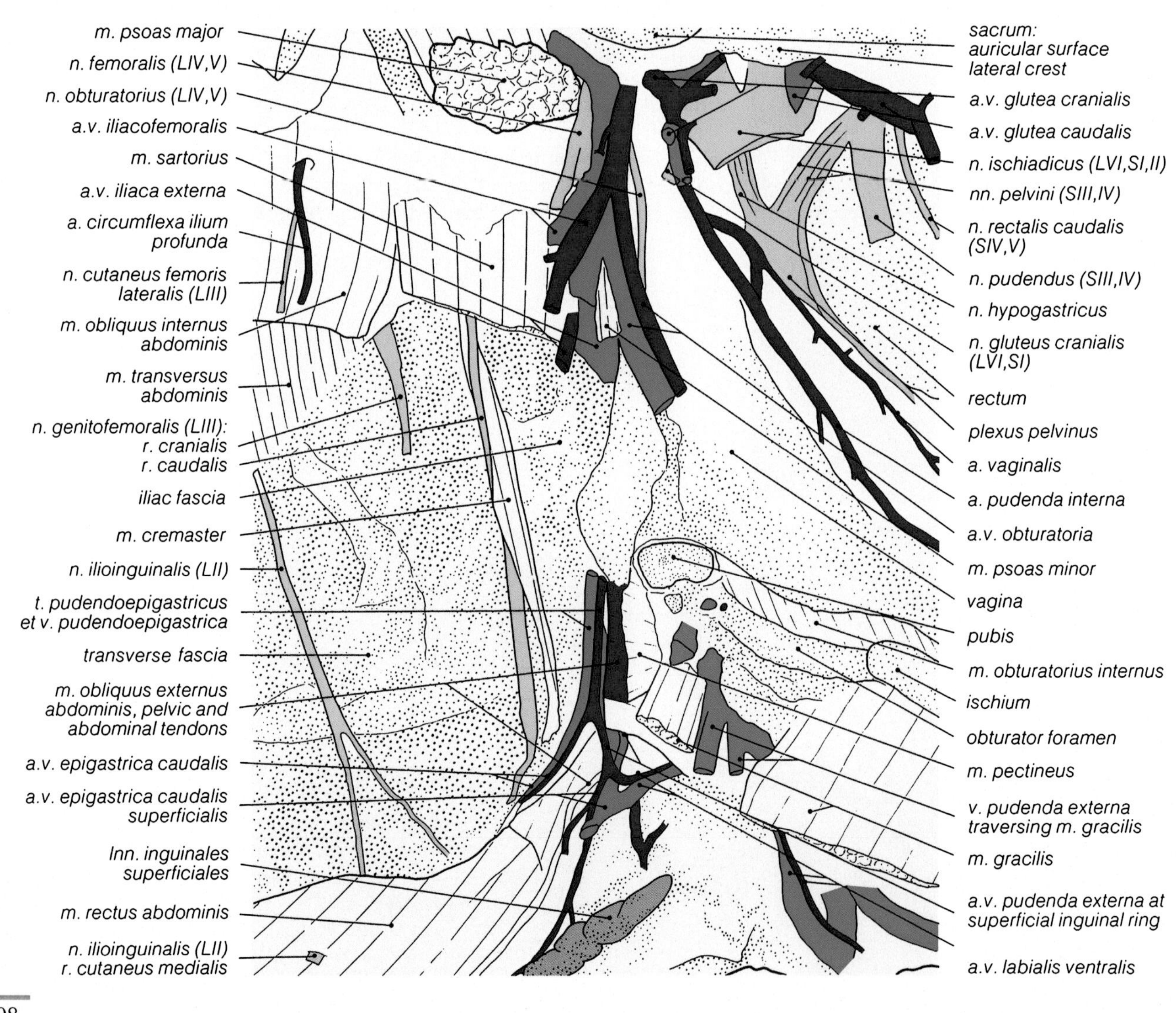
m. psoas major
n. femoralis (LIV,V)
n. obturatorius (LIV,V)
a.v. iliacofemoralis
m. sartorius
a.v. iliaca externa
a. circumflexa ilium profunda
n. cutaneus femoris lateralis (LIII)
m. obliquus internus abdominis
m. transversus abdominis
n. genitofemoralis (LIII): r. cranialis r. caudalis
iliac fascia
m. cremaster
n. ilioinguinalis (LII)
t. pudendoepigastricus et v. pudendoepigastrica
transverse fascia
m. obliquus externus abdominis, pelvic and abdominal tendons
a.v. epigastrica caudalis
a.v. epigastrica caudalis superficialis
lnn. inguinales superficiales
m. rectus abdominis
n. ilioinguinalis (LII) r. cutaneus medialis
sacrum: auricular surface lateral crest
a.v. glutea cranialis
a.v. glutea caudalis
n. ischiadicus (LVI,SI,II)
nn. pelvini (SIII,IV)
n. rectalis caudalis (SIV,V)
n. pudendus (SIII,IV)
n. hypogastricus
n. gluteus cranialis (LVI,SI)
rectum
plexus pelvinus
a. vaginalis
a. pudenda interna
a.v. obturatoria
m. psoas minor
vagina
pubis
m. obturatorius internus
ischium
obturator foramen
m. pectineus
v. pudenda externa traversing m. gracilis
m. gracilis
a.v. pudenda externa at superficial inguinal ring
a.v. labialis ventralis

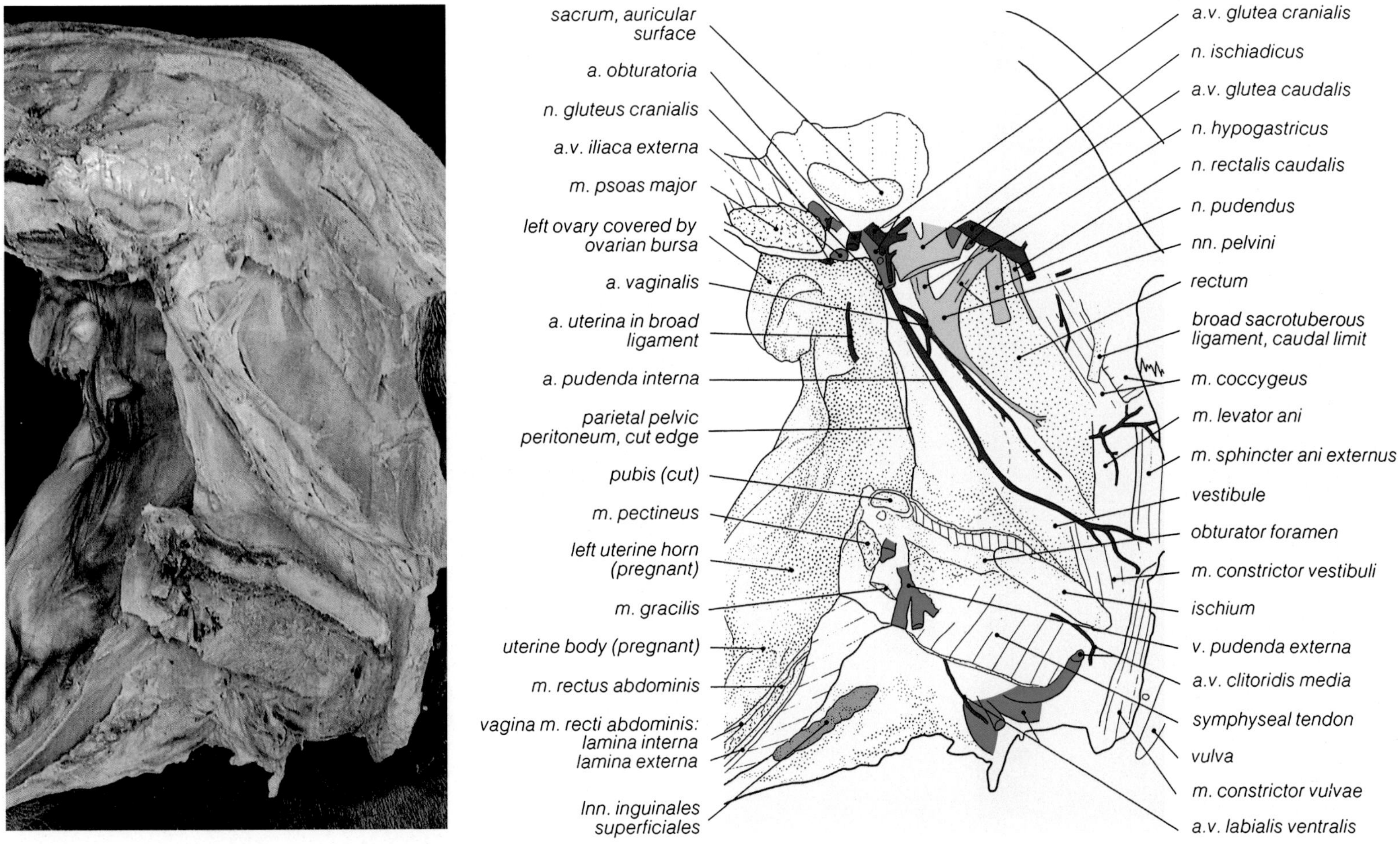

sacrum, auricular surface
a. obturatoria
n. gluteus cranialis
a.v. iliaca externa
m. psoas major
left ovary covered by ovarian bursa
a. vaginalis
a. uterina in broad ligament
a. pudenda interna
parietal pelvic peritoneum, cut edge
pubis (cut)
m. pectineus
left uterine horn (pregnant)
m. gracilis
uterine body (pregnant)
m. rectus abdominis
vagina m. recti abdominis: lamina interna lamina externa
lnn. inguinales superficiales
a.v. glutea cranialis
n. ischiadicus
a.v. glutea caudalis
n. hypogastricus
n. rectalis caudalis
n. pudendus
nn. pelvini
rectum
broad sacrotuberous ligament, caudal limit
m. coccygeus
m. levator ani
m. sphincter ani externus
vestibule
obturator foramen
m. constrictor vestibuli
ischium
v. pudenda externa
a.v. clitoridis media
symphyseal tendon
vulva
m. constrictor vulvae
a.v. labialis ventralis

Fig. 8.76 The contents of the pelvis of the pregnant mare: left lateral view. The remnants of the tuber coxae and the left lateral abdominal wall have been removed to expose the uterus and ovary. A broken blue line shows the approximate caudal limit of the peritoneal cavity.

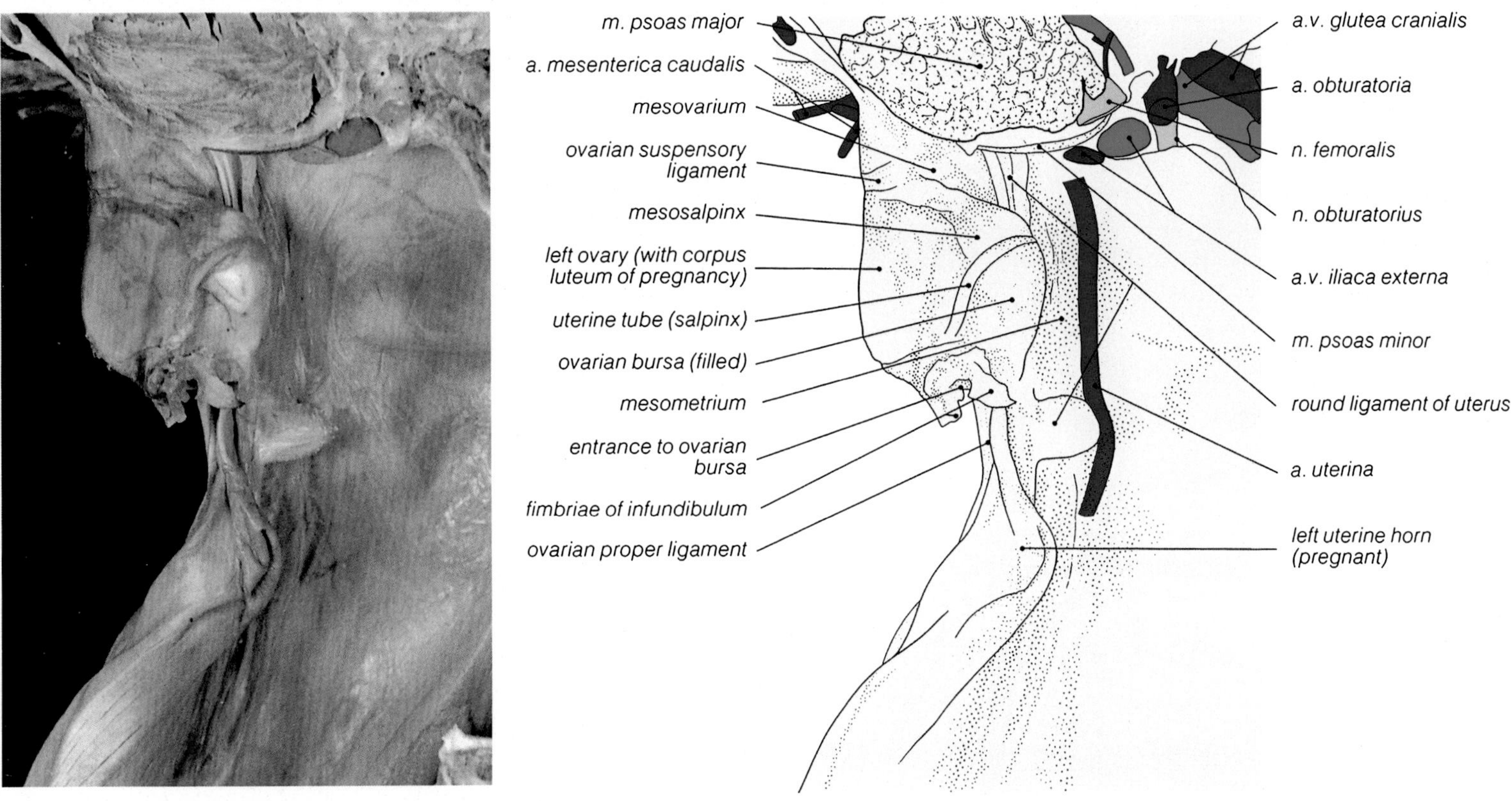
m. psoas major
a. mesenterica caudalis
mesovarium
ovarian suspensory ligament
mesosalpinx
left ovary (with corpus luteum of pregnancy)
uterine tube (salpinx)
ovarian bursa (filled)
mesometrium
entrance to ovarian bursa
fimbriae of infundibulum
ovarian proper ligament
a.v. glutea cranialis
a. obturatoria
n. femoralis
n. obturatorius
a.v. iliaca externa
m. psoas minor
round ligament of uterus
a. uterina
left uterine horn (pregnant)

Fig. 8.77 The left ovary of the pregnant mare: left lateral view. This is a closer view of a part of the specimen shown in Fig. 8.76. The ovarian bursa has been filled with cotton wool. The various parts of the broad ligament (mesovarium, mesosalpinx, mesometrium) are separately labelled.

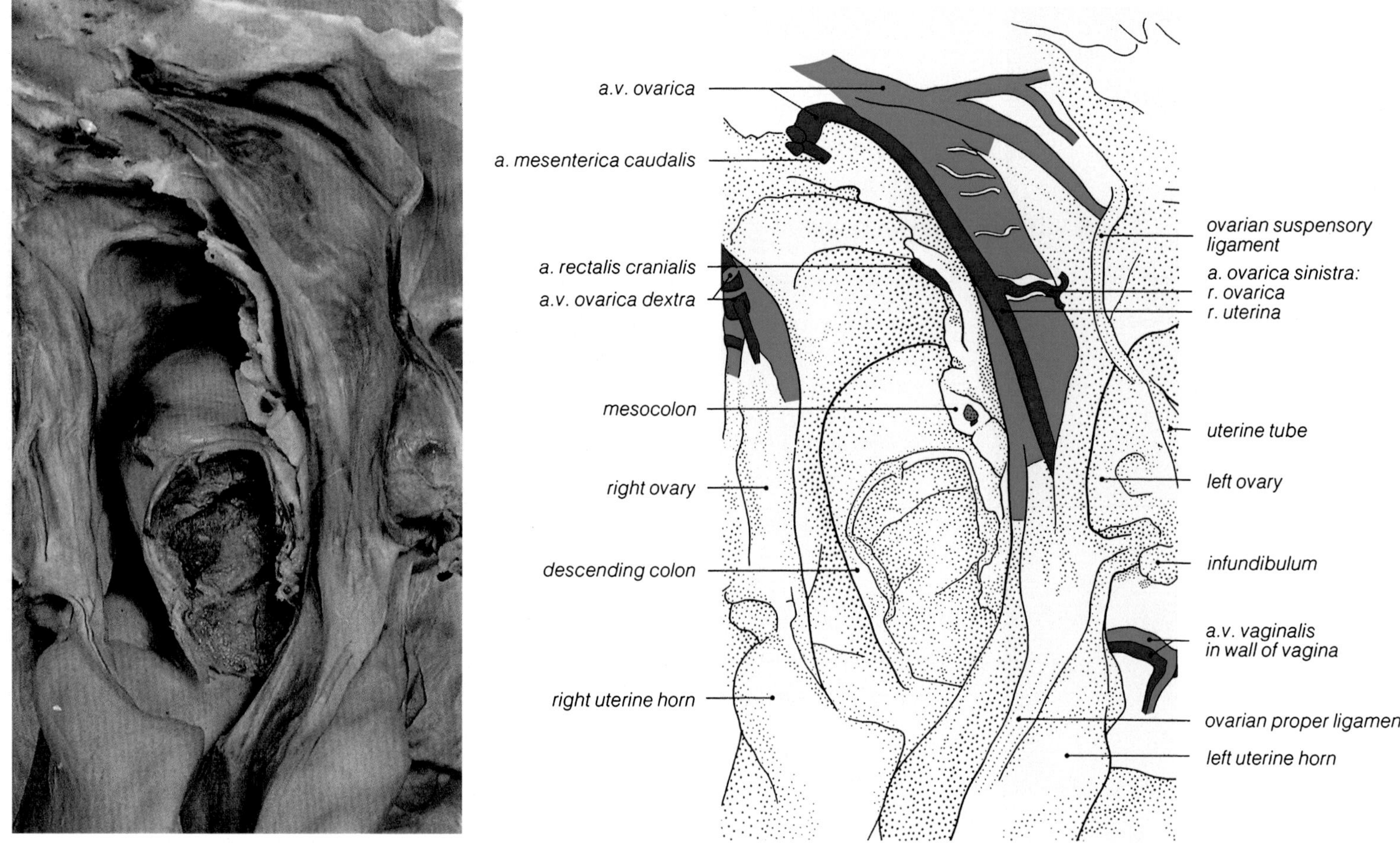
a.v. ovarica
a. mesenterica caudalis
a. rectalis cranialis
a.v. ovarica dextra
mesocolon
right ovary
descending colon
right uterine horn
ovarian suspensory ligament
a. ovarica sinistra:
r. ovarica
r. uterina
uterine tube
left ovary
infundibulum
a.v. vaginalis in wall of vagina
ovarian proper ligament
left uterine horn

Fig. 8.78 The left ovary of the pregnant mare: cranial view. Topographical relationships are shown in Fig. 8.57.

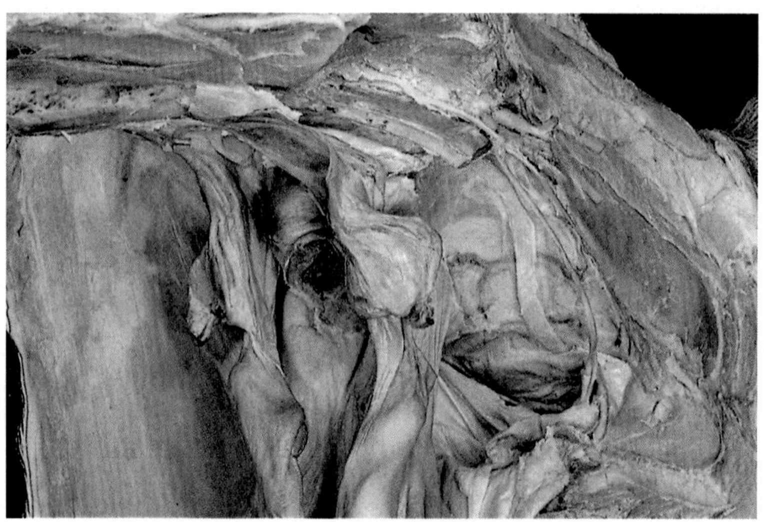

Fig. 8.79 The contents of the pelvis of the pregnant mare: left craniolateral view. The left ureter has been displayed. The apex of the empty urinary bladder is invaginated (see Fig. 8.83); its relationship to the occluded left umbilical artery is clearly seen.

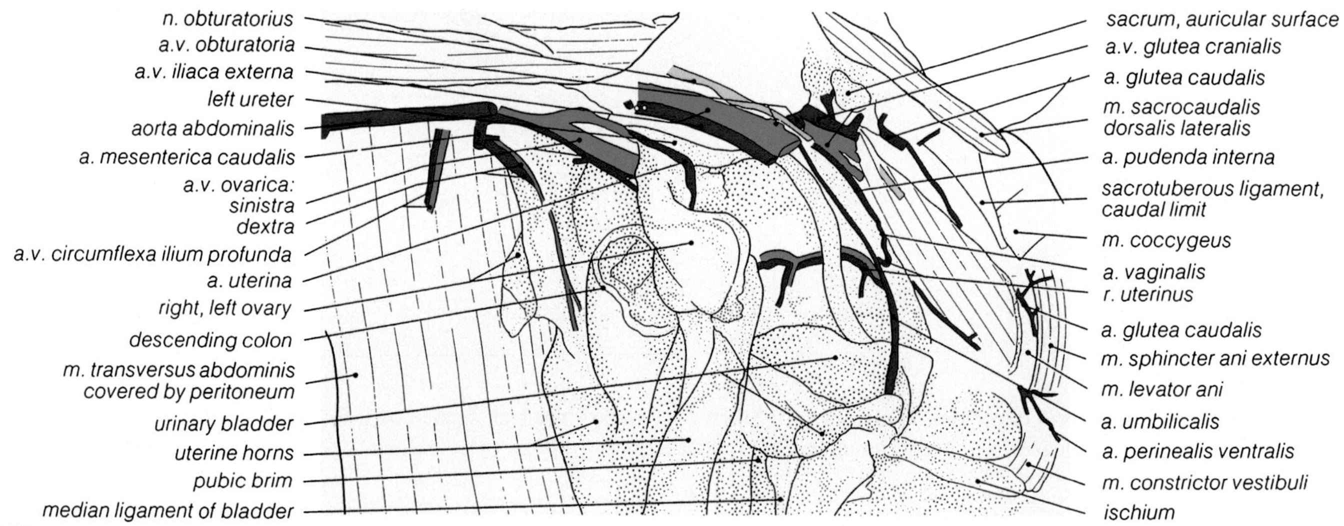
n. obturatorius
a.v. obturatoria
a.v. iliaca externa
left ureter
aorta abdominalis
a. mesenterica caudalis
a.v. ovarica:
sinistra
dextra
a.v. circumflexa ilium profunda
a. uterina
right, left ovary
descending colon
m. transversus abdominis covered by peritoneum
urinary bladder
uterine horns
pubic brim
median ligament of bladder
sacrum, auricular surface
a.v. glutea cranialis
a. glutea caudalis
m. sacrocaudalis dorsalis lateralis
a. pudenda interna
sacrotuberous ligament, caudal limit
m. coccygeus
a. vaginalis
r. uterinus
a. glutea caudalis
m. sphincter ani externus
m. levator ani
a. umbilicalis
a. perinealis ventralis
m. constrictor vestibuli
ischium

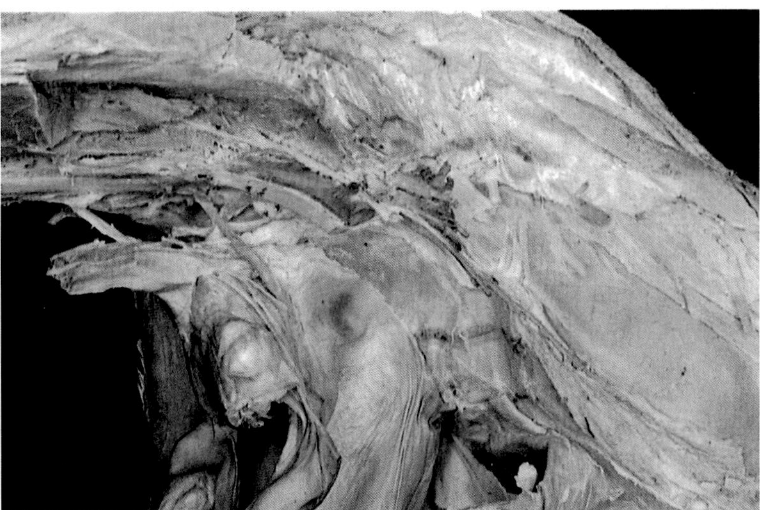

Fig. 8.80 Pelvic vessels and nerves of the pregnant mare: left lateral view. The origin of the external iliac artery has been revealed. The left ureter and umbilical artery have been removed.

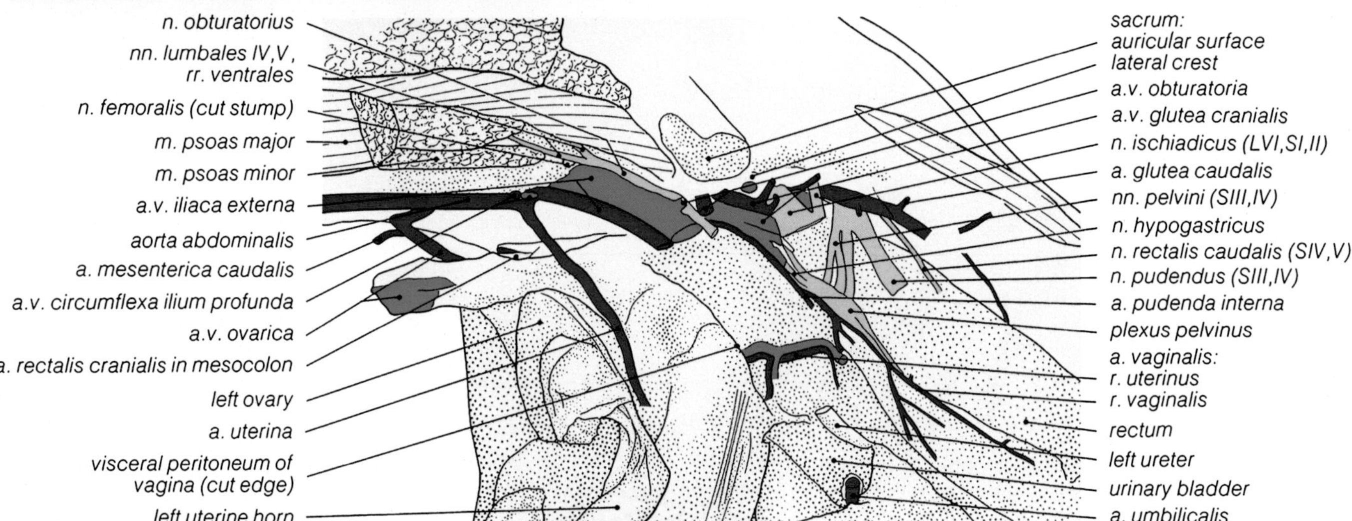

n. obturatorius
nn. lumbales IV,V, rr. ventrales
n. femoralis (cut stump)
m. psoas major
m. psoas minor
a.v. iliaca externa
aorta abdominalis
a. mesenterica caudalis
a.v. circumflexa ilium profunda
a.v. ovarica
a. rectalis cranialis in mesocolon
left ovary
a. uterina
visceral peritoneum of vagina (cut edge)
left uterine horn
sacrum:
auricular surface
lateral crest
a.v. obturatoria
a.v. glutea cranialis
n. ischiadicus (LVI,SI,II)
a. glutea caudalis
nn. pelvini (SIII,IV)
n. hypogastricus
n. rectalis caudalis (SIV,V)
n. pudendus (SIII,IV)
a. pudenda interna
plexus pelvinus
a. vaginalis:
r. uterinus
r. vaginalis
rectum
left ureter
urinary bladder
a. umbilicalis

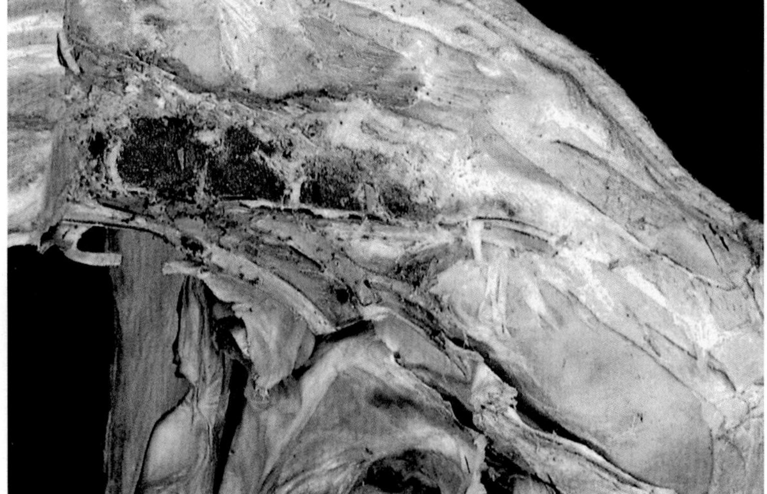

Fig. 8.81 Internal and external iliac vessels of the pregnant mare: left lateral view. The lumbar and sacral vertebral bodies have been cut away in the sagittal plane to display the iliac arteries and veins and the vessels arising from them.

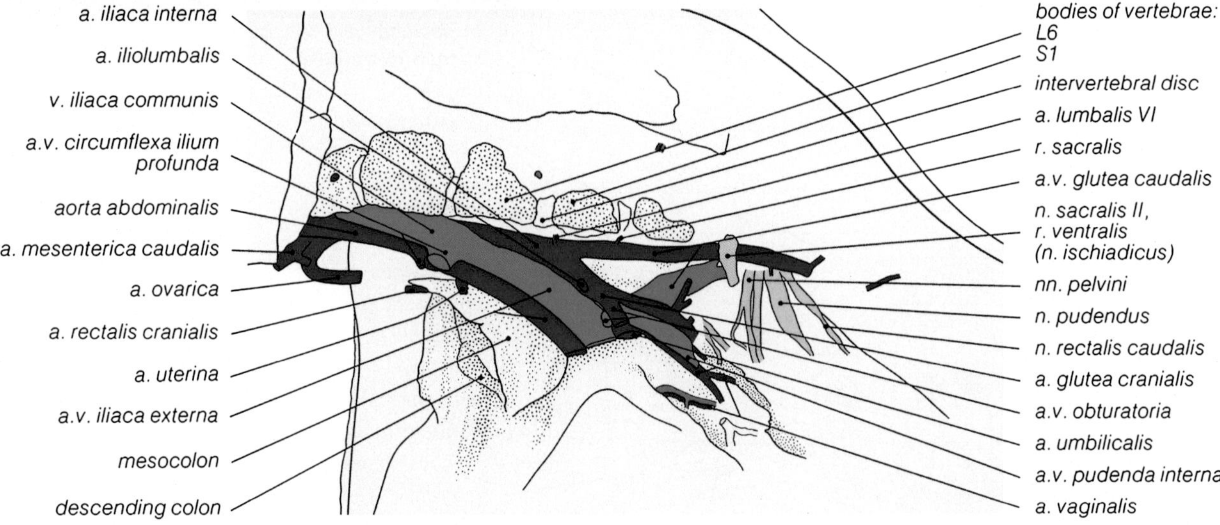

a. iliaca interna
a. iliolumbalis
v. iliaca communis
a.v. circumflexa ilium profunda
aorta abdominalis
a. mesenterica caudalis
a. ovarica
a. rectalis cranialis
a. uterina
a.v. iliaca externa
mesocolon
descending colon
bodies of vertebrae:
L6
S1
intervertebral disc
a. lumbalis VI
r. sacralis
a.v. glutea caudalis
n. sacralis II,
r. ventralis
(n. ischiadicus)
nn. pelvini
n. pudendus
n. rectalis caudalis
a. glutea cranialis
a.v. obturatoria
a. umbilicalis
a.v. pudenda interna
a. vaginalis

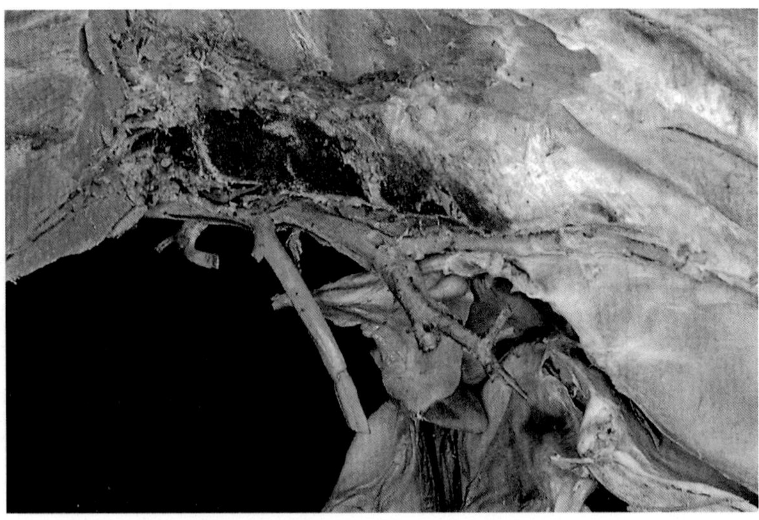

Fig. 8.82 Internal and external iliac arteries of the pregnant mare: left lateral view. The veins and nerves have been removed to show the arteries more clearly.

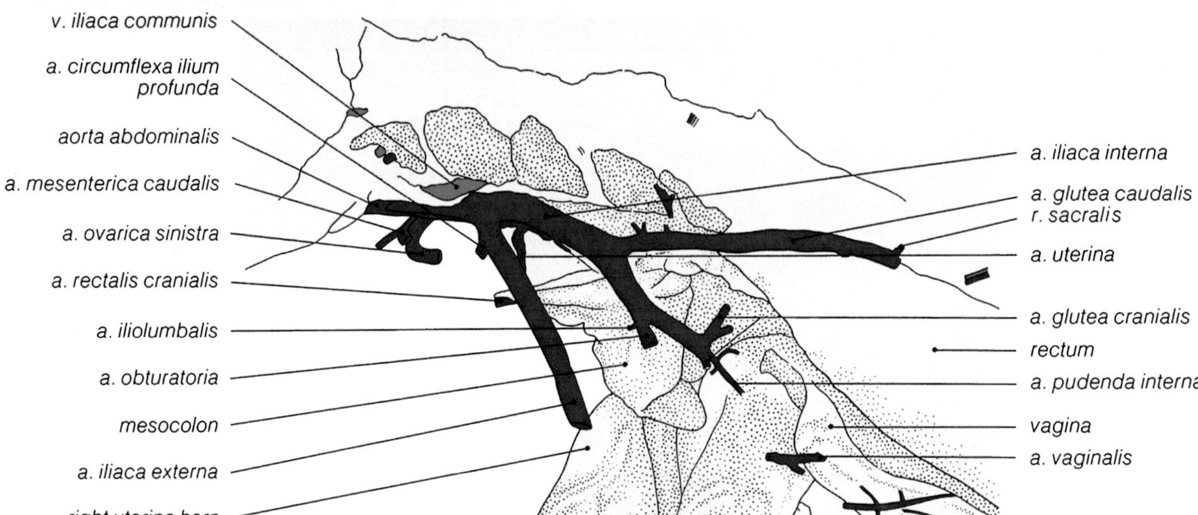
v. iliaca communis
a. circumflexa ilium profunda
aorta abdominalis
a. mesenterica caudalis
a. ovarica sinistra
a. rectalis cranialis
a. iliolumbalis
a. obturatoria
mesocolon
a. iliaca externa
right uterine horn
a. iliaca interna
a. glutea caudalis
r. sacralis
a. uterina
a. glutea cranialis
rectum
a. pudenda interna
vagina
a. vaginalis

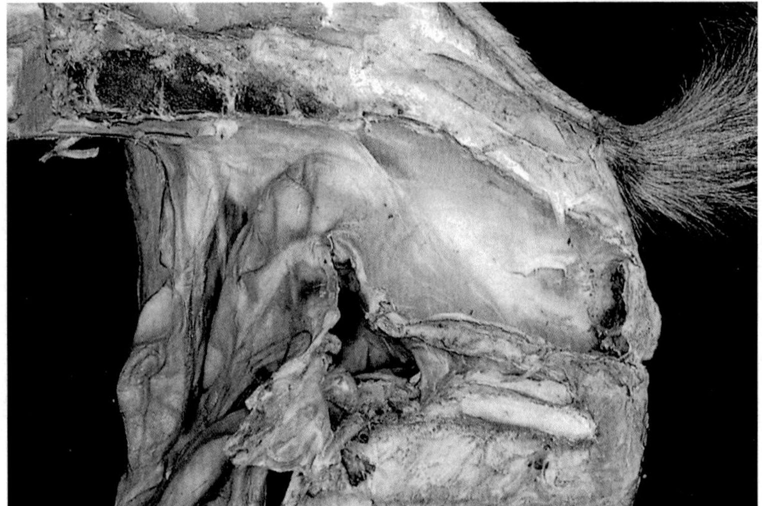

Fig. 8.83 Pelvic viscera of the pregnant mare: left lateral view (1). The rectum has been removed and the left ovarian vessels reflected ventrally to show the topography of the female tract in this mare at 100 days pregnancy. A broken blue line indicates the caudal limit of the peritoneal cavity on the wall of the vagina.

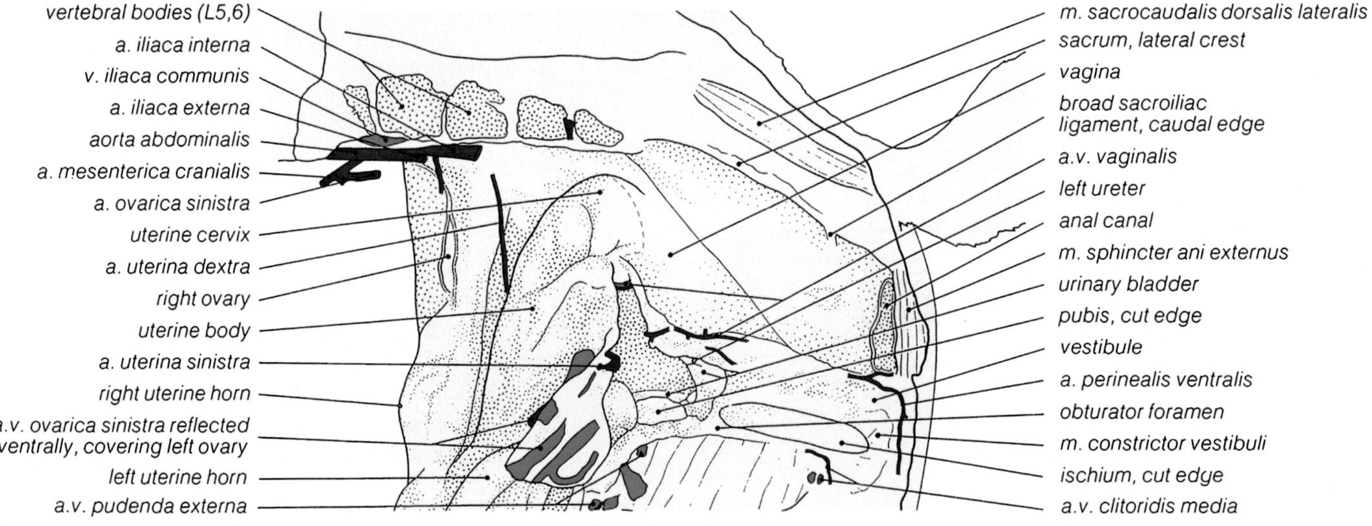
vertebral bodies (L5,6)
a. iliaca interna
v. iliaca communis
a. iliaca externa
aorta abdominalis
a. mesenterica cranialis
a. ovarica sinistra
uterine cervix
a. uterina dextra
right ovary
uterine body
a. uterina sinistra
right uterine horn
a.v. ovarica sinistra reflected ventrally, covering left ovary
left uterine horn
a.v. pudenda externa
m. sacrocaudalis dorsalis lateralis
sacrum, lateral crest
vagina
broad sacroiliac ligament, caudal edge
a.v. vaginalis
left ureter
anal canal
m. sphincter ani externus
urinary bladder
pubis, cut edge
vestibule
a. perinealis ventralis
obturator foramen
m. constrictor vestibuli
ischium, cut edge
a.v. clitoridis media

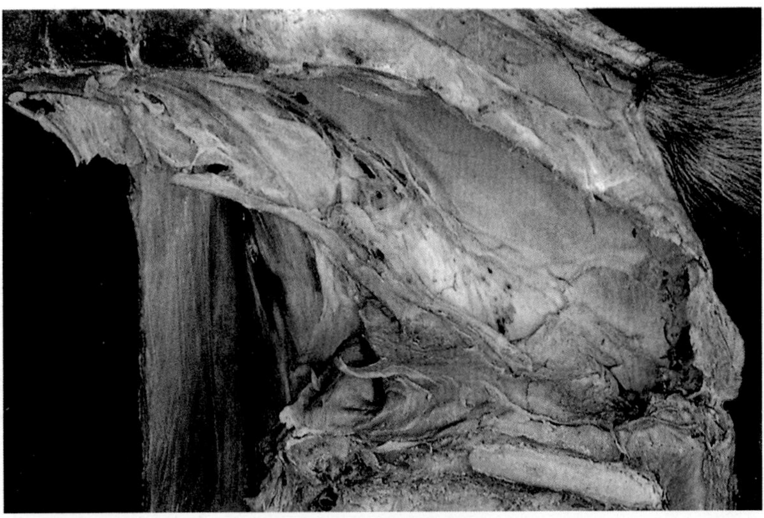

Fig. 8.84 Pelvic viscera of the pregnant mare: left lateral view (2). The female tract has been removed after incising the caudal vagina, to reveal the topography of the urinary bladder, urethra, and ureters. The bladder is empty and its apex is invaginated into the body of the organ.

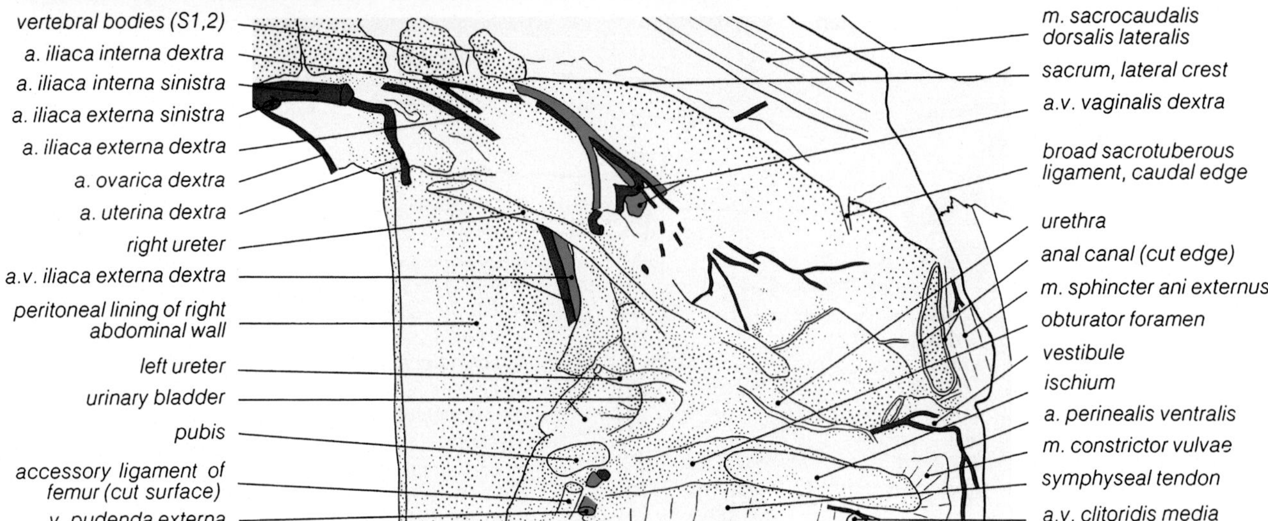
vertebral bodies (S1,2)
a. iliaca interna dextra
a. iliaca interna sinistra
a. iliaca externa sinistra
a. iliaca externa dextra
a. ovarica dextra
a. uterina dextra
right ureter
a.v. iliaca externa dextra
peritoneal lining of right abdominal wall
left ureter
urinary bladder
pubis
accessory ligament of femur (cut surface)
v. pudenda externa
m. sacrocaudalis dorsalis lateralis
sacrum, lateral crest
a.v. vaginalis dextra
broad sacrotuberous ligament, caudal edge
urethra
anal canal (cut edge)
m. sphincter ani externus
obturator foramen
vestibule
ischium
a. perinealis ventralis
m. constrictor vulvae
symphyseal tendon
a.v. clitoridis media

Fig. 8.85 Pelvic viscera of the pregnant mare: left lateral view (3). The urinary bladder and urethra have been opened. Wires have been inserted into the right and left ureteric orifices.

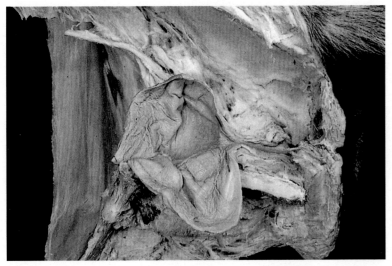

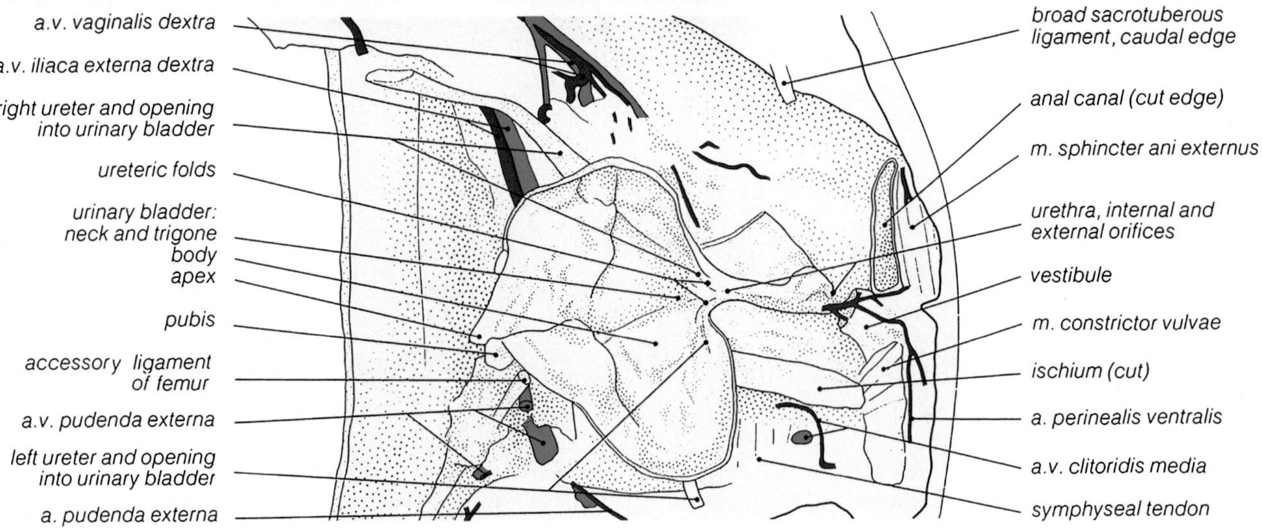
a.v. vaginalis dextra
a.v. iliaca externa dextra
right ureter and opening into urinary bladder
ureteric folds
urinary bladder: neck and trigone
body
apex
pubis
accessory ligament of femur
a.v. pudenda externa
left ureter and opening into urinary bladder
a. pudenda externa
broad sacrotuberous ligament, caudal edge
anal canal (cut edge)
m. sphincter ani externus
urethra, internal and external orifices
vestibule
m. constrictor vulvae
ischium (cut)
a. perinealis ventralis
a.v. clitoridis media
symphyseal tendon

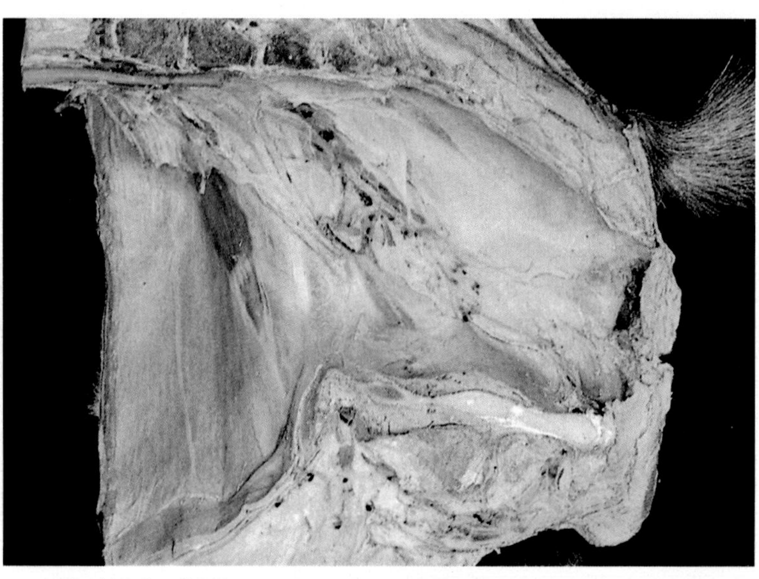

Fig. 8.86 The right pelvic wall of the pregnant mare: medial view (1). The viscera have been removed, but the peritoneal and retroperitoneal lining of the pelvic cavity have not yet been dissected. The left side of the abdominal and pelvic floor has been cut away.

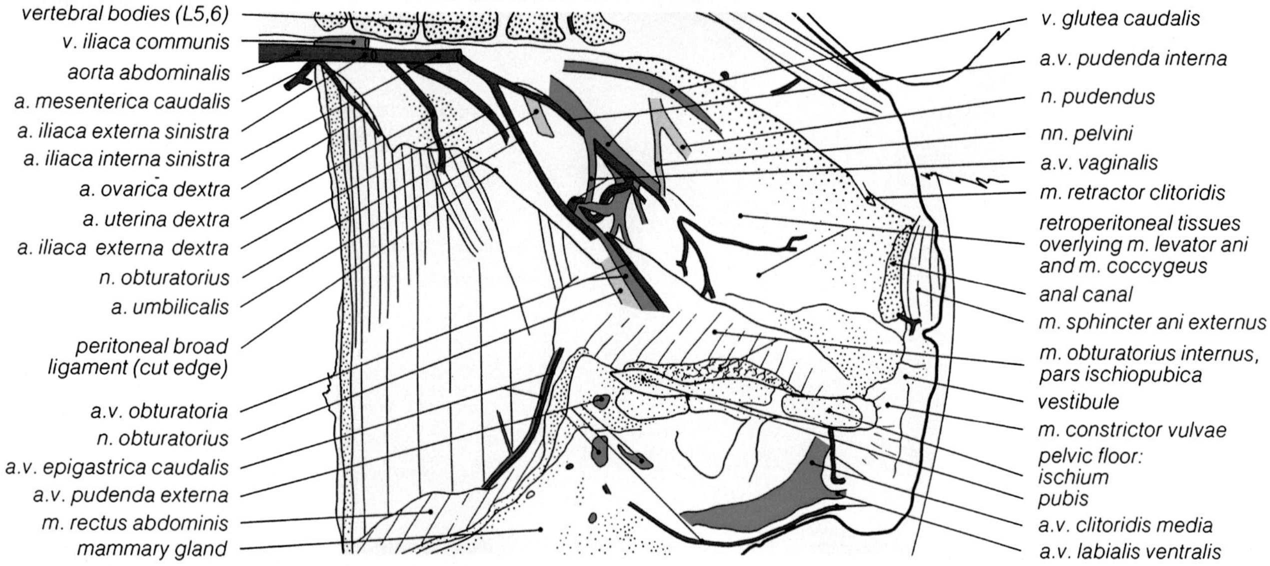

vertebral bodies (L5,6)
v. iliaca communis
aorta abdominalis
a. mesenterica caudalis
a. iliaca externa sinistra
a. iliaca interna sinistra
a. ovarica dextra
a. uterina dextra
a. iliaca externa dextra
n. obturatorius
a. umbilicalis
peritoneal broad ligament (cut edge)
a.v. obturatoria
n. obturatorius
a.v. epigastrica caudalis
a.v. pudenda externa
m. rectus abdominis
mammary gland
v. glutea caudalis
a.v. pudenda interna
n. pudendus
nn. pelvini
a.v. vaginalis
m. retractor clitoridis
retroperitoneal tissues overlying m. levator ani and m. coccygeus
anal canal
m. sphincter ani externus
m. obturatorius internus, pars ischiopubica
vestibule
m. constrictor vulvae
pelvic floor:
ischium
pubis
a.v. clitoridis media
a.v. labialis ventralis

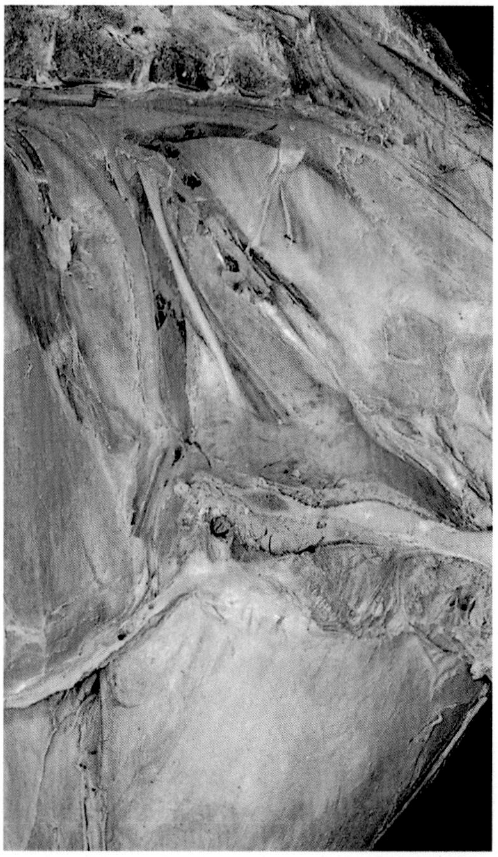

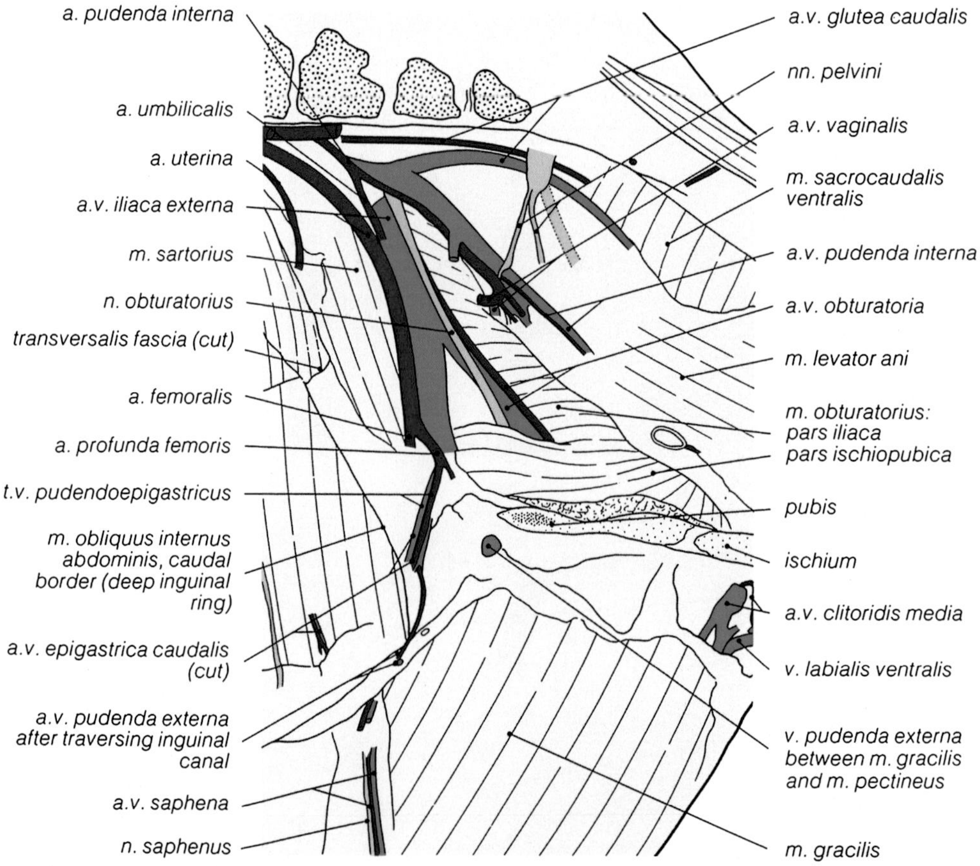

a. pudenda interna
a. umbilicalis
a. uterina
a.v. iliaca externa
m. sartorius
n. obturatorius
transversalis fascia (cut)
a. femoralis
a. profunda femoris
t.v. pudendoepigastricus
m. obliquus internus abdominis, caudal border (deep inguinal ring)
a.v. epigastrica caudalis (cut)
a.v. pudenda externa after traversing inguinal canal
a.v. saphena
n. saphenus
a.v. glutea caudalis
nn. pelvini
a.v. vaginalis
m. sacrocaudalis ventralis
a.v. pudenda interna
a.v. obturatoria
m. levator ani
m. obturatorius:
pars iliaca
pars ischiopubica
pubis
ischium
a.v. clitoridis media
v. labialis ventralis
v. pudenda externa between m. gracilis and m. pectineus
m. gracilis

Fig. 8.87 The right pelvic wall of the pregnant mare: medial view (2). The peritoneum and connective tissue have been removed to display the vessels, nerves and muscles of the pelvic wall. The rectus abdominis muscle and the mammary gland have been removed.

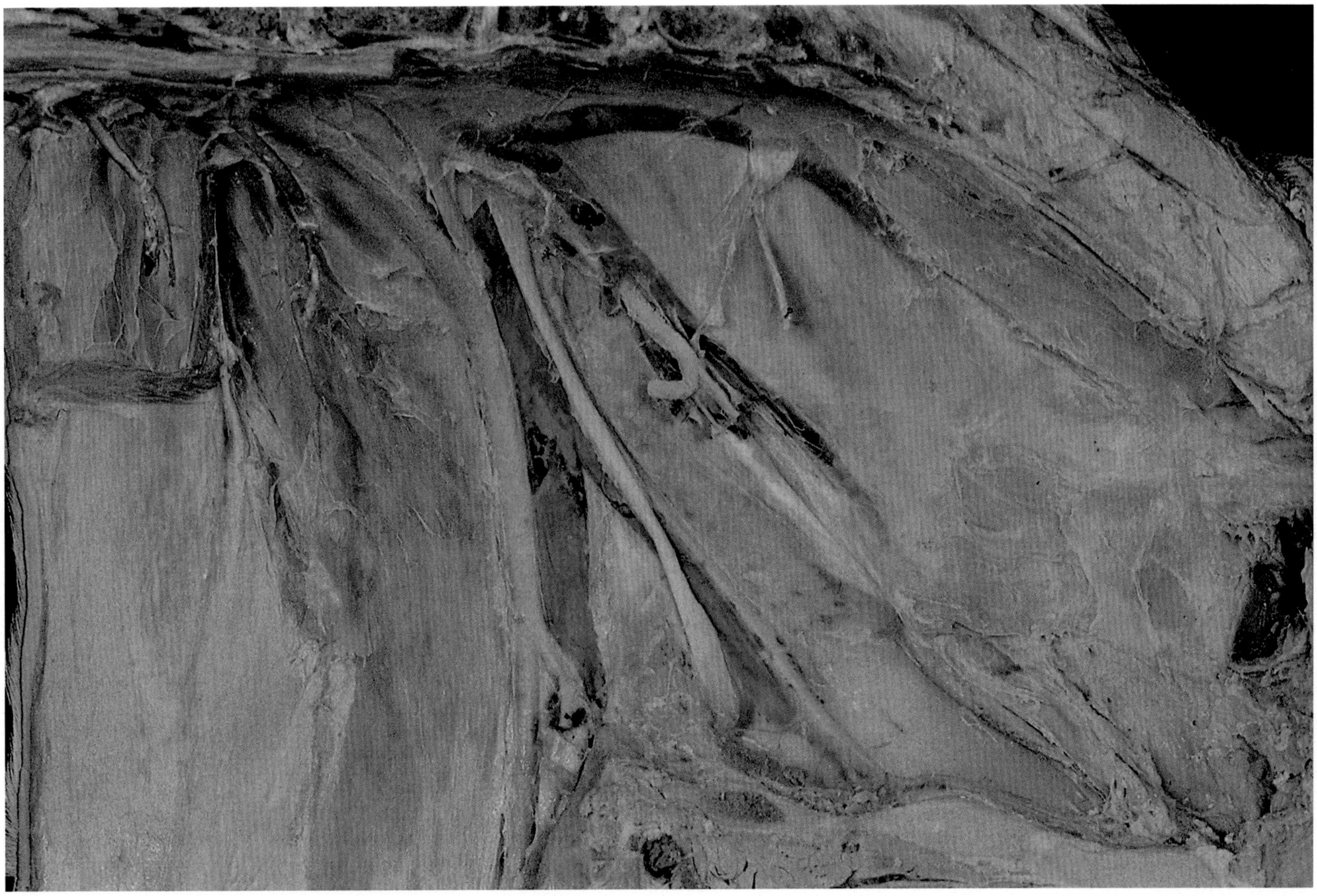

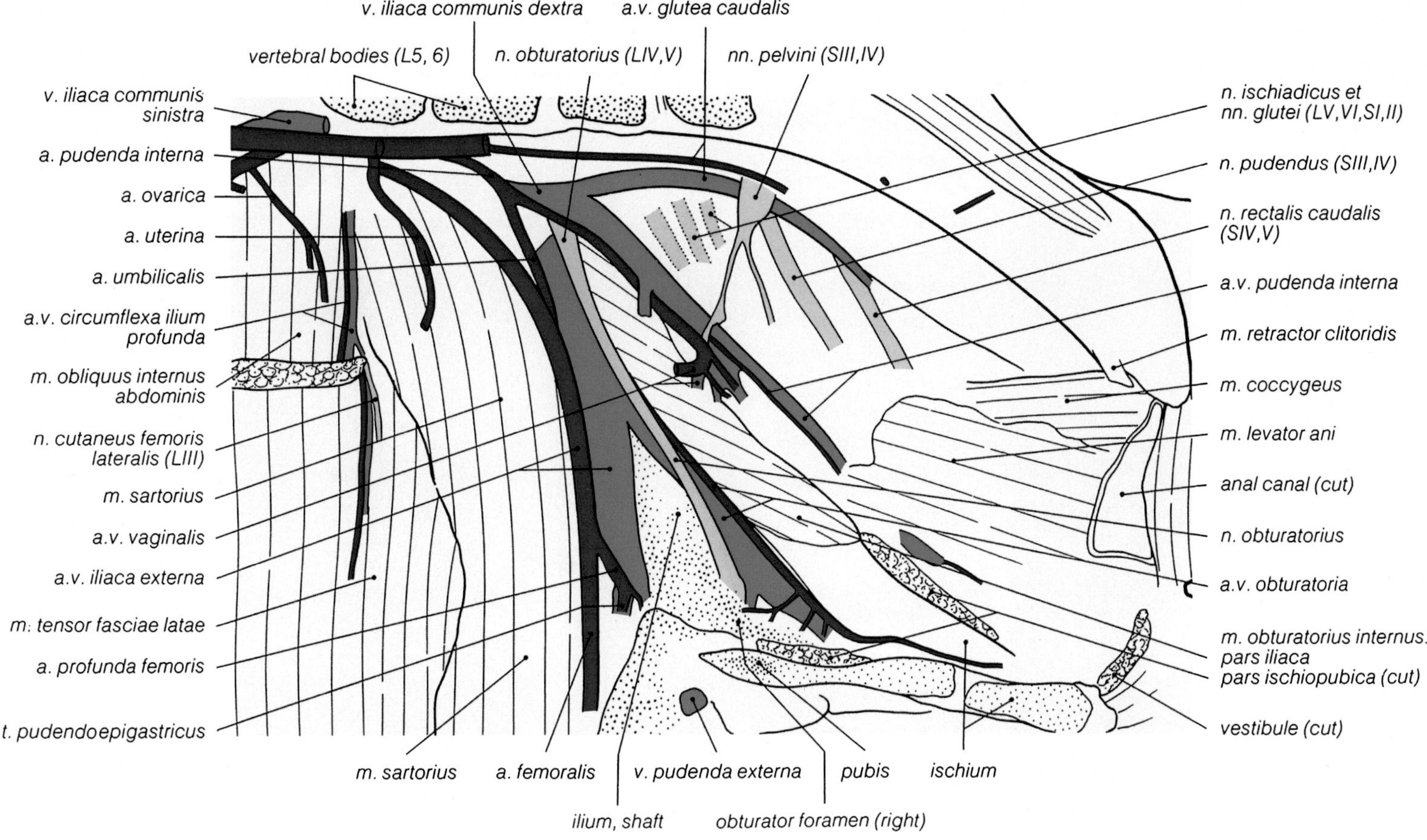
v. iliaca communis dextra
a.v. glutea caudalis
vertebral bodies (L5, 6)
n. obturatorius (LIV,V)
nn. pelvini (SIII,IV)
v. iliaca communis sinistra
a. pudenda interna
a. ovarica
a. uterina
a. umbilicalis
a.v. circumflexa ilium profunda
m. obliquus internus abdominis
n. cutaneus femoris lateralis (LIII)
m. sartorius
a.v. vaginalis
a.v. iliaca externa
m. tensor fasciae latae
a. profunda femoris
t. pudendoepigastricus
n. ischiadicus et nn. glutei (LV,VI,SI,II)
n. pudendus (SIII,IV)
n. rectalis caudalis (SIV,V)
a.v. pudenda interna
m. retractor clitoridis
m. coccygeus
m. levator ani
anal canal (cut)
n. obturatorius
a.v. obturatoria
m. obturatorius internus:
pars iliaca
pars ischiopubica (cut)
vestibule (cut)
m. sartorius
a. femoralis
v. pudenda externa
pubis
ischium
ilium, shaft
obturator foramen (right)

Fig. 8.88 The right pelvic wall of the pregnant mare: medial view (3). The abdominal wall has been resected. The ischiopubic part of the internal obturator muscle has been removed to display the position of the obturator foramen.

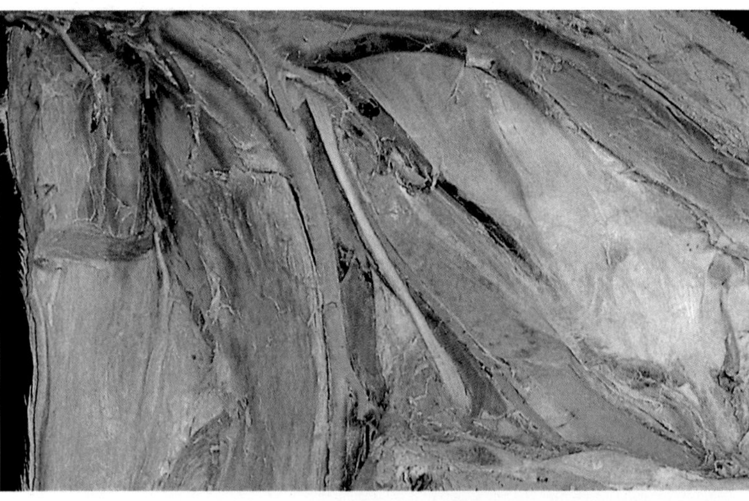

Fig. 8.89 The deep surface of the broad sacrotuberous ligament of the pregnant mare: medial view. The pudendal nerve disappears from sight in this medial view because it runs between superficial and deep laminae of the broad sacrotuberous ligament.

a.v. pudenda interna
a. umbilicalis
m. psoas minor
broad sacrotuberous ligament
a.v. iliaca externa
m. sartorius
n. obturatorius
a.v. obturatoria
ilium, shaft
obturator foramen
a. profunda femoris
t. pudendoepigastricus
pubis
a. femoralis
m. pectineus
v. pudenda externa

a.v. glutea caudalis
nn. pelvini
n. ischiadicus et nn. glutei
n. pudendus
a.v. vaginalis
n. rectalis caudalis
m. sacrocaudalis ventralis
m. coccygeus
origin from broad sacrotuberous ligament
lnn. anorectales
a.v. pudenda interna
m. levator ani, origin
a. perinealis ventralis
m. obturatorius interna:
pars iliaca
pars ischiopubica
lesser ischiatic notch
ischium

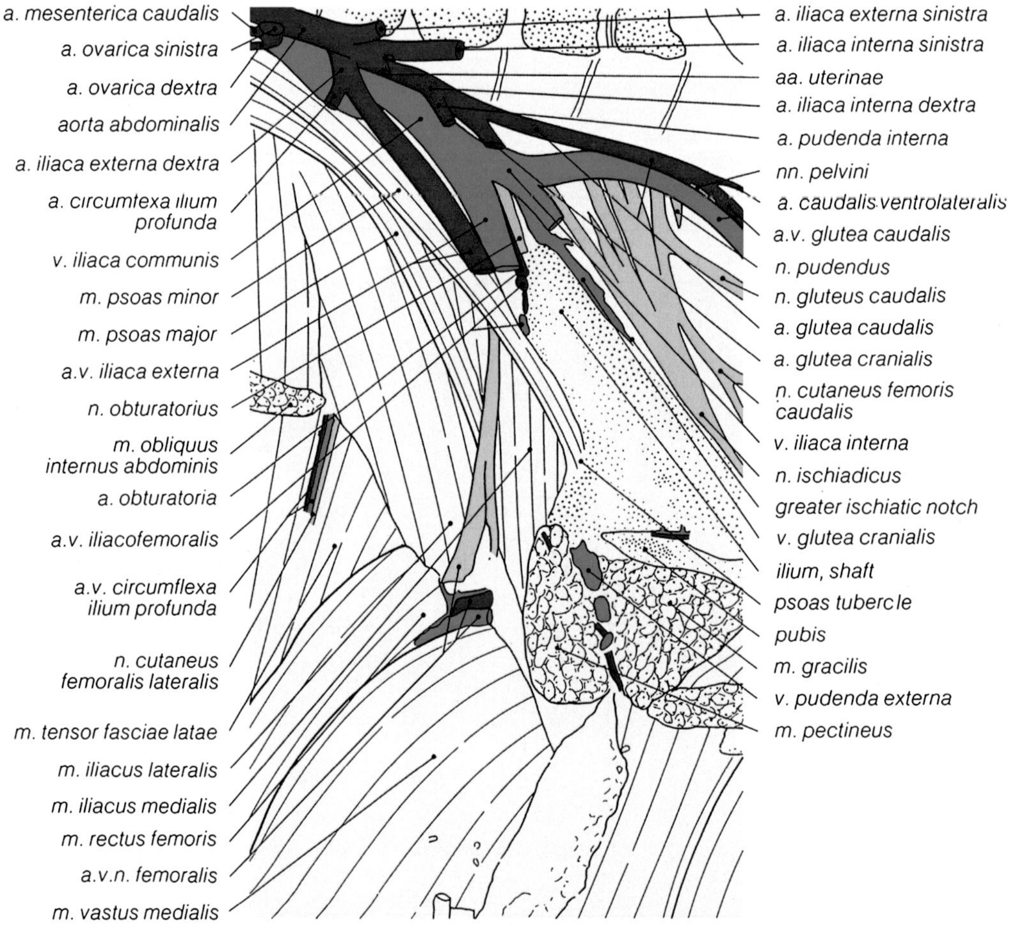

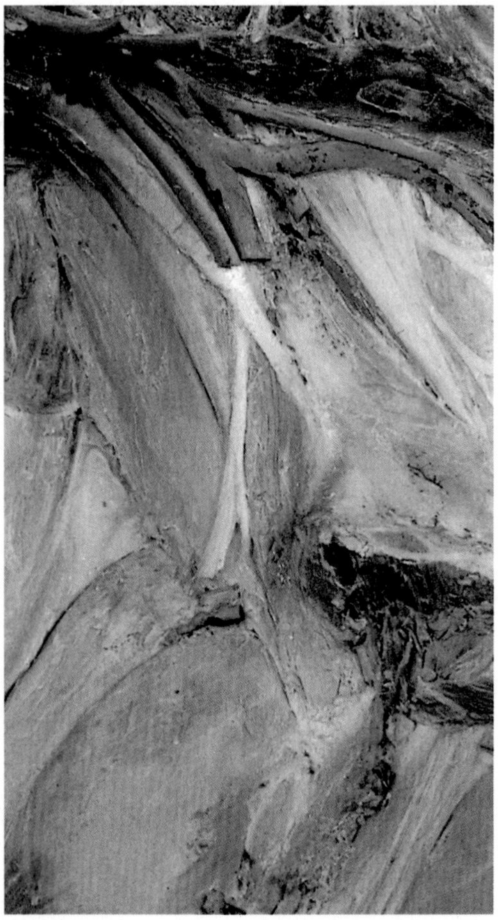

a. mesenterica caudalis
a. ovarica sinistra
a. ovarica dextra
aorta abdominalis
a. iliaca externa dextra
a. circumflexa ilium profunda
v. iliaca communis
m. psoas minor
m. psoas major
a.v. iliaca externa
n. obturatorius
m. obliquus internus abdominis
a. obturatoria
a.v. iliacofemoralis
a.v. circumflexa ilium profunda
n. cutaneus femoralis lateralis
m. tensor fasciae latae
m. iliacus lateralis
m. iliacus medialis
m. rectus femoris
a.v.n. femoralis
m. vastus medialis

a. iliaca externa sinistra
a. iliaca interna sinistra
aa. uterinae
a. iliaca interna dextra
a. pudenda interna
nn. pelvini
a. caudalis ventrolateralis
a.v. glutea caudalis
n. pudendus
n. gluteus caudalis
a. glutea caudalis
a. glutea cranialis
n. cutaneus femoris caudalis
v. iliaca interna
n. ischiadicus
greater ischiatic notch
v. glutea cranialis
ilium, shaft
psoas tubercle
pubis
m. gracilis
v. pudenda externa
m. pectineus

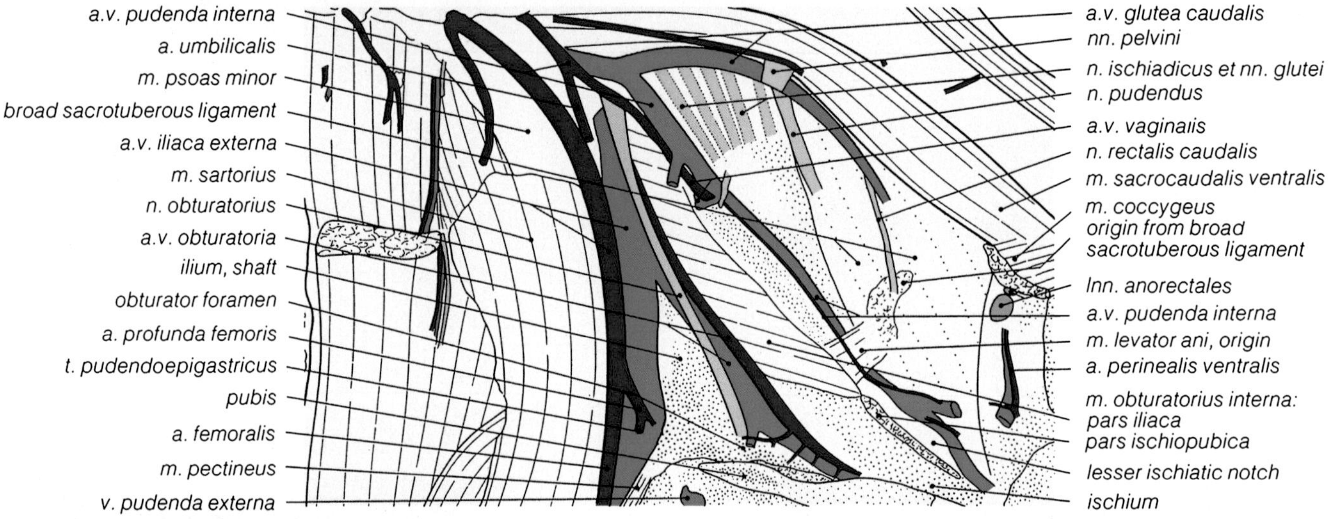

Fig. 8.90 Structures related to the shaft of the right ilium of the pregnant mare: medial view. The broad sacrotuberous ligament has been removed to show the nerves that pass through the greater ischiatic foramen and then run lateral to this ligament. The sartorius muscle has been removed to show the course of the femoral nerve and the iliopsoas muscles. Note that in this specimen the left and right uterine arteries arose from the internal iliac arteries.

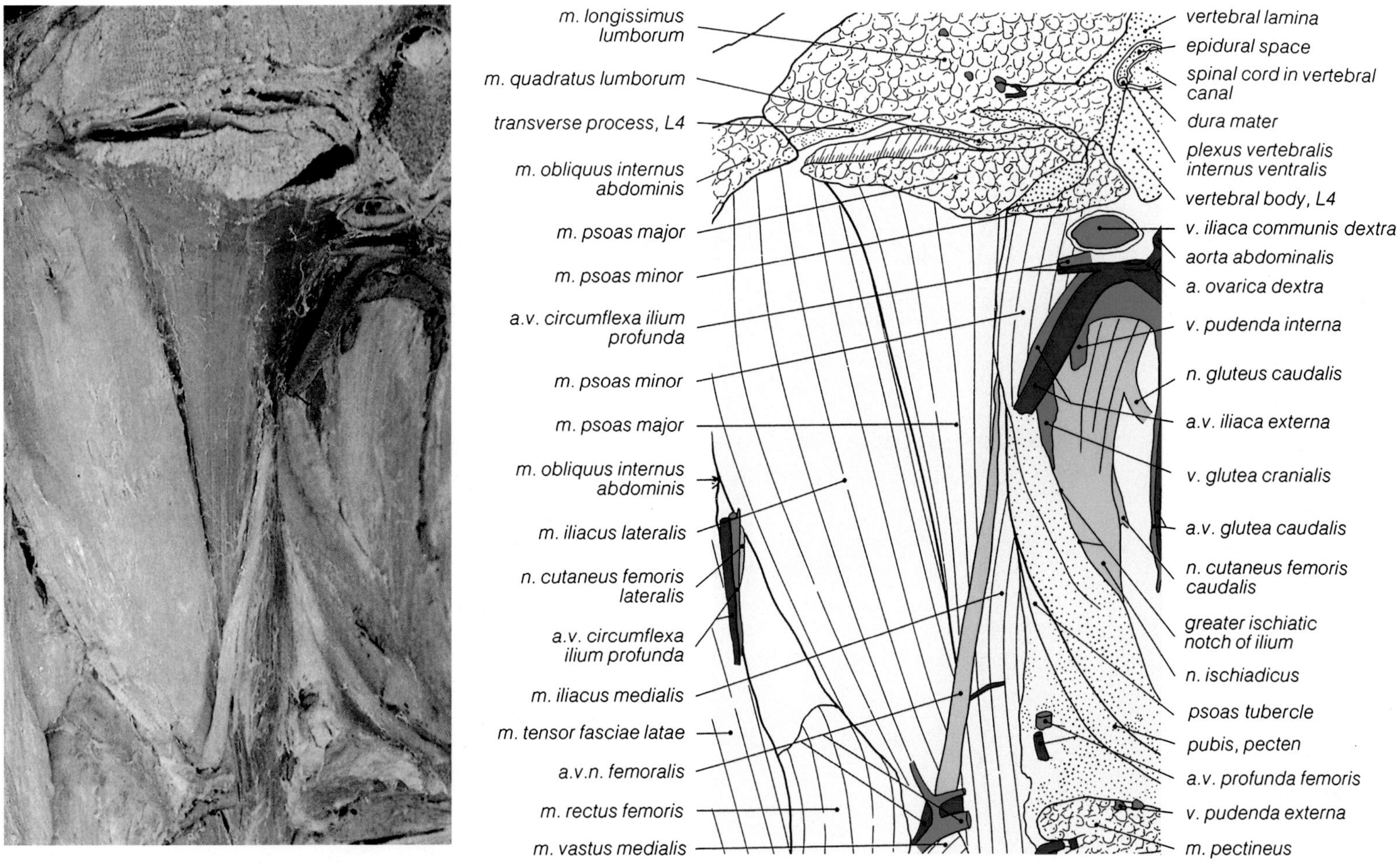

m. longissimus lumborum
m. quadratus lumborum
transverse process, L4
m. obliquus internus abdominis
m. psoas major
m. psoas minor
a.v. circumflexa ilium profunda
m. psoas minor
m. psoas major
m. obliquus internus abdominis
m. iliacus lateralis
n. cutaneus femoris lateralis
a.v. circumflexa ilium profunda
m. iliacus medialis
m. tensor fasciae latae
a.v.n. femoralis
m. rectus femoris
m. vastus medialis
vertebral lamina
epidural space
spinal cord in vertebral canal
dura mater
plexus vertebralis internus ventralis
vertebral body, L4
v. iliaca communis dextra
aorta abdominalis
a. ovarica dextra
v. pudenda interna
n. gluteus caudalis
a.v. iliaca externa
v. glutea cranialis
a.v. glutea caudalis
n. cutaneus femoris caudalis
greater ischiatic notch of ilium
n. ischiadicus
psoas tubercle
pubis, pecten
a.v. profunda femoris
v. pudenda externa
m. pectineus

Fig. 8.91 Structures related to the shaft of the right ilium of the pregnant mare: cranial view. The dissection is at the same stage as that shown in Fig. 8.90.

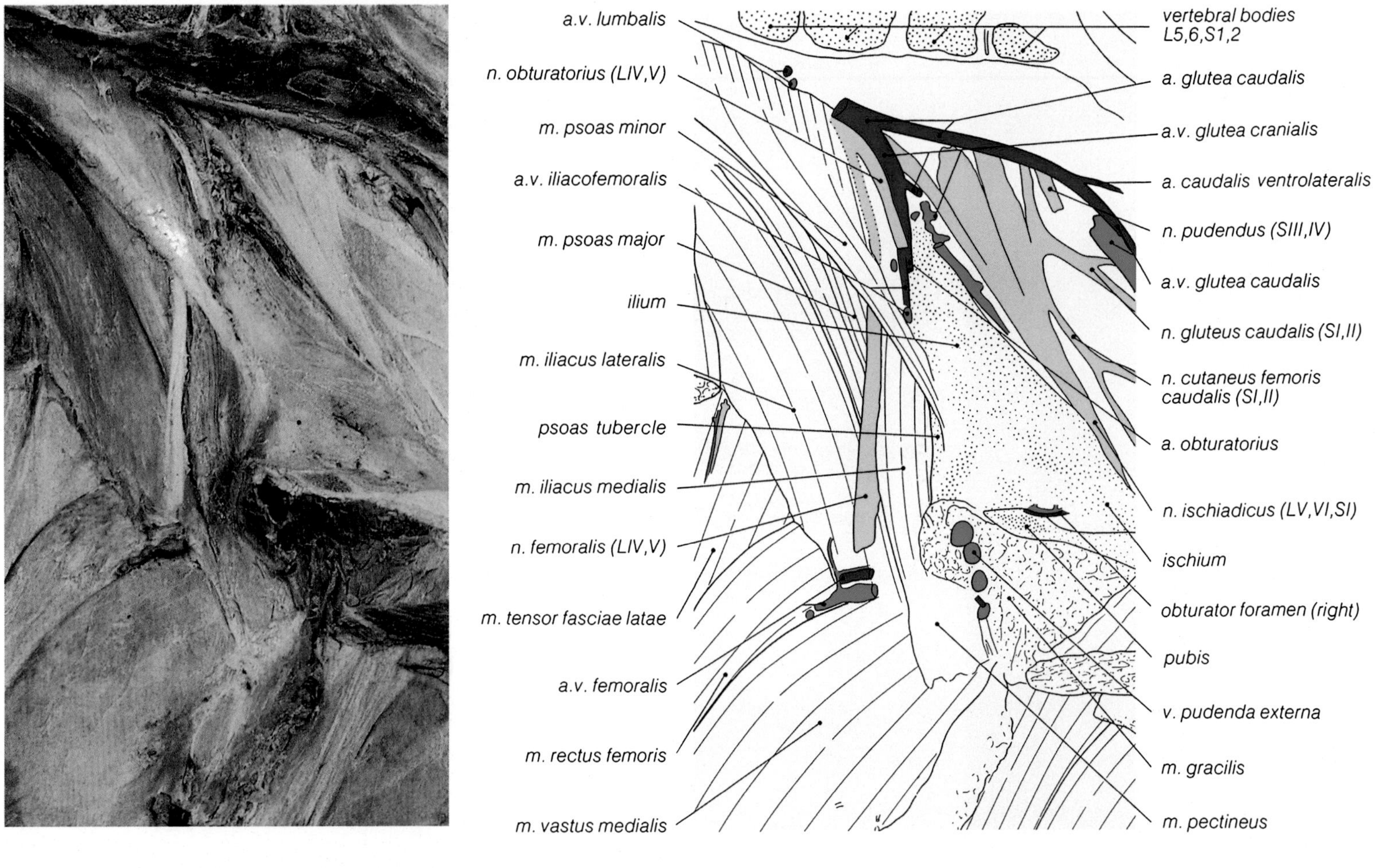

a.v. lumbalis
n. obturatorius (LIV,V)
m. psoas minor
a.v. iliacofemoralis
m. psoas major
ilium
m. iliacus lateralis
psoas tubercle
m. iliacus medialis
n. femoralis (LIV,V)
m. tensor fasciae latae
a.v. femoralis
m. rectus femoris
m. vastus medialis
vertebral bodies L5,6,S1,2
a. glutea caudalis
a.v. glutea cranialis
a. caudalis ventrolateralis
n. pudendus (SIII,IV)
a.v. glutea caudalis
n. gluteus caudalis (SI,II)
n. cutaneus femoris caudalis (SI,II)
a. obturatorius
n. ischiadicus (LV,VI,SI)
ischium
obturator foramen (right)
pubis
v. pudenda externa
m. gracilis
m. pectineus

Fig. 8.92 The right femoral nerve and cranial gluteal artery of the pregnant mare: medial view. The internal and external iliac vessels have been removed to show the emergence of the femoral nerve between the psoas major and minor muscles. The course of the nerve is indicated by a broken line.

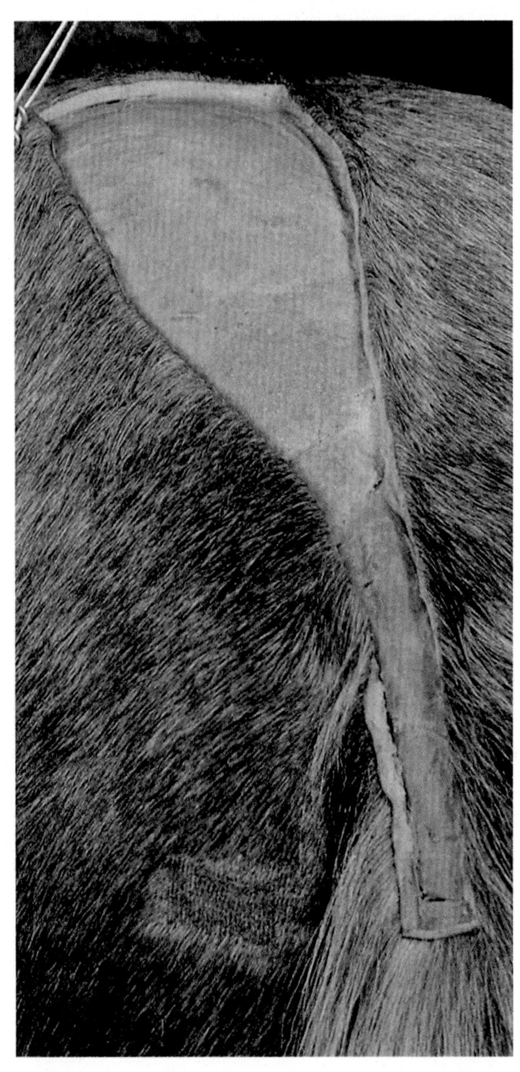

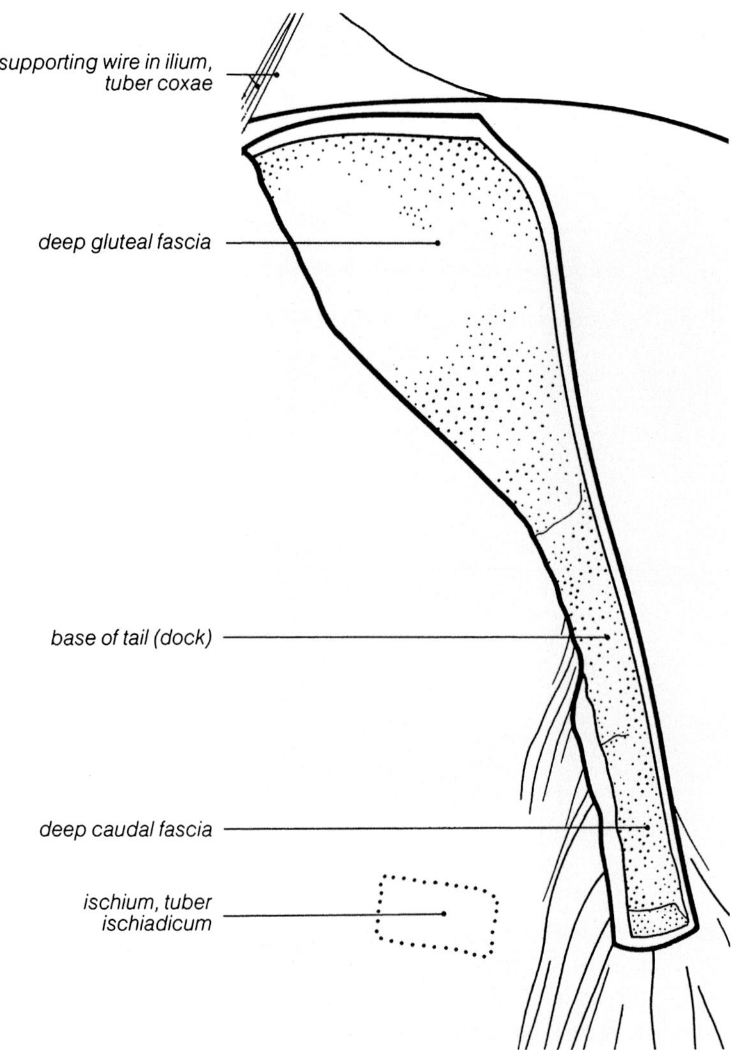
supporting wire in ilium, tuber coxae
deep gluteal fascia
base of tail (dock)
deep caudal fascia
ischium, tuber ischiadicum

Fig. 8.93 The gluteal and caudal fasciae, left caudal view. Figs. 8.93–8.103 show a series of dissections of sacral and caudal (coccygeal) vertebrae and nerves in a 2 ½ year-old horse. Here, the skin and superficial fasciae have been removed. Hair has been clipped over the principal bony landmarks.

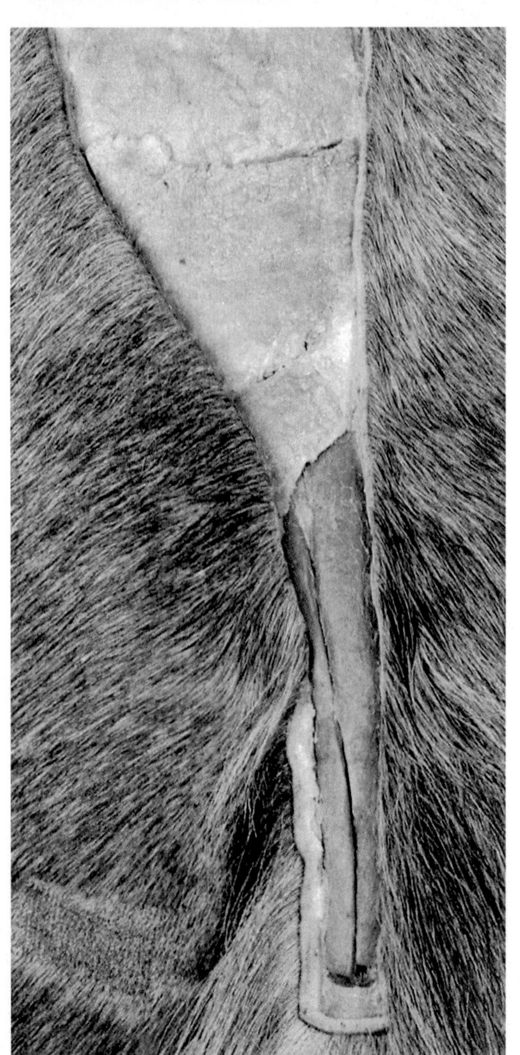

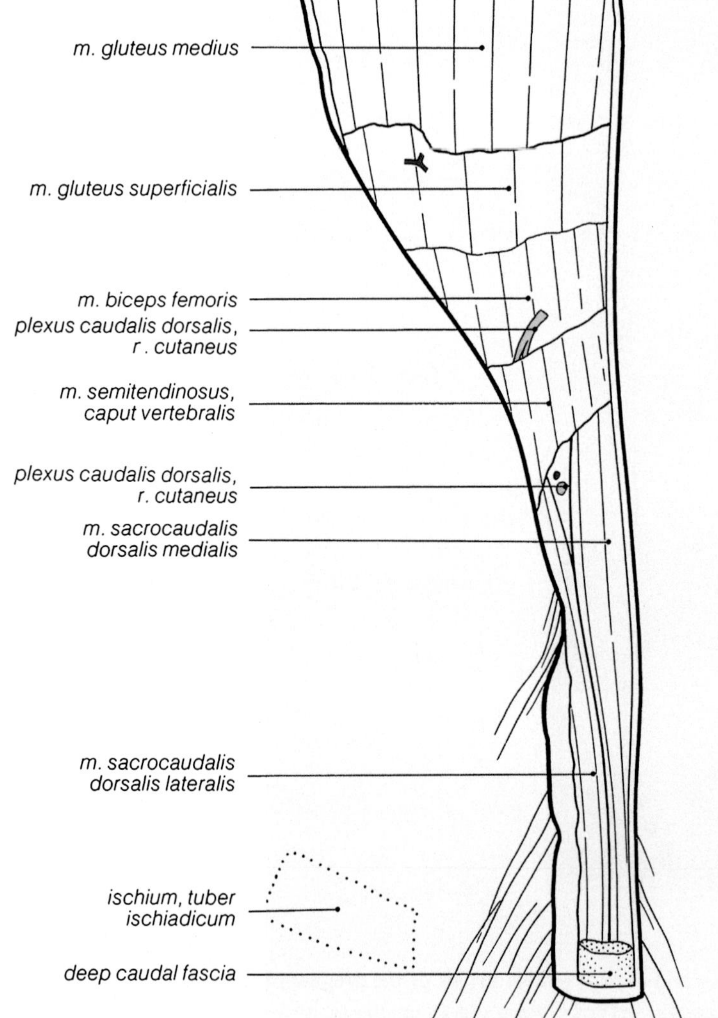
m. gluteus medius
m. gluteus superficialis
m. biceps femoris
plexus caudalis dorsalis, r. cutaneus
m. semitendinosus, caput vertebralis
plexus caudalis dorsalis, r. cutaneus
m. sacrocaudalis dorsalis medialis
m. sacrocaudalis dorsalis lateralis
ischium, tuber ischiadicum
deep caudal fascia

Fig. 8.94 Superficial muscles of the left sacral and caudal regions: dorsal view.

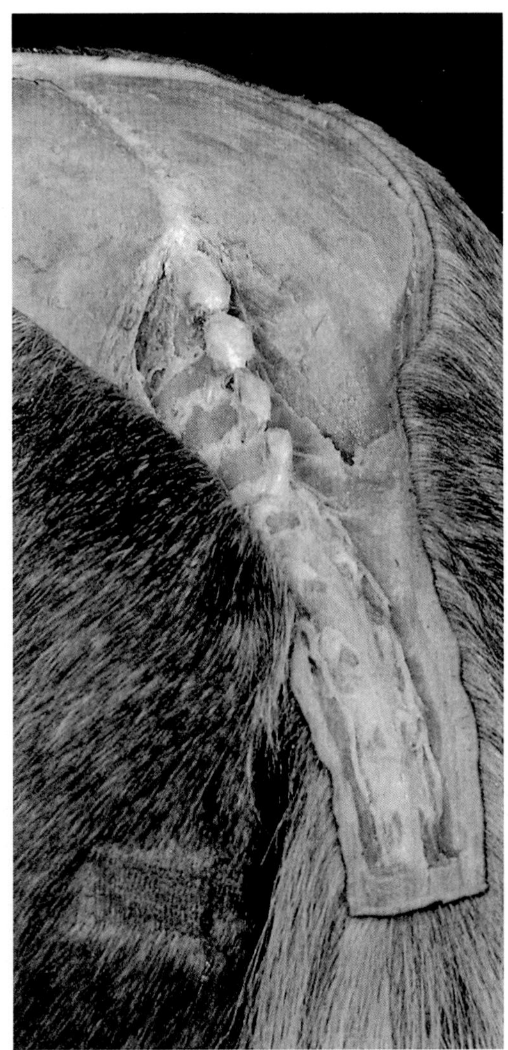

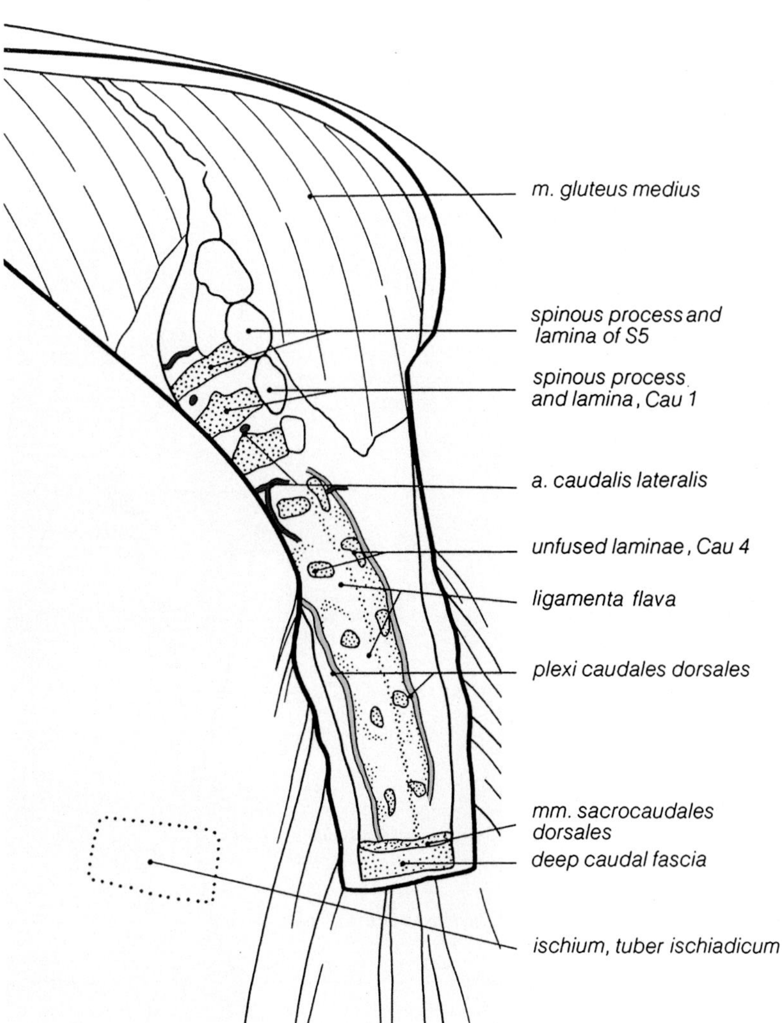
m. gluteus medius
spinous process and lamina of S5
spinous process and lamina, Cau 1
a. caudalis lateralis
unfused laminae, Cau 4
ligamenta flava
plexi caudales dorsales
mm. sacrocaudales dorsales
deep caudal fascia
ischium, tuber ischiadicum

Fig. 8.95 Structures of the sacral and caudal regions: left caudo-dorsal view. The epaxial muscle mass has been removed from the last two sacral and first seven caudal vertebrae.

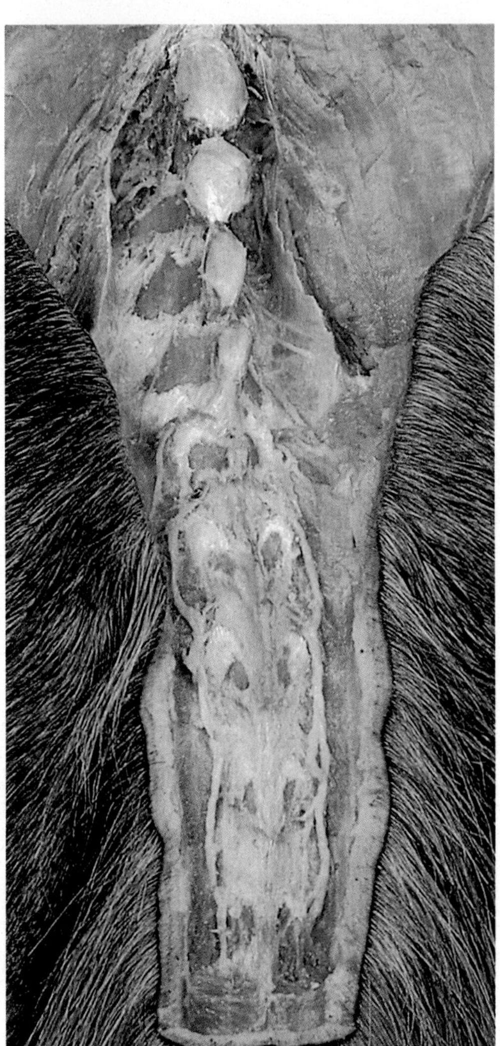

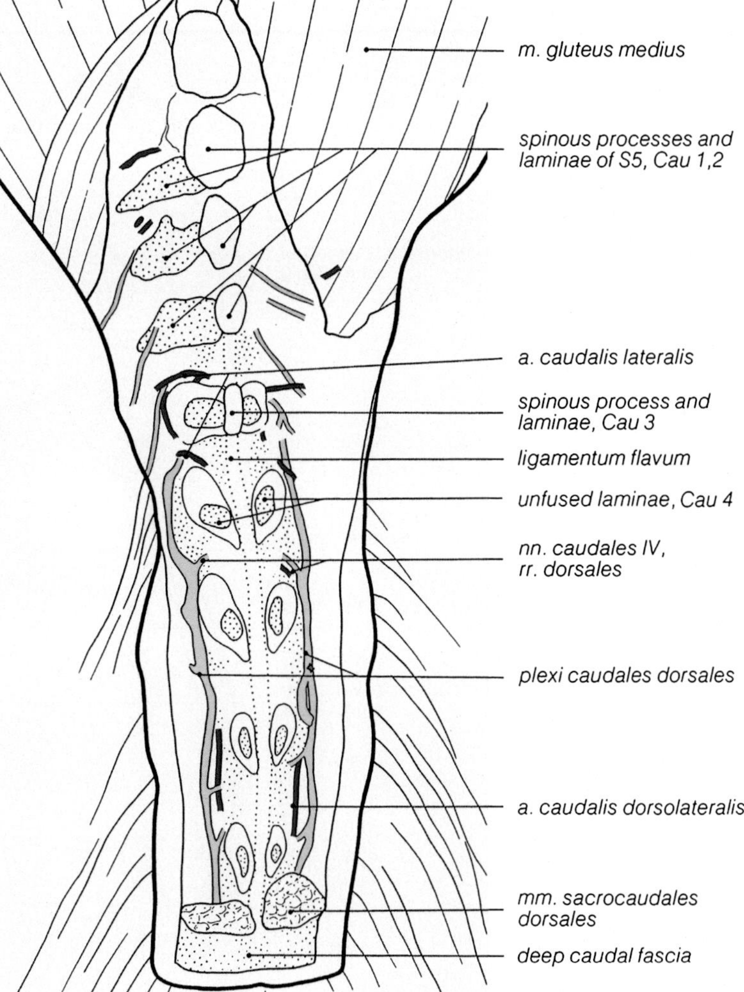
m. gluteus medius
spinous processes and laminae of S5, Cau 1,2
a. caudalis lateralis
spinous process and laminae, Cau 3
ligamentum flavum
unfused laminae, Cau 4
nn. caudales IV, rr. dorsales
plexi caudales dorsales
a. caudalis dorsolateralis
mm. sacrocaudales dorsales
deep caudal fascia

Fig. 8.96 Structures of the sacral and caudal regions: dorsal view. The epaxial muscle mass has been removed from the caudal sacral and first seven caudal vertebrae.

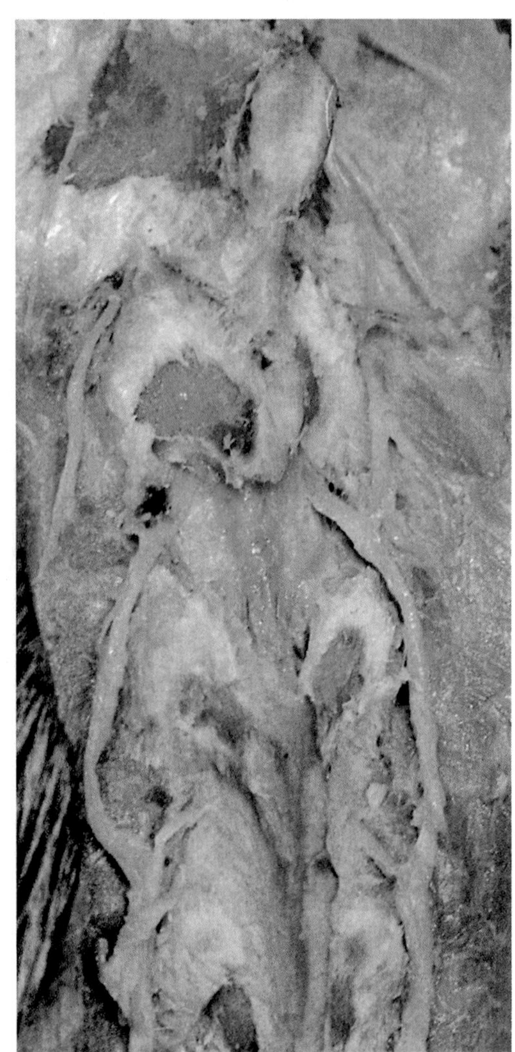

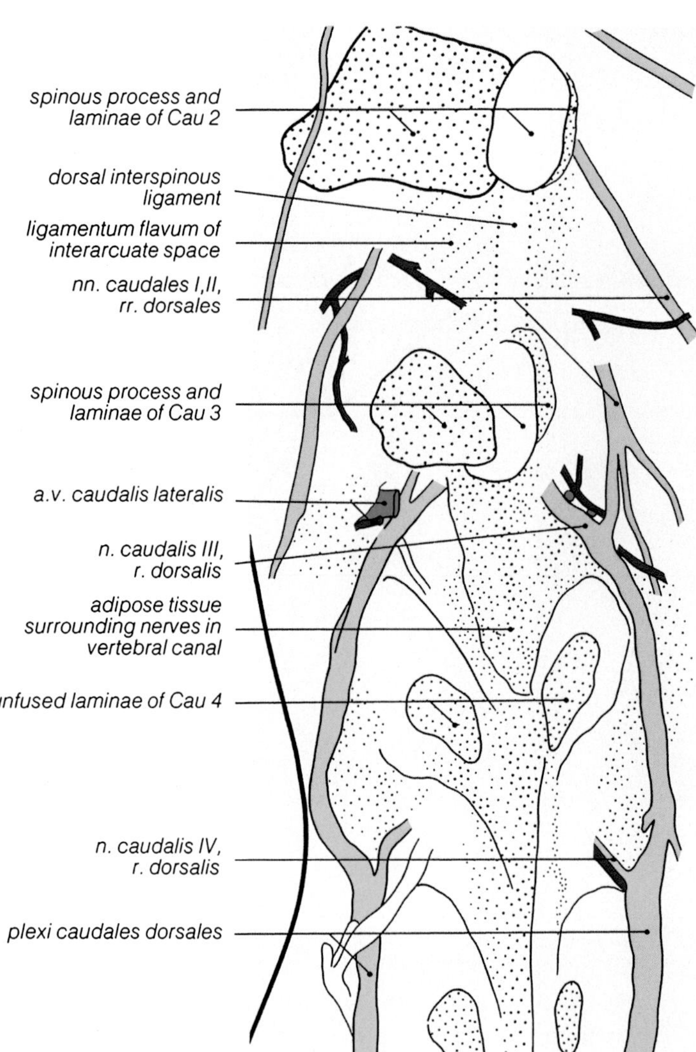
spinous process and laminae of Cau 2
dorsal interspinous ligament
ligamentum flavum of interarcuate space
nn. caudales I,II, rr. dorsales
spinous process and laminae of Cau 3
a.v. caudalis lateralis
n. caudalis III, r. dorsalis
adipose tissue surrounding nerves in vertebral canal
unfused laminae of Cau 4
n. caudalis IV, r. dorsalis
plexi caudales dorsales

Fig. 8.97 Structures of the caudal region: dorsal view (1). The ligaments have been removed from the interarcuate space between the spinal arches of third and fourth caudal vertebrae to expose the contents of the vertebral canal.

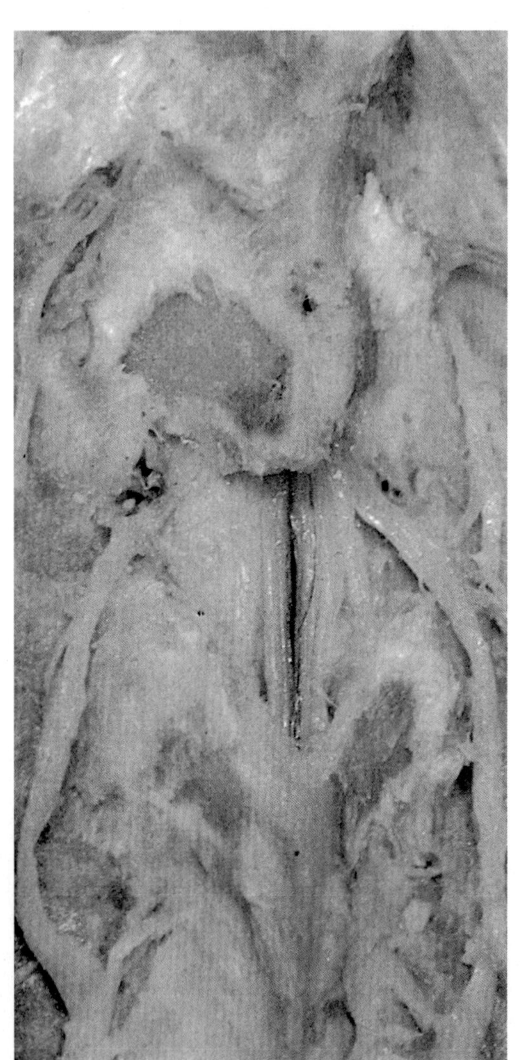

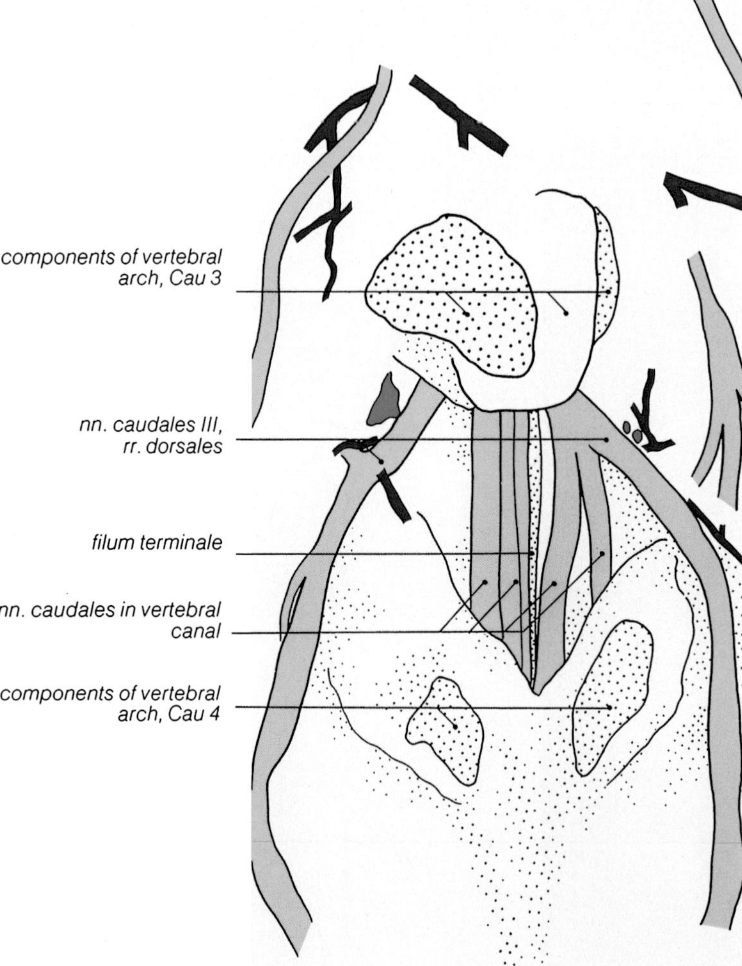
components of vertebral arch, Cau 3
nn. caudales III, rr. dorsales
filum terminale
nn. caudales in vertebral canal
components of vertebral arch, Cau 4

Fig. 8.98 Structures of the caudal region: dorsal view (2). The epidural adipose tissue of the vertebral canal has been removed from the interarcuate space to show the caudal nerves within the canal.

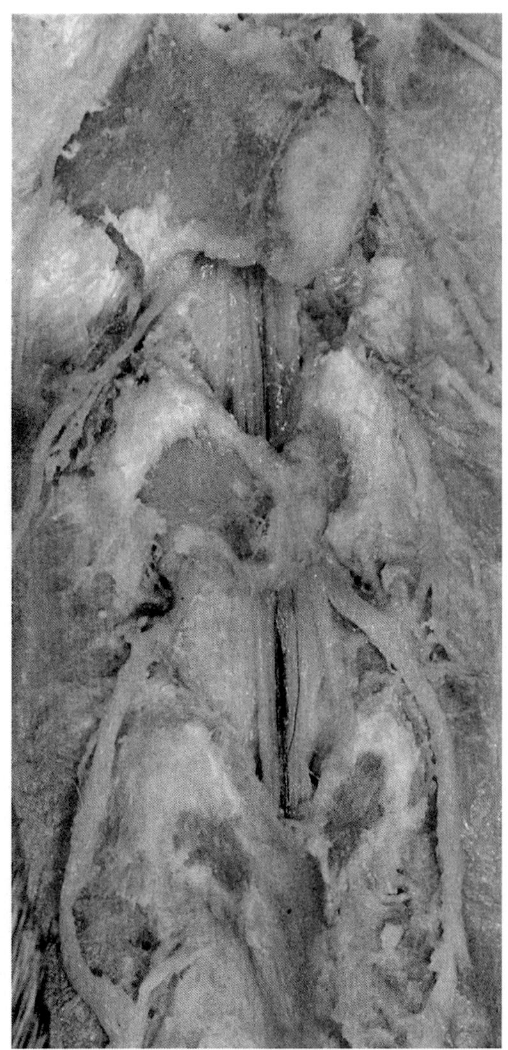

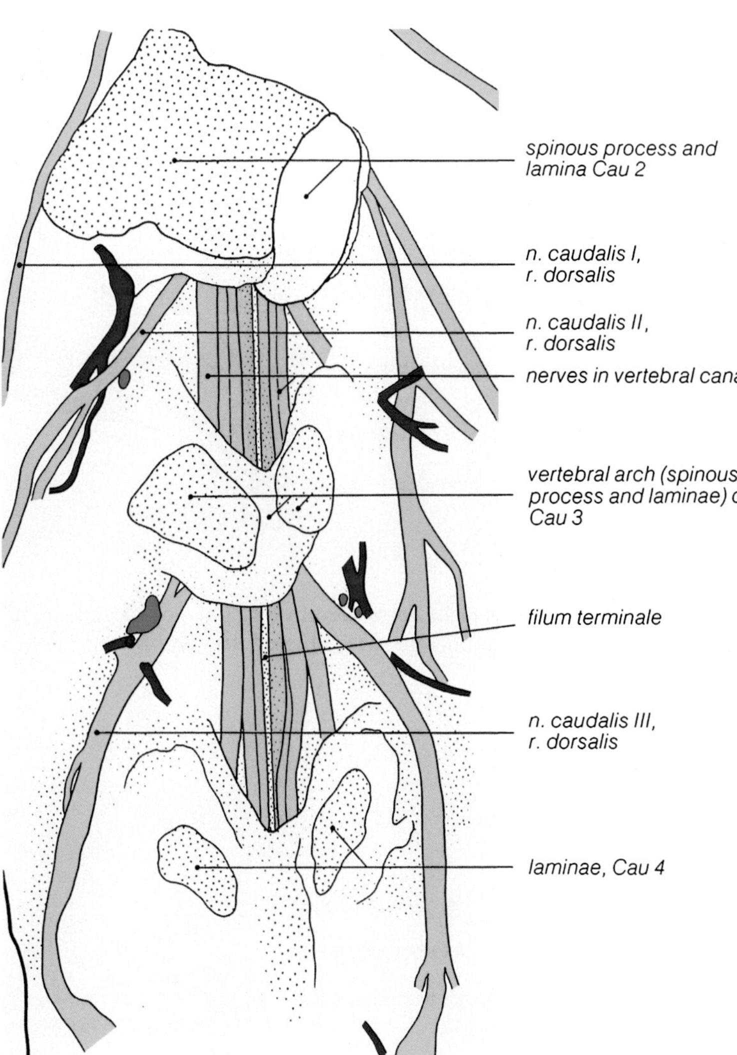
spinous process and lamina Cau 2
n. caudalis I, r. dorsalis
n. caudalis II, r. dorsalis
nerves in vertebral canal
vertebral arch (spinous process and laminae) of Cau 3
filum terminale
n. caudalis III, r. dorsalis
laminae, Cau 4

Fig. 8.99 Structures of the caudal region: dorsal view (3). The interarcuate spaces have been dissected and the adipose tissue of the vertebral canal removed to show the vertebral arch of the third caudal vertebra. In the fourth caudal vertebrae the laminae do not fuse and there is no spinous process.

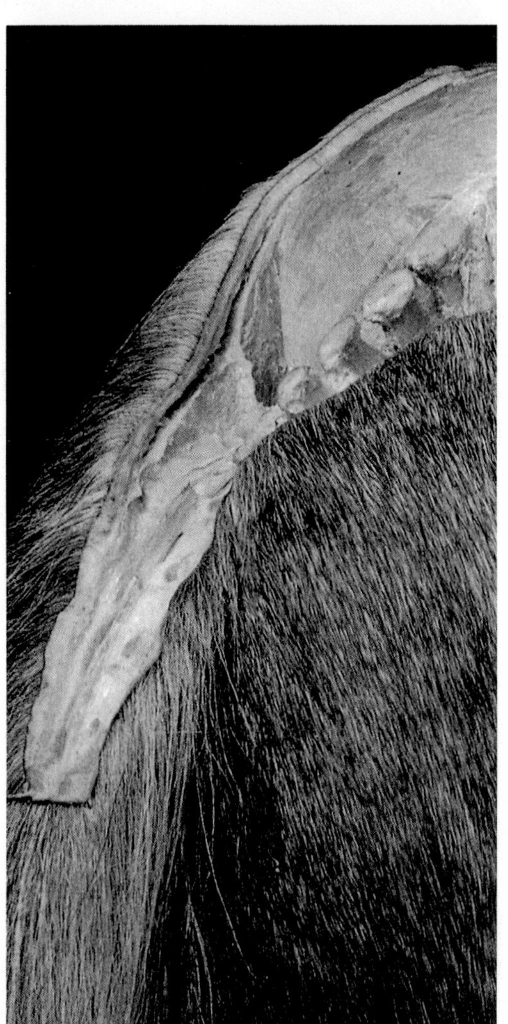

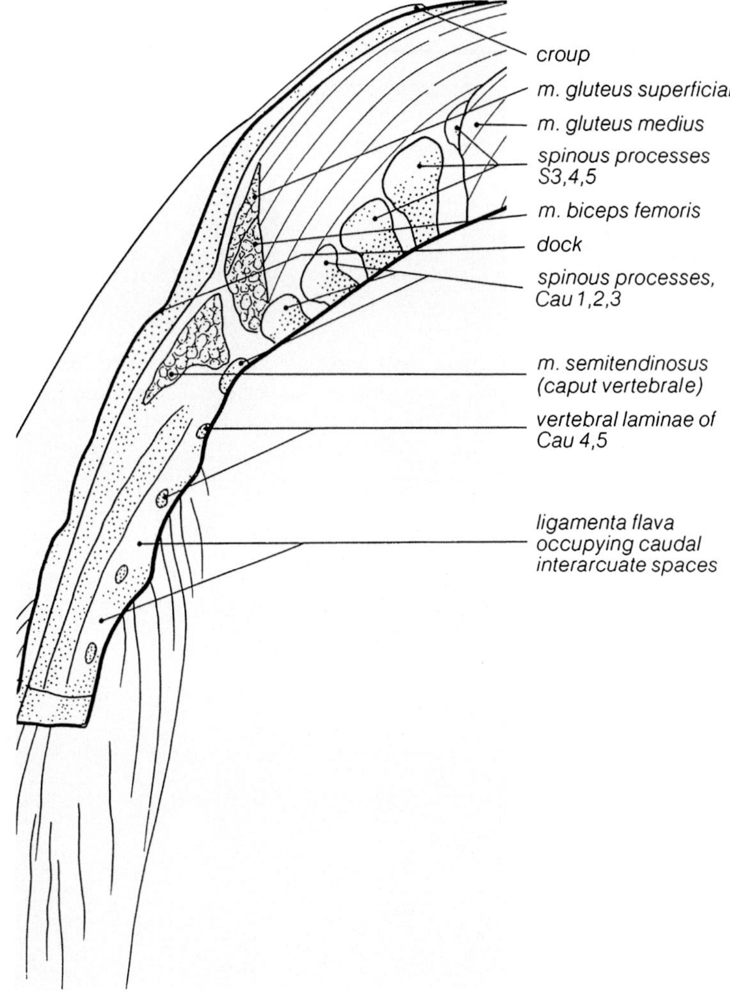
croup
m. gluteus superficialis
m. gluteus medius
spinous processes S3,4,5
m. biceps femoris
dock
spinous processes, Cau 1,2,3
m. semitendinosus (caput vertebrale)
vertebral laminae of Cau 4,5
ligamenta flava occupying caudal interarcuate spaces

Fig. 8.100 Topography of sacral and caudal vertebrae: right dorsocaudal view. The hamstring and caudal muscles have been removed from the vertebral arches and the positions of these arches are seen in relationship to the croup and to the dock (root of tail).

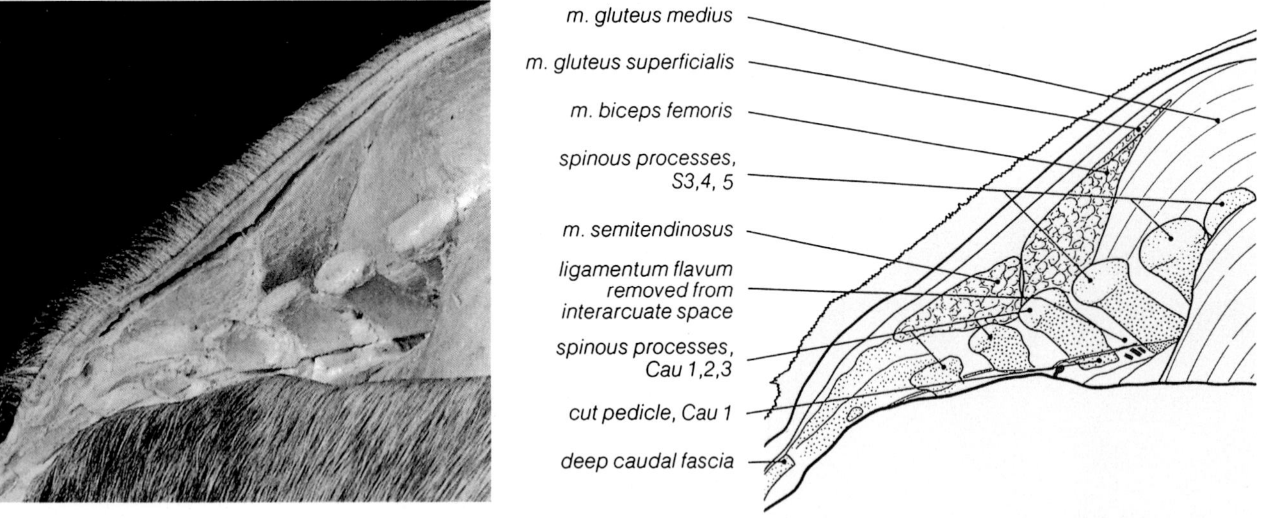
m. gluteus medius
m. gluteus superficialis
m. biceps femoris
spinous processes, S3,4, 5
m. semitendinosus
ligamentum flavum removed from interarcuate space
spinous processes, Cau 1,2,3
cut pedicle, Cau 1
deep caudal fascia

Fig. 8.101 Topography of sacral and caudal vertebrae: right dorsolateral view. The pedicles of the fifth sacral and the first three caudal vertebrae have been sawn through to display the caudal nerves by laminectomy (see Figs. 8.102 and 8.103).

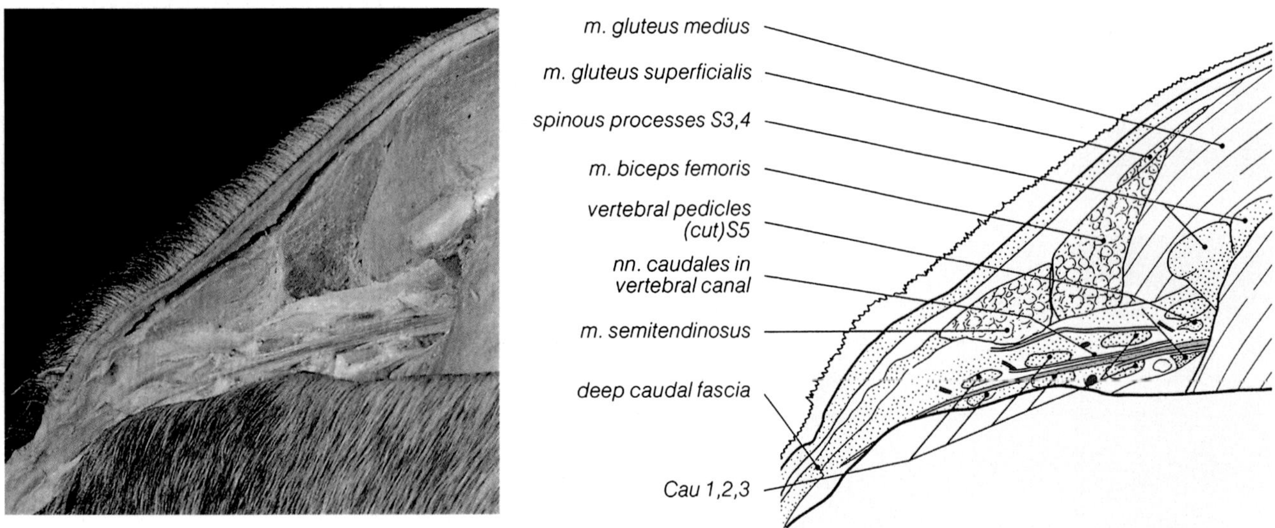
m. gluteus medius
m. gluteus superficialis
spinous processes S3,4
m. biceps femoris
vertebral pedicles (cut)S5
nn. caudales in vertebral canal
m. semitendinosus
deep caudal fascia
Cau 1,2,3

Fig. 8.102 Topography of caudal nerves and vertebral canal: right dorsolateral view. The vertebral laminae have been removed from the fifth sacral and first three caudal vertebrae to show the topographical position of the vertebral canal and its contents in relationship to the dock and the sacral spinous processes.

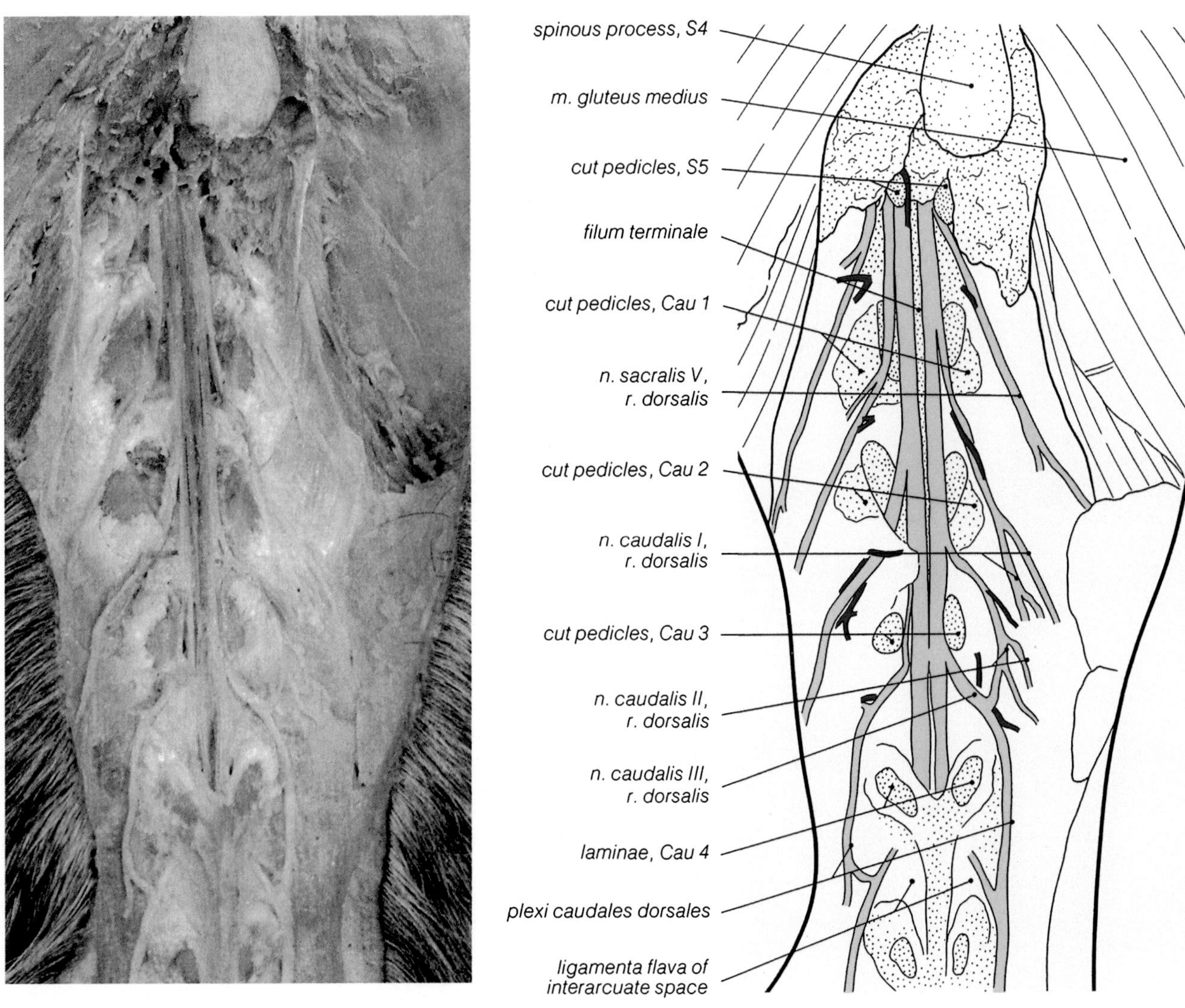
spinous process, S4
m. gluteus medius
cut pedicles, S5
filum terminale
cut pedicles, Cau 1
n. sacralis V,
r. dorsalis
cut pedicles, Cau 2
n. caudalis I,
r. dorsalis
cut pedicles, Cau 3
n. caudalis II,
r. dorsalis
n. caudalis III,
r. dorsalis
laminae, Cau 4
plexi caudales dorsales
ligamenta flava of
interarcuate space

Fig. 8.103 The caudal nerves: dorsal view. The arches of the vertebrae have been removed as indicated in Figs.8.101 and 8.102 and the spinal nerves have been dissected.

9. DIAGNOSTIC IMAGING OF THE HEAD, WITHERS, MANUS AND PES

Clinical considerations for diagnostic imaging

Radiography is a very useful diagnostic tool in equine medicine, particularly in the skull and the distal limbs, although higher-powered equipment will also enable images of the spine, proximal limbs and pelvis to be made. However, in order to be able to interpret radiological abnormalities appropriately, knowledge of normal radiological anatomy must be gained. In general, the distal limb of the equine animal is not too complex. In contrast, the head is extremely complex and so it is of paramount importance to have an atlas of normal radiographic anatomy, or a normal radiograph, available for comparison when attempting interpretation of this area.

The commonest clinical indication for radiography of the limbs is lameness, and the commonest causes of lameness in equine animals are tendon or ligament problems (tendinitis or desmitis), inflammatory conditions (such as laminitis affecting the laminae of the hoof) and trauma (soft tissue injuries and fractures). Although radiography will not demonstrate primary changes in the soft tissue structures, it may demonstrate secondary effects on the bones, such as degenerative joint disease or sclerosis (when the bone becomes dense and hard).

At least two views of the affected area should be taken (orthogonal projections) and, in the case of the limbs, the contralateral limb may also be imaged, to provide a control for comparison. In the distal limb, it is routine to take at least two additional oblique projections of the region of interest in order to assess as much of the region as possible.

Advanced cross-sectional imaging modalities, such as computed tomography (CT), allow appreciation of anatomy without superimposition from overlying structures. CT is of particular value in assessing bony structures, so is particularly useful in demonstrating incomplete fractures and for characterising comminuted fractures (in which the bone has been fragmented into multiple pieces). The lack of superimposition provided by CT is particularly useful in the head, although it is also used to demonstrate change in the limb bones. If appropriate equipment is available, CT may be performed in the standing animal, obviating the need for general anaesthesia.

The presence of cartilaginous epiphyseal (or growth) plates must be remembered when interpreting radiographs of the limbs in young horses. The following times of epiphyseal fusion have been determined radiographically:

- After birth, the distal epiphysis (lateral malleolus) of the fibula fuses with the tibia at about 3 months of age. The distal epiphysis of the ulna (lateral styloid process) fuses with the radius at a slightly later age (4–9 months).
- The distal metapodial epiphyses at the fetlock joints and the proximal epiphyses of the proximal and middle phalanges all fuse at about 6–9 months of age.
- The distal epiphysis of the radius fuses at 2–3 years and that of the distal tibia fuses considerably earlier (17–17.5 months).

Epiphyseal fusion is a gradual process. The epiphyseal growth plate stops producing new metaphyseal bone and becomes itself converted to bone, uniting the epiphysis with the shaft. The process can be traced radiographically or histologically until fusion is complete. Gross anatomical fusion, however, is 'complete fusion', when a standard maceration technique fails to separate the epiphysis from the shaft. For the horse, the results of some investigations by these three methods of study are summarized by Getty in Sisson & Grossman (1975, pp 272 & 298).

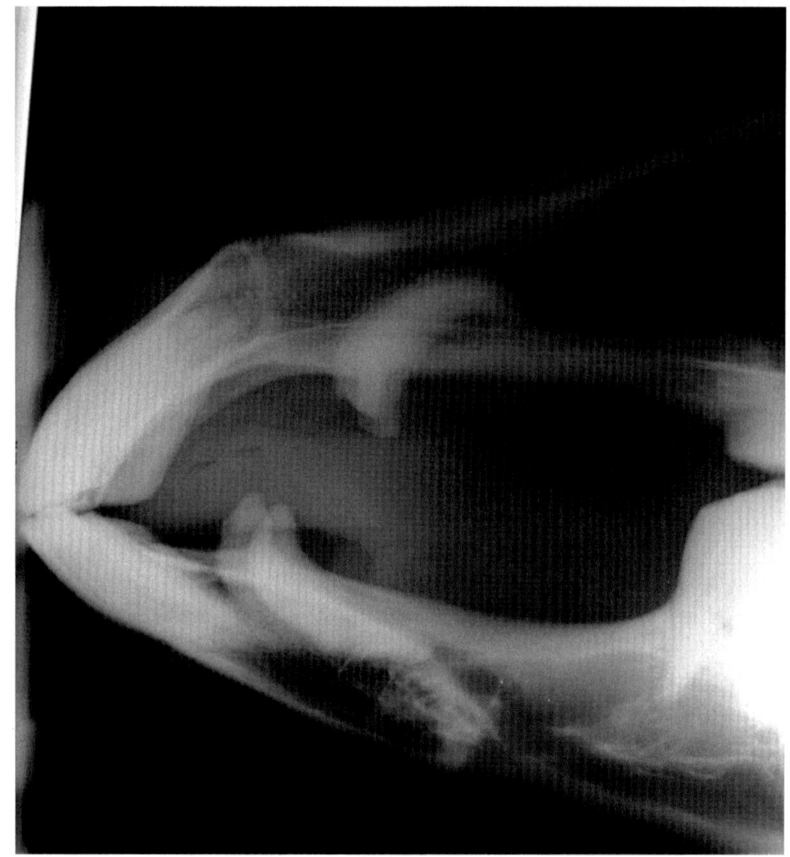

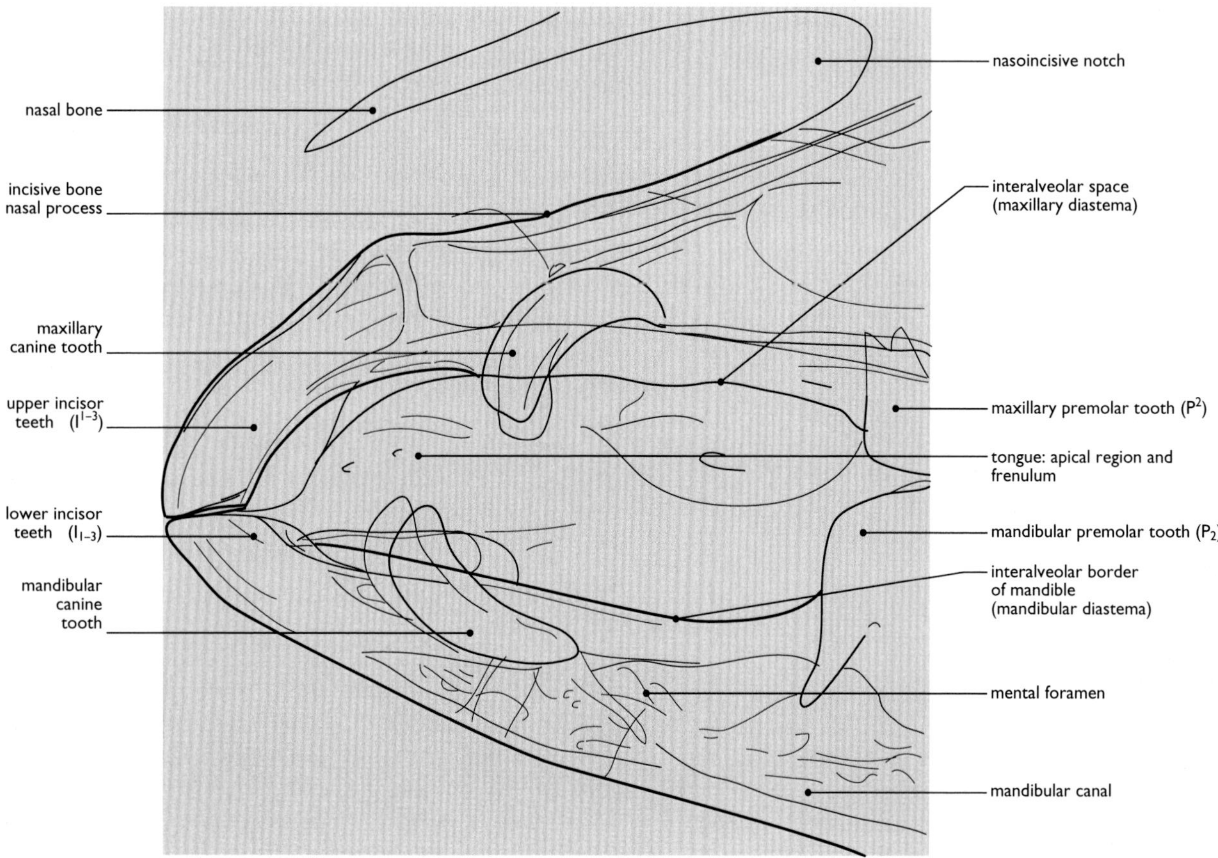
nasoincisive notch
nasal bone
incisive bone
nasal process
interalveolar space
(maxillary diastema)
maxillary
canine tooth
upper incisor
teeth (I^{1-3})
maxillary premolar tooth (P^2)
tongue: apical region and
frenulum
lower incisor
teeth (I_{1-3})
mandibular premolar tooth (P_2)
mandibular
canine
tooth
interalveolar border
of mandible
(mandibular diastema)
mental foramen
mandibular canal

Fig. 9.1 Radiograph of the rostral teeth: lateral view. The canine teeth are large in this horse (probably a male). The first premolar teeth (wolf teeth) are not present.

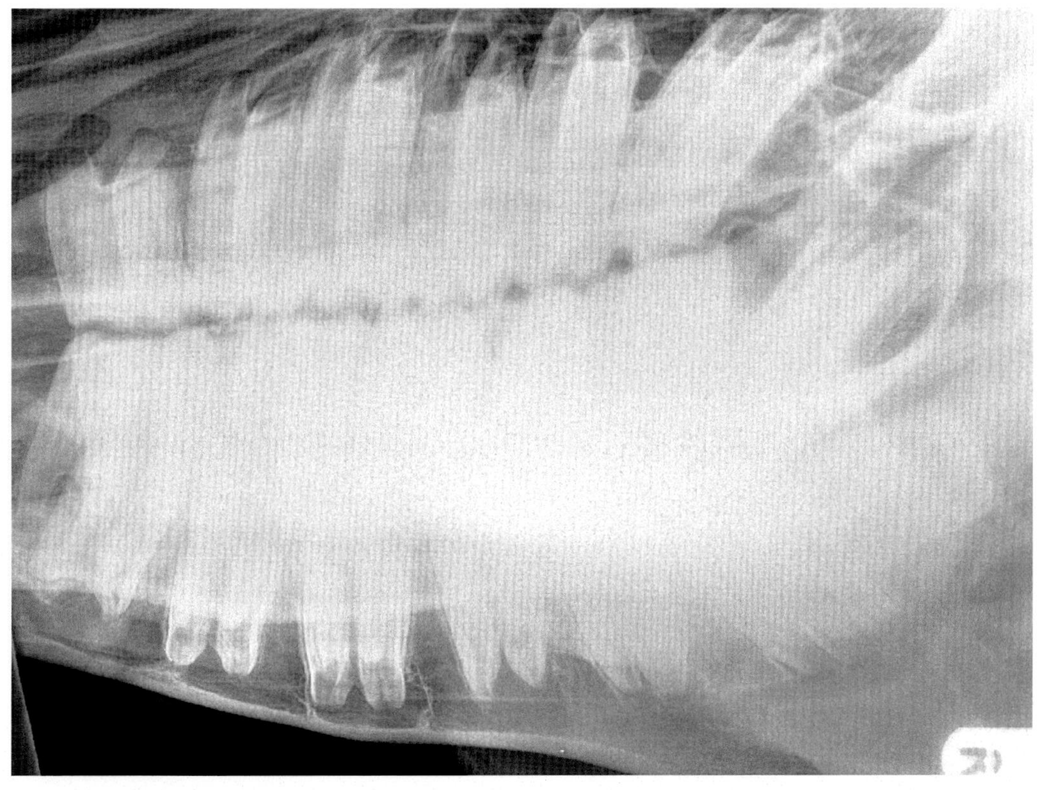

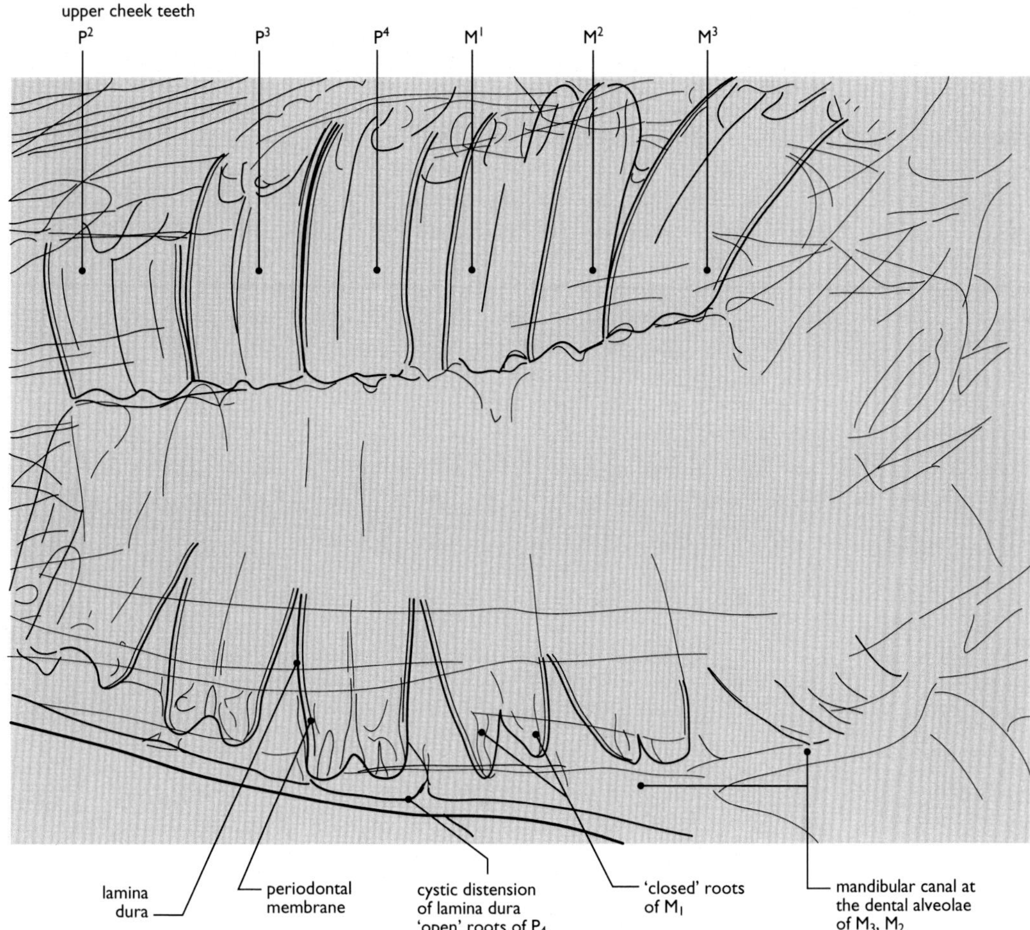
upper cheek teeth
P2
P3
P4
M1
M2
M3
lamina dura
periodontal membrane
cystic distension of lamina dura 'open' roots of P4
'closed' roots of M1
mandibular canal at the dental alveolae of M3, M2

Fig. 9.2 Radiograph of the cheek teeth: lateral view. Compare the roots of P_4 (erupts c. 4 y) with those of M_1 (erupts c. 9–12 m).

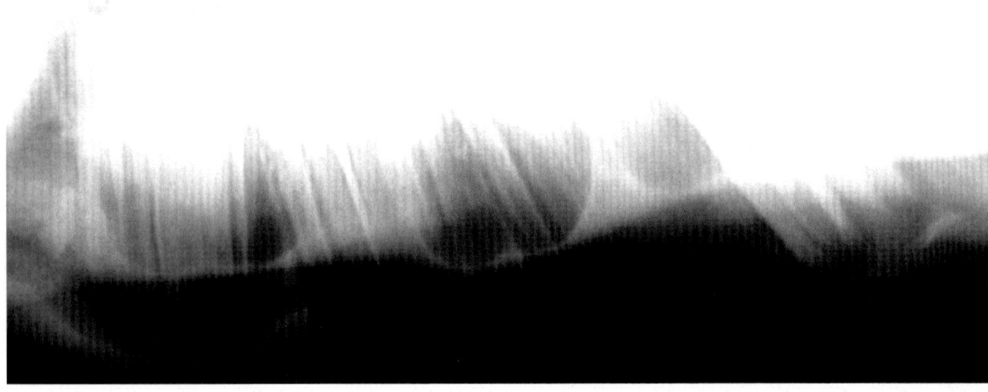

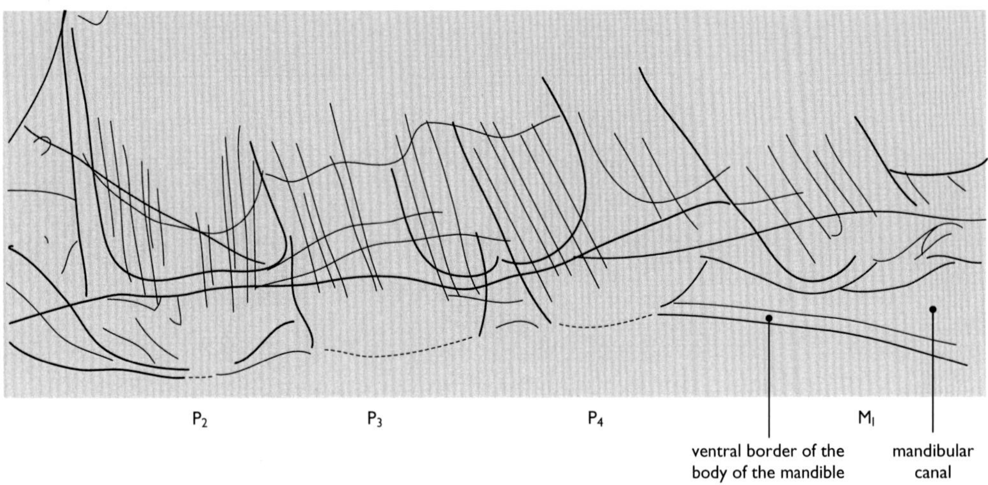
P_2
P_3
P_4
M_1
ventral border of the body of the mandible
mandibular canal

Fig. 9.3 Radiograph of the mandible: lateral oblique view. Dentally immature horse. The developing crowns of the permanent mandibular premolar teeth (P_2–P_4) lie beneath the roots of the temporary premolar teeth (p_2–p_4). They produce palpable bony prominences on the ventral borders of the mandibles in chronological sequence, between the ages of 1½ and 3–4 years. Each prominence disappears after each temporary premolar tooth is lost and the crown of the permanent premolar tooth comes into wear.

A similar developmental sequence of palpable prominences in the maxillary bone occurs, between the ages of 2 and 5 years, at the level of the infraorbital foramen, when the upper permanent maxillary premolar teeth (P^2–P^4) develop and eventually replace the temporary maxillary premolar teeth. At about 2 years of age, the palpable infraorbital foramen lies dorsal to the prominence related to p^3 and the developing P^3 tooth. At about 3½ years of age, all three maxillary prominences are in line with the supraorbital foramen. See Fig. 1.55 and compare the positions of p^2 and p^3 and the infraorbital foramen in the foal with those shown for P^2, P^3 and the infraorbital foramen in the adult horse (Fig. 1.44). None of these mandibular or maxillary bony prominences are seen in the horse at 6 years of age (Fig. 1.44).

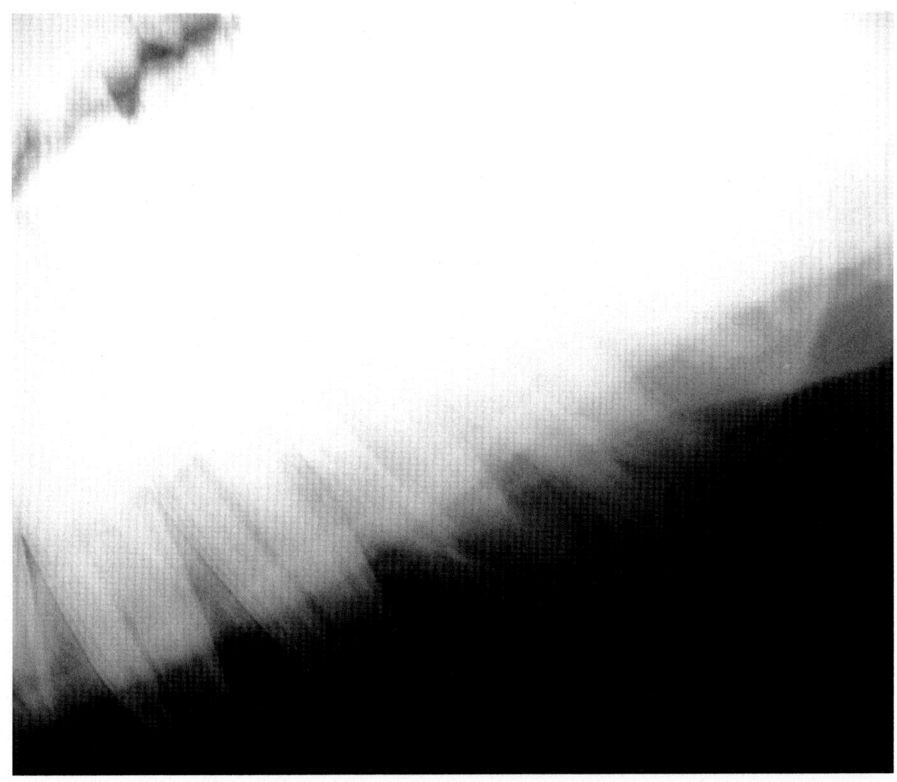

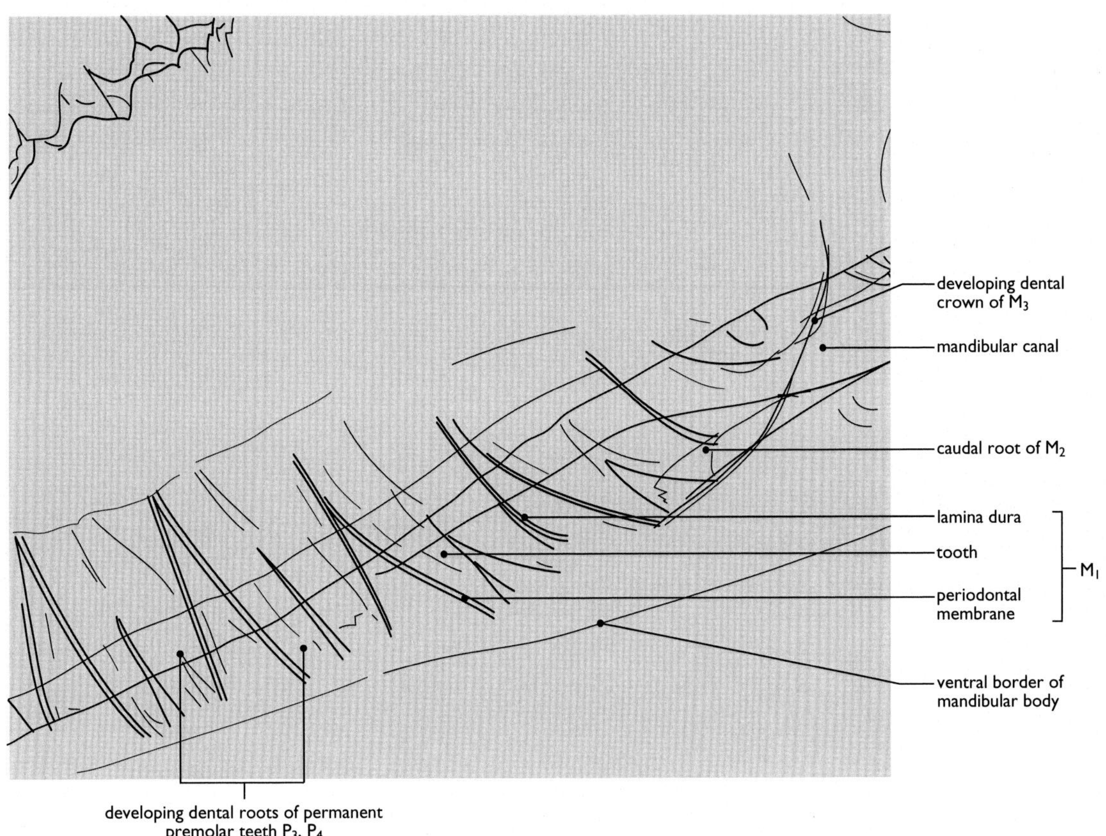
developing dental crown of M_3
mandibular canal
caudal root of M_2
lamina dura
tooth
periodontal membrane
M_1
ventral border of mandibular body
developing dental roots of permanent premolar teeth P_3, P_4

Fig. 9.4 Radiograph of the mandible of an older horse: lateral view. The third molar tooth erupts at c. 3.5–4 y. M_1 and M_2 erupt at c. 9–12 m and 2 y respectively.

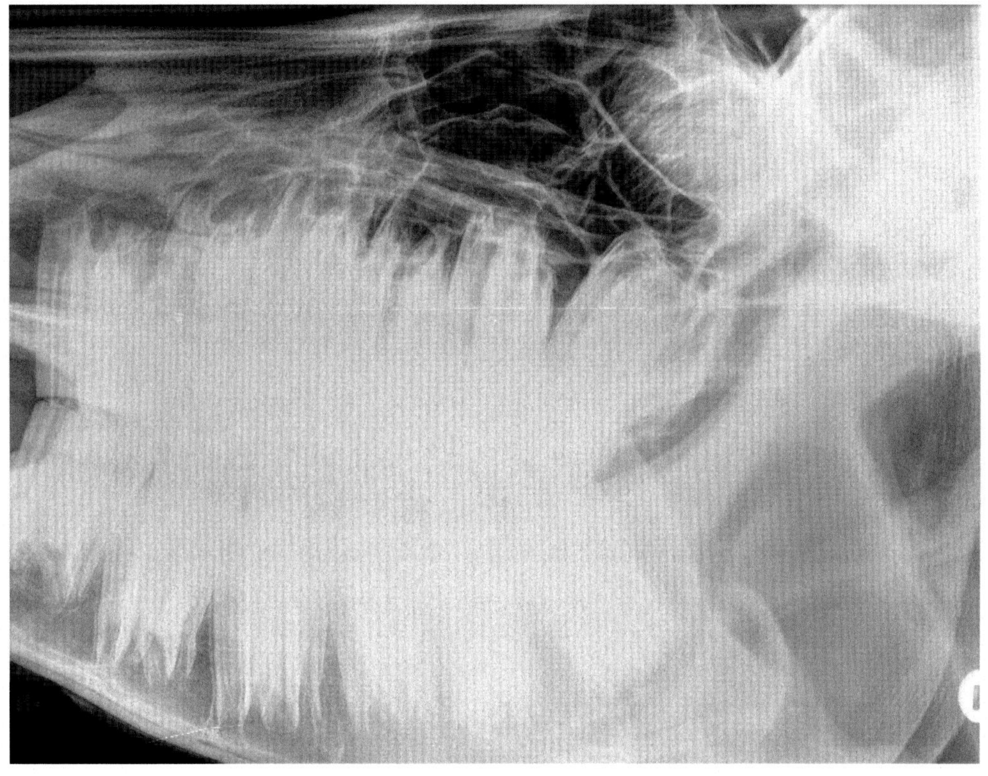

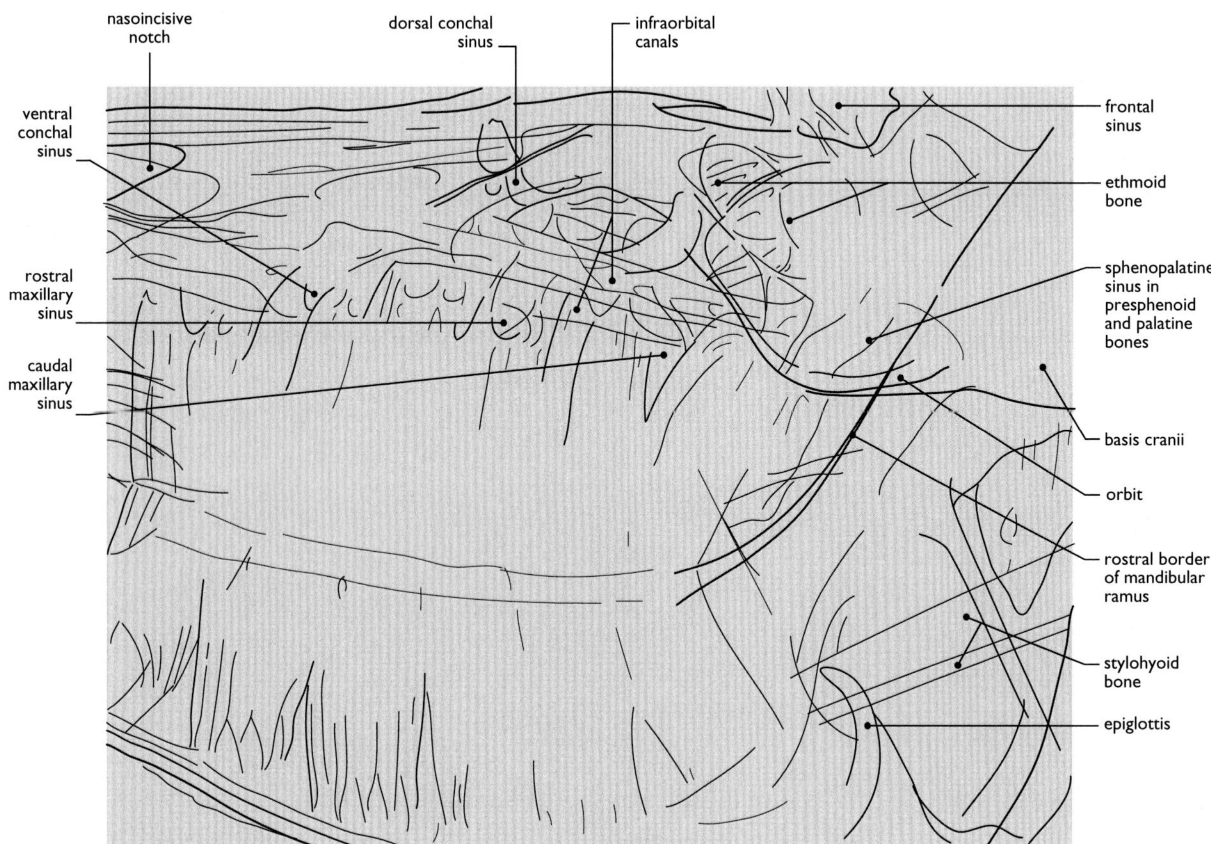
nasoincisive notch
dorsal conchal sinus
infraorbital canals
ventral conchal sinus
frontal sinus
ethmoid bone
rostral maxillary sinus
sphenopalatine sinus in presphenoid and palatine bones
caudal maxillary sinus
basis cranii
orbit
rostral border of mandibular ramus
stylohyoid bone
epiglottis

Fig. 9.5 Radiograph of the cheek teeth and nasal region: lateral view.

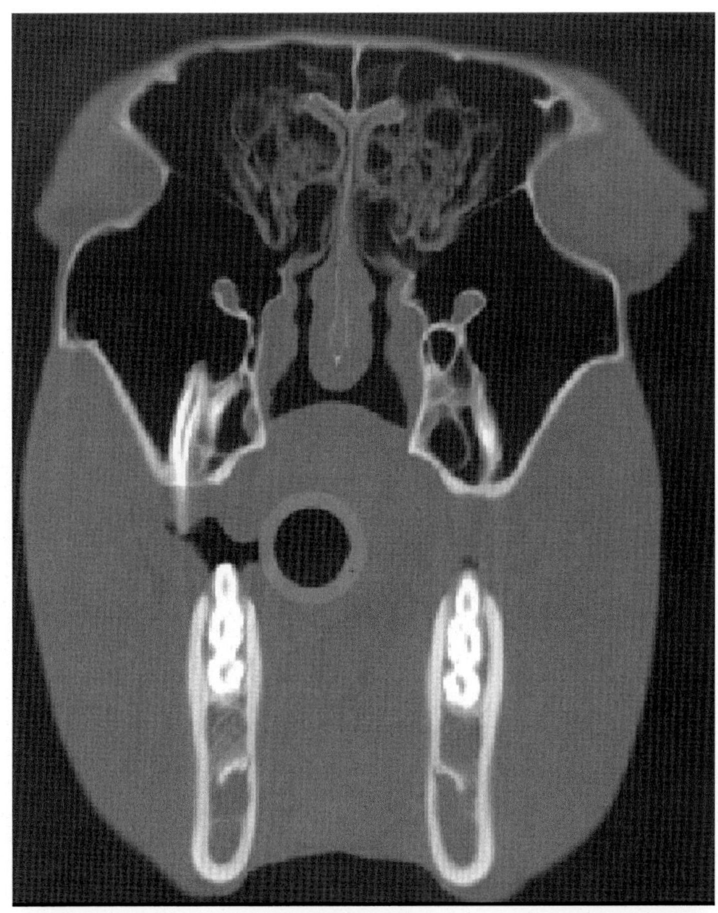

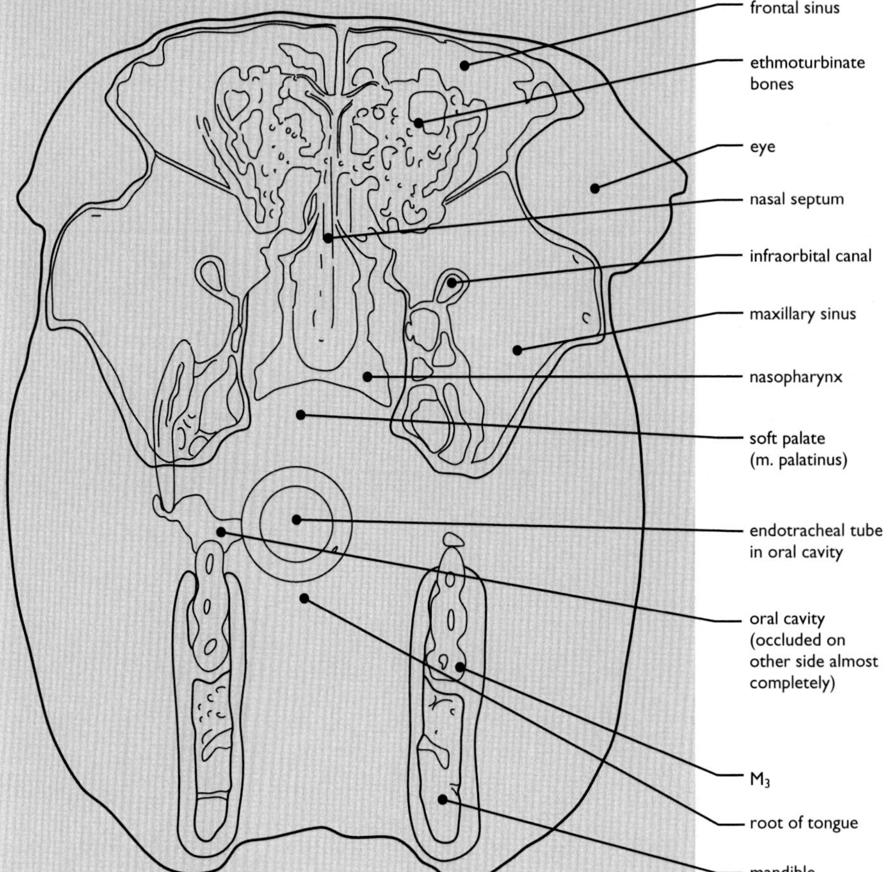
frontal sinus
ethmoturbinate bones
eye
nasal septum
infraorbital canal
maxillary sinus
nasopharynx
soft palate (m. palatinus)
endotracheal tube in oral cavity
oral cavity (occluded on other side almost completely)
M_3
root of tongue
mandible

Fig. 9.6 Computed tomography image of the head: transverse plane through the eyes. On the left side, the oral cavity has been almost obliterated by the buccal and lingual soft tissues. The third molar tooth shows as three parts because of its oblique orientation in the mandible (see Fig. 1.44). The most ventral part of the mandible forms the mandibular canal: this contains the inferior alveolar artery, vein and nerve, which supply the dental alveoli of the mandibular teeth. At the rostral termination of the canal, the mental foramen (Figs. 1.44, 1.12), the mental nerve gives off branches which supply the lower lip (labium) and chin (mentum). The nerve continues as a number of fine dental branches which run within the bone of the incisive part of the mandible to supply the canine and incisor teeth.

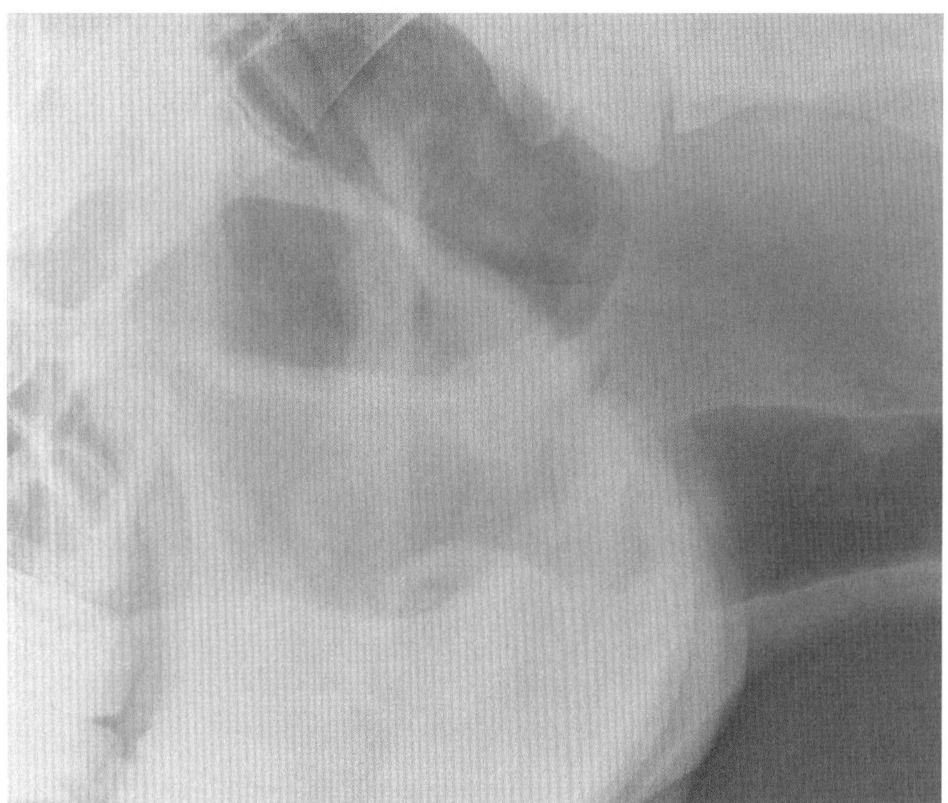

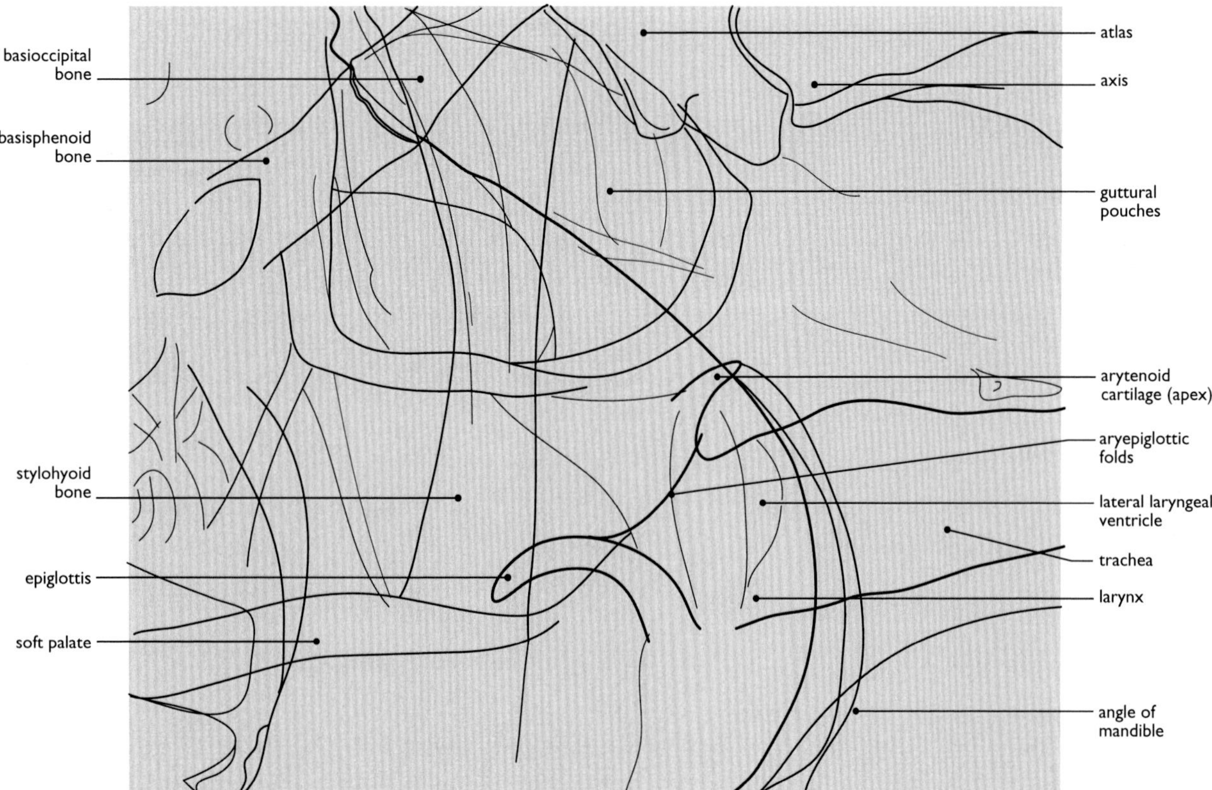
basioccipital bone
basisphenoid bone
stylohyoid bone
epiglottis
soft palate
atlas
axis
guttural pouches
arytenoid cartilage (apex)
aryepiglottic folds
lateral laryngeal ventricle
trachea
larynx
angle of mandible

Fig. 9.7 Radiograph of the laryngeal region: lateral view. The joint between the basisphenoid and basioccipital bones (basis cranii) is cartilaginous.

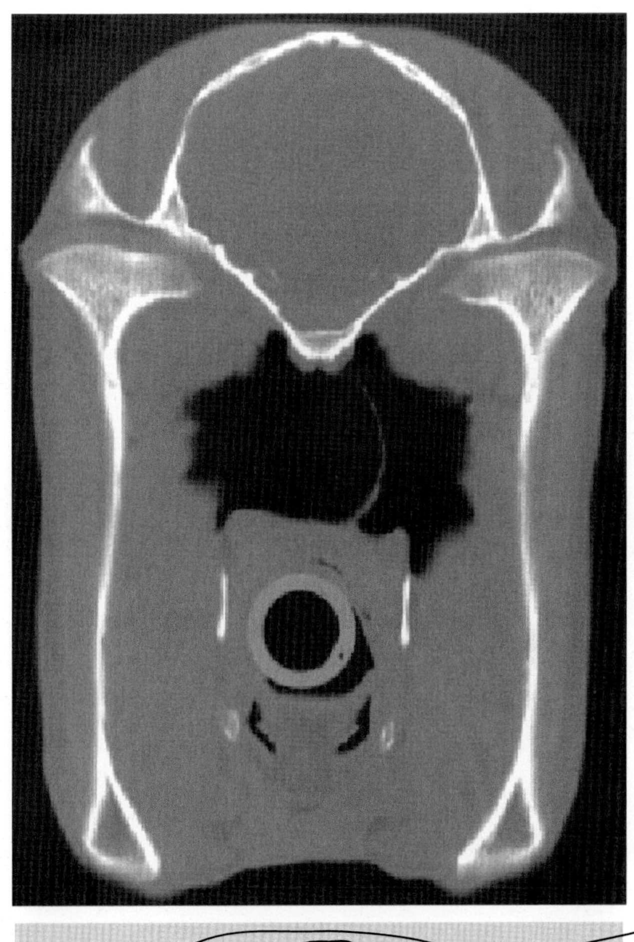

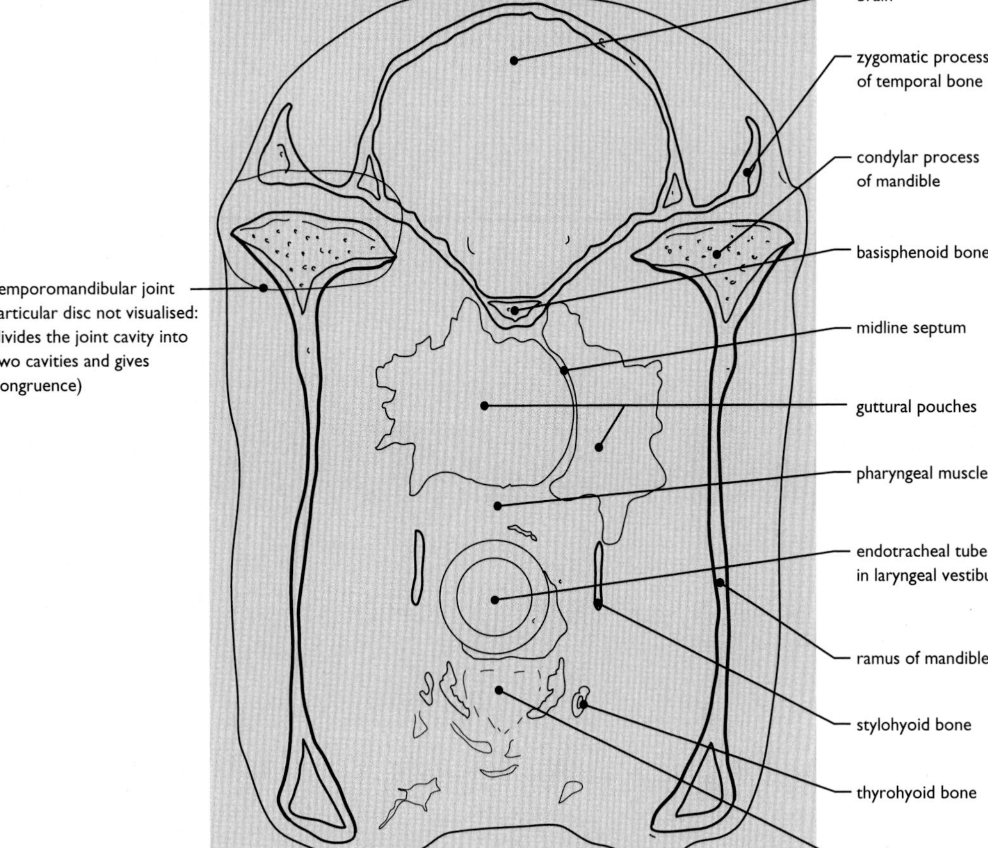
brain
zygomatic process of temporal bone
condylar process of mandible
basisphenoid bone
midline septum
guttural pouches
pharyngeal muscles
endotracheal tube in laryngeal vestibule
ramus of mandible
stylohyoid bone
thyrohyoid bone
epiglottis
temporomandibular joint (articular disc not visualised: divides the joint cavity into two cavities and gives congruence)

Fig. 9.8 Computed tomography image of the head: transverse plane through the temporomandibular joints. The guttural pouches lie between the basis cranii, the medial pterygoid muscles of the mandible, and the muscular wall of the pharynx. The temporomandibular joint has a hinge-like movement in which the articular disc participates. For mastication of coarse fibrous food, the mandibular cheek teeth are drawn transversely across the maxillary cheek teeth and this is accomplished by a rotatory action of the condyles in which one articular disc moves rostrally and the other moves caudally. It is thought that the medial pterygoid muscles (Fig. 1.15), acting singly, produce this important grinding action.

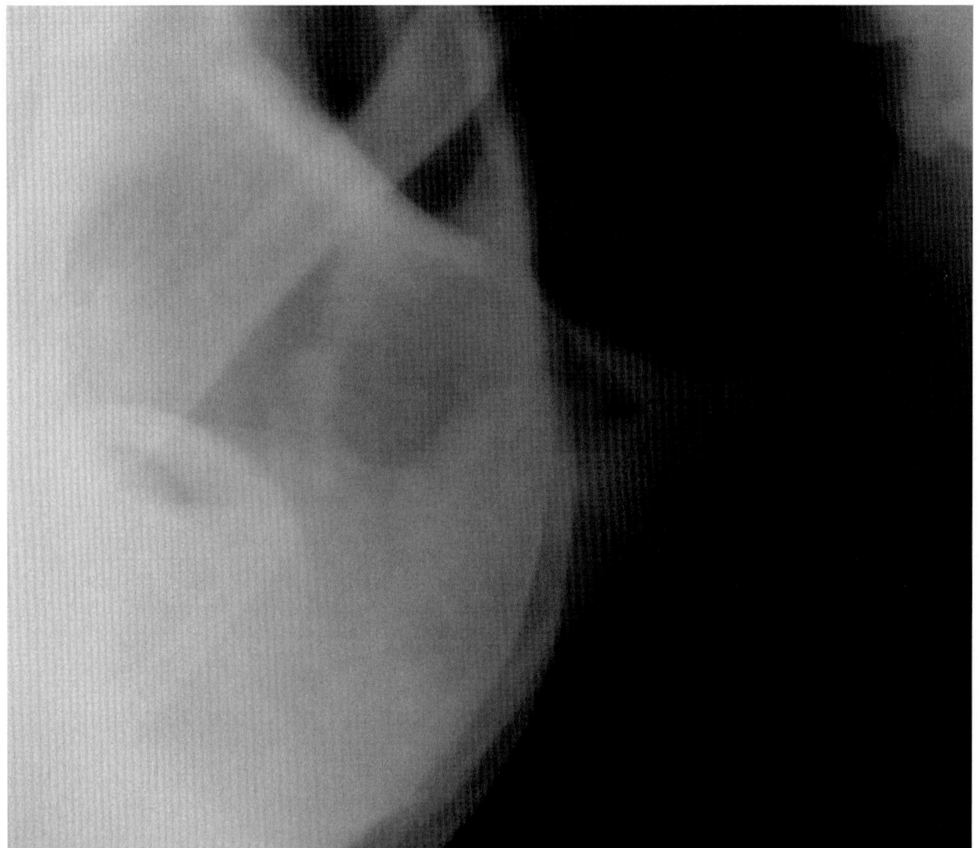

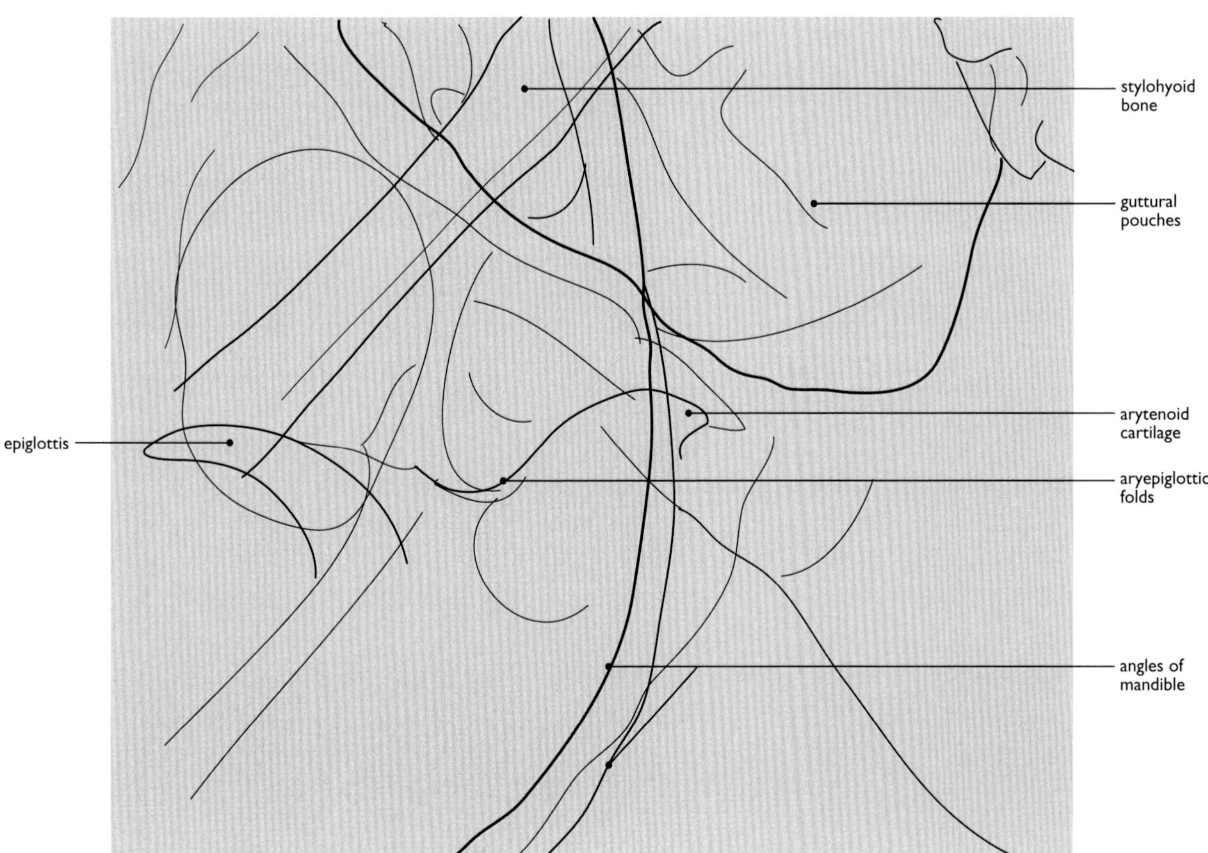
stylohyoid bone
guttural pouches
epiglottis
arytenoid cartilage
aryepiglottic folds
angles of mandible

Fig. 9.9 Radiograph of the laryngeal region: lateral view. The position of the larynx is well demarcated by the epiglottis, arytenoid cartilages, and the aryepiglottic folds.

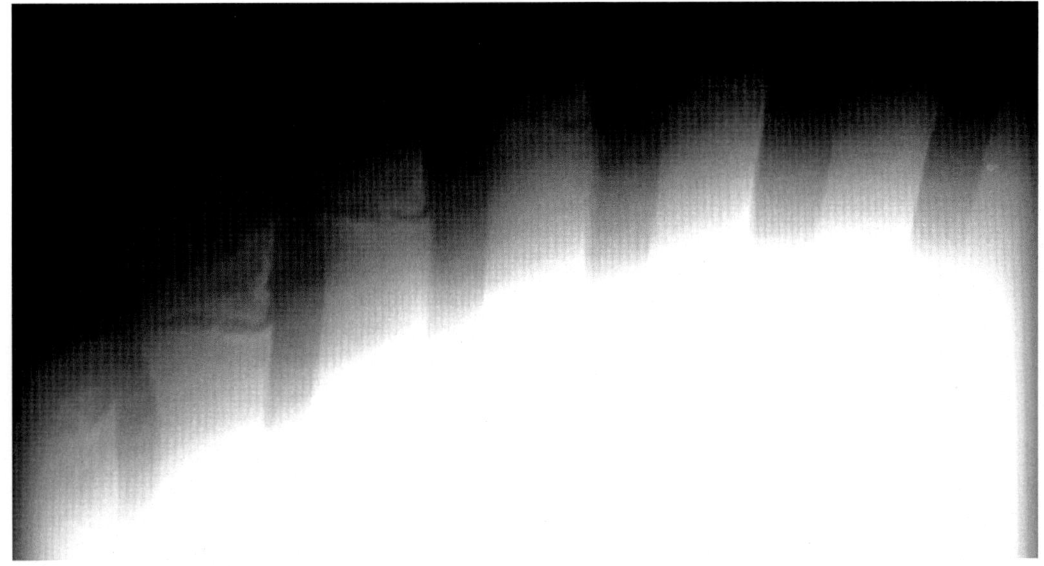

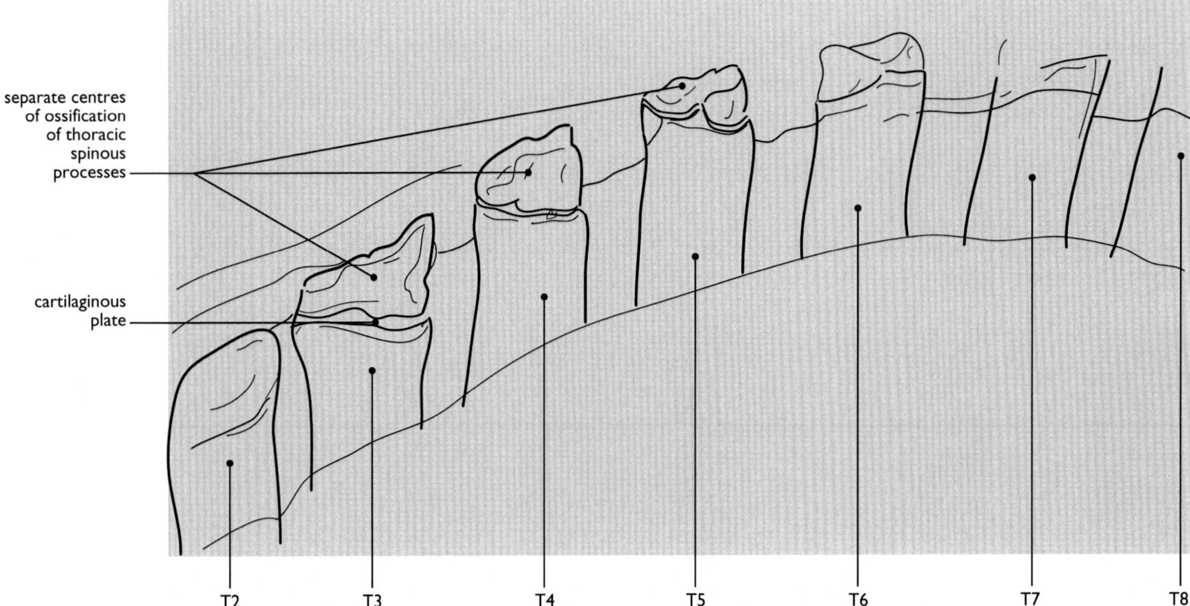
separate centres of ossification of thoracic spinous processes
cartilaginous plate
T2
T3
T4
T5
T6
T7
T8

Fig. 9.10 Radiograph of the summits of the spinous processes of thoracic vertebrae T2–T8: lateral view. Osteometry shows that the dorsal spinous processes of the fourth and fifth vertebrae, T4, T5, are the longest in the series. Radiography, however, shows that in the adult horse, during level standing, the highest point of the withers is usually formed by the spinous process of T6 or T7 (Butler et al 2008). The ends of the spinous processes of T2–T6 (T7, T8) show centres of ossification in yearlings. The cartilage is gradually replaced by bone until, by 10 y, the thin cartilaginous plates which join the ossified ends to the spinal processes begin to disappear. The cartilages at the dorsal tips persist for a much longer time (Ellenberger & Baum, 1943). The more ventral details in this radiograph are lost, due to superimposition of the scapulae, their cartilages, and the appendicular and axial muscles (Figs 3.2, 3.7 and 4.15).

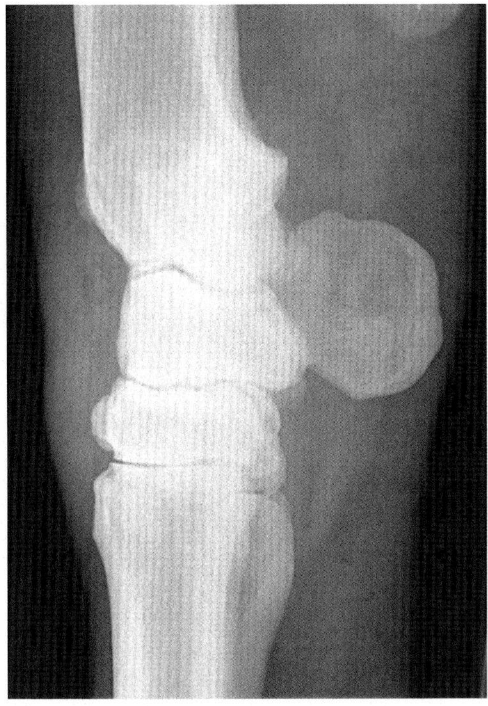

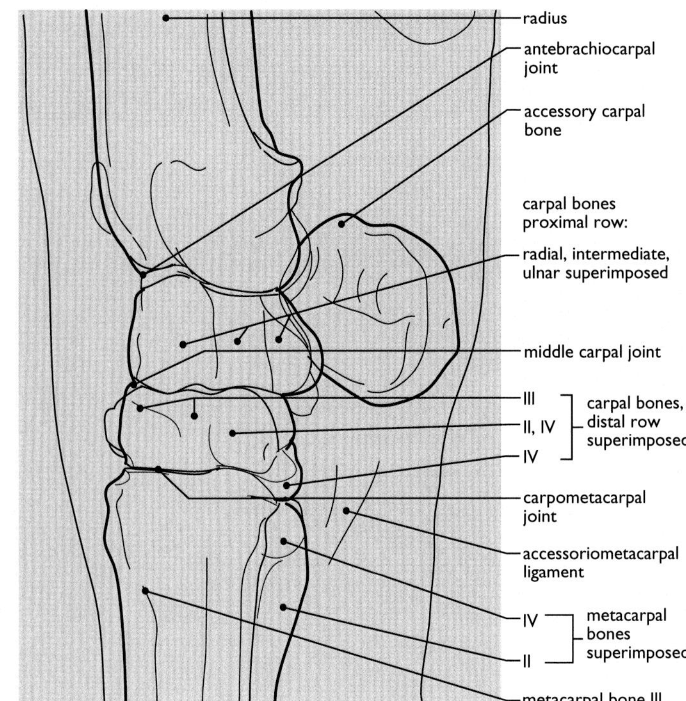
radius
antebrachiocarpal joint
accessory carpal bone
carpal bones proximal row:
radial, intermediate, ulnar superimposed
middle carpal joint
III
II, IV
IV
carpal bones, distal row superimposed
carpometacarpal joint
accessoriometacarpal ligament
IV
II
metacarpal bones superimposed
metacarpal bone III

Fig. 9.11 Radiograph of the carpus: lateral view. The accessory carpal bone can be assessed on this view. For the accessoriometacarpal ligament, see Fig. 3.38.

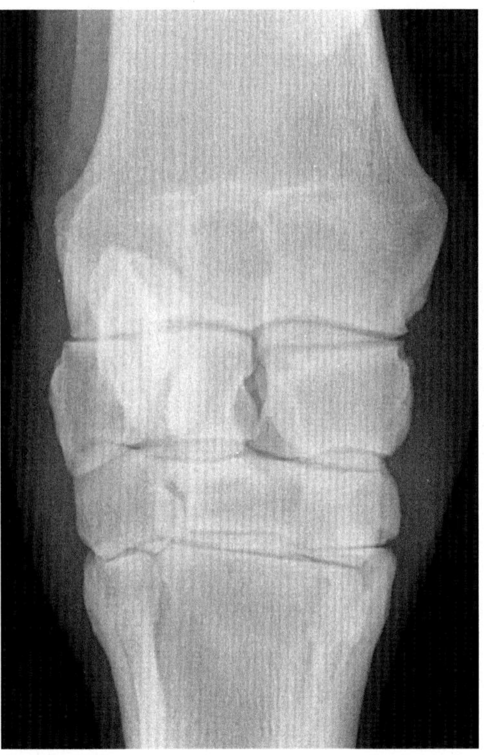

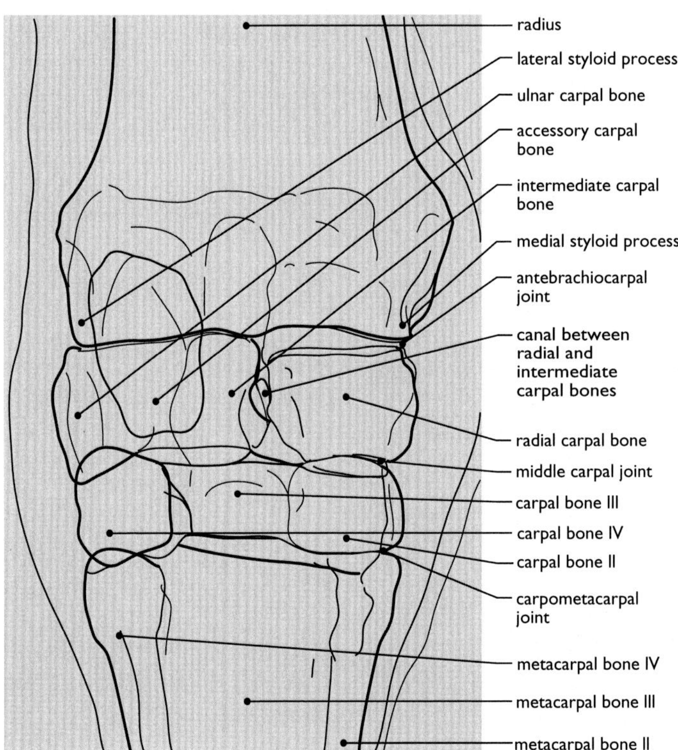
radius
lateral styloid process
ulnar carpal bone
accessory carpal bone
intermediate carpal bone
medial styloid process
antebrachiocarpal joint
canal between radial and intermediate carpal bones
radial carpal bone
middle carpal joint
carpal bone III
carpal bone IV
carpal bone II
carpometacarpal joint
metacarpal bone IV
metacarpal bone III
metacarpal bone II

Fig. 9.12 Radiograph of the carpus: DorsoPalmar (DP) view. The lateral styloid process of the ulna usually fuses with the radius during the first year of life.

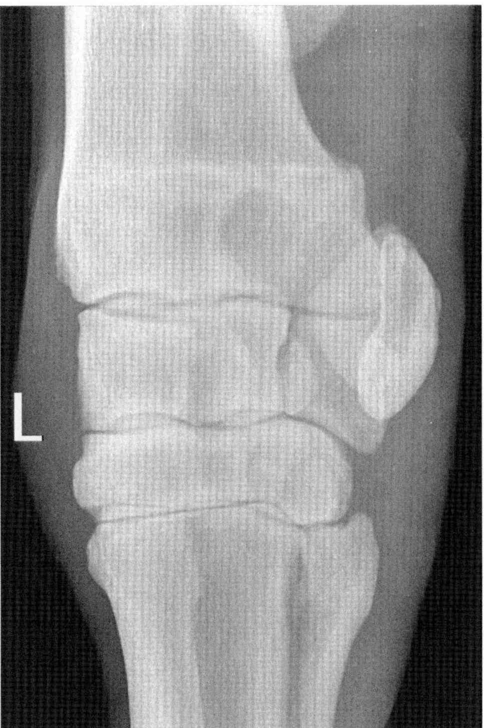

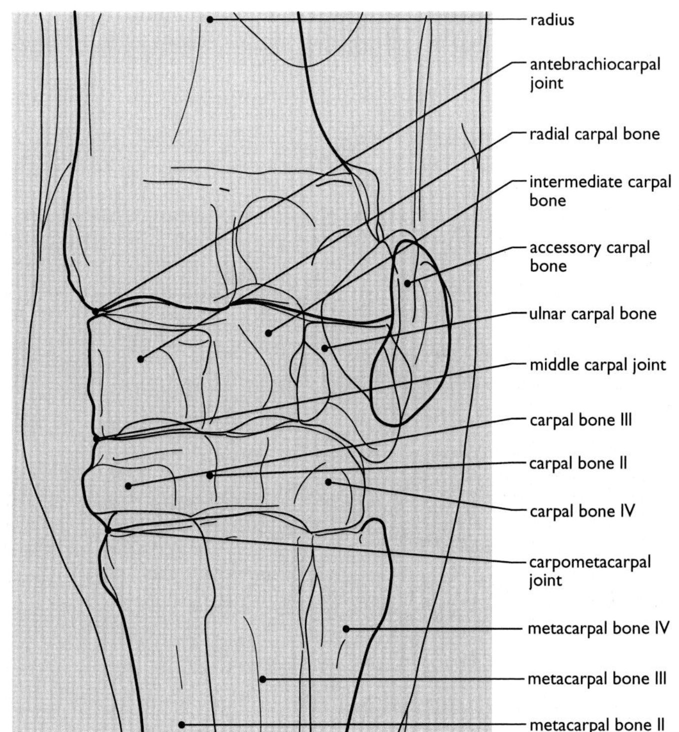

radius
antebrachiocarpal joint
radial carpal bone
intermediate carpal bone
accessory carpal bone
ulnar carpal bone
middle carpal joint
carpal bone III
carpal bone II
carpal bone IV
carpometacarpal joint
metacarpal bone IV
metacarpal bone III
metacarpal bone II

Fig. 9.13 Radiograph of the carpus: DorsoLatero-PalmaroMedial Oblique (DLPMO) view. The radial facet of carpal bone III, and the 4th carpal and metacarpal bones, can be assessed.

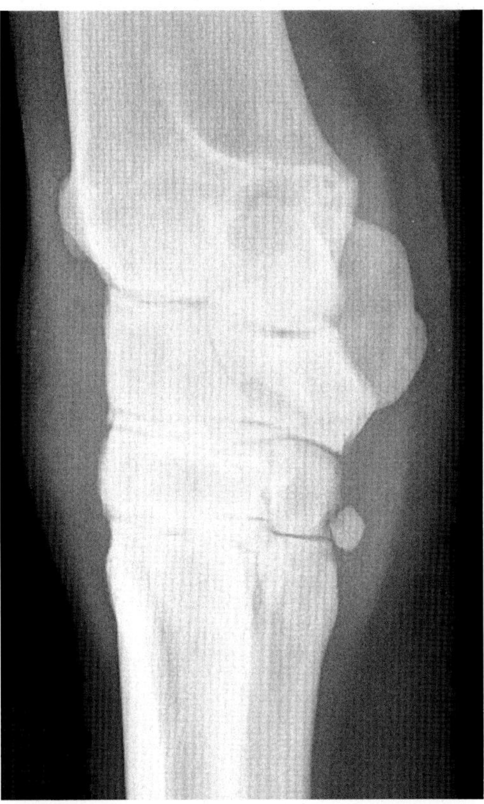

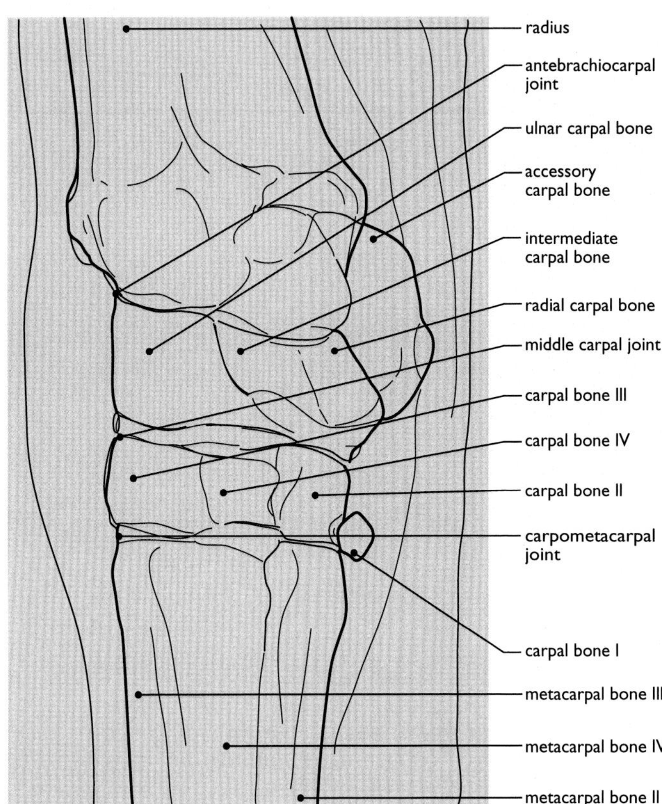

radius
antebrachiocarpal joint
ulnar carpal bone
accessory carpal bone
intermediate carpal bone
radial carpal bone
middle carpal joint
carpal bone III
carpal bone IV
carpal bone II
carpometacarpal joint
carpal bone I
metacarpal bone III
metacarpal bone IV
metacarpal bone II

Fig. 9.14 Radiograph of the carpus: DorsoMedio-PalmaroLateral Oblique (DMPLO) view. Carpal bone 1, embedded in the medial collateral ligament of the carpus (Fig. 3.13), is inconstant and sometimes unilateral.

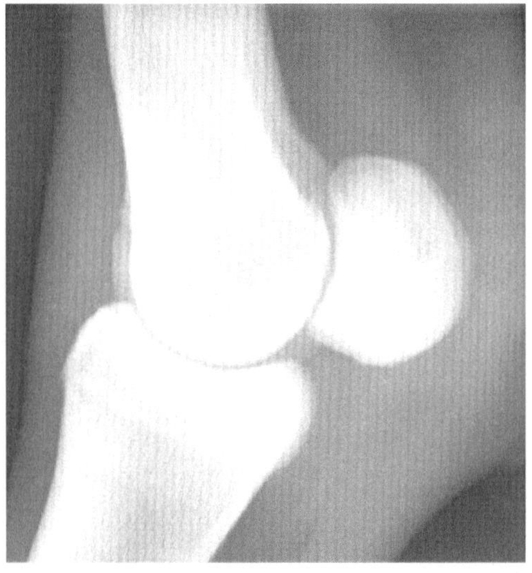

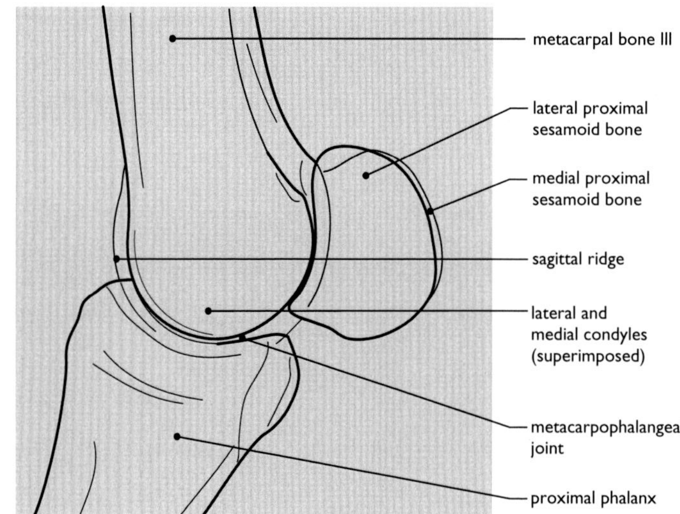
metacarpal bone III
lateral proximal sesamoid bone
medial proximal sesamoid bone
sagittal ridge
lateral and medial condyles (superimposed)
metacarpophalangeal joint
proximal phalanx

Fig. 9.15 Radiograph of the fetlock: lateral view.

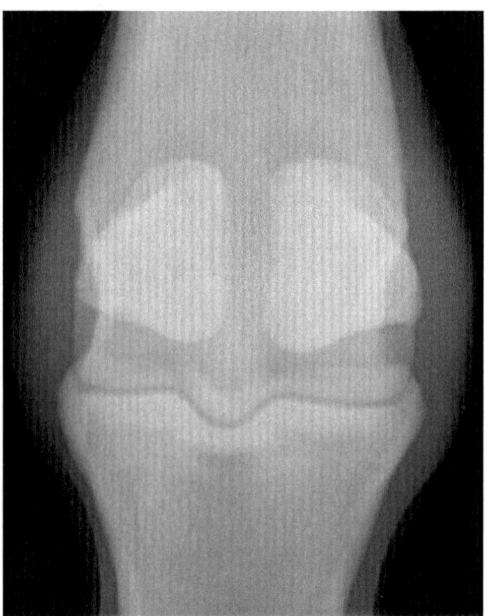

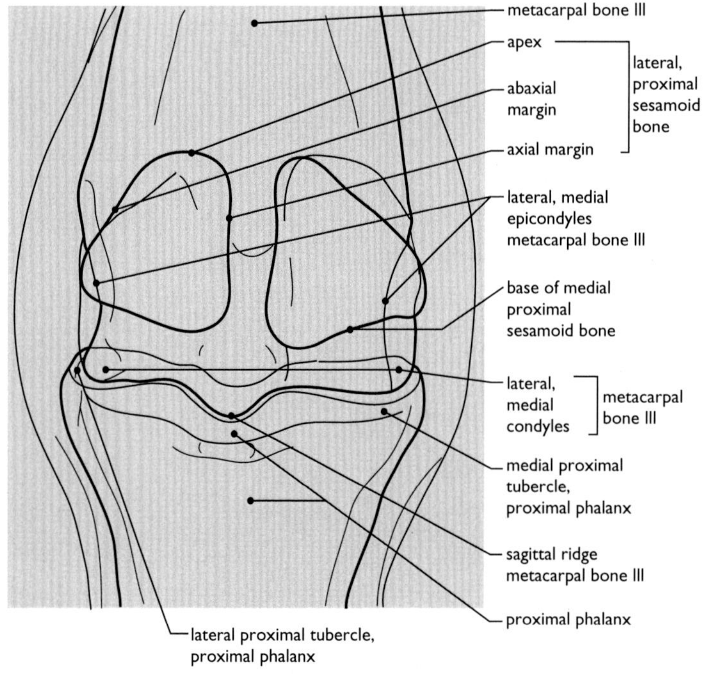
metacarpal bone III
apex
abaxial margin
axial margin
lateral, proximal sesamoid bone
lateral, medial epicondyles metacarpal bone III
base of medial proximal sesamoid bone
lateral, medial condyles
metacarpal bone III
medial proximal tubercle, proximal phalanx
sagittal ridge metacarpal bone III
proximal phalanx
lateral proximal tubercle, proximal phalanx

Fig 9.16 Radiograph of the fetlock : DorsoPalmar (DP) view.

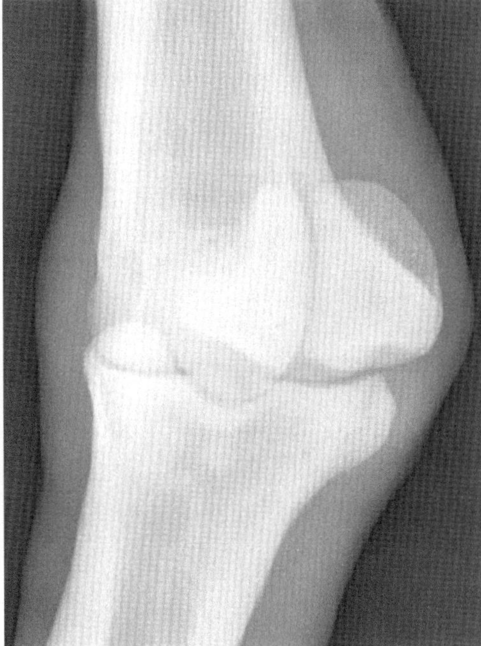

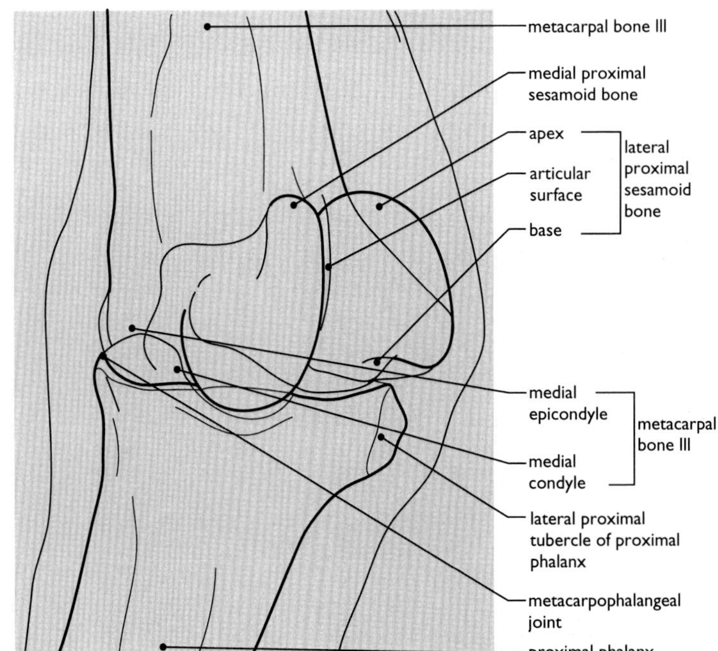
metacarpal bone III
medial proximal sesamoid bone
apex
articular surface
base
lateral proximal sesamoid bone
medial epicondyle
medial condyle
metacarpal bone III
lateral proximal tubercle of proximal phalanx
metacarpophalangeal joint
proximal phalanx

Fig. 9.17 Radiograph of the fetlock: DorsoLatero-PalmaroMedial Oblique (DLPMO) view. The lateral proximal sesamoid bone is highlighted.

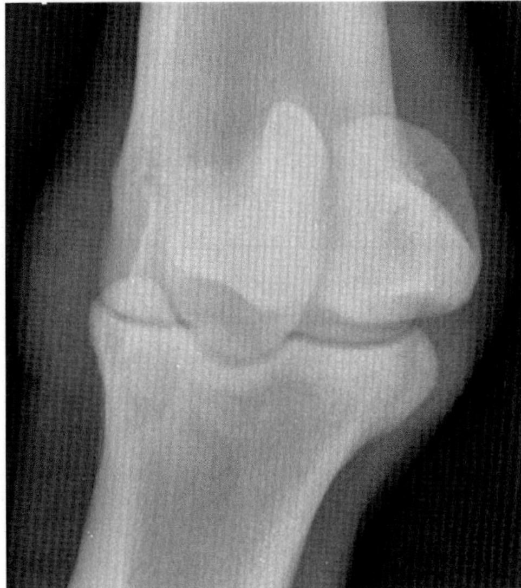

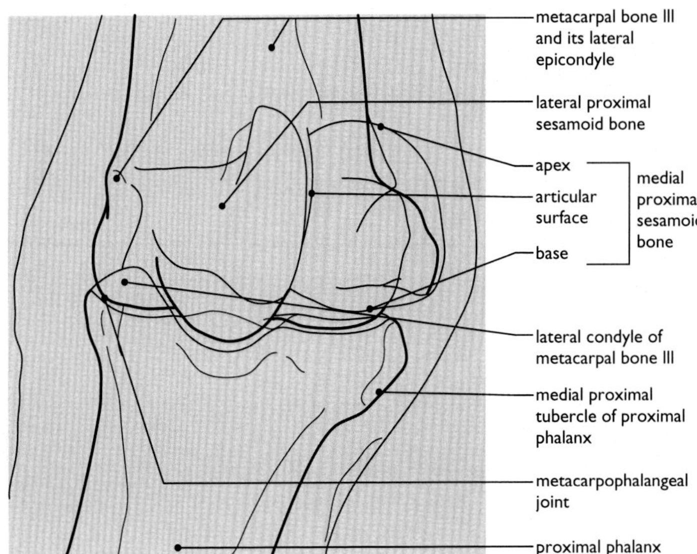
metacarpal bone III and its lateral epicondyle
lateral proximal sesamoid bone
apex
articular surface
base
medial proximal sesamoid bone
lateral condyle of metacarpal bone III
medial proximal tubercle of proximal phalanx
metacarpophalangeal joint
proximal phalanx

Fig. 9.18 Radiograph of the fetlock: DorsoMedio-PalmaroLateral Oblique (DMPLO) view. The medial proximal sesamoid bone is highlighted.

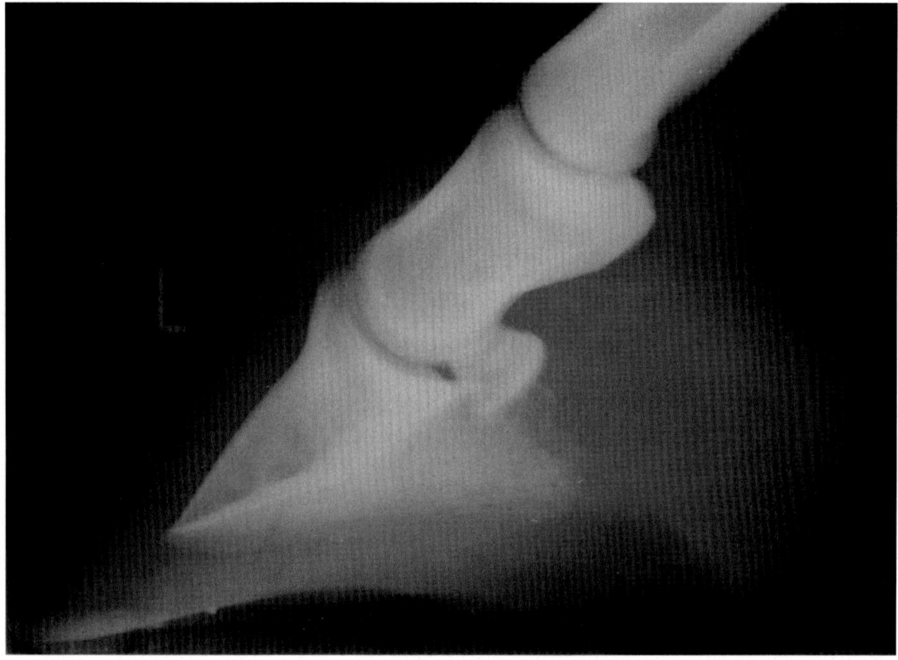

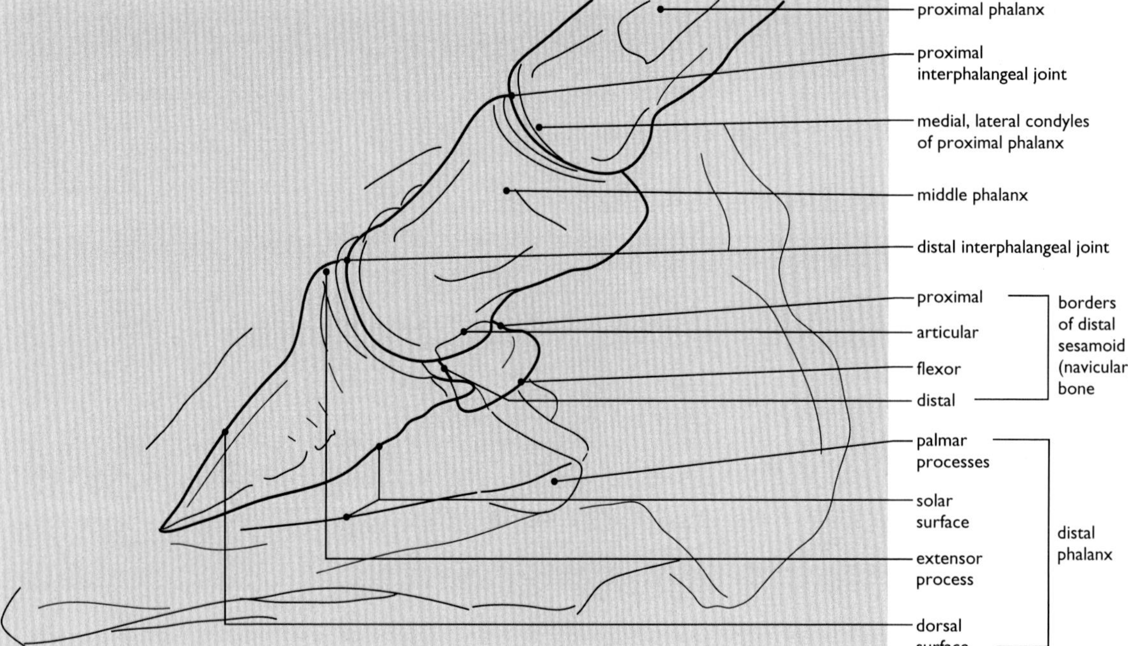
proximal phalanx
proximal interphalangeal joint
medial, lateral condyles of proximal phalanx
middle phalanx
distal interphalangeal joint
proximal
articular
flexor
distal
borders of distal sesamoid (navicular) bone
palmar processes
solar surface
extensor process
dorsal surface
distal phalanx

Fig. 9.19 **Radiograph of the digit and hoof: lateral view.**

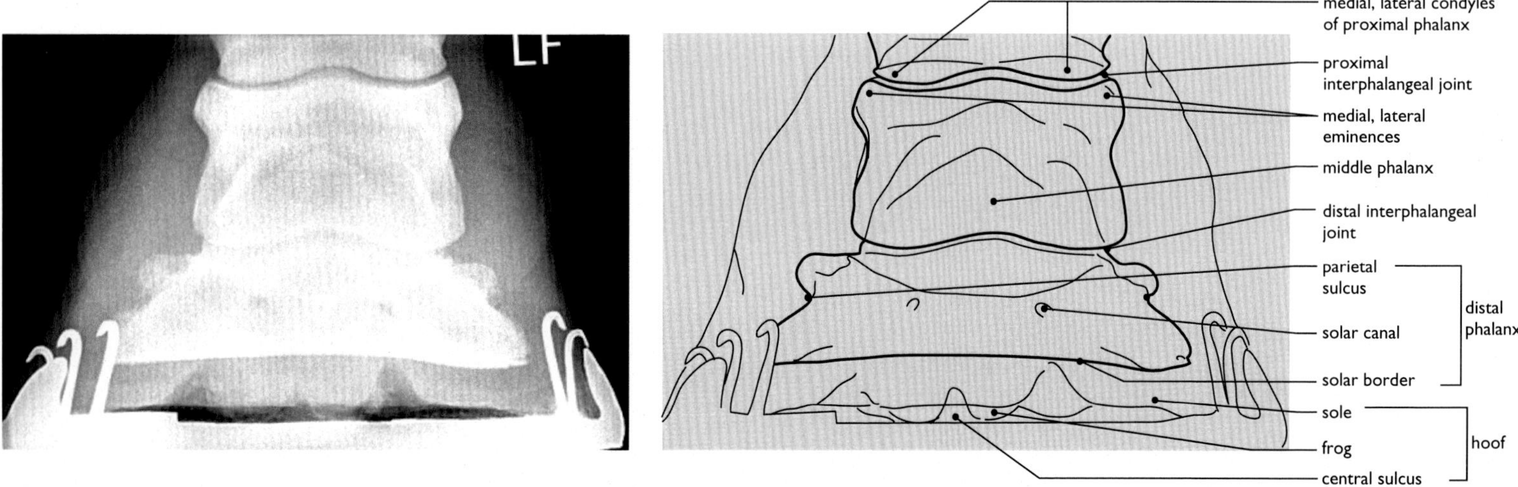
LF
medial, lateral condyles of proximal phalanx
proximal interphalangeal joint
medial, lateral eminences
middle phalanx
distal interphalangeal joint
parietal sulcus
solar canal
solar border
distal phalanx
sole
frog
central sulcus
hoof

Fig. 9.20 Radiograph of the digit and hoof: standing DorsoPalmar (DP) view. Mediolateral foot balance can be assessed on this view.

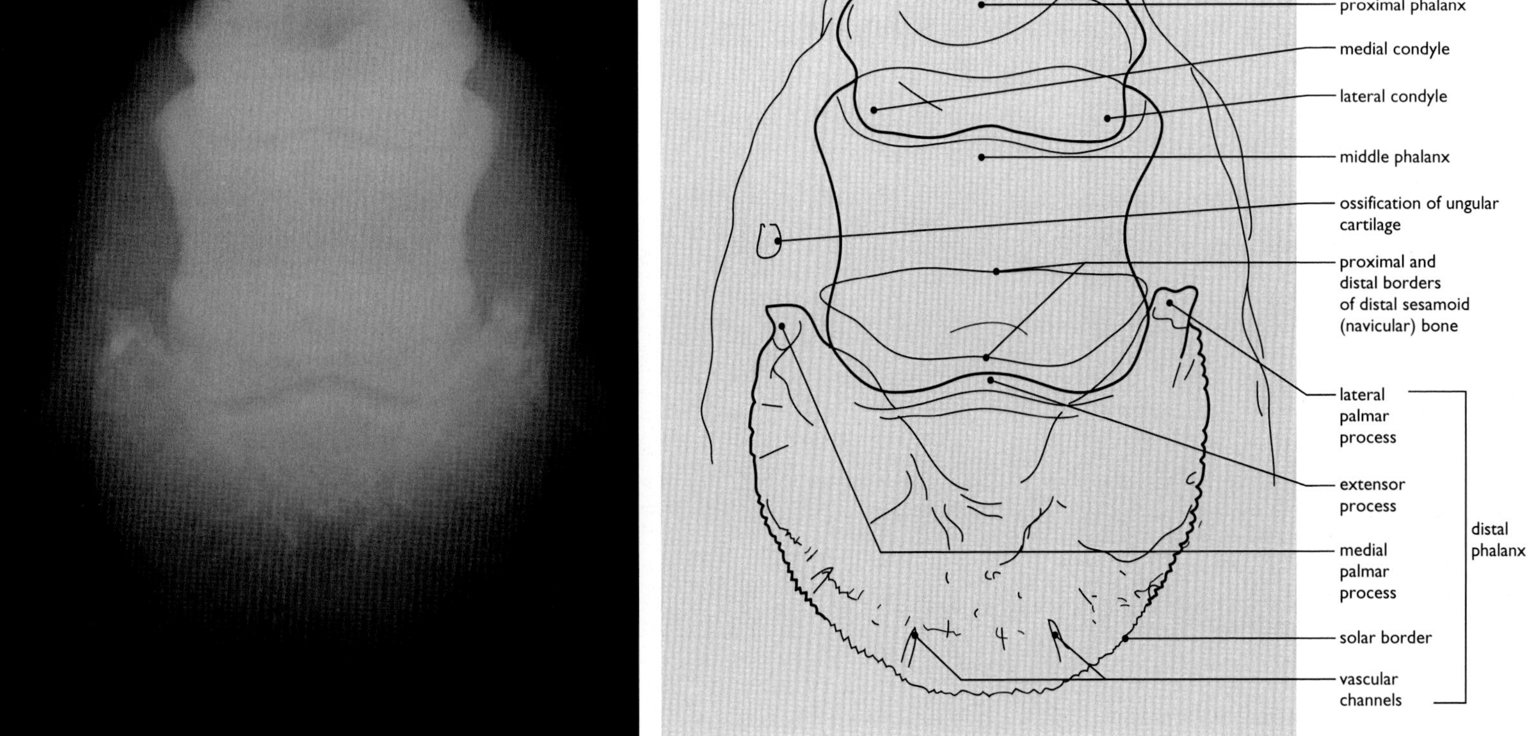
proximal phalanx
medial condyle
lateral condyle
middle phalanx
ossification of ungular cartilage
proximal and distal borders of distal sesamoid (navicular) bone
lateral palmar process
extensor process
medial palmar process
solar border
vascular channels
distal phalanx

Fig. 9.21 Radiograph of the digit: DorsoProximo-PalmaroDistal Oblique (DPrPDiO) view. Some ossification of the ungular cartilages is present. The distal sesamoid (navicular) bone is superimposed on the middle phalanx.

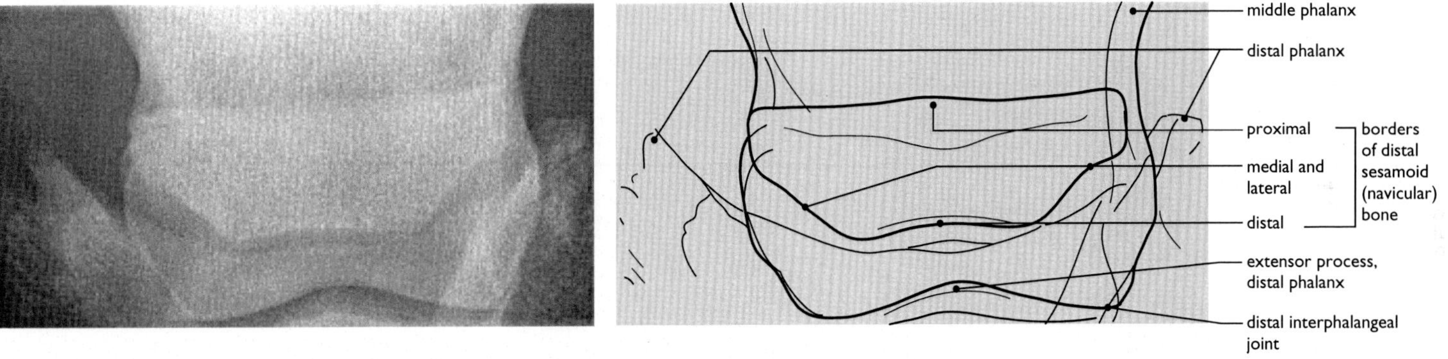
middle phalanx
distal phalanx
proximal
medial and lateral
distal
borders of distal sesamoid (navicular) bone
extensor process, distal phalanx
distal interphalangeal joint

Fig. 9.22 Radiograph of the digit: DorsoProximo-PalmaroDistal Oblique (DPrPDiO) view. This view shows the four borders of the distal sesamoid (navicular) bone.

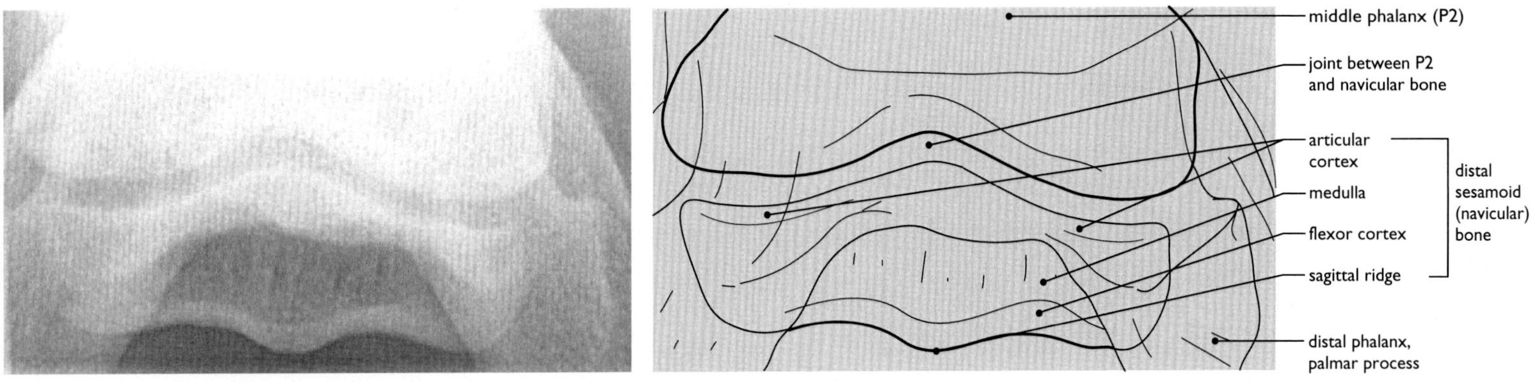
middle phalanx (P2)
joint between P2 and navicular bone
articular cortex
medulla
flexor cortex
sagittal ridge
distal sesamoid (navicular) bone
distal phalanx, palmar process

Fig. 9.23 Radiograph of the digit: PalmaroProximo-PalmaroDistal Oblique (PPrPDiO) view. Corticomedullary definition in the distal sesamoid (navicular) bone can be assessed.

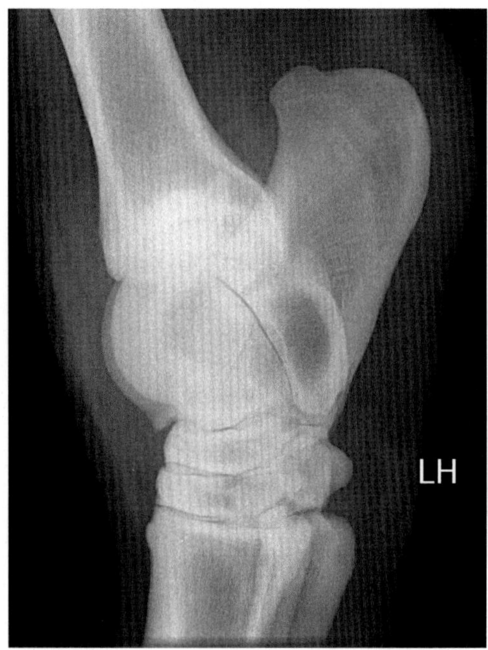

LH

tibia
calcaneal tuberosity
tarsocrural joint
calcaneus
medial
lateral
trochlear ridges of talus
talus
sustentaculum tali (calcaneus)
proximal intertarsal joint
central tarsal bone
centrodistal joint
tarsal bone IV
tarsal bones III, I and II
distal row
tarsometatarsal joint
metatarsal bone IV
metatarsal bone II
metatarsal bone III

Fig 9.24 Radiograph of the hock: lateral view.

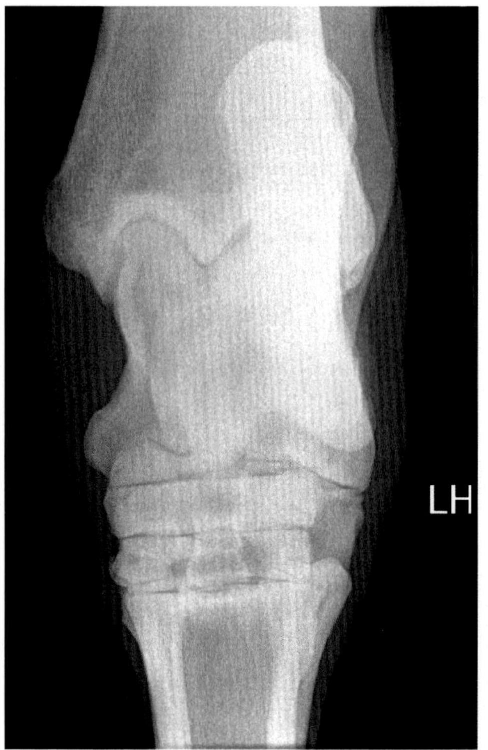

LH

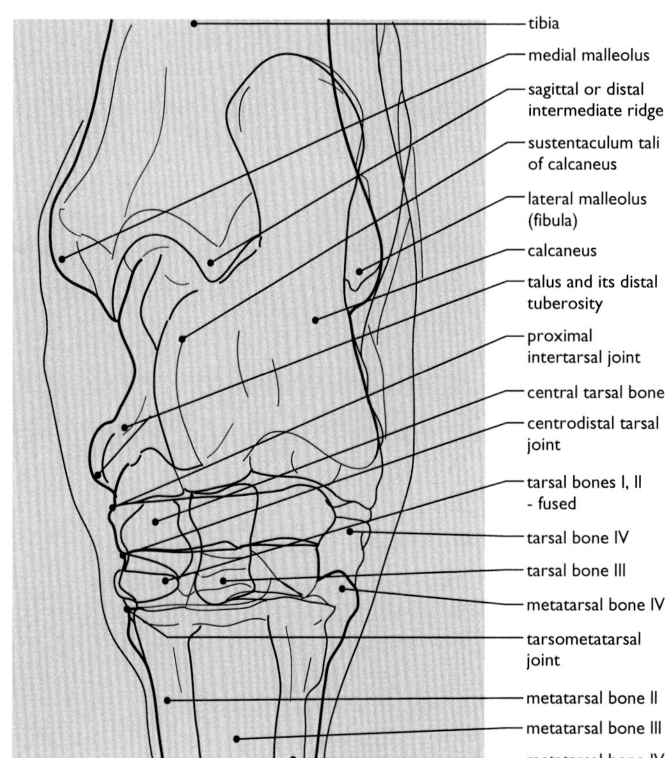

tibia
medial malleolus
sagittal or distal intermediate ridge
sustentaculum tali of calcaneus
lateral malleolus (fibula)
calcaneus
talus and its distal tuberosity
proximal intertarsal joint
central tarsal bone
centrodistal tarsal joint
tarsal bones I, II - fused
tarsal bone IV
tarsal bone III
metatarsal bone IV
tarsometatarsal joint
metatarsal bone II
metatarsal bone III
metatarsal bone IV

Fig. 9.25 Radiograph of the hock: DorsoPlantar (DP) view. The distal epiphysis of the fibula fuses with the tibia during the first year of life.

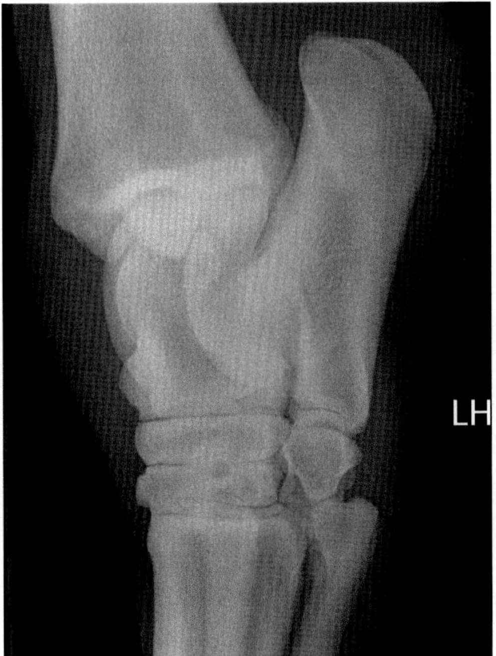

LH

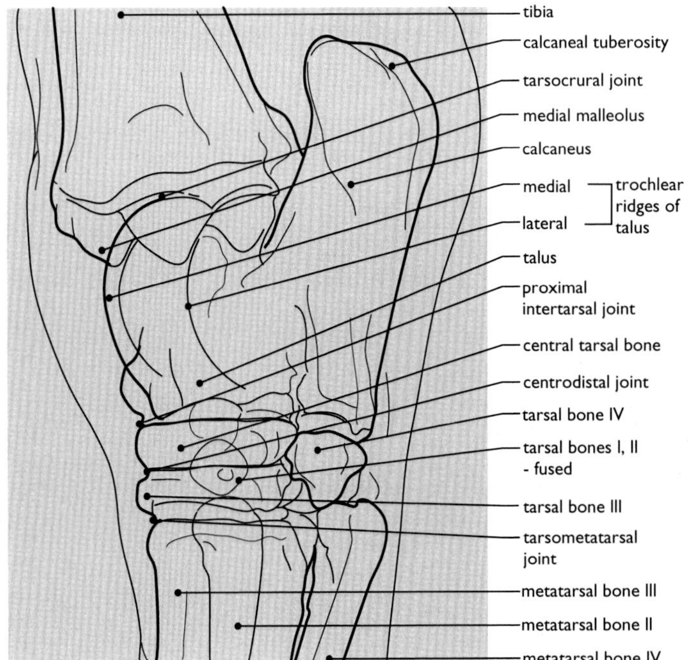

tibia
calcaneal tuberosity
tarsocrural joint
medial malleolus
calcaneus
medial
lateral
trochlear ridges of talus
talus
proximal intertarsal joint
central tarsal bone
centrodistal joint
tarsal bone IV
tarsal bones I, II - fused
tarsal bone III
tarsometatarsal joint
metatarsal bone III
metatarsal bone II
metatarsal bone IV

Fig. 9.26 Radiograph of the hock: DorsoLatero-PlantaroMedial Oblique (DLPMO) view. The calcaneal tuberosity can be assessed. (It should be completely fused to the calcaneus by 3y.)

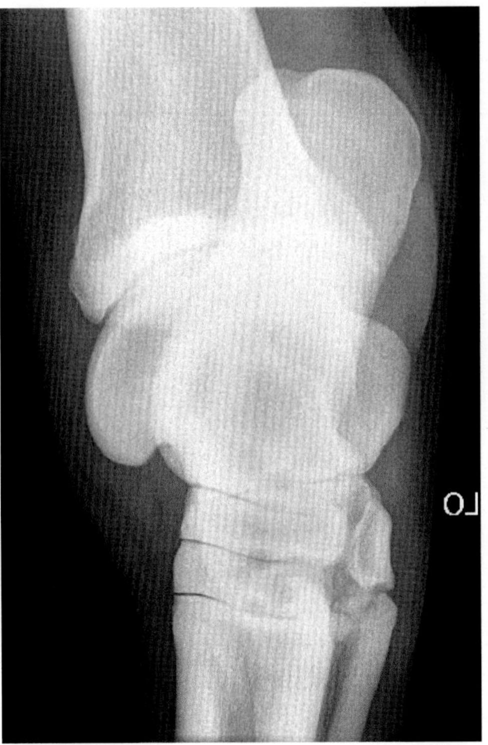

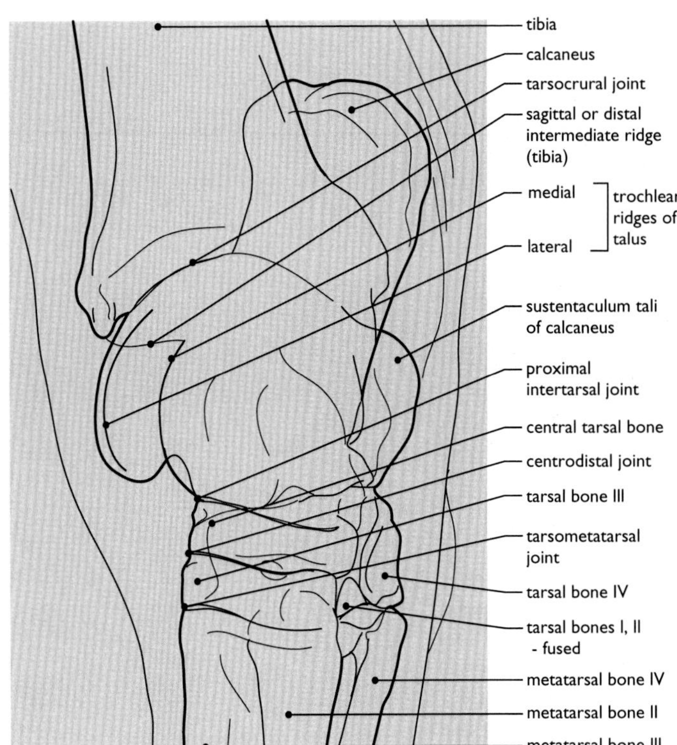

tibia
calcaneus
tarsocrural joint
sagittal or distal intermediate ridge (tibia)
medial
lateral
trochlear ridges of talus
sustentaculum tali of calcaneus
proximal intertarsal joint
central tarsal bone
centrodistal joint
tarsal bone III
tarsometatarsal joint
tarsal bone IV
tarsal bones I, II - fused
metatarsal bone IV
metatarsal bone II
metatarsal bone III

Fig. 9.27 Radiograph of the hock: DorsoMedio-PlantaroLateral Oblique (DMPLO) view. The lateral trochlear ridge of the talus can be assessed.

INDEX

References in this index are to page numbers, not to figures. The index lists the pages on which each structure has been labelled in the drawings that accompany the photographs.

In general. the names chosen for the labels to the drawings conform to the Anatomica Veterinaria (1983); the index lists these names as they appear in the labels.

Arteries, lymph nodes, muscles, nerves, veins and their trunks are indexed under the usual abbreviations (a., ln., m., n., v., t.), as in the labels. For most other structures the anglicized names are used, but the classical name has been retained where it is much more familiar than the anglicized form (e.g.corpus luteum).

A

abdominal tunic, yellow, 114-119, 122, 148-151, 192, 196-198, 202, 218, 276, 277, 280, 284-286, 289, 290-291, 301, 304, 306
abdominal wall, 164, 166, 168
accessory femoral ligament, 205, 219, 222, 223, 278, 280, 283-287, 289, 304, 305
acetabulum, 205, 219, 269, 279, 283, 285, 303-305
adrenal gland, 165, 172, 174, 175
alar nasal cartilage, 9, 11, 34, 35, 45
  cornu, 45, 46
  lamina, 45, 46
aneurysm, of a. mesenterica cranialis, 165
annular cartilage, 15, 16
annular ligaments, digital,
  distal, 249-253
  palmar, 233, 234
  plantar, 249-253
  proximal, 249-253
ansa subclavia caudalis, 124, 127, 134
antebrachial fascia, 83, 85
antebrachium, 75, 228, 230
anus, 279-281, 306, 313-316
aorta,
  abdominalis, 162-165, 179, 220, 224, 274, 275, 310-312
  arcus aorticus, 122-132, 134-138
  thoracica, 126, 128, 135-138, 156-159, 161-163, 165-172
aortic hiatus, 145, 159, 165, 171, 174
aortic valve, 110, 128, 129, 139
arachnoid villi, 42, 43
arcus plantaris profundus, 255
arteria/arteriae,
a. alveolaris mandibularis, 15, 25
a. angularis oculi, 11, 50
a. auricularis caudalis, 14-17, 20, 36
a auricularis rostralis, 50
a. axillaris, 63, 80, 84-86, 89, 91
a. brachialis, 89, 90, 92, 93
e. broncho-oesophagea, 130
a. buccalis, 36
a. bulbi penis, 288, 289
aa. caecales mediates et laterales, 165
a. carotis communis, 24-30, 61-64, 69, 78-81, 126-127, 130-134
a. carotis externa, 11, 14-25, 28, 31, 36, 37
a. carotis interna, 20, 24, 28, 30, 59, 69
a. caudalis femoris, 195, 201, 218, 219, 224, 276
a. caudalis lateralis, 319-322
a. cervicalis profunda, 66-71, 130
a. cervicalis superficialis, 60-65, 116-127, 132-137
a. circumflexa femoris laleralis, 203, 204, 205, 224, 280, 282, 284-286, 303
a. circumflexa femoris medialis, 196, 200, 201, 224
a. circumflexa humeri caudalis, 92
a. circumflexa humeri cranialis, 87, 88, 92
a. circumflexa ilium profunda, 179, 181, 192, 194-197, 220-224, 276, 277, 300-304, 310, 311, 315, 316
a. coeliaca, 161, 163, 165, 172, 174, 175
a. colica media, 165, 175
a. colica sinistra et dextra, 164, 165, 179, 181
a. collateralis radialis, 88, 94
a. collateratis ulnaris, 83-85, 240-243
a. coronaria dextra, 137-139
a. coronaria sinistra, 126-130
a. digitalis lateralis, 100, 101, 232-235, 240-243, 248-253, 262-265
a. digitalis medialis, 101, 233, 235, 241-243, 249, 251-253, 255-256, 258, 262, 263, 265
a. digitalis palmaris communis II, 99-103, 233, 235, 241-243
a. digitalis palmaris communis III, 240-243
a. digitalis plantaris communis II, 263, 265
  see also a. plantaris medialis
a. digitalis plantaris communis III, *see* a. plantaris lateralis
a. epigastrica caudalis, 220, 291, 300, 308, 314
a. epigastrica cranialis, 131
a. ethmoidalis externa, 42, 43, 46
a. facialis, 10-20, 25, 32-36, 50-53
a. femoralis, 195, 201-204, 208, 209, 218-224, 276-279, 282-285, 303, 314-317
a. gastrica sinistra, 161, 165, 172, 174, 175
a. glutea caudalis, 194, 196-201, 218-224, 276, 277, 302, 306-311
a. glutea cranialis, 197, 218, 219, 277, 302-311
a. hepatica, 165, 172-175
a. ileocolica, 165, 168
a. iliaca externa, 220-224, 303-306, 314-317
a. iliaca interna, 220-224, 312-314
a. iliacofemoralis, 220-224, 276-280, 302-308, 316
a. incisiva, 45, 47, 48
a. intraorbitatis, 49
a. intercostaiis dorsalis, 119, 132, 133, 136-138, 159, 165, 176, 180
a. intercostalis suprema, 70, 123-127, 129, 130, 138
a. intercostalis ventralis, 121, 131, 136-138
a. interossea communis, 87, 88
a. interossea cranialis, 87, 88, 94, 98-101
aa. jejunales, 165, 175
a. labialis mandibularis, 12, 13
a. labialis maxillaris, 11, 32, 36
a. labialis ventralis, 307-309, 314
a. laryngea cranialis, 30, 31
a. laleratis nasi, 11, 32, 36
a. lienalis, 159-163, 165, 175
a. lingualis, 16, 18, 20, 25, 30
a. lumbalis, 311
a. malaris, 52, 53
a. malleolaris caudalis lateralis, 221, 263
a. marginis solearis, 239
a. maxillaris, 16
a. mediana, 85, 86, 89, 90, 93-102
a. meningea,
  caudalis, 69
  rostralis, 43
a. mesenterica caudalis, 144, 165, 181, 300, 301
a. mesenterica cranialis, 165, 175
a. metacarpea dorsalis II, 97, 99, 101-103, 232-235, 240-243
a. metacarpea dorsalis III, 98-101, 232, 234, 240-242
a. metatarsea dorsalis III, 212-213, 221, 250, 253, 262, 265
a musculophrenica, 131
a. obturatoria, 196, 204, 205, 218-224, 276-277
a. occipitalis, 20, 24, 27, 30, 59
a. oesophagea, 178
a. ophthalmica, 52, 53
a. ovarica, 300, 301, 310, 312-317
a. palatina ascendens, 16, 20, 25
a. palatina major, 47, 48, 49
a. penis, 287, 294
a. perinealis ventralis, 219, 303, 310, 313
a. plantaris lateralis, 213
  see also a. digitalis plantaris communis III
a. plantaris medialis, 211, 214, 221
  see also a. digitalis plantaris communis II
a. poplilea, 220, 224
a. profunda femoris, 205, 220, 222, 223, 278, 282-285, 303, 315
a. pudenda externa, 220, 222, 275, 279-289, 313-317
a. pudenda interna, 197, 201, 204, 205, 218-220, 223, 224, 278
a. pulmonalis, 126-130, 138, 139
a. radialis, 83, 88-90, 95-106, 240-243
a. rectalis caudalis, 102, 240-243
a. rectalis cranialis, 165, 179, 181, 300, 301, 311, 312
a. renalis dextra, 171, 172, 174
a. renalis sinistra, 165
a. saphena, 193, 206, 213, 220, 222, 224, 290, 291
a. scapularis dorsalis, 66, 84, 118-124, 126-135
a. sphenopalatina, 47
a. subclavia sinistra et dextra, 126, 130, 133-137
a. sublingualis, 16, 20
a. subscapularis, 80, 84, 85
a. supraorbitalis, 52
a. suprascapularis, 79, 80, 84-86, 89-93
a. tarsea perforans, 212, 217
a. temporalis superficialis, 50-52
a. testicularis, 292, 293
a thoracica nxterna, 63, 65, 84, 85, 116, 118, 120, 122-127
a. thoracica interna, 116, 118, 120, 124-130, 133-137
a. thoracodorsalis, 80, 84, 85, 89, 90, 93
a. thyroidea cranialis, 27-31, 62
a. fibialis, 206-208, 211, 213-215, 221, 263
a. transversa cubiti, 86, 88-90, 94
a. transversafaciei, 11, 13-16, 36, 50, 51
a. ulnaris collateralis 89, 90, 93
a. umbilicalis, 220, 223, 224, 289, 310, 311, 315
a. uterina, 301, 308-311, 316
a. uterina dextra, 312-314, 316
a. uterina sinistra, 312, 314, 316
a. vaginalis, 220, 222, 310-316
a. vertebralis, 66, 69-72, 133-135, 138
artery, *see* arteria/arteriae
arytenoid cartilage, 30, 31, 56, 332
atlas, 70, 72, 332
  alar foramina, 69
  lateral vertebral foramina, 69, 72
  wing, 57, 69, 72, 271
atrioventricular valve,
  left, 110, 128-130
  right, 136-139
atrium,
  left, 126-139
  right, 128-130, 136, 137
auditory tube (orifice of),
  medial lip, 47
  in nasal pharynx, 49
auricular cartilage, 15, 16
axis,
  caudal articular process, 69
  dens, 69, 70, 72
  dorsal arch, 72
  dorsal spinous process, 69, 72, 271

B

basihyoid bone, 29
bile duct, 145, 172, 173
bladder, *see* urinary bladder
bone, *see under* individual names

broad ligament, 177, 184
bronchus,
  left, 128, 129
  right, 135, 137
buccal gland, 14, 15, 19
butbourethral gland, 288

C

caecocolic junction, 168, 169, 171
caecum,
  apex, 164
  base, 166-172, 176, 178
  body, 162-167, 178
  caecocolic orifice, 171
  ileal orifice, 171
calcaneal tendon, common, 187, 206-216
calcaneus, 186, 187, 211-217, 221, 342, 343
  sustentaculum tali, 246, 247, 342
  tuberosity, 186, 189, 191, 211-217, 221, 244-247, 262, 263
carotid sheath, 64, 65
carpal bones,
  IV, 74, 98, 227, 336, 337
  acccccory, 74, 75, 77, 83, 87, 88, 96, 97, 102, 103, 228-231, 240, 241, 271
  intermediate, 98
  radial, 83
  ulnar, 83, 98
  see also carpus
carpal canal, 75, 102, 103
carpal ligaments,
  lateral collateral, 83, 98
  medial collateral, 83
carpal pad *see* chestnut
carpus,
  bones, *see* carpal bones
  carpometacarpal articulation, 77
  extensor retinaculum, 86
  flexor retinaculum, 86
  radiocarpal joint, 77, 96-103
  synovial cavity and synovial sheath, 102, 103
cartilage, *see under* individual names
caudal fascia, 318, 319
caudal vertebrae, 318-322
caval foramen, *see* diaphragm
ceratohyoid bone, 29
cerebrum, 41, 42
  falxcerebri, 41, 42, 43
  gyri and sulci, 43
  location, 40
cervix, *see* uterus
chestnut,
  carpal pad, 231
  tarsal pad, 247
choanae, 47-49
chondrocoronal ligaments, 236, 237
chordae tendineae, 128, 137
coffin joint, *see* interphalangeal joint, distal
colon, ascending,
  diaphragmatic flexure, 158, 162, 164
  left dorsal, 144, 156-158, 160, 164, 180
  left ventral, 144, 156, 158, 160, 164, 180
  origin, 166
  pelvic flexure, 158, 169, 171
  right dorsal, 144, 166-173
  right ventral, 144, 166-171
  sternal flexure, 158
  transverse, 144, 161
colon, descending, 156-165, 274, 300, 301, 310
  hautra, 156
  mesocolon, 162-165, 170
  taenia, 157
conchal sinus, *see* frontal sinus. maxillary sinus
conus arteriosus, 126-129
corium, 226, 266, 267
cornea, 3, 35, 49, 50
coronary cushion, 236, 237
coronary groove, 136
coronary sinus, 138, 139
coronet, 228-236, 242, 243, 244-251, 253, 255, 262-264, 266, 268
coronoid process (mandible) 37, 38
corpus luteum, 309
  see also ovary
costal arch, 116, 118, 120, 122, 146
costal cartilages, 118-122
costochondral junction, 110, 118-121, 132, 133
costodiaphragmatic recess, 122
costomediastinal recess, 133, 141
cricoid cartilage, 28, 30, 31
cricothyroid ligament, 31
cricotracheal ligament, 31
crista terminalis, 136-138
cruciate ligaments (distal sesamoidean), 267
crural extensor retinaculum, 193, 206, 207
crural fascia, 193, 206-208
crus, 189-191
crus penis, 288, 289
cubital ligaments,
  lateral collateral, 94
  median collateral, 86

D

dental alveoli, 3, 32, 33, 37-39, 44-46
dentition,
  incisor(1, i), 4, 7, 45-48, 54
  molar (M), 4, 19, 23, 24, 32, 33, 37-39, 44, 46, 49
  premolar (P, p), 19, 21, 23, 32, 33, 37, 38, 44-47, 49, 54
  see also dental alveoli
diaphragm,
  aortic hiatus, 145, 159, 165, 171, 174
  caval foramen, 129, 145
  central tendon, 120, 122, 123, 132, 156, 158, 160
  costal attachments, 120, 122, 131, 151, 156, 158, 160
  costal part, 132-133
  costodiaphragmatic recess, 122
  crura, *see* lumbar part
  cupola, 112, 122
  lumbar part, 156-159, 161, 168, 170-172
  oesophageal hiatus, 157, 159-161, 172, 181
  sternal part, 131, 151, 156
diaphragmatic line of pleural reflection, 112, 122, 132
digital cushion, 236-239, 260, 261
dorsoscapular ligament, 81, 116
ductus arteriosus, 111, 142
ductus deferens, 275, 292, 293
ductus lymphaticus dexter, 133
ductus thoracicus, 68, 122-134, 138, 141
duodenum, 144, 145, 168-171, 173
dura mater, 43, 317

E

epidermis, (hoof), 237, 239
epididymis, 269, 270, 290-293
epiglottis, 5, 30, 31, 56, 330, 332, 333, 334
ergot (metatarsal pad), 235, 264
  ligament, 232, 233, 240, 241, 263-265
ethmoid bone, 41, 42, 43, 46-48, 331
  cribriform plate, 41, 43
  ethmoid nasal conchae, 49
extensor retinaculum (carpus), 86, 89, 90
extensor retinaculum (hock), 193, 206, 207, 211, 213

F

facial crest, 4, 6, 8, 10, 18, 32, 33, 37, 39, 46, 53
  see also maxilla, zygomatic bone
falciform ligament (liver), 183
falxcerebri, 43
fascia, *see under* individual names
fascia lata, 192
fascia transversalis, 291, 314
  see also transverse fascia
femoral fascia,
  medial, 289-291
  deep, 193
femoral ring, 269, 304
femoral triangle, 291
femorotibial joint, *see* stifle joint
femur, 188, 189, 208-210
  articular surface, 74, 202-205
  greater trochanter, 186, 188, 189, 197-204, 269, 272, 273, 276, 277
  lateral condyle, 198, 199, 215, 271
  lesser trochanter, 202, 203
  medial condyle, 198, 199
  third trochanter, 188-209, 272, 273, 276, 277
  trochlea, 186, 215, 272, 273
    tuberculum, 188, 198, 203, 204, 206-208, 210, 211
fetlock joint, *see* metacarpophaiangeal and metatarsophalangeat joints
fibula, 186, 187, 189, 190, 199, 271, 325
  see also tibia, lateral maileolus
filum terminate, 323
flexor retinaculum (carpus), 89, 90, 97, 102, 241
flexor retinaculum (hock), 211
foramen, *see under* individual names
foramen ovate (heart), 111, 142
fossa glandis, 274, 295, 296
frontal bones, 33, 37, 39-42, 44, 46-51, 53
  interfrontal suture, 41
  temporal line, 6, 8, 32, 33, 37, 40
  zygomaticofrontal process, 6, 8, 10, 11, 32, 33, 37, 39, 52, 53
frontal sinus, *see* paranasal sinus

G

ganglion aorticorenalia, 174, 175
ganglion cervicale medium, 25, 65, 68, 124-127
ganglion cervicothoracicum, 66-68, 123-125, 135
ganglion coel acum, 165, 172
ganglion stellatum, *see* ganglion cervicothoracicum
genital fold, 274, 275
genual joint, *see* stifle joint
gingiva, 44
  gingival margin, 3, 21, 39
glans clitoridis, 299
glans penis, 294-298
gluteal fascia, deep, 318
guttural pouch, 2, 3, 4, 5, 14-18, 28-29, 31, 56, 57, 110, 332, 333, 334
  lateral part, 15-17, 20, 22, 24, 25, 29, 269
  medial part, 16, 17, 20, 22, 24, 25, 27, 29, 186

H

heart, 110, 111, 123-130, 135-139, 270
  of foal, 141, 142, 270
hepatorenal ligament, 169
hock, *see* tarsus
hoof, 226, 227, 228-234, 236-239, 244-251, 254-261, 266, 268, 325
humerus,
  deltoid tuberosity, 58, 76-78, 86, 92, 112
  lateral epicondyle, 76, 87, 88, 92, 94, 112
  major tuberosity, 58, 86, 87, 91, 112
  medial epicondyle, 93
  musculospiral groove, 92
  surface features, 76, 112
hyoid apparatus, see individual bones

I

ileac orifice and papilla, 171
ileocaecal junction, 163
ileum, 125, 132, 144, 160-167
iliac fascia, 283-288, 304-308
iliopubic eminence, 304, 316, 317
ilium,
  gluteal line, 200, 202, 218, 219
  shaft, 186, 200, 202, 205, 225, 269, 278-283, 325
  tuber coxae, 145, 188-197, 202, 218, 269, 271, 272-279, 283, 302, 303
  tuber sacrale, 188, 189, 218, 269, 271, 277, 279, 283, 302, 303
  wing, 57, 201, 202, 269, 271
incisive bone, 3, 38, 44-47, 326
infraorbital canal, 38, 39
infraorbital foramen, 6, 8, 11, 22, 38, 39, 44-46
inguinal canal, 270, 275, 284-286
inguinal ligament, 290-293
inguinal ring,
  deep, 270, 274, 275, 282, 284-289, 307, 308, 304
  superficial, 269, 270, 275, 285, 290, 291, 306-308
interphalangeal joint,
  distal (coffin), 225, 226, 228-231, 236, 244, 246
  proximal (pastern), 225, 228-231, 233-235, 244-247
interspinous ligament, 68, 72, 320
intervenous tubercle, 137, 138
intestine, *see* caecum, colon, duodenum, ileurn, jejunum
ischiatic foramen,
  greater, 196, 201, 205, 277, 302
  lesser, 196, 205, 277, 278, 302
ischium, 188, 189, 223, 269, 278-287, 302, 318
  spine, 205

tuber ischiadicum, 188, 189, 192, 196, 200-204, 273, 278-285

J

jejunum, 144, 145, 162, 163
joint, *see under* individual names

K

kidney,
- left, 160-165
- right, 168-175

L

labiurn, mandibular, 6-9
- maxillary, 4, 6-9
- vulvae, 218, 299, 307

lacrimal bone, 38-41, 44, 50-53
lacrimal caruncle, 35
lacrimal duct, 3, 39
lacrimal lake, 35
large intestine, *see* caecum and colon
larynx, 2, 3, 5, 28-31, 56, 57, 110, 332
- laryngeal aditus, 29
- laryngeal pharynx, 29, 30
- laryngeal saccule, 31

ligament, *see under* individual names
- ligamentum arteriosum, 126-130

ligamentum flavum, 319-323
ligamentum nuchae, 67-69, 72
linea alba, 131, 145, 275, 300
lingual apex, 7
lingual papillae,
- filiform, 23, 26, 47
- fungiform, 21, 45, 47
- vallate, 47, 49

liver,
- caudate process, 145, 168-169, 183
- falciform ligament, 183
- left lateral lobe, 158, 160, 176, 180, 182
- left medial lobe, 160, 182
- left triangular ligament, 159, 176
- right coronary ligament, 168
- right lateral lobe, 167-169, 178
- right medial lobe, 167-169, 178
- right triangular ligament, 168, 176, 178

lung,
- left, cardiac notch, 121, 122
- left, caudal border, 120-123
- left, caudal lobe, 120-123
- left, cranial border, 120-123
- left, cranial lobe, 120-123
- left, dorsal border, 120-123
- right, accessory lobe, 125, 126
- right, cardiac notch, 132, 133
- right, caudal lobe, 132, 133
- right, cranial lobe, 132, 133
- right, dorsal border, 132, 133

lymph node,
- *see* lymphonodus/lymphonodi

lymphonodus/lymphonodi:
lnn. anorectales, 279, 280, 303, 306, 316
ln. axillaris, 80, 84, 85, 107
lnn. caecales, 163, 164, 168-170, 176
ln. cervicalis profundus caudalis, 62-65, 116, 118, 120, 122, 124, 133-137
ln. cervicalis profundus cranialis, 16-20, 24, 27, 59-62, 81
ln. cervicalis profundus medius, 62-64, 66
ln. cervicalis superficialis, 60-63, 78, 79, 81
lnn. colici, 166-171
ln. coxalis, 302
lnn. cubitales, 88, 89, 90, 93, 96
ln. hepaticus, 183
ln. iliacus medialis, 177
ln. inguinale profundum, 205, 278, 279, 282, 283, 303
lnn. inguinales superficiales, 278, 279, 282, 306-309
ln. ischiadicus, 196, 277
lnn. lienalis, 159, 160
ln. lumbalis aorticus, 174
ln. mandibulare, 13-15, 18, 20, 22, 24-29
ln. mediastinalis cranialis, 124, 134, 137
ln. mediastinalis medius, 130, 138
ln. parotideum, 14, 15
ln. popliteus, 195, 197, 200, 218
lnn. renales, 172, 174, 175
ln. retropharyngeus lateralis, 16, 17, 20, 24, 25, 57
ln. retropharyngeus medialis, 16, 17, 19, 20, 22, 25, 27, 29, 59, 62
ln. sternalis cranialis, 124, 126, 133-136
ln. subiliacus, 152, 181, 192, 196, 217, 300
ln. tracheobronchalis medius, 126-130, 135-138, 142, 170
ln. tracheobronchalis sinister, 124, 130, 142

M

mammary gland, 184
- lateral suspensory lamina, 304, 305
- *see also* scrotum, suspensory laminae

mandible, 3, 4, 16-22, 57, 331
- condyle, 8, 14, 37, 50, 51, 53
- coronoid process, 37, 38
- insertions, m. masseter, 14
- mental foramen, 8, 11, 13, 22, 37
- ramus, 8
- vascular notch, 13, 22

mandibular gland, 13-17, 19, 20, 22
- duct, 17-20

mandibular labium, 6-9, 54
manica flexoria, 235, 254
manus,
- bones, 228-231
- hoof, 236, 237

maxilla, 3, 4, 13, 32, 33, 37, 45, 47, 48-53, 57
- dental alveoli, 3, 32, 33, 38, 39, 44, 46
- lacrimal groove, 46
- tuberosity, 37, 38
- *see also* facial crest, zygomatic arch

maxillary labium, 6-9, 34, 35, 54
mediastinum,
- caudal, 135
- cranial, 127
- dorsal, 126, 130
- ventral, 128

mental foramen, (mandible), 18, 11, 13, 22, 37
mentum, 8
mesocolon, 162-165, 170, 274, 275, 300, 301
mesometrium, 309
mesosalpinx, 177, 184, 301, 309
metacarpal bones:
- II, 99-103, 227, 228, 230, 336, 337
- III, 98-103, 228-235, 240-243, 336, 337, 338, 339
- tuberosity, 99-101, 228, 229
- IV, 77, 99-103, 227, 228-235, 240-243, 336, 337

metacarpal fascia, deep, 98-101, 235
metacarpophalangeal joint, 228-231, 233-236, 240-242, 338, 339
metacarpus, 87, 88, 228-231
metatarsal bones:
- II, 187, 191, 213, 214, 216, 221, 228, 231, 244, 342
- III, 213, 214, 221, 244-247, 342
- IV, 187, 212-214, 221, 244-247, 342

metatarsal pad (ergot), 241, 245, 264
metatarsophalangeal joint, 244-251, 253, 255, 259-264, 267
metatarsus, 187, 191, 244-246, 259
mouth,
- angle, 47, 48
- labia, 6-9
- *see also* oral cavity

muscle, *see* musculus/musculi
musculus/musculi:
m. abductor digiti I longus, 86-90, 94, 97, 99-102
m. adductor, 195, 200-205, 207, 219-224, 278, 282
m. arytenoideus transversus 31
m. biceps brachii, 82, 85-93
- lacertus fibrosus, 86-93

m. biceps femoris, 192-194, 272, 273, 276-280, 318-322
m. biventer cervicis, 67
m. brachialis, 75, 85-87, 92, 93
m. brachiocephalicus, 59, 133
- *see also* mm. cleidobrachialis and cleidomastoideus

m. buccinator, 10-14, 18, 36
m. bulbospongiosus, 206, 279-289, 294-295
m. caninus, 10, 11, 13
m. capsularis, 203, 278-280, 284, 285
m. cleidobrachialis, 60, 61, 78, 79, 82, 87-90
m. cleidocephalicus, 10, 14, 16, 78, 79
m. cleidomastoideus, 36, 59-61
m. coccygeus, 279-281
m. complexus, 67
m. constrictor vestibuli, 29, 31
m. coracobrachialis, 86, 89-93
m. corrugator supercilii, 50
m. cremaster, 282-287, 290-293
m. cricoarytenoideus dorsalis, 30, 31
m. cricoarytenoideus lateralis, 31
m. cricopharyngeus, 15, 16, 19-22, 24-28, 62
m. cricothyroideus, 27-31
m. cutaneus colli, 58-60
m. cutaneus femoris, 194
m. cutaneus omobrachialis, 78, 79, 113, 147-149
m. cutaneus trunci, 78, 79, 83, 84, 113-117, 133, 147-151, 192
m. deltoideus, 78, 79, 86, 87, 148
m. depressor anguli oris, 11
m. depressor labii mandibularis, 10-13, 15, 18
m. depressor labii maxillaris, 15
m. digastricus, 14-21, 24-29, 36, 69
- pars occipitomandibutaris 14, 15
- venter rostralis 16, 17, 19

m. dilator naris apicalis, 34
m. extensor carpi radialis, 82, 88-91, 94, 98-103
m. extensor carpi ulnaris, 83, 87, 88, 94, 96, 97, 102
m. extensor digitorum brevis, 212-214, 217
m. extensor digitorum communis, 82, 86, 87, 92, 94, 98-101, 232-239
m. extensor digitorum lateralis, 87, 88, 94, 98-101, 193-195, 198-199, 202, 207-212, 214-216, 217, 218, 221
m. extensor digitorum longus, 193-195, 197-199, 202, 207-215, 217, 189, 248-255, 260, 262-265
m. fibularis (peroneus) tertius, 207, 210, 212-214
m. flexor carpi radialis, 82, 85, 86, 89, .90, 95-97, 102
m. flexor carpi ulnaris, 83, 85, 88-90
m. flexor digiti I longus 193-195, 202, 206-217, 221
m. flexor digitorum longus, 193, 206-209, 211, 213-217, 221, 263
m. flexor digitorum profundus, 87, 88, 94-103, 193, 194, 206, 209-216, 221, 232-239, 248-255, 260, 262-265
m. flexor digitorum superficialis, 95-103, 193-195, 207-215, 217, 220, 221, 232-235, 240-243, 248-255, 260, 262-265
m. frontoscutularis, 10-12, 14, 16, 50
m. gastrocnemius, 193, 195, 199, 200, 203-212, 215, 218, 224
mm. gemelli, 197, 201, 204, 205, 278-284
m. genioglossus, 26
m. geniohyoideus, 19, 21, 26
m. gluteus accessorius, 196, 302, 303
m. gluteus medius, 192, 194, 196, 201, 272-274, 276, 277, 318-322
m. gluteus profundus, 277, 278-287, 302, 303
m. gluteus superficialis, 192, 318-322
m. gracilis, 201, 205, 206, 211, 215, 219-223, 273, 278-283, 290, 291, 303-308
m. hyoglossus, 16-19, 25-29
m. hyopharyngeus, 20, 24-27
m. iliacus, 196-205, 218, 219, 222-224, 276, 277, 283-287, 302, 303
m. iliocostalis, 61, 62, 64
m. iliocostalis cervicis, 66, 67, 71, 81, 116, 118, 120, 124
m. iliocostalis lumborum, 150, 151
m. iliocostalis thoracis, 67-70, 81, 116-123, 132
m. iliopsoas, 204, 279, 280
- *see also* m. iliacus, m. psoas major

m. infraspinatus, 75, 78, 79, 86, 87, 91, 92
mm. intercostales externi, 81, 92, 114-119, 157
mm. intercostales interni, 116-119, 122, 133, 148-151, 157, 166, 167
m. intercostobrachialis, 148, 149
m. interosseus, 98-103, 232-235, 240-243, 248-255, 260-265
m. interscutularis, 12, 40
mm. interspinales, 67, 72
mm. intertransversarii cervicis, 67, 69, 71
m. ischiocavernosus, 205, 278-283
m. latissimus dorsi, 78-80, 84, 114-119, 148
m. levator ani, 279-281, 302, 305, 306
m. levator labii maxillaris, 10-13, 23, 34-36, 45-51
m. levator nasolabialis, 10-13, 36, 50
m. levator palpebrae superioris, 52, 53
m. levator veli palatini, 30
mm. levatores costarum, 71, 120
m. longissimus atlantis, 66

m. longissimus capitis, 10, 11, 16, 20, 59, 61, 66, 36
m. longissimus cervicis, 63-67, 118-124
m. longissimus lumborum, 151
m. longissimus thoracis, 63-69, 72, 81, 117-124, 133
m. longus capitis, 27, 29, 61-63, 66-70
m. longus colli, 62-71, 123-128, 130, 138
m. malaris, 10-12, 50
m. masseter, 5, 10-14, 32, 36, 44-53
m. multifidis cervicis, 68, 70
m. mylohyoideus, 15-21, 24, 26
m. obliquus capitis caudalis, 10, 11, 16-20, 25, 29
m. obliquus capitis cranialis, 10, 11, 16-20, 25, 29
m. obliquus dorsalis, 49, 52, 53
m. obliquus externus abdominis, 113-116, 118-122
'abdominal tendon', 154, 290
'pelvic tendon', 154, 290, 291
m. obliquus internus abdominis, 115-121, 150-155, 192-198, 218, 222-224, 276, 277
m. obliquus ventralis, 52, 53
m. obturatorius externus, 205, 283-286, 303-305
m. obturatorius internus, 201-205, 222-224, 277-279, 287, 288, 302-306
m. occipitohyoideus, 16, 19, 20, 25, 69
m. omohyoideus, 10-16, 20, 22, 24, 27-30, 36, 56, 59-62, 78, 79
m. omotransversarius, 59-66, 78, 79
m. orbicularis oculi, 12, 50-53
m. orbicularis oris, 11, 13
m. palatopharyngeus, 16-19, 24, 25, 28
m. parietoauricularis, 40
m. parotidoauricularis, 10-14
m. pectineus, 203-205, 209, 222, 269, 278-286, 290
m. pectoralis ascendens, 63, 80-86, 89, 90, 93, 113-116, 132-138, 147-149
m. pectoralis descendens, 60-63, 78-84, 132-138
m. pectoralis transversus, 60, 82, 84, 85
m. peroneus tertius *see* m. fibularis tertius
m. popliteus, 206-211, 215-217
m. psoas major, 165, 174, 222, 274, 275, 288, 289, 300, 303-306, 308-311
m. psoas minor, 132, 165, 172, 174, 175, 274, 288,, 289, 300, 304-306
m. pterygoideus lateralis, 15, 16, 18
m. pterygoideus medialis, 15
m. pterygopharyngeus, 18, 19, 24, 27, 28
m. quadratus femoris, 196, 197, 200, 205, 218, 219, 276-282
m. quadriceps femoris, 202, 203, 215
see also m. rectus femoris, m. vastus intermedius, lateralis, medialis
m. rectus,
dorsalis, 52, 53
lateralis, 52, 53
medialis, 49
ventralis, 52, 53
m. rectus abdominis, 116-122, 194, 202, 291, 301, 308
vagina m. recti abdominis, lamina externa, 309
vagina m. recti abdominis, lamina interna, 131, 300
m. rectus capitis dorsalis major, 67-69, 72
m. rectus capitis dorsalis minor, 70-72
m. rectus femoris, 192, 194-204, 218, 219, 276-280, 284, 285, 302-304
m. rectus thoracis, 81, 116-120
m. retractor bulbi, 49, 52, 53
m. retractor costae, 118, 120, 122
m. retractor penis, 206, 279-289
m. rhomboideus, 115-118, 133
m. rhomboideus cervicis, 61-63, 66, 81, 116-122
m. rhomboideus thoracis, 67, 68, 81
m. sacrocaudalis dorsalis lateralis, 200, 277, 279, 281, 283, 302-305, 312
m. sacrocaudalis dorsalis medialis, 283-287, 318-319
m. sacrococcygeus ventralis lateralis, 223, 279
m. sartorius, 200, 203-206, 220-224, 278, 279
m. scalenus dorsalis, 63, 64, 79, 80, 116-120, 133
m. scalenus ventralis, 61-64, 79-81, 116-120, 133
m. scutuloauricularis, 40
m. semimembranosus, 187, 192, 195-208, 215, 218-223, 276-278
m. semispinalis capitis, 63, 66, 67
m. semitendinosus, 56, 192-209, 218-223, 272, 273, 276, 277, 318-322
m. serratus, scapular origins, 87, 89-91
m. serratus dorsalis caudalis, 114-119, 149, 150
m. serratus dorsalis cranialis, 114-119, 149, 150
m. serratus ventralis cervicis, 59-63, 78-81, 84, 92, 93, 133
m. serratus ventralis thoracis, 63, 78-81, 84, 92, 114-119, 148
m. soleus, 194, 195, 202
m. sphincter ani externus, 278-281, 302-306
mm. spinalis et semispinalis thoracis et cervices, 67-70, 72, 117, 133, 151
m. splenius, 10, 11, 14, 36, 61-67, 81, 116-123, 133
m. sternocephalicus, 59-68, 71, 121, 133, 134
see also m. sternomandibularis
m. sternohyoideus, 10, 16, 24, 29, 30, 56, 59, 61-64
m. sternomandibularis, 10, 11, 14-16, 20-22, 36, 133
see also m. sternocephalicus
m. sternothyrohyoideus, 27-31, 63-68, 72, 81, 133
see also m. sternohyoideus, m. sternothyroideus
m. sternothyroideus, 63, 64, 134
m. styloglossus, 16-19, 24-28
m. stylohyoideus, 15-20, 24-31
m. stylopharyngeus, 20, 24-28, 31
m. subclavius, 59-63, 78-81, 84, 116-120, 129, 132-138
rn. subscapularis, 80, 84, 89-93
m. supraspinatus, 59, 61, 78, 79, 84-93
m. temporalis, 32, 33, 40-43, 51-53
m. tensor fasciae antebrachii, 78, 79, 83-90, 93, 114-119, 148, 149
m. tensor fasciae latae, 195, 222-224, 276, 277
m. tensor veli palatini, 18, 25, 30
m. teres major, 80, 84, 89-93, 149
m. teres minor, 87, 92
m. thyrohyoideus, 16, 25, 27, 62
m. thyropharyngeus, 16, 20, 24-28, 62
m. tibialis caudalis, 195-209, 211-217
m. tibialis cranialis, 193-195, 199, 202, 206, 214, 217, 221
m. transversus abdominis, 117-122, 150, 300
m. trapezius, 59, 61, 113-117, 133, 147-149
m. triceps, 78, 79
m. triceps brachii, 78-82, 86-93, 113-117, 147-149
m. triceps surae, 209, 214, 216, 217
see also m. gastrocnemius. m. soleus
m. ulnaris lateralis, *see* m. extensor carpi ulnaris
m. vastus intermedius, 200-204
m. vastus lateralis, 192-204, 218, 219, 276, 277, 302, 303
m. vastus medialis, 197-204, 222-224, 290, 291
m. vestibularis, 31
m. vocalis, 31
m. zygomaticoauricularis, 50
m. zygomaticus, 10-13, 50

N

nares,
see nostril
nasal bone, 11, 13, 32-38, 44-46, 50-53, 326
nasal, cartilage, dorsal, 45
nasal cavity, common ventral meatus, 3, 4, 34, 35, 45, 110
nasal concha,
dorsal, 3, 32-39, 43-49
middle, 47, 49
ventral, 3, 32, 39, 48, 49
see also ethmoid bone
nasal diverticulum, 3, 6, 8-13, 35, 45, 100
nasal meatuses, 42, 47, 48
nasal septum, 34, 47-49, 331
mucosa, 47
nasoincisive notch, 6-11, 32, 38, 44-46, 326
nasolacrimal duct, 9, 32-34, 46
nasomaxillary opening, 3, 46
nasopharynx, 29, 47, 48, 56, 110, 331
navicular bone, *see* distal sesamoid bone
nerve, *see* nervus/nervi
nervus/nervi:
n. abducens, 53
n. accessorius XI, 19, 20, 24, 30, 31, 59, 69
n. alveolaris mandibularis, 15, 17, n. auriculopalpebralis, 11-17, 36, 50-53
n. auriculotemporalis, 11-14
n. axillaris, 79, 80, 84, 85, 89-93
n. buccalis, 14-18, 22-24
n. cardiacus cervicothoracicus, 127-129, 134
nn. caudales, 319-322
nn. cervicales,
n. cervicalis I, 19, 20, 24, 69, 72
n. cervicalis II, 10, 14, 70, 72
n. cervicalis III, 59, 61, 68
n. cervicalis IV, 59-64
n. cervicalis V, 59-66, 70
n. cervicalis VI, 59, 66, 70-72
n. cervicalis VII, VIII, 71
nn. clunium caudales, 192
nn. clunium medii, 192
n. costoabdominalis, 148, 151
n. cutaneus antebrachii caudatis, 88-96
n. cutaneus antebrachii cranialis, 78, 79, 92
n. cutaneus antebrachii lateralis, 82, 91
n. cutaneus antebrachii medialis, 86-88, 240, 241
n. cutaneus colli (CII), 36
n. cutaneus femoris caudalis, 194-197, 200-204, 218, 224, 276-280, 302, 305
n. cutaneus femoris lateralis, 194-197, 219, 222, 223, 276, 277, 302
n. cutaneus surae caudalis, 193, 194, 197, 200-204, 208-215, 218-221
n. digitalis palmaris lateralis, 232, 233, 242, 243
n. digitalis palmaris medialis, 233, 243
n. digitalis plantaris lateralis, 248, 249, 262-265
n. digitalis plantaris medialis, 249, 263, 265
n. facialisVII, 10-18, 23, 36, 45
n. femoralis, 200, 203-205, 219, 223, 224, 278-289, 303-306
n. fibularis communis, 195-204, 207-213, 217, 218, 277
n. fibularis profundus, 195-204, 207-213
n. fibularis superficialis, 193-195, 199, 207-213, 216, 217
n. frontalis, 11, 12, 52, 53
n. genitofemoralis, 279, 282-286, 304-308
n. glossopharyngeus IX, 17-20, 24-30
n. gluteus caudalis, 194-201, 218, 277-281, 302
n. gluteus cranialis, 196, 197, 201, 205, 277-280, 302
n. hypogastricus, 219, 306-308
n. hypoglossus XII, 17-30
n. ilioinguinalis, 307, 308
n. infraorbitalis, 13, 18, 23, 32-36, 44, 45, 49
nn. intercostales, 114-119, 148-151, 159
n. intercostobrachialis, 78, 79, 114-119, 148, 149
n. ischiadicus, 196-205, 218, 219, 224, 277-279, 302-306
n. laryngeus caudalis, 27-31
n. laryngeus craniatis, 17-30, 62
n. laryngeus recurrens, 64-67, 124-130, 133, 134, 138
n. lingualis, 15-18, 21
nn. lumbales, 192
n. mandibularis, 18, 19, 25, 30
n. massetericus, 14, 51
n. medianus, 79, 80, 84-90, 93-97, 102
n. mentalis, 18-23
n. metacarpeus palmaris lateralis, 232, 233, 242
n. metacarpeus palmaris medialis, 243
n. metatarseus dorsalis II, 212-214, 221, 248
n. metalarseus dorsalis III, 213, 248-255
n. musculocutaneus, 79, 80, 84, 85, 93
n. mylohyoideus, 15, 17
n. obturatorius, 205, 220-224, 278-283, 287, 303-306, 309
n. oculomotorius III, 52, 53
n. olfactorius I, 47

n. opticus II, 47, 49
n. palatinus major, 49
n. palmaris lateralis, 95-103, 232, 240-243
n. palmaris medialis, 95, 96, 98, 99, 102, 103, 232, 233, 240-243
n. pectoralis caudalis, 79-85, 116-120
n. pectoralis cranialis, 84, 85
n. pelvinus, 219, 220, 304-311
n. peroneus, *see* n. fibularis
n. phrenicus, 63, 65, 81, 116-122, 128, 167, 168, 176, 180
n. plantaris lateralis, 211-215, 217, 221, 248, 249, 262, 264, 265
n. plantaris medialis, 211-215, 221, 249, 262-265
n. pudendus, 219-224, 279-289, 303, 305
n. radialis, 79, 80, 84, 85, 89-94
n. rectalis caudalis, 219, 279-281, 302, 303, 311
n. saphenus, 193, 204, 206, 219-222, 262, 263, 278, 279, 303
nn. spinates, 78, 79
n. splanchnicus, 159, 161, 163, 165, 171, 172, 175
n. subscapularis, 79, 80, 84, 85, 89-93
nn. supraclaviculares, 60, 61, 78, 79
n. suprascapularis, 79, 80, 84, 85, 89-93
nn. thoracici, 116-119
n. thoracicus lateralis, 79, 80, 84, 85, 116-120
n. thoracicus longus, 63, 116, 118, 120
n. thoracodorsalis, 79, 80, 84, 116, 118, 120
n. tibialis, 193-197, 200-211, 214-221, 263, 277
n. trochlearis IV, 53
n. ulnaris, 83-90, 93-103, 240-243
n. vagus X, 20, 25, 28-31, 69, 124-130, 133-137
  see also t. vagalis X dorsalis, t. vagalis X ventralis
n. vertebralis, 66, 67, 71
n. zygomaticus, 52
nostril,
  alar cartilage, 3, 9, 11, 34, 35, 45, 46
  alar fold of ventral concha, 9, 35, 45, 46, 48
  dorsal cartilage, 45
  dorsal commissure, 9
  lateral ala, 6, 8, 35, 45
  medial ala, 6, 35
  ventral commissure, 9
nuchal ligament, 56, 67-69, 72

O

obturator foramen, 269, 303, 306, 307, 316, 317
occipital bone,
  condyle, 70, 72, 186, 271
  jugular process, 69
  protuberance, 40, 70, 72
ocular angle,
  lateral, 35, 44
  medial, 4, 50
oesophagus, 3, 27-31, 56, 57, 63, 68
oesophageal hiatus, *see* diaphragm
olecranon, *see* ulna
olfactory bulb, 43
omentum, greater, 157-164, 269
oral cavity,
  vestibule, 7
  see also mouth
orbit, 2, 4, 33, 38, 39, 50
  foramina, 38, 39
oropharynx, 47, 48, 49
ovarian bursa, 301, 309
ovary, 177-181, 270, 300, 301, 309-312
  corpus lutem, 309
  infundibulum, 301, 309
  ligaments,
    proper, 300, 301, 309, 310
    suspensory, 301, 309, 310
  mesovarium, 300

P

palate,
  hard, 47, 48
  soft, 4, 5, 29-31, 47-49, 56
palatine bones, 3, 47-49
palatine glands, 24-31
palatine sinus, *see* paranasal sinus
palmar ligaments, proximal interphalangeal joint, 225, 226, 234, 235
palpebra, III, 4, 35
palpebral fissure, 6, 8, 49
pancreas, 161-163, 171-173, 179
  duct, 145, 173
panniculus adiposus, 147
panniculus carnosus, 147
paraconal interventricular groove, 130
paranasal sinus,
  frontal, 32, 33, 37-39, 41-44
  maxillary,
    caudal, 32, 33, 37-39, 46
    rostral, 32, 33, 37-39, 46
  palatine, 28
  sphenopalatine, 39, 47
parietal bones, 40-43
parotid gland, 10-13, 50-53
pastern joint, *see* interphalangeal joint, proximal
patella, 186, 188-190, 193-195, 197-199
  accessory cartilage, 207, 208
  ligament,
    intermediate, 74, 186, 188, 194-198
    lateral, 186, 187, 193-200, 206, 272
    medial, 186, 187, 198, 199, 206-208, 210
pelvic fascia, 308, 313
pelvis,
  bones, 146, 188-190
  see also ilium, ischium, obturator foramen, pubis
penis, 205, 206, 270, 274, 278-290, 294-298
  see also glans penis, crus penis
pericardium, 121-125
  see also sternopericardial ligament
perineal raphe, 295, 299
perineal region, 270, 290, 295, 299
periople, 228-234, 238, 239, 244-247
periorbita, 2, 44, 46, 52, 53
pes,
  bones, 244-247
  hoof, 256-261
phalanges, *see* manus, pes
pharyngeal recess, 53
pharyngeal wall, 28, 29
pharynx,
  laryngeal part, 3, 24, 27-31
  nasal part, 29
  oral part, 29
philtrum, 6, 7
pia mater, 43
pinna, 40, 41
plantar ligament, long (hock), 211-214
plantar ligaments, proximal interphalangeal joint, 225, 226, 250, 252, 253, 255, 256, 258, 259, 267
pleura, pleural reflection, diaphragmatic line, 120, 122, 132
pleural cavity, 125, 140
plexus brachialis, 63-66, 71, 79-81, 116-127, 133-135
plexus caudalis dorsalis, 318-323
plexus coeliacus, 165
plexus coronarius, 236-239
plexus intermesentericus, 172, 174
plexus lienalis, 159, 161, 163
plexus mesenterica cranialis, 175
plexus palmaris
plexus parietalis, 237-239, 261
plexus pelvinus, 305
plexus plantaris, 258, 261
podotrochlear bursa, 236, 238, 254, 255
'poverty line', 272, 273, 276
prepubic tendon, 269, 275, 304
prepuce, 270, 274, 289-291, 294-298
preputial orifice, 290, 294-298
pubic brim, 310
pubis, 222-224, 270, 300, 307-317
pulmonary valve, 110, 128-130
punctum lacrimale, 35
pylorus, 172, 179

R

radiocarpal joint, 77, 96-103, 337
radius, 74, 75, 77, 82, 94, 95, 325, 336, 337
  lateral styloid process, 86, 88, 98, 325
  lateral tuberosity, 58, 74, 76, 87, 88
  medial styloid process, 82, 86, 88, 97-102, 228, 231
rectum, 110, 269, 270, 274, 275, 303-312
rate carpi rinrsale, 93, 88, 98
retina, 3, 47, 75
ribs, 112, 118-122, 130-135

S

sacroiliac articulation, 273, 304
sacroiliac ligament,
  dorsal, 196, 218-222, 280, 302
  ventral, 304-306
sacrotuberous ligament, 194, 197, 200-205, 218, 219, 222, 276-281, 302-305, 316
sacrum, 188, 202, 279-281, 289, 310, 311, 318-322
salivary gland, *see* buccal, mandibular, parotid, palatine and sublingual glands
scapula, 56, 57, 58, 74, 75, 76, 112
  cartilage, 3, 56, 57, 87, 91, 93
  coracoid process, 91, 93
  spine, 91, 111, 145, 271
  supraglenoid tubercle, 91, 93
scrotum, 269, 270, 290-293
  dartos tunic and fascia, 291
  lateral suspensory lamina, 282-284, 290
  medial suspensory lamina, 283-287, 290, 291
  raphe, 290, 295
  septum (dartos), 291
  vaginal process, 269, 270, 278-282, 285
  see also mammary gland, suspensory lamina
scutiform cartilage, 6, 8, 10, 15, 16, 40-42, 50, 51
sesamoid bones,
  distal (manus), 230, 236
  distal (pes), 245, 246, 254, 255, 257, 260, 268
  proximal (manus), 225, 227, 229-233, 235
  proximal (pes), 245-247, 251, 252, 254, 255, 260, 267
sesamoidean ligaments,
  collateral, 250, 251
  distal sesamoidean, 250-255, 259-261, 267
  distal sesamoid impar, 236-239, 254, 255, 257
  intersesamoidean, 254, 255, 267
sinus communicans, 42, 43
sinus coronarius, 139
sinus occipitalis dorsalis, 43
sinus petrosus dorsalis, 43
sinus sagittalis dorsalis, 42, 43
sinus temporalis, 42, 43
sinus transversus, 42, 43
sinus urethralis, 274
sinus v. buccalis, 14, 36
sinus v. profunda faciei, 14, 36
sinus v. transversa faciei, 14, 36
sinus venarum cavarum
skull,
  bones, 7, 9, 37-46
  see also under individual names
small intestine,
  see duodenum, ileum, jejunum
spermatic cord, 270, 274, 291-293
sphenopalatine sinus, *see* paranasal sinus
spleen, 144, 145, 156, 157, 176, 180
splint bones,
  see metacarpals II & IV and *see* metatarsals II & IV
sternopericardial ligament, 123, 125, 131, 138
sternum,
  manubrium, 118, 121
  xiphoid cartilage, 131
stifle joint, 186, 194-199, 202, 206-211
  capsule, 208
  collateral ligament,
    lateral, 186, 195-199, 207
    medial, 186, 207, 208
  femoropatellar ligament, 197, 204
  see also femur, patella, tibia
stomach,
  cardia, 179
  fundus (saccus caecus), 159-164, 179-181
  greater curvature, 158-164, 176, 180, 181
  lesser curvature, 159-162, 181
  pylorus, 172, 179
stylohyoid bone, 15-20, 24-31, 57, 330, 332, 333, 334
subarachnoid cavity, 43
sublingual gland, 18, 19, 21
subsinuosal interventricular groove, 138
supraorbital adipose tissue, 40, 50
supraorbital foramen, 6, 32, 33, 37-39, 46-53
suprarenal gland, *see* adrenal gland
supraspinous ligament, 68, 70, 72
suspensory ligament, *see* m. interosseus

symphyseal tendon, 278, 283-287, 304-307, 313

T

talus, 186, 191, 210-214, 221, 244-247, 342
lateral trochlea, 186, 212-214, 342
medial trochlea, 210, 212-214, 244, 246, 247, 342
tarsal bones,
central, 221, 244-247
first and second (fused), 227, 246, 247, 342, 343
fourth, 227, 244-247, 342, 343
third, 186, 221, 244-247, 342, 343
see also calcaneus, talus
tarsal pad, *see* chestnut
tarsus,
bones, *see* tarsal bones extensor retinaculum, 207, 210, 212
flexor retinaculum, 75, 211, 216
superficial structures, 193
surface features, 191, 244-247
tarsocrural joint, 186, 211-214
tarsometatarsal articulation, 244-247
temporal bone, 2, 50, 52
mandibular fossa, 37
see also zygomatic arch
temporal line, 41, 50
see also frontal bone temporal fossa, 32, 41
temporomandibular joint, 5, 10, 14, 16, 36, 57
tendo calcaneus communis, 206-216
testis, 269, 270, 290-293
thoracic vertebrae, 58, 70-72, 78, 79, 149, 271
thoracolumbar fascia
thymus, 121-126, 132-137
thyrohyoid bone, 19, 20, 24-31, 333
thyroid cartilage, 20, 25-31
thyroid gland, 27-31, 56, 62, 66-70
tibia, 342, 343
crest, 189, 193
extensor suicus, 189, 190, 272
lateral condyle, 189, 190, 195, 272
lateral malleolus, 186, 193, 212-214
medial malleolus, 191, 193, 212-214, 262, 263
tuberosity, 186, 189, 193-195, 197, 215
tibial extensor retinaculum, 210-215
tongue, 3, 4, 18, 19, 1, 50, 56
see also lingual apex, lingual papillae, individual muscles
tooth, *see* dentition
trachea, 3, 27, 56, 57, 62-71, 110, 127, 133-136, 332
transverse fascia, 155, 177, 274, 275, 308
truncus,
t. bicaroticus, 124, 134, 138
t. brachiocephalicus, 4, 13-130, 136-139
t. costocervicalis, 4, 15, 134-138
t. linguofacialis, 27, 28
t. massetericus, 14
t. pudendoepigastricus, 222-224, 284, 304
t. pulmonalis, 123-130, 138, 139
t sympathicus, 30, 123-127, 134, 138, 172-176
t. trachealis, 62, 64, 121-123
t. vagalis X dorsalis, 126-130, 158, 163, 168, 180
t. vagalis X ventralis, 126-130, 158, 163, 168, 180
t. vagosympathicus, 27-30, 62-64, 125, 126, 133
tuber coxae, *see* ilium
tuber ischiadicum, *see* ischium
tuber sacrale, *see* ilium
tunica albuginea (testis), 290, 291
tunica dartos, *see* scrotum
tunica vaginalis, *see* vaginal process

U

ulna, olecranon, 74, 76-78
see also radius, lateral styloid process
umbilical cord, 270, 285, 295
umbilicus, 295
ureter, 172, 174, 175, 274, 275, 288, 301, 313
urethra, pelvic, 313
urethral process, 274, 294-298
urinary bladder, 274, 275, 288, 300, 312-313
see also vesicular ligaments
uterine tube, 177, 300, 301
infundibulurn, 300, 301
uterus,
cervix, 312
non-pregnant, 177
pregnant, 178, 179, 181, 300, 301, 309, 310

V

vagina, 145, 269, 270, 300, 305-312
vagina m. recti abdominis, *see* m. rectus abdominis
vaginal process, 269, 270, 275, 278, 279, 282-285, 290-293
vasa efferentia lymphatica, 133, 134
vein, *see* vena/venae
vena/venae,
v. alveolaris mandibularis, 25
v. angularis oculi, 11, 32
v. axillaris, 63, 65, 80, 84, 85
v. azygos, 135-138, 168-171, 176, 178
v. brachialis, 89, 90
v. buccalis, 14-19, 36
v. caudalis femoris, 195, 201, 218, 219
v. cava caudalis, 159, 167-175, 274, 275
foramen, 129
v. cava cranialis, 65, 126, 127, 133, 136-139
v. cephalica, 65, 78-85, 95-101, 116-127, 133, 134, 240-243
v. cephalica accessoria, 60, 82, 86, 89, 90
vv. cerebri dorsales, 42
v. circumflexa femoris lateralis, 203, 204, 205, 224
v. circumflexa femoris medialis, 196, 200, 201, 224
v. circumflexa ilium profunda, 179, 181, 192-197, 220-224, 276, 277, 300-304, 310, 311
vv. circumflexa penis, 279, 281-289
v. clitoridis media, 313, 314
v. colica dextra, 164
v. collateralis ulnaris, 83-85, 230-243
v. cordis magna, 128, 130
v. cordis magna dextra, 136-139
v. coronalis, 248, 249
v. costocervicalis, 127, 128, 135-137
v. digitalis dorsalis communis II, 213, 221, 249, 262, 263, 265
v. digitalis lateralis, 232, 233, 240-242, 248-253, 262-265
v. digitalis medialis, 233, 241, 243, 248-255, 262-265
v. digitalis palmaris communis II, 232, 233, 7, 15-243
v. digitalis palmaris communis III, 233, 240-243
v. digitalis plantaris communis III, 248
see also v. plantaris lateralis
v. dorsalis nasi, 11, 32
v. dorsalis penis, 206
v. epigastrica caudalis, 220, 291, 300, 308, 314
v. epigastrica cranialis, 113, 131
v. facialis, 10-20, 25, 32, 33, 36
v. femoralis, 195, 201-204, 218-224, 278-285, 303, 316, 317
v. glutea caudalis, 277, 302, 306-311
v. glutea cranialis, 302-305, 308-311
v. ileocolica, 168, 176
v. iliaca communis, 300, 3011, 311, 312
v. iliaca externa, 220, 222-224
v. iliaca interna, 220, 223, 224
v. iliacofemoralis, 277, 278, 280, 302-308
v. intercostalis, 136, 159, 176
v. intercostalis dorsalis, 138, 142
v. interossea communis, 87, 88, 94
v. interventricularis paraconalis, 126
v. jugularis externa, 10, 14, 36, 59-68, 78-81, 116-127, 133-135
v. labialis communis, 13, 18, 36
v. labialis mandibularis, 18
v. labialis maxillaris, 18
v. labialis ventralis, 307-309, 314
v. lateralis nasi, 32, 36
v. lienalis, 159, 163
v. lingualis, 25, 28
v. linquofacialis, 10-13, 16-24, 27, 36, 59, 61
v. malleolaris caudalis lateralis, 221
v. marginis solearis, 239
v. masseterica, 36
v. masseterica ventralis, 36
v. maxillaris, 10-20, 24, 25, 36, 61
v. mediana, 83-90, 93-102, 240-243
v. metatarsea dorsalis II, 212-214, 221, 263-265
v. obturatoria, 277, 278-287
v. occipitalis, 19, 20, 24, 27, 30, 36, 61
v. oesophagea, 178
v. ovarica, 179, 300, 301
v. palatina major, 47, 48
v. perinealis ventralis, 219
v. phrenica cranialis, 178, 180
v. plantaris lateralis, 212, 213, 221
see also v. digitalis plantaris communis III
v. poplitea, 224
v. portae, 172, 174, 175, 179
v. profunda faciei, 14, 15, 18, 23, 36, 53
v. profunda femoris, 205, 222, 278, 282, 283, 303
v. pudenda externa, 220, 222, 275, 279-289, 302, 303, 316, 317
v. pudenda interna, 197, 201-205, 218, 220, 223, 224, 294, 295
v. pudendoepigastricus, 284, 285, 304
v. pulmonalis, 126-130, 160, 168, 170
v. radialis, 83, 88-90, 95-102, 240-243
v. saphena lateralis, 192-195, 206-214, 220-224, 262, 289-291
v. saphena medialis, 206-214, 224, 262, 263, 314
v. sphenopalatina, 47
v. sublingualis, 15-21, 28
v. subscapularis, 80, 84, 85
v. suprascapularis, 79, 80
v. tarsea perforans, 212, 217
v. testicularis, 290-293
v. thoracica externa, 84, 85
v. thoracica interna, 148, 149
v. thoracica superficialis, 78-80, 83-85, 113-115
v. thoracodorsalis, 80, 84, 85
v. tibialis caudalis, 193, 214, 263
v. tibialis cranialis, 221
v. transversa cubiti, 86, 88-90, 94
v. transversa faciei, 11-18, 23, 36, 50
v. umbilicalis, 182-184
v. vaginalis, 222
v. vertebralic, 72
v. vorticosa, 52, 53
ventricle,
left, 126-130, 136-139
right, 130, 135-139
vertebra,
caudal, 318-322
cervical, 56, 58
lumbar, 146, 271
sacral, 188, 271
thoracic, 78, 79, 271
see also atlas, axis
vesicular ligament (urinary bladder)
laterial, 184, 274
median, 184, 300
vestibule (vaginal), 312
vomer, 47-49
vulva, 218, 270, 299, 307

W

withers, 57, 58, 76, 325
see also thoracic vertebrae
wolf tooth (P_1), 21, 23

X

xiphisternum, 131

Y

yellow abdominal tunic, *see* abdominal tunic, yellow

Z

zygomatic arch, 6, 8, 10-12, 22, 33, 50, 51
see also zygomatic, maxillary and temporal bones
zygomatic bone, 44, 47-53
zygomaticofrontal process, 50-53